Operative Surgery
and Management

Operative Surgery and Management

Edited by

G. Keen MS FRCS

*Surgeon, Bristol Royal Infirmary
and Frenchay Hospital*

Second edition

WRIGHT

Bristol
1987

Published under the Wright imprint by
IOP Publishing Limited,
Techno House, Redcliffe Way, Bristol BS1 6NX

First edition, 1981
Second edition, 1987

British Library Cataloguing in Publication Data

Operative surgery and management.——2nd ed.
 1. Surgery, Operative
  I. Keen, G.
  617′.91   RD32

ISBN 0 7236 0836 9

Printed in Great Britain at
The Bath Press, Avon

Preface to the Second Edition

Since publication of the first edition in 1981, progress in surgery continues to accelerate, and current conventional treatment may become obsolescent more rapidly than at any other previous period of surgical development.

The introduction of potent H_2 antagonists, the rapid advance in surgical endoscopy, the development of percutaneous dilatation of atheromatous arterial stenoses, together with continuing reappraisal of the contribution of radiotherapy and cytotoxic agents in the management of malignant disease, have significantly modified practice in many branches of surgery. The impact of the laser awaits full assessment. Nevertheless, a thorough understanding of the principles of operative surgery remains essential in the training of those who will see many advances or changes in fashion during their surgical careers. Furthermore, the majority of patients throughout the world will rely for many years to come on conventional surgical operations in the anticipated long absence of highly expensive equipment and technical support in their countries.

With this in mind, the chapters have been expanded and brought up to date where this has been necessary, and several further chapters introduced.

Many of the original illustrations have been retained, but Peter Cox and Paul Bodenham have added further artwork for which I am most grateful.

I wish to thank again the many contributors and to acknowledge the support and encouragement of the managing, editorial and production staff of John Wright in the preparation of this second edition.

G. K.
1987

Preface to the First Edition

The increasing elaboration of surgical care, with the emphasis on critical and objective assessment of this care, has established a clear need for an up-to-date textbook of operative surgery. The days when an individual or a handful of contributors could write such a book are gone, and I have been fortunate to secure the co-operation of over fifty surgeons, each an authority, or having particular interest in his subject.

The complete field of operative surgery, with the exception of ear, nose and throat and ophthalmic surgery, is covered. Bearing in mind the long and comprehensive training required in surgery, I have, in addition to the traditional topics, included sections on neurological, reconstructive, thoracic, neonatal and cardiovascular surgery. Each author has presented the main features of his subject, emphasizing the indications for and the techniques of important surgical operations. A full discussion of postoperative care and of the management of complications is included.

The book is intended for trainees and residents in general surgery who are preparing for higher professional qualifications and, having regard to those who will find the book useful, each contributor has avoided highly controversial methods of treatment. It is hoped that it will also serve as a useful handbook for the practising surgeon.

The text has been illustrated by several medical artists, but I wish to express my particular gratitude to Mrs Clare Burford, Mr Frank Price and Mr Peter Cox, who undertook the greater part of this work.

I would like to thank the managing and editorial staff of John Wright & Sons for their continued encouragement and support in the preparation of this textbook.

G. K.
1981

List of Contributors

F. Ashton ChM FRCS
Professor of Surgery,
University of Birmingham,
and Hon. Consultant Surgeon,
United Hospitals,
Birmingham
The abdominal aorta and its peripheral branches 505

J. D. Atwell FRCS
Consultant Paediatric and Neonatal Surgeon,
Wessex Paediatric Surgical Centre,
Southampton
General Hospital, Southampton
Surgery of the newborn 893

J. S. Bailey BA FRCS
Consultant Cardiothoracic Surgeon,
Groby Road Hospital, Leicester
Perfusion techniques in cardiac surgery 552

R. N. Baird ChM FRCS
Consultant Surgeon, Bristol Royal Infirmary
The adrenal gland 495
Abdominal aortic aneurysms 544

J. C. Baldwin MD
Assistant Professor of Cardiovascular Surgery,
Stanford University School of Medicine,
Stanford, California
Cardiac transplantation 963

W. A. Baumgartner MD
Associate Professor of Surgery,
Johns Hopkins University,
Baltimore, Maryland
Cardiac transplantation 963

R. H. R. Belsey MS FRCS
Emeritus Consultant Thoracic Surgeon,
Frenchay Hospital, Bristol
Oesophageal reconstruction 97

Sir Roy Calne MA MS FRCS FRS
Professor of Surgery,
University of Cambridge
and Hon. Consultant Surgeon,
Addenbrooke's Hospital, Cambridge
Transplantation of the liver and pancreas 951

J. A. S. Carruth MA MB FRCS
Senior Lecturer in Otolaryngology,
Southampton University.
Consultant Otolaryngologist,
Southampton University Hospitals
Lasers in medicine and surgery 31

A. B. Cassie FRCS
Consultant Surgeon, Burnley Hospital Group,
Lancashire
Suture material and the healing of surgical wounds 3

L. R. Celestin FRCS
Consultant Surgeon, Frenchay Hospital,
Bristol
The small intestine 199

C. A. C. Charlton MS FRCS
Consultant Urological Surgeon,
Bath Health District
The kidney and ureter 435

Denton A. Cooley MD
Surgeon in Chief, Texas Heart Institute,
Houston, Texas
and Clinical Professor of Surgery,
University of Texas Medical School,
Houston, Texas
The aortic arch 618

M. J. Cooper MS FRCS
Senior Lecturer in Surgery,
University of Bristol
and Hon. Consultant Surgeon,
Bristol Royal Infirmary
The spleen 179
The liver 186

Contents

Gynaecology and Neonatal Surgery

Transplantation Surgery

Introduction

Chapter one

Suture Material and the Healing of Surgical Wounds

A. B. Cassie

The behaviour of wounds, whether surgical or traumatic, is now largely predictable. Many of the multifactorial influences on healing (Forrester, 1976) can be moderated by the exercise of surgical science and to that extent a healed, uncomplicated wound is the only acceptable outcome. Yet wound complications such as infection, disruption, herniation and chronic discharging sinus are by no means uncommon. One important factor is the selection of suture material and its method of use. Dogma in regard to materials and methods may fail to acknowledge newer understanding of the healing process or take advantage of the choice and performance of suture materials now available.

Consideration must therefore be given to some of the factors that influence wound healing and pertain particularly to the conduct of the surgical exercise in relation to suture material.

WOUND HEALING

Wound strength is dependent on the apposition and healing of the fascial layers (or in gut, the collagen-supporting layer, the submucosa). No other layers exhibit equivalent strength. Preliminary fibrinous adhesion occurs within 24 hours but insignificant wound strength results, until the formal healing process begins.

Three phases of healing are commonly recognized in a fascial or aponeurotic wound in the animal model.

The lag phase extends from the 1st to the 4th day. An inflammatory response follows haemostasis with the assembly of the components for collagen synthesis. Yet temporary collagenolysis may predominate. At this stage wound strength is entirely extrinsic and reliant on sutures.

The proliferative phase follows from the 5th to the 20th day. This reflects the laying-down of collagen lattice in a ground substance by fibroblasts. There is rapid increase in wound strength to 30 per cent of that before injury.

The remodelling phase is a continuous process from day 21 to approximately 1 year and embraces the constant absorption and replacement of collagen more appropriately orientated to the lines of stress. Fibroblast regression occurs and the wound then appears stable. Approximately 70 per cent of pre-wound strength is recovered, but to achieve this, pro-

longed extrinsic support from suture material may be required, varying with the tissue. Some structures heal rapidly, small intestine and bladder being examples of organs which regain their normal bursting strength within 3 weeks. Stomach heals more slowly (Van Winkle and Hastings, 1972), achieving 50 per cent strength in 14 days. Colon heals much less quickly requiring 100 days to achieve normal bursting strength, due partly to the large mucosal content of collagenase which results in a large net loss of collagen in the first 6 days after injury. Infection, ischaemia and foreign material may increase this loss. Skin also appears to heal quickly but the elasticity in surrounding skin appears to buffer wound stress and the underlying fascia augments strength. Skin itself recovers slowly achieving 70 per cent recovery in 120 days. Late wound suture (after 4–7 days as an 'open' wound) and resuture (after dehiscence) form sound scars with quicker healing than after primary suture as the components for healing are already organized. Tissues such as tendons and joint capsules require prolonged support to secure sound healing (Scholz et al., 1972).

The healing of surgical or traumatic wounds is dependent on the interplay of two contrary groups of influences—the disruptive forces and the healing computation. Their interplay formulates the outcome of the healing equation and determines success or failure. In any situation where surgical intervention is required this must be taken into account before the correct decision regarding suture technique and material can be made.

THE DISRUPTIVE FORCES

Lythgoe (1960) demonstrated that the majority of acute wound failures, 'the burst abdomen', result from the cutting-out of intact suture material, thus signifying that the tissues had failed to hold the suture placement. As we see later, the type of suture used in a particular situation can influence this debility, for the greater the tissue reaction to the suture the more likely are oedema and inflammatory response to weaken the tissue bite. Premature absorption of suture material appears to be influential in only a minority of 'burst abdomens' but important in late wound weakness and herniation (Bucknall and Ellis, 1981). Dudley (1970) has noted the pressure of a suture on tissues is inversely proportional to the diameter of the suture material, but consideration has also to be given to the augmented tissue reaction should excessive bulk of suture material be used. Howes (1940) described the augmented strength of wounds sutured with large tissue bites. A sufficient number of sutures is required to distribute tension reasonably without ischaemia. A maximum zone of inflammatory reaction with oedema and a resultant weak area was recognized to lie in the 0·5 cm adjacent to the wound edge (Adamson et al., 1966). One-layer closure perhaps affords an appropriate economic compromise to this paradox. Total quantities of material are reduced by avoiding multi-layer closure, but sufficient strength is gained by deeper bites of appropriate strength suture. There is theoretical and experimental evidence to support this technique (Dudley, 1970). Mathematical calculations on the suture length required for any wound to allow for oedema and to avoid with certainty an over-taut wound were formulated by Jenkins (1976), who showed that the suture length used must not be less than four times the length of the wound to be sutured. Suture material must lie at right angles to the line of tissue fibres if the risk of tearing out is to be diminished. Ischaemia must be avoided. An adequate supply of oxygenated blood is necessary for tissue healing.

There are many detrimental factors such as the particular disease, distension, coughing, obesity, debility, malnutrition, medication and age, which require individual assessment when determining the suture technique to be used.

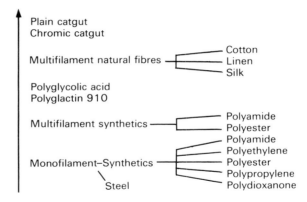

Fig. 1.1. Diagrammatic scale of tissue reaction to suture material.

secure healing. The advent of modern 'inert' synthetic suture materials has done much to reduce tissue reaction (*Fig.* 1.1). Catgut is a foreign protein and the well-known reaction to this has been much reduced by chroming. The naturally occurring non-absorbables, silk, linen and cotton, evoke a major response. Multifilament (braided) synthetics produce a lesser response, but compare still unfavourably with the minor tissue reaction to the monofilament synthetics and steel. Tissue reaction is proportional to total quantity of any given suture material. Excessive knotting and long 'ends' may constitute a local suture excess and may be counterproductive in terms of total wound security.

THE HEALING COMPUTATION

The assimilation and compounding of the necessary elements for wound repair may be influenced by factors which modify both the structure and the time required to complete the process. This complex summation of responses, the healing computation, is accountable when the surgeon elects a particular technique or chooses a particular suture material. Sutures must be as strong as the tissues to be apposed, and must take into account progressive loss through absorption or reaction with tissues after placement. The rate of suture strength loss, if present, and the relative predictable rate of gain of intrinsic wound strength through healing, must be compatible, as must the tissue reaction to the suture. The choice of material must aim at harmony with biological events.

Introduction of a suture immediately causes further injury, with consequent inflammatory response. The design of the needle and the mechanical abrasiveness of the suture need to be considered. The previously noted inflammatory response in the 0·5 cm adjacent to the wound edge also occurs in the needle track and this response should be minimal to promote

INFECTION

The association between infection and the suture material used in a wound has been an important consideration in the surgeon's mind since Lister's antiseptic technique allowed the safe introduction of catgut to the surgical wound. Elek and Conen (1957) showed that the virulence of staphylococci is enhanced 10 000 times when a foreign body is included in the wound. Silk and the other *natural* braided or twisted non-absorbable materials are pre-eminent in establishing, augmenting and maintaining infection, and resolution may be achieved only when such a suture is removed or rejected by the patient. All synthetics of monofilament profile are less conducive to infection and indeed infected wounds are known to heal satisfactorily in the presence of these materials. Accordingly they are chosen when potential infection is recognized and suture removal is then only rarely required. The multifilament (braided) synthetics are less than satisfactory in the presence of infection although their individual meritorious characteristics and their superior knotting and handling qualities may maintain their usefulness. These induce more tissue reaction and their introduction into infected material is known to pick up organisms which lodge in the braid (Katz et al., 1981; Durdey and Bucknall, 1984). Further, the capillary action of braided material may draw surface infection along the suture track and, once established, infection may require suture removal before eradication is achieved. Catgut, particularly plain, although simulating a monofilament produces much tissue reaction and should not be used in the presence of infection where enzymes will accelerate its digestion. Polyglycolic acid (Dexon), although braided, is less reactive than catgut and may have some local antibacterial action (McGeehan et al., 1980).

Infection, when established, disrupts the healing process. Tissue oedema and collagenolysis result in loss of wound strength, and necrosis, disruption or late herniation may result. Patients with incisional hernias frequently have had sepsis—56 per cent in the series of Bucknall and Ellis (1981), 88 per cent in the series of Fischer and Turner (1974). Surprisingly, and fortunately, infection delays the normal loss of strength of the synthetic monofilament absorbable polydioxanone at 28 days after an initial acceleration of loss (Durdey and Bucknall, 1984). In the presence of infection simple taping of wounds to provide approximation, if need be with removal of all buried sutures, may accelerate healing (Brunius, 1969).

During the lag phase of wound healing wound strength is dependent entirely on sutures. No purpose is served in using a strength of material greater than that of the tissues approximated (bearing in mind the known loss of suture strength due to absorption). Douglas (1949) pointed out that it is the loop strength that must be considered in judging this adequacy. The loop strength is approximately the sum of the linear tensile strength plus the knot strength and equates with the practical demand that will be made on a suture when tied in the wound. Tensile strength of suture material is usually measured using the Instron tensiometer. Knot security has attracted considerable study. Monofilaments generally have a low coefficient of friction and the knot may slip, nylon being particularly hazardous, and Prolene a little less so. Braiding provides a striking rise in security. Polyester has a very secure knot, but snags the tissue. Teflon coating and polybutylate coating improve the drag but lessen the knot security. Catgut notoriously 'swells' the knot loose. Polyglycolic acid (Dexon) produces a secure knot but a careful technique to lay the knot accurately is required.

Occasional problems with healing may result from faulty suture technique such as over-tightening of sutures with resultant oedema and ischaemic or infected devitalized tissues. Many surgeons would agree that surgical techniques and expertise in placement of sutures are in every way as important as the selection of sutures themselves.

It is now appropriate to look at the qualities of suture materials which influence their selection for individual procedures.

ABSORBABLE SUTURES

Catgut

This is produced from the submucosa of sheep's intestine or the serosa of beef intestine. Split into ribbon which may be chrome tanned to delay absorption, it is twisted under tension and dried to promote adhesion and finally polished to achieve a monofilament profile. Plain cargut induces a marked inflammatory response with tissue oedema and leucocyte encasement, which are obvious within 24 hours, but chroming moderates this response.

Homogenized collagen, derived from the Achilles tendon of cattle, became an alternative sterile source of suture in plain and chromic form. Stiffer than catgut, it has mainly been used in ophthalmic surgery where tissue reaction to the material is possibly less than to catgut. Catgut absorption is by proteolytic enzymatic digestion, and is usually absorbed in 80–120 days although it has been found in wounds after 3 years. Haxton (1963) reported little catgut strength in wounds after 8–9 days, and variability and unpredictability, particularly with infection, are hallmarks of catgut. On gastric and duodenal mucosa such digestion may be functionally complete within 24 hours (Cassie, 1973) and similar early functional loss is reported in terminal ileum (Everett, 1970). Catgut should be avoided when infection is predictable and in sites where healing is slow such as linea alba. Handling of the material is, however, excellent and it does not snag the tissues or drag, and furthermore the laying of knots is accurate though they are prone to 'swell' loose. Swelling of catgut also exposes more material to elicit a tissue reaction. These excellent handling characteristics have hindered the acceptance of synthetic absorbables with better tissue response but poorer handling qualities. Sterilization of catgut is either by gamma radiation or ethylene oxide. It is packaged in a fluid which retains its ideal handling characteristics.

Polyglycolic Acid (PGA) Sutures (Dexon)

A synthetic suture produced by the polymerization of glycolide to PGA, the extruded filaments are stretched and then braided to attain high-tensile strength (Howes, 1973). PGA is insufficiently flexible in monofilament form for general surgical use and braiding is necessary. Straight pull tensile strength is about 1·2 times greater than catgut, but knot pull strength is even better. PGA loses 28 per cent of strength on knotting, whereas plain catgut loses 53 per cent and chromic catgut 40 per cent. PGA retains strength on wetting, but plain and chromic catgut both lose strength when wet. Thus in the tissues PGA has the advantage of an initial wet knot strength 1·4 times that of chromic catgut and twice that of plain. PGA knot slippage is rare, it does not swell, and it is reported to retain strength in the tissues for approximately the same period as chromic catgut.

Its greater initial strength would appear to leave an advantage at the end of 14 days although it has the disadvantage of braiding in respect of infection. Abdominal wound closure trials initially indicated favourable comparison with monofilament nylon and steel (Leaper et al., 1977), but subsequent trials have disputed this. (Pollock et al., 1979; Bucknall and Ellis, 1981). The early absorption of PGA makes it quite unsuitable for sites where healing is slow, particularly in the orthopaedic fields—tendons, ligaments, arthrotomies and capsular repairs (Scholz et al., 1972).

Absorption is by hydrolysis from the 10th to the 120th day after implant and is uniform and predictable. Unaffected by collagenases it is less directly susceptible to infection than catgut. Knot security of PGA is excellent but knots may be more difficult to lay and a high degree of tissue drag due to braiding is present. Some alleviation of this can be obtained by wetting the suture before use. Coating the suture with a water-soluble lubricant agent, poloxamer 188 (Dexon Plus), provides some improvement to drag but adversely affects knot security. Sterilization of PGA is by ethylene oxide.

Polyglactin 910—Coated Vicryl

Derived from glycolic and lactic acids, the suture is prepared from a copolymer of glycolide and lactide. The braided filaments are coated with a mixture of copolymer and calcium stearate to reduce drag and the average strength of polyglactin 910 is greater than PGA, particularly after 14 days. Some samples of PGA lose all strength after 21 days, but polyglactin 910 always retains some strength at this time (Craig et al., 1975). Absorption commences at 40 days and is complete between 60 and 90 days after implantation (Conn et al., 1974). As with PGA there is a mild-to-moderate inflammatory response to implantation. There is very little difference in handling qualities to those discussed for PGA. The coating has made drag less tiresome but does not appear to have significantly influenced knot security. It suffers the disabilities of a braided suture. Sterilization is by ethylene oxide.

Polydioxanone (PDS)

Polydioxanone (PDS) is a new polymer—a polyester of paradiaxanone which is melt extruded into monofilaments of any size. It is distinguished by flexibility which is uniquely retained in monofilament form. The strength of PDS at implantation is greater than that of all commonly used monofilaments other than steel (Ray et al., 1981). Seventy per cent of strength is retained at 2 weeks, 50 per cent at 4 weeks, 14 per cent at 8 weeks. Absorption is by hydrolysis; it starts at 90 days and is completed in 6 months. In the tissues only a mild reaction—mainly macrophages and proliferating fibroblasts—occurs. Handling properties compare favourably with those of catgut (Berry et al., 1981), and the laying of knots has not proved difficult. Security is good although a fourth throw is advisable. The monofilament profile makes it particularly suitable for potentially infected suture lines although the presence of infection appears to accelerate loss of strength initially. At 28 days this loss of strength is retarded and it remains stronger than in a non-infected wound, with obvious advantages (Durdey and Bucknall, 1984). It has proved safe also in the biliary system (Hoile, 1983) and would appear to offer considerable merit for use in colonic anastomoses. Satisfactory performance has been reported in muscles, tendon fascia, stomach and colon (Lerwick, 1983).

It is sterilized by ethylene oxide.

The generally agreed performance of absorbable sutures is measured by retained breaking strength.

NON-ABSORBABLE SUTURES

Sutures are termed 'non-absorbable' when no enzymatic or dissolution process is actively involved by their presence in the tissues. Many non-absorbable sutures do eventually fragment and multi-filament nylon and silk lose most of their strength by fragmentation in the first 6 months.

Natural Silk

This is derived from thread spun by the larva of the silkworm by degumming of the surface silk albumin layer. The filaments are then twisted or braided, forming a multifilament.

Silk has always found favour because of its excellent handling characteristics. It knots well, allowing ends to be cut short. Unfortunately, it promotes a marked tissue response because of its foreign protein content and fibrous encapsulation is found after 2–3 weeks in tissues. Braiding induces capillary attraction. With infection, organisms may be harboured in the interstices. Waxing and silicone coating reduce drag but also reduce knot security, and three throws are always necessary (Holmuno, 1977). Silk loses 20 per cent of tensile strength when wet, an effect also counteracted by waxing. Fragmentation occurs and all strength is lost after 6 months. Despite these drawbacks, its fine handling qualities have established its position as a yardstick of performance. It is not weakened by boiling or autoclaving. Normally, it is sterilized by gamma radiation.

Cotton

Cotton is a cellulose suture of vegetable origin, manufactured by twisting the seed hairs of long-fibre Sea Island or Egyptian cotton. It is therefore a multifilament suture and its properties are similar to those of silk. Surprisingly, though, it gains strength when wet. It ranks as a rather weak suture. It is cheap.

Linen

Long staple flax fibres are twisted to produce linen thread. Linen has similar properties to those of cotton but is stronger and gains strength when wet. It has maintained favour in gastrointestinal surgery.

Synthetic

Polyamides

These are better known as nylon and are manufactured in mono- and multifilament forms. Nylon is comparatively inert in monofilament form producing a very modest tissue reaction, but braided nylon stimulates more tissue reaction than the monofilament and fragments and loses its strength within 6 months. The monofilament form loses only 16 per cent of its strength in the first year. The braided suture handles well and has good knot security. The monofilament has poor handling characteristics and poor knot security due to a low coefficient of friction and a 'memory' which inclines the knot to untie. Braided nylon may prove troublesome in the presence of infection and may require removal, but the monofilament is usually sufficiently inert to allow healing of an infected wound. Normally sterilized by gamma radiation, it can tolerate autoclaving (up to three times) without degradation.

Polyesters

These materials enjoy a high and permanent tensile strength and induce only modest tissue reaction. Generally available as braided materials, they enjoy good knot security and have found favour in the cardiovascular field. Unfortunately, strands tend to adhere making it difficult to handle or lay the knot. The application of a coating of PTFE (polytetrafluoroethylene) or polybutylate attributes smoothness but knot security then requires particular care. Polyester is now available as a monofilament in the finer gauges (Novafil) with reasonable handling properties and knot security. It appears to offer gauged elasticity and recoil which may be helpful qualities.

Special developments of polyester have been engineered to meet the requirements of vascular surgery where its permanence and strength find merit. Endeavours to encourage engagement of Dacron (polyester) arterial grafts to host tissues have centred on the development of a polyester velour with a specialized filamentous wall. Fibrous tissue ingrowth has not attracted endothelial proliferation so that only a false intima has resulted. Polyester is also produced as a mesh, felt and knitted fabric with uses in general surgery as well as in cardiovascular repair. Knitted fabrics and meshes conform particularly well to required shape without wrinkling, thus lending themselves well to repairs of defects and hernias. Polyester is normally sterilized by gamma radiation but can be autoclaved.

Polyethylene

This is a strong suture material available in monofilament form. There is, however, a progressive loss of strength in the tissues with eventual fragmentation. Tissue reaction is minimal and handling is less difficult than nylon. It presents a soft surface which contributes to the excellent knot security and the ease of handling.

It is also produced as a mesh for use in general surgery. Sterilization is by gamma radiation or ethylene oxide. It melts at 132 °C so that autoclaving is not possible.

Polypropylene (Prolene)

Polymerized propylene is a synthetic suture which is a monofilament and retains its strength permanently. Tensile strength is high—similar to nylon—but it does not fragment or weaken. It is among the most inert of sutures, infected wounds accomplishing healing in its presence. The handling characteristics are less tiresome and hazardous than those of nylon. The absence of a 'memory' and the inclination to untie, found in nylon, facilitate its use, knots being secure on the third throw. It is available as a knitted mesh for defect repairs which has been used in repair of prolapse of rectum (Keighley et al., 1983). When used to suture blood vessels blood loss is much less than is the case with polyester sutures. The vivid blue dye facilitates visualization, but avoidance of instrumental damage is very important as weakness and fracture may be induced. Sterilization is by ethylene oxide or autoclaving.

METALLIC SUTURES

Stainless steel is as traditional as silk in the suture armamentarium. It is an alloy of steel with molybdenum, chromium and nickel, and is usually monofilament, although a braided product is available for specific requirements. More steel is now being used with the advent of sophisticated applicators and stapling guns. Monofilament steel is extremely strong and almost inert and infected wounds heal in its presence. Shouldice et al. (1961) reported excellent results with minor infection rates in a review of 28 000 hernias repaired with steel wire. Metal fatigue may occasionally occur and result in fracture, and kinking accelerates this. Knot security is high, but the knot itself may produce irritation and discomfort and long ends must be avoided. The dermis is not insensitive on its deeper aspect so that inversion and burying of the knot are required. Handling of metallic sutures requires a special technique but need not be regarded as a drawback. Mechanical suturing devices now exploit the advantages of steel. Sterilization is by autoclaving.

STERILIZATION OF SUTURE MATERIALS

Three methods of sterilization are employed: gamma radiation, ethylene oxide and autoclaving. Each may affect the suture material properties to some degree (*Table* 1.1).

Table 1.1. Sterilization of suture material

	Autoclave	Ethylene Oxide	Gamma Radiation
Catgut		†	*
Vicryl		*	
PGA		*	
PDS		*	
Steel	*		
Silk			*
Cotton	†	*	
Linen	†	*	
Polyester	†		*
Polyethylene		†	*
Polyamide	†		*
Polypropylene	†	*	

* Method of choice.
† Alternative.

Gamma Radiation

A monitored dose (2·5 Mrad) is used to avoid deterioration of material, which can occur if the dose is excessive. Linen, cotton, PGA, polyglactin 910 and polypropylene are damaged at the required dosage. This method has the manufacturing advantage of applicability to the packaged material.

Ethylene Oxide

The poisonous nature of this gas, together with the requirement for the packages to be opened prior to sterilization, makes this choice less attractive. It is the selected method in the treatment of PGA, polyglactin 910, PDS, polypropylene, linen and cotton. It can be used in catgut and polyethylene sterilization.

Autoclave

This is readily available but weakens catgut, PGA, polyglactin and polyethylene. Silk, linen and cotton may be autoclaved but lose some strength. However, polyesters, nylon, polypropylene and metals will tolerate at least three autoclaving procedures.

SOME OPERATIVE IMPLICATIONS

Many guidelines are seen to emerge, but there are no rules.

General Abdominal Closure

Suture material strength is measured in relation to the cross-sectional area. Generally metals are strongest, natural fibres and materials weakest and synthetics intermediate in strength. Accordingly, suture size will depend on the disruptive forces, the tissue resistance and the material employed. The interface between suture and tissue provide resistance to 'cutting out'. Synthetics at implantation, or steel, may be disproportionately strong, and the temptation to use a finer grade of suture may be counter-productive if the interface reduction results in cutting out or tissue strangulation. In the case of an absorbable suture the percentage strength remaining before anticipated intrinsic wound strength recovers adequately must always be kept in mind when suture gauge is selected.

Supportive sutures should avoid the area of maximum tissue reaction in the 0·5 cm adjacent to the wound. The '1 cm plus' bite achieves this and secures the mechanical advantage of a musculo-aponeurotic buffer to the suture (Leaper et al., 1977). Coaptation of the wound is sought by uniform support from an adequate number of sutures rather than reliance on fewer sutures, which may be under excessive tension, increasing ischaemia. Adequate length of continuous suture is a suture:wound ratio of 4:1. As advocated by Jenkins (1976) it is required if 'cutting out' is to be avoided, and this concept makes allowance for the appropriate depth of tissue bite. A reduction in the incidence of dehiscence and late herniation following the introduction of one-layer closure (mass ligature) must reflect these factors. The Smead-Jones suture technique has succeeded in retaining anatomical accuracy (Jones et al., 1941; Higgins et al., 1969; Goligher et al., 1975). Anatomical difficulties where suture direction is parallel to anatomical fibres—as in tendon or posterior rectus sheath closure—may be overcome by techniques of looping or traversing the suture, thereby off-setting part of the load at right angles to fibre direction.

The selected suture material must be capable of providing support so long as this is required. Chromic catgut can no longer be regarded as reliable in the abdominal wall (Goligher et al., 1975), modern synthetics or steel achieving better performance. Monofilament steel is generally too cumbersome and produces more pain. Where absorbable sutures are required PDS appears to offer strength and durability that are superior to those of polyglycolic and polyglactin 910, both of which have probably too short a life-span. Where healing potential is impaired for any reason, the long-term advantage of a monofilament unabsorbable suture must weigh in its favour.

Intestinal Anastomosis

The cut tissue reactive margin which influences general closure techniques has not been defined in stomach or in bowel. Essentially the bite must include submucosa to achieve security. Tissue reaction to catgut and its premature absorption have imposed some limitations on its use unless reinforced by a non-absorbable seromuscular suture layer. Catgut entering the lumen of stomach fails by digestion early in a small percentage of cases. Similarly, there are hazards in ileum and jejunum so that its use in right hemicolectomy, ileorectal anastomosis and oesophago-jejunostomy may be unwise (Everett, 1970). Tanner (1951) described ulceration in the stomach where continuous braided non-absorbable sutures had been used as a through-and-through stitch, and this complication may also occur when interrupted non-absorbable sutures erode through on to the mucosa (Kalima and Asp, 1973). The synthetic absorbables appear to be safe in stomach and in small intestine for use on the haemostatic layer. Silk, linen and cotton thread are not reported to have untoward consequences on the invaginating layer in small intestine, their handling attributes allowing easy invagination, although a synthetic monofilament would theoretically be preferable.

Large bowel anastomosis has consistently been less secure in surgical practice. Clinical leakage is reported to carry a mortality of 22 per cent. Goligher et al. (1977) reported loss of integrity, radiological or clinical, at the suture line in up to 58 per cent of cases dependent on whether anastomosis was high or low and on whether a one- or two-layer inverting suture was employed. Surgical technique is paramount and well demonstrated by the dramatic increase in fistulas and other complications when an everting instead of inverting suture is employed (Goligher et al., 1970). Matheson and Irving (1976) achieved the exceptionally low leakage rates in colo-rectal anastomosis of 6 per cent, using interrupted braided nylon, and it is to be noted that these sutures did not penetrate the mucosa. The suture material itself may have significant influence. It is known that the collagen content of the colon remains lower than that in small intestine after injury, and that collagenase, present in mucosa, increases after surgery. Breakdown of collagen predominates in the first 4 days, and synthesis is marked in the 2nd week. General and local factors are important, but particularly so is infection, which accelerates collagenolysis. Good mechanical and antimicrobial preparation will help, but the nature of the suture material in such an infected site is of great importance. Braided material which penetrates the lumen draws in organisms and potentiates infection (Katz et al., 1981). Infected anastomotic lines and micro-abscesses appear to delay collagen formation and catgut and PGA begin to lose strength by the 8th day. Colonic strength (collagen) requires 10–14 days. It would appear wise to avoid catgut sutures as sole support. Monofilaments, inert and unreactive, Prolene, nylon or PDS should be used in at least one layer (Durdey and Bucknall, 1984).

Stapling guns are particularly useful in rectal and oesophageal surgery. In the rectum there has been no significant advantage in regard to sepsis or leakage. They permit restorative surgery at a low level where technical access was previously difficult and hazardous (Waxman, 1983). Intraoperative testing for leakage is advisable. The incidence of late stenosis may, however, be higher after stapled anastomosis (see Chapter 2).

Bladder

Healing of a bladder wound is complete in 21 days and occurs with any suture material. Multifilaments may induce calculi, although the rapid disappearance of polyglactin 910 and PGA in the bladder (within 28 days) appears to obviate this problem.

Biliary Tree

Unabsorbable sutures may act as a nucleus for recurrent stone formation, and absorbable sutures have proved safe. PDS has proved safe (Hoile, 1983) and is more acceptable as a monofilament.

Skin Closure

It is apparent that the position of the suture is as important to the incidences of wound infection as the nature of the material. In controlled trials (Pickford et al., 1983) stainless steel clips which did not penetrate the dermis into subcutaneous tissue produced significantly less wound infection than the widely used and established interrupted monofilament suture which did penetrate. Similar improved results are reported with sutureless closure—effected by an adhesive polyurethane membrane—although a subcutaneous stitch to fat layers may be required (Eaton, 1980; Tinckler, 1983). Skill is required to avoid misalignment, gaping and inversion (Bunker, 1965), but reduced infection is achieved. The sutureless wound is also easily managed and there are economies. The continuous subcuticular suture using synthetic absorbables has proved valuable, helps to avoid ischaemia and the cosmetic result is good. Fiennes (1985) has described a safe technique using interrupted subcuticular sutures of polyglactin with an inverted knot for abdominal closure. The inconvenience, delay and expense of awaiting suture removal may thus be avoided.

Economies

Cost can no longer be ignored. A universal procedure such as skin closure may cost £10·00 (1985) using steel clips in a disposable applicator, 61 pence using blue nylon and needle. A disposable circular stapling device used in colo-rectal anastomosis costs £83·00, a hand suture £2·00.

Suture Size

Metrication is resolving the diverse and illogical system of sizing which becomes acceptable only through familiarity. The metric gauge recognizes the smaller of the 'limit' figures for a particular size. This figure is multiplied by 10 to give the metric gauge. Thus a suture of diameter range 0·30–0·33 mm would be classified as no. 3 metric.

The Needle
The needle track histopathology resembles that described in relation to any surgical wound and similar consequences may be expected. Trauma must be minimized. The design of needles which are swaged to sutures attempts to achieve a maximum technical efficiency with minimum tissue trauma. The range of needles and points endeavours to achieve specific objectives within these requirements and has commanded as much interest as the sutures they carry.

REFERENCES

Adamson R. J., Musco F. and Enquist I. F. (1966) The clinical dimensions of a healing incision. *Surg. Gynecol. Obstet.* **123**, 515.

Berry A. R., Wilson M. C., Thomson J. W. et al. (1981) Polydioxanone—a new synthetic absorbable suture. *J.R. Coll. Surg. Edinb.* **26**(3), 170–172.

Bentley P. G., Owen W. J., Girolami P. L. et al. (1978) Wound closure with Dexon (P.G.A.) mass suture. *Ann. R. Coll. Surg. Engl.* **60**, 125–127.

Brunius U. L. F. (1969) Wound healing impairment from sutures. *Acta. Chir. Scand.* Suppl. 395.

Bucknall T. G. and Ellis H. (1981) Abdominal wound closure—comparison of monofilament nylon and polyglycolic acid. *Surgery* **89**(6), 672–677.

Bunker T. (1975) Problems with Op.-site closure. *Ann. R. Coll. Surg. Engl.* **65**, 260–262.

Cassie A. B. (1973) Catgut and polyglycolic acid. An evaluation in the human stomach. *R. Coll. Surg. Engl.* **59**(1), 69–72

Conn J., Oyasu R., Welsh M. et al. (1974) Vicryl (polyglactin 910) synthetic absorbable sutures. *Am. J. Surg.* **128**, 19–23.

Craig P. H., Williams J. A., Dausk W. et al. (1975) A biologic comparison of Polyglactin 910 and polyglycolic acid synthetic absorbable sutures. *Surg. Gynecol. Obstet.* **141**, 1–10.

Cronin K., Jackson D. S. and Dunphy J. E. (1968) *Surg. Gynecol. Obstet.* **126**, 1061.

Douglas D. W. (1949) Tensile strength of sutures. *Lancet* **2**, 497.

Dudley H. A. F. (1970) Layered and mass closure of the abdominal wall. *Br. J. Surg.* **57**, 664.

Durdey P. and Bucknall T. E. (1984) Assessment of sutures for use in colonic surgery, an experimental study. *J. R. Soc. Med.* **77**, 472–476.

Eaton A. C. (1980) Controlled trial of Op. Site skin closure technique. *Br. J. Surg.* **67**, 857–860.

Elek S. D. and Conen P. E. (1957) The virulence of *Staphylococcus pyogenes* for man: A study of the problems of wound infection. *Br. J. Exp. Path.* **38**, 573.

Everett W. G. (1970) Suture materials in general surgery. *Prog. Surg.* **8**, 14.

Fiennes A. G. T. W. (1985) Interrupted subcuticular polyglactin sutures for abdominal wounds. *Ann. R. Coll. Surg. Engl.* **67**, 121.

Fischer J. D. and Turner F. W. (1974) Abdominal incisional hernias. A 10 year review. *Can. J. Surg.* **17**, 202–204.

Forrester J. C. (1976) Surgical wound biology. *J. R. Coll. Surg. Edinb.* **21**(4), 239–249.

Goligher J. C., Lee D. W. G. Simpkins K. C. et al. (1977) A controlled comparison of one and two layer techniques of suture for high and low colo-rectal anastomosis. *Br. J. Surg.* **64**, 609–614.

Goligher J. C., Morris E., McAdam W. A. F. et al. (1970) A controlled trial of inverting versus everting intestinal suture in clinical large bowel surgery. *Br. J. Surg.* **57**, 817–822.

Goligher J. C., Irvin T. T., Johnston D. et al. (1975) A controlled trial of three methods of closure of laparotomy wounds. *Br. J. Surg.* **62**, 823–827.

Haxton H. (1963) The absorption of catgut in human abdominal wounds. *Br. J. Surg.* **50**, 534.

Holmuno D. E. W. (1977) Knot properties of surgical silk. Model study. *Br. J. Surg.* **64**, 677–678.

Higgins G. A., Anthowiak J. G. and Esterlyn S. H. (1969) A clinical and laboratory study of abdominal wound closure and dehiscence. *Arch. Surg.* **98**, 421–427.

Hoile R. W. (1983) The use of a new suture material (P.D.S.) in the biliary tree. *Ann. R. Coll. Surg. Engl.* **65**, 167–171.

Howes E. L. (1940) Immediate strength of sutured wound. *Surgery* **7**, 24.

Howes E. L. (1973) Strength studies of polyglycolic acid versus catgut sutures of the same size. *Surg. Gynecol. Obstet.* **137**, 15.

Jenkins T. P. N. (1976) The burst abdominal wound: A mechanical approach. *Br. J. Surg.* **63**, 873.

Jones T. E., Newell E. T. and Brubaker R. E. (1941). The use of alloy steel wire in the closure of abdominal wounds. *Surg. Gynecol. Obstet.* **72**, 1056.

Kalima T. V. and Asp K. (1973) Suture line ulcers after gastric surgery. *Ann. Chir. Gynaecol. Fenn.* **62**, 370.

Katz S., Mordechai I. and Mirelman D. (1981) Bacterial adherence to surgical sutures. *Ann. Surg.* **194**, 35–41.

Keighley M. R. B., Fielding J. W. L. and Alexander-Williams J. (1983) Results of Marlex mesh abdominal rectopexy for rectal prolapse in 100 consecutive patients. *Br. J. Surg.* **70**, 229–232.

Leaper D. S., Pollock A. V. and Evans M. (1977) Abdominal wound closure: a trial of nylon, polyglycolic acid and steel sutures *Br. J. Surg.* **64**, 603.

Lerwick E. (1983) Studies on the efficiency and safety of polydioxanone monofilament absorbable suture. *Surg. Gynecol. Obstet.* **156**(1), 51–55.

Lythgoe J. P. (1960) Burst abdomen. *Postgrad. Med. J.* **36**, 388.

Matheson N. A. and Irving A. D. (1976) Single layer anastomosis in the gastro-intestinal tract. *Surg. Gynecol. Obstet.* **143**, 619–624.

McGeehan D., Hunt D., Chaudhuri A. et al. (1980). An experimental study of relationships between synergistic wound sepsis and suture materials. *Br. J. Surg.* **67**, 636–638.

Pickford I. R., Brennan S. S., Evans Mary et al. (1983) Two methods of skin closure in abdominal operations: controlled clinical trial. *Br. J. Surg.* **70**, 226–228.

Pollock A. V., Greenall, M. J. and Evans M. (1979) Single layer mass closure of major laparotomies by continuous suturing. *J. R. Soc. Med.* **72**, 889–893.

Ray J. A., Doddi N., Regula D. et al. (1981) Polydioxanone (P.D.S.) A novel monofilament synthetic absorbable suture. *Surg. Gynecol. Obstet.* **153**, 497–507.

Scholz K. C., Lewis R. C. and Bateman R. O. (1972) Clinical failure of polyglycolic acid surgical suture. *Surg. Gynecol. Obstet.* **135**, 525–528.

Shouldice E. E., Glassow F. and Black N. (1961) Sinus formation following infected herniorrhaphy incisions. *Can. Med. Assoc. J.* **84**, 568–569.

Tanner N. C. (1951) Operative methods in the treatment of peptic ulcer. *Edin. Med. J.* **58**, 279.

Tinckler L. (1983) Surgical wound management with adhesive polyurethane membrane. A preferred method for routine use. *Ann. R. Coll. Surg. Engl.* **65**, 257–259.

Van Winkle W. and Hastings J. C. (1972) Consideration in the choice of suture material for various tissues. *Surg. Gynecol. Obstet.* **135**, 113–126.

Waxman B. P. (1983) Large bowel anastomosis II. The circular staplers. *Br. J. Surg.* **70**, 64–67.

Chapter two

Mechanical Stapling in Surgery

D. J. Leaper

HISTORICAL BACKGROUND

Surgeons have always been innovators, which has probably arisen from the needs of their profession, and had this not been the case it is unlikely that our surgical research and development would have led to the high standards of surgery expected today. The Hungarian surgeon Professor Humer Hultl was no exception to the rule, being the first to produce and successfully use a mechanical linear stapler for distal gastrectomy. He was a great teacher and a typical example of this was in his training of young surgeons in surgical techniques using corpses which were made to 'bleed' at incision by using a pump in place of a heart. Among other original ideas he introduced asepsis and an iodine skin preparation, face masks and rubber gloves to his hospital in Hungary.

In 1908 Professor Hultl presented his 'tissue-closing device', which he had produced with the instrument maker Victor Fischer, to the Hungarian Surgical Society. It was a heavy device weighing 5 kg, and used steel wire staples which allowed a double row of staples to be placed at each side of a line of transection across a viscus. A later version was lighter but still took about 2 hours for its assembly with staples in place prior to use.

Aladar von Petz presented another linear stapling device to the Hungarian Surgical Society in 1921. It was still large in size but much lighter and employed two parallel rows of silver wire staples. The instrument of von Petz soon enjoyed widespread popularity and, although further modifications have been made in Japan, the Soviet Union, Europe and North America, the B-closure of staples (allowing haemostasis but avoiding necrosis), the staggered double row of staples and basic technology are unchanged. The Russians made further major developments in stapling techniques at the Institute of Experimental Surgical Apparatus and Instruments in Moscow. Their instruments were designed in the early 1950s for use in vascular and bronchial surgery and included the first end-to-end and side-to-side anastomotic devices which have been modified and developed, with the linear stapling instruments, into the versatile precision instruments currently available for many fields of surgery.

PRESENT INSTRUMENT RANGE (*Table* 2.1)

Stapling devices which are currently available in the United Kingdom are of three basic types: linear, side-to-side and end-to-end staplers.

Linear Staplers

The early American Auto Suture old-style TA instruments with disposable loading units have been replaced by the similar but more refined stainless steel Premium TA instruments (*Fig.* 2.1). In turn these are being supplanted by totally disposable units (*Fig.* 2.2). Two parallel staple lines are placed with lengths of approximately 30, 55 or 90 mm by the TA 30, TA 55 or TA 90 guns respectively, which may be chosen to fit the appropriate length of viscus to be closed. For example, the TA 30 may be used to close an

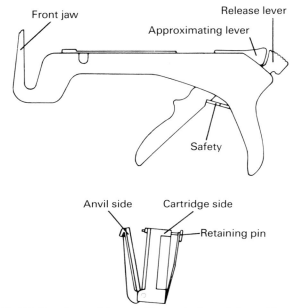

Fig. 2.1. Premium stainless steel linear stapler and disposable cartridge.

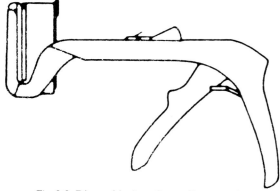

Fig. 2.2. Disposable Auto Suture linear stapler.

Table 2.1. List of currently available stapling instruments (*Note: Manufacturer's instructions must always be read*)

1. Linear Staplers	Place two parallel staggered staple lines	
Auto Suture TA	Premium stainless steel instrument and disposable cartridge Three staple line lengths (30, 55, 90 mm) Three staple sizes (vascular TA 30, 3·5, 4·8 mm)	*Fig.* 2.1
	Completely disposable instrument Three staple line lengths (30, 55, 90 mm) Three staple sizes (vascular TA 30, 3·5, 4·8 mm)	*Fig.* 2.2
Ethicon Proximate LS	Completely disposable instrument Three staple line lengths (30, 60, 90 mm) Staple height adjustable for tissue thickness	*Fig.* 2.3
2. Side-to-side staplers	Place four parallel staple lines and knife blade simultaneously divides tissue between two double lines	
Auto Suture GIA 50	Premium stainless steel instrument and disposable cartridge With or without knife blade	*Fig.* 2.4
	Completely disposable instrument With or without knife blade	*Fig.* 2.5
3. End-to-end (side) staplers	Place two concentric rings of staples and circular knife blade simultaneously advanced for inverting anastomosis	
Auto Suture EEA	Stainless steel instrument and disposable cartridge Three sizes of cartridge (diameters 25, 28, 31 mm)	*Fig.* 2.6
	Completely disposable instrument—straight Three sizes of head (diameters 25, 28, 31 mm)	*Fig.* 2.7
	Completely disposable instrument—curved Four sizes of head (diameters 21, 25, 28, 31 mm)	*Fig.* 2.8
Ethicon Proximate ILS	Completely disposable instrument Four sizes of head (diameters 21, 25, 28, 31 mm) Adjustable staple height mechanism	*Fig.* 2.9
Auto Suture EEA	Stainless steel purse-string device Stainless steel sizers	*Fig.* 2.10
Ethicon Proximate	Disposable purse-string device (PSD) Disposable tissue-measuring device (TMD)	*Fig.* 2.11 *Fig.* 2.12

enterotomy and the TA 90 may be used to fashion a new lesser curve in Billroth-I gastrectomy. Different sizes of staples are also available to accommodate varying thicknesses of tissue: the 3·5 mm staple (coded blue) is suitable for closing small bowel whereas the 4·8 mm staple (coded green) is necessary for closing a thickened pylorus in Heineke–Mikulicz pyloroplasty. An even smaller staple (coded white) is available for vascular closures with the TA 30.

The Ethicon Proximate linear stapler (*Fig.* 2.3) is a totally disposable instrument which also fires two parallel rows of staples and allows parallel jaw closure to ensure even tissue compression prior to firing. This last feature was present in the old-style Auto Suture

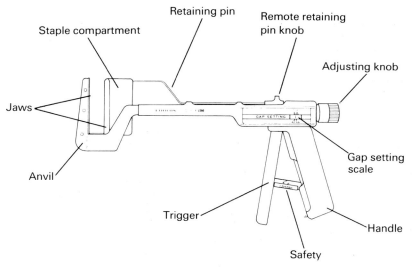

Fig. 2.3. Disposable Ethicon Proximate linear stapler.

TA instruments and has been reintroduced with the latest disposable units. The Proximate linear stapler is available in three lengths—30, 60 and 90 mm—and also allows an adjustment in each instrument for two staple heights—3·5 and 4·8 mm.

Side-to-side Staplers

The Auto Suture GIA instrument is unique in being able to place four 50 mm staple lines simultaneously with tissue division between the staples by a knife blade making side-to-side intestinal anastomosis, for example, a single manoeuvre. The old-style GIA instruments have been replaced by similar stainless steel Premium instruments with a simpler disposable loading unit (*Fig.* 2.4). There is also a completely

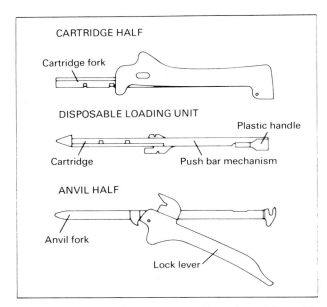

Fig. 2.4. Premium stainless steel side-to-side stapler and disposable loading unit.

disposable GIA now available which, like the Premium GIA, allows an even tissue compression and contains 50 per cent more staples (*Fig.* 2.5). All GIA instruments can be supplied without the knife blade for use in making Koch ileal reservoirs for example.

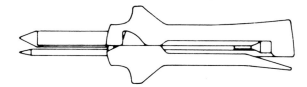

Fig. 2.5. Disposable side-to-side stapler.

End-to-end Staplers

The Russian SPTU gun, which allowed an inverting intestinal anastomosis with a single row of staples, has now been replaced by the Auto Suture EEA range and the Ethicon Proximate ILS instruments which provide a double row of staples (*Fig.* 2.6). The stainless steel Auto Suture EEA gun (*Fig.* 2.7) is presented with three sizes of disposable cartridges—of 25, 28 and 31 mm diameter (coded white, blue and green respectively)—which place two concentric rings of staggered staples on firing while a circular knife blade simultaneously divides tissue inside the smallest circle of staples. Completely disposable units are also available and in the curved range, useful for oesophageal and low rectal anastomoses, there is a fourth cartridge size of 21 mm (*Fig.* 2.8).

The Ethicon Proximate ILS instruments are completely disposable and have four cartridge sizes available—21, 25, 29 and 33 mm (*Fig.* 2.9). The staple height can be adjusted for varying tissue thickness in end-to-end anastomoses from 1 to 3 mm by using a separate disposable spring-loaded device (TMD) which allows intestinal tissue thickness to be measured prior to setting the tissue gap with the adjusting

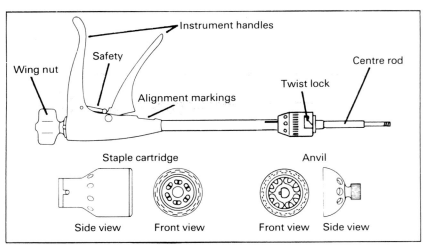

Fig. 2.6. Stainless steel end-to-end stapler and disposable cartridge.

knob on the ILS. The TMD also has a scale printed on it for determining the diameter of cartridge required for anastomosis and, although crude, is probably safer than using the EEA sizers which can damage bowel if over-enthusiastic attempts are made to insert them into small-diameter bowel lumens.

All the current stapling instruments employ stainless steel staples which are closed in tissue in the same B-closure pioneered in the von Petz instruments. Haemostasis is thereby achieved without tissue necrosis. There is little question that surgeons, as in so many new operations and techniques, need to go through a 'learning curve' period. This may be achieved using fresh abbatoir bowel, that from the pig is particularly suitable, with simulating jigs such as those available at the anastomosis workshops at the Royal College of Surgeons of England. Stapled anastomoses are easier and quicker to fashion once expertise has been attained. Such anastomoses rarely bleed and tend to function quicker allowing a reduction in hospital stay. However, over-use of stapling instruments presents a high financial burden despite any reductions in theatre and inpatient time which may be accrued and, although surgeons in training should be aware of their advantages, stapling instruments will never replace traditional hand-sewn anastomotic techniques which remain the mainstay of training programmes. The light manoeuvrable

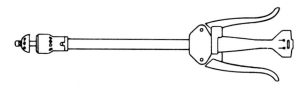

Fig. 2.7. Disposable Auto Suture straight end-to-end stapler.

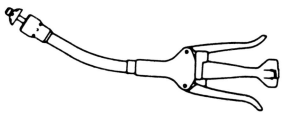

Fig. 2.8. Disposable Auto Suture curved end-to-end stapler.

disposable instruments do facilitate access in difficult areas—transabdominal oesophageal and low rectal anastomoses are the classic examples. The usual clinical criteria for success apply to any anastomosis whether hand-sewn or stapled. A stapled anastomosis in ischaemic bowel, for example, is no less at risk of leakage with attendant fistula and subsequent stricture formation.

Other stapling devices are available which allow individual staples to be placed rapidly in fascia, after laparotomy, or in skin. Staples in fascia (Auto Suture) are closed in a B-configuration and are delivered by a disposable unit which may be gas powered for even greater speed, whereas staples in skin (Auto Suture, Ethicon, Davis & Geck, and the 3Ms Company) are rectangular shaped and may be easily removed later with simple extractor devices. Auto Suture also manufacture a device for simultaneous division and ligation of tissue (the LDS). Any amount of tissue which can be placed into the LDS jaws can be safely division-ligated. The units are disposable and are also available gas powered which helps to avoid damage to tissues, the greater omentum being divided along the greater curve of stomach, for example, by inadvertent jerking manoeuvres.

STAPLING PROCEDURES IN GENERAL SURGERY (GASTROENTEROLOGY)

The first stapling instruments used in the United Kingdom to any extent were the inverting circular end-to-end, or end-to-side, anastomosing devices. Their use is now widespread for sphincter-saving operations for carcinoma of the rectum and they have saved many patients from permanent colostomies after abdomino-perineal resection. Even obese males may be suitable for low anterior resection using stapling instruments. For the same advantage of increased access circular staples may allow total gastrectomy with a Roux-en-Y oesophago-jejunostomy through the abdomen and avoiding a thoracotomy. The usual clinical criteria for a safe anastomosis must be followed, however; an inadequate anterior resection risks suture line recurrence and an ischaemic oesophago-jejunostomy risks leakage. Stapled anastomoses in such circumstances offer no advantage to

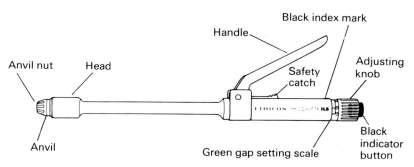

Fig. 2.9. Disposable Ethicon, proximate end-to-end stapler.

the patient. Following the reported, more widespread use of stapling instruments, particularly from the United States, the linear and side-to-side staplers are becoming increasingly favoured even within the financial restraints of the National Health Service. They will never replace traditional general surgical procedures, however, unless some definite benefit is achieved. *Table* 2.2 lists the range of procedures, with examples, which can be performed; some are specialized and full details and description are not within the scope of this chapter. (The reader's attention is drawn to the bibliography and reference list.)

Some of the most common stapling procedures are now described with each of the three types of instrument in detail.

Table 2.2. Range of procedures possible in gastroenterological surgery (some require all three types of stapling instrument)

1. *Linear staplers—linear everting terminal staple line*
   Closure duodenal stump (Polya gastrectomy)
   Closure rectal stump (Hartmann's procedure)
   Closure enterotomy (Heineke–Mikulicz pyloroplasty)
   Prior to resection (new lesser curve in Billroth-I gastrectomy)
   End-to-end anastomosis (triangulation)

2. *Side-to-side staplers*
   a. Linear inverting anastomosis with transection:
      Side-to-side enteroenterostomy (gastroenterostomy)
      Bypass enteroenterostomy (palliative ileocolostomy)
      Functional end-to-end (ileocolic anastomosis after right hemicolectomy)
   b. Linear staple line without transection (no knife):
      Enteric reservoirs (Kock pouch, ileal pouch or reservoir)
   c. Linear staple line with transection:
      Closure of viscus (small bowel resection)
      Gastrostomy and reverse gastric tube

3. *End-to-end staplers—circular inverting anastomosis*
   Low anterior anastomosis (closure of Hartmann's)
   Postgastrectomy anastomoses (Roux-en-Y, Billroth-I gastroduodenal)
   Transection of varices
   Gastropexy (morbid obesity)

Low Anterior Resection

Many colostomies have been avoided since the more widespread use of the circular stapling devices, and anterior resection is probably their commonest application overall. It must be emphasized again that these instruments only facilitate surgery by making a difficult operation technically more feasible; they cannot make what would be a palliative resection into a curative resection.

The rectum is mobilized in the usual way and prior to resection of a low rectal cancer the stump may be irrigated with a cytotoxic solution per anum using a right-angled non-crushing clamp placed under the cancer. Stay sutures placed at three or four equidistant points in the seromuscular layer of the proposed rectal stump enable the rectum to be more gently and easily manipulated after resection. The proximal colon should be mobilized perhaps more than in conventional anterior anastomosis, thereby ensuring that there will be no tension on the stapled anastomosis, and that one or two loops of redundant colon fill the pelvis, thereby lowering the risk of a pelvic collection which may become infected. The colon ends for anastomosis should be prepared after resection by clearing excessive extramuscular tissue or appendices epiploicae 1·0 cm from the edge; this prevents too much tissue being inverted into the circular stapling device which can be a cause of technical anastomotic failure. The bowel edges must be viable and if there is doubt should be re-prepared. Purse-string sutures may be placed using a modified Furness clamp (*Fig.* 2.10) or a disposable device (*Fig.* 2.11). Alternatively these may be placed by hand, and have to be on the rectal stump in any case because of poor access, using a strong slippery monofilament suture (2/0 polypropylene is ideal). A continuous technique taking 2 mm bites 5 mm apart, going 'inside out' with each loop, ensures an inverted anastomosis and avoids excessive tissue being incorporated into the gun at firing. Passing one of the EEA sizers per anum can push a low rectal stump higher into the pelvis making the placement of a purse-string suture much easier.

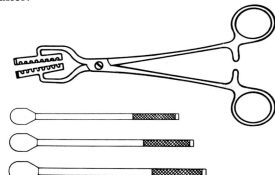

Fig. 2.10. Stainless steel purse-string device (*top*) and stainless steel sizers (*bottom*).

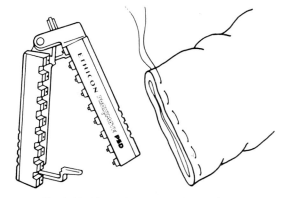

Fig. 2.11. Disposable purse-string device.

The appropriate-sized (judged using EEA sizers or Ethicon TMD; *Figs.* 2.10, 2.12) circular stapler can now be passed per anum fully closed and well lubricated ensuring, as with *all* stapling devices, that the safety catch is on. The abdominally sited surgeon can guide this manoeuvre with a hand in the pelvis.

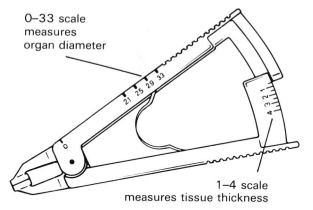

Fig. 2.12. Disposable tissue-measuring device.

0–33 scale measures organ diameter

1–4 scale measures tissue thickness

After opening the gun the purse-string sutures can be tied as tightly as possible onto the centre rod, the distal suture first (*Fig.* 2.13). The instrument may then be closed, to a marker on the Auto Suture EEA gun or to a pre-set tissue thickness using the Ethicon ILS gun (gauged using the TMD device, *Fig.* 2.12) and fired. There is an unquestionable 'feel' to the firing of staples and tissue division, accompanied by an audible 'clunk' caused by division of a plastic washer in the ILS. Supporting the head of the gun at firing prevents inadvertent movement. The instrument is opened by two or three turns of the wing nut and then rotated 360° prior to 'button-holing' the

anvil out of the stapled anastomosis which is facilitated by a non-crushing tissue forceps (*Fig.* 2.14).

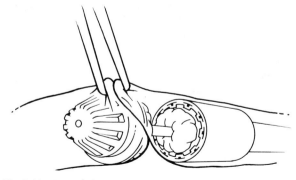

Fig. 2.14. Method of 'button-holing' a fired and opened end-to-end stapler out of an anastomosis.

Anastomotic integrity may be checked by examining the two 'doughnuts' of tissue in the stapling head for completeness (these should be sent for histology to ensure clearance of cancer in appropriate operations). Some surgeons also fill the pelvis with sterile isotonic saline and check the anastomosis for leaks by insufflating air from below per anum. A further check may be made by Gastrografin enema on the 10th postoperative day (*Fig.* 2.15).

Complications after stapled low anterior anastomosis probably lessen with the operator's experience. Leakage is slightly less than after hand-sewn low anterior anastomosis being apparent clinically in 3–10 per cent of cases and radiologically in 10–20 per cent. Suture line recurrence is between 5 and 10 per cent, although more than 30 per cent has been reported, and may be kept lower by adequate cancer clearance particularly of the rectal 'mesentery'. This in turn may be detrimental to the blood supply of the rectal

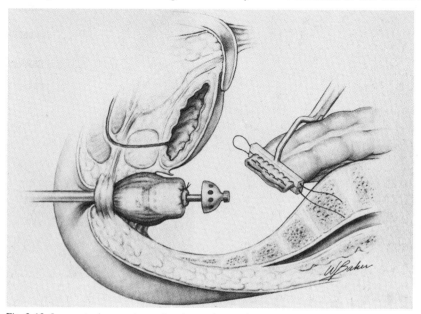

Fig. 2.13. Low anterior anastomosis using end-to-end stapler and modified Furness clamp.

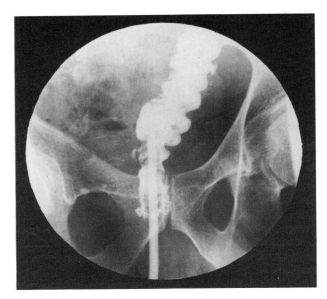

Fig. 2.15. Gastrografin enema of low anterior anastomosis on the 10th postoperative day showing no leak. (The staples lie over the symphysis pubis.)

stump with an increased risk of leakage. Stenosis (5–10 per cent) is probably secondary to subclinical leakage followed by secondary intention healing and scarring. Stenoses usually respond to simple dilatation. Haemorrhage from the suture line, around 1 per cent, is kept low by the B-configuration of staple closure. If a modified anastomosis using the GIA instrument is performed the suture line is more prone to bleeding and should be visually checked. Incontinence, 1–2 per cent, relates only to very low anterior resection although up to 30 per cent of patients complain of a temporary poor control or impaired sensation.

Circular Stapling Devices in Upper Gastrointestinal Surgery

The same principles, using circular staplers, apply to Roux-en-Y oesophago-jejunostomy after a proximal gastrectomy. *Figure* 2.16 shows a satisfactory result of a total gastrectomy and *Fig.* 2.17 shows no leakage of Gastrografin after a proximal gastrectomy with stapled oesophago-gastrostomy during a swallow performed on the 6th postoperative day. The anastomosis in *Fig.* 2.16 is an end-to-side oesophago-jejunostomy which is formed by passage of the circular stapler through the open jejunum without the anvil. The centre rod can then be passed through a separate stab enterotomy without the need for a jejunal purse-string prior to reattaching the anvil for the anastomosis and later closing the end jejunostomy separately. The avoidance of a purse-string on the stomach is equally useful for stapling together

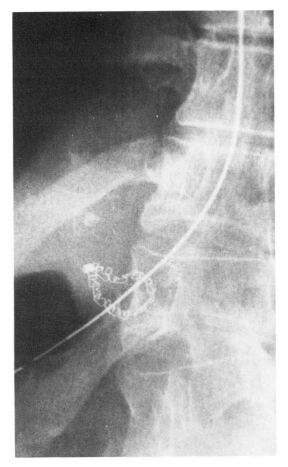

Fig. 2.16. Stapled end-to-side oesophago-jejunostomy-en-Y after transabdominal total gastrectomy. (A nasogastric tube passes through the anastomosis.)

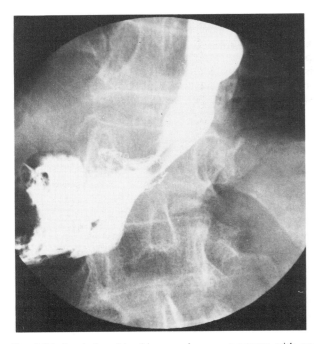

Fig. 2.17. Stapled end-to-side oesophago-gastrostomy with no leakage of swallowed Gastrografin on the 6th postoperative day. (The staples at the anastomosis are clearly seen.)

an oesophago-gastrostomy as in *Fig.* 2.17 (just as on the rectal side for closing a Hartmann's procedure colostomy).

Bleeding oesophageal varices may be controlled by oesophageal transection if medical therapy or injection sclerotherapy fails. It is a relatively easy technique requiring gastrotomy and mobilization of the lower oesophagus to pass a closed circular stapling device into the lower oesophagus. After opening the jaws a tight purse-string ties the full thickness of oesophagus around the centre rod prior to closure and firing. A complete transection and stapled anastomosis are achieved in one (*Fig.* 2.18).

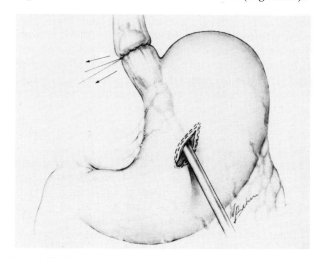

Fig. 2.18. Transgastric oesophageal transection for bleeding varices using end-to-end stapler.

The circular devices may also be used to fashion a Billroth-I anastomosis. Several modifications are possible and a posterior gastroduodenal anastomosis is shown in *Fig.* 2.19 through a separate gastrotomy after closure of the proximal stomach with a linear stapler.

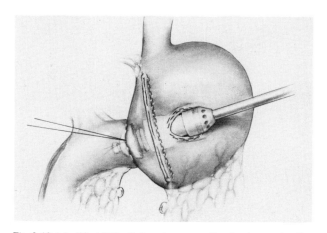

Fig. 2.19. Modified Billroth-I gastrectomy. Proximal resection line closed by linear stapler and continuity restored by posterior gastro-duodenostomy using end-to-end stapler.

Complications after upper gastrointestinal stapled anastomoses are leakage (2 per cent) and bleeding (1 per cent); technical failures, usually resulting in stenosis, should be less than 5 per cent. Stenosis is more common after oesophageal transection for varices but usually responds to dilatation.

Examples of Stapling Using Linear or GIA Instruments

The linear stapling devices may be used to close bowel either prior to resection, as in formation of a duodenal stump in Polya gastrectomy (*Fig.* 2.20), or to close an enterotomy, as in Heineke–Mikulicz pyloroplasty (*Fig.* 2.21). Inversion of a closed duodenal stump or reinforcement of a pyloroplasty may be performed with conventional sutures but is unnecessary. The use of stay sutures or atraumatic tissue forceps ensures that the whole tissue line to be closed

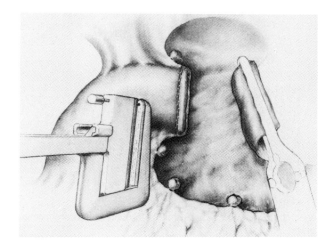

Fig. 2.20. Closure of duodenal stump with linear stapler.

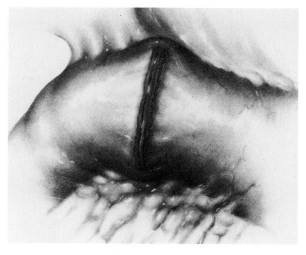

Fig. 2.21. Heineke–Mikulicz pyloroplasty fashioned with linear stapler.

stays in the jaws of the linear stapler otherwise it tends to slip out on tightening the jaws leaving an imperfect stapled line. This is most important for the technique of end-to-end bowel anastomosis by triangulation where an everting anastomosis is performed with three applications of a linear stapler (*Figs.* 2.22 and 2.23).

The GIA instrument allows a wide, rapidly performed side-to-side anastomosis in one manoeuvre.

Gastroenterostomy (*Fig.* 2.24) and bypass entero-enterostomy are made simple. The two forks must be inserted separately into each segment of bowel to be anastomosed fully and evenly to ensure the maximal anastomotic lumen. The anastomosis should always be fashioned on the antimesenteric border of small bowel to avoid damage to supplying vessels. Prior to closure of the enterotomies made for the GIA forks, the staple line should be inspected for haemorrhage, particularly on a gastric side if present, and persistent bleeding can be easily stopped by a simple under-running suture. The functional end-to-end anastomosis gives a wide stoma after an intestinal resection (*Figs.* 2.25 and 2.26). The GIA forks are placed in the afferent and efferent bowel loops away from the mesentery and after firing a wide stoma is achieved. The enterotomies may be closed with a linear stapler prior to resection. Anastomoses

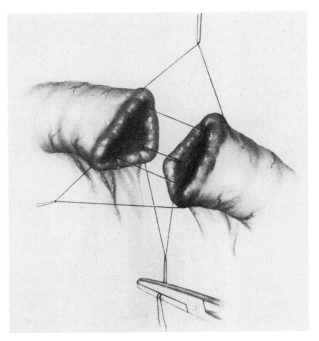

Fig. 2.22. Preparation of intestinal ends for anastomosis by triangulation.

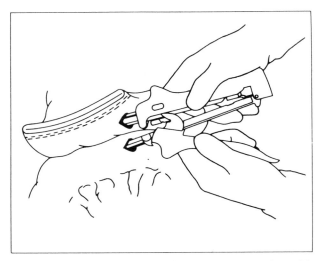

Fig. 2.24. Gastroenterostomy fashioned by GIA side-to-side stapler in one manoeuvre.

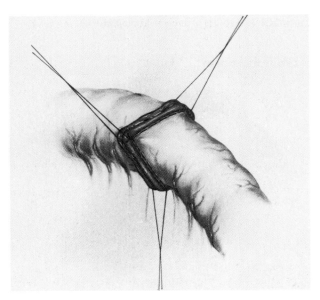

Fig. 2.23. End-to-end anastomosis completed in triangulation following three applications of a linear stapler.

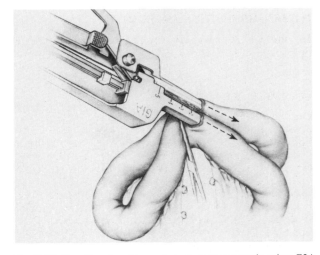

Fig. 2.25. Functional end-to-end stapled anastomosis using GIA side-to-side stapler.

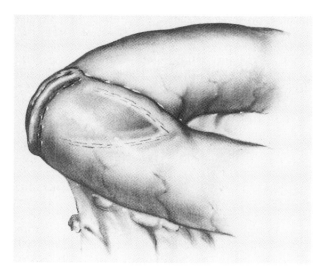

Fig. 2.26. Completed functional end-to-end stapled anastomosis after application of linear stapler. (Note wide stoma.)

formed by the GIA instrument may be reinforced with additional sutures at each end but these are usually unnecessary. The modifications using the GIA stapler devised for gastric and intestinal pouch surgery seem endless and the reader is referred to the specialist texts and atlases listed at the end of this chapter.

When a combination of stapling instruments is used in gastrointestinal surgery a good blood supply should be ensured by keeping at least 2·5 cm between the two staple lines. It is possible to fire knife-bearing instruments (circular and GIA stapler) through another staple line. The existing staples are either pushed out, or pushed aside, or cut through by the knife leaving an acceptable new suture line.

STAPLING TECHNIQUES IN OTHER BRANCHES OF SURGERY

In pulmonary surgery stapling techniques reduce operating time and blood loss. Peripheral open lung biopsy, segmental resection for carcinoma or bullas, and closure of lung lacerations is a simple procedure with single or multiple applications of linear staplers. Similarly bronchial stump or major vessel closure with the linear stapler is simplified and there are many reports of a reduced risk of stump fistula.

In vascular surgery the use of stapling techniques has not become a common procedure. Many of the earlier Russian developments were aimed at this field. Large vessels can be closed with linear staples, for exclusion of large artery aneurysm for example, with a low risk of erosion or vessel rupture. The possibility of a transluminal device which may close vessels or even fashion an anastomosis is attractive but probably a long way ahead.

Ileal conduits and flaps can be made in urological surgery and linear staples may be used in gynaecological practice to close the vaginal vault and to divide the round and broad ligaments The problem of stainless steel eroding through the vaginal vault is abolished by the use of copolymer absorbable staples which are being introduced.

Stapling techniques have an established place in general surgery particularly in low anterior anastomosis and transabdominal gastrectomy, and are ideally suited for fashioning pouches or Koch reservoirs. The reduction in operating time and, more controversially, the chance of safer surgery must be weighed against their substantial cost. Surgeons in training will need to learn, or at least be aware of, the range of surgical techniques possible but stapling techniques must never be allowed to supplant traditional teaching of conventional suture methods. Finally, it must be remembered that all the techniques described in this chapter are only superficially covered. Full manufacturer's instructions and precautions must be followed to the letter in order to avoid the disasters which may follow misuse.

Acknowledgements

The author is grateful to Auto Suture UK Ltd and Ethicon Ltd for permission to reproduce *Figs.* 2.1–2.14 and 2.18–2.26.

FURTHER READING

Dorricott N. J., Baddeley R. M, Keighley M. R. B. et al. (1982) Complications of rectal anastomoses with end-to-end anastomosis (EEA) stapling instrument. *Ann. R. Coll. Surg. Engl.* **64**, 171–174.

Forrester-Wood C. P. (1980) Bronchopleural fistula following pneumonectomy for carcinoma of the bronchus. Mechanical stapling versus hand suturing. *J. Thorac. Cardiovasc. Surg.* **80**, 406–409.

Fraser I. (1982) An historical perspective on mechanical aids in intestinal anastomosis. The surgeon's library. *Surg. Gynecol. Obstet.* **155**, 566–574.

Goligher J. C. (1979) Recent trends in the practice of sphincter-saving excision for rectal cancer. *Ann. R. Coll. Surg. Engl.* **61**, 169–176.

Heald R. J. (1979) A new approach to rectal cancer. *Bri. J. Hosp. Med.* **22**, 277–281.

London I. M. R., Gear M. W. L. and Kilby J. O. (1982) Stapling instrument in upper gastrointestinal surgery: a retrospective study of 362 cases. *Br. J. Surg.* **69**, 333–335.

Ravich M. M. and Steichen F. M. (1972) Technics of staple suturing in the gastrointestinal tract. *Ann. Surg.* **175**, 815–837.

Ravich M. M. and Steichen F. M. (1984) Surgical stapling techniques. In: Surgical Clinics of North America, Volume 64: W. B. Saunders Co., Philadelphia
Robicsek F. (1980) The birth of the surgical stapler. *Surg. Gynecol. Obstet.* **150**, 579–582.
Steichen F. M. and Ravitch M. M. (1973) Mechanical sutures in surgery. *Br. J. Surg.* **60**, 191–197.
Steichen F. M. and Ravich M. M. (1984) *Stapling in Surgery*. Chicago and London: Year Book Medical Publishers.
United States Surgical Corporation (1980) Stapling techniques. *General Surgery*, 2nd ed.
Waxman B. P. (1983) Large bowel anastomoses. II. The circular staplers. *Br. J. Surg.* **70**, 64–67.

Chapter three

The Use and Hazards of Surgical Diathermy

J. P. Mitchell

DESCRIPTION OF THE EQUIPMENT

Surgical diathermy operates by producing an alternating current with wavelengths in the radio frequency range. This current passes through the patient's tissues from the active electrode, which may be of various shapes, to the indifferent electrode, which is usually a metal or foil plate approximately 10×15 cm in size. As this current passes through the tissues there is a heating effect beneath each electrode. The indifferent electrode has a large contact area and therefore heating is reduced to a minimum and is dissipated rapidly (*Fig.* 3.1). The active electrode is always small, in the form of a needle, a blade,

lar to that of a simple radio transmitter oscillating at a frequency between 400 kHz (kilocycles) and 3 MHz (megacycles). The oscillator used in earlier diathermy machines incorporated the standard spark-gap principle which produced consistently a frequency of around 500 kHz. This gave excellent coagulation, but would cut only by increasing the intensity to a high-power output. Even then, the burned tissues adhered to the active electrode which had to be cleaned at frequent intervals. Early in the 1950s valve oscillators were introduced and these increased the frequency range up to 3 MHz which immediately improved the quality of cutting but was found to give poor coagulation. Consequently,

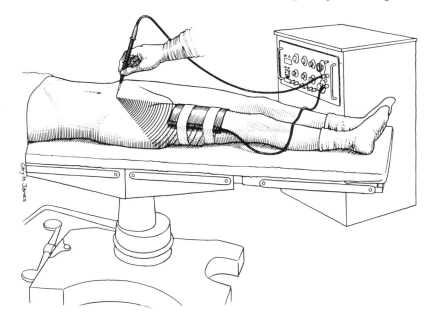

Fig. 3.1. Diagrammatic representation of the passage of a diathermy current through the body from a diathermy machine, via the active electrode to the large metal plate electrode.

a button, or a pair of forceps, and consequently there is concentration of heat in the tissues adjacent to the electrode. This heat is sufficient to cause coagulation in the same way as boiling water coagulates the white of an egg. If the intensity of current is increased then charring of the tissue will occur and this is described as 'fulguration', which may be associated with a crackling noise as the gases of hydrolysis are ignited by a spark. With further increase of intensity an arc can form between the tissues and the electrode, producing a cutting effect (electro-section). (*Fig.* 3.2.)

The circuit of a surgical diathermy machine is simi-

machines produced from 1960 and for the next decade were often constructed with two circuits—the cutting circuit operated by a valve oscillator, while the coagulating circuit had a spark-gap oscillator. Diathermy generators of increased power output were designed, ultimately reaching a maximum of about 1 kW for some of the Continental machines. This increased available power is now considered to be unnecessary and potentially dangerous, particularly when used on small children.

Early in the past decade it became apparent that the reason for the quality of coagulation or cutting

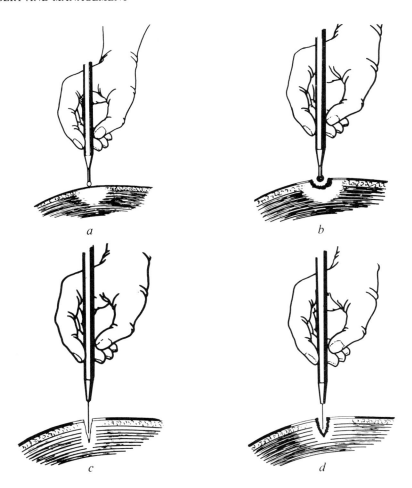

Fig. 3.2. A diagrammatic comparison of the three major surgical effects of diathermy. *a*, Coagulation—haemostasis with only a small amount of tissue damage. *b*, Fulguration—haemostasis with charring and deep-tissue necrosis. *c*, Cutting with a valve or transistorized oscillator, which shows minimal surrounding tissue damage. *d*, Cutting with a 'blended' current which gives a moderate degree of surrounding tissue coagulation.

depended not so much on the frequency of oscillation but on the wave form presented by the diathermy machine and, in this respect, a smooth sine wave gave perfect cutting while an interrupted burst of current would provide excellent coagulation, depending on the frequency of these bursts and the length of gap between each burst. The spark-gap machine gave bursts of damped oscillation at a frequency of approximately 10 kHz. When this interruption of current was superimposed on the sine wave oscillation, the machine was found to be capable of producing coagulation of equal quality to the spark-gap machine. In order to provide an adequate intensity of current, the amplitude of each wave had to be increased in proportion to the length of each burst of current. It was therefore possible for the new machines to dispense with the double circuitry and immediately the diathermy machine became much more compact. The use of transistors as oscillators rather than valves has also made the equipment more reliable and portable.

Blending the Current

In the older twin-circuit diathermy machines the blender switch brought both circuits into action at the same time, with the result that the active electrode was producing a cutting effect as well as a coagulating effect as it passed through the tissues. The power output was the summation of the normal power output of the two circuits together. Today, the solid state transistorized diathermy machines can produce the effect of a blended current from a single circuit merely by taking the setting halfway between the pure sine wave for cutting and the repeated short bursts for coagulation so that the patient is only subjected to the normal power output of a single circuit.

Earthing

It is the practice in the United Kingdom that every piece of electronic equipment should be connected to earth. In addition, any metal equipment in the theatre is earthed to the floor. Considerable expense has been incurred in preparing antistatic mattresses for operating tables, the surgeon's aprons, and the staff footwear, to avoid build-up of electrical potential, which could otherwise discharge in the form of a spark of static electricity. In the humid atmosphere of the United Kingdom such discharge sparks are probably hypothetical.

The disadvantage of earthing a diathermy machine is that it will continue to operate even though the indifferent electrode is not connected to the patient, the return circuit of the diathermy current being carried through any piece of metal in contact with the patient, or even though the antistatic mattress on the table top. Consequently, when the patient is not making adequate contact with the indifferent electrode there is a serious risk of a thermo-electrical burn at the site of any metal contact, such as the leg stirrups, arm rest, anaesthetic screen, or even the table top itself (*Fig.* 3.3). If the output circuit of the diathermy

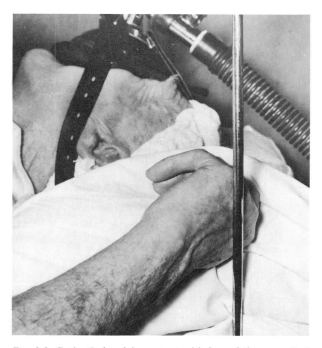

Fig. 3.3. Patient's hand in contact with bar of the anaesthetic screen.

is no longer earthed the current will fail to operate when the indifferent electrode is not in actual contact with the patient. Even turning up the intensity of the current cannot produce any coagulation or cutting, provided that the overall power output of the machine is restricted to reasonable limits (i.e. 400 kW). Only when the plate is placed in contact with the patient will the function of the machine be effective.

However, it should be appreciated that if the indifferent electrode is left accidentally on top of the diathermy cabinet, or is allowed to drop onto the pedestal of the table, the 'isolation' is lost and the circuit immediately becomes earthed, creating its own pathway from the patient (*Fig.* 3.4).

One American manufacturer has patented the principle of monitoring contact of plate to patient by measuring the potential difference between the input and output leads.

Variety of Diathermy Machines

The diathermy generator is a sturdy piece of equipment and will last for many years. Consequently operating theatres may be found equipped with valve oscillating machines, double-circuit spark and valve machines, transistorized solid state diathermies and in some theatres even an old spark-gap generator may occasionally be used. This variety of machinery is liable to be confusing for the nursing staff and its operation should be clearly understood by the surgical staff, because should staff forget to place the indifferent electrode of an earth-free transistorized diathermy on the patient and leave it lying in contact with some earthed object, such as the cabinet of the machine, a metal table top or, worse still, hanging on the radiator, this will immediately earth the circuit and the active electrode will function, while any metal contact with the patient can still give rise to a thermo-electrical burn. It is therefore important that the surgeon should appreciate which type of circuitry is incorporated in the diathermy machine until such time as we have passed through the transition period from earthed circuits to earth-free circuits. This transition period is liable to be 20 or 30 years in view of the durability of diathermy machines and the impecunious state of hospitals.

Monitoring

There are two major factors responsible for thermo-electrical burns in association with the use of surgical diathermy: (1) the inadvertent activation of the diathermy current and (2) failure to apply the indifferent electrode correctly.

Spark-gap oscillators make a clearly audible buzzing noise when the set is operating, but valve oscillators and transistorized diathermy oscillators can function silently. Their only audible noise is the click of the relay switch as the diathermy starts and finishes. It is therefore possible for the operating electrode to be activated accidentally without anyone hearing a noise from the diathermy set. An assistant may have left his or her foot on the foot switch unintentionally. The foot switch itself may become jammed in the 'on' position beneath the pedestal of the operating table or beneath the wheel of a trolley (*Fig.* 3.5). These foot pedals operate with an extremely light touch and almost any contact may activate the foot switch. For this reason all diathermy machines should be equipped with an added noise of operation. This should be an acceptable hum which

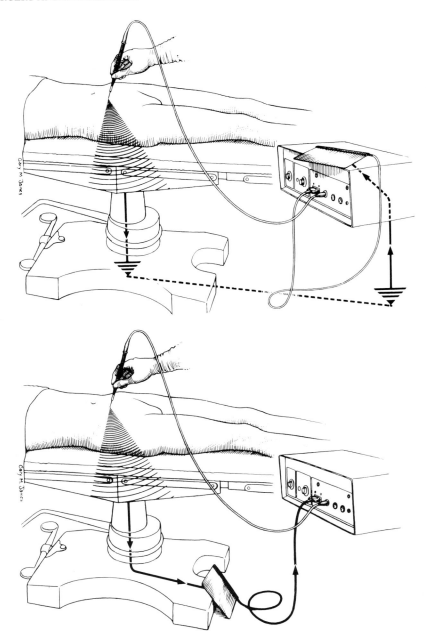

Fig. 3.4. *Top*, Return path of diathermy current to earth, resulting from the indifferent electrode being left on the top of the diathermy cabinet in an isolated circuit.

Bottom, Return path of diathermy current when the indifferent electrode is resting on the pedestal of the table using an isolated circuit.

is clearly audible above the extraneous noise of any routine operating theatre.

The problems of the diathermy indifferent electrode have already been enumerated in relation to earthed and earth-free circuits. It therefore remains the duty of both the medical and nursing staff to ensure that the diathermy plate is attached satisfactorily to the patient. Despite the monitoring devices currently available, inadequate contact with the patient's skin can under certain circumstances cause a thermo-electrical burn. No contact cream is necessary, but the plate should make even contact throughout its entire surface. In order to ensure that the plate is in electrical continuity with the diathermy generator, its cable is designed to have an internal circuit, so that if any point between the plate and

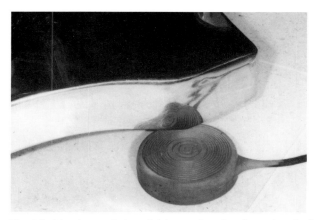

Fig. 3.5. The foot switch pedal jammed under the pedestal of the operating table.

operation it is advised that all machines are monitored in order to avoid confusion.

Today a wide variety of plate electrodes is available on the market, varying considerably in cost. Self-adhesive electrodes are popular and very convenient for use, but it should be appreciated that they can cause serious thermo-electrical burns if the manufacturer's instructions are not observed to the letter. The packages must be stored correctly and must not be out of date, otherwise the adhesive may not be reliable. The contact cream must still be moist, otherwise the current will not be transmitted evenly over the whole of the contact surface. The self-adhesive electrode must not be placed in any position where pressure is likely to occur, such as for example under the buttocks or anywhere between the patient and the table surface, otherwise uneven contact will occur and the electrode will dry out simply from pressure squeezing out the lubricant. The simple and cheap aluminium foil electrode (*Fig.* 3.6) is equally effective and can be re-used four or five times within the same operating list. It has an adequate area of contact and a similar foil electrode can be used even with small babies by wrapping the baby in the foil and applying the monitored clip-on terminal. Wrapping the baby in foil also helps to reduce any heat loss or fluid loss from the body surface.

the diathermy machine is disconnected then an alarm will sound. This alarm should be an intolerable noise which, at the same time, inactivates the circuit of the machine. This second type of monitor is, of course, not essential in the newer diathermy machines with an earth-free circuit, since the diathermy will be non-operational when the patient is not in contact with the indifferent electrode. However, for the sake of uniformity and consistency in

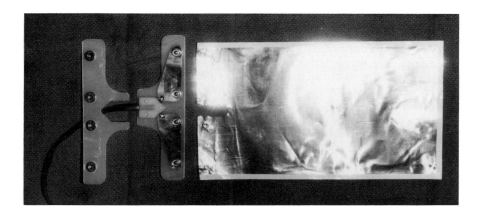

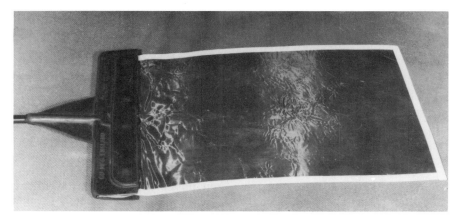

Fig. 3.6. 'Driplate' aluminium foil electrode. Note twin terminals for continuous circuit monitor.

INDICATIONS FOR SURGICAL DIATHERMY

In 90 per cent of operative procedures surgical diathermy is the method of choice for haemostasis of smaller vessels. It is used at all stages in open operative procedures and only larger vessels need to be tied. The cutting diathermy current may be used in place of a sharp knife but it should be remembered that even the pure sine wave cutting current will leave some burnt or coagulated tissue at the margin of the wound. If the surgeon is excising neoplastic tissue he or she may believe the blended current will give added security against the spill of tumour cells, as this will provide coagulation at the site of the cut to a depth of 0·5 mm.

There is now an increasing range of endoscopic surgery, carried out via a wide variety of endoscopes, not only in the urological field but also in the gastro-intestinal tract, and within the peritoneal cavity (via the laparoscope). In most circumstances the operation is performed in air, but in the urinary tract the diathermy functions under water. Here, distilled water should be used, as saline would produce dispersion of the current throughout the whole area of contact of the saline-filled cavity.

Much as diathermy will not function effectively in saline, so it cannot function beneath a pool of blood, as the current will flow throughout the whole of the pool of such an electrolytic solution.

There are scarcely any contra-indications to the use of surgical diathermy in any open surgical procedure, with the exception of circumstances where a channelling effect can occur. If the organ to which diathermy is being applied is held away from the body and its attachment is by a pedicle narrower than the diameter of the organ concerned, then the passage of the current through the pedunculated part will concentrate its intensity so that coagulation at the narrowest point may occur. The current will pass with greatest intensity where there is the highest concentration of electrolytic solution, and this can very well be the blood vessel supplying the organ, which might go into spasm and thrombose, resulting in ischaemia. The best example of such circumstances is the haemostasis required after the excision of a hydrocele (*Fig. 3.7*). The testis may then be suspended for inspection, and bleeding vessels coagulated. If the cord remains narrow and the testis is not in contact with the rest of the body, then there is a serious risk of thrombosis of the main testicular artery. Similarly, diathermy should never be used on a finger or on the penis. Several disasters have occurred from the use of diathermy in circumcision.

The presence of a cardiac pacemaker is no longer a contra-indication to the use of surgical diathermy. Urologists have frequently operated on elderly patients who have pacemakers, with no reported ill effects. Theoretically, the earlier pacemakers, controlled by an external inductance field, could be affected by surgical diathermy but this type of pace-

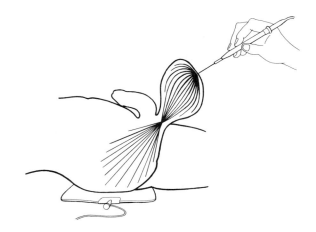

Fig. 3.7. The channelling effect which can concentrate sufficient heat to thrombose vessels in a narrow pedicle, such as in the cord when diathermy is applied to the testis.

maker is rarely found in use today. Nevertheless, two precautions are advisable:

1. To inform the Department of Cardiology that their patient with a pacemaker is about to undergo surgery with the use of diathermy.
2. To ensure that the active and indifferent electrode cables are well away from the region of the pacemaker itself.

Metal implants in the body, such as steel plates, screws, etc., are no contra-indication to the use of diathermy. However, when operating in the region of a metal implant the diathermy electrode should not be allowed to come into contact with the metal as the current would immediately arc from the electrode onto the metal of the implant.

COMPLICATIONS OF SURGICAL DIATHERMY

Most solutions used for skin preparation are made up in a solvent which is flammable. Surgical diathermy should never be used until this solution has had time to evaporate, and any pools of 'prep' solution, such as in the umbilicus or the vagina, must be thoroughly mopped up. One of the commonest causes of litigation today, where diathermy is involved, has been superficial burns from flammable 'prep' solution which has ignited in the vagina at the time of cervical curettage (*Fig. 3.8*).

The thermo-electrical burn can be due to a variety of causes, the return of current through earth to stray contact points on the operating table, inadequate application of the plate electrode so that it makes too small an area of contact, and inadvertent activation of the circuit so that the active electrode is alive and possibly resting near the patient's skin (*Fig. 3.9*).

Explosion from flammable anaesthetic gases is today a remote risk, since flammable gases are rarely used in open circuits. This may, however, increase

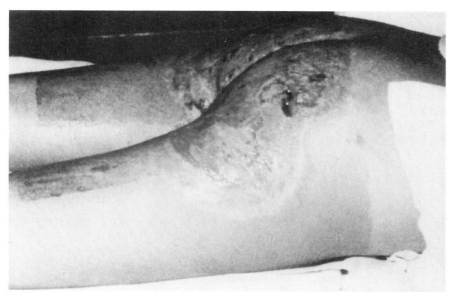

Fig. 3.8. Cutaneous burns of buttocks due to conflagration of the preparation solution.

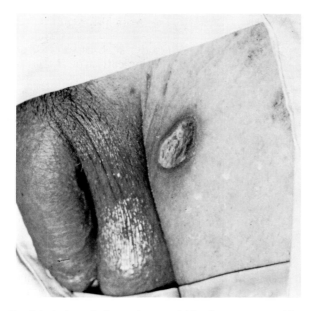

Fig. 3.9. A deep diathermy burn, resulting from an exposed junction of an active electrode lead.

the risk on those exceptional occasions when ether is the anaesthetist's choice, and the old habit of consulting the anaesthetist before switching on the diathermy should not be discarded.

In summary, diathermy is used in nearly all surgical operations. Its dangers are very real, with important medico-legal implications. A thermo-electrical burn or a conflagration on the skin surface is always due

to a fault in technique, and it is therefore the duty of surgeons and theatre staff to have a working knowledge of the principle of surgical diathermy.

PURCHASING A NEW DIATHERMY MACHINE

When purchasing a new diathermy machine it is most important to test the machine in use to see that it provides the facilities required by all the surgeons who will use the machine. Servicing facilities must be checked to ensure that costs of servicing and any delays are minimal. It may be that arrangements have already been made within the hospital for servicing other diathermy equipment. This would inevitably mean that purchasing from the same manufacturer would have some advantage in the cost of maintenance. Lastly, it is important to assess the cost of any disposable parts, such as leads and indifferent electrodes. The high cost of some disposable self-adhesive electrodes has already been mentioned (*see* p. 27).

Illustrations
Figures 3.1–3.3, 3.5–3.7 and 3.9 are taken from Mitchell J P., Lumb G. N. and Dobbie A. K. (1978) *A Handbook of Surgical Diathermy*, 2nd ed. Bristol, John Wright.

Figure 3.4 is taken from Mitchell J. P. (1984) *Endoscopic Operative Urology*. Bristol, John Wright.

Figure 3.8 is taken from Mitchell J. P. (1984) *Urinary Tract Trauma*. Bristol, John Wright.

FURTHER READING

This chapter deals only with the use of diathermy in general but for specific application in certain specialties, the reader is referred to the following literature:

Mitchell J. P., Lumb G. N. and Dobbie A. K. (1978) *A Handbook of Surgical Diathermy*, 2nd ed., with chapters by Harris P. and Smart G. E. Bristol, John Wright.

Mitchell J. P. (1984) Surgical diathermy in urological endoscopy. In: *Endoscopic Operative Urology*. Bristol, John Wright, Chap. 6.

Mitchell J. P. (1982) Surgical diathermy in urological practice. In: Chisholm G. D. and Williams B. I. (eds) *Scientific Foundations of Urology*, 2nd ed. London, Heinemann Medical, Chap. 100.

Chapter four

Lasers in Medicine and Surgery

J. A. S. Carruth

'If you don't need a laser, don't use one.' These words of Dr Leon Goldman, one of the fathers of laser surgery, must never be forgotten. A laser should only be used when it can be shown clearly that it can perform a specific medical or surgical task better than established conventional techniques. Almost any operation could be performed by using a laser, or a combination of lasers, but in this chapter an attempt is made to show not just that lasers can be used in certain clinical situations, but why they should be used and the advantages they offer to both doctor and patient.

Since the first laser was produced by T. H. Maiman in 1960, a large number of laser systems has been developed with a vast range of industrial, scientific and military uses. Within the last 20 years, the use of lasers in medicine and surgery has been extensively researched, and several are now in regular clinical use in a number of disciplines, while others are being researched and evaluated.

THE LASER

A laser (*light amplification by stimulated emission of radiation*) produces coherent light—an intense beam of pure, monochromatic light, which does not diverge, and in which all the light waves are the same length and travel in step in the same direction.

The name of the laser is taken from the lasing medium, which in most medical lasers is a gas. The lasing medium is contained in the laser tube, which has a fully reflective mirror at one end and at the other a partially reflective mirror which allows access to the laser beam.

The lasing medium is excited electrically to produce an inversion of the normal population ratio of excited:non-excited particles which normally has a large excess in the non-excited state. An excited particle will decay to the low-energy ground state with the release of a photon—a quantum of radiant energy or light particle. If this photon strikes an excited particle it stimulates it to emit an identical photon. Photons released by these collisions are reflected back into the lasing medium from the mirrors, with a rapid build-up of light energy in the tube—the cascade effect. The beam is emitted through the partially reflective mirror.

The absorption of the laser beam by body tissues and its effects on them are determined by the wavelength of the coherent light, and as each laser pro-

duces one wavelength it has one main clinical role, and to change role one must change laser.

MEDICAL LASERS

Carbon Dioxide (*Fig.* 4.1)

The carbon dioxide (CO_2) laser produces infra-red coherent light at a wavelength of 10 600 nm which is absorbed by water and, therefore, by body tissues which contain 70–90 per cent water.

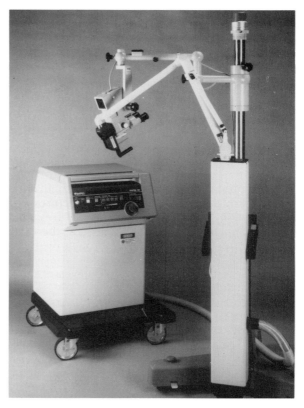

Fig. 4.1. Carbon dioxide laser mounted on an operating microscope.

Intracellular water absorbs the energy and is boiled, causing the cells to rupture, releasing non-viable cell contents into the beam where they are carbonized and fall as 'soot' around the laser wound. This instantaneous cell vaporization takes place at the relatively low temperature of 100 °C and, as tissues conduct heat poorly, there is an extremely thin

31

layer of damaged cells between the laser wound and adjacent, normal tissues. As a result healing is not complicated by oedema and is rapid and remarkably pain free. It has been shown experimentally that there is less contracture of a mucosal wound cut by laser than of one cut by scalpel or diathermy.

Tissue destruction is immediate—an advantage over cryotherapy—and dissection is relatively bloodless as the beam seals vessels of up to 0·5 mm in diameter. The beam also seals lymphatics possibly reducing the spread of tumour cells via this route.

The CO_2 laser is a high-precision, bloodless, light scalpel and much of the work is carried out under the operating microscope or colposcope, which provide a well-illuminated, magnified operative field. The working beam is aimed by a coaxial, low-powered, visible helium neon laser controlled by a micro-manipulator on the laser delivery head. By choosing appropriate power and exposure settings for the beam on the tissues, the amount of tissue destruction for each activation of the laser can be determined accurately. In addition, the beam does not denature the tissues through which it is passing and, as there are neither blood nor instruments in the wound, the progress of dissection can be followed with great accuracy. A sucker is needed to remove the vapour of tissue destruction, but otherwise no instruments are needed and this is of great value in surgery, where access is limited. At present the CO_2 beam cannot be transmitted via a flexible fibre but stainless steel mirrors may be used to reflect the beam into inaccessible areas.

Argon

This laser produces blue/green coherent light which will pass through clear and colourless structures without absorption, but is absorbed by structures which have its complementary colour red. It is, therefore, possible to treat vascular lesions through overlying, clear, normal tissues.

This laser is used primarily for blood vessel coagulation, although at high power levels, slow, thermal tissue destruction can be performed. It lacks the precision of the CO_2 laser and there is some spread of heat into adjacent tissues.

In the coagulation of blood vessels a precisely localized lesion of the vessel can be created by delivering an exactly calculated dose of energy without any mechanical contact with the vessel and with no spread of thermal or electrical energy to adjacent structures. The laser can be used to control both normal and abnormal vessels and also acute haemorrhage.

The beam can be transmitted via a flexible fibre and it is used with the operating microscope, slit lamp, handpiece and via the biopsy channel of a flexible endoscope.

Neodymium YAG

This laser produces infra-red coherent light at a wave-length of 1060 nm which is deeply absorbed in the tissues without colour or tissue specificity. At high power levels, thermal tissue destruction can be performed with, in many cases, better haemostasis than with the CO_2 laser. However, with the deep penetration of the beam into the tissues, there is a significant risk of thermal damage to adjacent structures even beyond the organ being treated. When tumour is removed with this laser there are three layers of damage. First, a layer which is vaporized; second, a layer of damage which will slough; and, third, a layer of damaged cells which are replaced by fibrous tissue, but without loss of physical integrity, and so in the treatment of a hollow viscus there is only a very small risk of perforation. The beam can be transmitted via a flexible fibre, and much of the work with this laser has been carried out via a flexible fibre-optic endoscope. In the control of haemorrhage from upper gastrointestinal ulcers, it appears that this laser will prove to be better than the argon laser, as it causes damage and fibrosis to the perivascular tissues allowing larger vessels to be controlled. This laser can be used to control normal and abnormal vessels and to carry out sutureless microvascular anastomosis.

The pulsed Nd YAG laser is being evaluated at present for the fragmentation of both renal and biliary stones by photo-acoustic effects. It is also being used in ophthalmology to create precisely controlled lesions in the eye using very short pulses of energy.

Krypton

This laser is used in ophthalmology, similarly to the argon laser for retinal photocoagulation.

Ruby

Much of the early medical research work was carried out with this pulsed laser, but it has been largely replaced by the more controllable continuous wave lasers. It is still used in the treatment of some pigmented skin lesions and blue and black tattoos.

Dye

The wavelength of the argon-pumped dye laser can be tuned over a significant range of the spectrum and it has been suggested that it may prove to be better than the argon laser for the selective destruction of blood vessels in the skin. Its main use at present is in the activation of intra-tumour haematoporphyrin derivative in photoradiation therapy for malignant disease.

Gold Vapour

This pulsed laser produces red light at the appropriate wavelength for activation of haematoporphyrin derivative in photoradiation therapy, and at much higher power levels than can be produced by the dye laser.

Safety

Although the lasers used in medicine and surgery are much less powerful than many used in science and industry, all those used therapeutically are in the highest power class and their use 'requires extreme caution'.

In Britain, the safe use of medical lasers is controlled by the Health and Safety at Work Act, the British Standards Code BS4803 and the *Guidance on the Safe Use of Lasers in Medical Practice*, recently produced by the Department of Health and Social Security. The codes insist on the appointment of a local laser safety officer who will produce local codes of safe practice for each laser, in each clinical situation.

The main risk with all lasers is damage to the eyes of the patient or a member of the operating theatre personnel. It is extremely unlikely that the eyes of a member of the operating theatre personnel could be exposed to the direct beam, but the beam could be reflected back into the operating theatre from an instrument or retractor and all in the theatre must be provided with appropriate, fully laser-proof eyewear. Securely fixed protective covering will be provided for the eyes of the patient.

The eyes of the surgeon are protected by the optics of the operating microscope when the CO_2 laser is used in this mode and, with the argon laser, shutters which close when the laser is activated are provided on the microscope and slit lamp. With the neodymium YAG laser a filter may be incorporated into the endoscope, but for all other uses the surgeon must also wear laser-proof eyewear appropriate to the laser being used.

There are certain other specific hazards, such as anaesthetic tube ignition when the CO_2 laser is used in laryngology, and the anaesthetist must use one of a number of 'laser-proof' techniques in this situation.

CLINICAL USE OF LASERS IN MEDICINE AND SURGERY

This review of the use of lasers in medicine and surgery must, of necessity, be brief and although all the statements are supported by references, these are not included in the text and a guide to further reading is provided at the end of the chapter.

Cardiovascular

Some exciting research and very early clinical work are in progress on the use of lasers in the transluminal disobliteration of obstructed vessels. Using the argon and neodymium YAG lasers transmitted via flexible fibres, either under radiographic control or under direct vision using a fine viewing fibre, it has been shown that both thrombus and atheroma can be destroyed without significant risk of distal embolization or of vessel perforation.

An alternative approach to the revascularization of the heart is to create a multiple perforation of the myocardium into the ventricle using a high-powered CO_2 laser. The channels remain patent and become endothelialized allowing blood to diffuse directly into the myocardium from the ventricle, but the perforations close on the surface of the heart. It has been shown that these channels can support the myocardium in dogs in which coronary arteries have been tied and early clinical work is in progress.

Intracardiac laser surgery can be used to relieve some forms of valvular stenosis and laser irradiation can cause shortening of the chordae tendinae to relieve valvular incompetence.

Chest Medicine

Many patients with 'untreatable' carcinoma of the bronchus die in extreme distress from obstruction of one of the major air passages by tumour. Both the CO_2 and Nd YAG lasers have been used to provide palliation of these patients by the removal of the obstructing tumour. The Nd YAG laser can be used via a flexible fibre-optic bronchoscope, whereas the CO_2 laser must be used with a rigid instrument. In theory the Nd YAG laser should be able to provide palliation in patients with peripherally situated lesions, but in practice palliation can only be achieved regularly in patients with obstruction of the trachea and main bronchi. Many workers use the Nd YAG laser with a rigid 'scope which allows better suction and removal of necrotic tumour fragments with forceps.

Photoradiation therapy (*see* p. 35) offers enormous potential for the palliation of advanced cases of bronchial carcinoma and for the diagnosis and treatment for cure of early cases.

Dermatology

The CO_2 laser may be used to cut the skin but with no particular advantage over the scalpel, except in patients with a haemorrhagic tendency and in the removal of multiple lesions such as warts or condylomata accuminata.

The argon laser is now the treatment of choice for the hitherto untreatable port-wine stain. The blue/green beam passes through the clear epidermis without significant absorption or thermal damage and is then absorbed by the blood in the network of abnormal capillaries in the outer dermis, causing thermal damage and thrombosis. The thrombosed vessels are then replaced over a period of months by fibrous tissue with a marked reduction in the colour of the birthmark, but the epidermis returns to normal and there should be no scarring. Certain features of the birthmark may be used to predict a good response and a wide range of treatment techniques have been described. In patients with a good prognosis, a satisfactory result can be obtained in about 80 per cent of cases and with a 'low-power technique' the incidence of scarring should be less than 2 per cent.

Gastroenterology

The mortality from upper gastrointestinal haemorrhage remains high in those patients who continue to bleed and in those who rebleed. A number of uncontrolled and controlled trials have been performed to show the value of the argon and neodymium YAG laser in the control of the acute bleed and in the prevention of rebleeding, and it appears that the Nd YAG laser will prove to be the better in this field. The laser energy is delivered by a quartz fibre introduced via the biopsy channel of a flexible endoscope and the acute bleed can be controlled in 70–100 per cent of cases, but only one series has claimed that the laser can control bleeding from oesophageal varices. One of the most valuable predicting signs for rebleeding is a visible vessel in the ulcer crater and, if these cases are treated by laser photocoagulation, a significant reduction in the incidence of rebleeding can be achieved. A reduction in mortality has also been reported.

The neodymium YAG laser can be used to provide palliation by removing obstructing oesophageal carcinoma to relieve dysphagia.

Gynaecology

With a greater understanding of the natural history of pre-malignant conditions of the cervix, there has been an increasing tendency to treat these lesions by local destruction under the microscopic control of the operating colposcope. To destroy these lesions with electrocautery requires a general anaesthetic and although cryotherapy can be performed without anaesthesia, many believe that the tissue removal lacks precision. Precise vaporization of appropriate cervical lesions can be performed by CO_2 laser with excellent results, and a large majority of women can tolerate the technique without anaesthetic. Post-operative complications are minimal and, as there is no scarring of the cervical canal, the women are able to have children. If the lesion necessitates a cone biopsy, it has been shown that this can be performed by CO_2 laser with advantages over the conventional 'cold knife' technique.

In the performance of pelvic reconstructive surgery, the lack of tissue reaction with the CO_2 laser offers potential advantages, but more research is needed before its role in this field is established. Another area of research is endometrial ablation with the neodymium YAG laser for menorrhagia.

Neurosurgery

Lasers offer the neurosurgeon true 'no touch' surgery, and as there is no shock impact when the laser beam strikes the tissues, surgery can be performed without mechanical or thermal trauma to vital areas of the central nervous system.

The CO_2 laser can be used to perform precise incisions in the brain and spinal cord. In the removal of tumours, the capsule is incised with this laser, the centre of the tumour is then exenterated allowing the capsule to be drawn medially to be vaporized. The CO_2 laser is also used to create precise lesions of the spinal cord for the control of pain.

The argon laser can be used to photocoagulate both normal and abnormal vessels, and some exciting research work is in progress on the control of aneurysms and vascular malformations.

The Nd YAG laser is used to exenterate vascular tumours but there is some risk of thermal damage to adjacent structures. This laser is being used to perform sutureless microvascular anastomoses with excellent long-term patency.

Ophthalmology

This was the first specialty in which lasers were used and it remains in the forefront of laser usage. One of the main causes of blindness in the Western world is diabetic retinopathy, in which new vessels develop in front of the plane of the retina. The argon and krypton lasers are used to perform photocoagulation to destroy areas of avascular retina which are thought to be the stimulus to new vessel growth. Laser photocoagulation may also be used to create chorioretinal adhesions around retinal tears to prevent detachment.

The argon laser may be used to reduce the abnormal intra-ocular pressure in both acute closed-angle glaucoma, by creating a hole in the iris and, in chronic simple glaucoma, by trabeculectomy improving the drainage through the trabecular network.

The pulsed Nd YAG laser is used to create precise lesions within the eye, using very short pulses of energy, to remove opaque intra-ocular structures such as the posterior lens capsule after the removal of a cataract. The use of the CO_2 laser via an intra-ocular probe is also being researched.

Otolaryngology

All the features of tissue removal by CO_2 laser make it of the greatest value in surgery to the larynx, particularly in children. The ability to remove tissue with precision, no bleeding, no postoperative oedema, and reduced scar formation with contracture, are unique to this modality. These features make the CO_2 laser the treatment of choice for juvenile laryngeal papillomatosis, in which the larynx of a child becomes filled with frond-like viral warts which recur after removal until the condition remits, often at puberty. These children require scores of procedures to keep the airway open and the CO_2 laser reduces the morbidity of each procedure, and gives the child the longest disease and symptom-free interval. A tracheostomy can be avoided in the vast majority of cases.

Research is in progress on the role of the CO_2 laser in the field of post-traumatic laryngeal stenosis and early vocal cord carcinoma. Lesions of the mouth and tongue can be removed with precision, low blood loss and minimal postoperative morbidity.

The use of the argon laser under the operating microscope to perform delicate surgery to the middle ear is being evaluated.

Urology

After treatment of tumours of the bladder by electro-surgical techniques, recurrence is common particularly when multiple tumours have been treated. This recurrence is blamed on the multifocal nature of the disease, and the possibility that viable tumour fragments are released and become implanted in the dome of the bladder.

The neodymium YAG laser can be used, via a cystoscope, with an Albarren bridge to direct the fibre into all parts of the bladder, to destroy the exophytic part of the tumour without releasing viable fragments and also to destroy tumour within the bladder wall without the risk of perforation or damage to adjacent viscera. The technique can be tolerated without the need for a general anaesthetic and postoperative catheterization is not needed.

The CO_2 laser can be used to treat superficial lesions of the external genitalia and may prove to be of value in the treatment of urethral stricture. Some exciting research work is in progress on the destruction of urinary stones using the pulsed Nd YAG laser.

Photoradiation Therapy

This technique represents a new and unique approach to the treatment of many forms of localized malignant diseases. It has been shown that haematoporphyrin derivative (HPD), after an intravenous injection, is taken up by all body tissues and is then selectively retained by malignant tissues. The mechanism for this retention remains uncertain, but it is thought to be due to the abnormal tumour circulation.

If tumour containing HPD is exposed to blue/violet light it will fluoresce and some exciting work is in progress on the detection of early carcinoma of the bronchus using a fluorescent bronchoscopic technique. A krypton laser is used to provide the blue light and an image intensifier to identify the areas of fluorescence. A similar technique can be used to identify malignant foci in multifocal bladder disease.

If tumour containing HPD is exposed to red light at a wavelength of 630 nm, which is the optimal wavelength for tissue penetration and activation of the HPD, singlet oxygen is produced by energy transfer from the excited porphyrin molecule and this transient, highly reactive state of the oxygen molecule is cytotoxic causing destruction of tissues containing HPD, but surrounding normal tissues are left undamaged.

In the development of the technique, many light sources were used, but it became apparent that the argon pumped tunable dye laser provided the best source of this light at appropriate power levels which could be transmitted down a flexible fibre. Recently, work has begun with the pulsed gold vapour laser which appears to be at least as good as the dye laser and much higher power levels are available.

A number of clinical trials have been performed and are in progress on tumours of the skin, head and neck, bronchus, bladder, eye and other sites. Some very encouraging early results have been obtained and when this technique has been fully investigated, it must represent an important modality for the treatment of many forms of malignant disease.

We are only at the beginning of the laser age, and in medicine and surgery lasers have already turned science fiction into science fact. With further research many more exciting developments can be anticipated.

FURTHER READING

Andreoni A. and Cubeddu R. (1984) *Porphyrins in Tumour Phototherapy*. New York, Plenum.

Andrews A. H. and Polanyi T. G. (1982) *Microscopic and Endoscopic Surgery with the CO_2 Laser*. Bristol, John Wright.

Arndt K. A., Noe J. M. and Rosen S. (1983) *Cutaneous Laser Therapy*. Chichester, John Wiley.

Atsumi K. (1983) *New Frontiers in Laser Medicine and Surgery*. Amsterdam, Excerpta Medica.

Bellina J. H. and Bandieramonte G. (1984) *Principles and Practice of Gynaecologic Laser Surgery*. New York, Plenum.

Choy D. S., Stertzer S., Rotterdam H. Z. et al. (1982) Transluminal laser catheter angioplasty. *Am. J. Cardiol.* **50**, 1206.

Fleischer D. and Brown S. G. (1983) Endoscopic laser therapy for upper gastro-intestinal carcinoma. In: Fleischer D., Jensen D. and Bright-Asare P. (eds.) *Therapuetic Laser Endoscopy in Gastro-intestinal Disease*. The Hague, Martinus Nijhoff.

Hetzel M. R., Millard F. J. C., Ayesh R. et al. (1983) Laser treatment for carcinoma of the bronchus. *Br. Med. J.* **286**, 12.

Jain K. K. (1983) Lasers in neurosurgery: a review. *Lasers Med. Surg.* **2**, 217.

Mirhoseini M., Muckerheide M. and Cayton M. M. (1982) Transventricular revascularisation by laser. *Lasers Med. Surg.* **2**, 187.

Rothenberger K., Pensel J., Hofstetter A. et al. (1983) Transurethral laser coagulation for treatment of urinary bladder tumours. *Lasers Med. Surg.* **2**, 255.

Simpson G. T. and Shapshay S. M. (1983) The use of lasers in otolaryngologic surgery. *Otolaryngol. Clin. North Am.* **16**(4).

Abdominal Wall and Gastroenterology

Chapter five

Abdominal Access and Closure

H. A. F. Dudley

ACCESS TO THE ABDOMINAL CAVITY

Appropriate access to the abdomen is critical to the correct performance of all abdominal procedures. How often has one seen a surgeon struggling to perform a procedure in the belly merely because he or she has inadequate exposure? In this regard, the so-called 'incision of indecision'—vertical and centred on the umbilicus—is not in itself adequate for a full abdominal exploration.

Though one can have every sympathy for both surgeon and patient in the former's desire to produce minimum disfigurement and the latter's to have as small a surface blemish as possible, incisions should be designed primarily for the job on hand and only secondarily for their ultimate appearance. The end-result is determined as much by good surface suture technique as by direction and position and, in a few cases, by the patient's employment—especially models of either sex—where the patient's economic future hangs on there being the best cosmetic result. This having been said, skin incisions can often be directed in creases to make for minimal scarring even though the underlying abdominal wall is cut according to the best exposure.

The following general anatomical points should be noted:

1. In a vertical incision the amount of lateral retraction is closely related to the length of the incision. Thus if a lateral structure such as the spleen is to be approached through a vertical incision, then the cut must be of considerable length—certainly greater than 17 cm and probably in excess of 20 cm in the adult.

2. The diaphragm is horizontal in the midline where its tendon passes directly backwards behind the xiphoid. To obtain maximum exposure of structures which are immediately below the diaphragm, such as the hiatus, a vertical incision must be carried up to the xiphoid or this structure split or excised.

3. If further exposure is required above this point a marginal gain can be made by either excising or splitting the xiphoid, which is usually a flexible structure, However, if a wide exposure is required of the immediately supradiaphragmatic structures then a full-length sternal split must be used because of the rigidity of that bone.

4. If exposure requires either a primarily muscle-cutting incision or a muscle-cutting extension, then no hesitation need be felt. Though muscle-cutting incisions are said to be more prone to incisional hernia than are muscle-splitting ones, I doubt if this is true provided sound closure techniques are used.

Incising the Abdominal Wall

With proper anaesthetic technique the abdominal wall is a flaccid structure at the time of incision. It is best stretched by the fingers of the surgeon's left and the assistant's right hands as the incision is made. I do not like to see this done by direct contact between the gloves and skin; I prefer a gauze pack to intervene and in any case this gives a slightly better grip.

Opening the Peritoneum

In an intact abdomen it is extremely difficult to injure an underlying structure while opening the peritoneum. If a small fold of peritoneum is picked up between two artery forceps or between a pair of artery forceps and dissecting forceps it can be opened quite safely by a gentle touch of the scalpel. Air immediately enters the peritoneal cavity and the underlying structures fall away. It is unnecessary to pick up a fold big enough to allow it to be pinched between finger and thumb because as long as the cavity is closed this will not displace anything underneath. However, matters are considerably different when the abdomen is being re-entered. Because there is a high incidence of adhesions to the inner aspect of any laparotomy wound and because further tramlining incisions may result in necrosis of the band of skin so enclosed (*Fig.* 5.1), it is always better to start from the rule that the same incision should be reopened. There may on occasions be exceptions to

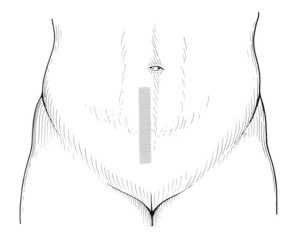

Fig. 5.1. Zone of skin at risk if two incisions are 'tramlined'.

this but they are relatively few. Nevertheless great care must then be taken to avoid injuring an adherent structure; to plough into the omentum is a surgical mess if not exactly a surgical crime.

One helpful manoeuvre is to make the new incision a little longer than the old in whatever direction is judged most useful and thus to find an entry point that is likely to lead directly into an adhesion-free part of the peritoneal cavity. More usually it will be necessary to carry sharp dissection down to the deepest fascial layer of the wound and then to dissect laterally so as to expose the plane between adhesions and inner aspect of the parietal peritoneum. This is greatly helped if it is possible to grasp the edge of (say) the posterior rectus sheath with artery forceps and turn it back on itself (*Fig.* 5.2). Not only does

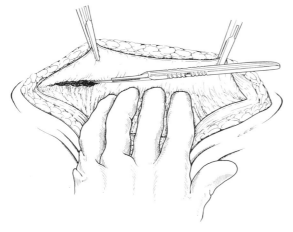

Fig. 5.2. Abdominal re-entry. Note the turned back inner peritoneal surface held under tension.

this put the tissues on the stretch but it also usually exposes the plane. Sharp dissection is then continued until at a varying distance from the wound the peritoneal cavity is entered. Once this has been done it is usually quite easy to work around the whole circumference of the wound until everything has been freed. Caution must still be observed while doing this as it is easy, the more the structures are freed, to hasten the pace or to draw a hidden loop of bowel up into the plane of dissection. Disaster may follow for it is truly clumsy to damage a hollow structure while re-entering the abdomen. It should be a rule that to make a proper re-exploration of the abdomen, it is necessary to free all parietal adhesions; once more there may be exceptions but the axiom is a sound one.

Dealing with Adhesions

The same precautions as for abdominal re-entry apply. Adhesions often tent up loops of bowel and it is all too easy to cut in the wrong plane. Putting structures on the stretch by gentle retraction with the left hand, or less satisfactorily the assistant's

hand, and the precise use of the knife—not scissors, which are a relatively clumsy instrument for this purpose—is the key to success. A special but important case is when the right upper quadrant must be re-explored after gallbladder surgery. Here it is necessary accurately to enter the plane between the undersurface of the liver and any adherent structures—omentum, duodenum or transverse colon; it is very easy to wander off into either the liver substance or the gut. The mass of soft tissues below the liver is drawn downwards and to the left and the knife used delicately to enter the plane at the edge of the liver. The best place to start is usually laterally because it is most probable that the adhesions are least marked at this point. As the dissection proceeds the hepatic edge is rolled back by a broad retractor such as a Deaver and it is surprising how easy it usually is to stay in the appropriate plane until, as the late Dr Cattell of the Lahey Clinic used to say, 'bile flows from the depths of the incision to indicate that the surgeon is deep enough!'

GENERAL ASPECTS OF HEALING AND THE CHOICE OF SUTURE MATERIALS

Wounds heal after the initial inflammatory phase by the deposition and orientation of fibrous tissue which is initially rapid but is not complete in a fascial layer until at least 8–10 months have elapsed. It can therefore be argued that it is necessary to 'support' wound apposition for at least that length of time. It would then follow that in the abdominal wall nonabsorbable sutures should always be used. However, matters are not probably quite so simple as that. Certainly in the initial stages—say the first 2–3 weeks—the sutures do ensure mechanical support against distractive forces and are thus critical to the prevention of wound dehiscence. Their role thereafter is more problematic and in that they are increasingly embedded in a collagen matrix, they may become progressively less significant. However, in that it is difficult to know what the slope of the initial healing curve is going to be for an individual patient and how this may be interfered with by sepsis it is, at the present time, better to continue to use monofilament absorbable sutures to close the laparotomy wounds. Clinical experiments are in progress to assess both polyglycolic acid (Dexon, Vicryl) and the newer synthetic monofilament polydioxanone (PDS) but the wise surgeon will await their outcome before abandoning what has, for many, become standard practice. It is worth mentioning that closure of the abdominal wall by the techniques described below has an acute failure rate of about 1 in 500 (though the incidence of incisional hernia is probably higher) and any new technique must live up to the same level of performance.

Sepsis obviously slows down the healing process and has a variable effect on the dissolution rate of absorbable sutures. Tryptic digestion of catgut is markedly accelerated and this partly accounted in the past for the very bad results that were obtained with abdominal wall closure using this material. Synthetic absorbables are relatively unaffected by the presence of sepsis and if they prove satisfactory in the uninfected wound then there will be no contra-indication to their use when sepsis is likely or inevitable.

The other side of this coin is whether sutures potentiate sepsis. It is certain that organisms can lodge in the interstices of braided material and thus produce an intractable infection which will not subside until the suture is removed or extruded. It is equally certain that infected wounds that contain monofilament non-absorbables can heal even with the sutures *in situ*. Midway between these two states, some wounds closed with monofilament may produce small sinuses up to 5 years or more after they have been made. One possible explanation is that there are certain types of organism more capable of adhering to a monofilament and even etching its surface and it is these which account for the small incidence of stitch sinus seen with such materials.

The upshot of all this is that braided material, though easy to handle, is probably not the right material for abdominal wall closure; that monofilament nylon or Prolene (though the latter is not very easy to knot securely) remains the material of first choice today. Steel was considered a good material at one time, before the advent of synthetic monofilaments, but it is demanding to use. Furthermore its stiff knots sometimes give rise to pain by prodding the subcutaneous tissues from within.

TECHNICAL FACTORS IN ABDOMINAL WALL CLOSURE

Incisions in the abdominal wall are, because of its function as a dynamic corset for the abdominal organs and as a muscle of respiration, defaecation and micturition, subject to more early distractive forces than those in any other part of the body. Anything additional that paroxysmally raises intra-abdominal pressure such as coughing and straining to sit up or get out of bed, also puts distractive tension on a laparotomy wound. Also, temporary intestinal dysfunction after laparotomy often leads to a variable degree of distension which is in effect distraction from within. In consequence closure of the wound must have, from the moment it is done, sufficient extrinsic strength to withstand these forces and keep the edges apposed until in the fullness of time intrinsic strength is restored. This means in turn that sutures must be inserted in such a way that they do not 'cut out'.

Though surgeons are conventionally taught that fine neat suturing with delicate materials is best for tissue healing, in the abdomen this is not the case. In order to reduce the force per unit area at the

suture–tissue interface a big bite of relatively coarse material is required (*Fig.* 5.3). No. 1 metric gauge inserted at least 1 cm back from the wound edge is suitable. It should penetrate all fasciomuscular layers of the abdominal wall which are usually about 1 cm thick. Sutures inserted by this technique pass through tissue which is outwith the 'healing zone', which is subject to collagenolysis and softening; hence they retain a good grip.

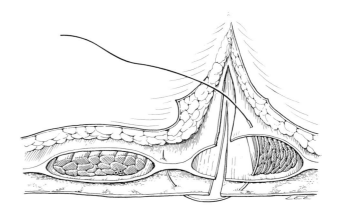

Fig. 5.3. Taking large bites in mass closure. (Reproduced from Dudley H. A. (1983) *Rob & Smith's Operative Surgery: Alimentary Tract and Abdominal Wall*, Vol. 1, 4th ed. London, Butterworths.)

In passing it should be noted that sutures for 'mass closure' should never include the skin. The latter plays no part in the integrity of the abdominal wall and has quite different physical properties from the underlying fascial layers. Even in resuture of an acutely disrupted (burst) abdomen, the same rule applies.

Continuous or Interrupted Sutures?
Provided a mass closure technique is used, there does not seem to be any evidence to suggest that one technique is preferable to another. Proponents of continuous closure point to its slight advantage in speed, to the fact that only two knots are formed (or one if a looped double suture is used) and thus the risk of sinus formation is numerically reduced. Those who support interrupted closure believe it to be intrinsically more secure, more fail safe in that it is not dependent on a single knot, and a technique that must be mastered to deal with the difficult case. Though I espouse the latter view, I do not feel strongly about it. Continuous suturing should always be used in a patient with ascites so as to make a watertight closure.

Loose or Tight Suturing?
Jenkins, the original exponent in the UK of mass closure, favoured a relatively loose closure to allow 'take-up' for abdominal distension without fear of cutting out. More recent work by Pollock does not

support this view. Obviously there is no call for surgeons to brace themselves against the end of the operating table and to pull as if in a tug of war; the aim should be a firm closure which 'feels right' rather than a deliberately floppy one.

Closing the Peritoneum

Like skin, peritoneum does not play a part in the structural security of the abdominal wall. Thus to suture it does not protect against burst or incisional hernia, except in so far as it is fused with the posterior rectus sheath (but not the linea alba). For this reason, many have advocated not incorporating it into closure sutures. There is support for this from experimental work which suggests that more adhesions will occur if there is a probably ischaemic suture line facing inwards towards omentum and viscera. I am not very impressed that this is the case in humans but there may be a marginal effect. The author's view is that peritoneum should be closed if this is easy, but no anxiety need be felt in not including it if to do so is going to be difficult. The serosal surface denudation will rapidly reconstitute itself.

Skin Closure

There are no adequate data to tell us what is the best method of skin closure. The abdomen is creased horizontally by our upright posture and tendency to bend forward and thus transverse incisions give the best cosmetic results however they are closed. Clips save time but are difficult to insert at the upper end of vertical incisions or at the thoraco-abdominal border where the skin tends to turn in. My advice is to use any method that works well in your hands. Continuous subcuticular sutures are probably contra-indicated in vertical wounds. The current (expensive) vogue is for staple 'guns' which are automated versions of the old Michel clips and, in my view, not as good.

Delayed Primary Closure

A wound which is heavily contaminated is left open so that the conditions for bacterial multiplication are rendered unfavourble. If the wound is then closed after 3–4 days, healing is not delayed—the preparatory phase has taken place with the wound open and the reparative phase is only just beginning. The same principle can be applied to the abdomen and was indeed introduced early in this century by Wilkie for the heavily contaminated appendix wound. Statistical proof of its utility is not easy to come by and in some hands the incidence of abdominal wall sepsis is so low that the addition of delayed primary closure is unlikely to add anything. However, I think it is a useful option to remember for the occasional case when faecal contamination has occurred. The abdominal wall closure is made in the usual manner. The skin and subcutaneous tissues are lightly packed with dry gauze. This is removed by soaking it free after 3 days. If the wound is healthy and there is only minimal exudate, closure can be achieved with tape or sutures according to the surgeon's preference.

INCISIONAL HERNIA

The use of the techniques and suture materials already described will keep the rate of wound disruption very low. However, the prevention of incisional hernia is more difficult. Recent studies from Hughes and his colleagues in Cardiff and from Ellis in London attest to the late occurrence of incisional hernia up to 8 or 10 years after the laparotomy. Presumably this reflects the dynamic nature of collagen even in what appears to be a totally quiescent scar. Another study has suggested that a further factor is that mass closure may contribute to this because it deposits a larger band of collagen than more meticulous layered closure but this is not supported by animal evidence. Nevertheless, though there may be an 'inevitable' incidence of incisional hernia this will be kept to a minimum by proper technique and the avoidance of infection. There is no hard evidence that other classic measures such as supporting the abdomen with a corset or avoiding excessive straining in the early postoperative period make any contribution.

POLYPROPYLENE MESH IN WOUND MANAGEMENT

With advances in surgical aggression towards severe and formerly fatal intra-abdominal sepsis and necrosis, such as is found in necrotizing pancreatitis, late gunshot wounds and complicated postoperative situations, there is emerging a group of patients who require repeated re-exploration of the abdomen and free drainage of what is often widespread purulent peritoneal exudate. To meet this need and, in addition, to avoid the wound complications which are prone to occur when attempts are made to suture the abdominal wall over distended bowel, the technique of either leaving the abdomen completely open or of suturing in a sheet of polypropylene mesh has been developed. The author prefers the latter because it allows free drainage but yet controls the abdominal contents. Moreover, when the need for further exploration is over, the mesh can sometimes be left as a buttress, granulations allowed to grow through it and split skin then applied. The last is wise if the inner surface of the mesh is not in direct contact with bowel because if this is the case late fistulization is common and any further surgery will almost certainly be associated with damage to the gut. Thus every effort should be made to achieve omental interposition if the mesh is to be permanent.

Technique

At the end of the laparotomy the wound is allowed to assume its own shape and the omentum positioned as well as possible in its depths. A sheet of polypropylene mesh is then pressed into place with its edges everted and tacked down with interrupted no. 1 nylon sutures inserted at 1·5 cm intervals through all layers of the abdominal wall deep to the skin. The mesh is trimmed back to within 1 cm of the suture line. A gauze dressing is applied and can be changed as often as necessary to soak up secretions.

When next the patient needs to be returned to the operating room it is a simple matter to remove the sutures and gently peel the mesh away. Some have recommended that for ease of re-entry a zip fastener is incorporated in the mesh but I like to remove the old piece and insert a fresh sheet because it is frequently dirty and choked with coagulum at the time of re-exploration.

Should the mesh be removed? Opinions differ about this and experience is still developing. If there is satisfactory omental interposition between mesh and gut then there is no need to remove it and the wound can be closed, once granulations have formed, by split-skin grafting. Direct contact between mesh and intestine can lead to late fistula formation and the mesh is better out. It should be removed by very careful horizontal blunt dissection and the area then grafted.

INDIVIDUAL INCISIONS (*Fig.* 5.4)

Paramedian Incisions

The theoretical advantages of paramedian incisions are twofold. First, they offset a vertical incision to

one or other side so making access to a lateral structure such as the spleen or the gallbladder that much easier (though it should be emphasized that it is only necessary to make a median incision a few centimetres longer to achieve the same effect). Second, they are supposedly more secure in that the rectus should act as a buttress particularly if the 'lateral' modification (*see below*) is used. Whether this is truly the case—given that the basic cause of early dehiscence is probably the insinuation of omentum or coils of bowel at a point where sutures have cut out or

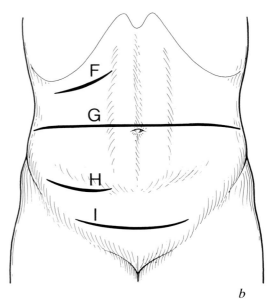

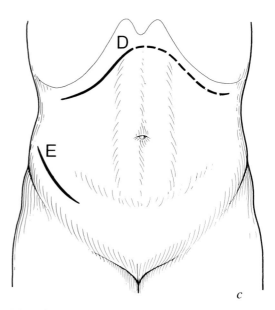

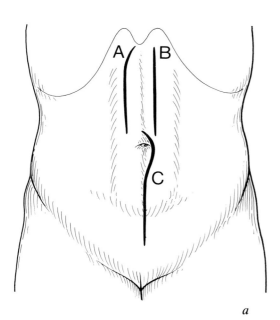

Fig. 5.4. *a*, Common vertical abdominal incisions. A, Right paramedian with Mayo–Robson extension. B, Left paramedian. C, Midline skirting the umbilicus. *b*, Transverse incisions. F, Modified Kocher's for gallbladder surgery. G, Transverse para-umbilical. H, Lanz. I, Pfannenstiel. *c*, Marginal incisions. D, Half or full rooftop. E, Lateral incision (Dowden) for appendectomy.

broken—is doubtful though impressive series of paramedian incisions without rupture are on record. Late hernia should be prevented, or at least reduced in incidence, by a sound rectus interposition though there is currently no numerical proof of this. The only small disadvantage of a paramedian incision is that it is slightly more finicky to make.

The essential points are few. Particularly in a muscular individual the skin incision for a conventional paramedian incision should be sited over the medial aspect of the bulging transverse convexity of the rectus so as to avoid a tedious dissection between the anterior sheath and the muscle which, of course, has to be accepted if the lateral approach is used. In the lower abdomen the incision should not be taken over the symphysis. This does not improve the exposure and the scar rubs against overlying clothing. Often this leads to keloid change which is distressing to the patient. Instead the skin incision should be stopped about 2 cm proximal to the bone and the underlying rectus sheath incised all the way down to the pubis.

The rectus sheath is incised through the whole length of the wound and then, if the rectus is to be displaced, picked up on the medial side and held vertically in the tips of fine haemostats. A few strokes of the knife then separate the sheath from the underlying muscle, bleeding points being coagulated at the tendinous intersections. Once the linea alba is reached, the plane is bloodless and the muscle belly is separated round onto its posterior aspect. In the upper abdomen it is not usual to encounter any further bleeding but subumbilically the inferior epigastric is nearly always present coursing upwards lateromedially to cross the linea semicircularis. Sometimes it can be displaced laterally but more usually it must be divided either between fine ligatures or after coagulation.

Rectus splitting is quicker and easier than rectus displacement (*Fig.* 5.5). A few vessels have to be coagulated but these do not usually cause much difficulty. It is arguable that the buttress of the muscle is lost but unless the incision is sited laterally this is not probably of great importance.

The posterior rectus sheath and its fused underlying peritoneum are picked up with two haemostats and incised with a knife blade held horizontally. In a patient who has not had a previous laparotomy there is certainly no danger of injury to a viscus because the moment the most minute hole has been made, air rushes in and gut moves away from the inner aspect of the parietal peritoneum. The small nick can then be enlarged upwards and downwards with either knife or scissors. Upwards towards the xiphoid the right or left aspects of the falciform ligament are encountered. If the incision has been made to the left of the midline it is very unlikely that the operator will want to undertake any extensive surgery in the right upper quadrant and the ligament can be ignored. On the right, however, it may be desirable to ligate and divide the ligament which in addition to the umbilical artery usually contains a small terminal branch of the internal mammary. The fat is pushed away by blunt dissection and the vessel coagulated. The peritoneum can then be incised upwards as far as the cupola of the diaphragm.

Below the same principle applies. The parietal peritoneum in the midline spreads out over the bladder and care must be taken to identify the peritoneum exactly and to incise only it rather than the underlying bladder wall. Blunt gauze dissection is best used to push the bladder down. Usually when operating down into the pelvis through any form of incision it is wise to have the bladder emptied by a catheter.

Closure of a paramedian incision follows the same principle as for a median incision—a single layer of monofilament can be used excluding the rectus if it has been displaced only minimally. Some will prefer to use a layer each in the anterior and posterior sheaths and this is quite acceptable provided that deep bites are taken. Experience of reopening these incisions (all too often in my own practice!) convinces me, however, that it is unnecessary to exclude the rectus muscle belly from the closure as loosely tied sutures do not strangle so I personally no longer displace the muscle laterally out of the way of the sutures.

The lateral paramedian incision is, as its name implies, an exaggeration of the conventional incision

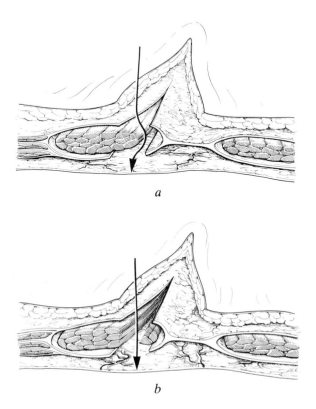

a

b

Fig. 5.5. Rectus displacement (*a*) and rectus splitting (*b*) in a paramedian incision.

in which the anterior and posterior sheaths are incised in their lateral thirds so increasing the buttress effect of the muscle (*Fig.* 5.6). The incision does not otherwise differ in principle from the conventional. Closure is in two layers with a running suture which must perforce take somewhat smaller bites than is usual. It is said that synthetic absorbable sutures are adequate for this purpose but long-term results are not at the moment to hand.

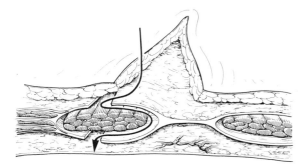

Fig. 5.6. Path of dissection in a lateral paramedian incision.

Midline Incisions

The generation of surgeons who worked predominantly with catgut and did not use mass closure was taught to regard a vertical midline incision as prone to rupture and late hernia. This view was supported by the high incidence of hernia after gynaecological surgery using subumbilical midline incisions. However, the reasons for the malign association between the linea alba and catgut or fine closure have already been described—to reiterate, the recovery of tensile strength to resist distractive forces in the abdominal wall is slow and catgut has lost too much of its strength before the abdominal wall has recovered its integrity. Mass closure with non-absorbables has changed all this. I suspect that the majority of surgeons who need to use vertical incisions in the abdomen will now prefer to enter the peritoneal cavity through the midline. It is speedy, relatively bloodless and allows the exploration to range from one side to the other. If a stoma is required the incision is well clear of this.

The incision is so well known that it does not need detailed description. The knife passes through skin and subcutaneous tissue to expose the linea alba as precisely as possible in the midline (*Fig.* 5.7). The fibres from both rectus sheaths can be seen decussating in the midline and both exposure and closure are easier if the flat of the knife's belly is used to push back the subcutaneous fat so as to clear about 1 cm of the glistening surface of the fascial layer. With the structures on the stretch the knife then cuts through the linea onto the extraperitoneal fat. Unlike in a paramedian incision there is a well-formed extraperitoneal space and it is unusual to enter the peritoneum direct. The variable amount of fat is swept laterally by blunt dissection, carrying with it a few

small vessels, some of which may have to be coagulated. The peritoneum is then exposed, picked up and incised in the usual manner.

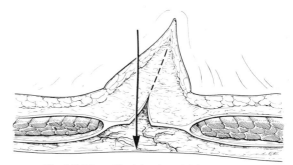

Fig. 5.7. Line of incision for midline exposure.

The Umbilicus

Most surgeons will skirt the umbilicus (*see Fig.* 5.4*a*) but some cut straight through it. The disadvantage of the latter is that it can be quite difficult to secure accurate skin apposition but otherwise it seems to do little harm.

Upward Extension

The xiphoid is best split rather than bypassed. Otherwise upward extension is as described.

Downward extension

The skin incision is carried down as far as the mons pubis but not into it. The linea can be incised right down to the pubic bone.

Closure

This is the incision which the original work on mass closure was done. Either interrupted or continuous nylon or polypropylene may be used.

Kocher's Incision (*see Fig.* 5.4*b*)

This incision has two advantages: it runs parallel to the edge of the liver so allowing this organ to be retracted uniformly upwards and to the right in order to expose the gallbladder; packing away the subhepatic structures—hepatic flexure, transverse colon and gastroduodenal junction—is easy. Its major disadvantage in my view is that its exact direction is conditioned by the obliquity of the costal margin and if the angle is narrow the line intersects with the midline acutely. A subsequent vertical incision then incurs the slight but real risk of necrosis of the bridge between the two. It is also quite difficult to carry out a good general exploration of the abdomen through a right upper quadrant incision. It used to be further said that Kocher's incision was prone to incisional hernia, perhaps because of division of one or more intercostal nerves. Certainly the latter does take place and in this respect the incision is in principle unattractive, but dehiscence relates more to suture material and technique than to the nature of the incision.

The author's personal preference for biliary tract surgery can be summarized as follows:

1. Narrow costal angle and/or the possibility of an extensive exploratory procedure within the biliary tree or resection of an ampullary tumour. Vertical midline or right paramedian incision with a 'hockey stick' at the upper end (Mayo–Robson, *see Fig.* 5.4*a*).

2. Wide costal angle and/or cholecystectomy with or without duct exploration being envisaged. The right half of a rooftop incision is slightly different from a classic Kocher's incision because it does not slavishly follow the costal margin except at its lateral end (*see Fig.* 5.4*c*). As it passes medially it curves more horizontally to intersect the midline more or less at a right angle. It divides the rectus sheath and the rectus muscle and can be extended to the left by cutting the left rectus sheath and, if necessary, the left rectus muscle belly. The flat muscles are all incised in the same line—across the external oblique but in the line of the internal oblique and transversus. It is a mistake to carry the incision too far laterally as these muscles become rapidly more thick and vascular, and as they turn posteriorly round the curve of the abdominal wall, little additional exposure is gained. On incising the peritoneum, the falciform ligament is seen to the left and the fundus of the gallbladder usually presents in the wound.

Rooftop Incision (*see Fig.* 5.4*c*)

This is not strictly a 'bilateral Kocher's' though it takes the same general form. It is in effect a transverse but slightly convex upwards incision suitable only for patients with wide costal angles. It is ideal for wide exposure of liver and hepatobiliary tree and also for the pancreas, in the latter particularly when it is necessary to débride the retroperitoneum both to the right and the left of the midline. The further advantage of this incision is that, provided it is sited sufficiently high in the epigastrium, there is no 'overhang' of its upper margin and one can look backwards along the horizontal central tendon of the diaphragm towards the hepatic veins on the right and the hiatus on the left.

There is little special about the way the incision is made. It passes through all layers of the abdominal wall in the same line and divides both recti transversely. In the midline the falciform ligament must be ligated and divided and if the ligatures are left long and held in haemostats they can be used to retract the upper and lower margins of the wound.

Closure is with a single layer of sutures deep to the skin and there is little tendency to herniation. This is a particularly appropriate wound if there is a need to insert polypropylene mesh because its edges do not retract and the ultimate result, in contrast to a vertical incision, is a strong abdominal wall whether the mesh is removed or not.

Access to the Appendix (*see* Chapter 18)

Pfannenstiel's Incision (*see Fig.* 5.4*b*)

The subumbilical horizontal approach is not often indicated in general surgery though it is widely used in gynaecology. It gives an excellent cosmetic result and sufficient exposure for most pelvic procedures on the uterus and adnexa. Disruption and hernia are almost unknown.

The skin incision is in the suprapubic crease. The flaps are dissected upwards and downwards to expose the anterior face of the rectus sheath. The space between the recti is then entered and the areolar tissue split for as far as is judged appropriate superiorly and down to the pubic symphysis. There being no posterior rectus sheath at this level the extraperitoneal fat and peritoneum are next encountered and are opened vertically in the usual way.

Closure

A running suture of PDS may be used in the peritoneum. A similar suture unites the anterior rectus sheath.

Modification

A wider exposure can be obtained by dividing the rectus muscle bellies transversely but this is rarely necessary.

Chapter six

Hernias

D. A. Griffiths

THE INGUINAL CANAL

The adult inguinal canal is approximately 4 cm long and lies between the deep and superficial inguinal rings running obliquely between the muscles of the abdominal wall above the medial part of the inguinal ligament. The male canal contains the spermatic cord, the ilio-inguinal nerve, testicular vessels and cremasteric fascia, and the female canal contains the round ligament. The anterior wall of the inguinal canal is formed by the external oblique aponeurosis which separates medially at the external ring. The posterior wall is formed from the transversus abdominis and the transversalis fascia and is strengthened medially by the conjoint tendon. The internal oblique muscle arches over the spermatic cord from the inguinal ligament laterally to the conjoint tendon medially.

The inferior epigastric artery lies at the medial border of the deep ring, the spermatic cord curving laterally around it to leave the abdomen and enter the inguinal canal. The floor of the canal is formed by the recurved inguinal ligament and lacunar ligament. The spermatic cord and any inguinal hernial sac are covered by the extraperitoneal areolar tissue, transversalis fascia, cremasteric muscle derived from the internal oblique, external spermatic fascia derived from the external oblique, the superficial fascia and the skin. The iliohypogastric nerve does not run in the inguinal canal but is exposed when the canal is opened, lying in front of the internal oblique a little away from its lower border.

THE FEMORAL CANAL

The adult femoral canal is approximately 1·25 cm long and is the medial of the three compartments of the femoral sheath formed by a prolongation into the thigh of the transversalis fascia. The femoral ring, 1·25 cm wide, is bounded laterally by the femoral vein, posteriorly by the pectineal muscle and pectineal fascia over the superior pubic ramus. The femoral ring is limited medially by the lacunar ligament and anteriorly by the inguinal ligament. The femoral canal contains lymph vessels and nodes, and its function may be that of accommodating the distended femoral vein. The inferior epigastric artery crosses the upper lateral margin of the ring and when an abnormal obturator artery arises from it, it descends along the medial margin of the femoral artery, where it may be damaged during femoral hernia repair.

When there is a femoral hernial sac present it progressively enlarges by descending down the femoral canal and then passes anteriorly through the saphenous opening and the cribriform fascia covering it. Further enlargement may cause the sac to retrace its course upwards superficially to the deep fascia and laterally when it may ascend as high as the inguinal ligament. When a femoral hernia is dissected the sac is found to be covered by fat and lymphoid tissue, transversalis fascia, cribriform fascia and skin.

THE SURGERY OF HERNIA

A hernia is described as the abnormal protrusion of an organ or part of an organ through a congenital or an acquired aperture in the surrounding structures; the commonest hernias are the protrusion of abdominal organs through a gap in the abdominal wall. Hernias may occur naturally as the result of anatomical weaknesses or the presence of congenital sacs, or may occur as the result of abnormal pressures. They may follow surgical incisions which breach and weaken the structure of the abdominal wall or which may damage the nerves of the abdominal wall. Five per cent of the population of the United Kingdom have hernias at one time or another: 80 per cent of hernias are in the inguinal region, 10 per cent of hernias are incisional hernias secondary to surgical operations, 5 per cent are umbilical hernias and 1 per cent are epigastric hernias. Femoral hernias are six times more common in women than in men, although inguinal hernia is still more common in women than is femoral hernia (*Fig.* 6.1).

Inguinal Hernia

There are two varieties of inguinal hernia—the oblique or indirect inguinal hernia, the common variety, and the direct inguinal hernia. The indirect inguinal hernia enters a peritoneal sac which travels along the inguinal canal and may enter the scrotum, whereas a direct inguinal hernia occupies only the medial part of the inguinal canal and does not follow the oblique course taken by the spermatic cord. It projects from the abdominal cavity through the inguinal triangle of Hesselbach, which is bounded medially by the rectus muscle, laterally by the deep epigastric vessels and below by the inguinal ligament. Although it may emerge through the superficial inguinal ring, it rarely descends into the scrotum.

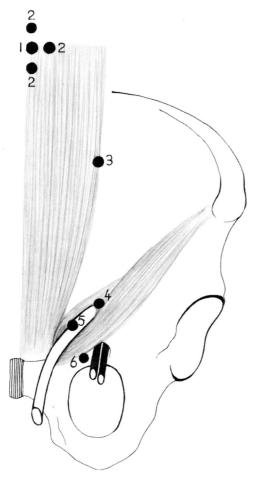

Fig. 6.1. Abdominal hernias. 1, Umbilical. 2, Para-umbilical. 3, Spigelian. 4, Indirect inguinal. 5, Direct inguinal. 6, Femoral.

Indirect Inguinal Hernia

Of the inguinal hernias, the majority are indirect and only 15 per cent are direct, although there are combinations of both varieties. Inguinal hernia can occur at any time of life and usually presents as an obvious bulge or a reducible swelling, which subsides when the patient lies down and increases in size when standing. The deep inguinal ring appears at the end of the 2nd month of fetal life as an outgrowth of the processus vaginalis. The 'U'-shaped ring of the transversalis fascia begins to develop about the 5th month and the valvular design of the inguinal canal is established at the 7th month. Descent of the testes usually takes place during the 7th to 8th month of intra-uterine life and the processus vaginalis normally closes before or soon after birth, though it may remain patent throughout life. The pressure valve effect of the deep inguinal ring is capable of protecting an open processus vaginalis often for months or years against the onset of a hernia, and the obliqueness of the inguinal canal plays an important part in the strength of the inguinal region. Surgeons need to understand this in the reconstruction of the canal following herniotomy.

Symptoms

The patient with a simple inguinal hernia usually presents with a lump in the groin which may have presented recently or have been present for months or years. Apart from a dull ache and occasional discomfort, most patients do not complain of many symptoms when the hernia is uncomplicated, unobstructed and reducible.

Differential Diagnosis

Preoperative differentiation into indirect or direct hernias is often very straightforward. A simple way to distinguish these varieties is to place the finger over the midpoint of the inguinal ligament and if this controls the hernia it is likely to be indirect. An inguinal hernia presents above and medial to the pubic tubercle, and this differentiates it from the femoral hernia which is found below and lateral to the pubic tubercle. Inguinal hernias have been classified into complete and incomplete varieties, the complete hernia entering the scrotum, usually containing bowel. Incomplete hernias may be found at any distance in the inguinal canal and may contain omentum or intestine or both. Associated problems such as hydrocele of the cord or of the testis may be present. There may be symptoms of chronic urinary obstruction, chronic cough, raised intra-abdominal pressure due to obesity, ascites or chronic intestinal obstruction, and these problems must be dealt with before the hernia is repaired, otherwise the risk of recurrence of the hernia is high.

Conservative Treatment

The conservative management of hernias using a truss is very rarely recommended. Few patients are unsuitable for hernial repair using local anaesthesia and in any event a truss rarely, if ever, controls a hernia effectively or for any length of time. In previous generations trusses were designed for both inguinal and femoral hernias but the use of a truss to control a femoral hernia is condemned.

There are many dangers associated with the use of a truss. A large number are not prescribed by surgeons but are purchased by the patient through a mail order advertisement, and most surgeons have seen patients using an inguinal hernia truss to attempt the control of femoral hernia, saphenous varix or a mass of lymph nodes. An important practical problem is the increasingly long surgical waiting list which may confront a working man who has a hernia, and in these circumstances it is tempting to advise that a truss be worn until surgery is undertaken. This is, of course, a counsel of defeat and when such symptomatic treatment is recommended it must be recognized that it is very bad surgical practice which may, however, be forced on the patient by circumstances.

In elderly patients, with a large recurrent direct inguinal hernia with a wide neck and in no danger of strangulation, a truss is sometimes supplied.

Operation

It is important to mark the side for repair prior to surgery at the time of shaving the abdomen, pubis and the scrotum. To avoid injury to the bladder, it is recommended that the bladder is emptied either naturally or with a catheter prior to operation. Operation may be performed under general or local anaesthesia and many are performed under local anaesthesia as day cases in hospital. After preparing the skin the surgeon stands on the side of the hernia and an incision is made approximately 2 cm above the inguinal ligament from the anterior superior iliac spine to the pubic tubercle. The superficial vessels are ligated and divided. The membranous layer of fascia is freed from the external oblique aponeurosis. It is important not to cross the midline as this may interfere with the venous return from the penis and scrotum, producing postoperative swelling. When the external oblique aponeurosis has been cleaned, it is incised from the external ring laterally and upwards in the line of the incision, separating its fibres (*Fig.* 6.2). The inguinal canal is exposed and

the cut ends of the external oblique aponeurosis are separated and held apart with a self-retaining retractor. Great care is taken to avoid injury to the iliohypogastric and ilio-inguinal nerves, for their involvement may contribute towards postoperative pain and anaesthesia in this area. The spermatic cord is identified and elevated and the cremasteric muscles separated to expose the testicular vessels, vas deferens and the hernial sac. The cremasteric fascia is carefully separated with a knife initially and then with a swab or finger, and the sac is freed as far as the deep inguinal ring (*Fig.* 6.3). In complete indirect hernias there is no need to trace the sac into the scrotum; it may be divided and left open distally. This obviates the dissection required to remove the sac from the scrotum, reducing the risk of subsequent haematoma formation. The residual scrotal part of the inguinal sac does not seem to cause later trouble.

The superfluous adipose tissue around the spermatic cord, which can be quite prominent in some patients, is excised. When the inguinal hernial sac is completely cleaned, it is opened and the contents examined, when adherent omentum or bowel is freed and replaced in the peritoneal cavity (*Fig.* 6.4). The

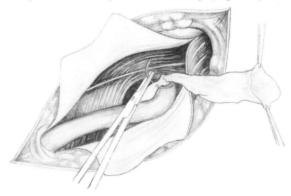

Fig. 6.4. Inguinal hernia. Following opening of the sac and reduction of its contents the hernial neck is transfixed.

sac is then held with clips, twisted and transfixed at the base with linen or a silk suture and the excess sac excised. Some surgeons fix the sac remnant superiorly using a suture deeply placed behind the internal oblique muscle in order to point the sac away from the inguinal canal, but this is not recommended for such fixation may lead to weakness elsewhere, predisposing to the formation of a further sac.

The procedure described, herniotomy, is adequate in children and in young adults with a congenital preformed inguinal hernia sac, and in these patients no further repair is necessary. However, in the majority of patients with an indirect inguinal hernia some form of repair is required.

Repair of the Inguinal Canal (Herniorrhaphy)

Bassini originally described suturing the divided transversalis fascia to the inguinal ligament, and

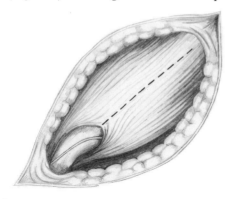

Fig. 6.2. Inguinal hernia. Line of incision of the external oblique muscle.

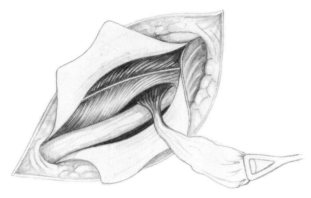

Fig. 6.3. Inguinal hernia. Dissection and isolation of the sac.

recent authors have modified this to the suturing of the conjoint tendon to the deep margin of the inguinal ligament. This operation has been criticized as being unphysiological but there is little doubt that the Bassini operation or its variations has been used by the majority of surgeons in the majority of instances of successful inguinal herniorrhaphy. There have been many variations of this operation and Halsted placed the spermatic cord subcutaneously by repairing all layers of the inguinal canal posterior to the inguinal ligament, but this is not recommended. Gallie and McArthur strengthened the posterior wall using fascial strips. When it does not appear possible to repair the posterior wall of the inguinal canal with native tissue, many alternatives have been suggested using nylon mesh, silver wire, tantalum gauze, Dacron patches and even portions of whole skin. The modern advent of the nylon darn (Moloney, 1958) has gained favour with the majority of surgeons.

The Bassini Method of Repairing Inguinal Hernias

Following removal of the sac, the spermatic cord and ilio-inguinal nerve are held away by retracting the lower leaf of the external oblique downwards. The conjoint tendon and the inguinal ligament are cleared of fascia and the muscles and tendons elevated forwards. Four or five interrupted sutures are inserted at 5-mm intervals between the conjoint tendon above and the inguinal ligament below (*Fig.* 6.5). It is

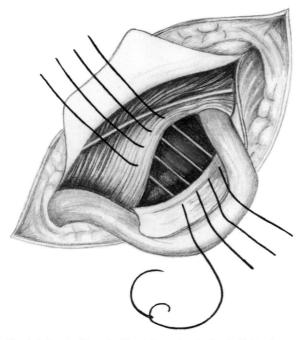

Fig. 6.5. Inguinal hernia. Bassini repair, placing individual sutures between the conjoint tendon and inguinal ligament.

important that deep bites are taken of the inguinal ligament and the sutures should not be tied until all have been placed. Care should be taken to protect

the femoral vein which lies deep to the inguinal ligament.

Although in the past numerous hernias have been repaired using catgut, this material is not recommended, reliance being placed on non-absorbable materials such as nylon or stainless steel.

Whichever suture material is used, ultimate success depends on adequacy of surgical technique complemented by adequacy of the tissues that are sutured. A common error is to tie these sutures too tightly, which results in strangulation of the tissues or the cutting out of the sutures. When the procedure is completed, the conjoint tendon should abut firmly against the medial aspect of the deep inguinal ring (*Fig.* 6.6). If it proves impossible to approximate the conjoint tendon to the inguinal ligament by sutures tied without undue tension, then some other form of reconstruction should be advised. The spermatic cord is placed back against the strengthened posterior wall of the canal, the external oblique is repaired using a simple continuous suture and the skin wound is then closed (*Fig.* 6.7).

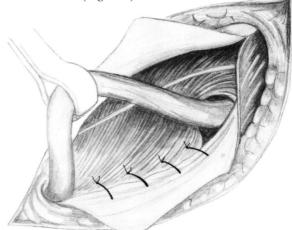

Fig. 6.6. Inguinal hernia. Bassini repair; after tying the sutures the conjoint tendon should fit snugly around the exit from the abdomen of the spermatic cord.

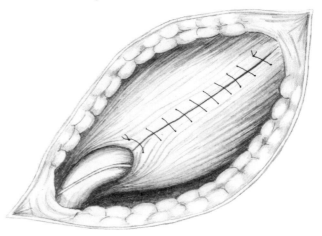

Fig. 6.7. Inguinal hernia. Closure of the external oblique aponeurosis.

Operative Variations

Following herniorrhaphy, some advocate closing the external oblique muscle by overlapping, which is said to strengthen the inguinal canal. It is difficult to see how this can, in fact, have any effect on recurrence, for it is not the anterior wall of the canal which requires strengthening but, of course, the posterior wall.

Tanner Slide Repair

It may prove impossible to bring the conjoint tendon down to the inguinal ligament. Tanner popularized a slide repair which has been used by many surgeons and in which the anterior sheath of the rectus muscle is incised for 5 cm over the muscle which releases the conjoint tendon which can then be brought down to reach the inguinal ligament. The rectus sheath defect is compensated and protected by the fleshy rectus abdominis muscles. However, if it is not possible to perform this procedure, especially where there has been previous surgery, a large posterior defect may require alternative techniques.

Fascial Repair

A large defect may be closed with fascia obtained from the iliotibial tract of the fascia lata (Gallie) or from the external oblique aponeurosis (McArthur). The Gallie repair (*Fig.* 6.8) is undertaken using strips

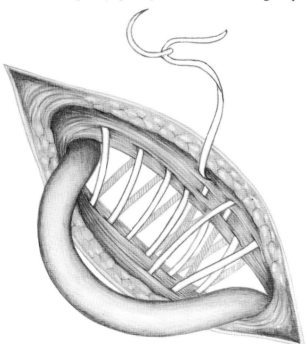

Fig. 6.8. Inguinal hernia. Gallie repair using strips of fascia lata.

of iliotibial fascia from the thigh which are obtained either under direct vision via a long incision or better still by using a fasciotome. These strips are threaded through the eye of a large Gallie needle which then pierces the fascial strips to anchor the fascial structure. Smaller strips of fascia may be obtained from the external oblique and used in the McArthur repair, and these are left anchored at the medial end of the fascia. The weak posterior wall of the inguinal canal is closed with narrow bands of fascia in a lattice fashion between the conjoint tendon and the inguinal ligament. The disadvantage of the Gallie repair is that the donor site may be painful and there may be muscle herniation at a later date. Furthermore, the thick Gallie needle may often leave large holes in the aponeurosis.

Nylon Darn

The success of this method of inguinal hernia repair has been achieved by the relative ease of the procedure and by the very low recurrent hernia incidence (Moloney, 1958). The inguinal hernia sac is transfixed and the posterior wall of the direct or indirect inguinal hernia is closed with a layer of monofilament nylon. The lattice work starts at the medial end of the posterior wall as near as possible to the pubic tubercle, the anchoring knot being tied very carefully and the free end of the suture held in a clip. The atraumatic monofilament nylon is then loosely sutured between the fascia of the conjoint tendon or the internal oblique fascia and the deep leaf of the inguinal ligament. Criss-cross back-and-forth sutures are placed without tension between these two structures. The lateral end of the pattern is shaped very much like a sun-burst around the deep inguinal ring and the suture is then brought back to the pubic tubercle. The criss-cross pattern is completed by tying the suture to the original knot and the wound is closed in the usual way. The nylon prevents recurrent hernia by acting as a matrix for strong fibrous union which gives an acceptably low recurrence rate of less than 1 per cent (*see Fig.* 6.22).

Associated conditions of the inguinal region may be treated at the same time as repair of the hernia, for example removal of a lipoma, hydrocele of the cord, hydrocele of the testis, spermatocele, epididymal cysts or varicocele. Haemostasis in inguinal hernia repairs is mandatory, as is replacing the testis in the correct anatomical position in the scrotum. Postoperative pressure bandaging of the scrotum or a scrotal support often helps to reduce postoperative pain and swelling.

Recurrent Inguinal Hernia

The problem of recurrent inguinal hernia plagues every surgeon. The aetiology of recurrence may be related to postoperative problems such as excessive coughing, straining at stool or excessively at work, but many instances of recurrent inguinal hernia may be traced to faulty technique. Certainly, during the re-exploration of recurrent hernia, it is not uncommon to find that the sac has been missed altogether or that the repair has torn away from the inguinal ligament. Multiple recurrent hernias are frequently found at operation and whenever an orifice is left in the posterior wall, which allows the passage of the spermatic cord, there is clearly a potential for recurrent hernia. Removal of the spermatic cord and orchidectomy with ablation of the inguinal canal offer the best chance of repair and are from time to time advocated in elderly patients. However, younger men are unlikely to agree to this radical treatment and other methods should be recommended. Closure of the deep inguinal ring with interrupted nylon sutures and approximation of the conjoint tendon to the inguinal ligament will often close the canal, but in recurrent hernia it is likely that some form of posterior reconstruction as outlined above will be required. Alternatively the pro-peritoneal approach and repair may be tried.

The Pro-peritoneal Approach

This approach to the inguinal hernia has gained popularity recently and is useful especially in the repair of recurrent inguinal hernia. This method of approaching the inguinal canal is made through the lower midline or transverse abdominal incisions. It is difficult to perform in infants and in obese patients and the abdominal wall needs to be very relaxed and adequate surgical assistance for retraction needs to be available. The inguinal canal is approached through a transverse incision 3 cm above the inguinal ligament. The three aponeurotic muscle layers are incised in the same direction and the muscle fibres retracted. The peritoneum is pushed away and carefully preserved. The posterior wall of the inguinal canal is inspected. The indirect sac where present is excised and the defect repaired and the spermatic cord is retracted laterally. The hernial defect margins are sutured together from the inside, and the deep inguinal ring can be further narrowed by placing one or two lateral sutures.

Direct Inguinal Hernia

These hernias most commonly occur in the elderly, in obese patients and in those with chronic urinary obstruction. Direct inguinal hernia is never congenital and operative cure is frequently difficult, recurrence not being at all rare. If this hernia repair is contemplated some form of posterior reconstruction is inevitable. The exposure is the same as that for indirect inguinal hernia, dividing the external oblique muscle. A sac, if present, is separated from the cord but particular care must be taken not to injure the bladder which lies extraperitoneally at the medial side of the sac, to which it may be adherent. If the sac is large and with a narrow neck, it should be opened and its contents returned to the abdomen, following which the sac is twisted and sutured. How-

ever, the direct inguinal hernia sac is usually broad-mouthed and does not require separate attention.

The associated muscles are usually thin and atrophic and the large posterior defect in the inguinal canal is usually not amenable to a direct repair such as that of Bassini. Some form of reconstruction is advisable.

Sliding Hernia (Hernia *en glissade*)

In a sliding hernia some or all of the contents lie outside the peritoneal sac and this is frequently a portion of colon or caecum, or a portion of the bladder. These organs are not reducible in the usual way as the sac forms part of the peritoneal covering of these organs. It is important to recognize this condition and to treat it adequately, otherwise the large bowel or bladder may be damaged and the likelihood of recurrence of the hernia is high under these circumstances. It is not possible to remove the sac in the usual way. The most appropriate method is an incision in the peritoneum at a distance of 3 cm from the bowel, which leaves a fringe of peritoneum, and this incision extends to the neck of the sac (*Fig.* 6.9).

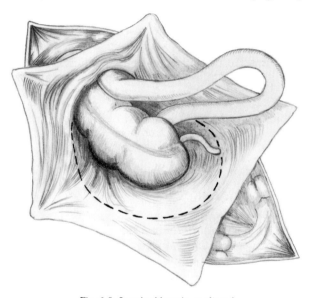

Fig. 6.9. Inguinal hernia *englissade*.

The bowel, which is then free from the sac, is recovered with peritoneum and replaced within the abdominal cavity (*Fig.* 6.10). It is then necessary to repair the sac where it has been incised before dealing with it in the customary way. Following this procedure the hernia is repaired.

Irreducible and Strangulated Hernia

1. *Irreducible Hernia (Incarcerated)*

An irreducible hernia is often tender but this may be on account of frequent attempts to reduce it.

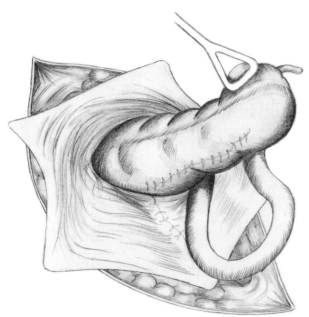

Fig. 6.10.

Figs. 6.9, 6.10. Inguinal hernia *en glissade*. The retroperitoneal caecum is mobilized by creating a cuff of peritoneum which is then sutured posteriorly to peritonealize the organ, following which the sac is repaired and dealt with in the usual manner.

There is sometimes a dragging pain which from time to time is colicky, but if this is associated with nausea and vomiting intestinal obstruction should be suspected. An apparently irreducible hernia may reduce readily when the patient lies down or is under anaesthesia. In any event a hernia which is apparently irreducible should be submitted to early surgical reduction and repair.

2. *Strangulated Inguinal Hernia*

A previously irreducible inguinal hernia may proceed to strangulation but more often than not strangulation occurs in a previously readily reducible hernia or more rarely may appear spontaneously in a patient with no previous symptoms.

Symptoms

The hernia is tense, tender and irreducible. Associated with this the patient will complain of central, colicky abdominal pain accompanied by nausea and vomiting. These are the signs of intestinal obstruction and if untreated will proceed to strangulation of the hernial contents with serious consequences for the patient.

Treatment

Early surgery is always indicated. However, in those patients who have experienced prolonged vomiting with associated fluid and electrolyte loss, it is most important to replace these losses intravenously. Prior to anaesthesia, decompression of the stomach and bowel via a nasogastric tube is mandatory and catheterization of the bladder must be performed before surgery is attempted to avoid injury to that structure. General anaesthesia with adequate muscle relaxation is used by most surgeons although in severely debilitated patients with cardiopulmonary problems, local anaesthesia may be safer. The strangulated hernia is approached through an oblique groin incision over the swelling and the inguinal canal may be opened by extending the external inguinal ring laterally. The sac is isolated, opened carefully and the contents inspected. Any fluid present is cultured. The bowel adjacent to the deep constricting ring must be seen and this is important as otherwise unrecognized necrotic constriction rings may be replaced into the abdominal cavity. Doubtful bowel may be left between warm saline towels for a few minutes in order to assess recovery. Reduction of the hernial contents can be accomplished by stretching or enlarging the neck of the sac with a finger or cutting under direct vision. Extension laterally is safer in indirect inguinal hernia as this avoids injury to the inferior epigastric vessels.

If during induction of anaesthesia the contents of an irreducible hernia reduce into the abdominal cavity, it is important that the original contents of the sac are reclaimed and examined. This is best achieved by grasping adjacent bowel with forceps and exteriorizing the small bowel through the hernial sac for inspection. The bowel contained within an obstruction or strangulated hernia should be carefully examined, and the mobilized bowel covered with warm saline packs and inspected for viability. If the bowel shows peristalsis and has a shiny peritoneum with pulsating blood vessels, it can be considered viable. Non-viable bowel lacks lustre, is dark purple in colour and has no pulsating blood vessels and is immobile. Gangrenous bowel is black with an offensive odour and is readily recognizable. Difficulties arise at the whitish constriction rings of otherwise healthy bowel. If the rings are too wide to invaginate with interrupted catgut sutures, this area should be excised. Methods of assessment of strangulated bowel and of bowel resection are described in Chapter 17.

COMPLICATIONS OF HERNIA REPAIR

The complications, apart from the general postoperative problems such as deep venous thrombosis and respiratory problems, are specific to the hernia. The local problems are haemorrhage with haematoma formation in the wound or scrotum, infection in the wound, undiagnosed indirect sac or undiagnosed femoral hernia, scrotal oedema and penile oedema following incisions which cross the midline, damage to the femoral vein and deep epigastric vessels, damage to the ilio-inguinal and iliohypogastric nerves producing pain in the wound, damage to the testicular vessels leading to testicular atrophy, and damage to the venous and lymphatic drainage in the scrotum which may lead to hydrocele formation. All of these complications can be avoided by careful attention to surgical detail. Scrotal oedema which often occurs following hernial repair may be alleviated by bandaging the scrotum with a turban bandage or wearing a scrotal support. Delayed stricture following reduction of partially ischaemic bowel may present with intestinal obstruction weeks or months after the hernia operation.

The complication of hernial repair that is most disturbing to the esteem of the surgeon is recurrence.

Return to Work
Return to work has in the past been postponed for at least 3 months, but there are reports where full activity has been achieved by the 4th week in heavy manual workers (Iles, 1972).

It has been estimated that over 75 000 inguinal hernia operations are carried out each year in England and Wales. This means that over 3·5 million working days are lost because of the usual delay in the return to work. There appears to be no correlation between the time of return to work and recurrent hernia rates. The author advises a shorter 4–6-week maximum convalescence before returning to work.

The average length of stay in hospital following a routine hernia repair is 3–8 days. Return to automobile driving should be delayed until the wound has healed. This usually takes about 10 days and after this time the reflex actions in an emergency situation will not be influenced by the fear of pain.

INGUINAL HERNIA IN CHILDREN

Inguinal hernia in children is always associated with a patent processus vaginalis. Most inguinal hernias present in the first few months of life and have a high incidence of incarceration. Over two-thirds of inguinal hernias are right-sided, thought to be due to the later descent of the testes through the inguinal canal, and studies have shown that in about half of these patients there is a potential patent process vaginalis on the contralateral side. Bilateral hernias usually appear before 1 year. Male infants are affected nine times more frequently than female infants. The uncomplicated inguinal hernia presents as a scrotal or groin swelling when the infant cries or coughs. Frequently the hernia is not obvious when the clinician examines the child.

Irreducible or incarcerated inguinal hernia is common in children, there being a reported incidence of 5–25 per cent. Strangulation is rare and bowel resection is rarely necessary (Palmer, 1978). Initial treatment is conservative, taxis, sedation, gentle pressure on the sac and gallows traction being usually successful, but the hernia should be surgically treated during the same hospital admission. If there is no success at reduction within 4 hours emergency surgery is indicated. Good anaesthesia is required and the usual precautions against dehydration, electrolyte imbalance and temperature loss must be followed. The approach to the reducible and irreducible hernia is similar. The inguinal canal is rudimentary in the infant and the deep inguinal and superficial inguinal rings often overlie one another, and the external ring need not be enlarged in simple cases. The skin is prepared and incised transversely along a skin crease and the sac is found superior and medial to the spermatic cord. These structures are very delicate and need to be treated with care. The vas deferens and spermatic vessels are separated from the sac by blunt dissection with a swab. The delicate sac is exposed down to the scrotum, care being taken to avoid injury to the epididymis and testis. The bladder is frequently intimately related to the medial side of the sac. The sac is opened and the contents inspected. Invariably in irreducible hernias the sac contains small bowel.

Strangulation is extremely rare and may be due in part to the rich blood supply of the bowel. The sac is transfixed at its base and excised. Complications of irreducible hernia include testicular gangrene due to pressure on the vessels and iatrogenic undescended testis following surgery.

Closure of the deep inguinal ring is usually unnecessary although in very wide sacs the author closes the defect with one or two interrupted sutures. The wound is closed in layers and the testis is replaced in the scrotum in its correct anatomical position. The position is checked by palpation at the end of the operation. Exploration of the contralateral inguinal canal is advocated by some surgeons, but there is also the potential risk of damage to the vas deferens and testicular vessels. At present there are no diagnostic techniques which reliably identify the patent processus vaginalis. Peroperative peritoneal insufflation with oxygen through a cannula passed through the sac on the affected side may demonstrate a contralateral hernia of surgical significance in an older infant (Bulow, 1974).

FEMORAL HERNIA

Femoral hernia is caused by breakdown in the integrity of the transversalis fascia covering the femoral canal. The peritoneal sac contents emerge through the femoral canal, which is limited anteriorly by the inguinal ligament, posteriorly by the pectineal fascia and laterally by the femoral vein (*Fig. 6.12*). Femoral hernias are not congenital, they are rare in children, they are twice as common on the right side as the left side, they are twice as common in females as in males and they are twice as common in women who have had children than in non-parous women. Approximately one-half are strangulated when they present although only 20 per cent contain gangrenous bowel. Simple removal of the hernial sac results in a very high recurrence rate of 26 per cent, therefore surgical repair is necessary. Surgical repairs of femoral hernias are legion. They have been divided into the low and high approach. The low femoral hernia repair (Lockwood) is useful for non-complicated femoral hernias and the high surgical approaches are often reserved for cases where bowel obstruction is suspected.

The Lockwood or Low Femoral Hernia Repair

In view of the high morbidity of femoral hernias it is important that they are repaired as soon as possible

after diagnosis. It is necessary that the bladder is emptied prior to surgery as this often forms a medial boundary of the femoral canal and may be injured. A transverse or oblique incision is made over the hernia, and the many layers of fascia are cleared until the sac is found (*Figs.* 6.11, 6.12). The contents of the sac are inspected. This is usually omentum, and if unharmed is returned to the abdominal cavity. In cases of difficulty the constricting band at the neck of the sac is extended medially by gentle finger dissection or careful incision into the lacunar ligament. The sac is transfixed and excised (*Fig.* 6.13), and then the repair is performed by placing two or three interrupted non-absorbable nylon or silk sutures loosely between the pectineal and inguinal ligaments (*Fig.* 6.14). These are then tightened while a finger is placed over the femoral vein to prevent compression injury. The femoral canal exists to provide an expansion space for the femoral vein and it is important that the vein is not obstructed. The superficial fascia and skin are closed with sutures of choice.

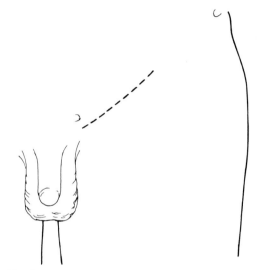

Fig. 6.11. Femoral hernia. Subinguinal or low approach.

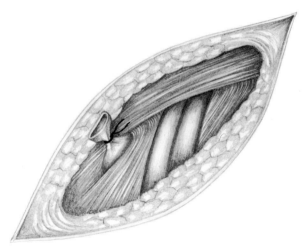

Fig. 6.13. Femoral hernia. Removal and ligation of the sac.

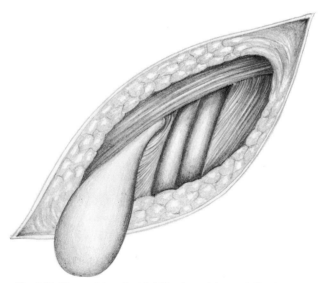

Fig. 6.12. Femoral hernia. Mobilization of the sac following emergence from the femoral canal.

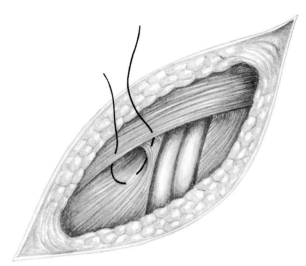

Fig. 6.14. Femoral hernia. Repair of the femoral canal.

Twenty per cent of strangulated femoral hernias contain dead bowel and it is impossible to resect bowel through a low femoral incision. In these circumstances, a separate abdominal incision should be made and the bowel resected through this incision. Offensive brownish staining fluid in the femoral sac usually means strangulation. As in all hernia surgery strict aseptic surgical practice should be employed, and if there is a large subcutaneous space this should be drained.

The High Surgical Approach

1. *The Lothiessen Repair*

The principle of this approach is to suture the conjoint tendon or inguinal ligament to the pectineal ligament. This repair has fallen out of favour because the inguinal canal is breached and needs to be repaired. The inguinal canal is opened as in an inguinal hernia repair, and the spermatic cord mobilized upwards. The posterior wall of the inguinal canal is incised and the femoral sac exposed. The sac is opened, the hernial contents inspected and replaced in the abdominal cavity. One advantage of this approach is that resection of the bowel may be carried out through this incision. The repair is in two phases: suture of the conjoint tendon or inguinal ligament to the pectineal ligament; and formal repair of the posterior wall of the inguinal canal.

2. *The McEvedy Repair*

This is a useful approach because the femoral hernia can be repaired and any necessary bowel resection performed through the same incision. The curved vertical incision follows the lateral border of the rectus and continues down to the pubic tubercle. An oblique incision in the skin crease above the medial half of the inguinal ligament is preferred by many surgeons, for the vertical pararectal incision may denervate the lower rectus muscle. The rectus is reflected medially. The femoral sac is approached by separating the extraperitoneal tissue and the femoral sac is drawn upwards. In difficult cases the incision can be extended downwards, the hernia being approached from the outside as well as inside. The hernia can be repaired from the abdomen with interrupted monofilament nylon sutures placed between the conjoint tendon and the pectineal ligament, or alternatively between the inguinal ligament and the pectineal ligament.

3. *The Midline Repair* (A. K. Henry)

This is a useful repair in bilateral femoral hernias. It is important that the bladder is empty and that good muscular relaxation is obtained. The surgeon stands on the contralateral side of the hernia. The recti are separated, the pre-peritoneal tissue retracted with care to avoid damage to the bladder and its veins. Aberrant vessels must be avoided or ligated. Retraction of the hernia is often eased by incising the iliopubic tract. The sac is opened and removed from the pre-peritoneal space. The repair is similar to that used in other approaches. The surgeon moves to the other side of the patient and repairs the second hernia or, if there is a weakness, reinforces the femoral ring.

PREVASCULAR HERNIA

There is a further hernia in the femoral region which causes difficulty in diagnosis and treatment. The prevascular hernia develops between the inguinal ligament and the femoral vessels. It is lateral to the inferior epigastric vessels and presents as a bulge in the femoral triangle. The prevascular hernia is usually asymptomatic and presents in the older age group.

Surgical treatment is difficult as it is impossible to close the defect. Excision of the sac will provide some relief.

UMBILICAL HERNIA

True umbilical hernia occurs in infants and children. This is a protrusion into the base of the umbilical cord and usually corrects itself as the child grows and the abdominal cavity increases in size. Adult 'umbilical hernias' are usually para-umbilical hernias which occur through defects in the linea alba, above, below or to one side of the umbilicus.

Infantile Umbilical Hernia

These usually resolve by the age of 3 years but if still present should be repaired. Best results are obtained by a semi-circular incision at the lower margin of the umbilicus, reflecting the skin superiorly and excising the sac. The linea alba defect is identified and closed with interrupted sutures of non-absorbable material, for example Prolene, silk or nylon. Care must be taken to make sure that the umbilicus dimples afterwards. This is easily achieved with a firm pad strapped to the skin on either side of the wound.

Adult Para-umbilical Hernia

There is an increased incidence of this hernia in Negroes, in obese patients and in those with hiatus hernia and with pelvic floor prolapses. Very large para-umbilical hernias may be surgically untreatable as the abdominal cavity may not be large enough to contain the replaced bowel. The Mayo operation for the adult para-umbilical hernia has been employed since 1899 and is a satisfactory way of treating the problem.

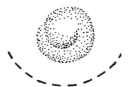

Fig. 6.15. Umbilical hernia. Subumbilical incision.

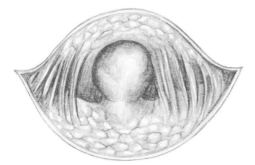

Fig. 6.16. Umbilical hernia. Mobilization and cleaning of the sac within the fat of the abdominal wall.

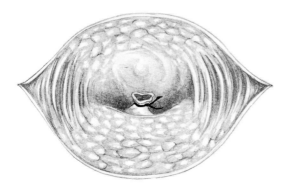

Fig. 6.17. Umbilical hernia. Following reduction of contents, the sac is transfixed and removed.

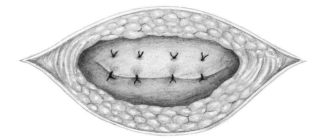

Fig. 6.18. Umbilical hernia. Mayo overlap repair.

subcutaneous tissue and vacuum drainage may be necessary. The recurrence rate in obese patients is about 5–7 per cent. Strangulated para-umbilical hernias carry a mortality of 15 per cent, which may increase to 40 per cent should bowel resection be necessary. Recent discussion on the aetiology and repair of para-umbilical and epigastric hernias emphasizes the importance of placing sutures obliquely across the wound to simulate the normal aponeurotic fibre pattern (Askar, 1978).

INCISIONAL HERNIAS

The problem of herniation through surgical incisions is well known and is the second most common form of hernia. The incidence varies from 4 to 7 per cent of abdominal operations. The defect is anticipated in those wounds which are associated with prolonged postoperative abdominal distension, wound haematoma, infection, burst abdomen, hypoproteinaemia, obesity, malignancy and multiple surgical incisions.

The symptoms are usually mild, producing an aching bulge which is accentuated on straining, e.g. lifting and coughing, and strangulation of the incisional hernial contents is very uncommon. The hernia is usually very obvious to the clinician and is at the site of a previous abdominal incision. The layers of the hernial sac consist of two or more of the abdominal wall layers but the minimal coverings may consist of skin and peritoneum. Sometimes the hernia may be multiloculated, and in long-standing cases there may be multiple adhesions between the contents and sac wall. The contents of the incisional hernia may consist of any intra-abdominal organ, but usually consist of omentum and bowel. The neck of the sac is wide and reduction of the hernia is readily produced by gentle pressure. Irreducible hernias may be painful but rarely cause obstruction or strangulation of bowel.

Management

1. Conservative

Many patients manage quite well with enormous incisional hernias, and this is especially the case in bedridden patients with cardiovascular and respiratory

The umbilicus is preserved by a subumbilical semicircular incision (*Fig.* 6.15). If there is gross infection of the umbilicus it may be wise to excise it completely by an elliptical incision. The neck of the sac is isolated and the sac reflected from the skin (*Fig.* 6.16). The sac is opened and the contents inspected. Often there is a multilocular sac with multiple loops of small bowel and omentum with adhesions. The sac is excised and the bowel replaced inside the abdominal cavity (*Fig.* 6.17). The margins of the linea alba defect are enlarged laterally, care being taken to avoid injury to the abdominal contents. This produces two flaps, superior and inferior, which are joined together in an overlap (*Fig.* 6.18). Interrupted Mersilene or monofilament sutures are placed through the upper flap 4–5 cm from its free edge, and then through the free margin of the inferior flap. When these are sutured the free margin of the upper flap is then sutured 4–5 cm away from the free margin of the inferior flap. The overlap repair produces a good sound wound. Often there is a large space in the

problems. Often the only covering of the bowel is peritoneum and skin, and bowel peristalsis is frequently observed. In patients with respiratory problems and large incisional hernias surgical reduction of the hernia might produce splinting of the diaphragm and be a disadvantage.

2. *Abdominal Support*

Symptomatic relief may be obtained by wearing a surgical corset. These vary from a simple roll of Tubigrip to a complicated tailor-made corset. The simplest are made of elastic material with a Velcro fastener. Two corsets are usually prescribed, one to be worn while another is cleaned.

3. *Surgical Repair*

Before surgical repair is undertaken the capacity of the abdominal cavity to receive the additional hernial contents must be assured. Simple reduction in weight often increases the abdominal capacity. Gradual staged increases in the abdominal volume have been achieved by weekly intraperitoneal insufflation of carbon dioxide through the laparoscope trocar. Preoperative preparation of the patient is essential to prevent recurrent herniation, and respiratory problems, chronic retention of urine and constipation must be dealt with before surgery. In upper abdominal incisions the stomach is emptied by nasogastric suction to avoid injury during the surgical procedure.

Methods of Repair

1. *Simple Closure*

a. Excision of redundant skin and fascia with approximation of as many layers as possible using non-absorbable sutures. The edges of the wound must be freshened and be of adequate strength.

b. Overlap of the wound edges will increase the strength of the repair. This is achieved in cases where the linea alba has been stretched, such as in divarication of the recti. The incision is carried through the linea alba. The two lateral flaps are sutured over and under each other as in the Mayo repair (*Fig.* 6.19).

c. Keel operation. This is suitable for large ventral hernias. The basic manoeuvre is the inversion of the rectus sheath, which strengthens the linea alba and approximates the muscles (*Fig.* 6.20). The aids to success in this operation are to excise the skin in a wide ellipse to prevent overlap and to clear the fatty tissues away from the rectus sheath. Postoperative ileus can be minimized by avoiding the peritoneal cavity. The inverting layers are approximated with at least three rows of non-absorbable sutures, and the large subcutaneous space is drained with a vacuum drain to prevent haematoma formation and infection.

d. Rectus muscle criss-cross for lower abdominal hernias. In this operation both rectus muscles are mobilized and crossed over to opposite pubic bones.

2. *Augmentation of the Defect by Synthetic or Natural Material*

Various materials such as fascia lata, polypropylene mesh and monofilament nylon darn have been successfully used to close large incisional hernia defects. All these methods require strict attention to asepsis, arrest of haemorrhage and prevention of damage to the bowel. Where possible the peritoneum is closed with catgut and the edges of the defect cleared of fat. When polypropylene mesh is used it is cut to shape and laid over the defect and the edges are attached to the aponeurosis with non-absorbable

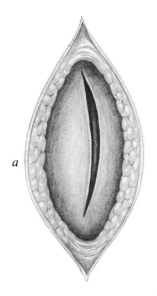
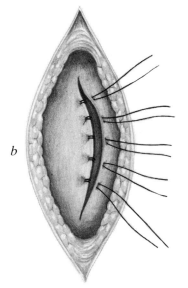
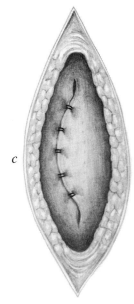

Fig. 6.19. Incisional hernia, repaired by the overlap technique.

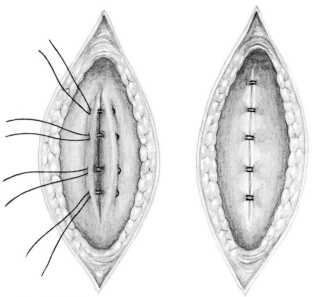

Fig. 6.20. Incisional hernia, repaired by the Keel operation.

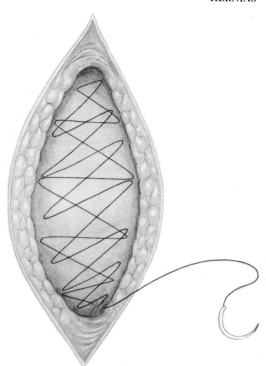

Fig. 6.22. Incisional hernia. The nylon darn technique may be used to repair incisional or inguinal hernias.

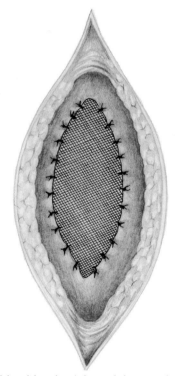

Fig. 6.21. Incisional hernia. A large defect may be closed using prosthetic mesh.

sutures, overlapping the edge by at least 2 cm (*Fig. 6.21*). The skin is closed over this with vacuum drainage of the subcutaneous space for 2–3 days (Drainer and Reid, 1972).

Nylon Darn (Fig. 6.22)
Once the edges of the aponeurosis have been cleared and closed with interrupted sutures the defect can be strengthened by darning with monofilament nylon. Each bite of the lateral suture margin must be adequate to prevent loosening of the darn. Large areas may be strengthened in this fashion (Moloney, 1958).

Postoperative ileus and abdominal distension must be avoided by attention to electrolyte and fluid replacement and nasogastric suction.

LESS COMMON HERNIAS

Obturator Hernia

This is a very uncommon hernia which is usually discovered at laparotomy for small bowel obstruction. There is no externally palpable swelling. The obturator foramen can be palpated by vaginal examination and the hernia may be palpated as a laterally placed swelling. An infrequent sign is pain or paraesthesia down the inside of the thigh to the knee due to compression of the obturator nerve.

Obturator hernias are seldom found in the dissecting room. They are more common in females, especially in pregnant women and women over 60, and the strangulated hernia may follow chronic constipation and cough. Partial strangulation, as in the Richter hernia, is not uncommon. Right-sided hernias are said to be more common and often contain terminal ileum. In suspected cases, early surgery is indicated as there is otherwise a very high mortality. The bladder is emptied and through a lower midline incision the pelvic cavity is explored. The obturator ring can be stretched by finger and the sac removed and the contents inspected. Bowel resection is undertaken where necessary. The obturator foramen is carefully closed by approximating the edges with interrupted non-absorbable sutures, but care must be taken to avoid damage to the obturator vessels or nerves. An alternative approach to the obturator hernia is across the retropubic space, opening the peritoneal cavity if necessary. The large obturator defect can be closed with Teflon or Dacron patches through this approach.

Epigastric Hernia

This uncommon hernia usually presents as a small, painful swelling in the midline of the epigastrium. The hernia consists of a protrusion of extraperitoneal fascia through the supra-umbilical area of the linea alba, and a small peritoneal process may accompany the fatty protrusion. Dragging epigastric pains and other gastrointestinal symptoms may be mimicked by an epigastric hernia, and these hernias are often more noticeable with the patient standing. The hernia is approached through an incision over the swelling and the sac is dissected and removed. The defect in the linea alba is usually small and can be approximated by two or three interrupted silk or nylon sutures.

Richter's Hernia

In Richter's hernia, which was first described in 1785, there is strangulation of part of the bowel wall. The bowel usually concerned is terminal ileum, although jejunum and colon may be involved. A knuckle of the antimesenteric border of the bowel is trapped in the hernia sac. If over two-thirds of the bowel wall are involved, complete intestinal obstruction develops. Fifteen per cent of strangulated femoral hernias are Richter hernias. The reduced bowel must be inspected and viability assessed.

Littré's Hernia

Littré's hernia is the name given to the rare hernia in which the sole content of the hernial sac, usually a femoral hernia, is an inflamed Meckel's diverticulum. This hernia is found in all age groups. It may present with faecal fistula although the diagnosis is usually made at operation for a tender groin swelling. The treatment is surgical removal of the Meckel's diverticulum and repair of the hernia.

Spigelian Hernia

This hernia through the semi-lunar line (Spigelian line) along the lateral border of the rectus abdominis is often misdiagnosed, especially when the only symptom is pain. The hernia is occasionally related to the vascular bundle and may consist of fat only when a small lump may be palpated. The treatment is surgical. The tender area is marked preoperatively and the deep fascia carefully explored, as the defect is often difficult to isolate. The anaesthetist may assist by increasing the intra-abdominal pressure to display the sac, which is excised after the contents have been inspected. The edges of the defect are defined, and closed with non-absorbable interrupted sutures.

Lumbar Hernia

These hernias present between the 12th rib and the iliac crest. They are often obvious, reducible with a wide sac and are associated with backache. Treatment is conservative.

Perineal Hernia

These hernias through the pelvic floor usually follow gynaecological and obstetrical trauma. They are associated with lax pelvic floor muscles and seldom present more serious symptoms than asymptomatic bulges.

Sciatic Hernia

This very rare hernia is produced by a protrusion of a peritoneal sac through the sacro-sciatic foramen. The diagnosis is made at operation for intestinal obstruction.

Maydl's Hernia

This rare hernia was first described in 1895. The W-shaped loop of bowel in the sac contains a strangulated intra-abdominal segment which may be missed unless the whole bowel is exposed.

Interstitial Hernia (Interparietal Hernia)

The interstitial hernia sac lies between the layers of the abdominal wall and may present without an external swelling. Occasionally the interstitial hernia is associated with an inguinal hernia. The sac may be found between the peritoneum and transversalis fascia or between the muscular layers of the abdominal wall, and is frequently associated with congenital deformities of the inguinal region and undescended testis.

The symptoms are those of bowel obstruction with an ill-defined mass above the inguinal ligament. The sac is often bilobed and must be fully exposed and identified before it is transfixed and excised.

REFERENCES

Askar O. M. (1978) A new concept of the aetiology and surgical repair of paraumbilical and epigastric hernias. *Ann. R. Coll. Surg. Engl.* **60**, 42–48.

Bulow S. (1974) Artificial pneumoperitoneum during inguinal herniotomy in children. *Acta Chir. Scand.* **140**, 127.

Drainer I. K. and Reid D. K. (1972) Recurrence-free ventral herniorrhaphy using a polypropylene mesh prosthesis. *J. R. Coll. Surg. Edinb.* **17**, 253–260.

Iles J. D. H. (1972) Convalescence after herniorrhaphy. *JAMA* **219**, 385–388.

Moloney G. E. (1958) Results of nylon darn repairs of hernias. *Lancet* **1**, 273–278.

Palmer B. V. (1978) Incarcerated inguinal hernia in children. *Ann. R. Coll. Surg. Engl.* **60**, 121–124.

Chapter seven

Inguinal Hernia Repair by the Shouldice Method

F. Glassow

Hernia repair is the most common operation in men. The recent upsurge in interest is motivated both by a genuine concern by all surgeons in improving results and by an increasing appreciation of the important socioeconomic implications of the operation.

In a 31-year association at the Shouldice Clinic, the author has performed more than 20 000 inguinal hernia repairs, of which more than 2000 were recurrent repairs. In the first 5 or 6 years the technique of the repair was being developed by the late Dr E. E. Shouldice. It has now become standardized.

Only elective inguinal repairs are considered here. There are many different operations for the repair of inguinal hernia, each with its own followers, and the operation here is a modified Bassini. At every operation the internal ring is routinely strengthened, as is the posterior inguinal wall, using a multilayered technique to achieve this. The recurrence rates recorded have remained consistently around 1 per cent for many years. However, an operation can be considered truly successful only when other surgeons around the world achieve comparable results using the same technique.

PREOPERATIVE ASSESSMENT

All medical conditions are carefully assessed and priorities judged. Many patients are in the older age groups so that cardiac, pulmonary and prostatic problems are common. Obesity is common, and these patients are encouraged to lose excess weight slowly before operation at a rate of about 0·5 to 1 kg a week. The operation is scheduled accordingly. Age in itself is no bar to operation, and 10 per cent of patients were over 70 years old. Older patients do just as well as the younger age groups and their recurrence rates are no different.

ANAESTHESIA

Local anaesthesia is used in more than 95 per cent of cases. A general anaesthetic is used only for children less than 12 years of age, for a few of the patients who have multi-recurrent hernias and, very rarely, for a very apprehensive patient.

A local anaesthetic is preferred for many reasons. It avoids the risks of general anaesthesia, and in some poor-risk and elderly patients it is the anaesthetic of choice. In Third World countries where first-class anaesthesia is less available it is ideal. Induction is quicker and the interval between operations in the operating theatres is lessened. It imposes a gentle technique on the surgeon because the patient is only interested in a painless operation at this stage. The surgeon is less likely to use tension with the repair. A conscious patient can be asked to cough to identify an evasive hernia or to test a repair. Patients can walk out of the operating theatre which boosts their morale preoperatively and subsequently has a great impact on their short hospital stay. They are ambulant throughout. Many patients specifically request local anaesthesia, and almost without exception, including those who previously had had a general or a spinal anaesthetic, state after operation that they prefer local anaesthesia. Immediate postoperative complications are fewer with the questionable exception of the degree of discomfort experienced in the first 24 hours. Catheterization is eliminated. (Nicholls, 1977; Makuria et al., 1982; Teasdale et al., 1982; Hashemi and Middleton, 1983).

A number of local anaesthetic agents are employed. Our experience is limited almost entirely to the use of 2 per cent procaine hydrochloride without adrenaline but recently I have been using 1 per cent and 1·5 per cent for the over-70 age group.

Premedication commences $1\frac{1}{2}$ hours preoperatively with oral administration of 200–250 mg sodium pentobarbital. Twenty minutes preoperatively 50–75 mg meperidine hydrochloride are given intramuscularly. A maximum of 150 ml of local anaesthetic solution may be used; 80–100 ml is initially injected as a subcutaneous regional infiltration in the line of the inguinal canal. A further 10–20 ml is used beneath the external oblique aponeurosis and a third injection of a similar amount is given around the internal ring, avoiding the inferior epigastric vessels. This volume of local has been used many thousands of times without adverse effects, given the adequate premedication cover described.

OPERATIVE TECHNIQUE

Skin Incision

Immediately after the subcutaneous local has been given the incision is made in the line of the inguinal canal. It is straight or slightly convex downwards. Pfannenstiel incisions are not used. A scar from a previous repair may require excision.

Cremaster Muscle

This structure is often ignored in descriptions of technique. It is identified surrounding the spermatic cord once the external oblique has been divided in the line of the inguinal canal. It is divided longitudinally along the cord so defining and mobilizing two separate leaves—one lateral, one medial. The lateral one is more bulky containing the cremasteric vessels, in its base, and the genital branch of the genitofemoral nerve. Once the cord is isolated and retracted laterally the third injection of local is given at the internal ring.

Internal Ring

All inguinal hernia repairs have two main components. The first is the dissection at the internal ring, the second the dissection of the posterior inguinal wall. This ritual attitude is very helpful when confronted by a very large primary hernia or by a difficult recurrent hernia. For example, all scrotal hernias are not indirect and a few are direct. Defining the inferior epigastric vessels will eliminate any such misdiagnosis.

High ligation of the indirect sac is standard practice and standard teaching, yet I do not regard it as vitally important (Glassow, 1965). I regard the complete freeing of the indirect sac from its fascial investments at the internal ring to be of equal or even greater importance. If this freeing is really complete, whether the sac is ligated high or low, the remaining ligated stump will retract out of sight within the internal ring. If the freeing is inadequate the stump remains adherent at the internal ring, and remains a potential hazard. The most obvious justification for this manoeuvre is that the recurrence rate achieved for primary indirect inguinal hernia repair is 1 per cent. Utilizing these same principles, the treatment of sliding indirect inguinal hernia is an extension of this argument, and converts a difficult operation into an easy one. Once identified the sliding hernia is simply freed completely at the internal ring and reduced within it without further treatment, even when large. The recurrence rate for sliding indirect hernia repair so achieved is also 1 per cent, and indeed few of these recurrences were sliding themselves (Ryan, 1956). Sliding hernias are nearly always indirect and left-sided, usually in men who are overweight and more than 50 years old. At this stage careful examination at the internal ring will detect the rare unsuspected interstitial hernia.

In the absence of an indirect inguinal hernia a peritoneal protrusion must be identified on the cord at the internal ring where it appears as a small whitish convex crescent. This eliminates the risk of missing an indirect hernia in cases in which the surgeon's attention may already be focused on an obvious direct inguinal hernia. The combination of an indirect and direct hernia is encountered in 8 per cent of men.

The two cremasteric leaves are now excised. This important step clearly demonstrates the whole posterior inguinal wall. If omitted a direct hernia may be missed.

Posterior Inguinal Wall and the Transversalis Lamina

The dissection and treatment of this layer constitute the second main component of any inguinal hernia operation and are of vital importance. Primary indirect hernia is twice as common as primary direct, yet recurrent indirect is less common than recurrent direct. This finding reflects the importance of the quality of the repair.

The repair performed here and described in detail later (p. 64) is based on an oblique linear division of the transversalis with subsequent overlap of the two leaves so obtained, both leaves being considered important. In the Cooper ligament repair (McVay, 1965; Halverson and McVay, 1970; Glassow, 1976a) the lower part of the transversalis, which is equivalent to the lower leaf just described, is not utilized because it is not attached to the inguinal ligament (Glassow, 1976b).

BILATERAL REPAIRS

One patient in 10 has a bilateral hernia on admission. Using local anaesthesia the repairs are staged 48 hours apart for several good reasons. A simultaneous bilateral repair would double the volume of local anaesthetic used. The timing of the second repair may be altered, for example in patients who have bilateral recurrent hernia or unilateral testicular atrophy, or in an elderly patient in whom the first repair was difficult, or in an extremely obese or tense individual. Occasionally, the patient decides on delay.

The external pudendal vessels should be preserved on one side at least to minimize prepuceal oedema.

Recurrence rates in simultaneous bilateral repairs are slightly higher, and tension may be a factor.

TESTIS

Orchidectomy is rarely performed and it is usually possible to preserve the testis even in patients who have multi-recurrent hernias. The patient who has a recurrent hernia is warned of the risks and a consent form for orchidectomy should be obtained in most cases. Testicular atrophy postoperatively is uncommon but, in recurrences where records are unavailable, the cord may lie subcutaneously and be easily damaged.

Patients of all ages welcome this conserving attitude.

SUTURE MATERIALS

Monofilament stainless steel wire gauge no. 34 is the suture material preferred. Occasionally no. 32 is needed for greater strength. Many surgeons use other non-absorbable sutures achieving excellent results. Absorbable sutures are unsatisfactory and their use is condemned. A continuous suture technique is used and is considered important because it distributes tension evenly. I have repaired many direct inguinal recurrences in patients in whom individual non-absorbable sutures were visible on either side of the neck of the hernia. It was considered that such ligatures were either inadequately placed or tied with uneven tension.

Although mesh is popular with some surgeons I have never used it even for the largest hernias. Indeed I have encountered it many times in repair of recurrent hernia and have often removed it.

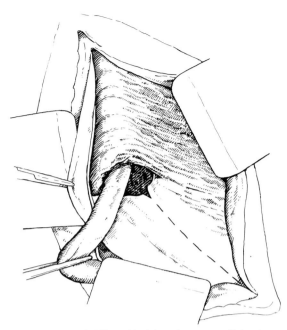

Fig. 7.1. Intended line of incision of transversalis lamina.

POSTERIOR INGUINAL WALL

Examination and Principles of Repair (Glassow, 1976c, 1978)

The assessment of the strength of the posterior inguinal wall is fundamental. This is accomplished first by inspection and then by testing its strength using a finger inserted at the internal ring deep to the transversalis plane. A direct inguinal hernia is obvious or will be demonstrated by this manoeuvre. In some cases only a weakness is present, but in either case a standard repair is applicable. The opening in the transversalis already made at the internal ring (*Fig.* 7.1) is extended medially towards the pubic bone over the centre of the direct hernia which is freed. If the transversalis is strong medially it may be left undivided, but attenuated excess transversalis may require excision. Firm transversalis of satisfactory quality can always be found even in the presence of a large direct or a recurrent direct hernia. A funicular direct sac is excised, although the more common diffuse direct sac is simply reduced.

The lower leaf of the divided transversalis should be wider than the upper (*Fig.* 7.2). In the subsequent repair it is carried upwards and medially beneath the upper leaf which is then brought downwards over it. This overlap is further strengthened by another immediately superficial to it bringing muscular structures medially to the inguinal ligament laterally.

Technique of Repair

In the reconstruction of the posterior wall four continuous lines of gauge no. 34 stainless steel wire are

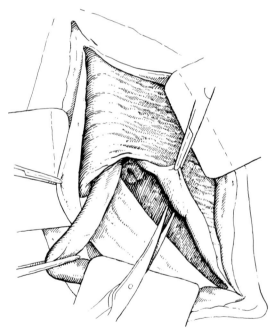

Fig. 7.2. Division of transversalis lamina.

inserted using only two separate sutures each being responsible for two lines. The first line starts medially at the pubic bone (*Fig.* 7.3) where it attaches the free edge of the lower transversalis flap to the posterior aspect of the lateral edge of the rectus, easily identified as a white border inserting onto the pubic bone. The suture should start as far medially as possible and be tied without tension. The entire free edge is now attached under the upper flap. After one or two small bites on the rectus it picks up the deep surface of the transversus and internal oblique as it travels laterally. Just medial to the internal ring the upper lateral ligated cremasteric stump is included in this first line, taking small bites without tension. At the internal ring the inferior epigastric vessels are avoided. After completion of this line of sutures it can be seen that quite a firm barrier has already been established and the defect or weakness eliminated. The suture is reversed and continues medially as the second line (*Fig.* 7.4). This brings the upper flap of divided transversalis downwards and laterally to the shelving surface of Poupart's ligament until it reaches the pubic bone again, where it is tied. This overlap strengthens the first layer and is particularly effective in the occasional case in which the first layer is of poor quality.

The third line (second suture) commences at the internal ring. Travelling medially (*Fig.* 7.5) it reinforces the subjacent lines, bringing the internal oblique and transversus lying medially to the deep surface of the inguinal ligament laterally. At the pubic bone it is reversed and travels laterally again utilizing the same structures. At the internal ring it is tied.

The repair should be performed without tension and relaxing incisions are never used. The spermatic cord should slide easily into the internal ring and the cord veins should not be engorged. The cord is replaced deep to the external oblique. The subcutaneous plane is separately closed eliminating dead space. Michel's skin clips are used.

Typically a primary inguinal repair takes about 40 minutes. A once recurrent repair might take 80 minutes while a more difficult multi-recurrent repair takes 2 or 3 hours.

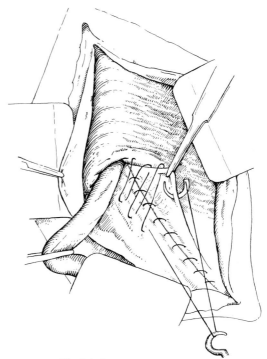

Fig. 7.4. Second line of sutures.

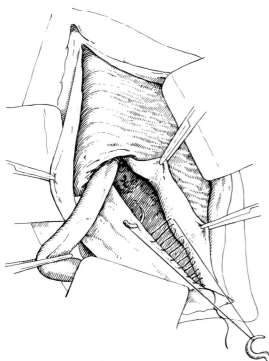

Fig. 7.3. First line of sutures.

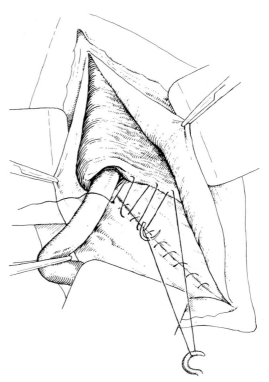

Fig. 7.5. Third line of sutures.

LENGTH OF HOSPITAL STAY AND ECONOMICS (Devlin et al., 1977)

Medical care costs continue to rise rapidly everywhere. Following surgery very early discharge from hospital is possible, consistent with an early return to work and good long-term results (Adler, 1977). A period off work of longer than 4 weeks is rarely authorized. A greater combined effort on the part of both surgeon and general practitioner would help to shorten longer periods allowed elsewhere. Patients may remain in hospital for 2 or 3 days because many live far away and earlier travel is inconvenient. In 1972 the average hospital stay in one large centre in Britain was 10 days but these periods are now very much shorter. One study showed that patients who were ambulant early did better in all respects than those kept in bed for longer periods (Palumbo and Sharpe, 1971). Many operations are now performed on an outpatient or day-care basis (Farquharson, 1955; Bellis, 1975; Ruckley, 1978; Goulbourne and Ruckley, 1979).

HERNIAS IN WOMEN

Groin hernias are approximately 25 times less common in women. While the inguinal:femoral ratio is 40:1 in men and only 3:1 in women, nevertheless inguinal hernia is also more frequent in women (Glassow, 1963). However, in women a primary inguinal hernia is almost always indirect. Primary direct hernia is very rare because the posterior inguinal wall is strong (Glassow, 1973). This is a good reason for performing a low operation for repair of a primary femoral hernia in women. However, recurrent direct inguinal hernia in women is more common than recurrent indirect suggesting an iatrogenic aetiology.

FOLLOW-UP

With the very large and ever-increasing number of repairs performed follow-up becomes increasingly more difficult, burdensome and expensive. Completely adequate long-term follow-up of very large series is impossible for a number of reasons, including shifting population, loss through death and indifference to correspondence. The argument that the patient who is lost to the follow-up may be the one who has a recurrence is unanswerable, but unlikely. All the evidence we can muster is to the contrary.

Of all recurrent hernias which followed a repair here, 50 per cent had developed at the end of 5 years, and 75 per cent at the end of 10 years, which indicates a minimum follow-up period of 10 years. If such rates are plotted graphically it is possible to predict eventual long-term recurrence rates if the rates for a shorter period are known.

RECURRENCES

The main criterion of success in any series of inguinal hernia repairs is the recurrence rate. As recently as 1977 a *British Medical Journal* Editorial quoted the recurrence rates for indirect hernias at 5–10 per cent, for direct hernias 15–20 per cent and for recurrent inguinal hernias 30 per cent (Editorial, 1977). A surgeon should aim at 1 per cent for repair of primary inguinal hernia, whether indirect or direct (Kirk, 1983).

DISCUSSION

It has been customary to give a general anaesthetic when repairing an inguinal hernia. It is hoped that this review has demonstrated how successfully such patients can be managed using local anaesthesia. Its indication and advantages have been intentionally described in detail in the hope that it may eventually become the anaesthetic of choice.

Emphasis is laid on the detailed appreciation of the anatomy of the inguinal canal, in particular the internal ring and the transversalis lamina. The technique used here has been carefully described and it is hoped that other surgeons may be persuaded of its efficacy. In our hands it has resulted in a short hospital stay, early return to a normal lifestyle and a recurrence rate of approximately 1 per cent for repair of primary inguinal hernia.

CONCLUSION

In 1971 Professor L. M. Zimmerman (Zimmerman, 1968) of Chicago wrote: 'The larger the series the more valuable are the figures offered and the percentage of patients returning for the follow up is also of great significance . . .'. Moreover, 'Hernia surgery demands meticulous technique, gentle handling of tissues, free anatomical exposure, accurate approximation of sutured structures, avoidance of tension and utilization of fine atraumatic needles and suture materials. The disregard of any of these attributes of good surgery will be reflected in a higher recurrence rate. With the same method the results will vary with the skill of the surgeon.'

I leave the most telling comment to the very end of this presentation because he put them more eloquently than I am able to do. Wakeley (1940) said: '. . . that so little interest is taken in the care of a hernia is a pity. The various operations are usually regarded as of minor importance and to be undertaken by a house surgeon, being beneath the dignity of a surgeon. A surgeon can do more for the community by operating on hernia cases and seeing that his recurrence rate is low than he can by operating on cases of malignant disease.'

Illustrations

Figures 7.1–7.5 were previously published in Nyhus L. M. and Condon R. E. (eds) *Hernia*, 2nd ed. (1978) Philadelphia, Lippincott, and have been modified.

Table 7.1. Primary inguinal herniorrhaphies, 1954–1982 (personal series).

Type of primary hernia	No. of repairs	No. of recurrences	% of recurrences
Indirect	10 893	79	0·7
Direct	5154	56	1·1
Combined indirect and direct	1023	6	0·6
Total	17 070	141	0·8

Table 7.2. Primary inguinal herniorrhaphies, 1954–1971 (followed to 1981; personal series).

Type of primary hernia	No. of repairs	No. of recurrences	% of recurrences
Indirect	6456	65	1·0
Direct	3179	42	1·3
Combined indirect and direct	718	5	0·7
Total	10 353	112	1·1

Table 7.3. Recurrent inguinal herniorrhaphies, 1954–1982 (personal series).

Type of recurrent hernia	No. of recurrences	No. of re-recurrences	% of re-recurrences
Indirect	1056	21	2·0
Direct	1468	42	2·9
Total	2524	63	2·5

Table 7.4. Recurrent inguinal herniorrhaphies, 1954–1971 (followed to 1981; personal series).

Type of recurrent hernia	No. of recurrences	No. of re-recurrences	% of re-recurrences
Indirect	628	12	1·9
Direct	776	32	4·1
Total	1404	44	3·1

Table 7.5. Inguinal herniorrhaphies (Shouldice repairs).

Name of surgeon	No. of repairs	No. of recurrences	% of recurrences
Barwell (UK)	1566	28	1·8
Berliner (USA)	1084	12	1·1
Burson (USA)	2000	70	3·5
Devlin (UK)	787	7	0·9
Dunn (USA)	2949	34	1·2
Shearburn (USA)	953	7	0·7
Wantz (USA)	2470	23	0·9
Total	11 809	181	1·5

REFERENCES

Adler M. W. (1977) Randomised controlled trial of early discharge for inguinal hernia and varicose veins. *Ann. R. Coll. Surg. Engl.* **59**, 251–254.

Bellis C. J. (1975) 16069 inguinal herniorrhaphies using local anaesthesia with one day hospitalisation and unrestricted activity. *Int. Surg.* **60**, 37–39.

Devlin H. B., Russell I. T., Muller D. et al. (1977) Short-stay surgery for inguinal hernia. Clinical outcome of the Shouldice operation. *Lancet* **1**, 847–849.

Editorial Br. Med. J. (1977) Activity and recurrent hernia. *Br. Med. J.* **275**, 3–4.

Farquharson E. L. (1955) Early ambulation with special reference to herniorrhaphy as outpatient procedure. *Lancet* **2**, 517–519.

Glassow F. (1963) Inguinal hernia in the female. *Surg. Gynecol. Obstet.* **116**, 701–704.

Glassow F. (1965) High ligation of the sac in indirect inguinal hernia. *Am. J. Surg.* **109**, 460–463.

Glassow F. (1973) An evaluation of the strength of the posterior wall of the inguinal canal in women. *Br. J. Surg.* **60**, 342–344.

Glassow F. (1976a) Inguinal hernia repair: a comparison of the Shouldice and Cooper ligament repair of the posterior inguinal wall. *Am. J. Surg.* **131**, 306–311.

Glassow F. (1976b) Short-stay surgery (Shouldice technique) for repair of inguinal hernia. *Ann. R. Coll. Surg. Engl.* **58**, 133–139.

Glassow F. (1976c) The Shouldice repair of inguinal hernia. In: Varco R. L. and Delaney J. P. (eds) *Controversy in Surgery*. Phildaelphia, W. B. Saunders, pp. 375–387.

Glassow F. (1978) The Shouldice repair of inguinal hernia. In: Nyhus L. M. and Condon R. E. (eds) *Hernia*, 2nd ed. Philadelphia, J. B. Lippincott, pp. 163–174.

Goulborne L. A. and Ruckley C. V. (1979) Operations for hernia and varicose veins in a day-bed unit. *Br. Med. J.* **2**, 712–714.

Halverson K. and McVay C. B. (1970) Inguinal and femoral hernioplasty: a 22-year study of the authors' methods. *Arch. Surg.* **101**, 127–135.

Hashemi K. and Middleton M. D. (1983) Subcutaneous bupivacaine for postoperative analgesia after herniorrhaphy. *Ann. R. Coll. Surg. Engl.* **65**, 38–39.

Kirk P. M. (1983) Which inguinal hernia repair? *Br. Med. J.* **287**, 4–5.

Makuria T., Alexander-Williams J. and Keighley M. R. B. (1982) Comparison between general and local anaesthesia for groin hernias. *Ann. R. Coll. Surg. Engl.* **64**, 238–242.

McVay C. B. (1965) Inguinal and femoral hernioplasty. *Surgery* **57**, 615–625.

Nicholls J. C. (1977) Necessity into choice: an appraisal of inguinal herniorrhaphy under local anaesthesia. *Ann. R. Coll. Surg. Engl.* **59**, 124–127.

Palumbo L. T. and Sharpe W. S. (1971) Primary inguinal hernioplasty in the adult. *Surg. Clin. North Am.* **48**, 143–154.

Ruckley C. V. (1978) Day case and short stay surgery for hernia. *Br. J. Surg.* **65**, 1–4.

Ryan E. A. (1956) Analysis of 313 consecutive cases of indirect sliding inguinal hernias. *Surg. Gynecol. Obstet.* **102**, 45–48.

Teasdale C., McCrum A., Williams N. B. et al. (1982) A randomised controlled trial to compare local with general anaesthesia for short-stay inguinal repair. *Ann. R. Coll. Surg. Engl.* **64**, 238–242.

Wakeley C. P. G. (1940) Treatment of certain types of external herniae. *Lancet* **1**, 822–826.

Zimmerman L. M. (1968) The use of prosthetic materials in the repairs of hernias. *Surg. Clin. North Am.* **48**, 143–154.

Chapter eight

Oesophageal and Gastric Carcinoma

K. Jeyasingham

The majority of malignant neoplasms of the oesophagus and stomach are epithelial in origin, and there the similarity between oesophageal and gastric carcinomas ends, except in so far as the presentations of adenocarcinoma of the cardia are indistinguishable from those of carcinoma of the lower oesophagus.

SURGICAL ANATOMY

The oesophagus is a midline hollow viscus commencing at the cricopharyngeal sphincter at the level of the 6th cervical vertebra (C6), entering the chest at the level of the suprasternal notch, traversing the posterior mediastinum and entering the abdomen through the oesophageal hiatus in the diaphragm to join the stomach at the cardia. During this course through three regions of the body it bears a close relationship to the trachea and pericardium in front, and the vertebral column posteriorly. It bears a close relationship to the vagus and its branches in its entire length and is not too distant from either pleural cavity during its thoracic course. For all practical purposes it is devoid of a serosal covering, but like other organs it does have a fascia propia.

The *blood supply* of the oesophagus is derived from the aorta and its major branches, directly as oesophageal branches or in common with branches to adjacent organs such as the pulmonary hilum, trachea and thyroid gland. The *venous drainage* is through tributaries draining into the azygos and hemi-azygos systems in the chest and via the thyroid veins in the neck and gastric veins in the upper abdomen.

The lymphatics of the oesophagus (*Fig.* 8.1) are distributed predominantly in the form of a submucosal plexus and a para-oesophageal plexus. Both plexuses receive lymph from all parts of the respective layers of the oesophageal wall. The plexuses communicate with each other through penetrating vessels which traverse the longitudinal and circular muscle walls. The para-oesophageal plexus drains into para-oesophageal lymph nodes which are situated on the surface of the oesophagus, and also into

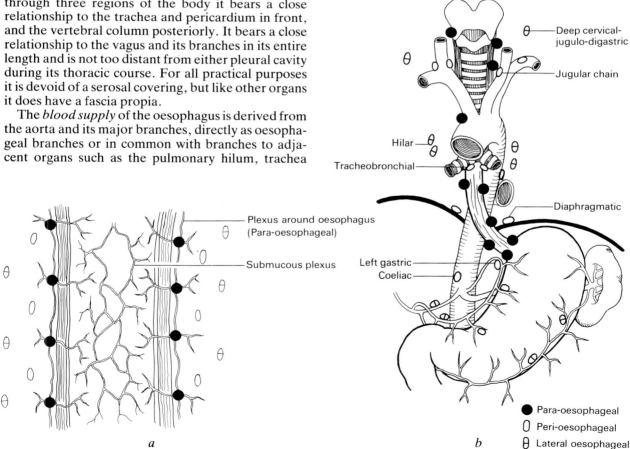

Plexus around oesophagus (Para-oesophageal)

Submucous plexus

Deep cervical-jugulo-digastric

Jugular chain

Hilar

Tracheobronchial

Diaphragmatic

Left gastric

Coeliac

● Para-oesophageal
◯ Peri-oesophageal
θ Lateral oesophageal

a

b

Fig. 8.1. *a*, Lymphatic drainage of the oesophageal wall. *b*, Distribution of lymph nodes in relation to regional drainage from the oesophagus.

peri-oesophageal lymph nodes situated in close proximity to the oesophagus. Lymphatics also drain from the peri-oesophageal nodes to the lateral oesophageal nodes, or directly from the para- to the lateral oesophageal nodes, skipping the perioesophageal group (Japanese Society for Esophageal Disorders, 1976 (*Table* 8.1).

Table 8.1. Lymph nodes of the oesophagus

Para-oesophageal nodes (on the wall of the oesophagus)	Cervical Upper thoracic Middle thoracic Lower thoracic
Peri-oesophageal nodes (in immediate apposition to the oesophagus)	Deep cervical Supraclavicular Paratracheal Subcarinal Para-aortic Diaphragmatic Left gastric Lesser curvature Coeliac
Lateral oesophageal nodes (located lateral to the oesophagus)	Posterior triangle of neck Hilar Superior pancreatico-duodenal and pyloro-duodenal Hepatic Greater curvature

Regionalization of the oesophagus has been adopted as an arbitrary mechanism of describing the exact location of the pathology in the organ. The cervical oesophagus commences at the cricopharyngeal sphincter and ends at the level of the sternal notch anteriorly and the lower border of the 2nd dorsal vertebra posteriorly. The upper thoracic oesophagus ends at the level of the aortic arch, azygos vein and tracheal bifurcation, while the middle thoracic oesophagus ends at the level of the inferior pulmonary vein. For practical purposes the upper and middle thoracic are together described as 'thoracic' oesophagus, while the lower portion together with the abdominal portion of the oesophagus are called the 'lower' oesophagus. The importance of such regionalization becomes more evident when appropriate surgical procedures are planned for lesions situated at different levels of the oesophagus (*Fig.* 8.2).

The stomach is a hollow viscus situated in the upper abdomen under cover of the left dome of the diaphragm and protected to a great extent by the costal margin of the chest cage. It bears a close relationship to the left lobe of the liver and the spleen and pancreas. Unlike the oesophagus it has a serosal covering over 90 per cent of its surface, the walls of which contain three distinct muscle layers. Like the oesophagus, the stomach is arbitrarily divided into three regions—upper (cardiac and fundus), middle (body) and lower (pyloric) (*Fig.* 8.3).

The blood supply of the stomach is received through branches of the left and right gastric arteries, branches of the gastro-epiploic arteries, and short gastric branches of the splenic artery. It is thus clear that the stomach receives all its arterial blood directly or indirectly from all three major divisions of the artery of the foregut—the coeliac axis. The venous

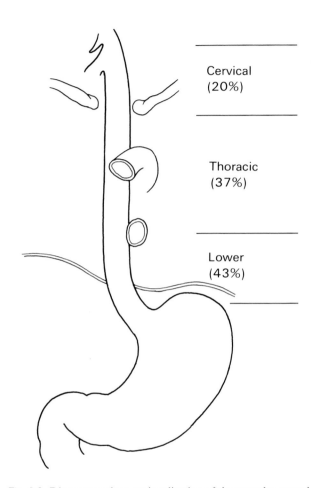

Fig. 8.2. Diagram to show regionalization of the oesophagus and the approximate distribution of carcinoma by region.

drainage from the stomach reaches the portal veins via the right and left gastric veins and the splenic veins. The lymphatics of the stomach are also disposed in the submucosal and subserosal plexuses with intercommunication but, unlike in the oesophagus the lymph nodes draining the stomach are distributed along the lesser and greater curvatures in the first tier of drainage, while the second tier of drainage is situated around the main arterial branches—the left gastric, splenic and gastro-epiploic. The third tier of nodes is located in a suprapancreatic position and around the superior mesenteric artery. Para-aortic and hepatic hilar nodes would constitute the fourth tier of nodes (Soga et al., 1979) (*Table* 8.2).

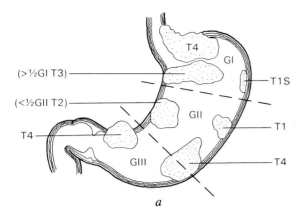

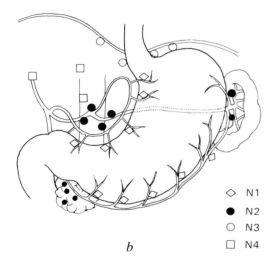

Table 8.2. Gastric nodes

N1 First tier or perigastric	Lesser curve ⎱of same Greater curve⎰segment
N2 Second tier	Left gastric
	Splenic hilum
	Left gastro-epiploic ⎱body and Oesophago-gastric ⎰fundus
N3 Third tier	Suprapancreatic
	Superior mesenteric
N4 Fourth tier	Para-aortic and pre-aortic
	Hepatic hilum

◇ N1
● N2
○ N3
□ N4

PATHOLOGY

By and large 90–98 per cent of all oesophageal carcinomas are squamous (epidermoid) carcinomas. The higher the tumour, the more closely it approximates the 98 per cent figure. About 1–9 per cent of the tumours are adenocarcinomas, the likelihood of this being about 9 per cent in the lower oesophagus (Gunnlaugsson et al., 1970).

Adenocarcinoma occurring in the lower oesophagus is commonly due to a tumour of the cardia of the stomach spreading upwards, occasionally due to adenocarcinoma arising in a columnar-lined lower oesophagus, and only rarely due to a truly oesophageal adenocarcinoma arising in the mucous glands of the oesophageal lining.

Primary malignant melanoma, mixed squamous and adenocarcinoma, muco-epidermoid carcinoma, adenoid cystic carcinoma and oat cell carcinoma and carcinosarcoma have all been reported in the oesophagus. Tumour spread is characterized by direct

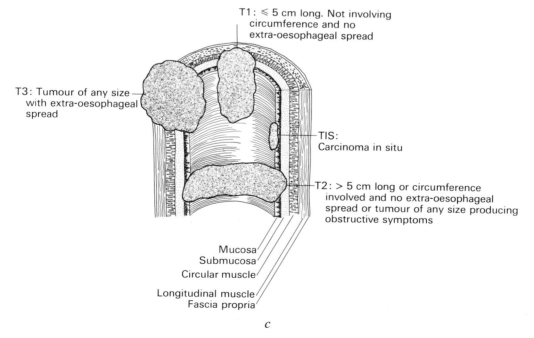

Fig. 8.3. *a*, T staging of gastric carcinoma. The interrupted lines show the demarcation of the stomach into the upper middle and lower regions. *b*, Lymph nodal drainage of the stomach in staging by nodes. *c*, T staging of oesophageal carcinoma (UICC).

infiltration through all layers of the oesophageal wall and into the lumen of the oesophagus. Based on the speed of proliferation, nature of direct progression, extent of trauma and ulceration of the surface and the proportion of fibrous stroma in the tumour, it assumes one of several morphological descriptions (*Table* 8.3). As the oesophagus has no serosal layer, direct spread into the adjacent organs occurs early. Depending on the location of the tumour the larynx, trachea, aorta and great vessels, azygos vein, pleura, pericardium, diaphragm and stomach are involved early in the direct spread of the tumour.

Table 8.3. Carcinoma of the oesophagus

Types of lesion
Ulcerative with undermined edges
Constrictive
Scirrhous infiltration
Diffuse-superficial
Polypoidal and necrotic
Rolled edge ulcer
Adenocarcinoma of Barrett's ulcer

Lymphatic spread occurs in different directions based on the flow of lymph in the submucosal plexus in a longitudinal or transverse manner and through penetrating lymphatics to the para-oesophageal lymphatic plexus. Tumour cell aggregates trapped in the submucosal lymphatics produce 'skip lesions'. These have been noted as far as 8 cm away from the outer edge of the primary tumour—an aspect that needs important consideration in deciding the upper limit of transection of the oesophagus (Burgess et al., 1951; Miller, 1962). The para-oesophageal plexus in turn drains into lymph nodes situated in para-oesophageal groups, peri-oesophageal groups and in lateral oesophageal situations. Spread through the bloodstream occurs late in oesophageal carcinoma and is often a terminal feature.

Gastric carcinoma is glandular in origin but depending on the rate of proliferation and extent of stromal tissue it may again take on one of several morphological forms (*Table* 8.4).

Table 8.4. Gastric carcinoma

Types of lesion
Polypoidal
Plaque like
Ulcerative and ulcero-cancer
Infiltrating
Linitis plastica

Because of the continuity of the oesophagus with the stomach, adenocarcinoma of the cardia often directly involves the lower oesophagus but the presence of the serosa delays direct spread into adjacent organs in the abdomen quite significantly. Lymphatic spread to regional nodes occurs early while submucosal spread of tumour does not appear to occur to the same extent as occurs in oesophageal carcinoma. The occurrence of subserosal nodules some distance from the outer limit of the primary tumour is, however, not uncommon. Bloodstream spread is again a feature of late disease. Extension of tumour from the pylorus into the duodenum does occur although a form of mucosal block appears to be exercised at the submucosal plane where the pylorus ends and the duodenum begins. It is not uncommon, however, to find direct infiltration of the first part of the duodenum by tumour of the pyloric antrum.

CLINICAL FEATURES

In the early stages, both oesophageal and gastric carcinomas are asymptomatic. The earliest symptom of oesophageal carcinoma is, however, painless dysphagia. Dysphagia is initially experienced with solids, and it gradually progresses, with short periods of remission, to dysphagia with liquids. Occasionally a patient presents with total dysphagia due to impaction of food at the neoplastic lesion. If painless dysphagia progresses to a stage of painful dysphagia one should suspect direct spread of tumour into the mediastinal structures. Progressive weight loss accompanies increasing dysphagia and is not necessarily due to extensive disease, a fact that needs to be borne in mind before denying surgical treatment to an emaciated patient. Blood loss in the form of haematemesis or melaena is not a common symptom, and anaemia is not a regular feature. Nausea and vomiting, cough, hoarseness, hiccups and halitosis are symptoms suggestive of oesophageal carcinoma. Excessive salivation is often a sign of obstructive pathology, and retrosternal oppression and shortness of breath may also accompany oesophageal carcinoma. Occurrence of cough induced by food would suggest recurrent laryngeal palsy or malignant tracheo-oesophageal fistula.

Physical examination, if it produces a positive sign, almost invariably indicates extensive disease. Palpable nodes in the neck or para-aortic area, hepatomegaly and pleural effusions are all features of late stages of the disease.

The clinical features of gastric carcinoma are even less specific than those of oesophageal carcinoma. Dysphagia, nausea, vomiting, anaemia, dyspepsia, anorexia, gaseous eructations with halitosis, are some of the symptoms noted in patients with gastric carcinoma. Persistent epigastric pain, unabated by food, is an important symptom which when present should draw a suspicion of gastric carcinoma. Melaena and haematemesis in the absence of an ulcer history should suggest a possible malignant cause. The physical presence of lymph nodal enlargement, hepatomegaly, ascites, abdominal mass and jaundice are all features of late disease.

INVESTIGATION OF OESOPHAGEAL AND GASTRIC CARCINOMA

The purpose of investigation in these diseases is manifold:

1. Diagnostic
2. Assessment of extent of disease
3. Assessment of physical status of patient
4. Grading of symptoms—dysphagia
5. Grading of performance status
6. Grading of nutritional status
7. Pathological staging of disease

Radiological screening of the patient is undertaken initially with liquid contrast medium with ciné or video recording or with serial exposure. The examination is carried from the buccal cavity through to the small bowel. This is then followed by double-contrast radiography, especially if the initial examination has not produced an obvious extensive lesion. Double-contrast radiography has in recent years contributed immensely to the detection of small lesions of the oesophagus and stomach, especially of the plaque-like and polypoidal varieties without any obstruction. When a lesion has been demonstrated on contrast radiography, in those centres where facilities are available for computed tomography the procedure is being increasingly employed to assess the length, the extent of infiltration of the organ, involvement of adjacent organs including the liver, and lymph node enlargement. The addition of a contrast medium to computed tomography adds a further dimension to the examination. Azygrography by the injection of a soluble contrast medium into the marrow of a rib on each side of the chest had been suggested as a useful investigation to detect extra-oesophageal spread, in the days prior to computed tomography, but has failed to gain popularity. Similarly, lymphangiography has no place, currently, in the investigation of oesophageal or gastric carcinoma.

Upper Gastrointestinal Endoscopy

This is the one investigation that has revolutionized the diagnosis, early detection and assessment of neoplasms of the oesophagus and stomach. A full and thorough examination of the entire pharynx, oesophagus, stomach and duodenum is carried out with full documentation of the appearances, both normal and abnormal. Suspicious areas are systematically biopsied and brushed. The size, extent and fixity of the tumour are assessed. The use of *intra vitam staining* of the mucosa to highlight suspicious plaques is a recent innovation (Monnier et al., 1985). The flexible slimline endoscopes have also enabled clinicians to look back at the cardia and fundus to pick up lesions that could easily have been missed otherwise.

Bronchoscopy

In carcinoma of the cervical and thoracic oesophagus, examination of the tracheobronchial tree is an essential prerequisite, in order to detect compression, infiltration and invasion with or without tracheo-oesophageal fistulation.

Haematological Assessment

This is carried out to detect anaemia, alterations in the blood picture, estimate the serum protein, and estimate the liver function tests, with special reference to the liver enzymes. Any alteration of the alkaline phosphatase, alanine transaminase and the aspartate transaminase to above normal levels would be highly suggestive of liver metastases in the presence of neoplasia, but could equally well be due to alcoholic liver damage in patients with oesophageal carcinoma.

Perfusion scan of the liver and bone is undertaken if the alkaline phosphatase has been known to be abnormal, but in the presence of a normal value the investigation could be immediately waived. Ultrasonography of the liver is an alternative procedure. In the presence of symptoms suggestive of brain metastases, a computed tomography of the head would be justified.

Mediastinoscopy and laparoscopy or mini-laparotomy are all investigations that could be appropriately employed if exploration with a view to resection is a contra-indication.

EARLY DETECTION OF OESOPHAGEAL AND GASTRIC CARCINOMA

The incidence of carcinoma of the upper gastrointestinal tract varies according to the region of the world under consideration. The routine screening of a whole population for detecting early carcinoma of the upper gastrointestinal tract is justified in parts of the world where there is a high incidence of oesophageal and gastric carcinoma such as the Orient. In the Western world, with the exception of parts of France, the incidence is such that routine screening of the general population is not an economic proposition. There are, however, groups of the population who would appear to be at high risk of developing oesophageal carcinoma and others for gastric carcinoma (*Table* 8.5).

Grading of Dysphagia

It is only by proper documentation of the pre-treatment grading of symptoms that one could assess the usefulness of any form of treatment, be it palliative or curative in intent. Such a grading scheme is seen in *Table* 8.6 which indicates inability to eat different types of food.

Table 8.5. High-risk population for oesophageal and gastric carcinoma

Oesophageal carcinoma
1. Heavy alcohol drinkers who also smoke
2. Patients with a long history of dyspepsia with oesophagitis
3. Patients with columnar-lined oesophagus
4. Patients with achalasia cardia with or without surgical treatment
5. Patients with corrosive strictures treated conservatively
6. Patients with scleroderma
7. Patients with long-standing diverticula not treated surgically
8. Patients with Plummer–Vinson syndrome
9. Patients with hyperkeratosis (tylosis)

Gastric carcinoma
1. Achlorhydric patients
2. Patients with pernicious anaemia
3. Patients with polypoid adenomas
4. Patients with chronic atrophic gastritis (alcoholic patients)
5. Patients who have undergone previous gastrectomy
6. Patients with Menetrier's disease

Table 8.6. Grades of dysphagia

0	Normal
1	Intermittent dysphagia to solids
2	Inability to eat solids
3	Inability to eat minced food
4	Inability to eat puréed food
5	Inability to drink liquids (or saliva)

Grading Performance

This could be achieved either according to the World Health Organization grading from 0 to 4 or on the Karnofsky scale from 9 to 0 under three groups A, B and C. They are both non-specific systems for assessment of performance status for each individual patient and can be usefully employed in routine follow-up for assessment of each patient after treatment (against his or her own norm).

Grading of Nutritional State

Patients with carcinoma of the oesophagus and of the stomach are progressively depleted of their nutritional requirements, which are reflected in the blood chemistry, total body compartment and in the cellular components of the blood. Apart from the deprivation of intake of nutrients, and the increasing demands of malignant cachexia, these patients often have impaired liver function from long-standing alcohol and tobacco abuse. The ability of any modality of treatment to correct the nutritional state of the patient is an important factor to be taken into consideration in the choice of the appropriate treatment.

Cardiological and Respiratory Assessment

Assessment of the cardiac and respiratory reserve of the patient has to be made both in the grading of the performance status as well as in the evaluation of his or her suitability to any specific modality of treatment. The presence of respiratory problems or of cardiac decompensation, while temporarily excluding surgical resection, may be a total contra-indication for chemotherapy or radiotherapy. The pre-treatment preparation of the patient should be aimed at controlling any cardiac decompensation by suitable therapy, and respiratory problems have to be adequately treated before a decision is made as to suitability or otherwise for surgical intervention.

Pathological Staging of Disease

Although pre-treatment investigations can greatly assist in assessing the extent of local and distant metastases, the final and conclusive procedure is documenting the exact extent of the primary lesion and of neighbouring structures. Without exploration, all pre-treatment staging is arbitrary. Non-exploratory treatment based on such staging is not comparable with post-exploratory treatment based on pathological staging of disease achieved by full assessment of the tumour, lymph nodes and neighbouring structures. Therefore randomized trials of non-surgical modalities such as radiotherapy and chemotherapy against surgical resection based on pre-treatment staging are already loaded unfavourably to surgery. Imaging techniques of staging of disease should ipso facto involve considerable numbers of invasive and time-consuming investigations, all of which could be far more expensive and demanding to the patient than surgical exploration, which, when feasible, almost always leads to a therapeutic procedure of a palliative or curative nature.

Numerous systems have been postulated for pathological staging of disease, all based on quantitating the extent of disease in the primary site (T) (*Fig. 8.3c*), in the lymph nodal distribution (N) and in distant metastases (M). The TNM staging of oesophageal cancer devised by the Union Internationale Contre le Cancer (UICC, 1982) and agreed on by the American Joint Committee on Cancer (AJCC) and numerous other national bodies, has certain drawbacks. The TNM system designed by the Japanese Society for Esophageal Disorders (1976) approximates closely to what the author has been using for some time now. However, for gastric cancers the system proposed by the UICC and agreed on by the AJCC would appear to be more rational when tumour can be designated as upper, middle and lower. The four-tier nodal system proposed by Soga et al. (1979) appears attractive in considering gastric carcinoma as one entity without compartmentalization. The author's own preference again has been for the latter system. Whichever TNM system one adopts, it is essential that each entity is precisely defined and that peroperative sampling be carried out in a prospective fashion (*Tables* 8.7, 8.8).

Table 8.7. Objectives of staging

Assessment of tumour extent	T
Nodal assessment	N
Distant metastases	M
Histological type	H
Allocation of region–site	S

TREATMENT OF OESOPHAGEAL CARCINOMA

Oesophageal carcinoma often presents at a stage when obstructive symptoms have been present for an average of 5 months, and tumour in existence several more months. The disease has now spread not only into the lumen and wall of the organ but also beyond the fascia propria and probably to distant lymph nodes and organs. Treatment at this stage, therefore, is unlikely to be productive in terms of long-term survival, but to the patient suffering from progressive dysphagia, loss of weight and increasing retrosternal discomfort, any treatment that alleviates these, and in doing so prolongs life, is likely to bring comfort, provided the treatment can be applied with a low morbidity and mortality, and does not occupy a great proportion of what life expectancy remains. Oesophageal carcinoma, at least in the Western hemisphere, is a disease of the elderly except in certain high-risk groups mentioned earlier (p. 73).

Surprisingly, elderly patients do tolerate surgical intervention well, but not radiotherapeutic or chemotherapeutic regimens, both of which carry far more debilitating systemic effects for much longer periods.

In recent years, with the widespread use of routine endoscopy of the upper gastrointestinal tract by an increasing number of endoscopists, for symptoms non-specific to oesophageal carcinoma, and with the development of routine screening endoscopy at regular intervals in high-risk populations, aided by brush cytology, lavage cytology or biopsy of suspicious areas highlighted by toluidine blue, it is likely that oesophageal carcinoma will be increasingly detected early in the disease, and the pessimism apparent in most reviews of the therapy of this disease will yield to a much healthier attitude towards it.

At present several modalities of treatment are available to the clinician dealing with this disease:
1. Chemotherapy
2. Radiotherapy
3. Surgery
4. Endoscopic procedures

Any one or a combination of such modalities may have to be employed in the management of each patient. The treatment has to be tailored to the needs of the patient, not vice versa. While randomized clinical trials of a multi-centred nature are essential for progress when new therapeutic vistas open up, the mature clinician managing the oesophageal cancer patient has to exercise judgement in the choice of an appropriate modality or combination of modalities in the first instance, and at later periods institute one

Table 8.8. Staging of oesophageal carcinoma by tumour and nodal extent

pT	Post-surgery tumour	pN	Post-surgery nodes
pT0	Tumour not found on resected specimen (biopsy positive)	pN0	Samples nodes all negative
pTIS	≤3 cm in any diameter Restricted to mucosa	pN1	*Submucosal* skip lesion in *same* region. *Para*-oesophageal nodes + of *same* region
pT1	<3 cm in any diameter Invading beyond mucosa but *no* invasion of fascia propria	pN2	*Peri*-oesophageal nodes + of *same* region *Para*-oesophageal node + of *adjacent* region *Submucosal* skip lesion on *adjacent* region
pT2	>3 cm in any diameter no invasion of fascia propria		
pT3	Any size >3 cm but involving *only* one region with extra-oesophageal spread	pN3	*Para*-oesophageal nodes + of *distant* region. *Peri*-oesophageal nodes + of *adjacent* or *distant* region. *Lateral* nodes of *any* region
pT4	*More* than one region involved with or without extra-oesophageal spread	pN4	Nodes *beyond* oesophageal groups involved
pTX	Means for assessment not available	pNX	Means for assessment not available

or other of the modalities during the remaining lifetime of the patient, if the need arises.

Chemotherapy

Single-agent chemotherapy and combination chemotherapy have both been evaluated. Among the drugs that have been studied—bleomycin, 5 fluorouracil, doxorubicin (Adriamycin), methotrexate, Cyclophosphamide, vindesine, cisplatin, mitomycin—single-agent activity and combination therapy have only produced a response rate ranging from 15 to 35 per cent and a median duration of response only in weeks, and almost unmodified survival (Gisselbrecht et al., 1983). Currently popular regimens are based on the synergism between adriamycin and 5 fluorouracil or between adriamycin and cisplatin.

Pre-treatment investigations, with the known toxicity of some of these drugs, should include a chest radiograph, creatinine clearance, serum bilirubin, full blood picture and an excretion pyelogram. The administration of cisplatin should be preceded by forced diuresis with mannitol.

Examples of combination chemotherapy are set out below:

Regimen I: Forced diuresis prior to cisplatin with mannitol 25 g in 1000 ml of 50 per cent dextrose in N/2 saline with 30 mg KCl.
Cisplatin 100 mg/m^2 on day 1 every 3 weeks.
5 Fu 1000 mg/m^2 in 2000 ml of 50 per cent dextrose in N/2 saline over 24 hours as an infusion on 4 days every 3 weeks.

Regimen II: 5 Fu 1000 mg/m^2 per day in one injection of 120 ml of fluid with cisplatin 100 mg/m^2 with forced diuresis every 3 weeks.

Regimen III: 5 Fu 600 mg/m^2 on day 1 and day 8.
Adriamycin 30 mg/m^2 on day 1.
Cisplatin 75 mg/m^2 on day 1 with forced diuresis and hydration.

Each course is repeated every 4 weeks.

Chemotherapeutic regimens are constantly changing, and varying response rates are being claimed by different investigators using different combinations. Although sporadic claims of complete response are recorded, no claims for cure have been made. In the context of the knowledge of histological confirmation of the presence of tumour cells at the time of resection after three cycles of chemotherapy, its role as a single-modality treatment can only be palliative. However, as a combination modality it has a role as a pre-surgery adjuvant with or without post-resection therapy based on whether there are widespread microscopic deposits at the time of resection.

Radiation Therapy

This modality has been a more popular form of palliation since the early 1960s when the results of surgical resection in extensive disease were proving to be poor. Relief of dysphagia is achieved for some considerable duration of time as most patients remain ambulant throughout the therapy until terminal disease and death. Since the publication of the Edinburgh results for patients treated in a 20-year period from 1948 to 1968 (Pearson, 1975) the curative potential of radiotherapy has been extensively explored. The Edinburgh results of that period have never been reproduced either in the same city or elsewhere, by Pearson or by others. Furthermore, palliation of dysphagia may not occur for several weeks after treatment has been completed. Stricture and tracheo-oesophageal fistulation rate is relatively high. Therefore, its place as a single-modality curative therapy is suspect.

Pre-resection irradiation has been applied with a view to local tumour shrinkage after preliminary laparotomy to exclude metastases (Guernsey et al., 1969; Groves and Rodriguez-Antunez, 1973) or after exclusion bypass of tumour, and staged resection. No significant improvement was achieved in any of these studies compared to surgical resection alone. In some of the more recently reported studies the deterioration and drop-off rate has been so high that results have been disappointing.

Radiotherapy as a single-modality treatment has, however, an important place in the treatment of hypopharyngeal (postcricoid) carcinoma where the response rate and cure rate have been high compared to those for other sites, especially taking into consideration the fact that the patient still has a voice, albeit a hoarse one, and is able to swallow satisfactorily. Some examples of dosage of irradiation with cobalt beam are given below.

Palliative

A total dose of between 3000 and 5000 rad is usually administered on a daily dose of 200 rad five times a week, for 3 weeks. The higher the total palliative dose, the longer the survival of the patient and the duration of symptomatic relief, but this may be a reflection of the general condition of the patient at the commencement of treatment and the ability of the patient to tolerate a higher dosage.

Curative

A total dose of 5000–6600 rad is divided into 20 fractions over 4–6 weeks through a portal of approximately 8 × 15 cm. The tumour margin is cleared by approximately 6 cm and if necessary by a separate portal for lymph nodal involvement not covered in the same field.

Pre-operative Irradiation

Dosage is limited to 2000–3000 rad in divided doses over 5–6 days followed by an interval of 10–14 days before proceeding to resection.

Palliative Irradiation to Bony Metastases

The total dose required for relief of pain is all that is necessary for control of symptoms of bony metastases occurring late after definitive treatment of the primary. Total dosage may vary from 600 to 1000 rad administered over 3–5 days.

Surgery

This modality has been the treatment of choice in the palliation of symptoms of oesophageal carcinoma since Torek's first oesophagectomy in 1913. In the 1960s and early 1970s there was a swing to other forms of therapy based on statistical data of 5-year survivals, and operative mortality and morbidity achieved from cumulative figures of several publications. The hopes rasied by claims for radiotherapy or chemotherapy as a curative modality were therefore explored and are still being explored as a single modality, or more rationally as an adjuvant to surgery. Examples of such adjuvant or multi-modality treatment are:

1. Preoperative radiotherapy and surgery.
2. Preoperative chemotherapy and surgery.
3. Preoperative chemotherapy followed by surgery and then by postoperative radiotherapy.
4. Preoperative radiotherapy and then surgery followed by postoperative radiotherapy.

The morbidity and mortality of oesophageal resections vary according to the experience and expertise of the team managing the patient. With proper assessment and preoperative preparation of patients, resectability rates of 80–90 per cent can be achieved, especially with increasing awareness and screening of high-risk populations. Morbidity and mortality of exploration are dependent on the preoperative preparation of the patients. Perioperative mortality rates of less than 5 per cent are being constantly achieved by teams dealing with substantial numbers of patients. Although the temptation does exist for every surgeon to take on this very demanding surgery, there is no place for the occasional oesophagectomist. One has to be a member of a team constantly dealing with oesophageal problems, both benign and malignant, to be able to achieve and guarantee the low mortality and morbidity of oesophageal surgery. Long-term survival with surgical resection can only follow early detection, and with stage I disease 5-year survivals of 80 per cent have been achieved (Nakayama and Kinoshita, 1975). The pessimistic attitude towards surgical treatment is based on the wrong assumption that because high mortality and morbidity are a rule with several smaller series, a few specialized teams dealing with the problem cannot improve on the results.

The objectives of surgery are:

1. To remove the oesophageal carcinoma, if resectable.
2. To reconstruct the upper gastrointestinal tract in one stage.

3. To bypass the tumour if found irresectable at exploration.
4. If preoperatively assessed as inoperable, or the patient found unsuited to major surgical resection, to establish a satisfactory oesophageal lumen for feeding purposes, by
   a. Endoscopic intubation—pulsion intubation.
   b. Operative intubation—traction intubation.
   c. Dilatation of the tumour alone.
   d. Endoscopic diathermy fulguration.
   e. Endoscopic photofulguration.
   f. Endoscopic insertion of intracavitary Selectron tubes.
5. When other modalities of treatment have previously been employed and the patient has obstructive symptoms warrranting surgical intervention, relief by pulsion or traction intubation.
6. When a complication such as fistulation has occurred following radiotherapy, to bypass the malignant or radionecrotic tracheo-oesophageal fistula with total exclusion of the fistula-bearing segment of mid-oesophagus from the rest of the upper gastrointestinal tract.

Curative surgical resection of oesophageal carcinoma is based on the concept that if all neoplastic tissue can be removed, then resection and reconstruction should lead to a substantial 5-year survival provided the operative mortality is low and the life expectancy of the patient is not short. Provided the tumour is contained within the fascia propria of the oesophagus, and submucosal spread has not occurred far, radical removal of the oesophagus by total or subtotal oesophagectomy with radical clearance of the lymph nodes draining the organ is a justifiable procedure. Some justification can also be applied to efforts to improve the cure rate by proceeding to an extended radical procedure if the tumour has invaded the peri-oesophageal tissues and local nodes in a fit, young adult. However, the same arguments would be untenable in the elderly patient in whom a shortened chance of survival should be preferred to the high morbidity and mortality that would ensue with an extended radical procedure.

Preoperative Preparation of the Patient

This is aimed at correction of any anaemia, attention to septic teeth, improvement of the cardiac and respiratory status, and correction of nutritional deficiencies. Although some nutrition can be maintained by the oral route, most patients require correction of hypo-albuminaemia, dehydration and electrolyte disturbances. The need for parenteral hyperalimentation over a short term has to be carefully weighed against the insertion of a thin nasogastric feeding tube past the neoplasm. There is increasing evidence to suggest that whichever route is employed, the impact on the serological and corpuscular components of blood may not be significantly different (Brister et al., 1984). In those patients who have failed to show satisfactory improvement it may be necessary to construct a feeding jejunostomy either before or at the time of surgery in order to continue hyperalimentation via the enteral route (*Fig.* 8.4).

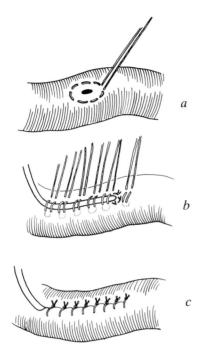

Fig. 8.4. Technique of construction of feeding jejunostomy for hyperalimentation pre- and postoperatively. *a*, Purse-string suture jejunostomy. *b*, Tunnelling of the small-bore tube. *c*, Final appearance.

Choice of Surgical Procedure

In oesophageal carcinoma this is dependent on the tumour location, the extent of spread and the objectives of the surgical intervention.

CARCINOMA OF THE HYPOPHARYNX AND CERVICAL OESOPHAGUS—LARYNGOPHARYNGO-OESOPHAGECTOMY

Resection here is achieved by removal of the larynx, lower pharynx, cervical trachea, one or both lobes of the thyroid gland and oesophagus. If the tumour is located in the hypopharynx only (postcricoid) the thoracic oesophagus can be conserved and a free graft of jejunum can be transferred by microvascular anastomosis of the jejunal vessels to the superior thyroid artery and internal jugular vein (*Fig.* 8.5). If tumour has extended on to the lower part of the cervical oesophagus, a total laryngopharyngo-oesophagectomy and gastric pull-up with immediate pharyngogastric reconstruction is the treatment of choice (*Fig.* 8.6).

If the stomach has been rendered unsuitable by previous surgery then a long segment of right or left

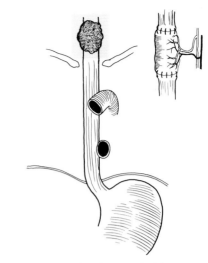

Fig. 8.5. Area of resection in postcricoid tumour prior to free jejunal autograft.

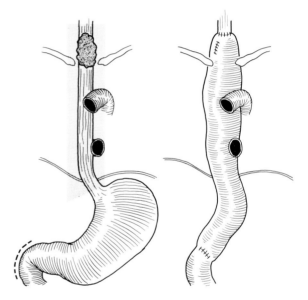

Fig. 8.6. Extent of resection when postcricoid tumour extends lower, needing total oesophagectomy with gastric pull-up.

hemicolon is brought up through the posterior mediastinum or retrosternally, to be anastomosed to the pharynx. As an alternative to the gastric pull-up the reversed (*Fig.* 8.7) *gastric tube* can be used, but except in the hands of a few it is often complicated by problems associated with suture line dehiscence. The operation of laryngopharyngo-oesophagectomy can be undertaken by two teams operating simultaneously, or by one surgical team performing the removal of the cervical tumour while the other mobilizes the stomach, colon or jejunum as the case may be. Microvascular techniques for free pedicle graft, being a well-established specialty procedure, would demand the services of a team constantly involved in small vessel surgery.

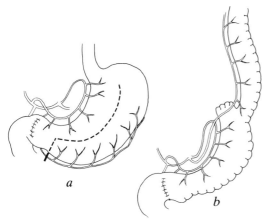

Fig. 8.7 *a*, Mobilization of the stomach retaining the blood supply derived from the left and right gastric arteries, and the anastomosis between the short gastric and gastro-epiploic arteries. Line of resection shown by interrupted line. *b*, Tube of greater curve after the Heimlich–Gavrileau fashion.

CARCINOMA OF THE THORACIC OESOPHAGUS

This is resected by total or subtotal oesophagectomy with cervical oesophago-gastric anastomosis via a laparotomy, right thoracotomy and cervical incision in one operation (McKeown, 1972), often erroneously described as a three-stage procedure. The procedure can be performed by the same operating team starting with a laparotomy, and having mobilized the stomach, closing the abdomen, turning the patient on the left side and performing a right posterolateral thoracotomy to free the tumour and resecting the tumour-bearing segment of oesophagus, before anchoring the oesophageal remnant to the pulled-up stomach and closing the chest with drainage. The patient is then turned on his or her back once again for dissection of the cervical oesophagus and completion of a total oesophagectomy and anastomosis to the stomach pulled up into the neck. The entire procedure can also be performed with the patient on his or her back right through the operation via a laparotomy, right anterolateral thoracotomy and a cervical exposure in which case either one or two teams could be operating at any one moment with considerable reduction in the time required (Royston and Dowling, 1976) (*Fig.* 8.8).

If the tumour is located in an area where clearance of tumour can be achieved with a 10-cm margin above the upper limit of tumour and the oesophagus tran-

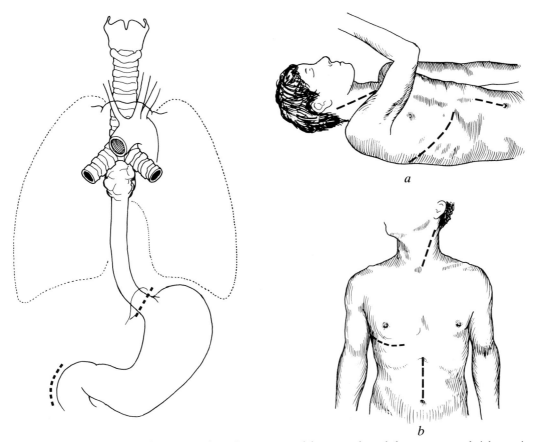

Fig. 8.8. Total oesophagectomy via a triple approach. *a*, Laparotomy, right postero lateral thoracotomy and right cervical approach requiring two turnings of the patient for the three incisions. *b*, Laparotomy, right anterolateral thoracotomy and left cervical exposure for synchronous surgery by two teams with the patient in the same supine position.

sected in the chest, then a subtotal oesophagectomy and intrathoracic oesophago-gastric anastomosis is performed high up in the apex of the chest (Franklin, 1942; Lewis, 1946). The operation is commenced with the patient on his or her back via a laparotomy for mobilization of the stomach, followed by closure of the abdomen and the patient being positioned in the left lateral decubitus for the right posterolateral thoracotomy.

CARCINOMA OF THE LOWER OESOPHAGUS

This is resected via a left thoracotomy, mobilization of the stomach through the diaphragm, mobilization of the tumour-bearing oesophagus both below and above the aortic arch with transection of the oesophagus in the apex of the chest for an intrathoracic oesophago-gastric anastomosis in a supra-aortic level, the stomach remnant being positioned either in the posterior mediastinum, medial to the aortic arch, or in the pleural cavity lateral to the aortic arch (*Fig.* 8.9).

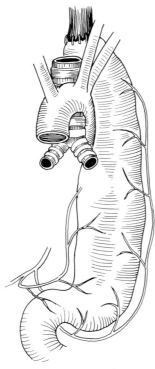

Fig. 8.9. A supra-aortic oesophago-gastric anastomosis after resection of a lower oesophageal carcinoma via a left thoracotomy.

PALLIATIVE RESECTION

Where carcinoma of the lower oesophagus is being resected purely as a palliative excision without any attempt at clearance of lymph nodal territory, a right thoracotomy and oesophagectomy can be performed without opening the abdomen, but by mobilizing the stomach through the oesophageal hiatus (Belsey and Hiebert, 1974).

In recent years, the procedure first described by Grey Turner (1936) for mobilization of the oesophageal carcinoma (and subsequently employed by Ong and Lee (1960) and Le Quesne and Ranger (1966) for freeing the normal oesophagus for a gastric pull-up without opening the chest) has been rejuvenated by Orringer (Orringer and Sloan, 1978; Orringer and Orringer, 1983; Kron et al., 1984; Orringer, 1984; Finley et al., 1985) in an almost single-handed fashion with the transhiatal eosophagectomy without thoracotomy. While enabling removal of the tumour, the procedure contravenes almost all the principles of radical surgery for malignancy, especially if spread has occurred beyond the submucosal and muscle layers of the oesophagus. Furthermore, it contributes little to the knowledge of proper pathological staging of the tumour at the time of surgery. Despite these drawbacks one has to concede that the procedure will have a place in the techniques available for removal of an oesophageal tumour if the operator is reluctant to enter the chest cavity, as was the case in Grey Turner's time. It may also gain application in the future as an appropriate procedure in the resection of carcinoma *in situ* (TIS) of the oesophagus.

Irresectable tumour of the oesophagus ascertained at the time of exploration can be appropriately bypassed depending on the stage at which irresectability is determined. The oesophagus is transected well clear of the tumour. The lower oesophageal remnant may be stapled and closed. The fundus of the stomach is then pulled up to reach the upper cut end of the oesophagus to which it is anastomosed in an end-to-side manner (*Fig.* 8.10).

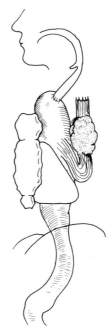

Fig. 8.10. Palliative end-to-side oesophago-gastric bypass of mid-oesophageal tumour found irresectable after mobilization of the stomach and exploration of the chest.

A malignant or radionecrotic tracheo-oesophageal fistula is a life-threatening complication, and even if the patient has only a short time left, the choking associated with saliva and food entering the tracheobronchial tree can be alleviated by a retrosternal bypass of the oesophagus with the stomach anastomosed to the transected cervical oesophagus, having excluded the thoracic part of the oesophagus from the rest of the alimentary tract (Orringer and Sloan, 1975). Surgery of this nature should be preceded by a thorough preparation of the chest with physiotherapy, etc. to overcome the effects of spillage into the tracheobronchial tree (*Fig.* 8.11).

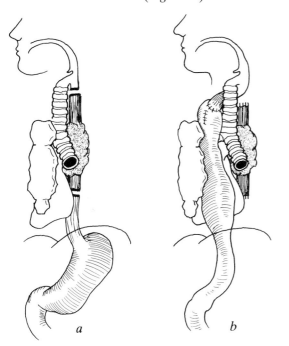

Fig. 8.11. Retrosternal bypass of irresectable oesophageal tumour with oesophago-tracheal fistula—by total disconnection and oesophago-gastric anastomosis in the neck.

Palliation of inoperable patients with oesophageal tumour by intubation (Souttar, 1924; Mousseau et al., 1956; Celestin, 1959) is effective if the tumour is located low in the chest. The higher the location of the tumour, the less satisfactory is the outcome of intubation, because of the proximity of the funnel of the tube to the glottic inlet. Operative intubation is performed by a laparotomy and gastrotomy with the traction technique described by Mousseau and Barbin for tumour of the cardia (Mousseau et al., 1956) and subsequently improved by Celestin (1959) for oesophageal and cardiac tumours (*Fig.* 8.12).

Pulsion Intubation: This was originally described by Souttar for mid-oesophageal tumour where the tube was introduced via the rigid oesophagoscope. Current techniques of pulsion intubation enable the placement of the funnelled tube over an introducer or mandril after passing a guide wire through the tumour and dilating it with bougies of the Eder–Puestow or the Celestin variety. Endoscopic intubation of oesophageal carcinoma has enabled patients who would otherwise have been unsuitable for general anaesthesia, to receive palliation (*Fig.* 8.13). Intermittent dilatation of neoplastic stricture of the oesophagus has been known to produce palliation of dysphagia for variable intervals of time, and can be resorted to if intubation is not tolerated or has been complicated by problems with the need for removal of the tube.

Endoscopic Photofulguration (laser fulguration): This is gaining popularity as a preferred form of enlarging the lumen of the oesophagus to palliate symptoms where the tumour is irresectable (McCaughan et al., 1984). Until sufficient experience is accumulated in the use of this modality of treatment, its place in the palliation of irresectable tumour will remain uncertain (*Fig.* 8.14).

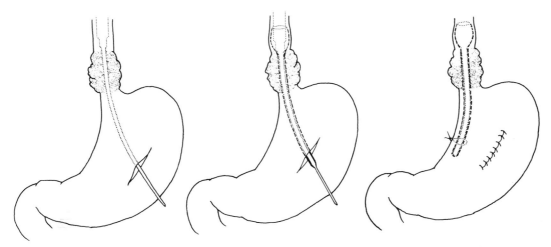

Fig. 8.12. Operative insertion of a Celestin tube by the traction method—for an irresectable carcinoma of the cardia or of the lower oesophagus with obstructive symptoms.

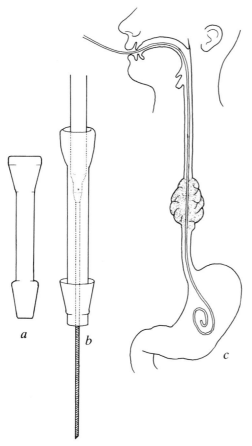

Fig. 8.13. Two types of prosthetic tubes suitable for pulsion insertion endoscopically over a guide wire. *a*, Atkinson tube. *b*, Celestin tube. *c*, Diagram showing a guide wire passing through an endoscopically dilated tumour.

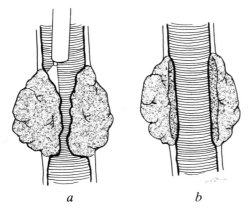

Fig. 8.14. Endoscopic photofulguration of oesophageal tumour that is not resectable. *a*, Before. *b*, After. Note that the lumen is re-established but most of the tumour is still there.

TREATMENT OF GASTRIC CARCINOMA

With the declining incidence and increasing pick-up of early gastric cancer, surgery offers the best chance of long-term survival in this disease. Overall resectability rates of nearly 80 per cent can be achieved with surgical exploration (Yan and Brooks, 1985), with an overall operative mortality of less than 5 per cent. With curative radical resection in stage I disease, 5-year survivals of 80 per cent have been achieved. If irresectability has been established after exploration, traction intubation or bypass surgery can be resorted to as a palliation of symptoms if dysphagia is a major one, as happens with tumour of the cardia. Radiotherapy and chemotherapy may still have a role to play in the palliation of symptoms of the primary disease or of metastases (Gunderson, 1976; Moertel, 1978; Yan and Brooks, 1985).

Principles in the Choice of the Surgical Procedure
(Jeyasingham et al., 1967; Jeyasingham, 1978)

As with carcinoma of the oesophagus, the choice of the procedure depends on the location and extent of tumour and the objectives of the surgical intervention.

Curative Radical Resection

This is aimed at total removal of all demonstrable tumour with the lymphatic field of drainage from the tumour, with an adequate margin of normal tissue. With carcinoma of the cardia, this would necessarily involve removal of the lower oesophagus, almost the entire lesser curve, a considerable proportion of the greater curve and omentum, spleen, tail of pancreas, with the lymph nodes in the subcarinal, para-oesophageal, diaphragmatic, left gastric and coeliac areas and in the splenic hilum (*Fig.* 8.15). A margin

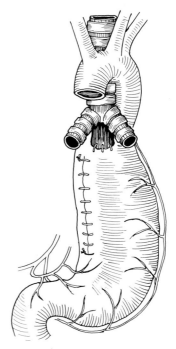

Fig. 8.15. A subaortic oesophago-gastric anastomosis for carcinoma of the cardiac end of the stomach.

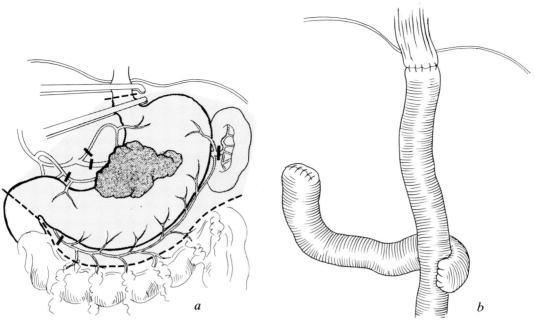

Fig. 8.16. *a*, Extent of resection in a radical total gastrectomy for carcinoma of the body of the stomach. *b*, Roux-en-Y reconstruction below the diaphragm if sufficient clearance can be obtained above the upper limit of tumour. If the tumour extends to within 10 cm of the diaphragm, a transthoracic approach with a subaortic anastomosis should be undertaken.

of diaphragm at the hiatus would have to be removed in continuity with the tumour. An extended radical procedure aimed at a curative resection of tumour of the cardia would involve a total gastrectomy in addition to the rest of the field described (Jeya-singham et al., 1967). For tumours of the body of the stomach, curative resection would involve a total gastrectomy removal of all omentum, in addition to all the areas described above (*Fig.* 8.16). A radical procedure in tumours of the pylorus should incorporate a subtotal gastrectomy with removal of all the

omentum and lymph nodes in the regional drainage of this area (*Fig.* 8.17). An extended radical procedure here would involve a total gastrectomy, splenectomy and removal of pancreas as a whole with the first part of the duodenum. However, such a procedure would carry a formidable mortality and morbidity that it would not be justified. Radical dissection is therefore limited to the spleen and body and tail of pancreas, and dissection of the pancreatico-duodenal nodes in addition to nodes in the coeliac and hepatic regions.

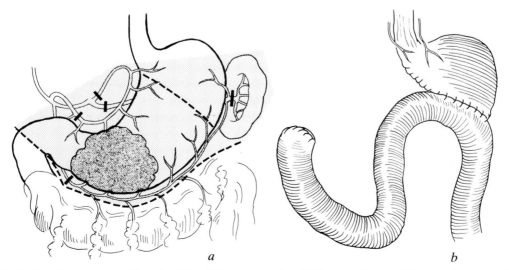

Fig. 8.17. Distal subtotal gastrectomy (*a*) and a Billroth-II reconstruction (*b*) for a carcinoma of the pyloric antrum. The stippled area indicates the extent of resection in an extended radical procedure which should include the spleen and body and tail of pancreas.

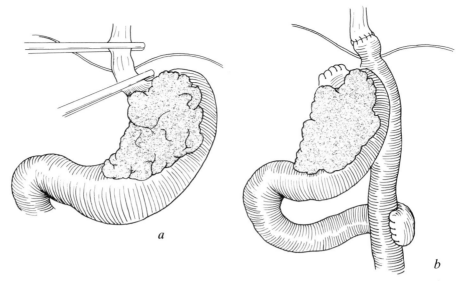

Fig. 8.18. Palliative bypass of carcinoma of the body or cardiac end of stomach by intrathoracic oesophagojejunal anastomosis and Roux-en-Y biliary diversion.

Palliative Oesophago-gastric Resection

This is aimed at removal of tumour with reconstruction of the upper alimentary tract with the knowledge that diseases has spread to adjacent organs or the third and fourth tiers of lymph nodes. In tumour of the cardia resection is achieved with subaortic oesophago-gastrostomy. With tumour of the body a total gastrectomy is justified provided the line of section does not go through macroscopic residual tumour. In tumours of the pylorus, palliative resection is achieved with a distal subtotal gastrectomy and a Billroth-II gastrojejunal anastomosis or with a defunctioning posterior gastroenterostomy. The involvement of adjacent organs such as the pancreas,

transverse colon or the left lobe of the liver should not deter from a palliative resection provided these areas can be resected without leaving obvious tumour behind.

If on exploration a tumour is deemed irresectable and if obstructive symptoms have been present, a *traction intubation* is done before closing the abdomen. If, however, dysphagia has not been a major symptom, biopsy of the tumour and sampling of the regional nodes are all that are performed at this stage. In patients who are considered unsuitable for surgical exploration, if dysphagia is a major problem endoscopic intubation or photofulguration can be performed without recourse to a general anaesthetic.

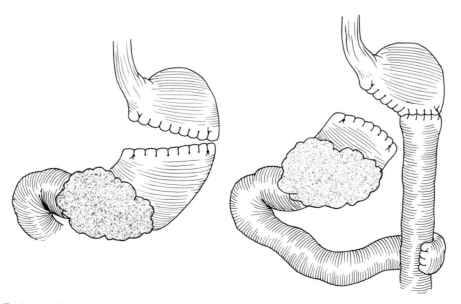

Fig. 8.19. Exclusion–diversion operation for an irresectable carcinoma of the pyloric antrum with obstructive symptoms.

Except in the tumour of the cardia, the results of such pulsion intubation are on the whole unsatisfactory.

OPERATIVE SURGICAL TECHNIQUE IN SPECIFIC PROCEDURES IN THE MANAGEMENT OF OESOPHAGEAL AND GASTRIC CARCINOMA

1. Mobilization of the Tumour-bearing Cervical Oesophagus in the Operation of Radical Pharyngolaryngo-oesophagectomy

With the patient in a supine position, anaesthetized with a standard endotracheal anaesthesia, a sandbag is placed under the chest between the scapulas, the neck being extended and the chin facing directly upwards. An incision is made obliquely on either side along the anterior border of each sternomastoid and joined in the skin crease with a curved transverse incision 2 cm above the sternal notch (*Fig.* 8.20). The incision is deepened through the platysma and flaps are elevated upwards, outwards and downwards. In order to facilitate elevation of the flaps over the posterior triangle of the neck, two short incisions are placed from the outer limits of the transverse portion extending to the anterior borders of the trapezius muscles on each side. Dissection of all the deep cervical chain of lymph nodes is completed, but both internal jugular veins are preserved, and both sternomastoid muscles are preserved (*Fig.* 8.21). The thyroid gland is mobilized with the trachea and larynx by control of the superior and inferior thyroid arteries and the thyroid veins. If the tumour is not extensive on one or the other side, the thyroid lobe of that side is preserved. If both lobes of the thyroid are removed, the parathyroids are identified and at least two of them are implanted into a muscle bed in one

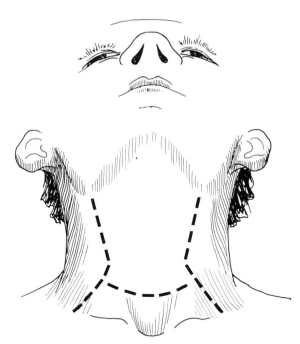

Fig. 8.20. Cervical incision in the operation of laryngopharyngo-oesophagectomy for postcricoid carcinoma.

of the sternomastoids. The trachea is now partially divided above the sternal notch and the anterior wall of the lower end attached to the skin edge here. An armoured endotracheal tube with a cuff is now passed into the lower end of the trachea in place of the previously sited endotracheal tube which is removed in readiness. Having gained control of the ventilation via the armoured tube, the posterior wall of the trachea is disconnected totally.

The hyoid bone is detached from its muscle anchorage to expose the epiglottis. The mucosa of the

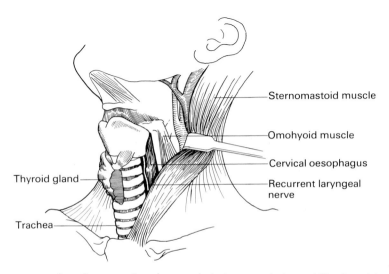

Fig. 8.21. Cervical exposure to show the more relevant anatomical structures during mobilization of the cervical oesophagus.

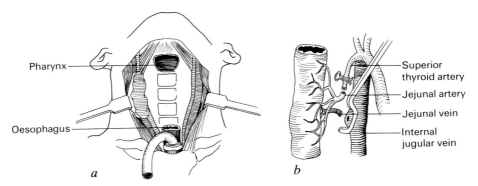

Fig. 8.22. *a*, Field of surgery after removal of postcricoid carcinoma. *b*, Free jejunal autograft ready for interposition, with vascular anastomosis to local vessels in the neck.

pharynx above the epiglottis is incised and stripped upwards and the incision is continued laterally to detach the lateral walls of the pharynx and finally the posterior wall is transected. The pharynx and larynx are then stripped off the prevertebral fascia down to the thoracic inlet with the tumour-bearing portion of cervical oesophagus. If the cervical oesophagus is being replaced by a pedicled free graft of jejunum, it is transected at the thoracic inlet level (*Fig.* 8.22). If on the other hand a gastric pull-up (*Fig.* 8.23) is planned, the entire viscus is covered in a pack and the operation field is covered with a sterile towel to await the next step in the procedure.

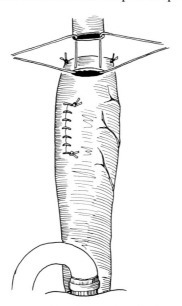

Fig. 8.23. Pharyngo-gastric reconstruction after laryngopharyngo-oesophagectomy.

2. Mobilization of the Normal Stomach via a Laparotomy for Gastric Pull-up in the Neck with Concomitant Removal of the Normal Oesophagus

This procedure is common to others such as mobilization of the stomach for transhiatal blunt oesophagec-

tomy and substernal defunctioning bypass of mid-oesophageal neoplasm with or without tracheo-oesophageal fistula. The abdomen is entered through a midline upper abdominal incision from xiphisternum to the umbilicus. If necessary the xiphoid cartilage is removed. The left triangular ligament of the liver is divided and the left lobe of the liver is gently retracted to the right. The stomach has to be mobilized with the minimum of handling of the organ, retaining the maximum amount of vascularity at the end of the procedure, and yet in such a manner as to enable the operator to position the fundus of the stomach at the level of the pharynx. The right gastric artery and the right gastro-epiploic artery are the only source of blood supply, but every attempt is made to preserve the collaterals at the termination of these vessels where they meet branches of the left gastric and left gastro-epiploic vessels. The epiploic branches of the gastro-epiploic arcade are divided commencing at a convenient point near the midline and proceeding towards the pylorus. Special care is taken here to preserve the gastro-epiploic vein which parts company from the artery to reach the groove between the neck and the uncinate process of the pancreas. The division of the omentum is then carried to the left towards the splenic hilum where special attention is paid to divide the vessels close to the spleen, thereby preserving every possible collateral channel that may carry some blood to the short gastric arteries. Ligation of the left gastric vessels is carried out close to the take-off before the bifurcation of the vessel, again preserving collateral channels (*Fig.* 8.24).

Extensive mobilization of the duodenum is achieved by Kocherization and dissection of the first and second parts from the posterior abdominal wall, freeing under these to reach the vena cava and aorta. The stomach is now freed from the subdiaphragmatic peritoneum and the oesophagus is freed from the hiatus. Dissection is carried upwards around the lower oesophagus. The hiatal margins are dilated with, if necessary, an anteriorly placed releasing incision to facilitate the next step in the procedure.

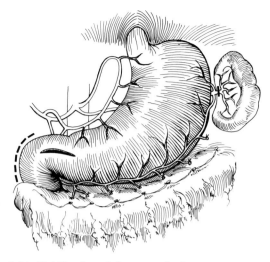

Fig. 8.24. Mobilization of the stomach via an upper abdominal incision in readiness for a gastric pull-up into the chest and as far up as the pharynx. Note the pyloroplasty incision and the Kocherization of the duodenum.

3. Dissection of the Normal Oesophagus without a Thoracotomy (*Fig* 8.25)

This technique is common to the gastric pull-up with removal of a normal oesophagus, as well as for blunt oesophagectomy without thoracotomy for palliative blind resection of neoplasia of the thoracic oesophagus. Blind finger dissection is done upwards, keeping close to the oesophagus as much as possible. Small oesophageal arterial branches are torn with the dissecting finger, but can be controlled with firm packing at a later stage. The cervical operator simultaneously dissects downwards, carefully avoiding the recurrent laryngeal nerve and avoiding damage to the back of the trachea. As the thoracic inlet is small, most of

the dissection has to be done from below and it will be necessary for the abdominal operator to pass an entire fist into the posterior mediastinum to reach the carina and back of the trachea from below. By gentle traction from above, and supportive assistance from below, the stomach is pulled up through the posterior mediastinum, bringing the duodenum and pancreas towards the midline in the epigastrium. The pylorus comes to be near the hiatus or above it. A pyloromyotomy or pyloroplasty has therefore to be completed prior to closure of the abdomen if any abnormality of this area is noted at this stage.

4. Pharyngo-gastric Anastomosis after Gastric Pull-up

The stomach is pulled up and the cardia is transected, stapled and oversewn with suture material. The highest point in the gastric fundus is now anchored to the anterior longitudinal ligament almost at the level of the atlas vertebra, and an end-to-side pharyngo-gastric anastomosis is completed. A nasogastric tube is introduced via the nose and left in the intrathoracic portion of the stomach.

The skin flaps are now approximated and the posterior wall of the trachea is finally anchored to the skin edges before closing the platysma and skin, with a Redivac drain in the neck.

5. Mobilization of the Stomach via a Midline Incision in the First Phase of a Total or Subtotal Oesophagectomy

This is carried out in exactly the same manner as in 2 above, except in so far as paying special attention to the lymph nodal clearance from the left gastric and coeliac areas.

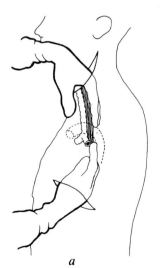
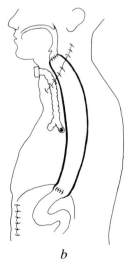

a   *b*

Fig. 8.25. Blunt oesophagectomy without thoracotomy. *a*, Diagrammatic representation of the bimanual dissection of the oesophagus from above and from below. *b*, The stomach pulled up into the neck and anastomosed to the pharynx in the operation of laryngopharyngo-oesophagectomy.

6. Right Thoracotomy and Mobilization of a Tumour-bearing Thoracic or Lower Oesophagus, as Part of a Lewis–Franklin Procedure or as Part of a Triple Procedure to Carry Out a Total Oesophagectomy

The patient is placed in a left lateral position and the chest entered through the 5th intercostal space. The lung is carefully retracted forwards. The azygos vein is dissected, ligated flush with the superior vena cava anteriorly and also posteriorly over the dorsal vertebral bodies without disturbing the intercostal veins. The intervening horizontal portion of the azygos vein is detached and left attached to the oesophagus. The pleura over the dorsal spine is incised longitudinally over the entire length of the chest cavity. Dissection is now commenced between the oesophagus and aorta posteriorly, and between the oesophagus and spine above the aortic arch. The oesophageal tumour is mobilized with a clear margin of the healthy tissue by keeping the dissection close to the aortic wall. Dissection is then continued between the oesophagus and trachea superiorly, and behind the right main bronchus and pericardium in the lower part. Once the oesophagus is encircled above the tumour, a sling is passed round it to enable easier dissection to free the tumour-bearing segment. All lymph nodes in the subcarinal and hilar areas are included with the peri-oesophageal tissues. Similarly, in the lower chest the pulmonary ligament is divided close to the lung and dissection is carried into the oesophageal hiatus (*Fig.* 8.26). Once the dissection of the entire length of the thoracic oesophagus has been completed, and then only, gentle traction is applied to deliver the stomach into the chest, ensuring that the organ does not undergo any rotation on its own axis. Dissection of the apex of the chest is now continued so as to free the cervical oesophagus from below.

7. Subtotal Oesophagectomy with a Thoracic Anastomosis

Once the mobilization of the oesophagus has been completed through the right chest, the stomach is transected obliquely at the cardia including a short length of the lesser curve, in order to remove some of the paracardiac lymph nodes with the oesophagus. The stomach remnant is stapled and oversewn. The fundus is then gently pulled up to the apex of the chest where it is anchored to the prevertebral tissues, making sure that the transection suture line is to the right and the fundus to the left. The oesophagus is transected with a clear 10-cm margin of normal oesophagus above the tumour, and an end-to-side anastomosis is completed, making an opening on the anterior surface of the stomach at a convenient point below the apex of the fundus. A nasogastric tube is then positioned into the intrathoracic stomach.

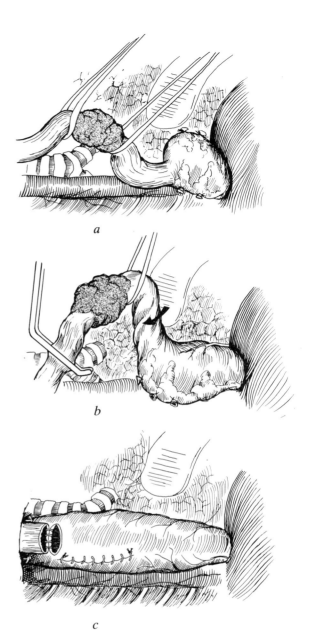

a

b

c

Fig. 8.26. Mobilization of the thoracic oesophagus via a right posterolateral thoracotomy for oesophagectomy and intrathoracic oesophago-gastric anastomosis. *a*, Step-by-step mobilization of stomach through the oesophageal hiatus without a laparotomy—as a purely palliative procedure. *b*, Delivery of a previously mobilized stomach into the chest by a pull-up technique. *c*, Stomach anchored to the apex of the mediastinum in readiness for end-to-side oesophago-gastric anastomosis.

8. 'Total' Oesophagectomy with a Cervical Anastomosis

The mobilized oesophagus and stomach are left intact and the chest closed with drainage. The patient is then turned over on to his or her back and the right side of the neck is exposed via an incision placed in the posterior triangle 2 cm above the clavicle. As an alternative procedure, the stomach can be transected in the chest as in 7 above, stapled and oversewn, and the oesophagus transected in the apex of the chest with a clear margin of normal oesophagus and anchored to the fundus at the uppermost point of its curvature with two or three anchoring sutures. This would then enable the oesophagus to be delivered into the neck at a later stage with the fundus of the stomach attached to it. The incision in the neck is retracted backwards and the middle thyroid vein may require ligation at this level. The carotid and jugular vessels are retracted laterally. The oesophagus is identified and the recurrent laryngeal nerve is carefully preserved alongside the trachea. Having dissected the oesophagus a sling is passed around it, and with gentle traction the oesophagus with the attached stomach is pulled up into the neck and if the cardia has not already been transected this is carried out now, followed by transection of the oesophagus at an appropriate length. Having performed a 'total' oesophagectomy, the remnant of the oesophagus is now anastomosed in an end-to-side fashion to the fundus of the stomach and the entire area is allowed to gently drop back into the mediastinum with a nasogastric tube in position. The incision in the neck is then closed without drainage.

9. Mobilization of Tumour-bearing Lower Oesophagus for Supra-aortic Oesophago-gastric Anastomosis for a Lower Oesophageal Tumour via a left Thoracotomy (also applicable for Cervical Anastomosis)

With the patient placed in a right lateral position an incision is made over the 7th rib on the left side and the chest entered through the bed of the resected 7th rib and a divided portion of the back end of the 6th rib. As an alternative, the chest may be entered through the 6th interspace with portions of the 6th and 7th ribs being excised posteriorly. The lung is retracted forwards after division of the pulmonary ligament close to the lung attachment, retaining all the lymph nodes in this ligament with the oesophagus. An incision is placed in the pleura overlying the descending aorta and dissection commenced above the hiatus in a subadventitial plane of the aorta, continued upwards controlling each of the oesophageal branches from the descending aorta by ligation and division. Dissection is then carried to a subaortic level where temporarily dissection is discontinued. An incision is then made anterior to the oesophagus in the sulcus between the pericardium and oesophagus, and with blunt dissection all the tissues around the oesophagus are separated from the fibrous pericardium, entering the right pleural cavity in order to retain all the peri-oesophageal tissues within the field of dissection. The downward dissection is continued to reach the diaphragm where all pericardiac fat is removed with the oesophageal segment. Dissection upwards is continued behind the pulmonary hilum

taking all the subcarinal lymph nodes and any visible hilar lymph nodes that may be situated posteriorly. The back of the bronchus and the pulmonary artery are bared. The inferior pulmonary vein covered by the pericardium is also cleaned thoroughly. At the level of the aortic arch the right and left vagi are disconnected distal to the left recurrent laryngeal nerve. In order to dissect the oesophagus above the aortic arch a second incision may have to be placed in the 4th interspace with division of the back end of the 5th rib. If dissection, however, is carried out through the previously made 6th interspace exposure, then adequate separation of the ribs can be achieved by mere division of the back end of the 5th rib and 5th and 6th intercostal bundles, and retracting the rib cage further.

Having passed a sling around the oesophagus above the tumour, an incision is made in a longitudinal manner in the pleura above the aortic arch. The superior intercostal vein is doubly ligated anteriorly and posteriorly and divided between these ligatures. The oesophagus is identified. A finger is passed from below the aortic arch to dissect around the aortic arch close to the media but taking great care not to traumatize the recurrent laryngeal nerve. The oesophagus is then cleared from under the aortic arch by careful blunt dissection, preserving the azygos vein on the right and ensuring that the back wall of the trachea is not damaged. Having carried the blunt dissection to a supra-aortic level, the supra-aortic oesophagus is encircled with a sling of rubber and dissection is then carried through under direct vision to the apex of the chest. Special care is exercised not to damage the thoracic duct. If a supra-aortic intrathoracic anastomosis is contemplated the dissection comes to a close at this stage. Mobilization of stomach through an incision in the diaphragm is then commenced as for tumour of the cardia.

10. Mobilization of the Oesophagus and Stomach for Carcinoma of the Cardia in the Operation of Oesophago-gastrectomy for Carcinoma with a Subaortic Anastomosis (*Fig.* 8.27)

Having mobilized the oesophagus as for a lower oesophageal carcinoma, ensuring that dissection around the oesophagus is carried out in a subadventitial plane of the aorta, the hiatus is defined. The diaphragm is then incised in a radiate fashion, taking the incision in the diaphragm to the hiatus where a cuff of diaphragmatic muscle is excised with the oesophagogastric junction, controlling phrenic branches of the aorta on either side and inserting two stay sutures at the anterior ends of the divided hiatus for later reconstruction. If, however, a peripheral detachment is carried through which gives adequate exposure for mobilization of the entire stomach right out to the duodenum, an incision is made from under the sternum, carried through to a point on the diaphragm under the costal margin close to the apex of the

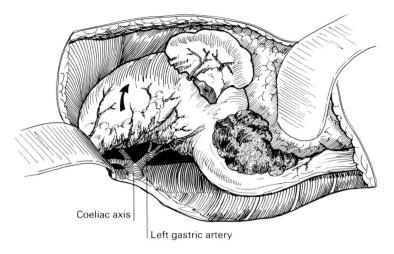

Coeliac axis

Left gastric artery

Fig. 8.27. Mobilization of the oesophagus and stomach for a carcinoma of the cardia via a left thoracotomy in preparation for a subaortic anastomosis. The stomach and spleen with the tail of the pancreas have been rotated forwards to expose the coeliac axis and its main branches.

spleen. Mobilization is then commenced at the splenic flexure of the colon taking the gastrocolic omentum along its avascular attachment to the colon all the way along the transverse colon, detaching the lienorenal ligament, freeing the posterior aspect of the splenic hilum, controlling the splenic vessels and taking with the spleen the tail of the pancreas by cross-clamping the pancreas and dividing between the clamps, suturing the pancreas with interrupted non-absorbable sutures, reflecting the spleen forwards to carry the dissection upwards, controlling the short gastric vessels and reaching the diaphragmatic hiatus to expose the descending aorta at the point where it passes through the median arcuate ligament. At this stage the gastrohepatic omentum is detached close to the liver, controlling the communicating branch between the left hepatic artery and the left gastric artery. Having rotated the stomach and oesophagus forwards the pancreas is retracted downwards and the left gastric artery and coeliac axis are exposed, dissecting away all the lymph nodes in this area towards the stomach and controlling the left gastric artery after identifying the hepatic branch of the coeliac axis, so that this vessel is not damaged. The dissection in the gastrocolic omentum is now carried through towards the gastro-epiploic arcade to reach it at a convenient point chosen well clear of the tumour in the stomach, allowing approximately 10 cm of clear stomach. The stomach is then transected taking almost the entire lesser curve after dissociating the right gastric anastomosis with the branches of the left gastric artery on the lesser curve and dividing the gastro-epiploic arcade at a chosen point. The transected stomach is stapled and oversewn, and attention is now directed towards the oesophagus which has been mobilized up to the subaortic level

behind the pulmonary hilum in a manner similar to that in 8 above.

A non-crushing clamp is applied at a point chosen with a clear margin of at least 10 cm of oesophagus above the tumour and the oesophagus is then transected below this clamp. The stomach is pulled up through the hiatus or the divided hiatus to be brought up into the chest ensuring that there is no rotation of the organ in its long axis. The pylorus is inspected at this stage and if there is any abnormality a pyloroplasty or pyloromyotomy is carried out. The oesophagus is then anatomosed in an end-to-side fashion to the gastric remnant and a Ryle's tube is positioned in the intrathoracic part of the stomach. The diaphragm is repaired (in a manner similar to that described in Chapter 22), reconstructing the hiatus around the gastric remnant. No attempt is made to anchor the stomach remnant to the margins of the hiatus but the stomach is anchored to the parietal pleura with a few interrupted sutures along its length in the chest. The left chest can then be closed with drainage and as the right pleura has been opened, that too is drained with a separate tube inserted between the stomach remnant and the back of the pericardium.

11. Mobilization of the Oesophagus and Stomach via the Right Chest and Oesophageal Hiatus for Palliative Resection of Tumour in the Thoracic or Lower Oesophagus

The procedure for entering the chest and mobilizing the oesophagus is exactly as was described for the Lewis–Franklin operation, but having divided the pulmonary ligament the dissection is carried down to reach the oesophageal hiatus where the margins of the hiatus are defined first, and entry into the peritoneal cavity is established initially in an anteromedial position avoiding damage to the ascending branch of the left gastric artery. The index finger is then passed into the peritoneal cavity and the left gastric artery is hooked up with the finger to be delivered into the hiatus where it is controlled with a clamp, divided between clamps, and ligated. Upward pull on the oesophagus and stomach with the sling now delivers branches of the short gastric vessels which are dealt with in a similar fashion. Sequential division of the remaining short gastric branches delivers more and more of the greater curvature to bring the gastro-epiploic arcade into view. From thence onwards the epiploic branches of the gastro-epiploic arcade are systematically divided until almost the entire length of the stomach is delivered into the chest. Delivery of the stomach into the chest is facilitated by dilatation of the hiatus using the index finger of each hand to stretch the muscular fibres. The gastrohepatic omentum is also divided during the course of the delivery of the stomach. The pylorus comes to lie almost at the level of the hiatus or just below it but the exposure would be totally inadequate to carry out a pyloroplasty if it was required. However, it is possible by digital invagination of the stomach to achieve sufficient dilatation of the pyloric sphincter, provided there is no fibrous scarring in the area.

It is worth noting that this procedure does not enable a thorough dissection of the lymph nodes along the lesser curve of the stomach, nor the collection of nodes around the coeliac and left gastric artery that are frequently involved by tumour in the lower or thoracic oesophagus. It is a purely palliative procedure. Having delivered a sufficient length of stomach a tube of greater curve with the vascular arcade of the gastro-epiploic vessels is fashioned sufficient to enable an end-to-side oesophago-gastric anastomosis after resection of the oesophagus with a clear 10-cm margin above the tumour. With this technique no difficulty is encountered in bringing the fundus of the stomach or end of the gastric tube to a level high enough for apical intrathoracic anastomosis or a cervical anastomosis if that was required.

12. Mobilization of the Tumour-bearing Stomach in Proximal Subtotal Gastrectomy with Oesophago-gastric Anastomosis via a Left Thoracolaparotomy

This procedure is carried out through a left-sided thoracolapartotomy incision of which the anterior end is completed first with an opportunity to explore the abdomen before completing the rest of the incision. An initial exploratory laparotomy would reveal if a radical procedure was feasible or whether some form of palliative procedure would be justified. The incision is placed over the level of the 8th rib and carried across the costal margin towards the umbilicus. The abdominal part of this incision is deepened

through to the peritoneum and exploration of the upper abdomen is undertaken through this part of the incision. Having ascertained resectability, the incision is carried through into the chest where the chest cavity is entered through the bed of the resected 8th rib and continuity of the operative field is achieved by detaching the periphery of the diaphragm from its costal attachment.

Mobilization of the stomach is commenced by detaching the colonic attachment of the gastrocolic omentum along its avascular plane all the way from the splenic flexure to the hepatic flexure. The entire omentum is detached and retracted upwards with the stomach, dissection then being continued upwards towards the splenic hilum where the splenic vessels are dissected and divided between ligatures, the tail of the pancreas clamped and divided between clamps to be included in the field of dissection, the pancreas being controlled with interrupted non-absorbable sutures. Having detached the spleen, tail of pancreas and stomach from the posterior abdominal wall, the cardia is mobilized with a cuff of diaphragm around the oesophago-gastric junction, the gastrohepatic omentum is detached controlling the gastric branch of the left hepatic artery which communicates with the left gastric artery. The entire stomach and spleen are rotated forwards and upwards to expose the coeliac axis and left gastric artery after retraction of the pancreas downwards. A thorough dissection of the lymphatic drainage reaching the coeliac lymph nodes is carried out to remove all visible tissue of a lymphatic nature. The dissection is further carried towards the pylorus where the pancreatico-duodenal lymph nodes are removed for histological examination. A tube of greater curve is now constructed, retaining the gastro-epiploic arcade but removing the weight of the omentum by ligation and division of the epiploic branches of the arcade over the extent of the omental detachment followed by transection of the stomach with a full 10-cm clearance of normal healthy stomach from the lower edge of the tumour taking the entire lesser curve and reconstructing the tube in two layers either by sutures or by stapling, and oversewing the stapled line. The entire mass of viscus detached is now wrapped in a gauze pack and swung upwards, without axial rotation, oesophageal dissection having been performed earlier as in mobilization of the lower oesophagus. A clamp is applied approximately 10 cm away from the upper margin of the tumour of the stomach. The oesophagus is then transected and an end-to-side oesophago-gastric anastomosis is completed after pulling the tube of stomach up into the chest through the hiatus. This having been achieved a Ryle's tube is now positioned in the stomach remnant, the diaphragm is reattached to the costal margin ensuring total isolation of the abdominal from the pleural cavity. The entire incision is then closed with drainage of the chest cavity ensuring layer by layer closure of each of the two portions.

13. Distal Subtotal Gastrectomy with Billroth-II Gastrojejunal Anastomosis for Tumour of the Pylorus

A midline upper abdominal incision is made with the patient lying supine. The incision may have to be extended below the level of the umbilicus on one or other side of this structure. Initial exploratory laparotomy is performed to ensure resectability and extent of resection required for control of tumour. A subtotal gastrectomy for tumour of the pylorus would not include resection of the spleen and tail of pancreas. However, if an extended radical subtotal gastrectomy is anticipated then mobilization of the spleen and tail of pancreas is required for adequate clearance of lymph nodes in that area. The left lobe of the liver is retracted after division of its triangular ligament. Mobilization of the entire gastrocolic omentum is achieved by detachment of the omentum from the transverse colon, the mobilization being continued towards the greater curve of the stomach, detaching the anastomosis between the left and right gastro-epiploic arcades at a point estimated to be well clear of the tumour. The gastrohepatic omentum is detached close to the liver to expose the coeliac axis with its main branches. A thorough clearance of the lymph nodes in this area is achieved before identifying the three individual branches and ligating the left gastric artery close to its origin. The dissection is now concentrated on the first part of the duodenum to free the posterior aspect of the duodenum to gain an adequate margin of the first part of the duodenum away from the outermost border of the tumour. The gastro-epiploic arcade is then divided close to its origin from the gastroduodenal artery. The duodenum is transected well clear of the tumour and closed either by stapling or by suture in two layers. The stomach is then transected obliquely extending the line of resection upwards towards the lesser curve so as to take almost all the left gastric lymph nodal distribution. The transection line is partially closed towards the lesser curve end and a Billroth-II type gastrojejunal anastomosis is completed in a retrocolic fashion. As an alternative a Roux-en-Y anastomosis is achieved with the vertical limb looped on itself to enable an end-to-side gastrojejunal anastomosis and add to the reservoir of the stomach remnant.

An extended radical subtotal gastrectomy would include the splenic hilum, tail of pancreas and the involved lymph nodes in that area as part of the region of resected tissues.

14. Total Gastrectomy and Roux-en-Y Anastomosis for a Tumour of the Body of the Stomach

The procedure as for distal subtotal gastrectomy is carried out with disarticulation of the xiphoid cartilage of the sternum for adequate exposure. The left triangular ligament of the liver is divided and retracted as before. Dissection is carried out to free the oesophagus in its intra-abdominal course, carrying the dissection around the oesophagus and into the gastrohepatic omentum. Dissection is then commenced again at the attachment of the gastrocolic omentum to the transverse colon from which it is totally detached, dissection being continued across its attachment and splenic flexure into the posterior abdomen where the lienorenal ligament is divided and the spleen and tail of pancreas are dissected away from their bed. Control of the pancreas by double clamping and division is achieved to remove the tail and body of the pancreas with the spleen and splenic vessels. The stomach is retracted away from the liver upwards and to the left to expose the coeliac axis and left gastric artery which are dealt with in a similar fashion to the previous operation. The gastrocolic vessels are divided at their point of origin from the gastroduodenal, and the right gastric artery controlled close to the first part of the duodenum. Having done this, sufficient mobilization of the first part of the duodenum is achieved to enable transection of this structure with an adequate margin of normal tissue, the duodenum then being stapled and oversewn or sutured in two layers. The stomach is retracted downwards, dissection continued up to the hiatus to free a length of intrathoracic oesophagus which is delivered into the abdomen. Transection of the oesophagus is achieved with a clamp controlling the oesophagus and the entire mass of viscera is removed. The jejunum is now mobilized to create a Roux-en-Y anastomosis or a looped Roux-en-Y anastomosis as in the previous section. Closure of the abdomen in both procedures is achieved with drainage of the duodenal stump area.

15. Techniques of Oesophago-Gastric Anastomosis

The ideal anastomosis is end to side with a clear-cut end of the oesophagus joined to a definitive opening made on the stomach remnant, well clear of any suture lines. The strength of such anastomosis depends on the one hand on the oesophageal mucosa and submucosa, and on the other hand on the gastric seromuscular coat. The gastric mucosa is fragile and tends to bleed on handling, while the oesophageal muscle coats tend to tear if grasped with a pair of forceps. Handling of these structures has therefore to be done with extreme care so as not to cause any damage. The success of any oesophago-gastric resection is dependent on the integrity of the anastomotic sites involved in the reconstruction. Breakdown of anastomosis may occur early due to technical faults, and late as a result of poor tissues, inadequate vascularity and inadequate healing.

A single layer of interrupted sutures inserted meticulously at 3-mm intervals with the material passing through all coats of each viscus and the knots tied on the lumen, is the technique preferred by the author (*Fig.* 8.28). Stainless steel wire of no. 38 gauge

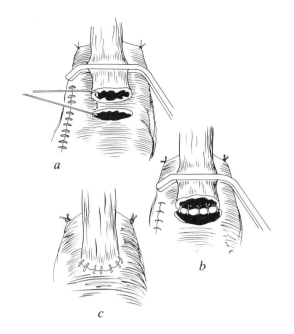

Fig. 8.28. Author's own preferred anastomotic technique: end to side, interrupted, all coats sutures using no. 38 stainless steel gauge wire mounted on an atraumatic needle.

mounted on an atraumatic needle is the author's choice for the suture material. The posterior layer is completed first, the two corners are rounded in turn and then the anterior layer is completed. The last stitch on the anterior layer is tied with a knot to the exterior. A three-layered ink-welling technique (*Fig.* 8.29) can be used with interrupted non-absorbable sutures such as polyester or Prolene, while the original technique described by Sweet (1945, 1950) is still the most popular. Anastomotic

stapling guns can also be used to achieve a two-layered stapled anastomosis. In the hands of the occasional oesophageal surgeon, this instrument has contributed to a safer operation, at some compromise to the gentle handling of tissues (*Fig.* 8.30).

16. Pyloroplasty

As to whether a pyloroplasty should be routinely performed after transection of the oesophagus is a question that has vexed more than one generation of surgeons. If the pylorus appears scarred from previous disease, a pyloroplasty is performed routinely. If the pylorus is healthy, the golden rule that the author has adopted is as follows: if the greater part of the stomach is preserved in the reconstruction then pyloroplasty is done routinely, especially if the pylorus comes to lie at the hiatus level or above it. This avoids an embarrassing manoeuvre if the pyloroplasty was not performed initially and came to be necessary in the long-term post-resection follow-up. If, however, a greater part of the stomach is removed and only a tube of stomach is retained, then a pyloroplasty is not performed as hypotonicity and delayed emptying of the gastric remnant are rarely noticed. In these patients the pylorus is usually situated well below the hiatus at the end of the operation, and is easily exposed if a pyloromyotomy should be required at a later date.

ROUTINE POSTOPERATIVE MANAGEMENT

1. Nasogastric decompression is continued for 48 hours and if the gastric aspirate or jejunal aspirate shows signs of receding, the tube is removed after that interval of time.

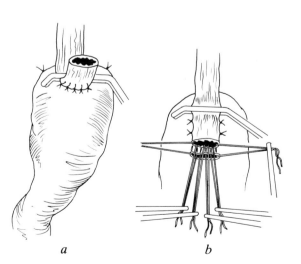

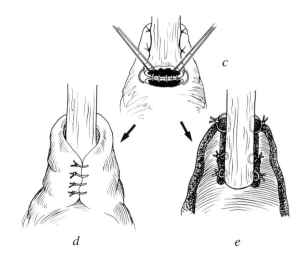

Fig. 8.29. Anti-reflux techniques in oesophago-gastric anastomosis, *a–c*, Stages in an end-to-side anastomosis with a 5 cm length of oesophagus anchored to the anterior surface of the stomach at three levels. *d*, Total 'fundoplication' wrap of stomach remnant around the oesophagus in the Nissen fashion. *e*, 'Ink-welling' of the oesophagus into the stomach in the Ottosen–Søndergaard fashion.

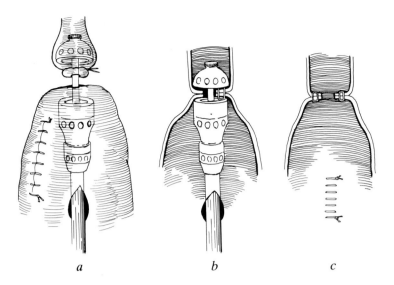

Fig. 8.30. Diagrammatic representation of an oesophago-gastric anastomosis achieved with a stapling device.

2. 'Nil by mouth' is the rule for 24 hours after surgery and then 30 ml of water are allowed every hour for the next 24 hours. On the 3rd postoperative day 60 ml are allowed every hour, increasing by 30 ml each day until free fluids are established after 5 days from surgery.

3. Parenteral nutrition is maintained with only crystalloids being allowed in the first 24 hours after surgery. A central venous line is maintained for the purposes of parenteral nutrition and once the post-operative circulatory state has been stabilized for 24 hours, total parenteral nutrition is established until such time as the patient is taking free fluids orally. Prolonged total parenteral nutrition has not been found necessary unless a complication has super-vened.

4. By the end of the 1st week the patient is permit-ted sloppy food by mouth and by the 8th day boiled fish and minced meat are permitted.

5. The intercostal tubes are removed once oral fluids have been commenced and drainage has ceased, and lungs fully expanded. In the event of the slightest suspicion of a 'leak', at least one inter-costal tube is retained until the false alarm has passed on.

6. Systemic antibiotics are commenced on the morning of the operation and continued for 5 days, as a prophylactic measure.

7. Subcutaneous low-dose heparin is administered routinely for 5 days or until the patient is fully mobile.

8. Chest physiotherapy is commenced in the re-covery room, and continued 4-hourly for the first 3 days, and then twice daily throughout the patient's hospital stay.

9. The chest is monitored daily with erect radio-graphs to ensure full expansion of the lungs and no accumulation of any fluid within the pleural cavities.

10. The need for routine intermittent positive pressure ventilation varies according to the practice of the individual department but is not employed by the author.

11. A pre-discharge barium meal screening is per-formed on the 10th to the 12th day after surgery.

12. From the time the patient is extubated, he or she is nursed on an inclined bed of approximately 15° with wooden blocks under the head end of the bed, to prevent inhalation of refluxed gastric or intes-tinal contents. Prior to discharge the patient is instructed that this should be followed for life, if the oesophago-gastric junction has been resected in the course of the surgery.

13. Instructions are given on the need to restrict the quantity of each meal, the need to avoid un-necessary stooping, bending or heavy lifting, and the need to stay upright for at least 3–4 hours after meals, before retiring to bed. Patients are advised against 'nightcaps'.

COMPLICATIONS FOLLOWING OESOPHAGO-GASTRIC RESECTION

1. *Dehiscence of the anastomosis or of a gastric suture line* is the most significant complication. The earliest sign may be a sharp pain in the side of the chest or epigastrium. A minor elevation of the body temperature and pulse soon occurs, and if the inter-costal tubes have already been removed, there is peripheral circulatory shut-down associated with an intrathoracic accumulation of fluid and air. De-hiscence occurring during the first 24–72 hours should be confirmed by contrast radiography and rectified surgically by return to the operating theatre and

closure of the dehiscence. Delayed dehiscence is treated conservatively with nil orally, pleural or peritoneal drainage, intravenous antibiotics, and parenteral nutrition, and jejunostomy should be considered.

2. *Respiratory complications* are common in view of the age groups involved, and may be prevented by meticulous nursing and preventative physiotherapy. When they supervene, treatment is carried out actively to counteract any sputum retention, inhalation and bronchopneumonia or atelectasis.

3. *Haemorrhage* occurring in the immediate postoperative period is usually associated with extensive dissection or with a slipped ligature, commonly of the left gastric or splenic artery. Immediate return to the operating theatre and arrest of haemorrhage are performed.

4. *Phlebothrombosis and pulmonary embolism* are not uncommon in the elderly age groups, and with the prolonged state of underhydration and disturbance of coagulability in malignant disease. Active anticoagulation is instituted with heparin in the first instance and warfarin after the 1st week.

5. *Myocardial infarction* and congestive cardiac failure are common causes of postoperative mortality and morbidity.

6. *Delayed problems associated with oesophagogastric resection* are those of deficiency states such as anaemia, problems of acid and biliary reflux, gastrointestinal hurry and 'dumping'. In resection of the cervical oesophagus, specific problems associated with removal of the thyroids or parathyroids may complicate the picture.

7. *Herniation of abdominal contents* through the repaired hiatus or diaphragm is an uncommon but not rare complication which may occur in the early or long-term follow-up of such patients, and will require surgical intervention.

REFERENCES

Belsey R. and Hiebert C. A. (1974) An exclusive right thoracic approach for carcinoma of the middle third of the oesophagus. *Ann. Thorac. Surg.* **18**, 1–15.

Brister S. J., Chiu R. L. J., Brom R. A. et al. (1984) Clinical impact of intravenous hyper-alimentation on esophageal carcinoma: is it worthwhile? *Ann. Thorac. Surg.* **38**, 617–621.

Burgess H. M., Baggenstoss A. H., Moersch H. J. et al. (1951) Carcinoma of the esophagus: clincopathologic study. *Surg. Clin. North Am.* **31**, 965.

Celestin L. R. (1959) Permanent intubation in inoperable cancer of the oesophagus and cardia—a new tube. *Ann. R. Coll. Surg. Eng.* **25**, 165–170.

Finley R. J., Grace M. and Duff J. H. (1985) Esophagectomy without thoracotomy for carcinoma of the cardia and lower part of the oesophagus. *Surg. Gynecol. Obstet.* **160**, 49–56.

Franklin R. H. (1942) Two cases of successful removal of the thoracic oesophagus for carcinoma. *Br. J. Surg.* **30**, 141–146.

Gisselbrecht C., Calvo F., Mignot C. et al. (1983) Flurouracil (F) Adriamycin (A) and Cisplatin (P) FAP. Combination chemotherapy of advanced esophageal carcinoma. *Cancer* **52**, 974–977.

Groves L. K. and Rodriguez-Antunez A. (1973) Treatment of carcinoma of the esophagus and gastric cardia with concentrated pre-operative irradiation followed by early operation. *Ann. Thorac. Surg.* **15**, 333–338.

Guernsey J. M., Doggett R. L., Mason G. R. et al. (1969) Combined treatment of cancer of the esophagus. *Am. J. Surg.* **117**, 157–161.

Gunderson L. L. (1976) Radiation therapy; results and future. In: *Clincs in Gastroenterology*, Vol. 5. London, W. B. Saunders, pp. 743–776.

Gunnlaugsson G. H., Wychulis A. R., Roland C. et al. (1970) Analysis of the records of 1,657 patients with carcinoma of the esophagus and cardia of the stomach. *Surg. Gynecol. Obstet.* **130**, 997–1005.

Japanese Society for Esophageal Disorders (1976) Guidelines for the clinical and pathologic studies for carcinoma of the esophagus. *Jap. J. Surg.* **6**, 79–86.

Jeyasingham K. (1978) In: Franchini A. et al., Clinica e terapia del carcinoma esofageo. *Dal Bollettino delle Scienze Mediche.* Organo Della Societa E Scuola Medica Chirurgica Di Bologna.

Jeyasingham K., Beligaswatte A. M. L. and Sandrasegara F. A. (1967) Carcinoma involving the oesophagus. *Ceyl. Med. J.* **12**, 187–201.

Kron I. L., Cantrell M. D., Johns M. E. et al. (1984) Computerised axial tomography of the oesophagus to determine suitability for blunt oesophagectomy. *Ann. Surg.* **200**, 173–174.

Le Quesne L. P. and Ranger D. (1966) Pharyngo-laryngectomy with immediate pharyngo-gastric anastomosis. *Br. J. Surg.* **53**, 105–109.

Lewis I. (1946) The surgical treatment of carcinoma of the oesophagus with special reference to a new operation for growth of the middle third. *Br. J. Surg.* **34**, 18–31.

McCaughan J. S., Hicks W., Laufman L. et al. (1984) Palliation of esophageal malignancy with photoradiation therapy. *Cancer* **54**, 2905–2910.

McKeown K. C. (1972) Trends in oesophageal resection for carcinoma. *Ann. R. Coll. Surg. Engl.* **51**, 213–218.

Miller C. (1962) Carcinoma of the thoracic oesophagus and cardia. A review of 405 cases. *Br. J. Surg.* **49**, 507–522.

Moertel C. G. (1978) Chemotherapy in gastro-intestinal cancer. In: *Clinics in Gastroenterology*, Vol. 5. London, W. B. Saunders, pp. 777–793.

Monnier P., Savary M. and Anani P. (1985) Endoscopic morphology of 'early' esophageal carcinoma. In: De Meester T. R. and Skinner D. B. (eds.) *Esophageal Disorders: Pathophysiology and Therapy*. New York, Raven Press, pp. 333–346.

Mousseau M., le Forestier J., Barbin J. et al. (1956) Place de l'intubation a demeure dans le traitement palliative du cancer de l'esophagi. *Arch. Mal. Appar. Digest.* **45**, 208–216.

Nakayama K. and Kinoshita Y. (1975) Surgical treatment combined with pre-operative concentrated irradiation. Current concepts in cancer. Esophagus—treatment localised and advanced. *JAMA*, **227**, 178–181.

Ong G. B. and Lee T. C. (1960) Pharyngogastric anastomosis after oesophago-pharyngectomy for carcinoma of the hypopharynx and cervical oesophagus. *Br. J. Surg.* **48**, 193.

Orringer M. B. (1984) Transhiatal oesophagectomy without thoracotomy for carcinoma of the thoracic esophagus. *Ann. Surg.* **200**, 282–288.

Orringer M. B. and Orringer J. S. (1983) Transhiatal oesophagectomy without thoracotomy—a dangerous operation? *J. Thorac. Cardiovasc. Surg.* **85**, 72–80.

Orringer M. B. and Sloan H. (1975) Substernal gastric bypass of the excluded thoracic oesophagus for palliation of oesophageal carcinoma. *J. Thorac. Cardiovasc. Surg.* **70**, 836–851.

Orringer M. B. and Sloan H. (1978) Oesophagectomy without thoracotomy. *J. Thorac. Cardiovasc. Surg.* **76**, 643–654.

Pearson J. G. (1975) Value of radiation therapy. Current concepts in cancer. Esophagus—treatment. *JAMA*, **227**, 181–183.

Royston C. M. S. and Dowling B. L. (1976) A combined synchronous technique for the McKeown three-phase oesophagectomy. *Br. J. Surg.* **63**, 122–124.

Soga J., Kobayashi K., Saito J. et al. (1979) The role of lymphadenectomy in curative surgery for gastric cancer. *World J. Surg.* **3**, 701–708.

Souttar H. S. (1924) Method of intubating the oesophagus for malignant stricture. *Br. Med. J.* **1**, 782–783.

Sweet R. H. (1945) Transthoracic gastrectomy and esophagectomy for carcinoma of the stomach and esophagus. *Clinics* **3**, 1288.

Sweet R. H. (1950) *Thoracic Surgery*. Philadelphia, Saunders, pp. 271–279.

Turner G. G. (1936) Carcinoma of the oesophagus—the question of its treatment by surgery. *Lancet* **1**, 130.

Union Internationale Contre le Cancer. *TNM Classification of Malignant Tumours 1982*, edited by M. H. Harmer. Geneva, UICC.

Yan C. J. and Brooks J. R. (1985) Surgical management of gastric adenocarcinoma. *Am. J. Surg.* **149**, 771–774.

Chapter nine

Oesophageal Reconstruction

R. H. R. Belsey

Reconstruction of the oesophagus is indicated when the organ is congenitally defective, irreversibly damaged by inflammation or trauma, following resection for tumours, and in any situation where permanent restoration of normal swallowing cannot be achieved by more conservative methods.

INDICATIONS

The common indications are:
1. Congenital oesophageal atresia
2. Severe trauma
3. Peptic strictures of the oesophagus
4. Corrosive strictures
5. Certain functional disorders of the oesophagus
6. Following resection for tumours.

Congenital Oesophageal Atresia

Where no primary anastomosis is possible without tension owing to the extent of the defect. At the first stage the tracheo-oesophageal fistula is closed, a cervical oesophagostomy is performed on the left side of the neck, followed by a feeding gastrostomy. At the age of 12–18 months the oesophagus is reconstructed by an interposition procedure and the gastrostomy is closed.

Trauma

Primary repair of the oesophagus is usually possible when the organ has been breached by penetrating or closed crushing injuries. In certain cases repair may not be possible owing to the extent and severity of the trauma, or as a result of previous unsuccessful attempts at repair, and reconstruction is necessary. Following spontaneous rupture, in cases of delayed diagnosis with established mediastinitis, the only way to save the patient's life is by exteriorizing the infected remnants of the organ, leaving the patient with a temporary cervical oesophagostomy and gastrostomy. Three months later, when all the inflammatory complications have been controlled, reconstruction is carried out.

Peptic Strictures

Early, dilatable strictures can be managed by more conservative measures. In more advanced cases, where dilatation fails to relieve the dysphagia satisfactorily and where, owing to the secondary shortening of the oesophagus characteristic of peptic oesophagitis, no adequate anti-reflux procedure is possible, then resection of the stenosed segment and reconstruction are called for. Uncertainty regarding the pathology of the stricture and the possibility of malignancy are further indications for resection.

Corrosive Strictures

The strictures following corrosive burns of the oesophagus tend to be more extensive and tighter than peptic strictures, and respond less satisfactorily to conservative methods of treatment. In this situation the problem of bypass as against resection has been widely discussed but the preference for resection whenever possible is based on accumulating evidence that a significant percentage of these strictures will ultimately undergo malignant degeneration.

Functional Disorders

In cases of diffuse oesophageal spasm with multiple diverticular formation the propulsive activity of the organ may be so disorganized that only by reconstruction can the normal swallowing mechanism be restored. An equally radical approach may be indicated in cases of achalasia where previous surgery has failed. The fact that the whole oesophagus is abnormal in this condition and because of the observed 10 per cent incidence of malignant degeneration there should be consideration of resection in certain cases.

Tumours

Reconstruction following resection for tumours is more relevant to the management of malignant disease but certain extensive benign tumours such as leiomyomas may need resection.

TECHNIQUES FOR RECONSTRUCTION

Any acceptable technique must satisfy definite criteria:
1. Complete and permanent relief of the dysphagia, with no undesirable side-effects.
2. Acceptable operative morbidity and mortality rate.
3. Must permit reconstruction of the entire oesophagus when necessary.
4. Must be applicable to infants and children.
5. The technique should permit synchronous

resection and reconstruction in a single-stage procedure.

6. The technique must be suitable for communication to trainee surgeons of average ability.

Numerous reconstructive techniques have been devised in the past but only those that have withstood the test of extensive clinical trial will be described. Attempts at reconstruction with various prosthetic devices have proved catastrophic. Only by the interposition of a living, propulsive transplant can the criteria outlined be met. The techniques in common use are:

1. Intrathoracic oesophago-gastrostomy
2. Cervical oesophago-gastrostomy
3. Reversed gastric tube
4. Jejunal interposition
5. Colon interposition; right, transverse or left.

Intrathoracic Oesophago-gastrostomy

ADVANTAGES

1. Quick, technically simple operation, involving a single anastomosis.

2. May be applicable as a palliative procedure for malignant strictures, especially in cases where resection of the lesser curve of the stomach has been indicated for lymphatic involvement.

DISADVANTAGES

1. High incidence of anastomotic dehiscence and fistulas.

2. High risk of acute, fatal, postoperative aspiration pneumonitis.

3. Can lead to severe nutritional disturbances in children.

4. The main disadvantage of this technique is the high incidence, in 30 per cent or more, of recurrent peptic oesophagitis and stenosis above the anastomosis. It is therefore contra-indicated in the management of all forms of benign oesophageal obstruction, and in any patient who may survive the resection for more than 2 years. Attempts to construct an antireflux device at the anastomosis have largely failed as a long-term solution to the problem.

Cervical Oesophago-gastrostomy

Through the left thoraco-abdominal approach, the stomach is mobilized, retaining the right gastric and gastro-epiploic arteries; the cardia is divided and closed. After resecting 75 per cent of the intrathoracic oesophagus, the stomach is displaced upwards through the hiatus, through the mediastinal bed of the oesophagus deep to the aortic arch, and the highest point of the closed fundus is attached to the ligated stump of the oesophagus. A pyloromyotomy is routinely performed. After reattachment of the

diaphragm to its costal origin the chest is closed. Through a left cervical incision the upper oesophagus is mobilized and the attached fundus drawn up into the neck incision. The remainder of the oesophagus is trimmed back, the fundus opened and an end-to-end anastomosis is performed. No difficulty will be encountered in bringing the fundus to this level provided that the mobilization has been completed.

ADVANTAGES

1. The observed operative mortality is half that of the intrathoracic anastomosis.

2. The incidence of anastomotic fistulas is lower, but of greater significance is the fact that the patient will survive this catastrophic complication after treatment of the local infection or empyema which may result. The mortality rate of a fistula complicating an intrathoracic anastomosis is well over 50 per cent.

3. Late postoperative oesophagitis and peptic stenosis are rare following this method of reconstruction.

4. The procedure is technically no more exacting than the intrathoracic reconstruction.

5. There is accumulating evidence that the long-term results of total oesophagectomy for malignant strictures irrespective of the location of the tumour are superior in terms of avoiding recurrent dysphagia due to lymphatic spread.

DISADVANTAGE

1. The only significant disadvantage is that the technique cannot be employed if partial gastric resection is necessitated by lymph node involvement.

Reversed Gastric Tube

This technique was first devised by Gavriliu as the initial bypass procedure prior to staged resection of the oesophagus for malignant tumours, and later advocated as a method of reconstruction in the management of benign oesophageal lesions. Essentially a tube is constructed from the distal portion of the greater curve of the stomach with the vascular supply maintained through the short gastrosplenic arteries and left gastro-epiploic artery. When originally described, it was recommended that the spleen be resected well distally to the point where these arteries arise from the main splenic artery, but more recently surgeons have avoided resecting the spleen without detriment to the operation (*Figs.* 9.1, 9.2).

The pyloric sphincter and a short length of duodenum may be included in the tube to gain extra length when necessary. The distal end of the tube is then swung up through one of the available routes, intrathoracic, retrosternal or antethoracic, and anastomosed to the cervical oesophagus.

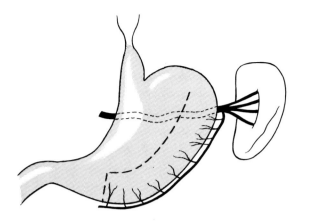

Fig. 9.1. Reversed gastric tube (1). The line of section of the greater curve of stomach, together with its supportive arterial supply from the splenic artery, is shown.

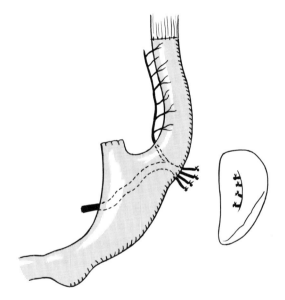

Fig. 9.2. Reversed gastric tube (2). The tube has been swung up for either intrathoracic or cervical oesophago-gastric anastomosis. Division of the short gastric vessels is optional but may facilitate mobilization.

ADVANTAGES

1. The only advantage of this technique compared with cervical oesophago-fundostomy, employing the intact stomach, may be the lesser diameter of the reversed gastric tube.

DISADVANTAGES

1. The extensive suture line from the region of the pylorus to the neck, irrespective of whether it is achieved by the stapling machine or by manual suturing techniques, is a potential source of danger from gastric fistulas.

2. The technique cannot be used following pre-

vious gastric surgery or where resection of the lesser curve has been necessary.

3. The reversed tube is in theory antiperistaltic and in practice has been found to be devoid of propulsive function on postoperative manometric studies.

4. There are few reports available on the late functional results.

End-to-end Oesophageal Anastomosis

Following the resection of short benign strictures, reconstruction by direct anastomosis may appear attractive. This can rarely be achieved without tension and the late results have proved disappointing. Mobilization of the lower oesophagus to relieve tension on the suture line usually creates severe reflux, with its attendant complications. This technique is rarely justified.

Jejunal Interposition (*see also* Chapter 10)

Reconstruction may be achieved by isoperistaltic pedicled transplants of upper jejunum.

ADVANTAGES

1. The active peristalsis of the transplant affords good functional results.

2. The technique is suitable for short reconstructions of the lower oesophagus.

DISADVANTAGES

1. The vascular anatomy of the jejunum may render it impossible to prepare a long transplant for total oesophageal replacement without leaving much redundant jejunum above the diaphragm, involving the necessity for 'tailoring' the transplant.

2. Jejunal interposition can rarely be used for reconstructions in infants or children owing to the fragility of the blood supply. Therefore, this method of reconstruction does not fulfil the criteria previously enumerated.

3. Evidence of alkaline oesophagitis above an oesophagojejunal anastomosis was observed by Allison.

Colon Interposition (*Fig. 9.3*)

Colon may be used for oesophageal replacement by one of three techniques:

1. Isoperistaltic transplant of terminal ileum, caecum and right colon supported by the middle colic artery.

2. Antiperistaltic transplant of transverse colon supported by the middle colic artery.

3. Isoperistaltic transplant of left colon and left half of transverse colon supported by the left colic artery.

The activity of the colon may not be peristaltic

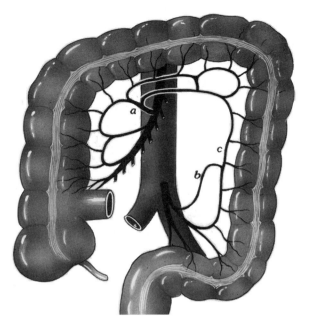

Fig. 9.3. Arterial supply of the colon. *a*, Middle colic artery. *b*, Left colic artery. *c*, Ascending branch of the left colic artery, the nutrient artery for both short- and long-segment colon transplant.

when compared with other parts of the intestinal tract, but it is certainly propulsive, with a highly developed sense of responsibility and direction. The use of antiperistaltic transplants can therefore be ruled out both on theoretical grounds and the observed unsatisfactory functional results in terms of the patient's ability to eat and drink with satisfaction. The practical choice lies between the use of left or right colon.

Left Colon Interposition

ADVANTAGES:

1. Left colon is less bulky than right colon.
2. It is more accustomed to propelling a solid bolus than right colon.
3. The left colic artery constitutes a robust vascular pedicle and anatomical variations are rare. The vascular anatomy of the ileocaecal region may be precarious.
4. Sufficient viscus is available to permit total oesophageal replacement, up to the pharynx, when indicated. Division of the left branch of the middle colic artery close to its origin effectively lengthens the marginal artery to support a long transplant.
5. Left colon interposition is applicable to infants and children.
6. The extended left thoracotomy approach, described later, permits synchronous single-stage resection and reconstruction through one incision, with the addition of a short neck incision for total replacement.

7. With an operative mortality rate of 5·5 per cent in a consecutive series of more than 350 reconstructions for all forms of oesophageal obstruction, on patients aged 6 months to 87 years, the technique compares favourably with other techniques for replacement.
8. Owing to the fact that the colon secretes benign mucus, anastomotic fistulas are rare (1 per cent) and will heal spontaneously with conservative treatment.
9. When no oesophageal resection is possible, relief of dysphagia can be effectively achieved by means of a bypass procedure with left colon.

LATE FUNCTIONAL RESULTS

1. Relief of dysphagia is satisfactory in 85 per cent of patients. In the remaining 15 per cent of cases, where colonic activity is inherently sluggish, the patient can eat normal food but must take the meal more slowly. With the passage of time, function slowly improves as the transplant begins to assume the apparent anatomy and function of the normal oesophagus.
2. In infants and children the transplant has been observed to grow at the same speed as the patient into adult life.

Oesophageal reconstruction with isoperistaltic left colon therefore satisfies the six criteria demanded of any technique to be acceptable. Operative details have been simplified to the extent that the method can be communicated to any resident or registrar of average ability, and with an adequate knowledge of human anatomy.

There are certain contra-indications to the use of left colonic interposition:

1. Intrinsic colonic disease. Mild diverticulosis with no history of previous inflammation is no contra-indication.
2. Mesenteric endarteritis, usually found in patients with severe systemic hypertension. If there is any doubt regarding the condition of the mesenteric vessels as revealed by palpation of the left colic artery and pulsation in the marginal artery, then colonic interposition is contra-indicated. In this situation, the alternative procedure of choice is reconstruction by means of cervical oesophago-gastrostomy, which can be achieved through the same incision at the same operative intervention.

TECHNIQUE

1. *Preoperative Preparation:* The general preparation of the patient consists of the elimination of all dental sepsis, thoracic physiotherapy to correct aspiration bronchitis when present, and correction of anaemia. If the nutritional state of the patient is poor, a period of gastrostomy feeding for 2–3 months prior to the major intervention may be advisable.

Opinion varies regarding the optimum local preparation for the colon. In the author's opinion preparation should aim at an empty, dry colon. This can best be achieved by placing the patient on a low residue diet for 2 weeks prior to surgery, by prohibiting all aperients, enemas and washouts, and by placing the patient on restricted fluids for the last 24 hours. Traditional methods of preparation have been found to result in a fluid bowel content which increases the risk of wound contamination. There is no convincing evidence that the routine use of antibiotics prior to operation has any influence on the incidence of postoperative wound infection and the practice has been abandoned by the author, although many advise antibiotic bowel preparation.

2. *Anaesthesia:* The anaesthetist must be alerted to the probable presence of aspiration bronchitis and the necessity for frequent suction toilet of the airway during the operation. One-lung anaesthesia is of no assistance to the surgeon as retraction of a partially inflated lung is easier than of an atelectatic lung.

3. *Exposure:* The standard incision for synchronous resection and reconstruction is the extended left lateral thoracotomy. With the patient in the right lateral position on the table, the left chest is entered through the 6th intercostal space. The incision is extended forwards in the line of the intercostal space, dividing the costal margin, to the lateral border of the rectus sheath. The posterior end of the 7th rib is divided beneath the erector spinae muscle and the 7th intercostal bundle is ligated and divided before inserting the rib spreaders.

The anterior margin of the diaphragm is separated from its costal origin for a distance of 15 cm, leaving a 1–2-cm fringe for reattachment later. The oblique muscles are divided in the line of the skin incision. Incising the peritoneum results in a T-shaped exposure affording good access to the upper abdomen.

4. *Preparation of the Colon Transplant:* The major abdominal procedures are completed before dissection of the mediastinum, to minimize blood loss. The probable length of the transplant will have been estimated from the preoperative investigations. The left colic and marginal arteries are examined. The greater omentum is dissected from the colon; the descending colon is mobilized by division of the lateral peritoneal reflection, thus improving access to the left colic artery. The marginal artery is divided distal to both branches of the left colic. Division of the colon is delayed until a later stage of the procedure when the length of the transplant has been finally determined.

5. *Pyloromyotomy:* A gastric drainage procedure is routinely indicated as both vagi will be divided when the oesophagus is resected. A simple pyloromyotomy has proved superior to a pyloroplasty as it is followed less frequently by duodenal reflux.

6. *Mobilization of the Oesophagus:* The stenosed segment of the oesophagus is dissected from the mediastinum. The cardia is divided and the stomach closed. The proximal point of oesophageal section will be indicated by the pathology of the stricture, but must be well above the upper limit of the inflammatory process, through normal oesophagus. When total replacement is necessary, the oesophagus is dissected from beneath the aortic arch by combined finger and sharp dissection after division of the two bronchial arteries and the branch passing to the oesophagus from the 4th intercostal artery above the arch. This dissection is facilitated by working close to the muscle layer of the organ.

7. *Isolation of the Transplant:* The colon transplant may be either a short segment, when an oesophago-colic anastomosis is undertaken at or distal to the level of the aortic arch, or a long-segment colon transplant, when oesophago-colic anastomosis is undertaken in the neck. Both short- and long-segment colon transplants are pedicled on both branches of the left colic artery and its accompanying veins. The omentum is separated from the splenic flexure of the colon and the left half of the transverse colon. An adequate length of colon is selected, the points of division determined and the marginal artery divided in the appropriate places. Distally this will be just below the point where the two branches of the left colic artery communicate with the marginal artery. When a short segment colon transplant is necessary the proximal division of the marginal artery is where the left branch of the middle colic artery and the marginal artery arising from the left colic artery meet (*Fig.* 9.4). However, when a long segment colon transplant is planned, the left branch of the middle colic artery is divided close to the bifurcation of the middle colic artery and the marginal artery at the point where it joins the right branch of the middle colic artery (*Fig.* 9.5). I have only rarely divided the main stem of the middle colic artery.

Following division of the appropriate vessels the colon is divided between occlusive clamps using either the scalpel or diathermy. When tailoring a long segment it is important to divide the colon as far proximally as possible towards or even at the hepatic flexure, to ensure that an adequate length of colon can be obtained. It is always possible to trim redundant or apparently ischaemic colon during the cervical part of the operation, which is more satisfactory than suturing too short a colon transplant in the neck under tension. The occlusive clamps are removed from the colon and the cut ends will usually bleed well, indicating an adequate vascular supply. Scybala are then milked from the isolated colon and the graft is temporarily returned to the abdomen.

8. *Reconstitution of the Colon:* The transverse and descending colon are now anastomosed end to end. The standard anastomotic technique used throughout

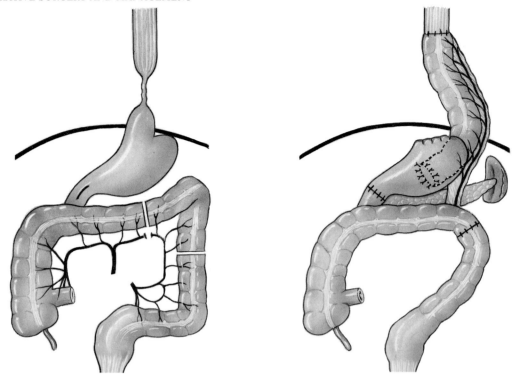

Fig. 9.4. Short-segment colon transplant. The segment is nourished by the ascending branch of the left colic artery. Pyloromyotomy is undertaken and oesophago-gastric anastomosis performed at the posterior aspect of the stomach, following which the colon transplant is passed into the chest via the hiatus.

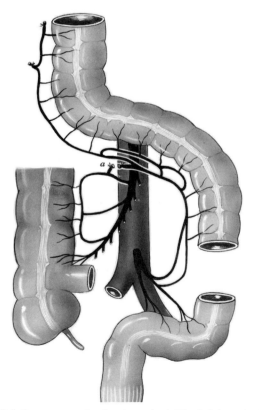

Fig. 9.5. Long-segment colon transplant. The left branch of the middle colic artery (*a*) has been divided and the colon segment is nourished by the left colic artery.

the procedure will be by a single row of closely spaced, interrupted, inverting, all-layer sutures of non-irritant suture material, with all but the last three sutures tied on the luminal aspect (*Fig.* 9.6).

The use of interrupted sutures is probably safer than a continuous suture when following the single-layer technique. The author's preference for mono-filament stainless steel wire, 38 SWG or 5/0, as the suture material for all intestinal anastomoses may be of less importance than the basic principle of avoiding impairment of tissue viability by the use of the mini-mal quantity of foreign material consistent with accurate tissue apposition. One of the major benefits of the wire technique is the elimination of any risk of anastomotic strictures.

9. *Cologastric Anastomosis* (*Fig.* 9.7): The design of this anastomosis is important. With the stomach turned over to the right, the point selected is on the posterior aspect, close to the greater curve, and one-third of the distance from the closed cardia to the pylorus distally from the fundus. Selection of this point ensures no tension on the pedicle and maintains a 6–10-cm segment of transplant in the high-pressure zone below the diaphragm, creating an anti-reflux mechanism similar in principle to that of the mark IV hiatal hernia repair (*see* Chapter 21). Cologastric anastomoses to the cardia have been observed to lead to reflux and peptic ulceration of the transplant. The single-layer anastomotic technique is employed.

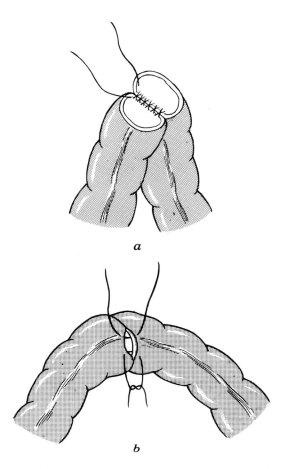

a

b

Fig. 9.6. Colo-colic anastomosis. This is undertaken using interrupted stainless steel wire sutures, the knots being tied within the lumen, with the exception of the final two or three anterior sutures which are tied outside the lumen.

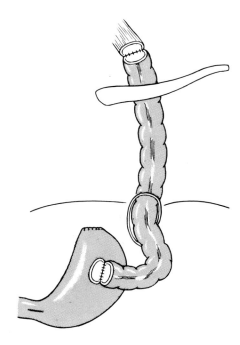

Fig. 9.7. Long-segment colon transplant. The cologastric anastomosis is undertaken on the posterior aspect of the stomach one-third of the distance between the closed cardia and the pylorus, following which the colon is passed into the thorax via the hiatus and thence into the neck. When the patient's oesophagus has been removed, the colon transplant follows the course of the oesophagus medial to the aortic arch and into the neck in place of the oesophagus. In patients with congenital oesophageal atresia, it is necessary to pass the upper colon into the neck through a tunnel created behind the anterior end of the 1st rib.

10. *Route for the Transplant:* The proximal end of the transplant is brought up behind the fundus of the stomach, through the hiatus into the mediastinum. Following resections for benign oesophageal lesions the ideal route is through the mediastinal bed of the resected oesophagus, deep to the aortic arch for total replacements. The advantage of this direct route is the avoidance of any kinking of the vascular pedicle and venous congestion of the transplant, which can lead to progressive fibrosis at its proximal end. The transplant may be brought up through the pleural cavity lateral to the aortic arch. The retrosternal route is chosen only when the mediastinum has been obliterated, as in a staged reconstruction or when a bypass procedure is planned; it involves the risk of kinking the vascular pedicle at the point where it turns back towards its origin at the lower end of the sternum. Obstruction of the venous return can be as deleterious to the viability of the transplant as interference with the arterial supply.

11. *Oesophago-colic Anastomosis:* This again is achieved by the one-layer technique. Inequality in the diameters of the colon and oesophagus can be met by simple 'tailoring' of the anastomosis. For total replacements the proximal end of the transplant is temporarily closed and loosely sutured to the stump of the resected oesophagus at the apex of the chest. The chest is then closed and the upper anastomosis performed through a separate cervical incision by the same technique. As this cervical incision communicates with the left pleural cavity it must not be drained.

12. *Anchoring the Transplant to the Diaphragm.* Before closing the chest any redundant transplant is drawn down and replaced in the abdomen. The seromuscular layer of the transplant is then sutured to the margin of the hiatus for half its circumference to prevent any subsequent prolapse into the pleural cavity, which could promote mechanical obstruction by kinking.

13. *Closure of the Diaphragm:* The diaphragm is sutured to the fringe on the chest wall created during the exposure for this purpose. With its nerve and blood supply intact, the diaphragm can now function normally.

14. *Closure of the Thoracotomy:* Closure is achieved by the standard technique after insertion of an intercostal catheter for the first 24–48 hours.

POSTOPERATIVE CARE

No oral intake is permitted for the first 48 hours. On the 3rd day oral fluids and soft solids, ice cream in particular, are allowed in small quantities. From this point progression to normal feeding is rapid, within 7 days when the wire technique has been employed for the anastomoses. Antibiotic therapy is given only on specific indications and not routinely. Thoracic physiotherapy should be administered vigorously to prevent postoperative atelectasis and control any residual aspiration bronchitis or pneumonitis.

Chapter ten

Replacement of the Oesophagus with Jejunal Interposition

A. J. Gunning

INTRODUCTION

Most obstructive lesions of the oesophagus requiring excision and replacement often occur at an age when eating and drinking are the major remaining pleasures in life. Most peptic strictures and other benign obstructive lesions of the oesophagus are at present amenable to conservative surgical procedures. Oesophageal replacement is usually performed for malignant disease of the gastro-oesophageal junction and the oesophagus, especially the lower third.

HISTORY

The concept of using the jejunum as a substitute for the oesophagus is not new. Its use for this purpose was first proposed by Wüllstein in 1904 after studies on the cadaver. He suggested both mediastinal oesophagojejunostomy and antethoracic oesophagoplasty by a continuation of a jejunal loop and skin tube. It was left to César Roux in 1907, however, to perform and publish—before he had completed the staged operation—the first successful operation on a human. He brought up a loop of jejunum subcutaneously on the anterior chest wall as far as the neck, anastomosed the lower end to the stomach and restored intestinal continuity by a Murphy button. The loop of jejunum so fashioned has since been known as a Roux loop. In 1908 Herzen performed a similar staged operation but anastomosed the distal end of the duodenojejunal segment by a T anastomosis to the loop, thus completing the Roux-en-Y as it is now known. By 1934 100 jejunodermato-oesophagoplasties and 36 jejuno-oesophagoplasties had been done. Morbidity and mortality were high.

INDICATIONS

In oesophageal obstruction it is the long-term functional results of reconstructive surgery that should be the surgeon's concern and target. Satisfactory oesophageal replacement should fulfil certain criteria as described by Belsey in Chapter 9. The jejunal loop is the best form of replacement and is indicated in four situations:

1. To restore continuity of the alimentary tract after total gastrectomy for carcinoma.
2. For benign lesions, e.g. strictures of the lower third of the oesophagus, unresponsive to dilatation and other conservative surgical operations.
3. For malignant lesions of the gastro-oesophageal junction and occasionally the lower third of the oesophagus (*Fig.* 10.4).
4. To short-circuit inoperable lesions of the gastro-oesophageal area (*Fig.* 10.3).

Fashioning a long loop is tiring and time consuming, often resulting in a loop that is redundant but which will not reach the site of resection. The anastomosis between oesophagus and jejunum can be difficult because of the thick and proliferative nature of the jejunal mucosa. Certainly the jejunum is now rarely used for total oesophageal replacement; another important reason is that even for carcinomas of the lower third of the oesophagus, the preference now is for total oesophagectomy, replacing the oesophagus with stomach or colon. This is not only for technical reasons, but because of the frequency with which oesophageal carcinomas produce skip lesions up the length of the oesophagus.

PREOPERATIVE MANAGEMENT

As most of the patients with gastro-oesophageal lesions are in the sixth or seventh decades they may also have cardiovascular and respiratory disease. Routine investigations are complemented by:

1. Chest radiographs, ECG, and a barium meal which will probably have been done before admission.
2. Oesophagoscopy and gastroscopy to determine the level and histology of the obstructing lesion.
3. CT scan to rule out liver, mediastinal and other intra-abdominal secondaries or disease, e.g. cholelithiasis.
4. All patients are given a syrup of nystatin and ampicillin or erythromycin for 48 hours three times a day.
5. Treatment of dehydration and anaemia. The value of preoperative intravenous feeding is debatable but may be useful in severe malnutrition.

ANAESTHESIA

After induction of anaesthesia a double-lumen endotracheal tube is passed to give one-lung ventilation to improve exposure by easy and gentle retraction of the lung. A loading dose of gentamicin, 80 mg, metronidazole, 500 mg, and flucloxacillin, 500 mg, is given with the induction of anaesthesia, and continued for 3 days postoperatively.

TECHNIQUE

The technical details for fashioning a Roux loop have not been bettered since the descriptions given by Roux (1907) and Allison and Da Silva (1953).

A left thoraco-abdominal incision is made through the bed of the 9th rib, but not across the costal margin. If greater thoracic exposure is required the posterior 2·5 cm of the 8th rib may be resected. The abdominal part of the incision is transverse and runs between the 9th and 10th costal cartilages, so avoiding actual cutting of costal cartilage. The transverse abdominal incision may be extended to the midline, but this is often unnecessary as on incising the diaphragm a wide exposure of the left upper abdomen is obtained. In cases of malignancy, the abdominal part of the incision is made first, and the operability of the carcinoma assessed, special care being taken to open the lesser sac to assess spread to the pancreas and posterior abdominal wall. In benign cases the diaphragm is incised circumferentially while in malignant cases it is divided radially to just above the hiatus. At this level the incision is converted into an inverted Y to enable excision of a segment of diaphragm and crura with the malignant tissue. The cut edges of the diaphragm are sutured to the edges of the costal incision, giving excellent exposure to the lower thorax and upper abdomen, which is further improved by the use of a self-retaining retractor. An assessment is made of the lesion and the probable length of the jejunal segment required is estimated. If the lesion is operable it is advisable to fashion the Roux loop first.

The jejunum immediately distal to the ligament of Treitz is identified. The jejunal mesentery is carefully inspected with the aid of transillumination and the pattern of its arteries and veins identified. The jejunum immediately proximal to the ligament of Treitz has a profusion of vessels with poorly defined arcades. Several centimetres distally the typically described jejunal vascular pattern of arterial arcades supplied at intervals by larger primary jejunal arteries is found. The veins accompany the arteries but often bifurcate at a different level. Because of this it is important to divide the arteries and veins separately. At least 20–35 cm of jejunum should be isolated.

The assistant holds as long a length of intestine as possible in his or her two hands so that with the mesentery it forms an outstretched fan. It is best to expose the vessels by incising only that layer of peritoneum nearer the surgeon and stripping down the fat, leaving the other layer of peritoneum intact until the loop is completed; this prevents glare from the transillumination source (*Fig.* 10.1).

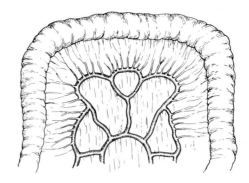

Fig. 10.1. Jejunal arcades in proposed loop. Vessel distribution improved by background illumination (*see text*).

From a point chosen for division of the intestine, the peritoneum is cut towards the root of mesentery, and the first primary artery and vein divided between ligatures—this means isolating a length of artery and vein and passing ligatures round the vessels. The ligatures nearer the root of the mesentery are divided. The ligatures nearest the intestine are held and with gentle traction towards the intestine the primary vessels are approximated towards the arcades, in order to maintain the vascular supply of the loop parallel to the intestine (*Fig.* 10.2).

The arteries and veins should be ligated sufficiently proximally to the bifurcation into arcades, in order to avoid obstructing the passage of blood along the bifurcation which now becomes a straight channel. However, these should not be ligated so far from the bifurcation that a blind pouch is created which may thrombose. The height to which the loop may be taken is not determined by the length of intestine, but by that of the free edge of its mesentery.

It is not necessary to divide the peritoneum nearer the surgeon at the bifurcation of the vessels, especially if the vasa rectae are long; rather the peritoneal incision is along the top of the arcade where it is nearest the intestine and then carried straight across to the top of the next arcade, which increases the effective length of the loop without impeding its blood supply. The primary arteries and veins supplying the other arcades are similarly isolated and

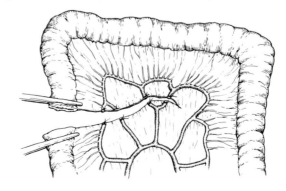

Fig. 10.2. Careful ligation and division of jejunal arteries. Veins not shown. (For technique *see text*.)

divided until the chosen main artery and vein supplying the isolated loop are reached. The peritoneal layer on the far side of the vessels is now cut. The ideal Roux loop is one that reaches to the point of anastomosis, without tension in its mesentery, without any surplus length and in a straight line. The straightness of the intestine depends on the length of its free mesenteric border being as nearly equal to the length of the gut. The effective length therefore depends on the exact technique of division of peritoneum and cellular tissue; the viability is governed by the care and accuracy of division of its vessels.

It is important that an estimate of the required length of loop should be made early for the risks are increased if vessels are divided unnecessarily and make too long a loop, or if a good loop is stretched a centimetre too far, and its draining vein occluded. It is frustrating and inadequate if the limits of resection of a carcinoma, or of a simple peptic stricture, are governed not by the dictates of pathology but by the available length of a poorly constructed loop.

The gut is now divided at the level chosen. In order that this may be done without sacrifice of any length of loop, one or two arteriae rectae above the point of section are divided close to the intestine to make a gap across which two narrow crushing clamps can be applied. The de Martel type of crushing clamp is useful as it can be easily threaded through the mesocolon. The loop is now dropped back into the abdomen to await the definitive resection of the lesion. It is therefore advisable that the loop be fashioned early in the procedure, and any doubts about its viability may be answered.

A partial or total gastrectomy or oesophagectomy is now completed. In benign disease of the gastro-oesophageal area the resection is conservative and most of the stomach may be left behind (*see* Chapter 8). In malignant disease a good clearance of the posterior mediastinum, diaphragm and diaphragmatic crura and as much of the stomach as deemed necessary is excised together with any glands around the coeliac axis. Occasionally splenectomy with or without the tail of the pancreas needs to be performed. It is prudent at this stage to check haemostasis in the posterior mediastinum and stomach bed. The resected end of the stomach is closed by staples or by suture (*see* Chapter 2). The proximal remaining oesophagus has a non-crushing clamp placed across it at least 5 cm above the resected end. In cases of malignancy the cut ends of the stomach and oesophagus are examined histologically by frozen section to check that the cut edges are free of neoplastic disease.

A hole is then made in the transverse mesocolon as far back as possible on the posterior abdominal wall, so that no ridge occurs here when the transverse colon is replaced. Through this hole, the Roux loop is threaded and passed up behind the stomach in the now widely opened lesser sac of peritoneum, through the hiatus and into the mediastinum. The loop is anastomosed side to end to the oesophagus using the

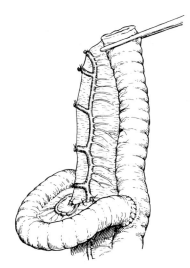

Fig. 10.3. Isolated Roux loop replacing resected lower oesophagus.

anastomosis stapler, which certainly makes the anastomosis easier and safer (*Fig.* 10.4) or by suture using 4/0 PDS interrupted full-thickness mattress sutures and 4/0 PDS continuous sutures for the mucosa. The open end of the jejunum can be closed by an inverting suture or staples.

In bringing up the loop care must be taken not to twist the loop and threaten its blood supply. The superior mesenteric vessels pass down in front of the

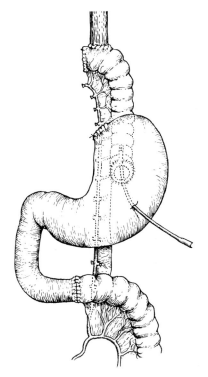

Fig. 10.4 Completed jejunal interposition. Gastrostomy tube in place (*see text*). Standard Roux loop used for bypass procedures.

third part of the duodenum and if reflected upwards would naturally lie to the right of the duodenojejunal flexure. The Roux loop should pass upwards to the right of the duodenal flexure.

The loop below the diaphragm is so arranged that it passes over to the left behind the fundus or remaining part of the stomach and reaches the greater curvature of the stomach in the region of the gastrosplenic omentum, and a point is selected on the loop that can be anastomosed to the posterior surface of the stomach without tension or kinking. The intestine is then divided at this chosen point. One or two arteriae rectae of the upper segment are divided flush with the intestine in order to free the circumference of the intestine and so facilitate the anastomosis to the stomach.

The intestine below the level of the section must then be freed so that it can be drawn down and reunited with the small length of jejunum attached to the duodenum by an end-to-end anastomosis below the transverse mesocolon (*Fig.* 10.4). This may mean the division of 6–10 arteriae rectae and even removal of a small section of the loop. The lower end of the loop is anastomosed end to side to the posterior wall of the stomach. For this purpose, it is wise to cut the end of the intestine obliquely so that it is not made to kink by necessity of turning abruptly forward to join the stomach.

At least 10–15 cm of loop should be below the diaphragm to avoid gasto-oesophageal reflux, by having the jejunal loop and its junction with the stomach all at the same intra-abdominal pressure. The loop passes over the back of the stomach so that as the stomach distends, it compresses the loop and helps to prevent reflux. The hole in the transverse mesocolon is closed above the duodenojejunal flexure. The stomach is sutured back to the diaphragm to reform the lesser sac. A gastrostomy is done on the anterior surface of the stomach.

Before inserting the gastrostomy tube a Tubb's mitral valve dilator is passed into the pyloric canal and the pyloric musculature stretched by opening the blades of the dilator. This avoids a pyloromyotomy or pyloroplasty. The gastrostomy tube is manoeuvred into the lower part of the isolated loop. It is used to decompress the loop of air in the postoperative period when the patient tends to swallow air, and also serves to prevent venous compression in a distended loop until peristalsis returns. A further advantage of a gastrostomy is that it is far more comfortable than a nasogastric tube and allows the patient to drink after the first 24 hours. The effect of being able to drink by mouth is a great relief and encouragement to the patient, even if most of the fluid so taken appears in the drainage bottle.

The diaphragm is reapproximated by a continuous suture and the loop in the chest fixed to the edges of the new or previous hiatus. The pleural cavity is drained with a tube and the mediastinum, behind the loop up to the anastomosis, with a Redivac drain which passes through the hiatus behind the stomach to emerge through the abdominal wall.

When at operation a carcinoma is found to be inoperable, the surgeon must decide whether to close the patient, to provide some form of intubation or to perform a bypass operation to relieve the obstruction. In the majority of patients intubation with a Celestin tube will suffice. In a few, however, the lesion may be so extensive that a tube will serve no useful purpose. In these patients it may be worth while using a Roux loop to bypass the obstruction.

A Roux loop fashioned as described above is brought up into the chest and anastomosed end to side to the oesophagus. The distal part of the loop is anastomosed to the duodenojejunal segment to complete the Roux-en-Y. The diaphragm is closed round the jejunum which is lightly sutured to the diaphragm (*Fig.* 10.3).

POSTOPERATIVE MANAGEMENT

These patients should, where possible, be nursed in the intensive care unit for the first 24–36 hours, particularly when there are possible respiratory or cardiac problems. The patient may drink after 24 hours and should be ambulatory after 36 hours when drainage tubes are removed. A Gastrografin swallow is done on the 3rd postoperative day to check on all the anastomoses and free passage through the stomach. If all is well the patient now progresses from nourishing fluids to light diet. The gastrostomy is spigoted but if abdominal discomfort proves troublesome, can be released to empty the stomach of gas and fluid. The gastrostomy tube is removed on the 7th–10th postoperative day.

COMPLICATIONS

Only those complications affecting the loop and their management are described.

Necrosis

Massive necrosis of the interposed loop has been variously reported in 2–25 per cent of patients. This incidence is higher in operations for malignant than for benign disease. Necrosis of the loop is due to compression, stretching or twisting of the vascular pedicle of the graft, causing venous congestion and thrombosis. It is essentially a failure of technique.

Necrosis of the loop may occur from day 1 up to 5 or 6 days postoperatively, and the diagnosis may not therefore be easy to make. The early signs are persistent tachycardia and/or arrhythmia, varying degrees of shock which become profound as the loop ruptures or the anastomoses dehisce and intestinal contents, saliva, etc. flood the mediastinum and the pleural cavity. The patient may rapidly deteriorate and die. A Gastrografin swallow may not always be helpful in these circumstances because, until the viscus ruptures or the anastomosis dehisces, there is no leak to be visualized and the radio-opaque medium passes readily through the loop. This state of affairs may persist until rupture on the 6th or 7th day. Once the diagnosis of necrosis of the loop has been made, and the patient can be resuscitated, the wound should be reopened and the gangrenous viscus removed. The stomach and distal oesophagus are closed.

The gastrostomy tube is left in place for feeding in the postoperative period. The closed-off oesophagus is drained by a T-tube through a side-wall cervical oesophagostomy. Thorough mediastinal and pleural toilet completes the intrapleural surgery. The pleural cavity and mediastinum are drained to allow full expansion of the lung to obliterate any possible space which may allow air or an empyema to collect. Intravenous antibiotic cover is started and continued for 5 days. In the immediate postoperative period the patient is treated by intravenous alimentation which is later replaced by gastrostomy feeding. At a later date—after 2–3 weeks—at further surgery the stomach is brought up to the cervical oesophagus.

Anastomotic Leak

An anastomotic leak usually occurs at the upper anastomosis and is due to partial necrosis of the suture line or faulty suture technique. Anastomotic leaks at the gastrojejunal anastomosis are rare. Necrosis at the upper end of the loop may not only be due to inadequate arterial supply, but may be caused by compression of, or poor drainage by, the veins. The fistula may vary from a few millimetres in size to complete dehiscence of the anastomosis and may present from day 1 to the 7th or 10th postoperative day. The leak, if small, may remain localized without giving rise to any symptoms and heal spontaneously, or may contaminate the postoperative fluid collection in the pleural cavity and lead to an empyema. By the time the empyema is diagnosed and drained the fistula may have healed.

If the leak is significant the patient will present with symptoms of mediastinitis—pain, tachycardia, or arrhythmia, dyspnoea and varying degrees of shock which may rapidly lead to death. A plain chest X-ray will show air and fluid in the pleural cavity and a Gastrografin swallow will confirm this disaster.

The treatment of an anastomotic leak will depend on the clinical state of the patient. If the leak is diagnosed soon after its occurrence and the patient's condition is satisfactory, the chest should be reopened and pleural and mediastinal toilet completed. If the leak is small an attempt may be made to resuture the area and drain the mediastinum and pleura to ensure complete expansion of the lung. It may be difficult to localize the leak once the chest is open and the method of filling the chest with sterile saline and asking the anaesthetist to blow down a large-bore

oesophageal tube sited just above the oesophagojejunal anastomosis will readily locate the leak by the bubbles of air escaping from the leak (Froggat and Gunning, 1966). With this 'conservative' surgical management, the leak will, with time, close. It has been found that the rate at which the leak will heal can be hastened by the endoscopic application of 20 per cent sodium hydroxide to the area of the leak (Gunning and Kingsnorth, 1978). The healing progress can be monitored by repeated Gastrografin swallows. The patient is fed parenterally for 1–2 weeks and then by gastrostomy feeds.

With large leaks, and the patient fit for surgery after resuscitative measures, the options are:
1. To repeat anastomoses, observing the rule of no tension, and to ensure that the blood supply to the oesophagus and loop is adequate.
2. Failing this, the procedure outlined above for gangrene of the loop should be performed.

Stenosis

Stenosis of the anastomosis between the oesophagus and the jejunum is rare and when present is usually the result of a small anastomotic leak leading to an abscess with subsequent fibrosis and contracture, causing stenosis. Endoscopic dilatation is all that is required. More commonly, stenosis is due to a recurrence of carcinoma in the remaining oesophagus. Dilatation with or without insertion of a Celestin tube may be necessary.

Pain and Discomfort

Pain is a later postoperative complication in some patients with an interposed jejunal loop and also occurs in those patients in whom it has not been possible to remove the oesophagus, as may occur in strictures with severe mediastinitis or in inoperable carcinoma. The pain and discomfort come on after meals, are usually situated in the left hypochondrium or retrosternally and may be present for many years after operation. The cause is difficult to define and treat. The most likely explanation is gastric dilatation associated with irregular peristalsis of the stomach. Pain from the oesophagus which has been bypassed is almost certainly due to spread of the carcinoma into the mediastinal structures.

Reflux

Reflux is not a problem with the interposed loop for reasons given earlier (*see* p. 108). Gastrojejunal ulceration has not been encountered.

Eating Disorders

There is a difference between children who have had an isolated loop and adults with the same loop. The former rapidly adjust to the altered anatomy, evidenced by their appetite, their weight and their development. In adults the amount of food taken without discomfort is limited in the first 12–18 months with resultant inability to gain weight or often enjoy food.

CONCLUSIONS

In spite of the difficulties in fashioning a jejunal loop, and the possible complications, the jejunum is, in the author's view, anatomically and physiologically the best replacement of the oesophagus for the following reasons:

1. It approximates the size of the oesophagus.
2. It retains a frequent effective peristaltic action.
3. Unlike the stomach, regurgitation is not a problem.
4. Gastrojejunal ulceration does not occur.
5. It is rarely affected by other diseases, e.g. carcinoma, ulceration or inflammation.

REFERENCES

Allison P. R. and Da Silva L. T. (1953) The Roux loop. *Br. J. Surg.* **41**, 173–180.

Froggat D. and Gunning A. J. (1966) Treatment of oesophageal perforations. *Thorax* **21**, 524–528.

Gunning A. J. and Kingsnorth A. (1978) Endoscopic treatment of oesophageal leaks. *Br. J. Surg.* **66**, 226–229.

Herzen P. (1908) Eine Modifikation der Roux'schen Oesophagojejuno-gastros. *Zentralbl. Chir.* **35**, 219.

Roux C. (1907) L'Oesophago-jejuno-gastromose: nouvelle opération pour rétrécissement infrouchissable de l'oesophage. *Sem. Med.* **27**, 37.

Wüllstein L. (1904) Ueber Antethorake Oesophagojejunostomie und Operationen nach gleichen Prinzip. *Dtsch. Med. Wochenschr.* **30**, 734.

Chapter eleven

Neuromuscular Disorders of the Oesophagus

G. Keen

The passage of food into the oesophagus depends on a well-coordinated oropharyngeal mechanism, and similarly the propulsion of food through the lower sphincter into the stomach is accomplished very satisfactorily if there is well-coordinated peristaltic activity. Disorders of motility and coordination of muscle contraction may affect the entrance of the oesophagus, the exit of the oesophagus, a localized segment or the whole of the oesophagus. The conditions to be discussed are:

1. Pharyngeal diverticulum
2. Achalasia of the cardia
3. Oesophageal diverticulum
4. Diffuse spasm of the oesophagus

1. PHARYNGEAL DIVERTICULUM

Surgical Anatomy

This is a false diverticulum consisting of the thick mucosal layer of the oesophagus lined by stratified squamous epithelium but with no external muscle coat. It herniates through a weak point posteriorly, the Killian–Jamison dehiscence, which is situated between the inferior pharyngeal constrictor muscle above and the cricopharyngeus muscle below (*Fig.* 11.1). The cause of this condition is unknown but

its occurrence in patients over the age of 50 years and rarely in younger people suggests that it is an acquired rather than a congenital condition. However, the constant site of origin of the diverticulum just between the cricopharyngeus muscle and the inferior constrictor pharynx suggests the possibility of an anatomical weak point in the muscular layers as well as some distal obstructive role of the cricopharyngeal sphincter.

The diverticulum is initially small and protrudes either to the left or to the right side, but with increase in size it becomes central. Because of the recurrent pressures involved, and the constant distension of the sac with food, there is rapid increase in size. Its neck overhangs the cricopharyngeus and the sac falls between the oesophagus and the vertebral column, compressing and deflecting the oesophagus anteriorly. Obstruction to swallowing follows and since the mouth of the diverticulum is above the cricopharyngeus, spontaneous emptying is often associated with aspiration into the bronchial tree in addition to regurgitation into the mouth. The chief complications are therefore nutritional and respiratory. Squamous-celled carcinoma may rarely develop within the diverticulum.

This condition is pre-malignant for much the same reason as is achalasia of the cardia, which is the persistent exposure of the mucosa to stagnant food carcinogens.

Oesophagoscopy is dangerous in this condition. It is good practice that oesophagoscopy, with the rigid or flexible instrument, should never be undertaken without excellent barium studies showing the whole of the oesophagus including the cervical portion. Neglect of this advice is the cause of occasional perforation of the pharyngeal pouch, for the oesophagoscope will tend to enter the pouch rather than pass into the oesophagus. When a pouch is not suspected, perforation is then inevitable and will be followed by the most serious complications of continuing leakage into the mediastinum, and mediastinitis.

The Operation

The two important and separate aims of operation are attention to the pouch and division of the cricopharyngeus muscle.

Position of the Patient

The patient lies on his or her back with the head

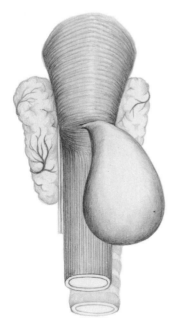

Fig. 11.1. Surgical anatomy of pharyngeal diverticulum.

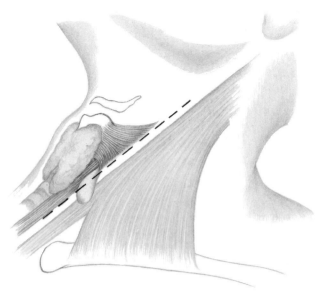

Fig. 11.2. Operative approach for excision of pharyngeal diverticulum.

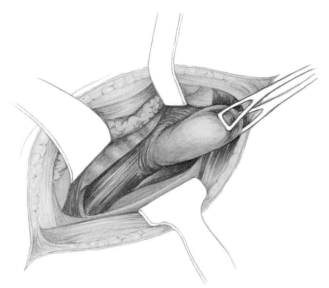

Fig. 11.3. Mobilization and cleaning of pharyngeal diverticulum. The transverse and constricting muscle distal to the diverticulum is well shown.

rotated to the right, the left arm by the side and a small pillow behind and between the shoulder blades. An incision 10 cm long in the line of the anterior border of the sternomastoid muscle, and with its centre at the level of the cricoid cartilage, is ideal for this operation (*Fig.* 11.2). The platysma muscle is incised, as is the deep fascia. The sternomastoid muscle is then retracted posteriorly with the carotid sheath and internal jugular vein. The thyroid gland is retracted anteriorly together with the larynx, and with swab dissection the sac is identified. It should then be cleaned down to the muscular neck, and to facilitate this procedure the pouch may be grasped with light tissue forceps. Care should be taken not to mistake the thyroid gland for the pharyngeal diverticulum. With the sac cleaned, the decision is made whether or not to excise it. Small pouches may be left undisturbed. Large pouches require excision and those of a size between these two extremes may be suspended (*Fig.* 11.3).

Excision of the Sac

It is wise at this stage for the anaesthetist to introduce a no. 30 Fr. gauge gum elastic or plastic bougie into the oesophagus to avoid surgical narrowing at this level, and when the bougie is in place the sac is excised. This may be undertaken either as an open procedure or over a vascular clamp, but in any event the sac must not be excised so enthusiastically that closure can be completed only by narrowing the oesophagus. Closure is undertaken using fine interrupted catgut sutures to the mucosa with a further row of fine interrupted Mersilene sutures to the muscle (*Fig.* 11.4).

Closure is also most elegantly and safely achieved by using the stapler.

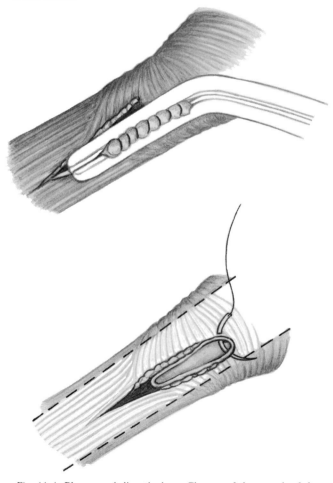

Fig. 11.4. Pharyngeal diverticulum. Closure of the mouth of the excised diverticulum may be undertaken with or without an occluding clamp but it is important that this closure is undertaken over a large intra-oesophageal bougie to prevent narrowing.

Diverticulopexy

Moderate-sized pouches need not be excised, for if cricopharyngeal myomotomy is adequately undertaken the suspended pouch will drain well. The dissected pouch is drawn up posteriorly to the pharynx and tacked by a series of interrupted fine sutures to the prevertebral fascia (*Fig.* 11.5).

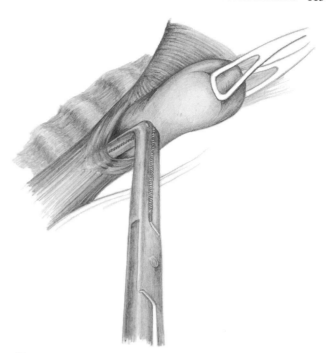

Fig. 11.6. Pharyngeal diverticulum. Cricopharyngeal myomotomy.

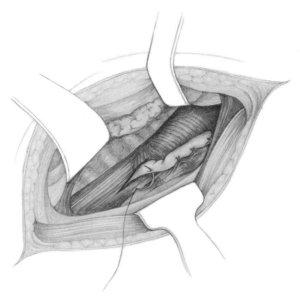

Fig. 11.5. Small pharyngeal diverticula may be sutured to the prevertebral fascia.

Cricopharyngeal Myomotomy

This is probably the most important part of the operation and for many patients pharyngeal diverticulectomy is unnecessary. Certainly no matter how thoroughly the pouch is removed, failure to deal with the cricopharyngeus muscle will result either in early postoperative fistula formation or in late recurrence of the pouch, together with its symptoms. A curved artery forceps is gently insinuated between the oesophageal mucosa and the cricopharyngeus muscle and passed slowly distally, opening and closing the instrument carefully (*Fig.* 11.6). The muscle readily separates from the underlying mucosa and is then cut with scissors (*Fig.* 11.7). It is advisable to cut this muscle for a length of at least 2 cm to ensure a satisfactory result. The platysma and skin are closed and a soft corrugated drain is passed down to the site of operation.

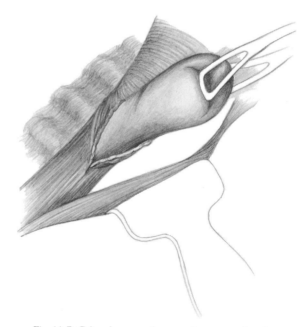

Fig. 11.7. Cricopharyngeal myomotomy completed.

Postoperative Management

The patient is allowed fluids in small amounts on the 1st and 2nd postoperative days, progressing to soft foods from the 3rd day onwards. A normal diet is resumed by the 7th day.

Complications

A combination of inadequate suture of the neck of the pouch and inadequate attention to the cricopharyngeus muscle is the cause of fistula formation. Although these salivary fistulas rarely cause mediastinitis, and tend to close spontaneously, this complication may be attended by the later recurrence of symptoms and of the pouch. Should the fistula fail to close, it is likely that the distal spastic obstruction of the cricopharnygeus muscle will need attention. In the presence of induration and sepsis, approaching the cricopharyngeus muscle from the contralateral side should be considered.

Other operations have been practised for this condition, one of which, the peroral diathermy excision of the septum or common wall between the diverticulum and oesophagus, was popular among some surgical groups. The effect of this procedure is to divide the cricopharyngeus muscle posteriorly, but of course this does not deal with the sac, which if large and dependent will continue to compress the oesophagus. This procedure appears to have no advantage over the operation described above and certainly is not free of the risks of cervical cellulitis, mediastinitis and recurrence. It is not recommended and is considered obsolete.

2. ACHALASIA OF THE CARDIA

This disease is characterized by (1) poor or absent oesophageal peristalsis and by (2) failure of relaxation of the lower end of the oesophagus.

Thus it is that any operation is usually palliative, for the disorder of motility cannot be overcome by surgery. Furthermore, the liability of up to 10 per cent of these patients to carcinoma of the oesophagus, whether or not the achalasia is surgically treated, invites both careful operation and close long-term follow-up.

Preoperative Investigations

Barium Swallow

The oesophagus may be almost normal in size or gigantic with a large sigmoid loop at the lower end, and between these two extremes there are many variations. The poor motility of the oesophagus associated with tertiary contractions and failure of relaxation of the lower end of the oesophagus with delayed emptying are characteristic of the condition. Certain drugs such as octyl nitrite and Buscopan (hyoscine butylbromide) will relax the lower end of the oesophagus in this condition, and if administered during the course of radiological study will demonstrate relaxation and emptying, confirming the diagnosis.

Oesophagoscopy

This is a most important investigation and should be conducted with great care. The oesophagus in this condition often contains a good deal of fluid and decomposing food material which may be readily aspirated into the lungs during the induction of general anaesthesia for oesophagoscopy. For this reason it may be advisable to undertake oesophagoscopy under local anaesthesia supplemented by intravenous diazepam while the patient reclines in a dental chair. Aspiration of oesophageal contents should be conducted using a wide-bore suction catheter, many

of the larger food particles requiring removal with biopsy forceps. It requires considerable patience to clear the oesophagus adequately but this is essential to obtain a good view of the whole of the interior of the oesophagus. Failure to do so and thus obtain excellent visualization of the whole of the interior of the organ will possibly allow a carcinoma to be overlooked. It is indefensible to undertake an operation for achalasia of the cardia in the presence of an undiagnosed carcinoma of the oesophagus.

Oesophageal lavage during oesophagoscopy, if attempted at all, should be undertaken with very great care, for it is only too easy for fluid and decomposing food to find their way into the air passages.

Treatment

Regular dilatation by self-bouginage is mentioned only to be discarded as a modern treatment. This method was introduced early in this century when operative treatment was either not available or was extremely dangerous, and it would be difficult nowadays to select the patient able to undertake self-bouginage who was otherwise unfit for corrective surgery. Regular dilatation at oesophagoscopy is of such limited benefit that it is not recommended, and furthermore it is in these patients that the risk of eventual perforation of the oesophagus during dilatation is unacceptably high.

Treatment with the Hydrostatic Bag

The treatment of achalasia by rupture of the constricting muscular fibres, using Negus' modification of Tucker's bag, has in the past been used with varying degrees of success. In some hands, nearly two-thirds of the patients treated with a hydrostatic dilator have been reported to have good to excellent results over an average follow-up period of about 10 years. Although few deaths have been reported there is good evidence that the complication rate is extremely high, and many patients have required surgical intervention because of inadvertent rupture of the distal oesophagus. While clearly a valuable form of treatment in some hands, this method is not without serious risk, and usually must be repeated to be effective. Hydrostatic dilatation was introduced as the natural successor to regular bouginage by the patient, and preceded the development of the safe, modern operation. With surgical procedures carrying minimal risk, forcible dilatation using the hydrostatic bag can no longer be seriously recommended as a method of treatment, although no doubt specialists in their use will continue to use these instruments for some time to come.

Operative Treatment

Many historic operations to relieve achalasia have been described, which usually involved destruction of the lower oesophageal sphincter with disastrous results. Although initially successful in relieving dysphagia, these procedures were often complicated by the development of severe reflux oesophagitis, and further dysphagia from this cause. For this reason, apart from the operation described by Heller (1913), the majority of these procedures have been abandoned. Von Mikulicz, in 1904, described four patients in whom he had dilated the cardiac sphincter and lower 5 cm of the oesophagus by introducing his hand into the stomach and then inserting the fingers into the oesophagus, gradually dilating it until the sphincter was ruptured. After dilatation, the stomach was closed. This became a popular operation in the first quarter of the present century but it is open to many obvious criticisms, the main complication, frequently fatal, being rupture of the lower end of the oesophagus followed by mediastinitis or peritonitis. Furthermore, digital dilatation failed to relieve the obstruction in over 25 per cent of the cases thus treated. It seems unlikely that this operation is practised today.

Oesophago-gastrostomy, undertaken by side-to-side anastomosis between the dilated oesophagus and the fundus of the stomach, was also practised early in this century, but although dysphagia was readily relieved the resultant severe reflux oesophagitis proved such a serious drawback that this operation was also abandoned.

HELLER'S OPERATION (EXTRA MUCOUS
OESOPHAGOCARDIOMYOMOTOMY)

This operation was first described in 1913 and Heller made two longitudinal incisions, an anterior and a posterior one, to ensure thorough division of all the constricting circular muscle fibres.

In 1923 Zaaiger modified this procedure, considering that an anteriorly placed incision through the coats of the oesophagus and stomach down to the mucous membrane was all that was needed to produce a cure.

Patients submitted to Heller's operation may be comparatively fit or in an extreme state of malnutrition and dehydration. Clearly this latter group of patients needs careful parenteral feeding and rehydration before an operation is contemplated, and in several instances of advanced wasting and dehydration the author has used preliminary feeding gastrostomy for several weeks to prepare the patient for operation.

The operation may be performed via the abdomen or using the transthoracic route. The transthoracic route has many advantages, not the least being the more ready access to the oesophagus and upper stomach, enabling the surgeon to undertake a more careful and complete oesophagomyomotomy. There is less likelihood of perforating the oesophageal mucosa via the thoracic approach than when using the more difficult exposure from the abdomen. Further-

more, the hiatus is more readily repaired following myomotomy from above than below.

The right lateral position is used with the left chest uppermost. The skin incision is made along the line of the 7th rib and reaches almost to the costal margin. The chest is opened through the bed of the 7th rib and, following retraction of the lung forwards and the diaphragm downwards, the oesophagus is mobilized from the hiatus as high as the inferior pulmonary vein and encircled with a rubber catheter (*Fig.* 11.8).

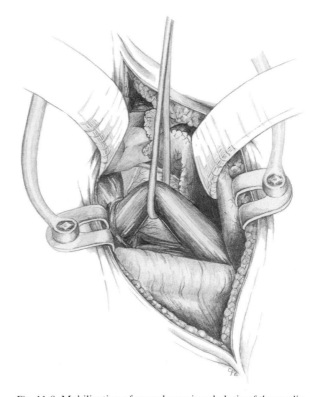

Fig. 11.8. Mobilization of oesophagus in achalasia of the cardia.

Although the oesophagus in many patients looks remarkably normal, it is usual that distal to the oesophageal dilatation the organ is very narrowed and the muscle is very thickened. The aim of myomotomy is to incise both the longitudinal and circular muscles of the oesophagus along its lower 10 cm, completely dividing the hypertrophied musculature above the pathological constriction and dividing the pathological constriction itself, allowing the mucosa to bulge freely through the incision, and it is important to avoid perforation of the mucosa (*Fig.* 11.9). It was formerly routine practice to divide the muscle over the upper 2 or 3 cm of the stomach in addition to dividing the oesophageal muscle, with a resulting 8–10 cm length of oesophageal and gastric mucosa, pouting through the incision. More recently, however, it is held that dividing the gastric muscle is both unnecessary and illogical for there seems to be no reason for the gastric muscle to hypertrophy and there is also no evidence that the neuromuscular

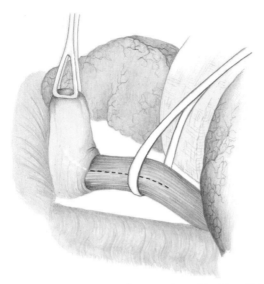

Fig. 11.9. Achalasia of the cardia, oesophageal incision. It is not considered necessary to continue this incision over the stomach; the constricting element terminates at the cardia.

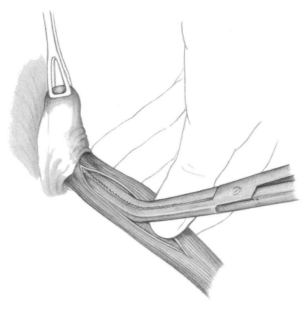

Fig. 11.10. Achalasia of the cardia. Blunt dissection separating the two muscle layers from the mucosa prior to extramucous oesophagomyomotomy.

incoordination involves gastric muscle. The mobilization of the hiatus and the disruption of the phreno-oesophageal ligament made necessary by such an extended myotomy may in some patients produce gastro-oesophageal reflux.

It is fortunate that the muscle layers of the oesophagus are separated from the submucous layer by a well-defined space which is amenable to blunt dissection and separation. The oesophagus is supported by the index finger and an incision is made longitudinally into the oesophageal mucosa using a scalpel or blunt-ended scissors until the oesophageal mucosa pouts into view. Either side of the mucosa, the muscle is then gently grasped using tissue forceps. A right-angled vascular clamp is then insinuated distally between the muscle layers and the mucosa, gently opening and closing the instrument, and when the muscle is readily separated from the mucosa it is then incised (*Fig.* 11.10). The instrument is again introduced and the procedure repeated down to the cardia. Although the muscle is readily separated from the mucosa of the oesophagus, it unfortunately becomes much more adherent at the cardia and over the stomach, and great care is required for it is in this situation that perforation of the mucous membrane is liable to occur. While dividing the muscle numerous small blood vessels in the muscular and submucous venous plexus will be divided and these will produce a certain amount of bleeding. The majority of this will cease with patient pressure using a swab, although some of these vessels may require ligation. Diathermy should be avoided in this area, lest the mucosa is inadvertently coagulated with the danger of later necrosis and fistula formation.

Following the completed myotomy the site of operation should be very carefully inspected for residual undivided constricting circular fibres, for if over-

looked these will eventually hypertrophy and cause further symptoms and recurrence of the condition (*Fig.* 11.11). Accidental perforation of the mucosa of the stomach or the oesophagus during this opera-

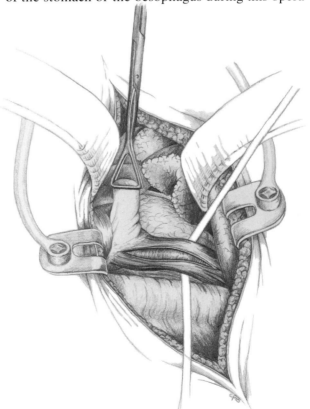

Fig. 11.11. Achalasia of the cardia. The bulging mucosa protrudes through the completed myotomy.

tion is a serious mishap. The mucosa is of the consistency of thin parchment and perforations are extremely difficult to repair using even the finest suture material. Nevertheless, attempts must be made to close these perforations. In the unhappy event of a small perforation becoming considerably larger during an attempt at closure the consequences must be assessed realistically, for clearly the fistula cannot be left to heal of its own accord. Resuture of the muscle layer over the perforation would, of course, vitiate the operation. In these circumstances it might be necessary to consider oesophago-gastrectomy with oesophago-gastric anastomosis at the level of the aortic arch, or short-segment colon replacement.

During myomotomy it is possible that associated manipulations at the cardia may result in the patient developing symptoms of gastro-oesophageal reflux with possible oesophagitis and stricture formation. Since it is impossible to predict which patients will develop gastro-oesophageal reflux following Heller's operation, it is the practice of some surgeons to perform an anti-reflux manoeuvre following the myomotomy (*Figs.* 11.12 and 11.13).

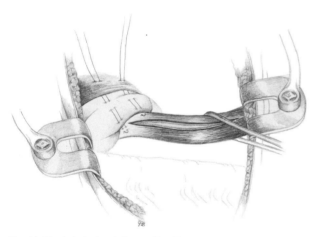

Fig. 11.12. Achalasia of the cardia. Should the hiatus be disturbed during this operation, repair of the hiatus should be undertaken.

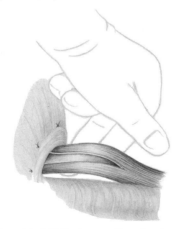

Fig. 11.13. Completed Heller's operation showing reduction and repair of cardia.

Complications: The important immediate complication, that of fistula formation, should be avoided if perforations of the mucosa are noted and dealt with at the time of operation. Should a fistula develop postoperatively, the safest method of dealing with this is to undertake immediate oesophago-gastrectomy.

Late Dysphagia: Dysphagia may recur from immediately postoperatively to more than 20 years following Heller's operation, and is due to one of three causes:

a. Failure to relieve achalasia: This is caused by the persistence of a few circular fibres that were not divided at the original operation. These few fibres hypertrophy over the years and will produce early or late recurrence. The diagnosis is made at barium meal examination when the typical appearance of achalasia of the cardia is again seen. The treatment of the condition is a further myomotomy, where the offending fibres are identified and divided.

b. Peptic stricture due to reflux oesophagitis: The occurrence of late dysphagia due to peptic stricture of the oesophagus was more commonly noted in the past, following Heller's operation, than it is now the operation is associated with an anti-reflux operation. These strictures are usually unresponsive to dilatation and often require surgical treatment, usually oesophago-gastrectomy or colon interposition.

c. Carcinoma of the oesophagus: Achalasia of the cardia is a pre-malignant condition. It is presumably due to the prolonged overexposure of the oesophageal mucosa to carcinogenic agents in food, which remain in the oesophagus for longer periods than in the normal oesophagus with rapid transit time. The development of dysphagia due to carcinoma of the oesophagus associated with achalasia of the cardia, either before myomotomy or after operation, is of very serious significance. These patients are accustomed to dysphagia and do not complain until the dysphagia is almost complete. In view of the large oesophagus, the carcinoma will have grown to a very large size before dysphagia is an important symptom, and it is almost invariably found that once diagnosed these tumours are inoperable.

Surgical Management of Very Advanced Achalasia of the Cardia

When the oesophagus is very dilated and the lower end is a sigmoid sump, it is clear that Heller's operation is unlikely to drain the oesophagus adequately. In these patients consideration should be given to the operation of oesophago-gastrectomy, excising the lower third of the oesophagus and the upper two-thirds of the stomach, and anastomosing the stomach to the oesophagus at the level of the aortic arch. An alternative procedure is to resect the lower 5 cm of the oesophagus and to rejoin the oesophagus to the cardia below the diaphragm.

Abdominal Approach to Achalasia of the Cardia

Although the author considers the thoracic approach a superior and safer approach for the performance of Heller's operation, some gastroenterological surgeons continue to favour the abdominal approach.

Through a left upper paramedian incision or a midline incision above the umbilicus the cardia and lower oesophagus may be readily identified, although excellent retraction and good relaxation anaesthesia are necessary. The left triangular ligament of the liver is divided, following which the peritoneum over the intra-abdominal oesophagus is incised, enabling a tape to be passed round the lower oesophagus. Using blunt and sharp dissection the lower 5–8 cm of the oesophagus can then be drawn into the abdomen. Care is taken to avoid damaging the anterior or left vagus nerve, and the procedure for extramucous oesophago-gastric myomotomy is identical to that when using the thoracic approach. In view of the difficulty of access via the abdomen, it is important to ensure that the oesophageal mucosa has not been perforated during this procedure and it is advisable to undertake an anti-reflux operation.

3. OESOPHAGEAL DIVERTICULUM

False diverticula may occur anywhere in the oesophagus and give rise to a variety of symptoms, including dysphagia, haematemesis and retrosternal pain. These diverticula are often associated with hypermotility of the oesophagus, the diverticulum being as it were a mucosal blow-out above a spastic area of musculature.

Surgical Treatment

It is dangerous to excise the diverticulum without attention to the spastic muscle at its neck, and such diverticula should be treated similarly to pharyngeal diverticula. The small diverticulum need not be excised, the operation being limited to an extensive extramucous oesophagomyomotomy below the diverticulum (*Fig.* 11.14). However, some of these diverticula are extremely large, reaching down almost to the diaphragm—so called 'epiphrenic diverticula'—and in these patients excision is inevitable. Nevertheless, very great care must be taken in closing the neck of the diverticulum and ensuring an adequate oesophagomyomotomy distally, for in the presence of residual obstruction the suture line will possibly give way with most serious consequences.

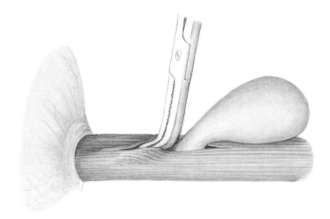

Fig. 11.14. Oesophageal diverticulum. Extramucous separation of oesophageal muscle.

4. DIFFUSE SPASM OF THE OESOPHAGUS

Hypermotility of the oesophagus or diffuse oesophageal spasm is often associated with hypertension of the lower oesophageal sphincter, and this condition may be associated with oesophageal diverticula. In these patients oesophageal motility studies demonstrate high-amplitude non-peristaltic contractions of the body of the oesophagus in response to swallowing, and pressures at the lower sphincter may be normal or elevated. The condition does not appear to be related to achalasia of the cardia. Pain is a more prominent symptom than is dysphagia, being typically substernal and often radiating through to the back, the neck or even into the arms, suggesting angina pectoris. The pain may be spontaneous or produced by eating. Oesophageal radiography will usually show advanced spasm of the whole oesophagus, the so-called 'corkscrew' oesophagus. In selected patients, extramucous oesophagomyomotomy of the whole oesophagus sometimes produces relief of symptoms, but the condition seems less amenable to good surgical relief than does achalasia of the cardia. Following myomotomy it may be wise to complete the operation with an anti-reflux procedure, as in the modified Heller's operation, to prevent gastro-oesophageal reflux and late stricture formation. Operation is best undertaken through the right side of the chest, when division of the azygos vein will expose the oesophagus from the thoracic inlet to the cardia (*Fig.* 11.15).

It is important in patients with diffuse oesophageal spasm to ascertain that their symptoms are not due to the irritation caused by gastro-oesophageal reflux, for in these patients repair of the hiatus hernia should cure the oesophageal symptoms.

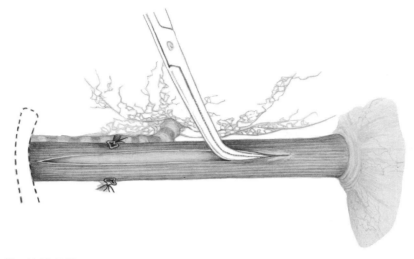

Fig. 11.15. Diffuse oesophageal spasm. Extensive extramucous oesophagomyomotomy.

FURTHER READING

Belsey R. (1966) Functional disease of the oesophagus. *J. Thorac. Cardiovasc. Surg.* **52**, 164–188.

Browne D. C. and McHardy G. (1939) A new instrument for use in oesophagospasm. *JAMA* **113**, 1963–1964.

Dohlman G. and Mattsson O. (1959). The role of the cricopharyngeal muscle in cases of hypopharyngeal diverticula: a cineroentgenographic study. *Am. J. Roentgenol. Rad. Ther. Nucl. Med.* **81**, 561–569.

Ellis F. H., Jr, Code C. F. and Olsen A. M. (1960) Long oesophagomyotomy for diffuse spasm of oesophagus and hypertensive gastroesophageal sphincter. *Surgery* **48**, 155–168.

Ellis F. H., Jr, and Olsen A. M. (1969) Achalasia of the oesophagus: major problems. In: *Clinics in Surgery*, Vol. 9. Philadelphia, Saunders, p. 221.

Ellis F. H., Jr, Schlegal J. F., Lynch V. P. et al. (1969) Cricopharyngeal myotomy for pharyngo-oesophageal diverticulum. *Ann. Surg.* **170**, 340–349.

Heller E. (1913) Extramuköse Cardioplastic beim chronischen Cardiospasmus mit Dilatation des Oesophagus. *Mitt. Grenzgeb. Med. Chir.* **27**, 141–149.

Kurlander D. T., Raskin H. F., Kirsner J. B. et al. (1963) Therapeutic value of the pneumatic dilator in achalasia of the oesophagus: long term results in 62 living patients. *Gastroenterology* **45**, 604–613.

von Mikulicz J. (1904) *Dtsch. Med. Wochenschr.* Jan-Feb.

Moersch H. J. and Camp J. D. (1934) Diffuse spasm of the lower part of the oesophagus. *Ann. Otol. Rhinol. Laryngol.* **43**, 1165–1173.

Negus V. E. (1950) Pharyngeal diverticula: observations on their evolution and treatment. *Br. J. Surg.* **38**, 129–146.

Payne W. S. and Clagett O. T. (1965) Pharyngeal and oesophageal diverticula. *Curr. Probl. Surg.* April, 1–31.

Payne W. S., Ellis F. H., Jr, and Olsen A. M. (1960) Achalasia of the oesophagus: a follow-up study of patients undergoing oesophagomyotomy. *Arch. Surg.* **81**, 411–417.

Payne W. S., Ellis F. H., Jr, and Olsen A. M. (1961) Treatment of cardiospasm (achalasia of the oesophagus) in children. *Surgery* **50**, 731–735.

Vinson P. P. (1934) Diverticula of the thoracic portion of the oesophagus: report of 42 cases. *Arch. Otolaryngol.* **19**, 508–513.

Wychulis A. R., Gunnlaugsson G. H. and Clagett O. T. (1969) Carcinoma occurring in pharyngoesophageal diverticulum: report of three cases. *Surgery* **66**, 976–979.

Chapter twelve

Peptic Ulcer: Resection Procedures

R. E. May

INTRODUCTION

'Peptic ulcer' is a term used to cover ulceration related to peptic secretions. It may occur in the oesophagus, stomach and duodenum. Less frequently it may be found in relation to a stoma or in association with gastric mucosa in a Meckel's diverticulum. Schwartz's 'No acid—no ulcer' has been the basic thesis of all those interested in peptic ulceration. The ulcer formula is one of auto-digestive power of gastric juice versus the resistance of mucus.

The evidence available in Britain generally shows that peptic ulcer has become a less frequent problem. Overall mortality and admission rates for gastric and duodenal ulcer have fallen in the past 20 years in England and Wales. This fall has been most obvious in men and has been particularly pronounced for duodenal ulcer in recent years. Perforation rates for gastric ulcer and duodenal ulcer have also fallen in men but not much in women. Similar findings have been recorded in the USA (Vogt and Johnson, 1980).

The management of peptic ulcer has changed radically in the past decade. Medical treatment has been strengthened by the discovery and availability of H_2 receptor antagonist drugs. The surgical management has also changed. Where partial gastrectomy was once favoured in the treatment of this common problem, recently more emphasis has been placed on the role of conservative surgery, and vagotomy in one of its many guises is used preferentially in the treatment of chronic duodenal ulcer. The treatment of gastric ulcer is more controversial.

In this chapter the indications for surgery are discussed. The various surgical procedures are described in detail as it is important that the surgeon in training should be familiar with a range of surgical procedures. The complications of these procedures and their management are also discussed.

GASTRIC ULCER

Gastric ulcer may be acute or chronic. Approximately 85 per cent of chronic gastric ulcers are found on or close to the lesser curve, the great majority being closer to the incisura angularis than to the cardia: 12 per cent are found in the antrum, 2 per cent of these in the pyloric canal. Only 3 per cent of chronic gastric ulcers are found at the cardia, whereas 15 per cent of gastric carcinomas are found in this situation. The greater curvature of the stomach, fundus and anterior and posterior walls are the site of only 5 per cent of benign gastric ulcers.

Interest has been focused on acute gastric ulcer as this may be the cause of painless gastrointestinal bleeding. There is no doubt that gastric irritants reduce the efficiency of the mucus barrier and may play an important role in many cases. It is clear, however, that other factors are concerned in the development of what are sometimes called 'stress ulcers'. Alterations in the gastric microcirculation giving local anoxia and loss of function of the mucosal barrier may then allow back-diffusion of hydrogen ions and this may initiate complicated local pharmacological responses (Jones, 1977).

Chronic gastric ulcer develops particularly in patients with chronic atrophic gastritis. This may be due to a primary pyloric sphincter dysfunction which facilitates duodenal reflux and results in a low-grade continuing disruption of the mucus barrier caused by the presence of bile and lysolecithin in the stomach. Secretin and cholecystokinin stimulate the secretion of pancreatic juice and bile into the duodenum. They also cause an increase in pyloric sphincter pressure which inhibits reflux of duodenal contents into the stomach. In patients with gastric ulcer this response to hormonal stimulation may be lacking. By reducing the efficiency of the normal protective gastric mucus barrier, bile may in turn reduce the threshold at which other gastric irritants may cause damage. The step between chronic gastritis and the formation of a chronic gastric ulcer remains a mystery.

Diagnosis

Diagnosis of a chronic gastric ulcer will depend on a complete medical history, clinical examination, usually followed by barium study and upper gastrointestinal tract endoscopy. Barium meal is still probably the commonest initial investigation although in many centres this has been replaced by endoscopy. Fibre endoscopy with its excellent optics and ever-increasing ease of manipulation has revolutionized the diagnosis of peptic ulceration. It will be required in every case of gastric ulcer to obtain a biopsy and histological confirmation of the nature of the ulcer.

Indications for Operation

1. *Relative:*
   a. Failure of medical treatment.
   b. Recurrent gastric ulceration.

c. Combined gastric and duodenal ulceration.

d. Haemorrhage.

Having established that the gastric ulcer is benign, the patient will initially be treated medically. This will involve general measures, including stopping smoking. Bed rest, possibly by reducing pyloric reflux, aids healing but is probably unnecessary if specific drug therapy is used as suggested below. Dietary precautions will involve reduction of fat as this tends to decrease biliary reflux. A proportion of gastric ulcers in some countries, for example Australia and the USA, is due to the consumption of anti-inflammatory drugs. These may act by altering the multiplication or maturation of surface epithelial cells by reducing bicarbonate secretion or altering mucus production and should be discontinued. This would be followed by specific therapy, for example carbenoxolone or H_2 blockers such as cimetidine or ranitidine may be given. More recently sucralfate, which acts by protecting the gastric mucosa from acid-pepsin attacks, has shown promise in initial trials, as has pirenzepine, which is a selective muscarinic anticholinergic drug.

There is no universal agreement on how many times a patient with a recurrence of gastric ulcer should be treated medically before being submitted to surgery. Many surgeons would advise operation after the first recurrence if it developed after as short an interval as a year. Finally, patients with combined duodenal and gastric ulceration have in the past tended to fare badly with medical treatment and have therefore been referred for surgery.

2. *Absolute:*

a. Perforation.

b. Suspicion of malignancy which cannot be excluded by combined clinical and radiological assessment, plus endoscopy and biopsy.

c. Anatomical organic deformity of the stomach owing to stenosing ulceration.

These complications and their management are discussed later in this chapter.

Preoperative Management of Gastric Surgery Patients

General

A full medical history and clinical examination are necessary to exclude disease in other systems. In particular, in any patient over 50 years of age a cardiovascular assessment is important and a baseline preoperative ECG is advisable. A chest radiograph, full blood count, urea and electrolytes are also useful baseline information prior to embarking on major surgery. If there is any history of liver disease or abnormal bleeding tendencies, in addition to the full blood count, a platelet count, prothrombin time and liver function tests should be performed.

Sputum retention is common after upper abdominal surgery and to minimize this, cessation of smoking for a minimum of 2 weeks preoperatively may pay handsome dividends. Heavy smokers must be told in no uncertain terms that failure to do this may result in serious postoperative chest infection and will compound their postoperative pain. Preoperative breathing exercises under the supervision of the physiotherapist will ensure better cooperation in the postoperative period.

Specific Measures

Gastric operations are associated with a high incidence of wound sepsis which is related to the underlying pathology (17 per cent with duodenal ulcer, 38 per cent with gastric ulcer and 56 per cent with gastric carcinoma). Most infections occurring after gastrointestinal surgery are caused by dissemination of organisms present in the lumen of the gastrointestinal tract at the time of operation (Gatehouse et al., 1978). As long ago as 1961, Burke demonstrated in animal studies that antibiotics were only effective in dealing with bacterial contamination for 3 hours following an operation, in other words in the immediate postoperative period. The author favours a single dose of antibiotic, for example a cephalosporin either intramuscularly with the premedication or intravenously with the induction of anaesthesia.

If a midline incision is to be used, it is particularly important that a thorough cleansing of the umbilicus be performed. A variety of organisms can be cultured from the umbilicus and in the elderly not infrequently calcified debris may be found. The chances of auto-infection from the skin may be reduced by thorough cleansing of the umbilicus with a skin disinfectant, e.g. 0·5 per cent chlorhexidine in 70 per cent spirit, and this may be carried out 1 hour preoperatively at the time of the premedication injection. Low-dose subcutaneous heparin (5000 units 8-hourly) may be used as a prophylaxis against deep venous thrombosis and pulmonary embolism in patients over 40 years. The first dose is given preoperatively and continued for 5 postoperative days. Its value has been disputed (Immelman et al., 1979) but in patients with a history of deep venous thrombosis or pulmonary embolism it would seem a sensible precaution.

Incision and Exposure in Gastric Surgery

The patient is placed in the supine position with the table tilted so that the head is slightly raised. A vertical upper abdominal midline incision is preferred by the author, and the incision should be made from the xiphisternum to the umbilicus. This incision is excellent for virtually all gastric surgery. Transverse or oblique incisions do not allow adequate exposure near the oesophageal hiatus in all patients. On occasion they may be combined with a vertical midline incision carried to the xiphisternum (an inverted T).

The midline incision is superior to the paramedian incision, first with regard to speed of entry which may be important, e.g. in cases of haemorrhage, and, second, closure of the abdomen is more secure as there is one good, firm fibrous layer for stitching as opposed to two rather flimsy fascial layers.

Having opened the abdomen, a retractor may be inserted to aid the initial careful laparotomy which must be carried out before starting any intra-abdominal procedure. Having confirmed the presence of the peptic ulcer, some surgeons favour the insertion of a self-retaining retractor either of the Balfour or Denis Browne variety. This is necessary in the absence of a second assistant but to prevent damage to the abdominal wall by pressure and dehydration a pack soaked in aqueous chlorhexidine (1 in 2000) is folded over the whole length of the incision on either side prior to insertion of the self-retaining retractor.

Choice of Operation for Benign Gastric Ulcer

1. Billroth-I gastrectomy.
2. Polya gastrectomy below a benign gastric ulcer (Kelling–Madlener operation).
3. Truncal vagotomy and drainage plus biopsy or resection of the ulcer.
4. Highly selective vagotomy plus biopsy or resection of the ulcer (see Chapter 13).

Partial gastrectomy has for many years been the most commonly performed operation for benign gastric ulcer. It had the advantage of removing at the same time the ulcer, the pylorus and the antrum. Thus the pathological lesion plus all the susceptible mucosa, as well as the site of the most favoured aetiological factors, are eliminated. Unfortunately, while this procedure has the advantage of giving a very low incidence of recurrent disease, the disadvantages are the mortality attached to a major procedure, and the problems associated with rapid gastric emptying. After gastric resection for gastric ulcer, the gastric remnant may be anastomosed to the duodenum or the jejunum. In the type 1 lesser curve gastric ulceration, the gastric remnant can with safety be anastomosed to the duodenum. In the type 3 (pre-pyloric ulcer) or the type 2 (combined gastric and duodenal ulcer or deformity) the acid secretion is often high and it is imperative to use a gastrojejunal anastomosis because the Billroth-I gastrectomy would be associated with a high incidence of recurrent ulceration. In general it may be said that approximately 70 per cent of gastric ulcers may be resected with a Billroth-I gastrectomy, in some cases coupled with a Pauchet manoeuvre. The latter is a modification of the Schoemaker operation.

Prior to the emergence of vagotomy in the treatment of gastric ulcer, the very high gastric ulcer presented a problem because of the high morbidity and mortality of resection. Kelling (1917–1918) and later Madlener (1923) described a 75 per cent gastric resection distal to the ulcer and anastomosis of the cut end of the gastric pouch to the first loop of the proximal jejunum. The benign ulcer which was left *in situ* would heal under these circumstances. Clearly if this procedure was contemplated, preoperative or peroperative gastric biopsy would be required to confirm that the ulcer was indeed benign.

In recent years vagotomy has been used increasingly in the treatment of gastric ulceration but until recently the results have been somewhat inferior to those of partial gastrectomy. The recurrence rate of gastric ulceration after vagotomy and pyloroplasty alone has been 5–13 per cent and for this reason in most centres partial gastrectomy has held pride of place in treatment with recurrence rates of 0–5 per cent. There are, however, as previously mentioned, other postgastrectomy symptoms occurring after Billroth procedure, although fewer than after a gastrojejunal (Polya) anastomosis. Many of the postprandial symptoms are attributed to lack of control of gastric emptying. The operative mortality of partial gastrectomy may be low in specialized units but the accepted world mortality is of the order of 2 per cent and may reach 4–5 per cent even in good units. In contrast the mortality of vagotomy is about 1 per cent.

In the past 15 years it has been suggested that vagotomy should be preferred to gastrectomy in selected patients with gastric ulcer (Kennedy et al., 1972), namely poor-risk patients, some patients with an ulcer high on the lesser curve in whom gastrectomy would be difficult and hazardous, and in many patients with a bleeding gastric ulcer. If vagotomy is used, multiple biopsies should be taken or the ulcer excised completely to establish that it is benign. Recently there have been several reports of series of either truncal vagotomy and drainage or highly selective vagotomy with excision of the ulcer (Cade and Allan, 1979; Duthie and Bransom, 1979). This procedure gains the security of a histological study of the full ulcer area, but by insisting on excision of the ulcer one of the advantages of conservative surgery has been abandoned. The symptomatic results have been good but the anticipated decreased recurrence rate of gastric ulcer does not seem to have been realized to date (Duthie and Bransom, 1979). The place of highly selective vagotomy in the treatment of gastric ulcer is further discussed (see Chapter 13).

Operative Technique

1. *Billroth-I Gastrectomy*

If the site of the gastric ulcer is not obvious and difficult to locate by palpation, a small suture may be placed into the serosal surface of the stomach over its superior border so that the mobilization can be performed without constant reference back to the site of the ulcer by palpation. If, however, the ulcer is adherent to the liver or pancreas, and is pinched off, this may leave a hole in the stomach which can be temporarily closed with a few stitches. The granulating base of the ulcer is left alone.

The stomach is initially mobilized at the greater curve by making an opening through an avascular area of the gastrocolic omentum. This hole is enlarged laterally in both directions by clamping, dividing and ligating the gastrocolic omentum on the colic side of the gastro-epiploic arch (*Fig.* 12.1).

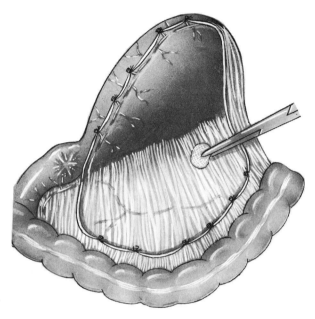

Fig. 12.1. Billroth-I partial gastrectomy. Initial mobilization of greater curvature of the stomach with preservation of the gastro-epiploic arch.

The transverse mesocolon is very closely applied to the back of the stomach and it is very easy to damage the middle colic artery unless the mesocolon is identified and pushed downwards away from the site of dissection as soon as the initial hole in the gastrocolic omentum is made. To the right, the dissection is taken to the inferior border of the pylorus, the main right gastro-epiploic vessels being ligated in this region. To the left, the site of resection on the greater curve of the stomach is estimated and the vessels are divided up to this level. For 2 cm above and below this position the vessels are individually ligated on the greater curve of the stomach as opposed to outside the gastro-epiploic arch. The right gastric vessels are then identified on the superior border of the duodenum running to the left in the free edge of the lesser omentum and are divided between artery forceps and ligated.

The filamentous lesser omentum is divided proximally, feeling for and preserving an accessory hepatic artery if it is present. The lesser curve is then cleaned over a 1-cm length, 2 cm proximal to the upper edge of the ulcer. This necessitates dividing the descending branches of the left gastric artery and its accompany-

ing veins, plus the nerve of Latarjet. This is best done by inserting a pair of blunt dissecting forceps through the lesser omentum directly on to the wall of the stomach. The tissue is then divided between two non-absorbable ties placed with the aid of an aneurysm needle. The duodenum may now be divided just distal to the pylorus. A Payr clamp may be used on the stomach and the duodenum may be held in a Lang–Stevenson or similar clamp. The pyloric end of the stomach is held and a further Payr clamp is applied at right angles to the greater curve approximately halfway along the greater curve. Prior to placing this clamp, the Ryle's tube if present in the stomach should be withdrawn into the fundus so that it will not be caught in the clamps. A Lang–Stevenson clamp is then applied parallel and just proximal to the Payr clamp. The stomach is divided halfway across between the clamps (*Fig.* 12.2). A curved

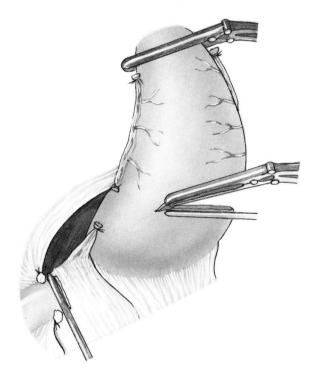

Fig. 12.2. Billroth-I partial gastrectomy. Partial division of stomach between clamps, prior to application of Parker–Kerr clamps to reconstruct the 'lesser curve'.

Parker–Kerr clamp is arranged to grasp the stomach from the tip of the Lang–Stevenson clamp and curving up to cross the lesser curve of the stomach about 1 cm above the ulcer. A second Parker–Kerr clamp is applied just distally and the stomach divided between these two clamps, thus removing the antrum and a piece of lesser curve, including the ulcer.

The new 'lesser curve' of stomach will be formed from the stomach in the Parker–Kerr clamp and this may be closed with an over-and-over 2/0 catgut atraumatic suture. This suture is tightened as the clamp is released and withdrawn. The first layer of

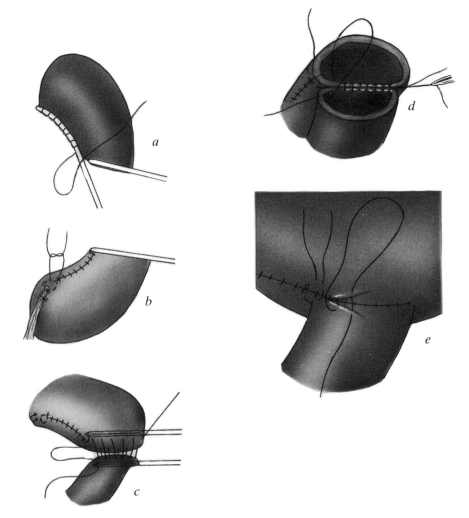

Fig. 12.3. Billroth-I partial gastrectomy. *a,* The gastric remnant is held by a Lang–Stevenson clamp (across the segment for duodenal anastomosis) and a Parker–Kerr clamp (over the newly fashioned lesser curve). *b,* The newly formed lesser curve is closed with a final continuous seromuscular suture, taking particular care to invert fully at the proximal end. *c,* The stomach and duodenum are approximated and a continuous posterior seromuscular suture is inserted, beginning at the greater curve. *d,* The duodenal and gastric clamps are removed and a continuous all-layers suture is inserted posteriorly and carried anteriorly to complete the anastomosis. *e,* The completed operation to show careful inversion at the junction of lesser curve and duodenal closure.

sutures may be invaginated by second seromuscular 2/0 catgut (metric 3·5) suture (*Fig.* 12.3*a,b*).

The distal part of the stomach included in the Lang–Stevenson clamp is then approximated to the duodenum held in a similar clamp. If there is any tension the duodenum may be mobilized by a Kocher manoeuvre. This initial posterior seromuscular Lembert suture is of 2/0 chromic catgut and is best inserted with clamps held a few centimetres apart, starting from the greater curve and working up to the lesser curve side of the stomach, and then the suture is tightened (*Fig.* 12.3*c*). The clamps are then removed. The posterior wall of the stomach and duodenum are then sutured with an all-layers 2/0 catgut suture again working from the greater to lesser curve aspect (*Fig.* 12.3*d*). Great care is taken at the upper border where the other suture line is encountered.

Good inversion is required and this may be best provided by one or two Connell sutures. The suture line is then completed across the anterior wall of the stomach and duodenum by an over-and-over inverting suture or, if there is no serious bleeding, by continuing the Connell suture. The original posterior seromuscular suture is then completed across the front of the stomach and duodenum. An extra catgut suture may help to support the critical angle and obviate any leak (*Fig.* 12.3*e*).

On completion of the anastomosis a systematic check of the abdomen should be made, having checked that the anastomosis is patent. The spleen should be checked for damage, the omental ties should be dry and the colon should be a good colour if the middle colic artery has not been damaged.

Sometimes a benign ulcer may be encountered on

the posterior wall of the stomach rather than on the lesser curve. The technique described above can still be performed by rotating the walls of the stomach so that the ulcer comes to lie at one edge. This edge is then held with a tissue forceps and the clamps are then applied from the other side in the manner already described and illustrated.

At the conclusion of the operation, a Ryle's tube is positioned in the stomach and the midline incision is closed in one layer with a continuous monofilament nylon suture taking at least 1 cm depth of tissue with 1 cm between the stitches (Jenkins, 1976; Pollock et al., 1979). The skin is closed with interrupted or continuous monofilament nylon (3/0).

POSTOPERATIVE COMPLICATIONS

(a) *Immediate:* Haemorrhage may occur from faulty haemostasis at the suture line in the stomach and in particular from the region of the refashioned lesser curve. Fresh blood in variable quantities will be aspirated up the Ryle's tube.

When haemorrhage does occur from the gastric anastomosis it often stops spontaneously and sedation of the patient coupled with some gentle gastric lavage with ice-cold saline may be all that is required. If the haemorrhage continues and the patient begins to show signs of decompensation despite blood transfusion, it may be necessary to take the patient back to theatre and to partially dismantle the anastomosis to find the bleeding point. Intraperitoneal haemorrhage may occur within the first 24 hours from unidentified damage to the spleen or the slipping of an omental tie. Bleeding from a damaged spleen is occasionally attributed to injudicious retraction. In fact, the end of even a deep retractor is seldom near the spleen. The damage usually results from vigorous traction on the greater curve of the stomach and adjacent transverse colon, tearing one of the small omental adhesions from the lower pole of the spleen. Under these circumstances further surgical intervention is required but splenorrhaphy rather than splenectomy should be attempted if possible (Cooper and Williamson, 1984).

(b) *Delay in Gastric Emptying:* There is always some postoperative oedema at the suture line and if the gastric mucosa is initially thickened there may be a delay in gastric emptying beyond the usual 3–4 days. Large quantities of bile-free gastric aspirate will be obtained. With patience this problem will usually resolve and in the meantime the electrolyte content in the gastric aspirate should be estimated and the appropriate fluid given as an intravenous supplement. Failure to be able to take a normal diet after 5 days will require intravenous hyperalimentation. A Gastrografin swallow may be undertaken to check gastric emptying. If a finger and thumb can be approximated across the stoma at the end of the operation drainage, in the author's experience, will always eventually occur.

(c) *Leakage from the Suture Line:* This may occur after a few days and is usually from the critical angle, i.e. the junction of the lesser curve closure and the gastroduodenal anastomosis. The patient may suddenly complain of upper abdominal pain or alternatively the general condition may insidiously deteriorate with equivocal abdominal signs. A straight radiograph is usually not very helpful because free gas is always present at this stage, but a Gastrografin swallow may confirm the diagnosis. Reoperation is required with excision of the necrotic tissue and conversion to a gastrojejunal anastomosis with closure of the duodenal stump. This complication carries a high mortality, partly because of delay in diagnosis.

REMOTE COMPLICATIONS

(a) *Recurrent Ulceration:* The incidence varies from 0 to 5 per cent in various series. The diagnosis is usually made by endoscopy as barium studies after gastric surgery are difficult and may be frankly misleading. Endoscopy also allows multiple biopsies to be taken. If malignancy can be excluded and if the stoma is patent, recurrent gastric ulceration may be treated by truncal or selective vagotomy rather than by further gastric resection.

(b) *Postgastrectomy Syndromes:* Following gastroduodenal anastomoses, the complications of dumping and bilious vomiting are rare. Diarrhoea, either continuous or episodic, also seems to be less frequent after a Billroth-I than after a Polya gastrectomy. Further discussion of these problems is found later in the chapter.

(c) *Deficiency States:* Many patients after gastric operations may develop deficiencies of iron, vitamin B_{12}, folic acid and other minerals and vitamins essential for bone development. Such deficiencies often develop insidiously and may not present as an obvious clinical syndrome for many years after the original operation. For this reason these deficiency states may escape detection until the patient is severely disabled.

Minor degrees of iron deficiency are extremely common after any gastric surgery. The cause of the iron deficiency is probably not due to diminution of the oral intake of iron but to a combination of impaired absorption and minimal increases in iron losses following gastric surgery. The majority of patients with chronic iron deficiency will respond to simple oral treatment with iron compounds. Instructions to take three tablets of iron 1 day a week on a regular basis will usually obviate the development of iron-deficient anaemia.

Examination of patients 5 years after partial gastrectomy for peptic ulcer shows that between 15 and 60 per cent of patients have low serum levels of B_{12}. This is the result of impaired absorption of vitamin B_{12} due to decreased production of intrinsic factor associated with gastric mucosal atrophy. Postgastrectomy vitamin B_{12} deficiency may be followed by all the complications associated with vitamin B_{12} deficiency from whatever cause.

Folic acid deficiency may also be found after major gastric resection and may be present in 6–12 per cent of patients if serum folic levels are estimated. Clinical manifestations of folic acid deficiency will take longer to become manifest.

(*d*) *Metabolic Bone Disease:* The detection and assessment of metabolic bone disease after gastric operations are more difficult than the assessment of haematological abnormalities. The two major metabolic bone diseases that have been studied are osteomalacia and osteoporosis. Osteomalacia is due to vitamin D deficiency and is probably rare but may occur if there is a poor oral intake of fat-containing foods or if there is malabsorption due to steatorrhoea. If present, extra-oral vitamin D may be given. Osteoporosis is more difficult to assess but where it occurs after gastric operations it is probably due to deficiency of calcium and protein. It appears that bones age earlier in patients after partial gastrectomy.

(*e*) *Malignant Change:* The majority of postgastrectomy patients have an abnormal mucosa when seen endoscopically. Some of these patients develop a mild or moderate dysplasia when the mucosa is examined histologically and it would seem that a proportion of these progress to a malignant change.

2. *Polya Gastrectomy*

As previously mentioned, Polya gastrectomy has in the past been advocated for the very high and benign gastric ulcer (Kelling–Madlener operation)—a 75 per cent gastric resection distal to the ulcer and anastomosis of the cut end of the gastric pouch to the first loop of proximal jejunum. The ulcer, which is left *in situ*, will heal. It has also been used for the treatment of type 2 gastric ulcer (i.e. combined gastric and duodenal ulcer). In both cases vagotomy, biopsy or excision of the ulcer has superseded Polya gastrectomy. The technique of this operation is described in the section on surgery of the duodenal ulcer (p. 127).

3. *Vagotomy and Drainage*

The technique of this operation is described later in this chapter (p. 132) and in Chapter 13. When using this operation for the treatment of gastric ulcer, either biopsy or excision of the gastric ulcer must be performed. Preoperative biopsy of the ulcer may be obtained endoscopically. It has been estimated that probably a minimum of 10 endoscopic biopsies are required from the circumference of the gastric ulcer to be certain of the true histology. A smaller number of biopsies may miss an early area of malignancy. Alternatively, or in addition, the ulcer may

be biopsied at the time of surgery through a gastrotomy. This biopsy may be taken with the aid of a sigmoidoscopic or oesophageal biopsy forceps which obviously obtain a larger piece of tissue for histological examination than one obtains with endoscopic biopsy forceps. Other surgeons excise the ulcer and this may be done by opening the stomach opposite the ulcer and excising the ulcer from the mucosal aspect, the defect being closed with catgut sutures. Alternatively, the ulcer-bearing area may be excised from the serosal aspect.

DUODENAL ULCER

Approximately 75–80 per cent of chronic peptic ulcers are found in the duodenum. More than 90 per cent of chronic duodenal ulcers are found in the first portion of the duodenum. In one postmortem series (Portis and Jaffe, 1938) 85 per cent were found within the first 2 cm of the duodenum, 10 per cent were within the next 3 cm, and the remaining 5 per cent were below the first 5 cm and above the ampulla of Vater. Of those ulcers occurring in the first part of the duodenum, 85 per cent are found on the posterior wall or to have extended from the posterior wall, and may subsequently completely encircle the duodenum. Multiple duodenal ulcers are said to occur in 10 per cent of cases and are usually seen on both anterior and posterior walls. Gastric and duodenal ulceration may occur in the same patient. The development of a duodenal ulcer after the healing of a gastric ulcer is a very rare event. However, Tanner (1954) and Johnson (1951) have noted that a duodenal lesion may well precede a gastric ulcer. Tanner found that the gastric ulcer was active and the duodenal ulcer inactive or healed in 80 per cent of patients, whereas in association with an active duodenal ulcer, the gastric ulcer frequently appeared to be an early lesion.

Diagnosis

Initially a full history must be taken from the patient, coupled with a complete physical examination. The first investigation used to be a barium meal but nowadays many clinicians will instead arrange an upper gastrointestinal tract endoscopy. In the past few years the instruments have become considerably smaller in diameter and these instruments may now be passed without the aid of intravenous sedation. Laboratory investigations have become less important. Gastric analysis is rarely performed, but the serum gastrin assay may be useful in the diagnosis of hypergastrinaemia, e.g. the Zollinger–Ellison syndrome.

Indications for Operation

1. *Relative*
   a. Failure of medical treatment is usually stated as an indication for surgical intervention. In the

past few years medical treatment has been revolutionized by the introduction of H_2 receptor antagonist drugs, e.g. cimetidine and ranitidine. There is no doubt that these drugs can reduce acid secretion as effectively as a surgeon. As a result, the referral rate for surgical treatment of duodenal ulcer has fallen to only half that of 8 years ago. These drugs are ideal for treating the patient who has periodic exacerbation of a duodenal ulcer, e.g. three times a year, but surgical treatment is needed for the patient who is constantly relapsing as soon as the drug is discontinued.

 b. Haemorrhage.

2. *Absolute*
 a. Perforation.
 b. Pyloric stenosis.

These conditions and their management are discussed later in this chapter.

Choice of Operations for Duodenal Ulcer
 1. Polya gastrectomy.
 2. Truncal vagotomy and drainage.
 3. Highly selective vagotomy (*see* Chapter 13).
The aim of any operation for duodenal ulcer is to try to reduce the excessive acid secretion and to try to do this as safely as possible, with the minimum of disturbance of the other normal functions of the stomach and duodenum. Acid secretion may be reduced surgically by vagotomy which will abolish the nervous secretion and will also reduce the antral release of gastrin. Alternatively, antrectomy will abolish gastrin-dependent acid production by the remaining parietal cells but they will still respond to nervous stimulation. Partial gastrectomy, however, will remove the gastrin-producing antrum and a variable number of parietal cells depending on the extent of the gastrectomy.

When partial gastrectomy is used in the treatment of duodenal ulcer, it should involve a gastrojejunal anastomosis, as gastroduodenal anastomosis is associated with a 15 per cent stomal ulcer rate. The Polya type of gastrectomy is an effective treatment of duodenal ulcer. The mortality rate is, however, higher than with vagotomy and drainage and there are other consequences following extensive gastric resection although the stomal ulceration rate is low.

Truncal vagotomy may reduce the gastric secretion by up to 70 per cent of maximum secretion, and thus in many duodenal ulcer patients acid secretion may be reduced to normal levels. Following the pioneer work of Dragstedt in the early 1940s, the operation was introduced but it was soon found that unless coupled with a drainage procedure gastric stasis with foul flatulence and vomiting became an incapacitating problem. This complication having been resolved, the operation of truncal vagotomy and drainage was found to be a safe procedure with a lower mortality (0·6 per cent) than gastrectomy. However, the recurrent ulceration rate was higher. Goligher found that the rate was twice as high. Other figures have varied from 1 to 15 per cent, and this may be due to an incomplete vagotomy.

Heineke–Mikulicz pyloroplasty is the commonest drainage procedure that is performed with vagotomy. A pyloroplasty has the theoretical advantage of preserving the continuity of the duodenal loop and hence the integrity of the various hormonal systems which act on the food as it passes. Occasionally, however, the duodenum may be so scarred as to render a pyloroplasty difficult and dangerous and then a gastroenterostomy is preferable. Tanner prefers an anterior juxtapyloric gastroenterostomy but the classic operation is a posterior gastroenterostomy to the most dependent part of the stomach. Vagotomy combined with antrectomy is a popular operation in the United States because it gives the most complete control of acid secretion. The stomal ulcer rate is the lowest of all procedures. However, the addition of a gastric resection brings the mortality nearer to that of partial gastrectomy, while in the survivors the morbidity is the sum of that of gastric resection and that resulting from vagotomy.

In 1948 bilateral selective vagotomy was described by Jackson, of Ann Arbor, and by Franksson, of Stockholm. This was a more logical procedure than truncal vagotomy because it spared the hepatic and coeliac branches of the vagus which supplied the extragastric viscera. Nevertheless, the whole of the stomach is denervated and the propulsive power of the antral musculature is weakened, hence a drainage procedure is required to avoid gastric stasis. Attempts by Burge in the late 1960s to carry out selective vagotomy without drainage in selected cases failed and were abandoned in favour of highly selective vagotomy.

Prospective randomized trials of truncal and selective vagotomy have shown that the latter leads to significantly fewer incomplete vagotomies and is followed by significantly less diarrhoea. Nevertheless, the overall Visick grading of selective vagotomy has not been significantly better than truncal vagotomy (Kennedy, 1973). Highly selective vagotomy or parietal cell vagotomy was introduced into clinical practice in 1970 by Johnston and Wilkinson of Leeds and by Amdrup and Jensen of Copenhagen. In contrast to other operations for duodenal ulcer, the motor nerve supply to the antrum and pyloric sphincter are left intact by the preservation of the nerves of Latarjet and the pyloric branch of the vagus. The vagotomy is thus confined to the acid-secreting part of the stomach, the parietal cell mass. The antrum, which is left innervated, is alkaline. The hepatic and coeliac branches of the vagus are also preserved.

1. *Polya Gastrectomy*
Although this operation is less frequently performed

for duodenal ulcer at the present time, it is described in detail as the technique forms the basis of the operation for resection of the distal half of the stomach for neoplasm.

The initial mobilization of the stomach is carried out in exactly the same way as for Billroth-I gastrectomy, namely that an opening is made through the gastrocolic omentum in the region of the midline. The posterior wall of the stomach is then identified. This is often adherent to the transverse mesocolon and the latter is separated by pushing it in a downward direction to the right and to the left of the midline, ensuring that the middle colic vessels will not be injured. The gastrocolic omentum is then clamped, divided and ligated in sections on the colic side of the gastro-epiploic arch. If tied in this area, fewer vessels need division and tying than if performed flush on the wall of the greater curve of the stomach. To the right this dissection is taken round to the pylorus. The main gastro-epiploic vessels are tied on the inferior border of the pylorus. To the left the dissection is taken up in the direction of the spleen. When 50 per cent of the greater curve of the stomach has been mobilized, the left main gastro-epiploic vessels are divided and the dissection is then taken right up onto the wall of the greater curve of the stomach. One or two of the short gastric vessels are then divided leaving a 3-cm length of the greater curve of the stomach clean and ready for subsequent resection.

Attention is then turned to the duodenum once again. The right gastric vessels which are usually small are identified and isolated and tied as they run to the left in the lesser omentum just above the duodenal bulb. The filamentous lesser omentum is then divided proximally, ensuring by palpation that an accessory hepatic artery, if present, is preserved. The duodenum is then divided between clamps. The first Payr clamp is placed across the duodenum just distal to the pylorus. The second Payr clamp may be placed across the pylorus or if the tissue is thickened a non-crushing clamp may be applied across the distal stomach. The important point is to ensure that no gastric antral mucosa remains attached to the duodenum.

The duodenal stump may be held up by the Payr clamp and inspected to ensure that it is sufficiently mobile to facilitate easy closure. Frequently, small additional blood vessels need to be ligated on the posterior wall or on the superior and inferior borders of the duodenum. These are divided flush on the wall of the duodenum to avoid damage to adjacent structures such as the common bile duct and the gastroduodenal artery. Closure of the duodenal stump may be further facilitated by performing a Kocher manoeuvre. The stump may be closed by an initial over-and-over suture including the clamp, using a 2/0 atraumatic catgut suture (*Fig.* 12.4). As the clamp is eased out the suture is gradually tightened; the suture line is then buried by inserting a purse-string

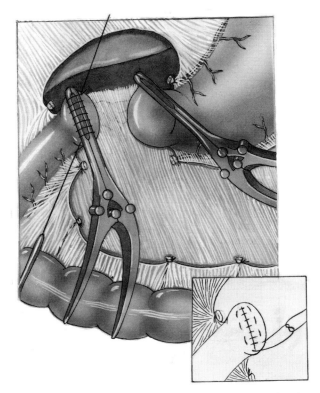

Fig. 12.4. Polya partial gastrectomy. The duodenum has been divided between clamps and the first row of duodenal closure sutures has been placed over the clamp. (Inset shows purse-string seromuscular closure of the duodenal stump.)

suture of 2/0 catgut. If there is sufficient tissue a second purse-string suture will provide a secure three-layer closure. The more difficult duodenal closure is discussed at the end of this section. The stomach is then inspected and the approximate level of resection is estimated. In the absence of pyloric or duodenal stenosis, a 60 per cent resection of the stomach is necessary in duodenal ulcer and will be achieved by placing the right hand on the anterior wall of the stomach, curving the tips of the fingers over the fundus. A resection of the stomach at the level of the base of the thenar eminence of the thumb will give a reasonable gastric remnant (*Fig.* 12.5). However, if the stomach is distended from preoperative obstruction and the same procedure is adopted, the gastric remnant which is left will shrink postoperatively and the patient will have an inadequate gastric reservoir, hence a larger gastric remnant must be left in these circumstances.

Having assessed the site of resection, the antrum of the stomach is held up, tensing the left gastric vessels as they run down close to the lesser curve of the stomach. These vessels are isolated at the level of the proposed resection, underrun and tied (*Fig.* 12.6). The second suture may be added after clamping and dividing the vessels. It is important that the left gastric artery is divided on the stomach wall rather than at its origin from the coeliac axis on the posterior abdominal wall. If this is performed the

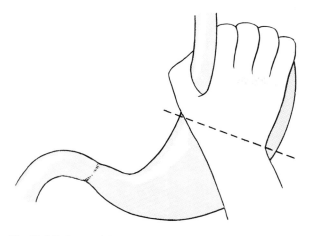

Fig. 12.5. Polya partial gastrectomy. Author's technique for assessing size of gastric remnant.

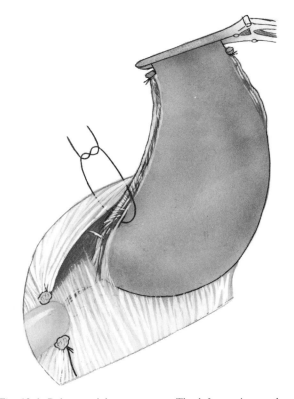

Fig. 12.6. Polya partial gastrectomy. The left gastric vessels are secured and divided close to the stomach. If the left gastric artery is dissected and divided at its origin, the coeliac branch of the vagus nerve will be unnecessarily damaged.

coeliac branch of the posterior vagus nerve may well be damaged. Having cleaned the greater and lesser curves of the stomach at the level of the resection, the stomach is held up and one half of the Lane twin gastroenterostomy clamp is applied, making sure that the nasogastric tube in the stomach is drawn back into the fundus to avoid it being trapped in the clamp. The other half of the twin clamp is applied to the

jejunum, the proximal end being about 5 cm from the duodenojejunal flexure. Before the clamp is applied the surgeon should demonstrate to the first assistant that he or she has indeed isolated the proximal jejunum in his or her hand by demonstrating the duodenojejunal flexure and the proximity of the inferior mesenteric vein. In this way the appalling error of an inadvertent gastro-ileostomy may be avoided. The jejunum is brought up in front of the transverse colon and the clamps united so that the proximal jejunum lies against the lesser curve and the efferent loop against the greater curve of the stomach (*Fig.* 12.7).

The two-layered 2/0 chromic catgut anastomosis is started with a posterior seromuscular Lembert suture joining the adjacent stomach and jejunum. The stomach is then held up and a Payr clamp is applied from the lesser curve to about 5 cm from the greater curve and the stomach is crushed about 1 cm distal to the seromuscular suture. A non-crushing clamp is then applied to the stomach to prevent contamination as the stomach is divided on the Payr clamp (*Fig.* 12.8). The small piece of stomach between the tip of the clamp and the greater curve is cut with care so that the layer nearest to the jejunum is cut 1 cm distal to the posterior seromuscular suture and the other layer is cut in a curved fashion so that the centre is about 2 cm longer. This will facilitate fashioning of the anastomosis (*Fig.* 12.9a).

The segment of stomach in the Payr clamp is then closed to form a valve. This may be achieved using an atraumatic suture and a sewing machine technique (*Fig.* 12.9a). This achieved, a 5-cm hole is made through all coats of the jejunum with diathermy to correspond with the hole in the gastric remnant. The posterior layers are then united with an all-layers 2/0 catgut suture, and the suture is then brought round on to the anterior layer where it is continued as an over-and-over inverting haemostatic suture to complete the inner layer (*Fig.* 12.9b,c). A Connell suture should not be used in this situation as it is not a haemostatic suture and any potential bleeding site will be masked by the clamps.

The Lane clamps are now unlocked, individually released and removed with care as the anastomosis is yet to be completed. This is achieved by continuing the original posterior seromuscular Lembert suture round and across the anterior gastric and jejunal walls back to the starting point. Having completed the anastomosis, it is inspected from the front and the back and any imperfections or bleeding points may be reinforced with an extra interrupted 2/0 catgut suture.

The anastomosis is checked with finger and thumb to make sure that it is patent. The transverse colon and omentum are then pulled over to the right so that the gastrojejunal anastomosis is sitting in front of the splenic flexure (*Fig.* 12.10). There should be no tension on the 5-cm long afferent loop but at the

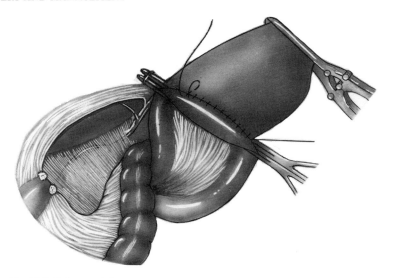

Fig. 12.7. Polya partial gastrectomy. Application of Lane gastrojejunostomy clamps.

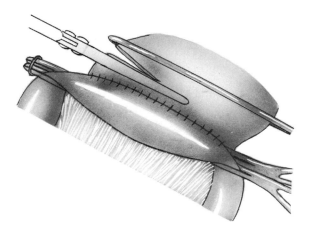

Fig. 12.8. Polya partial gastrectomy. The posterior seromuscular suture has been inserted, following which a Payr clamp and a non-crushing clamp are applied to the stomach, and the stomach is divided distal to the Payr clamp.

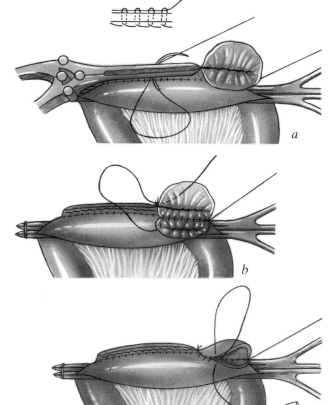

Fig. 12.9. Polya partial gastrectomy. *a*, The segment of stomach held by the Payr clamp is closed to form a valve using a sewing machine technique (*inset*). The small piece of stomach between the tip of the clamp and the greater curve is cut with care so that the lip nearest to the jejunum is cut 1 cm distal to the posterior seromuscular suture and the other lip is cut in a curved fashion so that the centre is about 2 cm longer, facilitating fashioning of the anastomosis. *b*, *c*, A jejunal opening is created to correspond with the gastric stoma and these are anastomosed with an all-layers continuous suture.

same time it lies snugly against the colon and the omentum plugs the gap, preventing all the interesting postoperative complications described by Stammers and Williams (1963).

Prior to closing the abdomen, a systematic check is carried out working from left to right. The spleen is visualized to exclude a minor tear and any blood is aspirated from the subphrenic space. The front of the anastomosis is examined again, and after the posterior layer has been checked any blood is aspirated from the lesser sac. The position of the Ryle's tube is checked so that it is lying in the middle of the gastric remnant. The omental ties in the colon and the colour of the omentum are checked. The latter may be slightly cyanosed if mobilization has been made outside the gastro-epiploic arch as described. This can be ignored; if omentum is grossly cyanosed it should be excised but this is only rarely necessary

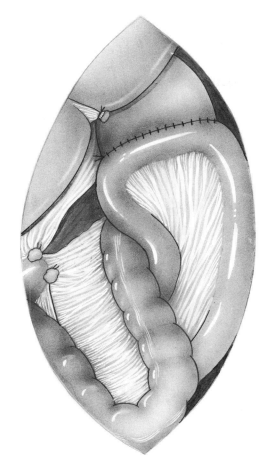

Fig. 12.10. Polya partial gastrectomy. The completed antecolic operation shows the stoma lying comfortably in front of the splenic flexure.

and usually in an obese patient. The pulsation of the middle colic artery and the colour of the transverse colon are also checked, as also is the duodenal stump. If the duodenal stump has been closed in three layers, as described, drainage is probably unnecessary, since the author has never seen such a stump leak. However, if the surgeon is relatively inexperienced or if the stump has been difficult to close, or if the closure has been in only one or two layers, drainage is mandatory. Ordinary corrugated rubber or tube drains have been used. The ends of the drain should be about 2–3 cm away from the stump. Tube drains have the advantage that if the stump does leak the duodenal contents, an irritant mixture of bile and pancreatic juice, may be tapped straight into a bag or bottle, thus avoiding contact with the skin. In recent years the author has used suction drains, e.g. Redivac, which have proved satisfactory. Finally, any blood is aspirated from the hepatorenal pouch and from below the diaphragm on the right, and the abdomen is closed in one layer as previously described. A similar 3/0 monofilament nylon suture is used for the skin.

SPECIAL POINTS OF TECHNIQUE

The contents of the stomach may be infected and before dividing the stomach it may be worth protecting the edges of the wound by packs or an impervious drape. A special towel which accommodates the handles of the clamp may be useful to prevent the sutures tangling in the instrument. All instruments used in the course of the anastomosis should be discarded before closure and the gloves should be changed, as these measures may reduce the chances of wound infection.

There has been much controversy in the past as to whether or not the anastomosis should be fashioned in an antecolic or retrocolic manner. The original Polya gastrectomy as described was a retrocolic anastomosis, and some believe that this is the only way to obtain a short afferent loop. However, if the technique already described is used, a 5-cm afferent loop is all that is required. Tanner has found no difference in the results of his antecolic and retrocolic operations and, since it is easier to construct and dismantle an antecolic anastomosis, the author strongly recommends the antecolic anastomosis when gastrectomy is performed.

The difficult duodenal stump is associated with a posterior penetrating ulcer eroding into the pancreas, and since these stumps are difficult to close, some would recommend that this situation is best treated by vagotomy rather than resection. However, if for some reason resection and closure of the duodenum are necessary, the following technique should be employed.

Having mobilized the antrum in the usual fashion, the stomach is pinched off the pancreas until the posterior ulcer crater is entered just distal to the pylorus (*Fig.* 12.11*a*). The ulcer crater may be at least 1 cm across and this will mean that the duodenum will have already been divided, possibly one-third to halfway round its full circumference. The stomach is then completely separated from the duodenum by dividing the anterior wall just distal to the pylorus. One is then faced with the situation shown in *Fig.* 12.11*b*. The posterior wall of the duodenum may be freed from the edge of the crater by inserting the index finger into the lumen of the duodenum and by placing a Babcock tissue forceps on the edge of the duodenal mucosa. By slight traction on the tissue forceps and sharp dissection the posterior wall of the duodenum may be mobilized off the pancreas. The plane of dissection lies close to the duodenal wall. There is often some oedema on the edge of the ulcer crater and this may facilitate the separation. The plane is often surprisingly avascular and by keeping close to the duodenal wall no damage will be done to the surrounding structures, such as the common bile duct. When it has been possible to free a 1-cm length of posterior wall of the duodenum, closure may be effected with an economical Connell suture of 2/0 atraumatic catgut (*Fig.* 12.11*c*). A Kocher

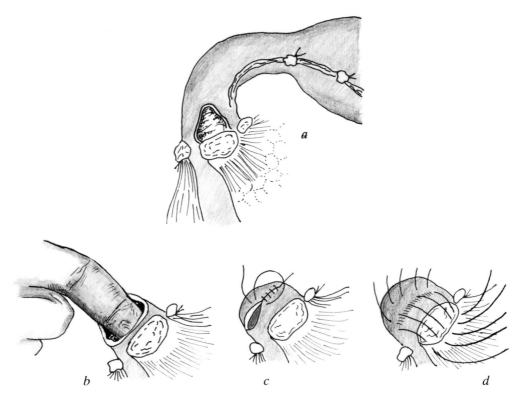

Fig. 12.11. Closure of the difficult duodenal stump. *a*, The ulcer is pinched off the pancreas until the posterior ulcer crater is entered just distal to the pylorus. *b*, The stomach is completely separated from the duodenum by dividing the anterior wall just distal to the pylorus. Dissection between the opened duodenum and pancreas may be facilitated by placing the index finger into the duodenal stump. *c*, *d*, The duodenal stump is closed by the use of a Connell suture and rolling the duodenum onto the ulcer crater where it may be held in place using a series of interrupted catgut sutures between the duodenal stump and the edge of the crater. This latter tissue is firm and fibrous and holds the sutures well.

manoeuvre may then be carried out if the duodenal stump is not sufficiently mobile and the second layer of closure may be achieved by rolling the duodenum on to the ulcer crater and inserting a series of interrupted 2/0 catgut sutures between the duodenal stump and the edge of the ulcer crater which is firm, fibrous tissue and holds the sutures well (*Fig.* 12.11*d*). There is no fear of damage to the pancreas. In such a closure the duodenal stump must always be drained.

2. *Truncal Vagotomy*

For any form of vagotomy an upper midline incision is the incision of choice which is taken from the umbilicus and extended up over the xiphisternum. The exposure of the stomach and hiatus may be improved by inserting a sternal lifting retractor which hooks under the xiphisternum and pulls it in an upwards and cranial direction (Goligher, 1974). The left triangular ligament of the liver may be divided, taking great care not to damage on of the inferior phrenic veins, and the left lobe of the liver is folded upon itself and tucked away to the right. In a more obese patient a self-retaining retractor may be required, and if it is used the wound edges should be protected with a pack soaked in aqueous chlorhexidine, as already described.

PROCEDURE

The abdominal oesophagus is more easily identified if a Ryle's tube is already in place. The surgeon holds the body of the stomach and pulls it downwards while at the same time placing the index and middle fingers either side of the lower oesophagus. The peritoneum is divided transversely over the cardio-oesophageal junction. Beneath this layer there is a condensation of connective tissue called the 'phreno-oesophageal ligament'. This is picked up in forceps and lifted off the oesophagus and again incised in a transverse fashion. A pair of scissors may then be placed under this layer and if opened the surface of the oesophagus is exposed. The tips of the scissors can slip into the posterior mediastinum. Failure to incise deliberately this fibrous layer ensures that the surgeon will be in the incorrect layer and makes subsequent dissection more difficult.

If the cardio-oesophageal junction of the stomach is grasped in the finger and thumb of the right hand and lightly pulled down, the anterior vagus is usually seen and can be palpated as a taut strand, usually towards the left border of the oesophagus. If elevated with a curved artery forceps it can be seen dividing inferiorly into its hepatic and gastric branches. The nerve is divided between two artery forceps. The proximal part is dissected off the oesophagus and is tied as high as possible to avoid missing any branches. The lower end is also clamped and divided and the intervening section sent for histology. The anterior oesophagus is then gently palpated to exclude any other vagal nerve. Occasionally the anterior vagus does appear to be in two trunks although the author has never seen this with the posterior trunk. The lower oesophagus is then encircled with the right thumb and forefinger, and the tissue behind and medial to the oesophagus is palpated between finger and thumb. The right vagus is usually palpated about 1 cm behind and medial to the lower oesophagus and is often thicker than the anterior vagus. Once identified, the nerve may be lifted on an aneurysm needle and dissected both upwards and downwards where it may be seen dividing into its coeliac and gastric branches. Again the nerve is clamped and divided and tied at its division into its principal branches. A final search is made to identify any other branches of the nerve that have been missed.

Haemostasis is then checked and the oesophagus and spleen inspected to make certain that neither has been damaged in the course of the dissection. Finally, some advocate suturing the divided phreno-oesophageal ligament with two or three absorbable sutures in the hope that this might fix the stomach and reduce the chances of gastro-oesophageal reflux, which may occur after vagotomy. What is probably more important is a gentle handling of the oesophagus and the minimal amount of mobilization compatible with identification and ligation of the vagal trunks. The left lobe of the liver is then replaced and a pack is placed between the left lobe of the liver and the upper stomach. This is left in place until the drainage procedure has been completed and the area is once again checked for haemostasis.

The drainage procedure which is then performed is described below. The Ryle's tube is checked to make certain that it is in the correct position, lying in the antrum, and the abdomen is closed in layers in the routine fashion.

Drainage Procedures

1. Heineke–Mikulicz Pyloroplasty

If this procedure is performed through a midline incision, and in particular if the patient is fat, it may be facilitated by initially performing Kocher's mobilization of the duodenum. The position of the pylorus is identified by palpation and a longitudinal incision is made with the cutting diathermy, or scissors, starting on the gastric side of the pylorus. Having incised down to the mucosa and entered the lumen of the stomach, any gastric juice is aspirated and a pair of

blunt dissecting forceps is inserted into the stomach and through the pylorus. The diathermy or scissors incision is continued through the pylorus by incising the tissue between the blades of the dissecting forceps. This will ensure that no inadvertent damage is done to the posterior wall of the stomach or duodenum. The total length of the incision should be 6 cm, extending approximately 3·5 cm on the gastric side and 2·5 cm on the duodenal side of the pylorus. It should be midway between the greater and lesser curves of the stomach and superior and inferior borders of the duodenum. The greater length on the gastric side is to allow for greater thickness of the gastric wall in making the alignment for closure of the pyloroplasty incision in the transverse direction (*Fig.* 12.12*a*).

The interior of the duodenum and stomach is inspected and a finger is inserted down the duodenum to make sure that there is no distal, stenotic segment. A tissue forceps is then applied to both sides at the midpoint of the incision. The tissue forceps are separated and traction on the stomach is relaxed. The incision becomes transverse and the two layers are sutured together to make a transverse incision line (*Fig.* 12.12*b*).

The technique of this closure is controversial. The traditional method is with a two-layer closure, which virtually eliminates the complication of leakage. The

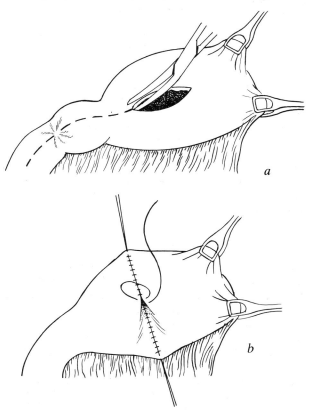

Fig. 12.12. Heineke–Mikulicz pyloroplasty. *a*, The stomach and duodenum are opened by a longitudinal incision across the pylorus. *b*, The longitudinal incision is closed transversely in two layers.

invaginated tissue does project into the lumen, but if done with all reasonable care this is never a problem and it certainly does not leave any permanent projection. If this technique is used an atraumatic 2/0 catgut suture may be used for the initial all-coats layer, having previously ligated any individual bleeding vessels on the edge of the incision. The second layer is a continuous seromuscular Lembert suture, again of 2/0 catgut. On completion of the anastomosis a finger and thumb are inserted on either side of the suture line to make sure that there is an adequate lumen through the anastomosis. Usually the tips of the thumb and two fingers may be passed through. The alternative technique is to use a one-layer closure, usually using a non-absorbable material such as silk or linen. While this has proved safe in the hands of more experienced surgeons, in reported series in which this technique has been used there has usually been some morbidity and mortality from an occasional leak which may be reduced to a minimum by meticulous attention to detail. Weinberg (1961) advocates using interrupted 4/0 surgical cotton sutures, the sutures being placed 3 mm apart and each suture being inserted so that the needle enters the serosa on one side about 3 mm from the cut edge and is directed obliquely through all layers to emerge at the cut edge of the junction of the submucosa and mucosa. The needle then enters the opposite layer of the incision at the junction of the mucosa and submucosa to emerge from the serosal surface 3 mm from the cut edge. With placement of the sutures in this manner, the corresponding layers are accurately approximated when the sutures are tied, thus reducing the possibility of emergence of mucosa into the serosal surface.

2. *Gastroenterostomy*

If the duodenum is grossly scarred and access is difficult, the easier drainage procedure to perform is a gastroenterostomy. This may be either antecolic and retrocolic. The advantage of an anterior juxtapyloric gastroenterostomy is that the anastomosis is close to the obstructing lesion and the anastomosis is between the alkaline-secreting gastric antrum and the jejunal mucosa. The anastomosis is simple to perform and is also easy to dismantle. In general, drainage through such an anastomosis is very satisfactory. Occasionally, however, although technically perfect there is a delay in satisfactory emptying through the stoma. Hence, if immediate drainage is imperative it may be better to perform a posterior gastroenterostomy.

A. ANTERIOR JUSTAPYLORIC GASTROENTEROSTOMY

The anterior wall of the gastric antrum is grasped with one of the Lane twin gastroenterostomy clamps. The anterior wall of the stomach is clasped towards the greater curve aspect and if held in the hand one can ensure that the mucosa does not slip out of the

grasp as the clamp is applied by the assistant. The omentum and transverse colon are lifted and the duodenojejunal flexure is identified. The other twin clamp is applied to the jejunum approximately 10–20 cm from the duodenojejunal flexure. The afferent loop should be as short as possible. The clamps are locked together so that the efferent loop of small gut is close to the pylorus. Before embarking on the anastomosis, one should check that there is no undue tension on the small bowel mesentery. The anastomosis is with two layers of 2/0 catgut, the initial suture being a continuous seromuscular Lembert suture uniting the adjacent gastric and jejunal walls. This suture line is usually about 7 cm long. An opening is then made between the jejunum and the gastric antrum, which is slightly shorter than the posterior suture layer. This incision with diathermy is usually made 5 cm long. The adjacent gastric and jejunal walls are then united with a running all-layers catgut suture. On the the anterior wall the layers are inverted using an over-and-over suture. A Connell suture must not be used in this situation because it is not haemostatic and any bleeding will be masked by the clamps. The inner suture layer having been completed, the clamps are removed and the posterior seromuscular suture is carried around the end and along the anterior walls to bury the all-layers suture.

B. POSTERIOR GASTROENTEROSTOMY

In this operation the jejunum is brought to the most dependent portion of the greater curve of the stomach. To do this an initial opening is made in the gastrocolic omentum and the lesser sac is opened. The mesocolon is inspected and an incision made parallel and to the left of the middle colic vessels about 8 cm long. The duodenojejunal flexure is identified and a loop of proximal jejunum is brought up through the hole in the mesocolon. The one half of the Lane twin clamp is applied to this proximal segment of jejunum as close as possible to the ligament of Treitz. The other half of the clamp is applied to a convenient part of the posterior wall of the stomach close to the greater curve. The two clamps are then locked together and the anastomosis is performed as with an anterior gastroenterostomy. On completion of this anastomosis the margins of the mesocolic defect are sutured to the stomach to prevent any small gut prolapsing through this hole and causing internal hernia (*Fig.* 12.13).

SUTURE MATERIAL

In all the anastomoses described in this chapter, two layers of 2/0 catgut have been used. This material seems to be very successful and the use of an outer layer of a non-absorbable suture, either as interrupted or continuous layer, seems to be quite unnecessary. It has been suggested that the use of a

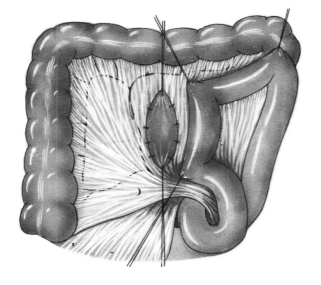

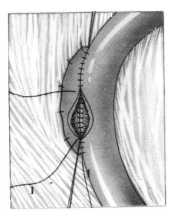

Fig. 12.13. Gastroenterostomy. An incision is made in the meso-colon parallel and to the left of the middle colic vessels, following which a two-layer anastomosis is undertaken. In this diagram the Lane clamps are not shown and the anastomosis is undertaken from below for the sake of clarity, although the author accomplishes this procedure on the other side of the mesocolon by passing the jejunum through the defect.

non-absorbable suture may be the cause of recurrent ulceration. There is, however, little evidence of this and it may be that as the ulcer enlarges, eroding through the wall of the bowel, if near an anastomosis, the suture material may eventually appear in the base of the ulcer. It does seem, however, that the use of non-absorbable sutures is unnecessary and hence the author advocates the use of atraumatic absorbable 2/0 catgut sutures on 30-mm needles.

The alternative would be a polyglycolic acid suture (Dexon) of similar strength. The most recent form of this suture (Dexon Plus) is much smoother than its predecessor and can be recommended as can PDS (polydioxanone).

Stapling devices have been available for some years to aid in the construction of a gastric anastomosis or to assist in closure of a duodenal stump. Certainly,

if either of these procedures were difficult, mechanical assistance would be more than welcome. Unfortunately, however, it is just in these circumstances that the rather bulky stapling devices cannot be used. For this, and possibly financial reasons, staplers have not in the past made the impact on gastric surgery that they have made on surgery of the rectum. Where they have been used on the stomach this has been as an alternative to suturing in the reconstruction of the lesser curve of the stomach in Billroth-I gastrectomy or for total closure of a gastric remnant prior to mobilization of the gastric remnant following resection of a carcinoma of the cardia.

In the future, stapling devices may become less bulky and be capable of use in the difficult reconstruction. If they can be shown to be more reliable than hand suturing, then their application may become more widespread, because certainly the cost of the stapling device and its maintenance are a fraction of that required to meet the extra hospitalization of a patient who has unfortunately developed an anastomotic leak.

POSTOPERATIVE

Management Following Gastrectomy and Vagotomy

General

The usual observations of vital functions are recorded in the recovery room. Initially half-hourly pulse and blood pressure should be taken for the first 4 hours and after this observations can be reduced to hourly for the next 8 hours. Effective relief of postoperative pain is essential so that early chest physiotherapy may be initiated.

Specific

1. The Ryle's tube is placed on free drainage and is in addition aspirated hourly for the first 12 hours. After this the tube is aspirated 4-hourly until removal. An accurate fluid chart recording all fluid input and output must be maintained. The Billroth-I anastomosis is smaller than a gastrojejunal anastomosis and it usually takes 3–4 days before it starts to drain. This is heralded by the appearance of bile in the gastric aspirate and a decrease in the volume of the aspirate, so that it becomes less than the input. The tube may then be removed. With a Polya gastrectomy the anastomosis is usually opened and is draining at 72 hours, and this is usually so following a truncal vagotomy and drainage.

2. Oral fluids in the volume of 25 ml hourly may be given from the 1st postoperative day. There is no point in increasing this volume until the stomach is emptying as it is merely aspirated up the Ryle's tube and acts as a gastric lavage, removing more hydrogen and potassium ions. A standard intravenous regimen is given until sufficient fluid may be

taken orally. Parenteral hyperalimentation is not as a rule required as the patients are usually taking sufficient calories orally by the 5th postoperative day.

It is important to convince all patients that they are capable of eating a normal diet prior to leaving hospital, otherwise they may continue to take a gastric diet indefinitely, the only restrictions being that where patients have had a gastrectomy or a vagotomy and drainage they should avoid eating citrus fruit (juice only) and nuts. This will avoid bolus obstruction developing due to a phytobezoar.

COMPLICATIONS OF POLYA GASTRECTOMY AND VAGOTOMY

Immediate

Haemorrhage may occur following Polya gastrectomy from faulty haemostasis at the suture line. Fresh blood will be aspirated up the Ryle's tube in variable quantities. This problem may be prevented by meticulous attention to detail when constructing the gastrojejunal anastomosis. When stitching the inner layer, each suture must be approximately 3 mm apart and the suture must be followed down to make certain that it is evenly spaced and a steady tension must be maintained on the suture by the assistant. These points are particularly important if the gastrectomy is being constructed with the aid of gastrectomy clamps which will, of course, mask any potential bleeding until after they are removed. Haemorrhage may also occur from the suture line of a pyloroplasty or a gastroenterostomy associated with total or selective vagotomy. The length of the suture lines are, however, smaller and this reduces the chance of significant haemorrhage.

When haemorrhage does occur, it fortunately often stops spontaneously and no active measures are required. If haemorrhage does continue and the patient begins to show signs of decompensation despite blood transfusion, reoperation will be required. In the case of bleeding from a Polya anastomosis, the site of the bleeding may be identified through a small gastrotomy above the suture line and the bleeding point may be under-run with a catgut suture. A similar technique may be employed with bleeding from a gastroenterostomy, but in the case of a pyloroplasty it is probably best to dismantle the suture line from one end until the bleeding point is identified and ligated.

Delay in Gastric Emptying

This rarely occurs after a Polya gastrectomy because the stoma is larger than with a Billroth gastrectomy. Sometimes, however, one may get the false impression of delayed emptying because large quantities of fluid are aspirated up the Ryle's tube. At the same time the patient says that he or she feels hungry and is having his or her bowels open. What has happened in these cases is that the Ryle's tube has slipped through the stoma into the efferent loop and the fluid that is being aspirated is a combination of gastric and pancreatic juice plus bile. The treatment is, of course, to remove the Ryle's tube and feed the patient.

Delay in gastric emptying following either truncal or selective vagotomy may occasionally be a problem, particularly if the patient has had preoperative pyloric stenosis. If problems are anticipated at the time of operation it may be wise to insert a double-lumen gastrostomy tube, e.g. Maurice Lee tube. One portion of the tube may be used for emptying the stomach and the other part of the tube may be threaded through the stoma into either the duodenum or, in the case of a gastroenterostomy, the jejunum. If the stomach is slow to empty any gastric residue may be aspirated from the gastric portion of the tube and returned down the jejunal tube. This prevents any electrolyte imbalance and in addition the patient may be fed enterally through the intestinal portion of the double-lumen tube. Unfortunately, however, this problem often occurs unexpectedly. Under these circumstances one may have to keep a Ryle's tube down until the gastric aspirate diminishes and the patient will require feeding parenterally. If the problem does not resolve within 10–14 days, re-exploration of the anastomosis may rarely be required.

Leakage from the Gastrojejunal Anastomosis

This is extremely uncommon after Polya gastrectomy but may occasionally occur following a one-layer pyloroplasty. This will require reoperation and refashioning of the suture line.

Duodenal stump rupture or leakage may occur often on the 3rd postoperative day following Polya gastrectomy. Prevention of this problem is discussed earlier in this chapter. If a drain is present the fluid escapes freely into the drainage bag and the patient's condition will remain stable and the problem may be treated conservatively. In the absence of a drain there will be flooding of the abdominal cavity with duodenal contents, mainly consisting, of course, of bile and pancreatic juice which will lead to a rapid collapse. In the event of such a leak, the stump must, of course, be repaired and the rest of the anastomosis checked to make sure that there is no distal obstruction.

Small Bowel Obstruction Secondary to Internal Hernia

Small bowel obstruction from adhesions may occur following any operation, but Stammers and Williams (1963) have described a number of cases of obstruction resulting from small bowel slipping behind the afferent and efferent loops of an antecolic gastrectomy. This problem may be prevented by the technique already described, using a short afferent loop. It may also complicate a retrocolic gastrectomy or gastroenterostomy if the hole in the mesocolon is not closed around the anastomosis.

Dysphagia

This may be an occasional complication following either truncal or selective vagotomy and develops 7–10 days after the operation. The patient feels as if food sticks behind the lower sternum and has to be regurgitated. The problem often persists for 7–10 days and then improves. The aetiology of this self-limiting dysphagia is ill understood but may represent a neuropraxia affecting the lower gullet or the result of some oedema around the hiatus following the oesophageal mobilization. The symptoms may be cured by persuading the patient to swallow a Hurst's mercury-filled bougie, after the pharynx has been sprayed with local anaesthetic.

Remote Complications

Recurrent Ulceration

The mean incidence of recurrent ulceration following vagotomy varies from 5 to 10 per cent. Truncal vagotomy has a higher incidence of incomplete vagotomy while selective vagotomy is a more reliable method of carrying out a complete gastric vagotomy, hence the incidence of recurrent ulceration is less. Polya gastrectomy has a mean incidence of approximately 3 per cent, while vagotomy and antrectomy have the lowest incidence of recurrent ulceration of about 1 per cent. The diagnosis of recurrent ulceration must be by endoscopy as barium studies following previous gastric surgery are usually unreliable.

In cases of recurrent ulceration, particularly if they recur soon after the original operation, the possibility of a Zollinger–Ellison syndrome must be considered, which of course can be confirmed by serum gastrin assay. If the patient has previously had a Polya gastrectomy the duodenal stump must be checked for retained gastric mucosa. If this is absent, the stomal ulceration may be treated by adding a selective or truncal vagotomy. On the other hand, where truncal vagotomy has failed, there are usually dense adhesions around the hiatus and further surgery in this region is hazardous. Accordingly, gastric resection is usually performed to cure the recurrent ulceration. While in the past the treatment of recurrent ulceration has always been surgical, medical treatment can now be attempted with H_2 receptor antagonists, apparently with some success.

Dumping

This syndrome, occurring 10–20 minutes after a meal, is associated with a feeling of fullness, weakness, sweating, palpitations and sometimes even faintness. The syndrome is thought to be caused by rapid emptying of hypertonic food into the jejunum. This exerts an osmotic effect within the lumen of the gut, resulting in an outpouring of fluid into the gut. It is possible, however, that there may be a hormonal component contributing to the syndrome. This syndrome occurs most frequently after Polya gastrectomy (21 per cent), but it may occur after any operation on the stomach in which a drainage procedure has been performed. It may therefore occur after truncal or selective vagotomy. Humphrey et al. (1972) reported an incidence of 18 per cent following truncal vagotomy and gastroenterostomy and 12 per cent following truncal vagotomy and pyloroplasty.

Fortunately, the frequency and severity of the attacks of dumping seem to decrease in the months and years after operation and dietary advice can be of help to patients. It should be suggested that they avoid sweet and starchy foods and should take their meals dry. A drink should be taken midway between meals. A relatively dry meal empties very much less rapidly from the stomach than does a fluid meal. Very rarely, if the symptoms are incapacitating and occur after a Polya gastrectomy, it may be possible to treat the patient by inserting a retroperistaltic loop between the gastric remnant and the duodenum. The results, however, as described by Alexander-Williams (1973), are not very encouraging.

Bilious Vomiting

The typical history of patients with bilious vomiting is that shortly after a meal they begin to feel uncomfortably distended, become nauseated and then vomit a large quantity of pure bile. After vomiting, the symptoms are relieved. In some patients the symptoms are present when they wake in the morning, the nausea continuing until they vomit spontaneously or induce vomiting. This symptom may occur after any form of gastric surgery, but is particularly common after Polya gastrectomy and vagotomy and gastroenterostomy. Originally this syndrome was thought to be due to afferent loop constriction but the evidence now points to the fact that it is the presence of bile in the gastric remnant which in some patients acts as an irritant and causes a gastritis and interferes with gastric emptying.

In order to cure these symptoms it is necessary to prevent bile refluxing into the gastric remnant. In the case of Polya gastrectomy, this may be achieved by converting the gastrectomy to a Roux-en-Y or 'Roux 19' anastomosis (Tanner, 1951), ensuring that the bile enters 19 in (48 cm) below the gastric remnant. It is more rarely a problem after Billroth-I gastrectomy but if so an isoperistaltic loop of jejunum may be placed between the gastric remnant and the duodenum, again preventing reflux of bile (Alexander-Williams, 1973).

Diarrhoea

Diarrhoea may occur after any gastric operation and may be either continuous or intermittent. Episodic diarrhoea is a common problem, particularly after operations associated with vagotomy. It may occur in 24 per cent of patients following truncal vagotomy and drainage, but the incidence of severe diarrhoea is only 5 per cent. The incidence of diarrhoea following selective vagotomy appears to be lower (18 per cent). In either case symptoms become much less troublesome with the passage of time and they may be helped by avoiding milk products and wet sweet foods. Continuous diarrhoea is a less common problem and appears to occur with equal frequency after gastric resection or after vagotomy with drainage. In the more severe cases investigation usually reveals a variable degree of steatorrhoea and this may be due to pancreatic exocrine insufficiency. It certainly may be worth giving patients pancreatic replacement to see whether it is of any benefit. If the problem is intractable the possibility of a reversed ileal loop might be considered. A rare but important cause of acute profuse diarrhoea is the development of gastro-jejunocolic fistula due to stomal ulceration, and this is dealt with later in this chapter (p. 142). Another rare cause is the Zollinger–Ellison syndrome, one feature of which may be diarrhoea. Finally, cases have been reported where the unfortunate patient has diarrhoea because the surgeon has inadvertently connected the gastric remnant to the ileum rather than to the jejunum. Once diagnosed, the remedy is obvious.

Deficiency States and Metabolic Bone Disease

These may occur following Polya gastrectomy or vagotomy and are described under the section on Billroth-I gastrectomies (p. 125).

COMPLICATIONS OF PEPTIC ULCERATION

In this section the management of the most common complications of peptic ulcer, namely haemorrhage, perforation and stenosis, is considered.

Haemorrhage

Bleeding from peptic ulceration is the most common cause of acute upper gastrointestinal tract haemorrhage. Most British series agree that around half the patients admitted have chronic peptic ulcers, duodenal ulcer outnumbering the gastric ulcer by 2 to 1. Before the days of widespread endoscopy, the incidence of bleeding from acute gastric erosions was assumed to be high. It now seems, however, to be less than previously supposed and most series in the UK report a frequency of less than 10 per cent. Other common causes of upper gastrointestinal tract bleeding revealed by endoscopy include evidence of oesophageal mucosal tears in the Mallory–Weiss syndrome (13 per cent) and reflux oesophagitis (10 per cent). Oesophageal varices are an infrequent cause of haemorrhage in the UK and the majority of workers report an incidence of around 2 per cent.

The role of drugs in the causation of acute upper gastrointestinal bleeding remains unclear. Aspirin and alcohol, either separately or together, may precipitate acute bleeding from the upper alimentary tract. Bleeding is usually from acute gastric erosions or sometimes from pre-existing chronic peptic ulcers. While there is no doubt that aspirin causes slight occult blood loss, in most individuals it probably only rarely produces major gastrointestinal bleeding. Phenylbutazone and indomethacin cause gastric ulcers which may bleed. Healing of the ulcers will occur when the drug is withdrawn. Contrary to the impressions of most surgeons, there is no good evidence that corticosteroids in ordinary doses cause either peptic ulcerations or gastrointestinal bleeding; these individuals are often taking other drugs that are known to precipitate bleeds such as aspirin, phenylbutazone and indomethacin.

Management of the Patient

When a patient presents with acute upper intestinal tract bleeding, two questions have to be answered. First, how much blood has the patient lost, and second, where is the source of bleeding?

1. BLOOD LOSS

An estimate of the blood loss may be made by taking a history, making an examination and by arranging some pathological investigations. With regard to history, haematemesis with melaena implies a considerably greater blood loss than melaena alone and the mortality is approximately twice as great. The volume of haematemesis can give some guide to the amount of blood loss but the patient's assessment of the volume is usually inaccurate. Bleeding associated with a feeling of faintness suggests rapid significant loss. On examination the obviously shocked patient with rapid pulse and low blood pressure has clearly lost several units of blood. When blood loss is less extreme, pulse rate, blood pressure and central venous pressure monitoring may be helpful in assessing the volume lost. It takes some hours for the blood to dilute and hence the haemoglobin level to fall after an acute bleed. However, if the bleeding is continued for some time the haemoglobin level is a useful guide. A low haemoglobin level soon after an acute bleed suggests previous occult bleeding.

2. SOURCE OF BLEEDING

While the history may indicate the cause of bleeding, in over 30 per cent of patients with peptic ulcer, no symptoms relative to the cause of the bleeding are found. There are usually no physical findings likely to be helpful in the diagnosis of bleeding peptic ulcers apart from possibly localized abdominal tenderness, but hyperactive bowel sounds may suggest rapid transit of blood through the gut.

3. INVESTIGATION

Investigation of the haemorrhage may be by fibre-optic endoscopy or barium radiology. Endoscopy provides a higher diagnostic yield than radiology although double-contrast barium radiology compares favourably with it in diagnosing chronic peptic ulcers (Scott-Harden, 1974). A high diagnostic yield is obtained with the endoscope, particularly if the investigation is carried out within 24 hours of the admission. This is due to the increase in diagnosis of acute superficial lesions that are undefined radiologically, but these rarely bleed severely. In patients with continued profuse haemorrhage, it may be difficult to detect the bleeding point by either method because of the presence of blood clot in the stomach. If the bleeding is obviously profuse and continuous, surgery will be required, which when performed immediately after endoscopy may be complicated by the presence of large quantities of air in the small gut, making exposure and subsequent closure more difficult.

Treatment

Resuscitation is the most important initial part of management. An estimate of the blood loss must be obtained and if the bleeding has been sufficient to bring the patient into hospital an intravenous infusion will be required. If clinical assessment suggests the blood volume to be depleted then transfusion of blood should be started. Similarly, patients with a haemoglobin below 10 g per cent usually require transfusion. Blood volume studies have shown that the loss in patients with upper gastrointestinal tract bleeding tends to be more severe than is suspected clinically (Tudhope, 1958). In the more difficult cases, and particularly in elderly patients, a central venous pressure line may be helpful in the initial assessment of the blood loss and also for guiding subsequent blood transfusion. It may also give early warning of further bleeds; fortunately four out of five patients stop bleeding spontaneously. It is important to recognize as early as possible patients with continuous or recurrent bleeding since the mortality rate of those who rebleed is four times higher. Rebleeding may be detected indirectly from frequent measurements of pulse and blood pressure and by regular examination of postural changes in pulse, blood pressure and central venous pressure. An indwelling nasogastric tube to detect early rebleeding has been suggested by some workers, but the author has found this unhelpful as it frequently becomes blocked with clot and fails to drain and merely contributes to the patient's discomfort.

The traditional method of treatment in the past has consisted of small doses of opiates to sedate the patient, ice cubes to suck and regular ingestion of antacids. H_2 receptor antagonists, however, will heal peptic ulcers and it was hoped that they might be useful in controlling acute bleeding from peptic ulcers, but as yet there are few results of any controlled clinical trials, and to date the figures suggest that bleeding from chronic ulcers may not be affected by treatment. Acute bleeding from gastric erosions may, however, respond to H_2 receptor antagonists and MacDougall et al. (1977) found that bleeding due to acute erosions in patients with hepatic failure was reduced from 53 per cent in controls to 4 per cent in the control group treated with H_2 receptor antagonists.

However, angiography may identify the bleeding point and allow a catheter to be introduced into the feeding vessel. Then haemostasis may be attempted, either by infusing vasopressin or by occluding the vessel with emboli. Vasopressin has been successful in only 25 per cent of patients, but embolization seems to have been more successful, although there have been no controlled trials.

An alternative approach is by way of the flexible endoscope. Cyanoacrylic glue has failed experimentally but electrocautery or laser beam might be expected to give more effective haemostasis. Several reports of large series show good initial control of haemorrhage by electrocautery with a low instance of rebleed, but randomized trials have yet to be published (Young, 1982).

SURGICAL INTERVENTION IN BLEEDING PEPTIC ULCER

There are in general four factors which have to be considered when contemplating surgery in patients bleeding from peptic ulcer.

1. *Quantity and Duration of Bleeding:* The most common indication for surgical intervention is either continued heavy blood loss or recurrent large haemorrhage. Jones et al. (1973) found that patients who suffered recurrent haemorrhage after admission had a fourfold increase in mortality rate, and they suggested that these patients should be submitted to early surgery in the hope of reducing this high mortality. There are no controlled trials to support this view but there are retrospective data by Jensen et al. (1972), who found that the mortality rate of patients with surgically treated bleeding gastric ulcers was 8 per cent compared with 18 per cent in the medically treated group. In general, however, one might say that a further significant bleed after hospital admission in conjunction with the other factors should be considered a possible indication for surgical intervention.

2. *Diagnosis:* Diagnosis will depend on history, examination and endoscopy. A patient with a history

of dyspepsia sufficient to warrant an elective operation should have surgery without waiting for further haemorrhage. Unfortunately, as already stated, a significant proportion of patients with bleeding chronic ulcers give no dyspeptic history and Johnston et al. (1973) found that this group had a higher mortality rate. Schiller et al. (1970) also observed that the mortality rate in patients with a dyspeptic history of more than 3 months was 7·5 per cent compared with 12 per cent in those with no such history, presumably due to the delay in diagnosis in such patients. Patients with ulcers without a dyspeptic history are just as likely to rebleed as those with such a history, and hence one should not be unduly influenced by a lack of dyspeptic history. This point stresses the importance of endoscopic diagnosis.

Endoscopy can confirm the diagnosis preoperatively except where massive bleeding obscures the view. Chronic ulcers, either gastric or duodenal, are more likely to give rise to bleeding, requiring surgery, rather than acute superficial ulcers. Acute erosive gastritis is strenuously treated medically in the hope that surgery may be avoided.

3. *Age of Patient:* Patients over the age of 60 have a less labile cardiovascular system and are less able to withstand the effects of bleeding and transfusion than the young. However, elderly patients always withstand operation less well. Nevertheless, an elderly patient presenting with a large bleed, who has been shown to have a chronic lesion, proved by endoscopy, and without any serious associated medical condition, is probably better operated on early rather than made to wait until he or she presents in extremis, having already had a large transfusion.

4. *Other Medical Conditions:* The prognosis of a patient with a bleeding peptic ulcer, who has important coexisting medical conditions such as cardiac or respiratory failure, is poor. If bleeding continues surgery may have to be contemplated, although clearly the risks would be considerable. Schiller et al. (1970) showed that delayed surgical treatment was associated with increased mortality but it is not clear whether this was due to unjustifiable delay or to the inevitable outcome in desperately ill patients, whom the clinicians were reluctant to recommend for surgery.

CHOICE OF OPERATION FOR BLEEDING PEPTIC ULCER

The aim of the emergency operation under these circumstances is to arrest the haemorrhage. Although important, a secondary consideration is the possibility of any sequelae as a result of the particular procedure. In the majority of cases the diagnosis will be made endoscopically preoperatively, but where this

is not possible a gastrotomy or duodenotomy may be necessary to identify the site of the bleeding.

Duodenal Ulcer: With bleeding duodenal ulcer the most frequently performed operation is underrunning of the ulcer with an atraumatic suture inserted as a Z stitch. The author uses 2/0 Dexon Plus or PDS which, although absorbable sutures, can guarantee retention of tensile strength until the ulcer has healed. The duodenotomy which has transgressed the pylorus is then closed as a Heineke–Mikulicz pyloroplasty and is followed by truncal vagotomy. This operation has the advantage over Polya gastrectomy of a much lower postoperative morbidity and mortality. Clark (1968) reported a postoperative mortality falling from 16 to 5 per cent on changing his operation from partial gastrectomy to vagotomy and pyloroplasty. Schiller et al. (1970) reported a similar drop from 14·3 per cent for Polya gastrectomy to 5·5 per cent with vagotomy and pyloroplasty. The recurrent bleeding rate is said to be no greater after vagotomy and pyloroplasty than after gastrectomy. Bleeding duodenal ulcers are almost invariably posterior penetrating ulcers and when Polya gastrectomy was the routine operation the mobilization of the duodenum and closure of the duodenal stump were more difficult than usual (*see* p. 128), and as a result of this there was an increased incidence of leakage from the duodenal stump which increased the postoperative morbidity and contributed to the mortality.

Control of the bleeding duodenal ulcer through a small duodenotomy, followed by highly selective vagotomy, may be used where the surgeon is particularly experienced in the procedure and where the patient's condition is satisfactory. However, if the surgeon is relatively inexperienced in the technique, it is probably better to do a good truncal vagotomy in a reasonable time rather than a prolonged procedure with a possibly incomplete highly selective vagotomy.

Gastric Ulcer: Where the bleeding ulcer is in the distal half of the stomach, Billroth-I gastrectomy is still the most commonly performed operation, but this procedure carries a higher mortality than simple underrunning of the ulcer coupled with truncal vagotomy and pyloroplasty. While sleeve resection of the lesser curve (Pauchet manoeuvre) will allow resection of a slightly higher gastric ulcer, it would seem that oversewing the ulcer with some form of vagotomy is mandatory for the high bleeding gastric ulcer. Truncal vagotomy will be the more speedy procedure and will be necessary if the patient's condition is poor. However, Johnston (147) has described the use of highly selective vagotomy under these circumstances. Clearly this could only be used by a surgeon who is skilled in the procedure which might well be more difficult under these circumstances because of the associated induration adjacent to the gastric ulcer. Once again a complete truncal vagotomy may be preferable to an incomplete highly selective vagotomy (*see* p. 147).

Perforation

The treatment of acute perforated ulcer in most hospitals is operative. Some surgeons use conservative treatment, and Taylor (1951) described a series with a mortality of 9·6 per cent. He recommended this treatment, however, only for those perforations where he considered there were good prospects of sealing off, such as the small duodenal perforation where there were signs of localization at the time they were first seen. He recommended that it should be instituted if some other factor such as heart or lung disease was present to contra-indicate surgery. This may account for only 5 per cent of all acute perforations.

The majority of perforations will be treated surgically and the procedure will depend on whether the ulcer is acute or chronic, and, second, on the site of the ulcer.

In the case of duodenal perforation where there is no history of indigestion and at operation where there is no sign of chronicity, the correct treatment is simple closure of the perforation with an omental patch. With acute ulcers 75 per cent have good results, 25 per cent relapse, and many require further surgery. In the case of perforation of a chronic ulcer, the story is very different with approximately 80 per cent developing recurrent ulceration and over 50 per cent requiring a second definitive procedure. Hence such patients should be treated by closure of the perforation combined with a definitive operation, providing they are fit enough to withstand a more lengthy procedure. This procedure should be either a truncal vagotomy and drainage or preferably a highly selective vagotomy if the surgeon performing the procedure has the necessary experience.

The mortality from perforation of a gastric ulcer is very much greater than that from duodenal ulcer when treated by simple suture and most of these deaths are due to reperforation. This problem can be prevented by carrying out a definitive procedure in all cases of perforated gastric ulcer. If the perforated ulcer is low in the stomach, then a Billroth-I gastrectomy may be performed without difficulty. The alternative is to excise the ulcer and combine this with either a truncal vagotomy and drainage or a highly selective vagotomy. It is clearly important that the ulcer should be excised for histological examination as Doll (1950) found that 8 per cent of gastric perforations proved to be due to unsuspected gastric carcinoma. Unfortunately, even when a gastrectomy has been performed for what turns out to be a perforated gastric carcinoma, the gastric resection is never radical enough for the malignant

process and in selected cases it may be necessary to reoperate on the patient to carry out a more extensive resection and couple this with local gland clearance.

Pyloric Stenosis and Hour-glass Contracture of the Stomach

Pyloric Stenosis

The term 'pyloric stenosis' is sometimes a misnomer as the obstruction is often in the duodenum. A degree of narrowing is a common occurrence following the healing of a juxtapyloric or duodenal ulcer. This narrowing is not necessarily reflected by clinical symptoms of obstruction or radiological evidence of delayed emptying. This slight narrowing may be fully compensated by muscular hypertrophy of the stomach. The development of clinical symptoms of pyloric obstruction is often due to an exacerbation of the ulcer with increased narrowing from oedema in the presence of an already compromised lumen. The resultant gastric stasis may result in gross electrolyte disturbances in addition to weight loss.

The initial procedure in these patients is to improve their general condition by rehydration and correction of their electrolyte and pH imbalance with appropriate intravenous infusions. The stomach is emptied each evening by the passage of a gastric tube. This has to be at least 32 Fr. gauge to remove some of the more solid material from the stomach. To pass this it may be necessary to spray the throat with Xylocaine (lignocaine) and to lay the patient flat and on his side to prevent aspiration of gastric contents. A Senoran's evacuator aids the gastric lavage. As the oedema resolves, the volume of gastric residue decreases and becomes cleaner. The bacterial count in the stomach will decrease and the chance of any wound infection following subsequent surgery will be reduced. In the case of malignant pyloric obstruction, the gastric lavage makes no difference to the volume of gastric residue.

The surgical management of duodenal stenosis has changed over the years. Originally partial gastrectomy was widely used. However, Ellis et al. (1966) reported the results of a series of cases treated by truncal vagotomy and drainage and showed that it was unnecessary to resect the distended stomach as it gradually returns to a normal size over the ensuing months. More recently Johnston has shown that these cases may be treated by highly selective vagotomy, the duodenal drainage being improved by either a duodenoplasty, not traversing and damaging the pylorus, or alternatively forcibly dilating the pylorus and adjacent duodenum with Hegar's dilators through a gastrostomy in the antrum (Johnston et al., 1973).

Hour-glass Deformity of the Stomach

Large chronic gastric ulcers may cause marked distortion of the stomach. This initially may represent a degree of spasm but is replaced by fibrosis as the ulcer heals. The ultimate result of this process may be the division of the stomach into two parts by a narrow zone of fibrosis and often some residual ulceration. This deformity is known as the 'hour-glass stomach'. It tends to occur more frequently in women and the symptoms resemble pyloric stenosis. The diagnosis may be made by barium studies but endoscopy will certainly be required to exclude malignancy. This is a rare surgical problem but when it occurs the treatment of choice is gastrectomy which relieves the obstruction and also removes the cause of the gastric ulcer.

Chronic Penetration of Adjacent Organs

Peptic ulcers as they enlarge may completely penetrate the wall of the stomach, duodenum or jejunum but may remain completely walled off from the peritoneal cavity by adhesions. Duodenal ulcer commonly penetrates into the pancreas and may rarely ultimately involve the common bile duct. Chronic gastric ulcers may penetrate the pancreas or the liver, while a stomal ulcer following partial gastrectomy may involve the chest wall or colon causing severe pain or a gastrojejunocolic fistula.

The management of the surgical problems presented has already been discussed with the exception of gastrojejunocolic fistula. Preoperatively patients may be emaciated following intractable diarrhoea and the consequent malabsorption. This may be improved by intravenous hyperalimentation and, while this is being achieved, endoscopy and biopsy may be carried out to exclude malignancy. If the ulcer is benign the possibility of a Zollinger–Ellison syndrome should be considered and serum gastrin studies will be required. If these results are normal, laparotomy will be necessary and the original gastric anastomosis will have to be dismantled and freed from the colon. If the hole in the colon is small it may be oversewn. If large, local resection will be necessary. A fresh gastrojejunal anastomosis can be fashioned following resection of originally involved tissue. To avoid further peptic ulceration a truncal or alternatively selective vagotomy should be added.

ULCEROGENIC TUMOURS OF THE PANCREAS (ZOLLINGER–ELLISON SYNDROME) (GASTRINOMA)

This syndrome was first described in 1955 and consists of a triad:

1. The presence of primary peptic ulceration in unusual locations, that is, in the second or third portions of the duodenum, upper jejunum or recurrent stomal ulcers following any gastric surgery short of total gastrectomy.

2. Marked gastric hypersecretion despite adequate or even intensive conventional medical or surgical therapy.

3. Identification of non-specific islet cell tumours of the pancreas.

The clinical syndrome may be that of severe diarrhoea or steatorrhoea but the symptoms are ordinarily those of a fulminating ulcer, which is intractable to the usual treatment. The diagnosis may be suggested by barium studies showing huge mucosal folds with considerable fluid retention in the stomach. The duodenum tends to be enlarged and irregular in appearance with one or more ulcers in an unusual location such as the second or third portion of the duodenum. Ulceration just beyond the ligament of Treitz is pathognomonic of an ulcerogenic tumour.

Barium studies after previous gastric resection may show multiple deep penetrating ulcers in the mesenteric border of the efferent loop rather than the usual marginal location. Gastric analyses are helpful, the resting juice usually being in excess of 60 per cent of the volume obtained following the augmented histamine study. Despite early optimism, a fasting basal gastrin estimation does not identify all patients. However, the discovery that a secretin infusion paradoxically raised gastrin levels in patients with a gastrinoma has become the single most valuable test available for confirming the diagnosis of Zollinger–Ellison syndrome. In 20 per cent of cases the syndrome is part of a multiple endocrine adenomatosis.

Approximately 70 per cent of the patients with ulcerogenic syndrome have multiple foci of gastrin-producing tumour and 60 per cent of these are malignant. The tumours may be single or multiple and they may be very small or reasonably large. Seventy-five per cent will have metastases to either the liver or regional lymph nodes by the time of surgery. A smaller percentage of patients will have either diffuse islet cell hyperplasia (Polak et al., 1972) or multiple benign adenomatosis.

Surgical Management

Once the diagnosis has been made, it is necessary to determine whether or not metastases are present. Ultrasound and isotope liver scans may be useful in confirming the presence of liver metastases. Gastrinomas are often vascular and arteriography has proved the most useful technique for their localization.

The management of this condition has changed in recent years. Prior to 1976 and the advent of H_2 receptor blocking drugs, nearly all patients underwent total gastrectomy, thus removing the target organ from the excess of circulating gastrin. However, it is now possible to control the gastrin hypersecretory state pharmacologically and the role of total gastrectomy, lesser resection and even laparotomy, has been reassessed (Mee et al., 1983). Effective control of the hypersecretion has promoted a conservative approach in those patients whose investigations have failed to localize the primary tumour or where there is evidence of metastatic disease. While gastrinomas are slow growing and symptoms may be controlled pharmacologically, the only hope of cure is resection of an isolated tumour. Suitable patients are subjected to exploratory laparotomy and, unless a localized tumour is found and resected, truncal vagotomy and pyloroplasty are performed to assist in the subsequent control of acid hypersecretion. Subsequently H_2 receptor antagonists are used to achieve a basal acid output of less than 5 mmol/hr. Total gastrectomy is reserved for patients in whom acid hypersecretion is not controlled pharmacologically. Chemotherapy is used when symptoms are due directly to the tumour and not to acid hypersecretion. 5-fluorouracil and streptozotocin have been helpful in producing relief of symptoms for over 12 months, but the long-term outcome is not known.

REFERENCES

Alexander-Williams J. (1973) Gastric reconstructive surgery. *Ann. R. Coll. Surg. Engl.* **52**, 1–17.

Amdrup E. and Jensen H. E. (1970) Selective vagotomy of the parietal cell mass preserving innervation of the undrained antrum. *Gastroenterology* **59**, 522–527.

Burke J. F. (1961) Effective period of preventive antibiotic action in experimental incisions and dermal lesions. *Surgery* **50**, 161–168.

Cade D. and Allan D. (1979) Long term follow-up of patients with gastric ulcers treated by vagotomy, pyloroplasty and ulcerectomy. *Br. J. Surg.* **66**, 46–47.

Clark C. G. (1968) Surgical aspects of gastrointestinal haemorrhage. *Postgrad. Med. J.* **44**, 590–593.

Cooper M. J. and Williamson R. C. N. (1984) Splenectomy: indications, hazards and alternatives. *Br. J. Surg.* **71**, 173–180.

Doll R. (1950) Perforated carcinoma of the stomach simulating perforated gastric ulcer. *Br. Med. J.* **1**, 215–218.

Duthie H. L. and Bransom C. J. (1979) Highly selective vagotomy with excision of ulcer compared with gastrectomy for gastric ulcer in a randomized trial. *Br. J. Surg.* **66**, 43–45.

Ellis H., Starer F., Venables C. et al. (1966) Clinical and radiological study of vagotomy and gastric drainage in the treatment of pyloric stenosis due to duodenal ulcer. *Gut* **7**, 671–676.

Franksson C. (1948) Selective abdominal vagotomy. *Acta Chir. Scand.* **96**, 409.

Gatehouse D., Dimock F., Burdon R. W. et al. (1978) Prediction of wound sepsis following gastric operations. *Br. J. Surg.* **65**, 551–554.

Goligher J. C. (1974) A technique for highly selective (parietal cell or proximal gastric) vagotomy for duodenal ulcer. *Br. J. Surg.* **61**, 337–345.

Humphrey C. S., Johnson D., Walker B. E. et al. (1972) Incidence of dumping after truncal and selective vagotomy with pyloroplasty and HSV without drainage procedure. *Br. Med. J.* **3**, 785–788.

Immelman E. J., Jeffery P., Benator S. R. et al. (1979) Failure of low dose heparin to prevent significant thrombo-embolic complications in high risk surgical patients: interim report of prospective trial. *Br. Med. J.* **1**, 1447–1450.

Jackson R. G. (1948) Anatomic study of the vagus nerves. *Arch. Surg.* **57**, 333.

Jenkins T. P. N. (1976) The burst abdominal wound, a mechanical approach. *Br. J. Surg.* **63**, 873–876.

Jensen H. E., Amdrup E., Christiansen P. et al. (1972) Bleeding gastric ulcer: surgical and non-surgical treatment of 225 patients. *Scand. J. Gastroenterol.* **7**, 535.

Johnston D., Lyndon P.J., Smith R. B. et al. (1973) Highly selective vagotomy without a drainage procedure in the treatment of haemorrhage, perforation and pyloric stenosis due to peptic ulcer. *Br. J. Surg.* **60**, 790–797.

Johnston D. and Wilkinson A. R. (1970) Highly selective vagotomy without a drainage procedure in the treatment of duodenal ulcer. *Br. J. Surg.* **57**, 289–296.

Johnson H. D. (1951) The present place of vagotomy in the treatment of peptic ulcer. *Ann. R. Coll. Surg. Engl.* **8**, 160–165.

Johnston S. J., Jones P. F., Kyle J. et al. (1973) Epidemiology and course of gastrointestinal haemorrhage in North East Scotland. *Br. Med. J.* **3**, 655–659.

Jones F. A. (1977) The pathogenesis and treatment of gastric ulcer. *Br. J. Hosp. Med.* 372.

Jones P. F., Johnston S. J., McEwan A. B. et al. (1973) Further haemorrhage after admission to hospital for gastrointestinal haemorrhage. *Br. Med. J.* **3**, 660–664.

Kelling G. (1917–18) Ueber die operative Behandlung des chronischen Ulcus ventriculi. *Arch. Klin. Chir.* **109**, 775–831.

Kennedy J. (1973) In: Cox A. G. and Williams J. A. (eds) *Vagotomy on Trial*. London, Heinemann, p. 95.

Kennedy T., Kelly J. M. and George J. D. (1972) Vagotomy for gastric ulcer. *Br. Med. J.* **2**, 371.

MacDougall B. R. D., Bailey R. J. and Williams R. (1977) H_2 receptor anatagonists and antacids in the prevention of acute gastrointestinal haemorrhage in fulminating hepatic failure. *Lancet* **1**, 617.

Madlener M. (1923) Uber pylorektomie bei pylorusfernem Magengeschwur. *Zentralbl. Chir.* **50**, 1313–1317.

Mee A. S., Ismail S., Bornman P. C. et al. (1983) Changing concepts in the presentation, diagnosis and management of the Zollinger–Ellison Syndrome. *Q. J. Med.* **52**, 256–267.

Polak J. M., Stagg B. and Pearse A. G. E. (1972) Two types of Z–E syndrome, immunofluorescent, cytochemical and ultrastructural studies of the antral and pancreatic gastric cells in different clinical states. *Gut* **13**, 501.

Pollock A. V., Greenall M. J. and Evans M. (1979) Single layer mass closure of major laparotomies by continuous suturing. *J. R. Soc. Med.* **72**, 889–893.

Portis S. A. and Jaffe R. H. (1938) A study of peptic ulcer based on necropsy records. *JAMA* **110**, 6.

Schiller K. F. R., Truelove S. C. and Williams D. C. (1970) Haematemesis and melaena with special reference to factors influencing outcome. *Br. Med. J.* **2**, 7.

Schwartz K. (1910) Ueber penetrierende Magen- und Jejunalgeschwure. *Beitr. Klin. Chir.* **67**, 96–128.

Scott-Harden W. G. (1974) Radiology of acute digestive tract bleeding. *J. R. Coll. Physicians Lond.* **8**, 365.

Stammers F. A. R. and Williams J. A. (1963) *Partial Gastrectomy*. London, Butterworths, pp. 49–53.

Tanner N. C. (1951) Operative methods in treatment of peptic ulcer. *Edinb. Med. J.* **58**, 279.

Tanner N. C. (1954) Surgical aspects of gastric and duodenal ulceration (excluding complications). *Postgrad. Med. J.* **30**, 124–131.

Taylor H. (1951) Aspiration treatment of perforated ulcers. *Lancet* **1**, 7.

Tudhope G. R. (1958) Loss and replacement of red cells in patients with acute gastrointestinal haemorrhage. *Q. J. Med.* **27**, 543–559.

Vogt T. M. and Johnson R. E. (1980) Recent changes in the incidence of duodenal and gastric ulcer. *Am. J. Epidemiol.* **111**, 713–720.

Weinberg J. A. (1961) Treatment of the massively bleeding DU by ligation pyloroplasty and vagotomy. *Am. J. Surg.* **102**, 158.

Young A. E. (1982) Stopping the haemorrhage from peptic ulcers. *Br. Med. J.* **284**, 530.

Chapter thirteen

Peptic Ulcer: Highly Selective Vagotomy

D. Johnston

In highly selective vagotomy (HSV), vagal denervation is confined to the acid-secreting part of the stomach, the parietal cell mass (PCM). The antral 'mill', pyloric sphincter and duodenum are left intact, so that gastric emptying is well controlled and reflux of bile into the stomach is minimized. Experience with HSV over the past 18 years has shown that the incidence of recurrent ulceration averages about 8 per cent (range 3–30 per cent), which is the same incidence as after truncal vagotomy (TV) with a drainage (D) procedure, while side-effects such as 'dumping', diarrhoea and bilious vomiting are significantly less common after HSV than after either TV + D or partial gastrectomy.

Nomenclature

Amdrup and I introduced this pylorus-preserving type of vagotomy in humans in 1969 (Amdrup and Jensen, 1970; Johnston and Wilkinson, 1970) and are in agreement that if the precise extent of the PCM is 'mapped' at operation, the procedure should be called 'parietal cell vagotomy' (PCV), while if anatomical landmarks only are used to determine what length of distal stomach shall be left innervated, it should be called 'highly selective vagotomy' (HSV) (Amdrup and Johnston, 1975). If a pyloroplasty is added routinely, as Holle originally suggested (Holle and Hart, 1967), then the operation should be called 'selective proximal vagotomy'.

INDICATIONS

Compared with *Polya partial gastrectomy (PG)* or *vagotomy combined with antrectomy (V + A)*, HSV has about one-quarter the operative mortality (0·3 vs 1·2 per cent), and produces significantly fewer side-effects and long-term metabolic sequelae (Johnston, 1975; Jordan, 1976; Sawyers et al., 1977; Dorricott et al., 1978). Moreover, gastric resection for peptic ulcer predisposes to the development of gastric carcinoma in the long term (Stalsberg and Taksdal, 1971; Schrumpf et al., 1977) probably because of the damaging effect of 'bile' on the gastric mucosa (Lawson, 1964). After HSV, reflux of bile into the stomach is less than after PG or V + A, and so the long-term incidence of gastric carcinoma may be lower. For these reasons, gastric resection should seldom be used in the initial surgical treatment of patients with duodenal ulceration, although it is still the mainstay of treatment for patients who develop recurrent ulceration after any type of vagotomy.

Compared with *truncal vagotomy* and *pyloroplasty (TV + P)* or *gastroenterostomy (TV + GE)*, which is still the most commonly used operation for duodenal ulcer in Britain, HSV is marginally safer (operative mortality 0·3 vs 0·6 per cent) and produces fewer side-effects and less loss of weight. Both HSV and TV + P have a mean incidence of recurrent ulceration of 5–10 per cent, which is significantly greater than the mean incidence of recurrence after PG (3 per cent) or V + A (1 per cent).

It cannot be emphasized too strongly that in spite of its apparent simplicity, TV + P is a *radical* operation, most of which is unnecessary. The vagal denervation of the gastric antrum in TV + P is unnecessary, for example, because, far from reducing circulating levels of gastrin, TV increases them significantly (Hansky and Korman, 1973). Destruction or bypass of the terminal antrum and pyloric sphincter (as in TV + P/GE) is thus also unnecessary, because when the gastric antrum is left vagally innervated, as in HSV, gastric emptying proceeds efficiently through an intact pylorus (Howlett et al., 1976). In contrast, the stomach is 'incontinent' of liquids after TV + P (McKelvey, 1970; Clarke and Alexander-Williams, 1973), while the pattern of emptying of solid food is also irregular (Buckler, 1967; Colmer et al., 1973; Donovan, 1976). The vagal denervation of the liver and biliary tract, pancreas and small intestine in the course of TV + P never had any logical basis, but was condoned in the past because it did not seem to do any harm. It is now known, however, that section of the hepatic vagal fibres causes the gallbladder to dilate, alters the chemical composition of the bile and leads to a significant increase in the incidence of gallstones in the human (Rudick and Hutchison, 1964; Parkin et al., 1973; Csendes et al., 1978). Likewise, section of the coeliac vagal branch, as in posterior truncal vagotomy, significantly impairs enzyme output from the pancreas in the human (Malagelada et al., 1974; MacGregor et al., 1977; Lavigne et al., 1979). Forty per cent of patients develop steatorrhoea after TV + P/GE, whereas after HSV faecal fat output is unaltered (Cox et al., 1964; Wastell and Ellis, 1966; Edwards et al., 1974). Finally, it should be emphasized that many of the vagal fibres that are cut in the course of a truncal vagotomy are responsible for inhibition, rather than stimulation, of gastric secretion (Kelly et al., 1964; Takita et al., 1971; Preshaw, 1973; Sjödin, 1974;

Becker et al., 1975; Stenqvist et al., 1978; Ahonen et al., 1979).

In summary, TV + P/GE fails to reduce serum gastrin, increases reflux of 'bile' into the stomach, destroys antropyloric control of gastric emptying and produces needless damage to the functions of the liver and biliary tract, pancreas and small intestine in the human. Clinically, too, the results of TV + P/GE are inferior to those of HSV (Stoddard et al., 1978), provided that the HSV is well done technically. For these reasons, TV/GE should no longer be used in the treatment of patients with duodenal ulcer, unless special circumstances such as massive haemorrhage or an unfit patient dictate that the operation should be completed in the minimum period of time. HSV is thus the treatment of choice for most patients who come to elective operation for chronic duodenal ulcer.

Elective Surgery for Duodenal Ulcer

Before surgical treatment is advised, medical treatment should have been shown to have failed, as judged by the patient's symptoms and by the finding of persisting ulceration at endoscopy. Patients themselves should be convinced of the need for surgical treatment, because of serious interference by the ulcer symptoms with their occupation or their leisure activities. Nowadays, a full course of cimetidine should usually be administered for at least 2 or 3 months, after which maintenance therapy (400 mg nocte or b.d.) may be continued for 6–12 months. However, cimetidine is far from being the 'specific' remedy many imagine it to be, and recent reports of gynaecomastia, lowered sperm counts and mental confusion in patients receiving cimetidine are disquieting. Moreover, when cimetidine therapy is stopped, 70–80 per cent of the ulcers recur within 1 year. Not all patients with recurrent ulceration after cimetidine therapy should be treated surgically, however. Duodenal ulceration, in contrast to gastric ulceration, remains a 'medical' disease which sometimes requires surgical treatment. It is thus particularly important to advise patients about their lifestyle; they should obtain sufficient rest and relaxation, stop smoking, moderate their alcoholic intake and eat at regular intervals. I try to avoid operating on young, neurotic people, particularly if they have been tattooed, have bad teeth and a poor work record, because, however treated, such patients tend to fare badly and to complain bitterly of any postoperative side-effects. Careful selection of patients for operation is as important as selecting the correct operative procedure and performing it well.

The author uses HSV in 99 per cent of patients who come to elective operation for chronic duodenal ulcer uncomplicated by pyloric stenosis (see below). Very rarely, in an elderly unfit patient, I would use TV + P. There is at present no established basis for the addition of antrectomy to selective gastric vagotomy in patients who are found to have gross hypersecretion of acid (>45 mmol HCl/hr) at the preoperative pentagastrin test, because neither Amdrup's group nor our own has found that such patients have a significantly higher risk of developing recurrent ulceration if treated by HSV alone. There are indeed authors who have found a correlation between preoperative acid output and recurrent ulceration after both TV +P and HSV, but since the incidence of *incomplete* vagotomy according to the results of the Hollander test 1 week after operation ranged in their series from 30 to 60 per cent, their conclusions probably do not apply to centres where the incidence of incomplete vagotomy is at more 'acceptable' levels (i.e. less than 20 per cent).

Obesity has not been a contra-indication to the use of HSV in my practice: we just have to work harder!

Pyloric Stenosis

A crucial question is, when should a drainage procedure be added to HSV? The patient's history gives the answer. If the patient has the classic, *clinical* features of 'pyloric' stenosis, with copious vomiting, weight loss and a succussion splash, he or she will unquestionably require either a drainage procedure or pyloric dilatation or duodenoplasty (Johnston et al., 1973; Kennedy, 1976; McMahon et al., 1976). About 10 per cent of duodenal ulcer patients in Britain belong to this category. However, many patients with duodenal ulcers vomit during exacerbations of their symptoms, but can eat normally during remissions. Such patients do not require the addition of a drainage procedure to HSV. Similarly, patients who lack the clinical features of pyloric stenosis, but who are found at operation to have gross scarring and distortion of the proximal duodenum, do not require the addition of a drainage procedure. Addition of a pyloroplasty in these circumstances significantly increases the risk of dumping without conferring any clinical benefit (Wastell et al., 1977; Amdrup et al., 1978).

Perforation

Patients with perforation of a *chronic* duodenal ulcer, if treated by simple closure of the perforation, have a 6 per cent operative mortality, a 70–80 per cent chance of developing recurrent ulceration and a 50 per cent chance of requiring a second, definitive procedure. Hence such patients should be treated by closure of the perforation combined with some form of vagotomy to cure the ulcer, provided that they are fit to withstand the more extensive operation and that the surgeon operating possesses the necessary skills. If these conditions are satisfied, the operative mortality is only 2 per cent, 5–10 per cent of patients develop recurrent ulceration and most of the others obtain a good clinical result. In the past, many surgeons were deterred from using definitive surgical treatment by the fear that the 20–30 per cent of patients who do *not* develop recurrent ulceration after simple closure of the perforation might have the quality of their lives impaired by the side-effects and long-term sequelae of PG or TV + D. The unnecessary use of HSV in a minority of patients does less harm than PG or TV + D, and several hundred patients with perforated duodenal ulcer have now been treated by HSV, with a mortality of 1 per cent (Johnston et al., 1973; Jordan and Korompai, 1976; Narbona and Charlo, 1977; Sawyers and Herrington, 1977; Amdrup and Skovgaard, 1978). No single method of treatment is appropriate for all patients with perforated duodenal ulcer. In my own practice, about 5 per cent of patients (the very unfit and those with sealed perforation) are treated conservatively, 25 per cent are treated by simple closure (these are mainly patients with perforation of an *acute* ulcer), while most of the remaining 70 per cent are treated by HSV, though a few elderly high-risk patients are still treated by TV + P because it is quicker and easier to perform than HSV.

Haemorrhage

The mean operative mortality of emergency partial gastrectomy for bleeding peptic ulcer is 16 per cent, whereas the mortality of emergency TV + P with under-running of the bleeding point is 8 per cent. Rebleeding is as common after PG as after vagotomy (13 per cent). Thus there is little doubt that direct suture of the bleeding point, combined with some type of vagotomy, is now the operation of choice for all patients with bleeding duodenal ulcer and probably for many patients with bleeding gastric ulcer. If the surgeon has extensive experience with HSV, there is no reason why HSV should not be used in preference to truncal vagotomy in the better-risk patients (Johnston et al., 1973; Johnston, 1977a). There is equally little doubt that the high-risk, severely shocked, elderly patients should continue to be treated by truncal vagotomy.

Gastric Ulcer

HSV, combined with excision of the ulcer through a gastrotomy, is being used increasingly in the surgical treatment of patients with gastric ulcer, and has obvious attractions in older, poorly nourished patients (Johnston et al., 1972; Johnston, 1977b; Duthie and Branson, 1979). The rationale for the use of HSV for gastric ulcer is that it blunts acid-pepsin attack on the gastric mucosa, speeds gastric emptying of liquids and diminishes reflux of bile into the stomach, whereas PG and TV + D increase bile reflux. Though outputs of acid and pepsin in patients with gastric ulcer are within normal limits, it is acid and pepsin nevertheless which breach the weakened mucosal defences, and so the 90 per cent reduction in basal acid output (BAO) and the 70–80 per cent

reduction in maximal acid output after HSV are effective in preventing recurrent ulceration in 90–95 per cent of patients. The possibility of missing an ulcer-cancer must, of course, be eliminated by preoperative endoscopy with multiple biopsy, and by frozen-section examination of the excised ulcer at the time of surgery. The results of HSV for gastric ulcer are at least as good to date as those of Billroth-I partial gastrectomy.

OPERATIVE TECHNIQUE

Two assistants are required, one to hold the stomach and the other to retract the liver. Good access to the upper abdomen and to the oesophageal hiatus is essential. A midline incision is used, extending from the xiphoid process to 3–4 cm below the umbilicus. The xiphoid is not excised. The edges of the wound are retracted by a self-retaining retractor. Access to the oesophagus is greatly improved if a metal hook is inserted under the xiphoid notch and strong traction exerted towards the head of the operating table. This upward retraction of the rib cage is rendered more effective if the table is tilted about 15° head up, which has the additional advantage of causing the other viscera to fall away from the stomach and oesophagus. The left lobe of the liver is next mobilized to the right by division of the left triangular ligament (beware the inferior phrenic vein). Access to the oesophagus is now complete. The diagnosis of chronic duodenal ulceration is confirmed, the stomach and oesophageal hiatus are assessed carefully, and a full laparotomy is carried out.

The next step is to mobilize the distal half of the greater curvature of the stomach by division of the gastrocolic omentum outside the gastro-epiploic arcades. The gastro-epiploic vessels are preserved so that interference with the stomach's blood supply will be kept to a minimum. Such mobilization of the greater curvature confers the advantage that the posterior nerve of Latarjet can then usually be seen, and this of course makes it easier to preserve. In addition, each of the major vessels entering the lesser curve on its posterior aspect can be ligated and divided precisely, close to the stomach, while the nerve is kept in view. Another advantage of this approach is that the stomach, which itself is the main 'retractor' in HSV, is easier to grip and pull upon if part of the greater curvature has been mobilized.

Contrary to popular belief, HSV is not a difficult operation. It does not, for example, involve any painstaking search for tiny nerve fibres, except on the oesophagus, where in any case a meticulous search for vagal fibres forms part of a well-conducted TV or SV. Another deterrent is the alleged complexity of the distribution of the vagal nerves to the stomach, but having studied and drawn the nerves at each HSV operation, the author is more impressed with their relative constancy than with their variability.

The anterior vagal trunk enters the abdomen in front of the oesophagus and runs downwards and to the right, giving off one or more large anterior gastric branches. It leaves the oesophagus near the cardia, gives off the hepatic fibres, and then runs downwards in the lesser omentum parallel to the lesser curvature and 1–2 cm from it, as the anterior nerve of Latarjet. This important nerve lies immediately beneath the peritoneum. It accompanies the descending branch of the left gastric artery, and terminates just distal to the incisura angularis, 5–7 cm from the pylorus, by passing across onto the anterior aspect of the antral region of the stomach, usually in the form of two major terminal branches (*Fig.* 13.1).

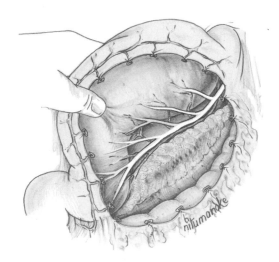

Fig. 13.2. Greater curvature has been mobilized by division of gastrocolic omentum to show the posterior nerve of Latarjet, which terminates on the antrum distal to the incisura. The terminal Y fork of the nerve is preserved and all the other branches to the stomach are divided. Mobilization of the greater curvature is normally much less extensive than that illustrated. Note also that the gastro-epiploic arcades are carefully preserved.

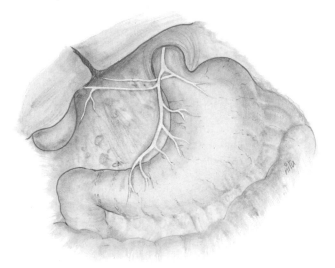

Fig. 13.1. Distribution of the anterior vagal trunk is shown. Note hepatic fibres and main continuation of trunk, the anterior nerve of Latarjet reaching the antrum distal to the incisura about 6 cm from the pylorus.

The posterior vagal trunk enters the abdomen behind or to the right of the oesophagus, gives off the large coeliac branch and a variable number of gastric branches, and then runs downwards in the posterior aspect of the lesser omentum as the posterior nerve of Latarjet. The course and distribution of this nerve to the posterior aspect of the stomach are similar to those of the anterior nerve of Latarjet to the anterior aspect. The anterior nerve of Latarjet is visible in 95 per cent of patients and even in the most obese its terminal branches can be discerned. Likewise, the posterior nerve of Latarjet is usually visible when the lesser sac has been opened (*Fig.* 13.2).

The surgeon should embark on the HSV dissection with an overall tactical plan in his head. The first major phase of the operation is to separate the lesser omentum, with its nerves of Latarjet, from the lesser curvature of the stomach between the incisura angularis and the cardia; and in the course of this dissection a delicate technique must be employed to avoid

damage both to the muscular wall of the stomach and to the nerves of Latarjet. The second major phase of the operation involves thorough mobilization of the distal 5–6 cm of oesophagus and clearance from it of all nerve fibres. The key questions are, first, how much of the distal stomach should be left innervated (i.e. where does the dissection begin on the lesser curvature), and second, how far proximally should the dissection be pursued on the oesophagus? While the answers cannot be absolutely precise, it may be stated as a rule of thumb that about 6 cm of stomach proximal to the pylorus should be left vagally innervated and that 6 cm of distal oesophagus should be cleared of all blood vessels and nerve fibres.

The anterior nerve of Latarjet is identified, and the position of its terminal branches noted. The nerve is rendered more obvious if the assistant exerts traction on the greater curvature. There is a 'crow's foot' arrangement of large veins (not of nerves) in the region of the incisura, and the major terminations of the nerve of Latarjet accompany the veins that form the 'toe' of the foot. The anterior part of the dissection begins just proximal to the point where these nerves pass across onto the musculature of the antral region. This point is usually 5–6 cm proximal to the pylorus. Hence, 5–7 cm of distal stomach are usually left innervated. Thus, one should identify the major nerves to the antrum and preserve them, rather than measure off an arbitrary length of the stomach and denervate the remainder.

The dissection begins at the chosen spot near the incisura on the anterior aspect of the stomach. The objective is to separate the lesser omentum from the lesser curvature between the incisura and the cardia by dividing all blood vessels and nerves that enter the lesser curvature from the lesser omentum. The blood vessels run in two distinct leashes, one of which passes to the anterior surface of the stomach and the other to the posterior surface. Each sizeable vessel is divided individually, and for this reason also it is an advantage to have secured access to the posterior aspect of the stomach.

The serosa overlying the vessels is divided by means of curved McIndoe's scissors, between the incisura and the cardia, along the line of the lesser curvature and well to the left of the nerves of Latarjet. The instruments can then be slid gently under the vessels, rather than having to be 'punched' forcibly through the serosa, which is surprisingly tough. Dissection begins near the incisura, about 2 cm proximal to the determined distal extremity of the dissection (this 2-cm segment is cleared at the *end* of the operation, because if it were divided at this stage the nerves of Latarjet would be at risk of injury by traction during the dissection). A curved haemostat, such as a Kilner or Roberts, is gently insinuated beneath each major vessel (*Fig.* 13.3), a ligature is passed, seized in the jaws of the haemostat, drawn under the vessel and the vessel is tied in continuity on the lesser omental side and then clamped close to the lesser curvature. The vessel is then divided (*Fig.* 13.4). This method is felt to be preferable to the application of two haemostats and division of the vessel between them, because it ensures that the vessel cannot slip from a clamp and retract into the fat of the lesser omentum where it cannot be pursued and clamped for fear that the nerves of Latarjet will be damaged. In addition, a haemostat placed on the lesser omental side may inadvertently crush one of the nerves of Latarjet or, when lifted up, may tent up a nerve and cause it to be trapped in the ligature.

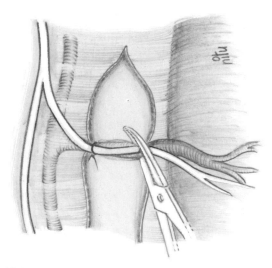

Fig. 13.4. Vessel is ligated in continuity on lesser omental side and clamped on lesser curve side. A fine-pointed haemostat is used and great care is taken to avoid damage both to the nerve of Latarjet and to musculature of the lesser curvature.

Each vessel should be ligated individually, because if large bites of tissue are taken the pedicle has a broad base and the ligature is more likely to slip when strong traction is exerted on the stomach during the oesophageal dissection. Loose areolar tissue between the blood vessels is clamped in a haemostat, coagulated with diathermy and then divided. My practice is to divide the anterior leaf of the lesser omentum in this way from near the incisura to the cardia and then to lay bare the anterior aspect of the oesophagus as far as the angle of His in like manner (*Fig.* 13.5). Alternatively, the entire oesophageal dissection may be left until later. The stomach is then turned over and the posterior leaf of the lesser omentum is dealt

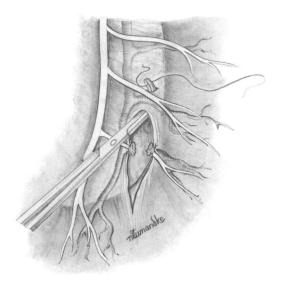

Fig. 13.3. Dissection of anterior leaf of lesser omentum. Note that each major vessel is separately under-run and ligated in continuity.

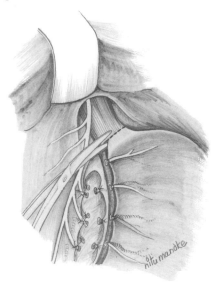

Fig. 13.5. Anterior leaf of lesser omentum has been divided and serosa overlying oesophago-gastric junction is being divided as far as the angle of His.

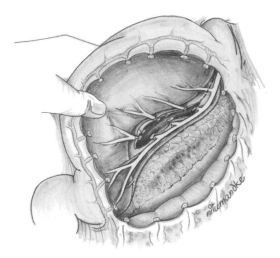

Fig. 13.6. Division of posterior leaf of lesser omentum has begun, leaving about 5 cm of pre-pyloric stomach innervated. Demonstration of posterior nerve of Latarjet in this way helps to prevent damage to it.

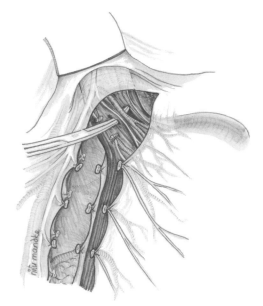

Fig. 13.7. Small vessels and nerves running down the anterior surface of the oesophagus in the meso-oesophagus are gently lifted by haemostat, seized in the forceps and destroyed by diathermy or else ligated with fine thread.

with similarly: the dissection begins at the incisura and is carried upwards to near the cardia (*Fig.* 13.6). One then returns to the anterior aspect of the stomach and if a breakthrough has not yet been achieved between front and back this is now done and the few remaining vessels and nerves entering the lesser curvature are divided. Separation of the lesser omentum from the stomach between incisura and cardia in this way is relatively straightforward, and ensures that vagal fibres cannot possibly enter the stomach between these two points. Thus the vagotomy of the parietal cell mass can only be incomplete either distally, at the antral end or on the oesophagus.

If only 5–7 cm of distal stomach are left innervated, there is little likelihood of the vagotomy being incomplete distally, because Amdrup and Jensen (1970), who routinely mapped the extent of the antrum at the time of operation, found that the boundary between parietal cell mass and antrum lay 8 or 9 cm on average proximal to the pylorus and seldom extended more distally than 6 cm from the pylorus. In addition, when the operative method described above was used in Leeds, only 3 out of the first 100 consecutive insulin tests 1 week after HSV were found to be positive and none was early-positive in the first hour after insulin. Thus the problem of incomplete vagotomy is, for the most part, a problem of missed vagal fibres on the oesophagus.

The next step is to expose the anterior surface of the oesophagus. The mobilized left lobe of the liver is drawn across to the right by means of a deep Kelly's retractor, and the serosa covering the oesophago-gastric junction is divided with long curved scissors (*see Fig.* 13.5). Small vessels are picked up in Roberts forceps, lifted off the muscle layer and coagulated with diathermy (*Fig.* 13.7). The Roberts forceps are then slipped gently across the surface of the lower

oesophagus, on the muscle layer and beneath the larger vessels and the anterior gastric branches of the anterior vagal trunk. These are then ligated in continuity proximally, clamped distally and divided. Division of these tissues frees the anterior vagal trunk, which remains out of harm's way above and to the left of the operator's scissors. The angle of His, 3 cm or so of upper greater curvature and the areolar tissue to the left of the oesophagus are then cleared of fat and blood vessels (*Fig.* 13.8).

The next and most difficult step is to expose the posterior and right lateral aspects of the oesophagus. It is still too early to pass a sling or tube around the oesophagus. The assistant grasps the body of the stomach and pulls it in both a distal and a vertical direction. The vessels and nerves entering the lower oesophagus and cardia are thus rendered taut and can be under-run, ligated in continuity and divided in the usual way (*Fig.* 13.9). The dissection is kept very close to the wall of the upper stomach and lower oesophagus to avoid damage to the nerve trunks and to their coeliac and hepatic branches. The danger to these structures is not as great as might be feared, because division of the vessels and nerves along the lesser curvature has allowed them to be swept upwards and to the operator's left. As the dissection proceeds it becomes possible to pass a soft rubber tube around the oesophagus. Traction on this tube further facilitates access to the posterior aspect of the oesophagus. At this stage, a leash of vessels passing from the lesser omentum to the upper part of the greater curvature is encountered and divided. Finally, the rubber sling is withdrawn and the operator grasps the oesophagus in his right hand and draws

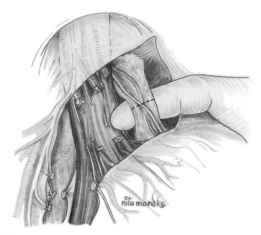

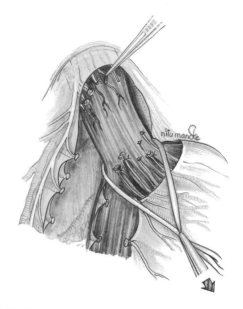

Fig. 13.8. This step is often carried out at the same time as division of the anterior leaf of lesser omentum. The serosa to the left of the oesophagus is divided and then fatty areolar tissue to the left of the oesophagus, which contains nerve fibres, vessels and lymphatics, is lifted up with the right index finger. The angle of His and the adjacent oesophagus and fundus of stomach are thoroughly cleared and in this way small nerve fibres running to the proximal 3 cm of fundus ('criminal' nerves of Grassi) are eliminated.

Fig. 13.10. The oesophagus is now fully mobilized and the operator can exert strong but gentle traction on it, and can also rotate it in order to reach fibres running down the posterior aspect. Small blood vessels and nerve fibres are picked up by dissecting forceps or in the tip of a haemostat, coagulated and divided. This is a painstaking exercise and the whole oesophageal part of the dissection may take 30 minutes. None the less, this is where vagotomies are usually incomplete and the complete 'skeletonization' of the distal 5–6 cm of oesophagus in this way ensures that few of the postoperative insulin tests will be positive and that the incidence of recurrent ulceration will be low.

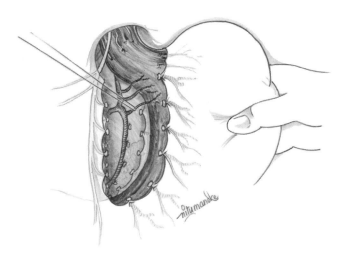

Fig. 13.9. Division of vessels and nerves to cardia and posterior aspect of oesophagus. Note that the assistant pulls the stomach downwards and at the same time elevates it. The operator stays very close to the muscle of lesser curvature and oesophagus in order to avoid vagal trunks and hepatic and coeliac branches.

it gently but firmly downwards (*Fig.* 13.10). He should be able to pass three or four fingers behind the oesophagus at this stage. This manoeuvre invariably reveals many more vessels and nerve fibres entering the oesophagus, particularly on the right lateral and posterior aspects. These are painstakingly ligated or coagulated and divided with fine curved McIndoe's scissors. It is obviously important not to perforate the oesophagus, but this is unlikely to happen if both the vessels and the nerves are lifted clear of the oesophageal muscle before being coagulated.

The importance of spending a long time (15–30 minutes) in ensuring that the vagotomy is complete on the oesophagus cannot be overemphasized. Postoperative insulin studies indicate that the distal extent of HSV vagally denervates the distal parietal cell mass in most patients (Johnston et al., 1973). More proximally, there can be no doubt about the completeness of the vagotomy between the incisura and the cardia. It is on the oesophagus that HSV may be and indeed often is incomplete. Some authors report that as many as 30–60 per cent of their patients have positive insulin tests 1 week after HSV, but such a high incidence of positive tests is of course not uncommon after TV and SV also (Johnston and Goligher, 1971). When the insulin test is early-positive 1 week after vagotomy the risk of recurrent ulceration is high (~20 per cent), whereas when the insulin test is negative soon after vagotomy the risk of recurrent ulceration is low (2–3 per cent).

If there has been a good deal of oozing around the oesophagus a fine suction drain is inserted which is withdrawn 1–2 days later. It should be added that all our patients receive low-dose subcutaneous heparin as an attempted method of prophylaxis of deep venous thrombosis. The linea alba is approximated with a running suture of monofilament nylon,

1 g of ampicillin powder is placed in the wound and the skin is closed.

POSTOPERATIVE CARE

Postoperative care is very simple. The nasogastric tube is withdrawn at the end of the operation and the intravenous drip is taken down at the same time. The patient is kept well hydrated before and during operation. On the day of operation only ice is given orally and on the 1st postoperative day 30 ml of water are given hourly. Since gastric emptying is better if the patient is upright, he or she is encouraged to sit up and by the 2nd postoperative day to get out of bed and walk a little. On the 2nd day the patient is given 60–90 ml of water per hour and by the 3rd day should be drinking fluids freely. Soup and custard are given on the 4th day and a light diet by the 5th day. The postoperative insulin test is done between the 5th and the 8th postoperative day. The patient is usually ready to go home 6–9 days after operation.

INTRAOPERATIVE TESTS FOR COMPLETENESS OF VAGOTOMY

The usefulness of such tests is debatable. Burge's electrical stimulation test (Burge, 1964) records an increase in intragastric pressure if an intact vagal fibre is included within the electrode which is placed around the oesophagus. Some authors, such as Amery and Allgöwer, have found a significant correlation between the finding of a positive Burge test after vagotomy and subsequent recurrent ulceration, but others have found the test less useful. In Grassi's test (Grassi, 1971) a pH-recording electrode is introduced into the stomach, which is stimulated to secrete acid by the intravenous infusion of pentagastrin. If the entire gastric mucosa is found to be alkaline after vagotomy, the vagotomy is complete: conversely, the finding of an acid area indicates an incomplete vagotomy, and also shows where the vagotomy is incomplete (Johnson and Baxter, 1977). Neither the Burge nor the Grassi test is completely reliable. However, both are probably useful in training surgeons to achieve a complete vagotomy, though their principal merit may be that they stimulate the surgeon to take great pains over the vagotomy in an attempt to 'defeat' the test.

POSTOPERATIVE COMPLICATIONS

Complications specific to HSV have been very unusual in our experience over the past 18 years. No patient has developed oesophageal perforation, in spite of the extensive oesophageal mobilization. Two or three per cent of patients require splenectomy because of operative trauma to the splenic capsule, but in recent years many small tears of the spleen have been treated conservatively, by temporary packing followed by suction drainage, without mishap.

Necrosis of the lesser curvature or fundus of the stomach occurs in approximately 1 in every 500 HSV operations, and caused death in 1 in 1000 (0·1 per cent; Johnston, 1975). In some cases it may be due to ischaemia, because the anastomotic network of blood vessels in the submucosa is much more sparse along the lesser curvature than in the anterior and posterior walls of the stomach. However, it seems likely that many cases of necrosis are also attributable to operative trauma to the gastric wall by diathermy, ligature or instrumental damage.

Gastric retention after HSV is unusual; less common, in fact, than after TV + D, as sophisticated studies of gastric emptying after HSV and TV + D have shown. Approximately 0·5 per cent of patients who have undergone HSV develop gastric retention and require the addition of a drainage procedure several months after the initial operation. This complication may be due to accidental damage to the nerves of Latarjet, cicatricial narrowing at the gastric outlet as the ulcer heals, or to other causes. The incidence of impaired gastric emptying is lower after HSV than after vagotomy combined with antrectomy (Dorricott et al., 1978).

The operative mortality of HSV is very low: 0·3 per cent in a survey of 5939 elective operations (Johnston, 1975).

HSV for Complications of Peptic Ulcer and for Gastric Ulcer

The operative techniques that are used in conjunction with HSV in patients with pyloric stenosis (Johnston et al, 1973; Kennedy, 1976; McMahon et al., 1976), haemorrhage (Johnston, 1977a) and gastric ulcer (Johnston et al., 1972; Johnston, 1977b) have been described in detail elsewhere and are felt to be beyond the scope of this brief review.

REFERENCES

Ahonen J., Hoepfner-Hallikainen D., Inberg M. et al. (1979) The value of corpus-antrum determinations in highly selective vagotomy. *Br. J. Surg.* **66**, 35–38.

Amdrup E. and Jensen H.-E. (1970) Selective vagotomy of the parietal cell mass preserving innervation of the undrained antrum. *Gastroenterology* **59**, 522–527.

Amdrup E. and Johnston D. (1975) Name of the new vagotomy. *Gastroenterology* **68**, 206–207.

Amdrup E. and Skovgaard S. (1978) Personal communication.

Amdrup E., Andersen D. and Høstrup H. (1978) The Aarhus County Vagotomy Trial. 1. An interim report on primary results and incidence of sequelae following parietal cell vagotomy and selective gastric vagotomy in 748 patients. *World J. Surg.* **2**, 85–90.

Becker H. D., Reeder D. D. and Thompson J. C. (1975) In: Thompson J. C. (ed.), *Gastrointestinal Hormones.* Austin, University of Texas Press, p. 437.

Buckler K. G. (1967) Effects of gastric surgery upon gastric emptying in cases of peptic ulceration. *Gut* **8**, 137–147.

Burge H. (1964) *Vagotomy.* London, Arnold.

Clarke R. J. and Alexander-Williams J. (1973) The effect of preserving antral innervation and of a pyloroplasty on gastric emptying after vagotomy in man. *Gut* **14**, 300–307.

Colmer M. R., Owen G. M. and Shields R. (1973) Pattern of gastric emptying after vagotomy and pyloroplasty. *Br. Med. J.* **2**, 448–450.

Cox A. G., Bond M. R., Podmore D. A. et al. (1964) Aspects of nutrition after vagotomy and gastrojejunostomy. *Br. Med. J.* **1**, 465–469.

Csendes A., Larach J. and Godoy M. (1978) Incidence of gall stones development after selective hepatic vagotomy. *Acta Chir. Scand.* **144**, 289–291.

Donovan I. A. (1976) The different components of gastric emptying after gastric surgery. *Ann. R. Coll. Surg. Engl.* **58**, 368.

Dorricott N. J., McNeish A. R., Alexander-Williams J. et al. (1978) Prospective randomized multi-centre trial of proximal gastric vagotomy or truncal vagotomy and antrectomy for chronic duodenal ulcer. *Br. J. Surg.* **65**, 152–154.

Duthie H. L. and Branson C. J. (1979) Highly selective vagotomy with excision of the ulcer compared with gastrectomy for gastric ulcer in a randomized trial. *Br. J. Surg.* **66**, 43–45.

Edwards J. P., Lyndon P. J., Smith R. B. et al. (1974) Faecal fat excretion after truncal, selective and highly selective vagotomy for duodenal ulcer. *Gut* **15**, 521–525.

Grassi G. (1971) A new test for complete nerve section during vagotomy. *Br. J. Surg.* **58**, 187–189.

Hansky J. and Korman M. G. (1973) Immunoassay studies in peptic ulcer. Peptic ulceration. In: Sircus W. (ed.) *Clinics in Gastroenterology*, Vol. 2. New York, Saunders, pp. 275–291.

Holle F. and Hart W. (1967) Neue Wege des Chirurgie des Gastroduodenalulcus. *Med. Klin.* **62**, 441–450.

Howlett P. J., Sheiner H. J., Barber D. C. et al. (1976) Gastric emptying in control subjects and patients with duodenal ulcer before and after vagotomy. *Gut* **17**, 542–550.

Johnson A. G. and Baxter H. K. (1977) Where is your vagotomy incomplete? Observations on operative technique. *Br. J. Surg.* **64**, 583–586.

Johnston D. (1975) Operative mortality and post-operative morbidity of highly selective vagotomy. *Br. J. Surg.* **62**, 160.

Johnston D. (1977a) Division and repair of the sphincteric mechanism at the gastric outlet in emergency operations for bleeding peptic ulcer. *Ann. Surg.* **186**, 723–729.

Johnston D. (1977b) Highly selective vagotomy with excision of the ulcer for gastric ulceration. In: Rob C. and Smith R. (eds) *Operative Surgery*, 3rd ed. London, Butterworths, pp. 142–149.

Johnston D. and Goligher J. C. (1971) The influence of the individual surgeon and of the type of vagotomy upon the insulin test after vagotomy. *Gut* **12**, 963–967.

Johnston D. and Wilkinson A. R. (1970) Highly selective vagotomy without a drainage procedure in the treatment of duodenal ulcer. *Br. J. Surg.* **57**, 289–296.

Johnston D., Humphrey C. S., Smith R. B. et al. (1972) Treatment of gastric ulcer by highly selective vagotomy without a drainage procedure: an interim report. *Br. J. Surg.* **59**, 787–792.

Johnston D., Lyndon P. J., Smith R. B. et al. (1973) Highly selective vagotomy without a drainage procedure in the treatment of haemorrhage, perforation and pyloric stenosis due to peptic ulcer. *Br. J. Surg.* **60**, 790–797.

Jordan P. H. (1976) A prospective study of parietal cell vagotomy and selective vagotomy-antrectomy for treatment of duodenal ulcer. *Ann. Surg.* **183**, 619–628.

Jordan P. H. and Korompai F. L. (1976) Evolvement of a new treatment for perforated duodenal ulcer. *Surg. Gynecol. Obstet.* **142**, 391–395.

Kelly K. A., Nyhus L. M. and Harkins H. N. (1964) The vagal nerve and the intestinal phase of gastric secretion. *Gastroenterology* **46**, 163–171.

Kennedy T. (1976) Duodenoplasty with proximal gastric vagotomy. *Ann. R. Coll. Surg. Engl.* **58**, 144–146.

Lavigne M. E., Wiley Z. D., Martin P. et al. (1979) A study of gastric, pancreatic and biliary secretion, and the rate of gastric emptying following parietal cell vagotomy. *Am. J. Surg.* **138**, 644–651.

Lawson H. H. (1964) Effect of duodenal contents on the gastric mucosa under experimental conditions. *Lancet* **1**, 469–472.

MacGregor I. L., Parent J. and Meyer J. H. (1977) Gastric emptying of liquid meals and pancreatic and biliary secretion after subtotal gastrectomy or truncal vagotomy and pyloroplasty in man. *Gastroenterology* **72**, 195–205.

McKelvey S. T. D. (1970) Gastric incontinence and post-vagotomy diarrhoea. *Br. J. Surg.* **57**, 741–747.

McMahon M. J., Greenall M. J., Johnston D. et al. (1976) Highly selective vagotomy plus dilatation of the stenosis compared with truncal vagotomy and drainage in the treatment of pyloric stenosis secondary to duodenal ulceration. *Gut* **17**, 471–476.

Malagelada J. R., Go V. L. W. and Summerskill W. H. J. (1974) Altered pancreatic and biliary function after vagotomy and pyloroplasty. *Gastroenterology* **66**, 22–27.

Narbona B. and Charlo T. (1977) In: Narbona B. and Charlo T. (eds) *Vagotomia Gastrica Proximal.* Valencia, Suc de Vives Mora-Artes Graficas, ch. 8.

Parkin G. J. S., Smith R. B. and Johnston D. (1973) Gall bladder volume and contractility after truncal, selective and highly selective (parietal cell) vagotomy in man. *Ann. Surg.* **178**, 581–586.

Preshaw R. M. (1973) Inhibition of pentagastrin stimulated gastric acid output by sham feeding. Fed. Proc. **32**, 410A.

Rudick J. and Hutchison J. S. F. (1964) Effects of vagal nerve section on the biliary system. *Lancet* **1**, 579–581.

Sawyers J. L. and Herrington J. L. (1977) Perforated duodenal ulcer managed by proximal gastric vagotomy and suture plication. *Ann. Surg.* **185**, 656–660.

Sawyers J. L., Herrington J. L. and Burney D. P. (1977) Proximal gastric vagotomy compared with vagotomy and antrectomy and selective gastric vagotomy and pyloroplasty. *Ann. Surg.* **186**, 510–517.

Schrumpf E., Serck-Hanssen A., Stadaas J. et al. (1977) Mucosal changes in the gastric stump 20–25 years after partial gastrectomy. *Lancet* **2**, 467–469.

Sjödin L. (1974) Inhibition of gastrin-stimulated canine acid secretion by sham feeding. *Scand. J. Gastroenterol.* **10**, 73–80.

Stalsberg H. and Taksdal S. (1971) Stomach cancer following gastric surgery for benign conditions. *Lancet* **2**, 1175–1177.

Stenqvist B., Knutson U. and Olbe L. (1978) The vagogastrone mechanism in man. *Scand. J. Gastroenterol.* **13**, 895–901.

Stoddard C. J., Vassilakis J. S. and Duthie H. L. (1978) Highly selective vagotomy or truncal vagotomy and pyloroplasty for chronic duodenal ulceration: a randomized, prospective clinical study. *Br. J. Surg.* **65**, 793–796.

Takita S., Sakakihara Y., Kushida T. et al. (1971) Clinical and experimental studies after several types of vagotomy. *Bull. Soc. Int. Chir.* **5/6**, 462–470.

Wastell C. and Ellis H. (1966) Faecal fat excretion and stool colour after vagotomy and pyloroplasty *Br. Med. J.* **1**, 1194–1197.

Wastell C., Colin J., Wilson T. et al. (1977) Prospectively randomized trial of proximal gastric vagotomy either with or without pyloroplasty in treatment of uncomplicated duodenal ulcer. *Br. Med. J.* **2**, 851–853.

Chapter fourteen

The Pancreas

R. C. N. Williamson

Besides their intimate anatomical relationship, the exocrine and endocrine portions of the pancreas (Greek: 'all flesh') possess complementary functions in the digestion, absorption and metabolism of food-stuffs. The symptoms and signs of pancreatic disease may be slow to develop because of the relatively inaccessible position of the gland and its functional reserve; the ultimate effects tend to be wide ranging and severe. Trauma and acute inflammation can both cause extravasation of powerful digestive enzymes from the pancreas, with potentially devastating local and systemic sequelae. Chronic parenchymal destruction (often by alcohol) produces combined exocrine and endocrine impairment, and the combination of steatorrhoea and diabetes mellitus is reproduced by surgical excision of enough functioning pancreatic tissue. Usually advanced by the time of presentation, exocrine carcinoma tends to be rapidly lethal. Islet cell tumours, though rare, are increasingly recognized and give rise to a variety of fascinating clinical syndromes.

In this chapter, a brief outline of the anatomy of the pancreas is followed by a discussion of the various pathological processes that can affect the gland, including modern methods of diagnosis and treatment. Lastly, the common pancreatic operations are described. Since the surgery of the pancreas frequently involves that of neighbouring abdominal viscera, the relevant chapters on the stomach, biliary tree and spleen should also be consulted.

SURGICAL ANATOMY

The pancreas is draped against the posterior abdominal wall by the peritoneum bordering the lesser sac and, along its inferior border, by the root of the transverse mesocolon. The head of the gland lies snug in the duodenal loop. It is connected by a slight waist at the neck to the body and tail of the pancreas, which pass to the left and gradually upwards, tapering gently to end at the splenic hilum. The uncinate process (Latin: 'hooked') arises from the lower part of the head and projects to the left, behind the superior mesenteric vein and artery but in front of the inferior vena cava and aorta. Anteriorly the pancreas is separated from the stomach by the lesser sac, and posteriorly the tail of the gland is related to the left kidney and adrenal. The common bile duct traverses the head of the pancreas in a groove that is palpable posteriorly.

The pancreatic head and duodenal loop share a common arterial supply (*Fig.* 14.1) derived from the gastroduodenal and superior mesenteric arteries via the anterior and posterior pancreaticoduodenal arcades. The distal part of the gland receives blood from branches of the splenic artery, which pursues a sinuous course along its upper border. In about 20 per cent of people, the main hepatic artery (or a large accessory branch) arises from the superior mesenteric artery and supplies the head of the pancreas. Venous drainage (*Fig.* 14.2) is by correspond-

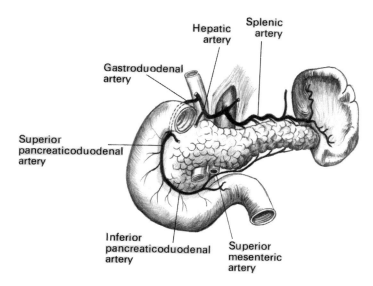

Fig. 14.1. Arterial supply to the pancreas.

155

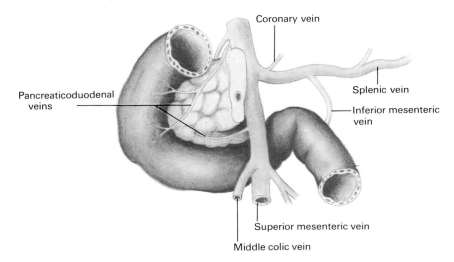

Fig. 14.2. Venous drainage of the pancreas.

ing veins entering the superior mesenteric and splenic trunks; these unite to form the hepatic portal vein directly behind the neck of the pancreas. The gastric (coronary) vein usually joins the portal vein close to its origin, and the inferior mesenteric vein enters the terminal part of the splenic vein. Pancreatic lymphatics accompany the blood vessels and drain to nodes in the region of the pylorus and along the superior border of the gland, thence to the coeliac and superior mesenteric chains.

Postganglionic sympathetic nerves and afferent fibres conveying pain sensation from the pancreas are relayed through the splanchnic nerves and coeliac plexus. Parasympathetic fibres from the vagus nerve provide a secreto-motor supply to the exocrine gland, and act in association with the duodenal hormones, secretin and pancreozymin (CCK-PZ). Besides water and electrolytes (notably bicarbonate), alkaline pancreatic juice contains proteolytic and lipolytic enzymes as inactive zymogens as well as enzymes capable of splitting carbohydrate and nucleic acids.

During embryological development, dorsal and ventral pancreatic buds grow separately from opposite sides of the duodenum at the junction of the foregut and midgut; subsequently the gland retains a dual blood supply from foregut (coeliac) and midgut (superior mesenteric) arteries. The dorsal pancreas forms most of the adult gland apart from the lower part of the head and uncinate process, which arise from the ventral moiety. In association with the primitive bile duct, the ventral pancreas rotates around the duodenum and fuses with the dorsal outgrowth during the 7th week (*Fig.* 14.3*a*). Following normal communication of the two ductal systems, the ventral pancreatic duct (of Wirsung) becomes dilated and acts as the final pathway for exocrine secretion from both the embryological parts of the gland (*Fig.* 14.3*b*).

The common bile duct usually joins the duct of Wirsung as the two ducts pierce the medial wall of the descending limb of the duodenum, forming a short common channel (ampulla of Vater). The ampulla is surrounded by the circular muscle sphincter of Oddi and opens at the summit of a small papilla, lying 8–10 cm distal to the pylorus. Alternatively, the two ducts enter the duodenum separately at the apex of this (major) papilla. When present, a minor or accessory pancreatic papilla projects into the duodenum about 2 cm proximally and drains the terminal portion of the dorsal pancreatic duct (of Santorini).

The exocrine pancreas is a compound racemose gland. Endocrine tissue is scattered throughout the pancreas in discrete islets of Langerhans, with a relative preponderance (about 70 per cent) in the body and tail. Islet cells elaborate insulin and glucagon and a number of other peptides, the function of which remains unclear, including pancreatic polypeptide (PP), vasoactive intestinal polypeptide (VIP) and somatostatin.

CONGENITAL PANCREATIC ABNORMALITIES

Annular Pancreas

Incomplete rotation of the ventral pancreas causes the rare condition of annular pancreas, in which the second part of the duodenum is encircled by pancreatic tissue. If the ring is complete and tight, the condition presents in early neonatal life with persistent vomiting, usually of bile-stained material; other congenital anomalies are commonly associated. The classic appearance of a 'double bubble' on plain abdominal radiography is produced by gaseous distension of both the stomach and duodenal cap. Annular pancreas may not cause symptoms until adult life, when gastric outlet obstruction supervenes. Barium meal and endoscopic examinations localize the site of obstruction to the second part of the duodenum.

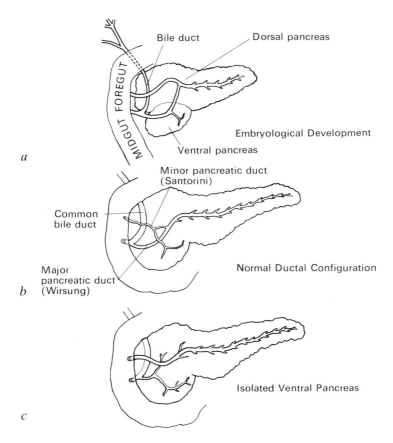

Fig. 14.3. Embryological development of the pancreas. The gland develops from dorsal and ventral pancreatic buds which fuse during the 7th week of intra-uterine life (*a*). The normal adult configuration of the pancreatic ducts (*b*) includes a communication between the Wirsung and Santorini systems. In isolated ventral pancreas or pancreas divisum (*c*) the two ductal systems remain entirely independent and the dorsal pancreas drains solely through the accessory papilla.

There may be associated pancreatitis or duodenal ulcer disease.

Since the annulus always contains a sizeable pancreatic duct, operative division of the ring has an unacceptable risk of pancreatic fistula. Moreover, the obstruction may not even be relieved, because the underlying duodenum is usually hypoplastic. Annular pancreas should therefore be circumvented by duodenoduodenostomy (where possible) or by duodenojejunostomy or retrocolic gastroenterostomy.

Ectopic (Aberrant) Pancreas

Islands of ectopic (aberrant) pancreas may occur in the wall of the small bowel at any point (including Meckel's diverticulum), but especially in the duodenum. These embryological rests are generally found within the submucosa and seldom give rise to symptoms.

Congenital Pancreatic Cysts

These are described later in this chapter (p. 162).

Pancreatic ductal anomalies

Though common, these are of uncertain clinical rele-

vance. The duct of Santorini and the accessory papilla may close or disappear during fetal life, leaving the major pancreatic ductal system to drain all the exocrine secretion. Alternatively, the duct of Wirsung may atrophy or remain very small, so that pancreatic juice escapes via the Santorini system. Virtual agenesis of either dorsal or ventral pancreas may even occur. Lastly, failure of fusion of the two ductal systems can result in the separate embryological components draining independently in the duodenum (*Fig.* 14.3*c*). Termed 'isolated ventral pancreas' or 'pancreas divisum',* this is normally discovered at endoscopic retrograde choledochopancreatography† (ERCP).

---

* The term 'pancreas divisum' is misleading, since it suggests physical separation of the two embryological moieties. 'Isolated ventral pancreas' is also used, but it is probably inadequate drainage of the *dorsal* portion that gives rise to symptoms.

† The pancreatogram obtained by cannulation of the major pancreatic papilla, as confirmed by the concomitant visualization of the biliary tree, is limited to the head and uncinate process. Cannulation of the minor papilla, though technically difficult, will establish the diagnosis.

Isolation of the dorsal pancreas from the papilla should protect against gallstone pancreatitis. However, the anomaly may be commoner in patients with recurrent idiopathic pancreatitis. Sometimes an exhaustive search provides no other explanation for persistent abdominal and back pain. Secretion studies may reveal a small volume of normal pancreatic juice, and biopsy of the tail may show periductal fibrosis. Arguably the narrow duct of the dorsal pancreas is unable to cope with most of the pancreatic secretion, and partial functional obstruction results. Both endoscopic and operative division of the accessory sphincter are technically demanding procedures and may not provide lasting benefit. An alternative approach is to amputate the pancreatic tail (preserving the spleen) and perform prograde pancreatography. Radiological or histological demonstration of obstructive pancreatitis may necessitate more extensive resection, since the duct is often too small for adequate drainage procedures.

PANCREATIC TRAUMA

Because the pancreas is placed deep within the upper abdomen, it is well protected against moderate external forces, and pancreatic trauma constitutes only 1–3 per cent of all abdominal injuries. As a corollary, the mortality rate is about 30 per cent. Serious pancreatic injury is encountered among automobile drivers involved in road traffic accidents, in which the gland is compressed against the vertebral column by the impact of the steering wheel (*Fig.* 14.4); seat belts should protect against this type of injury. Blunt trauma sufficient to disrupt the pancreas often damages adjacent viscera as well, and the resulting injuries, especially of major blood vessels, may prove lethal. Penetrating wounds of the pancreas almost

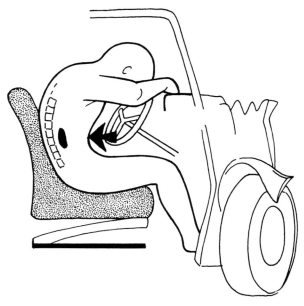

Fig. 14.4. Pancreatic trauma. The common mechanism of injury.

always involve neighbouring organs in addition. Generally knife wounds carry a better prognosis than those caused by bullets or shot and injuries from high-velocity missiles are lethal. The pancreas is at risk of operative trauma during splenectomy or occasionally gastrectomy (e.g. for penetrating ulcers), and pancreatitis is a recognized complication of endoscopic or surgical manoeuvres involving the sphincter of Oddi.

The prognosis and management of pancreatic injuries vary widely with the actual site of trauma to the gland. Injuries of the distal body or tail are usually the least severe, though they may be associated with damage to the spleen, stomach, diaphragm, left kidney or left colonic flexure. Trauma to the mid-pancreas (neck and proximal body) may be an isolated injury, typically a partial or complete fracture of the gland where it crosses the spine. There may be concomitant injuries of the liver, stomach, transverse colon or superior mesenteric vessels, however. Injuries of the pancreatic head are the most serious and the most difficult to manage. They often combine extensive destruction of the pancreas with duodenal trauma, which may also involve the bile duct and portal vein, liver, right kidney or right colonic flexure.

The clinical features of pancreatic trauma are sometimes slow to develop; they include hypotension, an abdominal mass and evidence of peritonitis. Repeated estimations of serum amylase should be obtained, and high amylase contents may also be detected in fluid obtained by diagnostic peritoneal lavage. Following resuscitation of the patient, any suspected pancreatic injury requires early laparotomy and thorough exposure of the entire gland, together with the duodenum and duodenojejunal flexure. Haematomas in the duodenopancreatic region should always be explored. The principles of treatment include control of haemorrhage by ligation and suture, search for ductal damage and leakage of pancreatic juice, resection of devitalized tissue and extensive drainage. For lesions to the right of the midline, internal drainage of the injured area into a Roux loop of jejunum may be a safer option than pancreatoduodenectomy. Lesions to the left of the midline (including fracture of the neck of pancreas) are best treated by distal pancreatectomy, with or without splenectomy.

The late complications of pancreatic trauma are external pancreatic fistulas, sometimes accompanied by intestinal contents, and pseudocyst formation. Detectable by serial scanning with ultrasound or computed tomography (CT), traumatic cysts need early operative intervention because of the risk of haemorrhage, rupture or infection.

ACUTE PANCREATITIS

This term embraces a range of conditions that vary in severity from mild and transient oedema of the gland to widespread pancreatic necrosis. The overall mortality rate is at least 10 per cent. The common presence of cholelithiasis* and the frequency with which small calculi can be recovered from the stools after an attack suggests that the passage of a small stone through the papilla may render the sphincteric mechanism incompetent, allowing duodenal reflux along the duct of Wirsung and thus intrapancreatic activation of the digestive enzymes.

Acute pancreatitis typically presents with epigastric pain of rapid onset, which radiates to the back and causes vomiting. Signs of peritonitis, often generalized in extent, may be accompanied by evidence of shock, dehydration, cyanosis or mild jaundice. Elevation of the serum amylase remains the single most valuable diagnostic test: levels usually exceed 1200 i.u./L (600 Somogyi units/dl), and hyperamylasaemia of this degree is seldom seen in the absence of pancreatitis. Equally common though, non-specific findings include an absolute neutrophilia and mild derangement of liver function tests. Blood-gas analysis often reveals a surprisingly low arterial Po_2. Initial hypocalcaemia ($<8\cdot0$ mmol/L) denotes a severe attack, though later reductions in serum calcium reflect the fall in albumin concentration. A high plasma fibrinogen content and methaemalbuminaemia may indicate severe (haemorrhagic) pancreatitis. Analysis of peritoneal fluid obtained by paracentesis (with or without lavage) may confirm the severity of pancreatitis and help to exclude other causes of peritonitis, such as perforated peptic ulcer or gangrenous cholecystitis. Likewise, plain abdominal radiographs may be of value in the differential diagnosis, besides showing certain characteristic features of pancreatitis such as distension of the duodenal cap or a 'sentinel loop' of jejunum.

Management

Management of acute pancreatitis is hampered by the lack of any specific treatment for the disease and by difficulty in predicting of the severity of the attack at the time of admission. The dominant requirement is rapid replacement of the large volumes of extracellular fluid sequestrated in the retroperitoneal pancreatic 'burn'. Several litres of intravenous fluid are often needed, including some units of plasma or plasma substitute; in these cases central venous pressure, haematocrit and serum urea and electrolytes must be carefully monitored. A nasogastric tube should be passed immediately to diminish upper

*In the UK, gallstones are present in over half the cases of acute pancreatitis, whereas in France and the USA alcoholism is commonly associated. Pancreatitis may follow abdominal trauma or operative procedures such as Polya gastrectomy, sphincterotomy and pancreatic biopsy. All series contain a proportion of 'idiopathic' cases, in which no definite aetiogical agent can be implicated.

alimentary secretion. Analgesia is best provided by parenteral administration of pethidine. Arterial hypoxaemia is countered by giving oxygen by face mask or, if necessary, by endotracheal intubation with assisted ventilation. Blood, calcium and vitamin supplements may be given intravenously. Antispasmodics are of doubtful value. Antibiotics are probably best reserved for septic complications. Steroids are contra-indicated. H_2 receptor antagonists may prevent stress ulceration and bleeding in a seriously ill patient.

With supportive measures many cases of acute pancreatitis will resolve within 2–5 days, allowing a gradual return to oral feeding (with a low fat diet), but persisting ileus should be managed by intravenous hyperalimentation. Agents that diminish exocrine secretion (e.g. glucagon) or inhibit pancreatic enzymes (e.g. aprotinin) do not appear to ameliorate established pancreatitis, probably because of the invariable delay (mean about 24 hours) between onset of symptoms and start of treatment.

Peritoneal lavage has been recommended in the early treatment of severe pancreatitis or for subsequent pancreatic abscess. It is carried out through a dialysis catheter introduced into the pelvis via a small incision sited either in the midline below the umbilicus or in one or other iliac fossa, avoiding any previous scars. Catheter placement is performed under local anaesthetic, using strict aseptic precautions; alternatively, the catheter can be left in situ following diagnostic laparotomy. Two litres of isotonic dialysate (Dialaflex 61) containing 8 mmol of potassium and 500 units of heparin are instilled into the peritoneal cavity over 10 minutes, and the fluid is allowed to drain by gravity thereafter. This cycle is repeated hourly for the next 3–4 days with daily bacteriological culture of the fluid. Respiratory embarrassment may necessitate the use of smaller volumes of fluid. Peritoneal lavage is well tolerated and helps to counter initial hypovolaemia, but its therapeutic value is unproven.

Operative treatment

Operative treatment of acute pancreatitis may be diagnostic, therapeutic or prophylactic. Since serum amylase levels are not always diagnostic of pancreatitis and hyperamylasaemia may accompany other upper abdominal catastrophes, laparotomy is mandatory if the diagnosis is in serious doubt. The findings in pancreatitis include bloodstained ascites, fat necrosis and marked peripancreatic and retroperitoneal oedema. It is safer to explore a case of acute pancreatitis than to treat a perforated gallbladder conservatively. Acute pancreatitis secondary to trauma always requires laparotomy.

There is no consensus regarding the best treatment of gallstones encountered at the time of diagnostic laparotomy. Cholecystectomy and choledocholithotomy are safe in the presence of mild or moderate pancreatitis. A calculus lodged at the ampulla is best disimpacted from above, since transduodenal sphincteroplasty can be technically difficult and represents a substantial escalation of the surgical attack. In the presence of haemorrhagic pancreatitis, operative procedures should be kept to a minimum, but cholecystectomy and T-tube drainage of the common bile duct may be necessary for cholangitis or biliary obstruction. Pancreatic débridement at this stage should be strictly avoided. Total or extended distal pancreatectomy is occasionally attempted in fulminating pancreatitis, but at least one-third of these patients die. The safety of an urgent endoscopic papillotomy requires further evaluation.

During the early convalescence from an attack the biliary tree should be thoroughly investigated for calculous disease (ultrasound scan, oral cholecystogram). If gallstones are confirmed, it is often wise to carry out cholecystectomy (and choledocholithotomy if necessary) during the same hospital admission to avoid the substantial risk of recurrent pancreatitis. In the absence of obvious gallstones or alcoholism, ERCP may be carried out, especially for recurrent pancreatitis, but this procedure should be delayed for 4–6 weeks after an acute attack.

Complications

There are many possible complications of acute pancreatitis. Chest infection, pleural effusion, venous thromboembolism, hypocalcaemia, diabetes mellitus, septicaemia and renal failure should be managed along standard lines. Pancreatic pseudocysts, which take several days to develop, are discussed later in this chapter (p. 162). Gastrointestinal haemorrhage from acute peptic ulceration can be lethal and should be treated conservatively if possible, using cimetidine and blood transfusion. Rarely, prolonged duodenal ileus may necessitate gastroenterostomy.

Pancreatic abscess is the commonest cause of death in patients who survive the acute phase of shock. Abscesses usually present in the 2nd or 3rd week of the disease with pyrexia, toxicity and a white cell count above $20 \times 10^9/L$. Ultrasound and CT scanning will help to delineate the abscess, which is usually extensive and multilocular. Prompt external drainage should be undertaken. The retroperitoneum is opened widely, pancreatic slough is removed piecemeal, three or four wide-bore tube drains are inserted and broad-spectrum antibiotic therapy is begun. Postoperative irrigation of the abdominal cavity may be beneficial. If the patient survives, the resulting external pancreatic fistulas usually close spontaneously, but permanent exocrine impairment may ensue. The mortality rate of pancreatic abscess varies between 35 and 75 per cent. Death results from uncontrolled sepsis (with or without bleeding) and multiple organ failure.

CHRONIC PANCREATITIS

This disease most commonly affects young or middle-aged men, who have a long history of alcohol abuse. Almost total destruction of the pancreas is compatible with minimal damage to the liver and vice versa. Pain is the dominant symptom. It is situated deeply within the epigastrium, radiates to the back between the shoulderblades and is sometimes relieved by sitting bolt upright. It tends to be severe and unrelenting and causes loss of weight. Swelling of the pancreatic head, with or without pseudocyst formation, may cause cholestasis of varying degree. In addition, progressive glandular destruction causes exocrine and endocrine impairment, which may become clinically apparent (steatorrhoea, diabetes mellitus) or detectable only as abnormalities of measured faecal fat output and glucose tolerance. Rarer complications include pancreatic ascites following internal rupture of a cyst, duodenal stenosis and gastro-oesophageal varices resulting from splenic vein thrombosis.

The preoperative diagnosis of chronic pancreatitis relies on an appropriate clinical history (especially in an alcoholic), demonstration of exocrine insufficiency, the presence of calcification or cysts and pancreatographic evidence of a disordered ductal system.

The symptoms and signs of chronic pancreatitis can mimic those of pancreatic cancer, and the differential diagnosis of these two conditions (*Table* 14.1) is as important as it can be difficult. Moreover, the two often coexist, since ductal occlusion by tumour causes distal obstructive pancreatitis, and pancreatitis itself, like other chronic inflammatory conditions, may predispose to cancer. Both conditions cause enlargement and destruction of the pancreas, and operative differentiation can also be confusing. The appearance of the common bile duct may be a useful guide, however; in carcinoma of the head of pancreas the duct is green, thin walled and translucent, whereas in chronic pancreatitis it is generally white, thickened and opaque, because of recurrent cholangitis.

Intractable pain and obstructive jaundice are the usual indications for operative treatment in chronic pancreatitis, but the management of this 'benign' condition can be one of the most difficult problems in surgical practice. Addiction has developed not just to alcohol but often to the opiates used to obtain analgesia, and this complicates assessment of suitability for operation, ability to withstand major surgical procedures and management of endocrine (and exocrine) insufficiency, created or aggravated by pancreatectomy. Major pancreatic resections should not be carried out on alcoholics who are continuing to drink, because of the serious risk of coma resulting from haphazard insulin medication after the patient has returned home. Splanchnicectomy, often performed as a definitive operation for pain, should be relegated to the role of an adjunctive procedure; similar benefit can often be obtained more readily by percutaneous coeliac plexus block. Transduodenal

Table 14.1. Investigations that help to differentiate between chronic pancreatitis and carcinoma of the pancreas

Diagnostic test	Common features	Chronic pancreatitis	Pancreatic cancer
Occult blood in stools	—	Usually negative	Often positive
Liver function tests	Obstructive jaundice (if head involved)	Obstruction often incomplete and fluctuates	Progressing unrelenting obstruction
Glucose tolerance test	Often diabetic	—	—
Analysis of duodenal juice	Findings often non-specific	Reductions in volume, bicarbonate and trypsin concentrations	Normal, or variable reductions
Plain abdominal X-ray	—	Pancreatic calcification in at least 30 per cent	Usually normal, occasionally punctate calcification
Barium meal/hypotonic duodenography	Distortion of stomach, widening of duodenal loop	Flattening of medial duodenal wall	Invasion of duodenal wall
Cholangiography (percutaneous transhepatic or endoscopic retrograde)	Obstruction of common bile duct, if pancreatic head involved	Smooth, tapering stricture, often incomplete	Abrupt and complete cut-off
Ultrasonography/CT scan	Enlargement of pancreas	Swelling often diffuse, calcification, cysts	Swelling often discrete, local invasion, hepatic metastases
Pancreatography (endoscopic retrograde)	Abnormalities of ductal system	Areas of stenosis and dilatation, 'chain of lakes', side-branch ectasia, cysts, internal fistulas	Invasion of duodenal wall, sharp cut-off pancreatic duct, ductal dilatation behind tumour
Selective arteriography (coeliac, superior mesenteric)	Pancreatic tumours outlined	Tumours smooth and avascular (cysts), fewer vessels supplying pancreas	Vascularity normal or increased, irregular tumours, obstruction of portal vein, hepatic metastases
Biopsy (histology, cytology)	—	Benign pancreatic tissue fibrosis	Adenocarcinoma (if correct area sampled)

sphincteroplasty of the major pancreatic duct may relieve a localized stricture in the pancreatic head, but seldom provides adequate ductal decompression in generalized pancreatitis. Attempts to obliterate the ductal system by injection of a rapidly setting acrylate glue should still be regarded as experimental. For practical purposes, therefore, the present choice of operation for chronic pancreatitis lies between extensive ductal drainage and resection.

Despite the probability that peripancreatitis contributes to the pain, drainage of obstructed ducts alone often provides dramatic and persistent improvement in symptoms. This is the optimal procedure for generalized pancreatitis with ductal dilatation, and it avoids the pancreatic insufficiency implicit in major resections. Long-term decompression is best achieved by longitudinal pancreatico-jejunostomy Roux-en-Y, after opening the duct widely throughout the strictured segment. Pancreatic calculi are removed and concomitant cysts are opened into the ductal system or separately drained. The Puestow procedure of inserting the filleted pancreas into the end of a Roux loop conveys no obvious advantage and makes haemorrhage less easy to control. End-to-side anastomoses between the transected pancreas

and a Roux loop tend to close eventually, unless the duct is greatly enlarged. If the left side of the pancreas is grossly diseased, distal* pancreatectomy may be combined with drainage of the proximal duct, but the duct should be opened for a short distance to increase the calibre of the pancreatico-intestinal communication.

Pancreatic resection is appropriate for those patients in whom either there is no ductal dilatation, or pancreatitis is essentially limited to one part of the gland, or previous drainage procedures have failed. Chronic inflammation of the left pancreas is readily treated by distal pancreatectomy, which normally includes splenectomy. Transection of the gland is carried out at the level of the portal vein or just to the right of this point, producing a 50–70 per cent pancreatectomy; this procedure usually avoids overt impairment of endocrine or exocrine function. More

* The term 'distal' is traditionally applied to that portion of the pancreas that lies to the left of the midline, although the 'distal' part of the pancreatic duct might be considered to be the terminal segment within the head of the gland. The terms 'left' and 'right' pancreas avoid this possible confusion, but are not in general usage.

extensive resections involving 80–95 per cent of the gland (subtotal pancreatectomy) may be necessary to remove the diseased segment, but cause varying degrees of pancreatic insufficiency. Sometimes the inflammatory process is limited to the head of the gland with relative sparing of the left pancreas, in which case pancreatoduodenectomy may be indicated. It may be possible to preserve the pylorus and duodenal cap and avoid the distal hemigastrectomy of a conventional Whipple's operation. Erosive gastritis does not appear to be a complication of this type of conservative proximal pancreatectomy, and the operation is less of a physiological insult. Occasionally either severe and generalized pancreatitis or the failure of lesser operative procedures necessitate total pancreatoduodenectomy. Permanent diabetes and malabsorption are the inevitable sequelae* which require lifelong treatment, but in this type of patient they are usually present to a greater or lesser extent before operation.

PANCREATIC CYSTS

These are traditionally classified as *true cysts*, which possess an epithelial lining, and *pseudocysts*, which do not. True cysts are congenital or neoplastic in origin, whereas pseudocysts occur in acute and chronic pancreatitis, trauma and sometimes carcinoma of the pancreas. The distinction becomes academic when true cysts are complicated by infection or haemorrhage that destroys the lining. It is of greater practical value to know whether a cyst is intrapancreatic or peripancreatic, and whether or not it communicates with the ductal system.

Congenital pancreatic cysts are usually small, intrapancreatic and silent, but they sometimes enlarge or become infected later in life. Rarely the pancreas is the site of *polycystic disease*, usually in association with the liver and kidney. *Cystic fibrosis of the pancreas* (mucoviscidosis) presents either with meconium ileus in neonatal life, or with steatorrhoea and recurrent chest infection in infancy and childhood.

Cystadenoma, though rare, is one of the commoner benign tumours affecting the gland and usually presents as a painless epigastric mass. It has a marked female preponderance. Complete excision should be performed where practicable; otherwise the cyst remnant should be covered by a Roux loop of jejunum. There is a strong tendency towards malignant change, although histological differentiation from *cystadenocarcinoma* can be difficult. Malignant neoplastic cysts may be sensitive to radiotherapy or chemotherapy.

By far the commonest cysts arising in and around the pancreas are those that accompany pancreatitis or trauma. At least 10 per cent of cases of *acute pancreatitis* produce encysted collections of fluid generally in the lesser sac but sometimes between the leaves of the lesser omentum or adjacent to the anterior surface of the gland. These (pseudo-) cysts cause pain, obstructive jaundice or an epigastric mass 1–2 weeks after admission, with renewed elevation in serum amylase levels. They may be detected by ultrasonography at an earlier stage, but many smaller cysts resolve spontaneously. Larger cysts may cause vomiting by anterior displacement of the stomach, as confirmed on lateral radiographs taken during barium meal examination. Other complications include erosion into adjoining viscera, perforation into the peritoneal cavity (pancreatic ascites) or chest (pleural effusion), and infection (pancreatic abscess). All cysts that fail to resolve should be drained, either externally if they are acute and thin walled or internally if it is possible to wait until they are mature. Percutaneous aspiration under ultrasonic guidance is an acceptable alternative, particularly if drainage becomes necessary within 1 month of the attack of acute pancreatitis.

The degenerative or retention cysts that arise in *chronic pancreatitis* are generally intrapancreatic and often communicate with the pancreatic ducts. Symptoms resemble those of the underlying disease. Cysts may be shown by pancreatic scans or ERCP, or by the operative finding of soft and fluctuant swellings in an otherwise hard and sclerotic gland. Besides confirming the presence of a cyst, needle aspiration permits introduction of contrast material to determine size, position and possible ductal communication. Cyst fluid should be sent for cytological examination to exclude malignancy. Treatment of the cyst must be combined with that of the associated pancreatitis. Localized disease may be suitable for resection, or cysts may be evacuated into the ductal system during pancreatico-jejunostomy. Discrete cysts within the head of the pancreas can be drained into the duodenum (*see* p. 171), though problems include damage to the bile duct and a lack of dependent drainage. Elsewhere in the gland, cysts may be treated by anastomosis to a Roux loop of jejunum.

Gastrointestinal haemorrhage is an uncommon but potentially lethal complication of a pancreatic pseudocyst, particularly in chronic alcoholic pancreatitis. The cyst enlarges and its contents digest the wall of neighbouring arteries, leading to pseudoaneurysms of the splenic or gastroduodenal arteries or their branches. These false aneurysms can rupture into the cyst or directly into the duodenum or pancreatic duct. Visceral angiography demonstrates the site of actual or potential bleeding. Elective resection of the cyst is the best option unless there is active bleeding, in which case transcatheter embolization with gelfoam is probably safer.

PANCREATIC FISTULAS

Besides occurring as a delayed complication of trauma, *cutaneous fistulas* may follow biopsy and

---

* Autotransplantation of islet tissue or the tail of pancreas is a potential method of avoiding diabetes that needs further evaluation.

resection of the pancreas and pancreatico-intestinal anastomosis, as well as planned external drainage of cysts or abscesses. Pancreatic fistula is one of the commonest and most serious complications of pancreatoduodenectomy.

Pure pancreatic fistulas usually discharge no more than 300 ml of greyish fluid per day and cause little excoriation of the surrounding skin, because the digestive enzymes are not activated. The pancreatic origin of a suspected fistula can be confirmed by the high amylase content (>5000 Somogyi units/100 ml) of the fluid. A fistulogram should be obtained and will often outline both the ductal system and any peripancreatic collection of fluid; alternatively ERCP may demonstrate the fistula.

Parenteral nutrition avoids the pancreatic stimulation that follows oral intake of food and counteracts the catabolic effect of protein loss. Most pure pancreatic fistulas close spontaneously with time, provided that there is adequate egress for any fluid collection and the underlying pancreatic disease is not too severe. Increasing pain or toxicity suggests the accumulation of infected fluid requiring proper drainage. If fluid loss is excessive or fails to diminish after prolonged conservative treatment, the fistula must be explored. Depending on the site of injury, either resection of the left pancreas or internal drainage of the leak into a Roux loop of jejunum will normally be appropriate.

The outpouring of dark or discoloured fluid rich in amylase indicates a *mixed* pancreatic fistula with concomitant leakage of bile or intestinal contents. Fluid losses and cutaneous inflammation are always much more severe, and there is a risk of secondary haemorrhage. Most of these patients require operation after a period of hyperalimentation.

Pancreatic ascites is an uncommon complication of chronic pancreatitis or trauma, in which progressive accumulation of fluid within the peritoneal cavity follows internal rupture of a communicating pancreatic cyst. Differentiation from ascites secondary to cirrhosis or carcinomatosis relies upon showing that the fluid obtained by paracentesis abdominis has a higher amylase content than serum. Endoscopic or operative pancreatography helps to localize the site of leakage from the duct, and treatment is again by distal pancreatectomy or pancreatico-jejunostomy (Roux-en-Y).

CARCINOMA OF THE PANCREAS

Already one of the commonest abdominal malignancies, pancreatic cancer is increasing in frequency. It remains virtually incurable. Over 70 per cent of carcinomas affect the head of the pancreas, and in these unrelenting jaundice and weight loss are the cardinal symptoms; abdominal and back pain are frequent but not invariable accompaniments. Vomiting suggests duodenal obstruction. Diabetes mellitus may develop *de novo* or deteriorate in an established diabetic.

Besides progressive icterus, there may be hepatomegaly, a palpable gallbladder, an epigastric mass, ascites or thrombophlebitis migrans. Half the patients have occult gastrointestinal bleeding. Tumours of the body and tail are notoriously silent and may elude diagnosis during several months of malaise and vague abdominal pain.

Summarized in *Table 14.1*, the diagnosis of pancreatic cancer rests on the demonstration of a solid pancreatic mass on scanning, radiological or endoscopic evidence of duodenal invasion, exclusion of common-duct stones in obstructive jaundice, obstruction of the pancreatic duct at ERCP and (unequivocally) detection of carcinoma cells after percutaneous needle biopsy, endoscopic aspiration of the duct or operative biopsy. Besides helping to discriminate from other causes of pancreatic enlargement, selective angiography delineates the arterial supply and venous drainage of the gland—valuable if resection is contemplated—and may demonstrate hepatic metastases.

Treatment

Surgery currently offers the only definitive prospect of cure in this disease, but macroscopically complete resection is feasible only for 10–20 per cent of tumours of the head and very seldom for tumours of the body or tail. Moreover, major resection for cancer carries an appreciable mortality rate (circa 20 per cent), especially in jaundiced patients, and long-term survival thereafter is exceptional. Yet matters can only improve, as modern diagnostic techniques offer the chance of earlier detection and adjunctive cancer therapy improves. In experienced hands pancreatectomy remains the optimal procedure for pancreatic cancer. Resection is also indicated for other cancers in this region that cause obstructive jaundice, namely carcinoma of the ampulla, terminal bile duct and descending duodenum. These tumours are generally slow growing and carry a much better prognosis. They are occasionally amenable to local excision, but adequate resection normally entails partial pancreatoduodenectomy (Whipple's operation).

The first step in any operation for pancreatic (or adjacent) cancer is to confirm the diagnosis, aided if necessary by frozen-section examination of tissue obtained by direct pancreatic biopsy or by sampling nodal or hepatic secondaries. In the absence of obvious metastases, the surgeon must next decide if the tumour is resectable, and this may involve a lengthy dissection. Adenocarcinomas of the left pancreas amenable to distal pancreatectomy are seldom encountered. Midline tumours of the gland usually involve the superior mesenteric artery and vein at an early stage. The common cancers of the head should be treated by pancreatectomy, unless there is encasement of the superior mesenteric pedicle, portal vein or aorta. Resection and grafting of major vascular structures or *en bloc* excision of involved adjacent viscera* (right kidney, transverse colon) are rarely indicated. In deeply jaundiced patients with resectable tumours, a two-stage procedure is advisable; the first stage is confined to the relief of the jaundice. Decompression of the obstructed biliary tree can also be obtained by means of a transampullary catheter inserted at ERCP or by percutaneous catheterization (see p. 000).

Resectable cancers of the head of the pancreas may be treated either by Whipple's operation or by total pancreatoduodenectomy. Partial resection of the gland usually prevents diabetes. The disadvantages are first that the pancreatico-intestinal anastomosis may be difficult to construct and thus may either leak or become occluded, and second that cancers may be multifocal or spread directly down the duct. In younger and fitter patients, and especially in those already diabetic, total pancreatectomy is probably the operation of choice. In older people with relatively normal glucose tolerance, or in those with a less favourable prognosis, the prospect of a modest gain in survival time is scarcely worth the extra misery of diabetes.

In most cases of pancreatic carcinoma resection is in any case impracticable, and efforts are directed towards obtaining a positive tissue diagnosis and palliating jaundice and pain. Biliary diversion is most easily achieved by fashioning a side-to-side anastomosis between the fundus of the dilated gallbladder and a loop of jejunum, provided there is no evidence of cholelithiasis and the cystic duct is not occluded by tumour. An entero-anastomosis below the cholecystojejunostomy may diminish entry of food into the gallbladder. Although recurrent jaundice can develop if carcinoma later spreads towards the porta hepatis, many patients die long before this occurs. The distance between the origin of the cystic duct and the superior edge of the tumour can be determined if necessary by needle cholecystography. If this distance is short or cholecystojejunostomy is otherwise inappropriate, bile should be rerouted through a choledocho-jejunostomy (Roux-en-Y). Complete transection of the bile duct with suture of the proximal end to the Roux loop has the theoretical advantage of being less liable to subsequent occlusion by submucosal spread of cancer than side-to-side anastomosis.

The possibility of late duodenal obstruction by direct invasion of the growth makes gastroenterostomy advisable in all but very advanced cases. H_2 receptor antagonists may be given postoperatively to prevent stomal ulceration and bleeding; truncal vagotomy is an alternative. Severe preoperative pain and evidence of marked pancreatitis distal to the cancer are indications to consider decompression of the obstructed pancreatic duct into the stomach or jejunum. Alternatively, intraoperative coeliac plexus

block may give a reasonable relief of pain. It is doubtful if postoperative radiotherapy or chemotherapy materially improves prognosis or quality of life.

ENDOCRINE TUMOURS OF THE PANCREAS

Neoplastic islet cells secrete normal pancreatic hormones (ortho-endocrine), hormones that are usually produced elsewhere (para-endocrine) or no hormones at all. Increased levels of circulating polypeptides can be detected by specific radio-immunoassay. Pancreatic apudomas* frequently secrete more than one humoral agent, though a single hormone dominates the clinical presentation. They may be part of a multiple endocrine neoplasia (MEN).

Non-functioning islet tumours may be benign or malignant, and their clinical features are those of an epigastric mass or a space-occupying lesion that distorts neighbouring organs. Whenever possible they should be completely excised, leaving a residuum of functioning pancreatic tissue. Growth rates are generally slow, and the prognosis is correspondingly better than for exocrine cancer.

The commonest ortho-endocrine tumour of the pancreas, and the first to be described, is insulinoma. The tumour is usually benign and solitary, causing episodic hypoglycaemia, which may masquerade as neurological or mental disease. Attacks are precipitated by fasting or exercise, characterized by low blood sugar and inappropriately high serum insulin levels, and relieved by intravenous glucose (Whipple's triad). Venous phase angiography provides the key to successful localization, since most islet tumours are hypervascular. Transhepatic cannulation of pancreatic veins allows direct sampling for insulin assay and may be valuable if localization proves difficult. Treatment is by enucleation or partial pancreatectomy. Blind resection may be unsuccessful and should be unnecessary with the modern diagnostic techniques. Occasionally diazoxide or chemotherapy may be needed for metastasizing malignant insulinoma.

The Verner–Morrison or WDHA syndrome† is caused by an islet cell tumour of the pancreas secreting VIP (vipoma). Profuse diarrhoea may precipitate severe hypokalaemia and dehydration, as suggested by the alternative term 'pancreatic cholera'. Diagnosis requires exclusion of other causes of secretory diarrhoea, demonstration of reduced gastric acid secretion and, if possible, accurate measurement of circulating VIP. Appropriate resuscitation with intravenous fluids should include bicarbonate to correct metabolic acidosis. Resection of a benign tumour

---

* Radical resections of this kind are sometimes termed 'regional pancreatectomy'.

* From the acronym APUD (amine precursor uptake and decarboxylation), used to describe the staining properties of endocrine cells that elaborate peptide hormones.

† Another acronym; watery diarrhoea, hypokalaemia and achlorhydria.

provides complete cure, but in the presence of metastases streptozotocin or prednisolone may control symptoms.

Glucagonomas are rare tumours that cause migratory necrotizing dermatitis and diarrhoea. Pure *somatostatinomas* or *pancreatic polypeptidomas* are both exceedingly rare, although these hormones may be encountered in other endocrine neoplasms of the pancreas.

The only common para-endocrine tumour is *gastrinoma*, which gives rise to the Zollinger–Ellison syndrome of intractable peptic ulceration and gastric hypersecretion. The excess acid may also cause diarrhoea. These tumours are often malignant, but death can also result from the virulent ulcer diathesis. Tumours are frequently multiple and may occur in extrapancreatic sites (e.g. duodenum). Peptic ulcers may be unusually large and affect atypical regions of the gut (e.g. distal duodenum, jejunum), but duodenal ulceration is usually normal both in site and size. The hallmark of the Zollinger–Ellison syndrome is failure of ulcer healing or early recurrence after standard medical or surgical treatment. The diagnosis is strongly suggested by finding a high basal output of gastric acid (>10–15 mmol/hr), which shows only a slight increase after pentagastrin stimulation. Radiological examination of the upper gastrointestinal tract may reveal prominent mucosal folds, luminal dilatation and large amounts of fluid. Marked elevation in fasting serum gastrin confirms the diagnosis, especially if levels rise sharply after infusion of secretin. Hypercalcaemia suggests an associated parathyroid adenoma; about 20 per cent of patients have MEN type I.

Both preoperative and operative localization of the primary tumour (and its metastases) can be difficult. Thus the standard treatment for Zollinger–Ellison syndrome is total gastrectomy. When possible, complete resection of tumour offers a reasonable surgical alternative. H_2 receptor antagonists usually produce dramatic improvement in symptoms, but these recur directly the drug is withdrawn. Chemotherapy or streptozotocin may provide remission in metastatic disease.

PREOPERATIVE AND OPERATIVE PRECAUTIONS

Since most operations on the pancreas are major undertakings, general preoperative precautions such as correction of anaemia and chest physiotherapy are especially important. Weight loss and malnutrition often complicate both pancreatic cancer and chronic pancreatitis, but preoperative nutritional support is of limited value in the presence of obstructive jaundice.

Pancreatic function should be assessed in the first instance by excluding glycosuria and hyperglycaemia or obvious steatorrhoea. Any evidence of pancreatic insufficiency should be checked by performing a glucose tolerance test and exocrine function tests, while on a normal diet. Psychiatric treatment may be valuable in patients with chronic pancreatitis who have problems of alcoholism or drug abuse.

As haemorrhage is sometimes unexpectedly severe during pancreatic surgery, cross-matched blood should always be available and monitoring of central venous pressure is wise. All major pancreatobiliary operations should be covered by prophylactic broad-spectrum antibiotics that are given parenterally, starting at the time of premedication.

Deeply jaundiced patients tolerate major operations poorly, though this is more often a serious problem in carcinoma of the head of the pancreas (or ampulla) than in chronic pancreatitis. If the serum bilirubin level exceeds 200 mmol/L, biliary decompression should be considered as a prelude to pancreatectomy. A fine polythene cannula may be introduced into a dilated biliary radicle at the time of percutaneous transhepatic cholangiography and left *in situ* thereafter; full antiseptic precautions must be observed and antibiotics are given. Problems include catheter displacement, sepsis and electrolyte loss. Endoscopic insertion of a flanged tube across the biliary stricture is a better option but one that requires considerable expertise. The author prefers to carry out a two-stage operation. If the first laparotomy confirms that resection is likely to be feasible, cholecystjejunectomy is performed; pancreatectomy is undertaken 3–4 weeks later.

Operations on jaundiced patients may be complicated by renal failure, especially if anoxia or hypovolaemia supervenes. The risk of the hepatorenal syndrome developing can therefore be minimized by skilled anaesthetic technique, but also by forced peroperative diuresis. Jaundiced patients should be catheterized after induction of anaesthesia and given 40–50 g mannitol during the surgical procedure. Hourly urinary output is measured during the operation and for at least 24 hours thereafter.

OPERATIVE DIAGNOSIS OF PANCREATIC DISEASE

Exposure of the Pancreas

Good access to this deeply placed organ is essential. Satisfactory exposure can be obtained through a long midline incision skirting the umbilicus, aided if necessary by the use of a sternal retractor. Just as good (and cosmetically often superior) is a bilateral subcostal incision or a curved transverse supraumbilical incision that divides both recti and is convex upwards. Particular attention must be paid to the stomach and duodenal loop, liver, spleen and biliary tree before approaching the pancreas. Thorough mobilization of the duodenum (*Fig.* 14.5) before insertion of the index finger through the epiploic

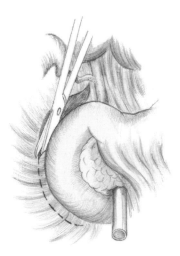

Fig. 14.5. Mobilization of the head of the pancreas. The peritoneum is divided on the lateral aspect of the duodenal loop (Kocher's manoeuvre).

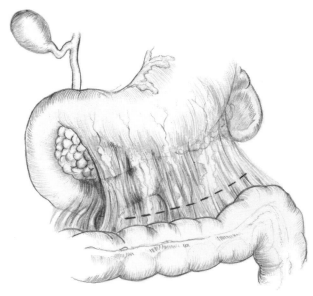

Fig. 14.7. Entry into the lesser sac. Division of the greater omentum and elevation of the stomach from its bed afford exposure of the neck, body and tail of the pancreas.

foramen facilitates palpation of the pancreatic head (and terminal bile duct), and its anterior surface can be directly inspected after clearing the overlying omentum (*Fig.* 14.6). Examination of the rest of the gland requires entry into the lesser sac after ligation and partial division of the gastrocolic omentum outside the gastro-epiploic arcade (*Fig.* 14.7). The filmy congenital adhesions passing from the front of the pancreas to the back of the stomach should then be separated. Incision of the peritoneum along the superior and inferior borders of the body of the pancreas allows the gland to be lifted forwards for systematic palpation throughout its extent.

Pancreatic Biopsy

Biopsy is generally carried out to exclude carcinoma, but sometimes to confirm the presence of chronic pancreatitis. Percutaneous fine-needle aspiration of the gland is increasingly performed to obtain a pre-

operative tissue diagnosis, usually during organ imaging. Cytological material can be obtained under direct vision at operation by fine-needle aspiration of any suspicious area of the gland. Direct pancreatic biopsy is usually superfluous if cancer can be confirmed by frozen-section examination of metastatic sites in the liver or adjacent lymph nodes. To obtain pancreatic tissue for histological examination requires either an incision into the gland or 'shave' biopsy of a superficial nodule or the use of Tru-cut or Menghini needles, which may be introduced transduodenally for lesions in the head. Even needle biopsy may occasionally cause pancreatitis or a fistula, but the finer the needle the lower the likely risk; these potential complications make deep incision biopsies hazardous in the presence of ductal obstruction. If there is much leakage of pancreatic fluid following biopsy and if no further procedure is anticipated, it is wise to cover the biopsy site with a Roux-en-Y jejunostomy.

Pancreatography

Satisfactory visualization of the pancreatic ducts helps to determine the best surgical procedure for chronic pancreatitis and, if ERCP is unavailable or unsuccessful, operative pancreatograms offer the only chance of obtaining this information (*Fig.* 14.8). Even if prior endoscopic cannulation has outlined the ductal system, operative radiographs may clarify equivocal findings. Pancreatograms may be obtained by injection of water-soluble contrast (e.g. Conray 420) from either end of the duct (depending on the operative approach). During transduodenal sphincteric surgery, for example, retrograde cannulation of the major (or minor) papilla is performed using

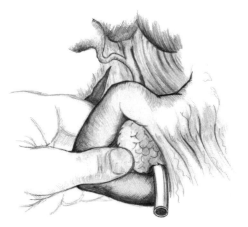

Fig. 14.6. Palpation of the head of the pancreas. The surgeon's left index finger is inserted through the epiploic foramen after thorough mobilization of the duodenum.

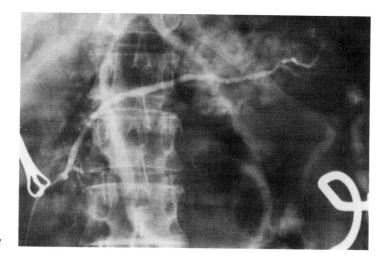

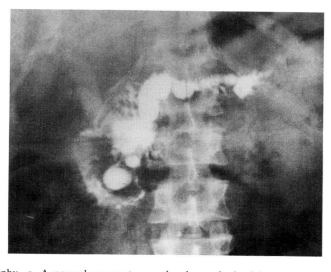

Fig. 14.8. Operative pancreatography. *a*, A normal pancreatogram has been obtained by transduodenal cannulation of the major pancreatic papilla. The Babcock forceps have been applied to the papilla to prevent leakage of contrast into the duodenum. Slight overdistension of the ductal system has led to parenchymal filling in the distal pancreas. *b*, Gross ductal dilatation is shown after introduction of contrast via a needle inserted into the pancreatic duct in the body of the gland. The dilated duct was readily palpable in this 29-year-old man with a 10-year history of alcohol abuse. Associated pancreatic cysts are shown, and the biliary tree and duodenal loop are outlined by previous peroperative cholangiography. The patient was treated by longitudinal pancreaticojejunostomy and choledochojejunostomy to relieve his obstructive jaundice.

a fine polythene cannula (*Fig.* 14.9*a*). Care must be taken not to overdistend the small pancreatic ducts by injecting more than 2 ml of contrast in the first instance. If distal pancreatitis predominates, prograde cannulation after caudal resection will define the ductal anatomy of the residual pancreas. If there is generalized inflammatory disease and a dilated ductal tree, the main duct may be felt as a softer area towards the upper surface of the sclerotic pancreas. Direct insertion of a needle into the duct will often permit introduction of contrast material in either direction (*Fig.* 14.9*b*). If the duct is impalpable or if needling fails to aspirate pancreatic juice, similar pancreatograms can be obtained by making a short vertical incision in the body of pancreas, deepening the incision to enter the main duct and inserting a

T-tube (*Fig.* 14.9*c*). Distal pancreatectomy or drainage is usually necessary thereafter. Lastly, any cysts in the region of the pancreas can be outlined radiologically after needle aspiration at the time of drainage. Operative cystography will demonstrate communications with the pancreatic ductal tree.

OPERATIONS ON THE AMPULLA

Transduodenal Sphincteroplasty

This operation is usually performed for calculi impacted in the transmural portion of the common bile duct or postinflammatory stenosis in this region (papillitis). These conditions may be encountered

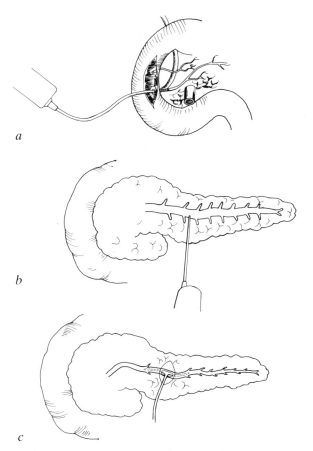

Fig. 14.9. Three methods of obtaining operative pancreatograms. Retrograde visualization of the ductal tree may be achieved by transduodenal cannulation of the major pancreatic papilla (*a*). A dilated pancreatic duct may be entered by direct needle puncture in the body of the gland (*b*). Alternatively, contrast may be introduced via a T-tube inserted into the duct through a short incision in the pancreas (*c*).

during biliary surgery following acute pancreatitis. Sphincteroplasty allows direct inspection of the orifice of the major pancreatic duct, which can also be incised and sutured, if appropriate (*see below*). Biliary strictures caused by chronic pancreatitis, however, are usually too long to be dealt with by incision from below.

After mobilization of the duodenal loop (Kocher's manoeuvre), the papilla can be palpated on the medial wall of the descending duodenum. A longitudinal duodenotomy is made opposite this point. Identification of the papilla is easier in the presence of inflammation, calculus or tumour, and in these circumstances incision or biopsy of the papilla may be appropriate. Localization of a normal papilla is assisted by intravenous injection of secretin (1 unit/kg), which rapidly produces an efflux of pancreatic juice from both pancreatic papillas (when present and patent). Alternatively, a soft polythene catheter (Jaques no. 8 Fr. gauge) may be passed through a supraduodenal choledochotomy down the bile duct and into the duodenum, aided by a small

incision in the sphincter if the catheter is held up at this point. The tip of the catheter is amputated, a grooved hernia director is impacted into its lumen and the catheter is withdrawn from above until the director enters the lower common bile duct. The subsequent placement of 3/0 or 4/0 chromic catgut sutures through the mucosa of the papilla is assisted by the groove in the director. The first stay sutures are inserted and tied at 10 and 12 o'clock on the circumference of the papilla, and a short incision is made between them. Another two sutures inserted near the apex of this incision are then tied and held in haemostats, and the process is repeated until there is a generous communication (>1·5 cm long) between the bile duct and the duodenal lumen. With this method of sphincteroplasty, haemorrhage is easily controlled and accurate mucosal coaptation can be achieved. The orifice of the major pancreatic duct can be seen on the lower lip of the papilla at about 5 o'clock. A polythene cannula (no. 4 or 5 Fr. gauge) can normally be inserted.

The duodenotomy is closed longitudinally in two layers, taking care not to narrow the lumen excessively when inserting the outer layer of interrupted 2/0 silk sutures. The choledochotomy is closed with one layer of chromic catgut sutures. T-tube drainage is optional if a wide sphincteroplasty has been created, but it will permit postoperative radiological studies if desired. A suction drain is inserted before closure of the abdomen.

Apart from duodenal leakage, the most worrying complication of biliary sphincteroplasty is acute pancreatitis, although this should be avoidable if the pancreatic duct is identified and care is taken to avoid damaging its orifice during the insertion of sutures.

Pancreatic Sphincteroplasty

The opening of the duct of Wirsung is routinely exposed during transduodenal (biliary) sphincteroplasty, though occasionally it can be seen to enter the duodenum independently of the bile duct. Scarring at and immediately behind this orifice is associated with generalized ductal dilatation in a few patients with chronic pancreatitis, for whom pancreatic or double sphincteroplasty is appropriate (synonyms: Wirsungoplasty, transampullary septectomy). This operation has also been advocated for certain patients with 'post-cholecystectomy syndrome', in whom injection of morphine/prostigmine reproduces symptoms and causes hyperamylasaemia (Nardi test). If the ductal orifice is stenosed, insertion of a lacrimal probe may permit cannulation and retrograde pancreatography. Stenosis is released by incising (or partly excising) the common septum between the terminal portions of the bile duct and pancreatic duct for a distance of 10 mm. The ductal mucosas are united with 5/0 chromic catgut sutures.

Sphincteroplasty of the minor (accessory) pancreatic duct (Santoriniplasty) may be carried out by a similar technique in patients with recurrent pancreatitis and an isolated dorsal pancreas. The orifice lies about 2 cm proximal to the major papilla. Identification is facilitated by intravenous secretin (*see above*) and the use of a magnifying lens.

Local Excision of Ampullary Tumours

Although partial pancreatoduodenectomy is ordinarily the operation of choice for carcinoma of the ampulla, in elderly people with small tumours it may sometimes be appropriate simply to excise the tumour locally by a transduodenal approach. A circumferential incision around the ampulla is deepened through the duodenal wall, using a diathermy knife, and a short cone of tissue is excised including the ampulla. The cut ends of the bile duct and pancreatic duct are then reattached to the duodenal mucosa, using interrupted sutures. In selected cases this procedure is well tolerated and may effect a cure.

Endoscopic Papillotomy

Like any other operation this procedure should only be undertaken by an experienced practitioner. The patient is admitted to hospital. Carriage of hepatitis B antigen is excluded, together with anaemia and hypoprothrombinaemia. Since blood transfusion is occasionally required, appropriate arrangements should be made preoperatively. The patient is starved for 6 hours, and endoscopy is performed with intravenous sedation (e.g. diazepam) and an agent to render the duodenum hypotonic (e.g. glucagon).

A side-viewing duodenoscope is passed through the pylorus and into the second part of the duodenum. The patient is rolled into the prone position, the papilla is identified with its covering fold of mucosa and the instrument is rotated until the lens is 'face-on' to the papilla. The bile duct is cannulated in a retrograde fashion and cholangiograms are obtained, using a water-soluble contrast agent such as Conray 420. Retrograde pancreatography may also be performed. If papillotomy is indicated, a diathermy catheter is inserted into the bile duct and placed under traction, so that its wire abuts against the roof of the ampulla. Cutting diathermy is used to make a 10–15 mm incision at 11 o'clock, and haemostasis is achieved by means of the coagulation current. Calculi may be retrieved from the bile duct by a balloon catheter, but small stones will often pass spontaneously, either at the time or during the next few days. Complications of papillotomy include bleeding, duodenal perforation and acute pancreatitis; emergency laparotomy is occasionally required.

PANCREATICOJEJUNOSTOMY

This operation is normally reserved for patients with generalized chronic pancreatitis, ductal dilatation and at least some residual pancreatic function. With slight modifications the operation may be used to decompress the distended duct distal to an irresectable carcinoma, to cover any leakage of pancreatic juice following biopsy or trauma, or to provide internal drainage of a pancreatic fistula. The present description will be limited to longitudinal pancreaticojejunostomy (Roux-en-Y), as performed for pancreatitis. If there are associated calculi in the gallbladder, cholecystectomy and operative cholangiography are performed. Obstruction of the common bile duct may be due either to concomitant ductal stones, which should be removed, or to chronic pancreatitis itself, in which case choledochojejunostomy may be required (*see Fig. 14.8*).

Accurate knowledge of pancreatic ductal anatomy is an essential prerequisite for pancreaticojejunostomy. There should be little hesitation in carrying out operative pancreatography if ERCP has been inadequate. If needle aspiration successfully locates the dilated ductal tree, the needle should be left *in situ* while opening into the duct (*Fig. 14.10*). Alternatively, a short vertical incision that partially traverses

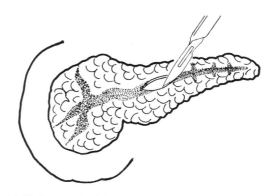

Fig. 14.10. Pancreaticojejunostomy. After the dilated pancreatic duct has been located by needle aspiration, a short incision in the anterior surface of the gland is deepened into the ductal system. Thereafter, the duct may be opened widely in each direction.

the body of the pancreas may be needed to demonstrate the position of an impalpable duct. In either case, one blade of a pair of angled scissors is inserted into the duct and the pancreas is opened along its axis in both directions. Adequate division of all strictures may require the pancreatic duct to be laid widely open virtually throughout its extent. Haemorrhage is controlled by diathermy or suture ligation. Pancreatic calculi are removed. Small cysts can often be opened into the ductal tree. The spleen is left intact.

When the ductal dissection is complete, an appropriate segment of upper jejunum is selected for creation of a Roux loop. Transillumination of the mesentery reveals the disposition of the arterial supply, and two or three vascular arcades are divided to allow sufficient mobilization of the loop (*Fig.* 14.11). The bowel is transected between clamps

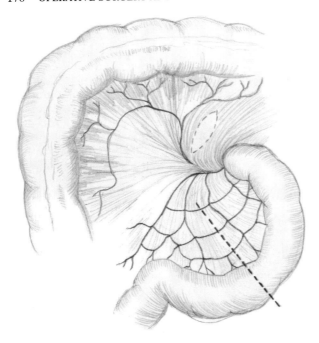

Fig. 14.11. Creation of a Roux loop of jejunum. Following transection of the upper jejunum (*see* broken line), division of two to three vascular arcades provides sufficient mobilization for the loop to be brought through a mesocolic window for pancreatic anastomosis.

applied 15–30 cm beyond the ligament of Treitz, and the distal cut end is closed and invaginated and brought through a window made in the transverse mesocolon to the left of the middle colic vessels. To construct the retrocolic pancreaticojejunostomy, interrupted silk sutures are first inserted between the anterior surface of the pancreas and the seromuscular layer of the Roux loop. The jejunum is then opened for a distance corresponding to the length of the previous pancreatic incision, and a running 2/0 Dexon or Vicryl suture is passed through all coats of the jejunum and the thickened pancreatic duct. Lastly, a layer of interrupted non-absorbable sutures is placed between the gland and the bowel. If the anastomosis is short or technically difficult, it may be splinted by a T-tube. The short limbs of the T lie in the pancreatic duct, and the long limb is brought through the anastomosis and out through the jejunum at several centimetres downstream, thence to the exterior via a stab incision in the overlying abdominal wall. Intestinal continuity is then re-established by end-to-side jejunojejunostomy 30 cm below the pancreatic anastomosis (*Fig.* 14.12). The mesocolic defect is sutured around the Roux loop. A suction drain is placed in the upper abdomen.

The main postoperative complications are haemorrhage and anastomotic leakage, but these are generally avoidable with careful operative technique. Exocrine and endocrine function are usually unaltered.

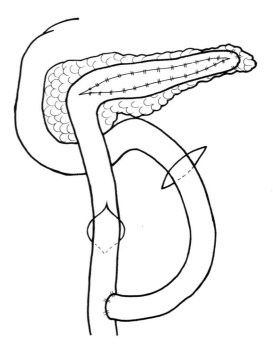

Fig. 14.12. Pancreaticojejunostomy. Diagram to show the final anatomical arrangement.

INTERNAL DRAINAGE OF PANCREATIC CYSTS

Cyst-gastrostomy (*Fig.* 14.13)

This operation may be chosen for symptomatic collections of fluid in the lesser sac, provided the posterior wall of the stomach is closely applied to the front of the (pseudo-) cyst and the gastrostomy can be sited low enough to provide dependent drainage. These criteria may partly be gauged by preoperative ultrasonography and contrast radiology of the upper gastrointestinal tract, but they should be confirmed by peroperative cystography. After inspection of the

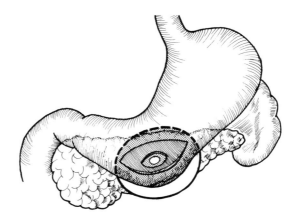

Fig. 14.13. Pancreatic cyst-gastrostomy. Through an anterior gastrotomy, an incision in the posterior wall of the stomach will enter an adherent retrogastric (pseudo-) cyst.

upper abdomen and palpation of the fluctuant retro-gastric swelling, a wide-bore needle is introduced through the great omentum and into the cyst. Some 30–50 ml of cyst fluid are withdrawn for bacterio-logical culture, cytological examination and amylase estimation. A similar quantity of 40 per cent Hypaque or Conray 420 is instilled to show both the anatomical relationship of the cyst and the presence or absence of loculi. After longitudinal incision in the anterior wall of the body of the stomach, the edges of the gastrotomy are retracted to reveal the posterior wall, which is incised for 5 cm. This incision is deepened into the cyst and fluid contents are evacuated by suc-tion. Digital exploration of the cyst cavity allows gentle division of trabeculas and removal of solid debris. The margin of the cyst-gastrostomy is over-sewn with continuous Dexon or Vicryl sutures, and the anterior gastrotomy is resutured in two layers. The abdomen is closed with drainage.

Cyst-duodenostomy

Small intrapancreatic cysts closely applied to the medial wall of the duodenum are sometimes suitable for direct drainage into the duodenal loop. If pan-creatic imaging and operative findings suggest this possibility, a longitudinal duodenotomy is made and a needle is inserted into the cyst. Aspiration of bile is an indication not to proceed, but to drain the cyst into a Roux loop of jejunum instead. Cystography will delineate both the cavity itself and any communi-cation with the pancreatic ductal system. If necessary, retrograde cholangiography via the papilla will out-line the exact position of the bile duct. If cyst-duodenostomy is considered appropriate, the needle is left in situ and a stab incision is made alongside, through the duodenal wall and into the cyst. The margins of the opening are sutured as for cyst-gastrostomy. The duodenum is closed in two layers.

Cyst-jejunostomy

The use of a Roux loop of jejunum is the most flexible method for internal drainage of pancreatic cysts and should be performed when either of the foregoing operations is impracticable. It is contra-indicated when the cyst wall is too thin to take sutures however, as in the peripancreatic collections that may compli-cate acute pancreatitis and require external drainage. After operative cystography, the cyst is opened near its lower pole and the contents are evacuated. A Roux loop of jejunum is created as in pancreatico-jejunostomy and is sutured directly to the cystotomy.

Whichever method of internal drainage is em-ployed, postoperative complications include infec-tion and reaccumulation of fluid, which may both be attributable to an inadequate stoma, and fistuliza-tion from a leaking anastomosis. Spontaneous haemor-rhage into the cyst (before drainage) or the upper alimentary tract (after drainage) may arise from arterial pseudoaneurysms. The bleeding, which may be catastrophic, is often extremely difficult to stop at operation, though insertion of a Foley catheter into the mouth of the vessel may apply sufficient tam-ponade to allow accurate suture ligation. If pseudo-aneurysms are shown on preoperative angiography, either the vessel should be ligated at operation or the cyst requires resection.

DISTAL PANCREATIC RESECTION

Hemipancreatectomy

Diseases of the body and tail of the pancreas may be amenable to cure by appropriate distal resection, usually including splenectomy. Such conditions include chronic pancreatitis that is largely confined to the left pancreas, trauma, fistulas, tumours and cysts. Distal pancreatectomy and splenectomy may also be performed as part of a radical lymphatic clear-ance during gastrectomy for carcinoma of the stomach.

Splenectomy is usually the first step after examina-tion of the pancreas. Division of the posterior layer of the lienorenal ligament allows the spleen to be mobilized into the wound for ligation and division of the short gastric vessels. If the spleen is torn during this manoeuvre, it should be removed after ligation of the splenic vessels at the hilum. Already partly mobilized with the spleen, the tail of the pancreas is further freed by dividing the peritoneum and underlying areolar tissue along its superior and in-ferior borders. As the dissection proceeds along the body of the pancreas, several small vessels must be secured by ligature or diathermy. The distal pancreas together with the spleen (if still attached) can now be lifted forwards and to the right, exposing the splenic vein coursing along its posterior surface. This vessel should be traced to its junction with first the inferior and then the superior mesenteric vein. The splenic artery is now dissected free and ligated just before it gains the superior border of the pancreas. The splenic vein is ligated immediately distal to the entry of the inferior mesenteric vein (*Fig.* 14.14). The body of the pancreas can then be gently elevated from the portal vein and its main tributaries.

The disposition of the great veins provides the key to safe pancreatectomy. In chronic pancreatitis, peri-glandular inflammation and dense fibrosis often make the dissection difficult and potentially dangerous. In these circumstances the middle colic vein (*see* Fig. 14.2) can be traced carefully downwards as a guide to the superior mesenteric and ultimately the portal vein.

A suitable site should now be chosen for transec-tion of the pancreas, usually where it crosses the por-tal vein (*Fig.* 14.15). Stay sutures are inserted into the superior and inferior borders of the gland on either side of this point. A non-crushing intestinal

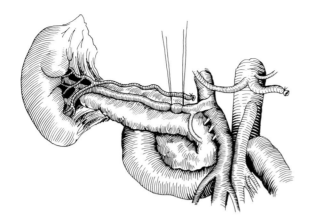

Fig. 14.14. Distal pancreatectomy. The spleen and body of pancreas have been mobilized upwards and to the right, exposing their posterior surfaces. The splenic vein is now divided between ligatures immediately beyond the entry of the inferior mesenteric vein. The splenic artery has previously been secured.

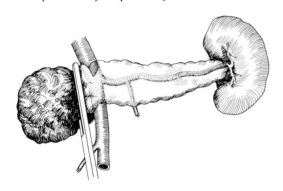

Fig. 14.15. Distal pancreatectomy. Transection of the pancreas in front of the portal vein completes the removal of the distal half of the gland. A non-crushing intestinal clamp limits bleeding from the proximal stump.

clamp is applied across the neck of the pancreas and the gland is divided by a scalpel to the left of the clamp, taking care to protect the subjacent portal vein. The distal pancreas and spleen are removed. Bleeding vessels are carefully oversewn with 3/0 silk sutures, and the clamp is removed to check haemostasis (*Fig.* 14.16). Interrupted silk sutures are placed to close off the ends of the amputated stump of pancreas. The pancreatic duct should be identified during closure of the stump and may be cannulated to allow pancreatography of the head.* A normal-calibre duct (2–3 mm) can best be closed with a silk transfixion stitch, but a thickened or dilated duct can often be grasped with a haemostat and encircled with a ligature. A suction drain should be placed to the splenic bed.

If the duct is very dilated, it may be sensible to combine distal resection with a limited longitudinal

---

* If operative radiographs are not required, transection of the pancreas may be performed using a gastrointestinal stapling gun.

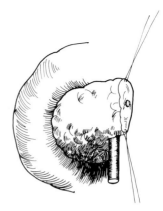

Fig. 14.16. Distal pancreatectomy. The head and uncinate process are left *in situ* following division of the pancreas just to the left of the portal vein.

pancreaticojejunostomy. The pancreatic duct is opened up for a few centimetres by incising the overlying glandular tissue. A Roux loop of jejunum is created for anastomosis to the spatulated duct, as previously described (pp. 169–170).

Postoperative complications are relatively uncommon, but include haemorrhage and infection in the splenic bed and sometimes a collection of pancreatic fluid. Persistent pancreatic fistula is unlikely to occur, provided there is no obstruction to the ductal system in the head of the pancreas. Pancreatic insufficiency seldom develops *de novo* after this operation.

Conservative Caudal Pancreatectomy

If the tail of the pancreas is relatively healthy, it can be dissected free from the splenic artery and vein and removed without the need for splenectomy and its attendant risks (*see* Chapter 15). This operation provides pancreatic tissue for histological examination and enables prograde pancreatography to be undertaken. It may therefore be of value in symptomatic patients with isolated dorsal pancreas or in those with suspected chronic pancreatitis but minimal changes on ERCP. The dissection can be tedious and bloody and is inappropriate in the presence of severe pancreatitis.

The pancreatic tail is approached through the lesser sac after ligation and division of the greater omentum. As in conventional distal pancreatectomy, the tail is mobilized by incising the peritoneum along its upper and lower borders. One or two retractors are placed within the lesser sac to displace the stomach and omentum. The tip of the pancreas is grasped by tissue forceps and elevated from its bed, taking care not to damage the subjacent splenic vein. The splenic vessels are closely applied to the posterior surface and may actually groove the gland. Several small arterial and venous branches need to be secured as they enter the pancreas (*Fig.* 14.17). Once the correct plane is established and developed, the dissection proceeds more easily. Ultimately the pan-

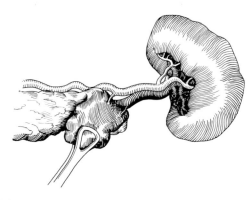

Fig. 14.17. Conservative caudal pancreatectomy. The pancreatic tail has been elevated and displaced to the patient's right. Several small branches of the splenic artery and vein need to be ligated and divided, but the parent trunks are preserved.

creas is transected and closed in the standard manner, and a suction drain is placed within the lesser sac.

Subtotal Pancreatectomy

This major operation is reserved for severe and generalized pancreatitis. It involves resection of 80–95 per cent of the gland, leaving a rim of pancreatic tissue within the duodenal loop. The residual pancreas is seldom sufficient to maintain normal exocrine and endocrine function. Since the duodenum and antropyloric mechanism are also preserved, diabetes and malabsorption should be less severe and easier to manage than after pancreatoduodenectomy. Obstructive jaundice suggests compression of the bile duct and is a contra-indication to subtotal pancreatectomy.

The initial operative steps follow those of left hemipancreatectomy, but the dissection is often particularly laborious owing to peripancreatic fibrosis. The gland is elevated progressively from left to right and mobilization is continued well beyond the midline, with individual ligature of the many vessels that pass from the medial borders of the head and uncinate process to the portal and superior mesenteric veins. At this stage a bougie is introduced through a supraduodenal choledochotomy to allow accurate localization of the terminal bile duct. The duodenum is mobilized, the pancreatic head is grasped by a hand placed from behind and the gland is transected from front to back within the duodenal cavity, by means of a diathermy knife (*Fig.* 14.18). The distal pancreas and spleen are removed. The remainder of the head is trimmed as required, preserving the bile duct and at least one (ideally both) of the superior and inferior pancreaticoduodenal arcades. If duodenal ischaemia develops, the operation must be converted into total pancreatoduodenectomy. The pancreatic duct is identified and closed by suture ligation as before. The incision in the common bile duct is sutured around a T-tube. The abdomen is closed with adequate drainage. During the recovery period, fluid balance and normoglycaemia must be maintained, and naso-

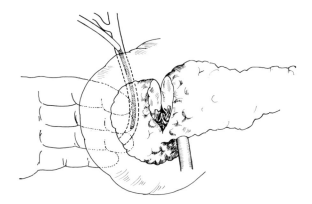

Fig. 14.18. Subtotal pancreatectomy. The head of the pancreas is divided at a safe distance from the common bile duct, while the organ is firmly grasped by the surgeon's left hand. The position of the bile duct is confirmed by the introduction of a metal bougie via a supraduodenal choledochotomy. Further resection of the pancreatic head is performed to complete an 80–95 per cent pancreatectomy, preserving a rim of glandular tissue within the duodenal loop to protect the pancreaticoduodenal arteries.

gastric intubuation is required until the passage of flatus. Exocrine status is assessed on resumption of oral feeding.

PROXIMAL PANCREATIC RESECTION

Whipple's Operation

Originally described by Dr Allen Whipple in 1935 for ampullary cancer, partial pancreatoduodenectomy is most commonly carried out for carcinoma of the head of the pancreas and is occasionally indicated for benign destructive disease of the proximal pancreas, as in trauma or chronic pancreatitis. It is the operation of choice for carcinomas of the ampulla, terminal bile duct and descending duodenum.

In operations for malignant disease, evidence of local invasion or metastases generally means that Whipple's operation should be abandoned in favour of palliative bypass. Preoperative tests including visceral angiography will indicate the likelihood of resectability. In palliative operations biopsies of the primary or secondary sites of tumour should be taken to establish a tissue diagnosis.

If the tumour mass is mobile and confined to the pancreatic head, an exploratory dissection is undertaken to assess resectability. After entry into the lesser sac, the superior mesenteric vein is traced to the inferior border of the neck of the pancreas. The duodenum is mobilized fully, and dissection within the free edge of the lesser omentum is undertaken to identify the (dilated) common bile duct, the hepatic artery with its right gastric and gastroduodenal branches and the portal vein, which lies posteriorly. The surgeon's left index finger is cautiously inserted alongside the portal vein from above and is introduced downwards behind the neck of pancreas (*Fig.*

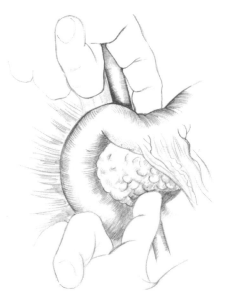

Fig. 14.19. Partial pancreatoduodenectomy. If the neck of the pancreas can be freed from the anterior surface of the portal vein, resection of the tumour is normally feasible.

14.19). If this finger makes contact with the right index, which is gently insinuated along the superior mesenteric vein from below, the portal vein is free of tumour anteriorly and resection is feasible.

Following ligation of the gastroduodenal artery close to its origin, four major structures require division; the order of dissection may be varied according to progress at different sites. Distal hemigastrectomy is performed by transecting the body of the stomach.* The supraduodenal bile duct is divided well above the tumour, and the gallbladder is removed. The neck of the pancreas is transected in front of the portal vein (*Fig.* 14.20). The pancreatic duct is frequently dilated at this point. Several vessels running from the head and uncinate process to the portal and superior mesenteric veins now require careful individual ligation, together with the inferior pancreaticoduodenal vessels. After dividing the ligament of Treitz and the vessels that supply the duodenojejunal flexure, the resection is completed by transecting the upper jejunum at a convenient point. The operative specimen is removed, and the jejunum is advanced through the transverse mesocolon.

Occasionally the surgeon may find towards the end of the resection that the tumour extends very close to the portal vein. It may be possible to clear the involved tissue by gentle blunt dissection, but sometimes it is safer to leave a rim of pancreas (or tumour) to protect the great veins. Alternatively, a short segment of portal vein can be resected en bloc. Upward traction on the mesentery will usually allow vascular continuity to be restored by direct end-to-end anastomosis.

* Truncal vagotomy and antrectomy are a reasonable alternative.

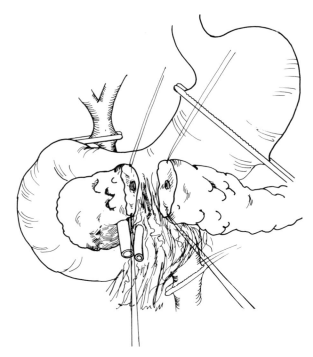

Fig. 14.20. Partial pancreatoduodenectomy. The operative specimen is removed after transection of the stomach, bile duct, pancreas and upper jejunum.

Several methods of reconstruction are possible. The author's preference is to start by joining the neck of pancreas to the upper end of jejunum (*Fig.* 14.21). The pancreatic duct (and overlying gland) are incised for 1–2 cm, so that a greater proportion of sutures will incorporate ductal mucosa; if the duct is grossly dilated, this step can be omitted. The end-to-end pan-

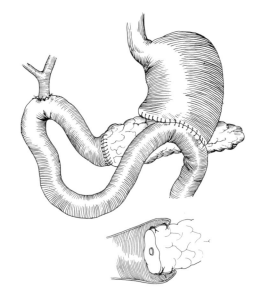

Fig. 14.21. Partial pancreatoduodenectomy. A convenient method for reconstruction. The *inset* shows the completed pancreatico-intestinal anastomosis, with invagination of a short sleeve of jejunum to protect the inner row of sutures.

creaticojejunostomy is carried out using two layers of interrupted 3/0 silk sutures. The first layer unites the cut surface of the pancreas and its duct to the full thickness of the jejunum. The jejunum is then invaginated for 1–2 cm to cover this anastomosis, and a second layer of sutures is placed between the seromuscular coat of the bowel and the pancreatic capsule. Alternatively an end-to-side pancreaticojejunostomy can be created (*Fig.* 14.22). A circular

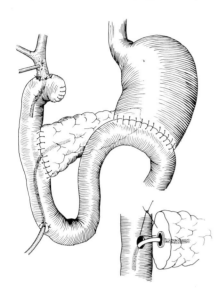

Fig. 14.22. Partial pancreatoduodenectomy. An alternative method for reconstruction. Gastrojejunostomy may be carried out either above or below the transverse mesocolon. The *inset* shows construction of the pancreatico-intestinal anastomosis.

disc of jejunal serosa and muscularis is excised, equal in size to the cut surface of the pancreatic neck. A tiny enterotomy is made in the centre of the denuded bowel. Direct mucosal apposition is achieved between jejunum and pancreatic duct, using a few interrupted 5/0 silk sutures. The pancreatic substance is sutured to the jejunal serosa, using 3/0 silk. If the pancreatic duct is narrow the pancreaticointestinal anastomosis may be splinted by a fine cannula, which is anchored to the jejunal mucosa with a catgut stitch. The tube is either brought out through the jejunum at a lower level and then exteriorized through the abdominal wall, or it is cut short and left within the bowel lumen, to be passed down the gut when the retaining stitch gives way.

The bile duct is joined end to side to the jejunum, either above or below the pancreas, depending on the type of pancreatico-intestinal anastomosis chosen (*Figs.* 14.21, 14.22). Care must be taken to ensure that the length of the jejunal incision corresponds to the width of the bile duct (which is usually dilated). One layer of interrupted 3/0 catgut sutures is employed. It is easier to insert the entire posterior row of sutures before tying any individual stitch. This anastomosis can be splinted by a T-tube which is inserted through a separate incision in the bile duct; one limb of the T-tube is placed through the choledochojejunostomy. These splinting tubes are generally removed about 10 days after the operation.

Lastly, a side-to-side gastroenterostomy is created, as after Polya gastrectomy (*see* Chapter 12), either above or below the transverse mesocolon. The GIA stapler can be used at this stage. At least two drains are placed in the region of the pancreatic anastomosis before wound closure.

Besides the complications attendant upon any operation of this complexity, leakage may occur from any of the three or four suture lines, but especially the pancreaticojejunostomy. If a pancreatic fistula develops, one drain may be used for irrigation of sterile saline to prevent local haemorrhage, and parenteral nutrition is instituted. Gastrointestinal bleeding may follow stress ulceration, but this risk is lessened by adequate gastric resection and by intravenous administration of an H_2 receptor antagonist during the recovery period. Late obstruction of the pancreatic anastomosis may cause progressive exocrine atrophy, but Whipple's operation seldom aggravates diabetes mellitus appreciably.

Conservative Proximal Pancreatoduodenectomy

The conventional Whipple's resection includes a distal gastrectomy, partly to widen the lymph node clearance for cancer and partly to reduce gastric acidity and prevent bleeding stomal ulcers in the early postoperative period. In resecting the head of pancreas for inflammatory disease, a radical excision is unnecessary and erosive gastritis might be avoided by retaining the pylorus and preventing bile reflux. This is the basic concept of the pylorus-preserving proximal pancreatectomy introduced by Traverso and Longmire in 1978. Early results appear very satisfactory. The operation may also be appropriate for less invasive tumours such as ampullary cancer.

The key to success lies in maintaining an adequate blood supply to the pylorus and stump of proximal duodenum that are retained in the body. The gastroduodenal artery can safely be ligated at its origin, but the right gastro-epiploic vessels should be carefully preserved. If the inflammatory changes in and around the head of pancreas are very severe, it may be better to carry out Whipple's operation than to struggle to retain the duodenal cap and its vessels of supply. In favourable cases, however, the first part of duodenum can be dissected free of the pancreas, and the bowel is transected 2–4 cm beyond the pylorus. The resection line should be carefully inspected to ensure that it is viable; it can be trimmed if necessary. Intestinal continuity is restored by end-to-side duodenojejunostomy (*Fig.* 14.23).

Total Pancreatoduodenectomy

Removal of the entire pancreas may be appropriate in a few cases of cancer or end-stage chronic pancrea-

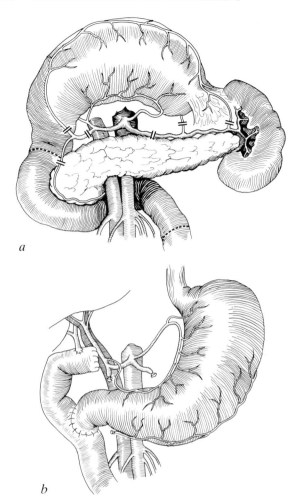

a

b

Fig. 14.23. Pylorus-preserving pancreatectomy. The duodenum is divided about 3 cm beyond the pylorus (*a*), and continuity is restored by end-to-side duodenojejunostomy (*b*). Total pancreatectomy is illustrated. Conservative proximal pancreatectomy can be performed by a similar technique but with preservation of the splenic artery and its branches and anastomosis of the distal pancreas to the upper jejunum.

titis, despite the permanent loss of function that ensues. The operation combines partial pancreatoduodenectomy with left hemipancreatectomy. The stomach and pylorus may be preserved in benign disease (*Fig.* 14.23). In chronic pancreatitis, the dissection will ordinarily proceed from left to right, and the correct plane in front of the great veins is established as before. In carcinoma, metastatic disease and involvement of the portal vein are excluded before subsequent dissection is carried out away from the panacreatic neck in each direction. Reconstruction is simpler after total than after partial resection, because the difficult pancreatico-intestinal anastomosis is no longer required.

Insulin must be given postoperatively, the dose being altered according to blood and urinary sugar levels. Before discharge patients are taught to manage their own diabetes. It is wise to allow patients

to become hypoglycaemic once or twice, so that they can learn to recognize the warning symptoms. They should be instructed to take regular meals and to carry sugar with them at all times. Careful outpatient supervision of diabetes is mandatory during the early postoperative weeks. Pancreatic enzymes are given by mouth as soon as feeding is resumed. A low fat diet is advisable, and enzyme supplements are adjusted to prevent steatorrhoea.

BYPASS FOR PANCREATIC CANCER

Cholecystojejunostomy

A distended healthy gallbladder that communicates with the bile duct by a wide cystic duct entering well above the site of tumour can readily be used for biliary diversion. After insertion of an Ochsner trocar and cannula into the fundus, the gallbladder is emptied by suction; if radiological visualization of the biliary tree is desired, contrast medium is instilled before evacuating all the bile. On withdrawal of the cannula the puncture site is grasped and sealed with Duval's forceps. A loop of upper jejunum is approximated to the gallbladder and short incisions are made in the adjoining viscera. A one-layer cholecystojejunostomy is fashioned using 2/0 chromic catgut sutures. Side-to-side jejunojejunostomy (enteroanastomosis) about 10 cm below this may limit entry of food into the biliary apparatus (*Fig.* 14.24).

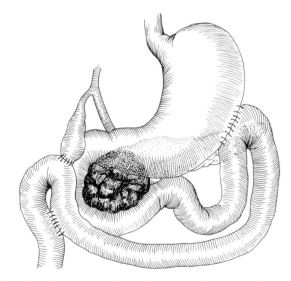

Fig. 14.24. Bypass procedures for irresectable pancreatic cancer. An entero-anastomosis below the site of the cholecysto-jejunostomy may decrease the entry of food into the gallbladder. An antecolic gastroenterostomy circumvents present or future obstruction of the duodenum.

Choledochojejunostomy

When the above procedure is unsuitable, jaundice should be relieved by end-to-side anastomosis between the transected common bile duct and a Roux loop of jejunum. The loop is brought up behind or in front of the transverse colon and is closed at its end. The dilated bile duct is dissected free and opened transversely. Bile is evacuated, and the duct is divided completely below a bulldog clip. The lower end is closed with catgut sutures, and the upper end is inserted into the Roux loop just below its apex, as after partial pancreatoduodenectomy. Intestinal continuity is restored as usual by end-to-side jejunojejunostomy about 30 cm downstream (*Fig. 14.25*).

Other Palliative Procedures

Biopsies should always be taken (if at all possible) to confirm the tissue diagnosis (*see* p. 166). Antecolic gastroenterostomy is carried out as for carcinoma of the stomach (*see* Chapter 12), in anticipation of duodenal invasion by tumour. To perform peroperative coeliac plexus block, 15–20 ml of 50 per cent alcohol are injected into the retroperitoneal tissues surrounding the coeliac ganglion on either side of the aorta and the vena cava at the level of the diaphragmatic crura. Neurolytic agents must never be injected if blood is aspirated into the syringe. Careful wound closure and antibiotic cover are advisable during palliative operations for pancreatic cancer.

An obstructed pancreatic duct may be drained into the Roux loop used for biliary diversion in a manner akin to pancreaticojejunostomy. A 2–3 cm longitudinal incision is made in the duct, and the anastomosis is splinted by a T-tube that is brought to the exterior. Alternatively, an intubated pancreaticogastrostomy is fashioned. The long limb of the T-tube is brought

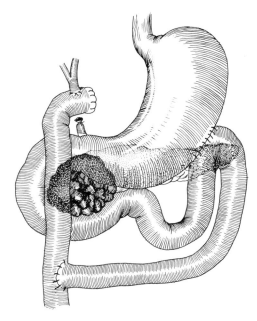

Fig. 14.25. Bypass procedures for irresectable pancreatic cancer. The bile duct has been transected well above the tumour, and its upper end is anastomosed to a Roux loop of jejunum; the lower end is tied off. Cholecystectomy has been performed.

through the posterior wall of the stomach and then obliquely through the anterior gastric and abdominal walls. About 10 cm of the tube (containing a few sideholes) should be within the cavity of the stomach. A few sutures are used to approximate the small posterior gastrostomy to the margins of the pancreatic defect. The tube can usually be clamped at 5 days and removed at 10 days postoperatively.

FURTHER READING

Bolman R. M. (1981) Surgical management of chronic relapsing pancreatitis. *Ann. Surg.* **193**, 125–131.

Braasch J. W. and Gray B. N. (1976) Technique of radical pancreatoduodenectomy with consideration of hepatic arterial relationships. *Surg. Clin. North Am.* **56**, 631–647.

Braasch, J. W., Vito L. and Nugent F. W. (1978) Total pancreatectomy for end-stage chronic pancreatitis. *Ann. Surg.* **188**, 317–322.

Bradley E. L., III. (1982) *Complications of Pancreatitis. Medical and Surgical Management*. Philadelphia, Saunders.

Brooks J. R. (1983) *Surgery of the Pancreas*. Philadelphia, Saunders.

Cameron J. L., Kieffer R. S., Anderson W. J. et al. (1976) Internal pancreatic fistulas: pancreatic ascites and pleural effusions. *Ann. Surg* **184**, 587–593.

Campbell R. and Kennedy T. (1980) The management of pancreatic and pancreaticoduodenal injuries. *Br. J. Surg.* **76**, 845–850.

Cohen J. R., Kuchta N., Geller N. et al. (1982) Pancreaticoduodenectomy. A 40-year experience. *Ann. Surg.* **195**, 608–617.

Colhoun E., Murphy J. J. and MacErlean D. P. (1984). Percutaneous drainage of pancreatic pseudocysts. *Br. J. Surg.* **71**, 131–132.

Cooper M. J. and Williamson R. C. N. (1983) The value of operative pancreatography. *Br. J. Surg.* **70**, 577–580.

Cooper M. J. and Williamson R. C. N. (1984) Drainage operations in chronic pancreatitis. *Br. J. Surg.* **71**, 761–766.

Corfield A. P., Cooper M. J. and Williamson R. C. N. (1985) Acute pancreatitis: a lethal disease of increasing incidence. *Gut* **26**, 724–729.

Cotton P. B. (1980) Congenital anomaly of pancreas divisum as cause of obstructive pain and pancreatitis. *Gut* **21**, 105–114.

Cotton P. B. and Williams C. B. (1982) *Practical Gastrointestinal Endoscopy*, 2nd ed. Oxford, Blackwell.

Fortner J. G. (1984) Regional pancreatectomy for cancer of the pancreas, ampulla, and other related sites. *Ann. Surg.* **199**, 418–425.

Heerden J. A. van., Edis R. J. and Service F. J. (1979) The surgical aspects of insulinomas. *Ann. Surg.* **189**, 677–682.

Hermann R. E. (1979) *Manual of Surgery of the Gall Bladder, Bile Ducts and Exocrine Pancreas.* New York, Springer-Verlag.

Huizinga W. K. J., Kalideen J. M., Bryer J. V. et al. (1984) Control of major haemorrhage associated with pancreatic pseudocysts by transcatheter arterial embolization. *Br. J. Surg.* **71**, 133–136.

Ihse I., Lilja P., Arnesjö B. et al. (1977) Total pancreactectomy for cancer: an appraisal of 65 cases. *Ann. Surg.* **186**, 675–680.

Ihse I., Toregard B.-M. and Åkerman M. (1979) Intraoperative fine needle aspiration cytology in pancreatic lesions. *Ann. Surg.* **190**, 732–734.

Jones R. C. (1978) Management of pancreatic trauma. *Ann. Surg.* **187**, 555–562.

Kivilaasko E., Lempinen M., Makelainen A. et al. (1984) Pancreatic resection *versus* peritoneal lavation for acute fulminant pancreatitis. A randomised prospective study. *Ann. Surg.* **199**, 426–431.

Lloyd-Jones W., Mountain J. C. and Warren K. W. (1972) Annular pancreas in the adult. *Ann. Surg.* **176**, 163–170.

Longmire W. P., Jr (1984) The vicissitudes of pancreatic surgery. *Am. J. Surg.* **147**, 17–24.

Malt R. A. (1983) Treatment of pancreatic cancer. *JAMA* **250**, 1433–1437.

Mayer A. D., McMahon M. J., Benson E. A. et al. (1984) Operations upon the biliary tract in patients with acute pancreatitis: aims, indications and timing. *Ann. R. Coll. Surg. Engl.* **66**, 179–183.

Moody F. G., Berenson M. M. and McCloskey D. (1977) Transampullary septectomy for post-cholecystectomy pain. *Ann. Surg.* **186**, 415–423.

Moossa A. R. (1980) *Tumours of the Pancreas.* Baltimore, Williams & Wilkins.

Morrow M., Hilaris B. and Brennan M. F. (1984) Comparison of conventional surgical resection, radioactive implantation, and bypass procedures for exocrine carcinoma of the pancreas 1975–1980. *Ann. Surg.* **199**, 1–5.

Nardi G. L. et al. (1977) Surgery for chronic pancreatitis. In: Malt R. A. (ed.) *Surgical Techniques Illustrated*, Vol. 2. Boston, Little, Brown.

Newman K. D., Braasch J. W., Rossi R. L. et al. (1983) Pyloric and gastric preservation with pancreatoduodenectomy. *Am. J. Surg.* **145**, 152–156.

Papachristou D. N. and Fortner J. G. (1981) Pancreatic fistula complicating pancreatectomy for malignant disease. *Br. J. Surg.* **68**, 238–240.

Prinz R. A. and Greenlee H. B. (1981) Pancreatic duct drainage in 100 patients with chronic pancreatitis. *Ann. Surg.* **194**, 313–320.

Sarr M. G. and Cameron J. L. (1982) Surgical management of unresectable carcinoma of the pancreas. *Surgery* **91**, 123–133.

Shi E. C. P., Yeo B. W. and Ham J. M. (1984) Pancreatic abscesses. *Br. J. Surg.* **71**, 689–691.

Thompson J. C., Lewis B. G., Wiener I. et al. (1983) The role of surgery in the Zollinger–Ellison syndrome. *Ann. Surg.* **197**, 594–607.

Thompson M. H., Williamson R. C. N. and Salmon P. R. (1980) The clinical relevance of isolated ventral pancreas. *Br. J. Surg.* **68**, 101–104.

Trapnell J. E. (1978) Subtotal pancreatectomy. *Br. J. Hosp. Med* **19**, 482–491.

Traverso L. W. and Longmire W. P. Jr (1978) Preservation of the pylorus during pancreaticoduodenectomy. *Surg. Gynecol. Obstet.* **146**, 959–962.

Tweedle D. E. F. (1979) Peroperative transduodenal biopsy of the pancreas. *Gut* **20**, 992–996.

White T. T. (1973) Surgical anatomy of the pancreas. In: Carey L. (ed.) *Diseases of the Pancreas.* St Louis, C. V. Mosby.

White T. T. and Slavotinek A. H. (1979) Results of surgical treatment of chronic pancreatitis. *Ann. Surg.* **189**, 217–224.

Williamson R. C. N. (1984) Early assessment of severity in acute pancreatitis. *Gut* **66**, 179–183.

Chapter fifteen

The Spleen

M. J. Cooper and R. C. N. Williamson

ANATOMY AND PHYSIOLOGY

Structure

The spleen is a friable and highly vascular organ. In a normal adult it weighs about 150 g and is 12 cm long; splenic size diminishes with age. Lying within the left hypochondrium, the spleen is protected from direct injury by the 9th, 10th and 11th ribs. Its diaphragmatic surface is smooth and convex. Its visceral surface is indented by gastric, renal, pancreatic and colic impressions.

Blood is supplied by the splenic artery, a sinuous vessel which runs along the upper border of the pancreas (*Fig.* 15.1). In the hilum of the spleen the artery

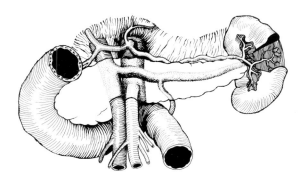

Fig. 15.1. Vascular anatomy of the spleen. The splenic artery arises as a branch of the coeliac axis and runs along the upper border of the pancreas to the splenic hilum. The artery branches before entering the splenic substance and forms segmental end arteries. The splenic vein runs deep to the pancreas to form the portal vein.

gives off about five short gastric vessels, together with the left gastro-epiploic artery, before dividing into four or five branches that enter the spleen. These terminal divisions are segmentally distributed; there is little blood flow between the various segments of the spleen. Blood leaving the spleen drains into the splenic vein, which runs deep to the pancreas towards the origin of the portal vein. The splenic vein accounts for some 40 per cent of portal blood flow.

Accessory spleens (splenunculi) are commonly situated near the splenic hilum within the gastrosplenic ligament. They are found in 20 per cent of the population.

Function

Although the spleen is not essential for life, it does have several important haematological and immunological functions. Atrophy or removal of the spleen produces long-lasting sequelae.

Haematological

In health splenic haemopoiesis is only important during intra-uterine life. Subsequently it may recur when the marrow capacity is exceeded, but in these circumstances red cell production is abnormal. Normal maturation and destruction of red blood corpuscles occur within the splenic cords. Surface craters and pits are effaced from new cells, and old cells are removed as they become effete. In humans the spleen acts as a storage site for iron and platelets, but not for blood.

Immunological

The spleen accounts for 25 per cent of the body's lymphoid tissue. Most lymphocytes are produced in the bone marrow, yet the spleen has an important though not indispensable role in both humoral and cell-mediated immunity. Circulating antigens are trapped and trigger IgM production in the germinal centres. The spleen is the major site of production of the opsonins, tuftsin and properdin, which are important in the phagocytosis of encapsulated bacteria.

Effects of Splenectomy

Haematological

There is an increase in the number of abnormal red cells in the circulation. Almost invariably there is leucocytosis and thrombocytosis, which peak at 7–10 days. Thrombocytosis results from increased platelet production and may persist for many years.

Immunological

The effect is age dependent, being maximal under 1 year. IgM levels fall and take 4 years to return to normal. IgA levels rise; IgG levels are usually unaffected. There is an immediate and prolonged reduction in the ability to opsonize encapsulated bacteria, with consequently impaired phagocytosis of these organisms. Splenosis or splenuncular hyperplasia may partially restore these functions.

Table 15.1. Indications for splenectomy

Traumatic rupture	Immediate
	Iatrogenic
	Delayed
	(Spontaneous)
Hypersplenism	Primary splenomegaly
	Secondary splenomegaly
Neoplasia	Hodgkin's disease
	Non-Hodgkin's lymphoma
	Leukaemia
	Massive haemangioma
With other viscera	Total gastrectomy
	Distal pancreatectomy
	Conventional splenorenal shunt
Other	To prevent graft rejection
	Splenic cysts
	Splenic abscess

INDICATIONS FOR SPLENECTOMY (*Table 15.1*)

Trauma

A ruptured spleen is the commonest serious injury to result from blunt abdominal trauma. Rupture follows a crush injury, a blow to the abdomen or left lower thorax, or a fall onto a protruding object. Penetrating injuries are relatively uncommon in the UK; they frequently cause mixed thoracic and abdominal injuries. A force sufficient to rupture the normal spleen will often produce associated injuries to the ribs and other internal organs. A pathologically enlarged spleen is more liable to traumatic rupture.

As many as 25 per cent of all splenectomies are the result of iatrogenic injury during other surgical procedures, particularly revision operations in the upper abdomen. Most of these injuries are capsular tears caused by the surgeon pulling on peritoneal attachments or adhesions, or sometimes by an assistant's over-enthusiastic use of a retractor. They can be avoided if care is taken to divide these attachments at an early stage in any laparotomy. Iatrogenic rupture has also been reported as a complication of various endoscopic procedures.

Delayed rupture of the spleen is often actually a delay in diagnosis. However, the development of a subcapsular haematoma or post-traumatic cyst may lead to rupture hours or weeks after the injury. The true incidence of the problem is unknown; its reported incidence varies from 2 to 35 per cent of all ruptures.

Spontaneous rupture is rare except as a complication of splenomegaly. The high mortality rate reflects late recognition of this condition.

Hypersplenism

This is defined as splenomegaly causing depression of one or more of the cell counts in the circulating blood. Reduced numbers of cells result from both pooling and excess destruction. The reduction may be generalized (pancytopenia) or specific to one element, e.g. platelets. Before splenectomy is undertaken for hypersplenism, it must be established that the excess cell destruction is taking place in the spleen and that the bone marrow can provide adequate haemopoiesis once the spleen has been removed. Splenectomy may be curative in hereditary spherocytosis and idiopathic thrombocytopenic purpura.

In many parts of the world splenomegaly and hence hypersplenism result from parasitic infestations such as malaria, schistosomiasis and leishmaniasis. Splenectomy may be required, but the effect on the host's immune mechanism must be carefully monitored and controlled.

Neoplasia

Lymphomas and leukaemias frequently infiltrate the spleen and can lead to gross splenomegaly. The underlying diagnosis is usually made by marrow or lymph node biopsy and should lead to treatment of the primary disease. Splenectomy is reserved for hypersplenism or pain or for purposes of staging the disease. The need for staging laparotomy in Hodgkin's disease is decreasing as the role of chemotherapy expands. Other primary and secondary tumours of the spleen are extremely uncommon.

With other Viscera

Splenectomy is an integral part of total gastrectomy or distal pancreatectomy for neoplasia. It facilitates the operation and permits a better clearance of the regional lymph nodes. However, the spleen can be preserved by careful technique when these organs are removed for benign disease, except in severe pancreatitis. Splenectomy may also be avoided during construction of a splenorenal shunt by the use of an H-graft. Splenic artery aneurysms can usually be treated by ligation without the need to remove the spleen.

Other Indications

Splenic cysts are rare. They may be congenital, degenerative, parasitic or traumatic. Although splenectomy is the recommended treatment at present, marsupialization may prove to be as effective without the immune consequences. Splenic abscess is best treated by early splenectomy and high-dose chemotherapy, but the results are poor.

MANAGEMENT OF THE RUPTURED SPLEEN

Diagnosis

This should be suspected when abdominal trauma is followed by the symptoms and signs of peritonism and shock. Difficulties arise in the unconscious or multiply injured patient, or when the bleeding is slight and contained within the splenic capsule.

The classic symptom is that of left hypochondrial pain, which is worse on moving and radiates to the left shouldertip (Kehr's sign). The physical signs are those of hypovolaemia and evidence of local injury. There is often grazing or bruising over the left side of the abdomen; abdominal and costal movement is reduced. Peritonism is initially confined to the left upper quadrant but will spread if the bleeding continues; there may be evidence of rib fractures. If the diagnosis is in doubt, abdominal paracentesis may confirm the presence of intraperitoneal blood.

The first priority is prompt resuscitation, with the establishment of adequate venous access and the cross-matching of blood. A chest radiograph will help diagnose rib fractures and associated pneumothorax or haemothorax.

Conservative Management

Initial management is aimed at restoring a normal circulating blood volume with blood and other intravenous fluids. Many younger patients respond well, with normalization of pulse and blood pressure. In these circumstances it is reasonable to treat them conservatively by careful observation and transfusion as required, with the aim of conserving the spleen. Cross-matched blood should always be available when pursuing a conservative policy, as deterioration can be sudden and unexpected. Urgent laparotomy is then indicated and may reveal other unsuspected internal injuries. Ultrasound and radio-isotope scans may confirm the diagnosis of splenic contusion or haematoma and enable the healing process to be monitored. A period of 10–14 days' inpatient observation is then advisable.

Emergency Splenectomy

Access should be gained through an upper midline abdominal incision (*Fig.* 15.2, *a–a*) since this can be readily extended (*a–c*) if other abdominal injuries are discovered. If the patient is bleeding heavily and access is difficult, a T-shaped extension (*b*) will quickly improve visibility. Initial assessment should be aimed at confirming that the spleen is the source of haemorrhage. This fact can be achieved by direct inspection or careful palpation; over-zealous handling at this stage can convert a reparable and minor injury into an irrecoverable pulp. Splenic conservation should be the aim, especially in the young, but if the spleen is shattered or bleeding profusely it should be removed at once to prevent exsanguination.

The spleen is drawn medially, and the left leaf of the lienorenal ligament is divided either with scissors (*Fig.* 15.3*a*) or with the fingers. Further careful traction will mobilize the spleen into the wound. The

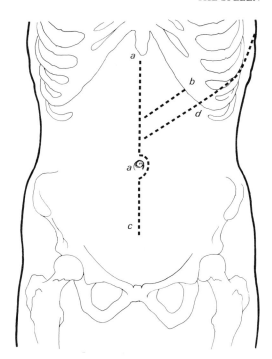

Fig. 15.2. Incisions used for splenectomy. The standard incision *a–a* can be extended as a T-piece (*b*) if access is difficult or be lengthened to *c* if other pathology is discovered. For large spleens a thoraco-abdominal incision (*d*) may be helpful.

vascular pedicle can then be compressed between finger and thumb to control the bleeding, while the extent of the injury is assessed. If repair is feasible it should now be undertaken (*see below*).

If total splenectomy is unavoidable the short gastric vessels should be tied and divided, care being taken not to damage the stomach wall (*Fig.* 15.3*b*). The splenic artery and vein are then identified between the pancreas and the spleen. These vessels should be doubly clamped and ligated without injuring the tail of the pancreas (*Fig.* 15.3*c*). Ideally the splenic artery and vein should be ligated individually in that order. If necessary it is permissible to clamp and tie the vascular pedicle *en masse*. The spleen can then be removed by dividing any remaining peritoneal attachments.

A thorough laparotomy should now be performed to exclude other associated injuries, before the abdomen is closed in the routine fashion. A drain should be left in the splenic bed.

Alternatives to Emergency Splenectomy

The role of a conservative (non-operative) approach has already been discussed, but even if a laparotomy is performed it is not always necessary to render the patient asplenic. If at laparotomy the peritoneal blood is completely removed it is often found that the haemorrhage has ceased. Particularly in young children it is important to conserve splenic function.

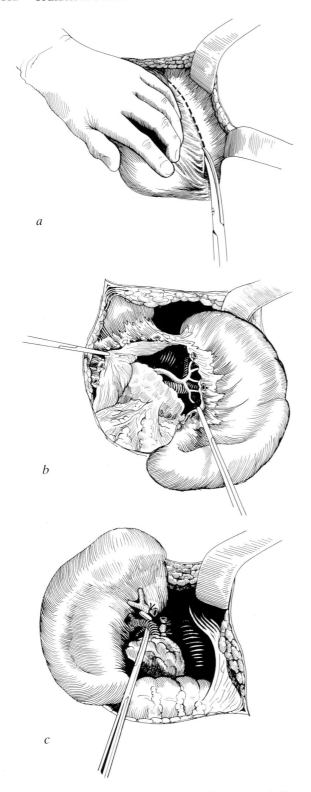

Fig. 15.3. Splenectomy. *a*, The spleen is displaced medially, and the lienorenal ligament is divided with scissors, allowing the spleen to be mobilized. *b*, The vasa brevia are divided between clamps. *c*, With the spleen pulled forward, the splenic artery and vein are identified and doubly ligated before division. The spleen can then be removed.

The following techniques are of proven value; many of them require splenic mobilization.

1. *Topical Applications*

Digital pressure combined with gelatin sponge, thrombin or microfibrillar collagen will usually suffice for simple lacerations. This approach is particularly applicable to iatrogenic injury during surgery. Packing off the spleen until the operation is completed will usually ensure that haemostasis has been secured.

2. *Splenorraphy*

Although the spleen has only a thin capsule, it is possible to suture it after all devitalized tissue has been removed (*Fig.* 15.4*a*); Teflon buttresses may help to prevent the sutures cutting through. The incorporation of omentum (*Fig.* 15.4*b*), cyano-acrylate adhesive or microfibrillar collagen into the mattress sutures will increase the haemostatic effect.

3. *Arterial Ligation*

Ligation of the main splenic artery does not lead to splenic infarction, since there is adequate inflow from the short gastric vessels. Arterial flow can be greatly reduced by ligating the splenic artery at the upper border of the pancreas. Topical applications or splenorrhaphy may then prevent residual haemorrhage. Although arterial ligation preserves the spleen, it does impair its function. Nevertheless the response to pneumococcal vaccination is much greater than in asplenic individuals.

4. *Partial Splenectomy* (*Fig.* 15.4*c*)

If one pole of the spleen is largely pulped and the other preserved, partial splenectomy may be appropriate. Most individuals have two primary lobar (intrasplenic) branches; the relevant vessel can thus be ligated before that portion of spleen is removed by a finger fracture technique. The cut surface of the organ is then secured with through-and-through sutures.

5. *Auto-transplantation*

If splenectomy is inevitable, some functional activity may be preserved by implanting a portion of splenic tissue. Experimental work suggests that 30 g of spleen should be inserted into a subperitoneal pouch under the diaphragm. This explant will develop a blood supply and the ability to respond to vaccination, but its capacity for pneumococcal clearance is very limited.

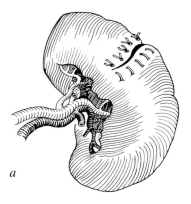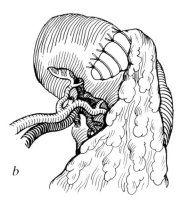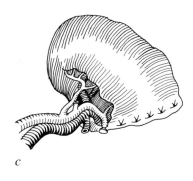

Fig. 15.4. Techniques of splenic conservation. *a*, Simple mattress suture of the splenic capsule. *b*, Incorporation of omentum beneath the interrupted mattress sutures. *c*, Partial splenectomy following ligation of the lower polar artery. The capsule is approximated with sutures.

ELECTIVE SPLENECTOMY

Technique

The operation is usually performed through an upper midline incision. In patients with a very large and adherent spleen a left thoraco-abdominal approach can sometimes be safer. On entering the abdomen the surgeon should perform a thorough laparotomy and make a careful search for splenunculi; these must also be removed if splenectomy is being undertaken for a blood dyscrasia.

If the spleen is very large or has many diaphragmatic adhesions, it is prudent to ligate the splenic artery at an early stage in the operation. After entry into the lesser sac and division of any adhesions, the artery is identified at the upper border of the pancreas and ligated with strong silk (*Fig.* 15.5).

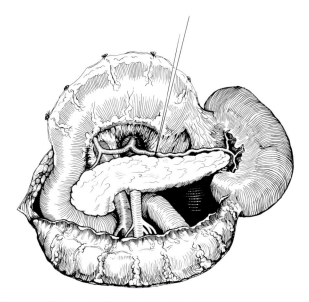

Fig. 15.5. If access is difficult or the spleen is very large, the splenic artery can be tied at the upper border of the pancreas to reduce haemorrhage.

The spleen is drawn away from the diaphragm and any adhesions are diathermied. Strong retraction of the wound edge will assist exposure. The left leaf of the lienorenal ligament is divided, and the spleen can now be gently mobilized with the fingers. The lienocolic attachments should also be divided at this stage. The splenic bed is then packed off, and the vasa brevia are divided to free the spleen from the stomach.

The main vascular pedicle is explored to identify the individual vessels, which should be doubly ligated and tied. The spleen can now be removed. Good haemostasis is important to prevent subphrenic haematoma and abscess formation, and a drain is placed in the splenic bed.

Alternatives to Elective Splenectomy

1. *Staging Laparotomy*

This is an invasive procedure with an appreciable complication rate: 30 per cent minor, 4 per cent major. It should be reserved for patients in whom local radiotherapy is likely to be the sole treatment as long as there is no abdominal dissemination. If a staging operation is required, partial splenectomy will avoid the risk of post-splenectomy sepsis; this risk approaches 10 per cent in children. Alternatively, patients (especially the young) should receive prophylactic penicillin after total splenectomy.

2. *Tropical Splenomegaly*

Splenectomy is performed to improve the cytopenia and reduce the risk of rupture, but it will also diminish the body's immune response to the parasite. In patients with malaria long-term chemotherapy may lead to a reduction in splenic size without the need for surgery. Alternatively segmental splenectomy (leaving 20–30 per cent) has been described, but whether regrowth will occur with time is unknown.

3. Hypersplenism

The prime indication for operation lies with proliferative disorders such as leukaemia, and here chemotherapy is the treatment of choice in the first instance. If splenectomy becomes unavoidable, however, the risk of postoperative sepsis is increased by the drug-induced immune deficiency.

Partial splenectomy has been achieved by arterial embolization under antibiotic cover, thus avoiding laparotomy. The treatment can be successful providing the operator aims for no more than a 35 per cent infarction at each attempt. The mortality rate is high but similar to that of laparotomy. Segmental splenectomy is clearly feasible, but the critical mass to retain is unknown. Portal decompression can be achieved by several techniques and should not involve splenectomy.

4. Splenic Cysts

If these are echinococcal (hydatid), splenectomy remains the treatment of choice. For other cysts an attempt should be made to preserve the spleen. Simple external drainage appears to be effective, but marsupialization into the peritoneal cavity may prove superior in the long term.

POSTOPERATIVE COMPLICATIONS

Haemorrhage

Severe bleeding from the splenic vessels should be prevented by doubly ligating them during splenectomy. Minor oozing from the splenic bed or diaphragmatic adhesions can be a problem, but this should be dealt with before the abdomen is closed. Otherwise development of a haematoma will predispose to subphrenic abscess.

Atelectasis

Minor degrees of collapse of the left lower lobe of the lung may be accompanied by a small effusion and chest infection. If fractured ribs exacerbate the problem, physiotherapy with or without intercostal nerve blocks should be considered to improve respiratory excursion.

Venous Thrombo-embolism

The risk of generalized venous thrombo-embolism secondary to the thrombocytosis is unknown, but it is probably small. Although anticoagulation is usually unnecessary, the administration of anti-platelet agents (e.g. asprin or dipyridamole) is probably a sensible precaution if the platelet count exceeds $800 \times 10^9/l$.

Ischaemic Heart Disease

The increase in whole blood viscosity and decrease in red cell deformability following splenectomy result in a two-fold increase in late deaths from ischaemic heart disease.

Other Risks

Damage to the gastric wall or pancreatic tail may lead to fistula formation; spontaneous closure will often ensue with conservative treatment. Postoperative nasogastric suction for 24 hours is a sensible precaution, but the risk of acute gastric dilatation is small.

Post-splenectomy Sepsis

This syndrome results from loss of the spleen's ability to promote phagocytosis of encapsulated bacteria; about 50 per cent of cases are due to infection with *Streptococcus pneumoniae*. Onset is insidious. The features are those of overwhelming infection, including rigors, abdominal pain, shock and disseminated intravascular coagulation. Overall only about 4 per cent of patients develop this complication after splenectomy, but the mortality rate is between 50 and 75 per cent. The risk of developing post-splenectomy sepsis is greatest in young children and is maximal within 2 years of the operation. Fortunately the risk is small following splenectomy for trauma (1–2 per cent), but it is substantial following resection for thalassaemia or acquired haemolytic anaemias (25 per cent).

Prophylaxis against post-splenectomy sepsis should be routinely considered. Antibiotics are effective, but they should probably be taken routinely for at least 3 years; patient compliance is a major problem. Immunization is likely to be better, although the response to vaccines is reduced after splenectomy and they do not cover all possible organisms. However, vaccines are available against 23 types of pneumococci as well as against *Haemophilus influenzae* and *Neisseria meningitidis*. They are ineffective in children under 2 years of age and of reduced value in those under 7 years. If splenectomy is a planned procedure, vaccination should be performed 1–2 months before operation.

FURTHER READING

Cooper M. J. and Williamson R. C. N. (1984) Splenectomy: indications, hazards and alternatives. *Br. J. Surg.* **71**, 173–180.

Dixon J. A., Miller F., McCluskey D. et al. (1980) Anatomy and techniques in segmental splenectomy. *Surg. Gynecol. Obstet.* **150,** 516–520.

Geary C. G., Clough V. and McIver J. E. (1980) Tropical splenomegaly. *Br. J. Hosp. Med.* **24,** 417–421.

Oakes D. D. and Charters A. C. (1981) Changing concepts in the management of splenic trauma. *Surg. Gynecol. Obstet.* **153,** 181–185.

Singer D. B. (1973) Postsplenectomy sepsis. In: Rosenberg H. S. (ed.) *Perspectives in Paediatric Pathology, Vol. 1.* 285–311. Chicago, Year Book Medical.

Chapter sixteen

The Liver

M. J. Cooper and R. C. N. Williamson

ANATOMY AND PHYSIOLOGY

Structure

The liver is the largest single organ in the body and weighs about 1500 g in the adult. It occupies the right hypochondrium and extends across to the midclavicular line on the left. It reaches up to the lower border of the right 5th rib and normally enjoys complete protection by the rib cage, although it may be palpable even in health.

Most of the liver surface is covered in peritoneum, but there is a large 'bare area' posteriorly lying in direct contact with the diaphragmatic muscle. The peritoneal reflections coalesce to form the suspensory ligaments of the liver. The coronary ligaments run across the diaphragm and surround the bare area, being known as the left triangular ligament at the extreme left. The falciform ligament hangs down from the umbilicus and contains the obliterated umbilical vein.

The liver is a segmented structure, each segment having its own vascular supply and biliary drainage. The organ can be divided into two lobes by a line joining the left margin of the gallbladder bed to the inferior vena cava (*Fig.* 16.1). Each lobe can be further divided into four segments, although the most useful subdivision is the splitting of the left lobe into medial and lateral segments by the umbilical fissure (*Fig.* 16.1). The traditionally named quadrate and

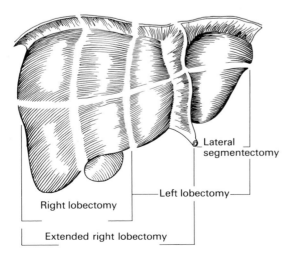

Fig. 16.1. Anatomical segments of the liver in relation to partial hepatectomy.

caudate lobes lie in the medial portion of the left lobe.

The liver has one blood supply from the hepatic artery and another from the portal vein. Most of the inflow (75 per cent) comes from the portal vein, but each vessel contributes 50 per cent of the oxygen supply. Just below the hilus of the liver each vessel divides into two lobar branches, which are segmentally distributed with little collateral association between segments. The junction of the hepatic ducts is at a higher level than the vessels. On the right the extrahepatic course of the blood vessels is very short, but on the left they run outside the liver to enter the umbilical fissure; the left medial segment is thus supplied by 'feedback' vessels. The hepatic veins have a very short extrahepatic course. They are three in number, but the middle hepatic vein frequently joins the left hepatic vein rather than draining directly into the vena cava. There are also three pairs of smaller veins which drain directly into the vena cava. The hepatic veins do not follow the same pathways as the portal triads but course almost at right angles to them.

There are many anomalies of vascular supply to the liver, which usually relate to the hepatic artery. In about 25 per cent of the population much or even all of the arterial blood comes from the superior mesenteric artery. Knowledge of such anomalies is important when undertaking hepatic resection.

Histologically the liver comprises reticulo-endothelial elements (Kupffer cells) and hepatocytes, which are endowed with a rich blood supply and are drained by the biliary system.

Functions

The functions of the liver are many, complex and incompletely understood. Sixty-five per cent of the body's reticulo-endothelial system is contained within the liver. This tissue is responsible for filtering and destroying bacteria absorbed from the gut and removing debris resulting from cellular breakdown. The liver detoxifies a great variety of endogenous and exogenous substances, including most drugs.

Hepatocytes play the dominant role in metabolism and storage of basic foodstuffs. Carbohydrates are stored as glycogen and released when necessary. Fats are metabolized, cholesterol is synthesized. The liver is the only source of albumin and alpha-globulin. It is a major storage site for vitamins, particularly those that are fat soluble (A, D, K); it also synthesizes many of the clotting factors.

A fundamental function of the liver is the formation and excretion of bile. About half the bile flow is dependent on the secretion of bile acids, which are manufactured in the liver and are reabsorbed (all but 3 per cent) in the terminal ileum; the remaining half derives from ductal secretion. Bile is the major excretory pathway for bilirubin, cholesterol, drugs and lipid-soluble metabolites. The formation of micelles in the gut aids the absorption of dietary lipids and also solubilizes water-insoluble compounds.

The most obvious sign of liver failure is jaundice, which reflects the accumulation of bilirubin in the tissues. Not all causes of jaundice are amenable to surgical treatment, and intensive investigation is required to determine the exact nature of the disease. Indeed, inadvertent laparotomy for some diseases (e.g. hepatitis) may be a danger to both the patient and the surgeon.

Resection of major portions of the liver is made possible by the ability of the organ to regenerate. Compensatory liver growth may be controlled in part by hormones delivered via the portal vein. Following resection both hypertrophy and hyperplasia occur until the liver is restored to near-normal size.

PERIOPERATIVE MANAGEMENT OF LIVER DISEASE

Investigation

Biochemical
Serial measurements of bilirubin, alkaline phosphatase and transaminase levels in the serum should indicate the extent and nature of the jaundice, including the presence of extrahepatic obstruction and concomitant damage to hepatocytes. Serum albumin is a good guide to the synthetic capacity of the liver and the nutritional state of the patient. Since the liver produces many of the clotting factors, the prothrombin time should be assessed; hypoprothrombinaemia often responds to administration of parenteral vitamin K. Produced by over 70 per cent of hepatomas, alpha-1-fetoprotein is a valuable tumour marker, although the test is not specific and there are many false negatives. Raised serum levels should return to normal after resection of hepatoma and may subsequently indicate recurrence. The measurement of serum bile acids and various dye excretion tests are not universally available but may help to determine hepatic reserve.

Ultrasound
This is undoubtedly the most useful screening test, being non-invasive, inexpensive and repeatable. Sensitivity is reduced by obesity, excess bowel gas or a high subcostal situation of the liver. Ultrasonography is most commonly employed to search for a dilated ductal system but can also detect cysts, abscesses and tumours; differentiation between primary and secondary neoplasms may not be possible. Resolution down to 15 mm is possible. Scans permit guided fine-needle aspiration for cytology.

Computed Tomography
This may be a useful adjunct to ultrasonography. It has a better resolution (10 mm) and can show malignant invasion of surrounding structures. However, it is less widely available and is more expensive.

Radionuclide Scanning
This technique has a poor resolution and can only report the presence of a 'filling defect', not its nature. It has been largely superseded. Postoperatively the excretion of Tc-HIDA may be used to determine the patency or otherwise of biliary-enteric anastomoses.

Cholangiography
Intravenous cholangiography is only feasible in the absence of jaundice and produces a poor-quality image. Introduction of the Chiba ('skinny') needle has made percutaneous transhepatic cholangiography (PTC) a safe procedure, although success is limited in the absence of dilated intrahepatic ducts. PTC is of particular value in determining the exact level as well as the nature of an obstructing lesion. Endoscopic retrograde cholangiopancreatography (ERCP) can similarly delineate the obstruction, but the failure rate is greater except in highly skilled hands.

Arteriography
Selective coeliac and superior mesenteric angiograms are a prerequisite for safe elective hepatic surgery. The examination has a high resolution (4 mm). Its most important function is to provide a road map for the surgeon by delineating the vascular supply, including anomalies. Late-phase angiography will demonstrate the portal vein. Thus neoplastic involvement of arterial and venous structures can be determined. More direct information on venous anatomy may be obtained by splenoportography, transjugular venography and venacavography but is rarely required.

Laparoscopy
This permits direct visualization of the liver and enables accurate biopsies to be taken of both involved and normal liver tissue. It avoids the potential problems inherent in percutaneous biopsy of hydatid cysts and haemangiomas.

Percutaneous Liver Biopsy

This is an invasive procedure with a risk of haemorrhage, sepsis and bile peritonitis; however, with care it is safe and carries a mortality rate of <0·02 per cent. It is most valuable in the diagnosis of diffuse liver disease, though accuracy is enhanced when insertion of the needle is guided by ultrasound or laparoscopy.

Preoperative Precautions

Certain measures are applicable to any patient with obstructive jaundice undergoing major surgery. Assessment of nutritional and clotting status should be made and corrected if possible. Vitamin K may reverse a clotting abnormality, but the serum albumin is unlikely to respond to parenteral nutrition if the liver is obstructed or diseased. Prophylactic antibiotics are essential, as sepsis is a major cause of death; they are also required for invasive diagnostic procedures such a PTC and ERCP. Percutaneous decompression of obstructive jaundice may improve liver function and postoperative recovery. This technique is most applicable to patients with hilar lesions, but at present the risk of cholangitis precludes it from general use.

Preoperative Precautions

Patients undergoing surgery for obstructive jaundice are prone to develop acute renal failure (the hepatorenal syndrome). This complication can be avoided by adequate preoperative hydration, the avoidance of hypotension and the use of mannitol to promote an osmotic diuresis. Introduction of bile salts into the lumen of the gut is also claimed to decrease the risk of hepatorenal syndrome, possibly by reducing endotoxin formation by intestinal bacteria. All patients should be rehydrated and catheterized before operation, so that the renal output can be increased and monitored. Great care must be taken with haemostasis, and the wound should be closed carefully as healing is impaired.

Postoperative Care

Jaundice may deepen after any major operation, because of further damage to the liver from surgical and anaesthetic trauma. Even when the serum bilirubin is normal at the outset, some degree of jaundice is almost inevitable after major resection but is usually mild and self-limiting. Even when severe, jaundice is often the result of hypotensive damage and should not be taken as an indication for further operation without proof of biliary obstruction. Clotting function may be severely deranged, requiring correction with vitamin K or fresh frozen plasma. Blood sugar levels must be monitored for the first 48 hours, since loss of glycogen stores can lead to hypoglycaemia. Nutritional status may be severely impaired, and the serum albumin requires careful monitoring; parenteral nutrition may be indicated after the biliary obstruction has been relieved.

CONGENITAL CONDITIONS OF THE LIVER

Biliary Atresia

The commonest cause of prolonged neonatal jaundice is extrahepatic biliary atresia. Uncorrected, this condition will lead to liver failure and death, with only a few infants surviving beyond 6 months. Between 10 and 20 per cent of patients have a short length of extrahepatic bile duct permitting a conventional mucosa-to-mucosa anastomosis. For the majority, however, a hepatic porto-enterostomy (Kasai operation) should be attempted. The operation should be undertaken within 60 days of birth; otherwise intrahepatic fibrosis will rapidly ensue and reduce the chance of cure. Even when undertaken early the operation is complicated by the development of cholangitis, cirrhosis and portal hypertension; long-term survivors are few. Recent interest has focused on the use of liver transplantation in this condition, particularly as this is not precluded by a previous Kasai procedure.

Congenital Cystic Disease

Cysts may be solitary or multiple. Multiple cysts are frequently associated with polycystic disease of the kidney. The cysts are often small and asymptomatic, being found incidentally at laparotomy or autopsy. If large they may cause pressure symptoms and require surgical treatment. Small cysts usually require no treatment, but they can be aspirated and often do not recur. Larger cysts may become infected or present as a result of bleeding or rupture. They can be aspirated and treated according to the contents. Cysts filled with clear serous fluid can be treated by deroofing into the peritoneal cavity. Bile would indicate the need for enteric drainage into a Roux loop. Rarely the cyst may have destroyed the whole lobe and a partial hepatectomy may be indicated.

Caroli's disease is congenital cystic dilatation of the intrahepatic ducts. It usually presents with recurrent upper abdominal pain and later cholangitis. The disease is often diffuse, in which case there is no specific therapy apart from antibiotics. Occasionally it is confined to one segment or liver lobe, and in these cases resection may be curative. Adequate surgical drainage of the cyst cavity has given excellent results.

Inborn Errors of Metabolism

Several inborn errors of hepatic metabolism are at present untreatable and lead to death at an early age. It has become apparent with increasing experience of liver transplantation in children that some of these problems are curable. Long-term follow-up is very limited, but transplants have been performed for Wilson's disease, alpha-1-antitrypsin deficiency, tyrosinaemia and Niemann–Pick disease. This group of indications for transplantation will undoubtedly increase.

HEPATIC TRAUMA

In the UK liver injury is usually the result of a road traffic accident and is frequently accompanied by other serious skeletal, thoracic or abdominal injuries. Penetrating trauma due to knives or bullets is uncommon. Stab wounds leave an obvious track and usually stop bleeding spontaneously. Low-velocity bullet wounds need only the removal of the foreign body and adjacent devitalized tissue, but parenchymal shattering after a high-velocity injury is often best treated by formal hepatic resection.

The primary treatment must be to resuscitate the patient and then fully to assess the injuries. Penetrating wounds should as a rule be explored, with débridement and control of the haemorrhage; tetanus toxoid should be administered, together with prophylactic antibiotics. The diagnosis of hepatic injury after blunt trauma is largely clinical. The commonest sign is abdominal tenderness, often progressing to guarding and rigidity; 25 per cent of patients have no specific abdominal signs or symptoms. Radiographs will show any associated chest or abdominal injuries. Abdominal paracentesis and lavage are reliable techniques for detecting intra-abdominal haemorrhage and are of particular value if the clinical signs are equivocal or the patient is unconscious. If operation is not performed soon after admission, then ultrasound scanning is useful to determine hepatic injury and the presence of a subcapsular haematoma. Laparotomy is indicated for continuing or major blood loss, as manifest by serial measurement of vital signs. Detailed management is considered later (p. 192).

Complications after treatment for hepatic trauma are common, affecting 56 per cent of patients with blunt trauma and 35 per cent of those with stab wounds. Sepsis is the major problem, notably within the chest. Biliary fistulas do occur but usually close spontaneously. The mortality rate is directly related to the number of organs injured. If the liver is the only injured organ it should only be 6 per cent, but if four organs are injured it will exceed 50 per cent; overall it will be between 10 and 20 per cent.

INFECTIONS OF THE LIVER

Amoebiasis

Infection results from the ingestion of *Entamoeba histolytica* in contaminated material, usually drinking water. Once established in the gut the parasites travel via the portal vein to the liver, most commonly the right lobe. As many as 70 per cent of patients may give no antecedent history of intestinal disease. Presenting symptoms are upper abdominal pain, fever and anorexia, with diarrhoea in only 30 per cent of cases. On examination the liver is enlarged and tender. The majority of patients are anaemic, but the liver function tests may be entirely normal. Stools should be examined for amoebas and the amoebic complement fixation test should be performed. Liver scans will demonstrate a cystic cavity.

Treatment is by metronidazole, which may be combined with percutaneous needle aspiration. Resolution is slow and should be followed by serial ultrasonography. Complete disappearance of the cavity may take up to 80 days. Surgical treatment is required for less than 10 per cent of patients and is prompted by failure of medical treatment or secondary bacterial infection; it consists of external drainage. The most dangerous complication is rupture into the pleural or peritoneal cavities; this occurs in 25 per cent of cases and has a mortality rate of 10–40 per cent.

Hydatid Cyst

This disease is endemic in many parts of the world but with the increase in world travel may present anywhere. Infection is usually with *Echinococcus granulosus*. The dog is the usual primary host, with humans being infected via dog faeces and acting as the intermediate host. Once ingested the eggs hatch and larvae burrow through the gut wall into the bloodstream. Seventy per cent of the larvas lodge in the liver, where they either die or develop into cysts. About 75 per cent of cysts are solitary and located in the right lobe.

Presentation may be delayed for months or years and is often incidental; symptoms are related to the size of the lesion. Occasionally a cyst will rupture, giving rise to abdominal pain and collapse. The cyst can be detected on plain radiographs but is best evaluated by scans; serological tests are now reliable.

Treatment is by surgical excision of the cyst. Great care must be taken not to spill daughter cysts into the peritoneum, as they are capable of growth at this site. The cyst is first aspirated and then injected with hypertonic saline to kill the scolices. The cyst wall can then be enucleated from the liver. An alternative technique is to use a metal cone which can be frozen onto the cyst wall before it is opened. Recent reports suggest that mebendazole may be used to treat patients medically. The major complication is rupture, which may be into the peritoneum, biliary system or pleural cavity.

Pyogenic Abscess

This is an uncommon disease which generally affects

the elderly and has a high mortality (at least 35 per cent). Most cases are secondary to biliary tract diseases, other causes being systemic septicaemia, trauma and pylephlebitis; some cases are cryptogenic. The commonest isolate is of mixed bowel flora. Common solitary organisms are *Escherichia coli*, *Staphylococcus aureus* and various anaerobes.

Presentation is often insidious. The features of the precipitating cause may mask the abscess. The patients are ill with fever, rigors, anorexia and general debility; pain will be right hypochondrial but may radiate to the shouldertip. The liver may be enlarged and tender. Blood tests are non-specific, and diagnosis is best made by ultrasound or CT scan.

Treatment involves broad-spectrum antibiotics and drainage. Often a catheter can be inserted percutaneously and guided by ultrasound, but if this technique fails open surgical drainage is mandatory.

NEOPLASMS OF THE LIVER

Benign

These are uncommon and often present incidentally or by mimicking biliary disease. The usual types are haemangioma, adenoma and focal nodular hyperplasia. The latter two forms are associated with oral contraceptive use and may regress when this drug is withdrawn. Up to 20 per cent of all these lesions present with intraperitoneal rupture and haemorrhage, which have an appreciable mortality rate. The treatment is surgical excision, which can be performed by wedge resection in most instances.

Hepatocellular Carcinoma

This tumour is uncommon in the UK, with fewer than 2 cases per 100 000 of the population per annum. Many causative agents have been identified, but chronic liver disease and hepatitis B virus infection seem to be the most important. In parts of the world where these are common, hepatoma may be the commonest intra-abdominal malignancy. Thus among the black population in Southern Africa there are up to 30 cases per 100 000 per annum. The presenting features are often vague, especially if they are superimposed on ill health from chronic liver disease. Most patients complain of malaise, weight loss, abdominal discomfort, unexplained fever or jaundice. The liver may be enlarged and tender, often containing a palpable mass.

Liver function tests may be disordered but are non-specific. Over 70 per cent of patients will have increased levels of alpha-1-fetoprotein. The tumour should be revealed by liver scanning, CT probably being the most helpful. Preoperative biopsy is best performed under direct laparoscopic vision as there is a risk of haemorrhage. Angiography is then important to assess arterial anomalies and resectability.

Ideally the treatment would be surgical resection, but this is only feasible for 10–20 per cent of patients and offers a mean survival rate of around 6 months. The palliative treatment of hepatic neoplasms is described below. There are few series of resections reported, but the 5-year survival rate is anticipated to be between 30 and 50 per cent. A more radical approach to irresectable tumour without extrahepatic spread is liver transplantation. This might be feasible for younger patients and should have a 30 per cent 1-year survival. Death resulting from tumour in the transplanted liver is common.

Cholangiocarcinoma

The treatment of extrahepatic cholangiocarcinoma is not within the bounds of this chapter, but about 30 per cent of these tumours arise at the hepatic duct bifurcation (Klatskin tumour) and are often intrahepatic. Presentation is almost invariably with obstructive jaundice. The systematic combination of ultrasonography, PTC and ERCP should demonstrate the lesion in virtually every case. Differentiation between cholangiocarcinoma and sclerosing cholangitis may be difficult, and fine-needle aspiration biopsy can be helpful. Arteriography, including venous phase studies, is important to determine vascular invasion and hence assess resectability.

Tumour resection should be the treatment of choice, but this is a major procedure that often involves either a hepatic split or partial hepatic resection. It is feasible in 20 per cent of patients at the most and has an operative mortality of 15–20 per cent. Figures are not available for 5-year survival, but at least resection is good palliation. Other palliative options, including insertion of an endoprosthesis, surgical intubation or biliary-enteric bypass, are described later.

Metastatic Cancer

This is by far the commonest liver tumour in the Western world. It is usually asymptomatic, but when advanced it results in hepatic pain, ascites, jaundice and a palpable mass; other features are those of generalized malignancy such as anorexia and weight loss. Serial assays of carcino-embryonic antigen (CEA) after colonic resection may enable detection of small metastases before symptoms develop. The poor prognosis of untreated metastatic disease is evident from mean survival rates of less than 3 months and a 1-year survival rate of less than 7 per cent.

The palliative options described later might be expected to prolong life. Perhaps 10 per cent of patients with hepatic metastases may be suitable for potentially curative resection, there being either a solitary metastasis or multiple deposits in a single segment. Though sparse, published data include an operative mortality rate of about 5 per cent and a 5-year survival rate of 20 per cent.

OTHER INDICATIONS FOR LIVER SURGERY

Cirrhosis

The management of ascites and portal hypertension is considered in Chapter 45. Those patients who are likely to die from liver failure are potential candidates for liver transplantation. In practice, patients with cryptogenic and alcoholic cirrhosis or chronic active hepatitis do badly following this procedure. Patients with primary or secondary biliary cirrhosis represent a better risk, since their liver function is more stable and the timing of transplantation can be better determined.

Sclerosing Cholangitis

This is a non-specific inflammatory condition which leads to multiple stricture formation and ultimately hepatic failure. It is often associated with inflammatory bowel disease. Concomitant gallstones are common, and the condition is easily confused with cholangiocarcinoma even on cholangiography. Operation is indicated to bypass distal obstruction, and for these patients the prognosis is good. If the disease is diffuse and intrahepatic, stenting is all that can usually be offered; hepatic transplantation has been employed in a few cases with good results.

Intrahepatic Stones

Although uncommon in the UK (0·5 per cent) intrahepatic stones are found in up to 15 per cent of biliary tract operations in the Orient. If they are associated with multiple extrahepatic stones they can be removed from below in the usual manner. However, they may be found in congenital intrahepatic cysts, or be impacted above ductal strictures, some of which are malignant. In such cases the cyst or proximal bile ducts must be decompressed into a Roux loop of jejunum unless the stones are peripherally placed, in which case partial hepatectomy is more appropriate.

Peliosis Hepatis

In this rare condition the liver contains blood-filled lacunar spaces, which appear as blue-black dots on the surface. Rupture with haemorrhage can be fatal.

Haemobilia

Haemorrhage into the biliary tract should be suspected whenever upper gastrointestinal bleeding is associated with jaundice or right hypochondrial signs and commoner lesions have been excluded. It may result from trauma, gallstones, hepatic tumours or hepatic artery aneurysms. Treatment is by exploration and drainage of the affected bile duct.

TECHNIQUES OF LIVER SURGERY

Access (*Fig.* 16.2)

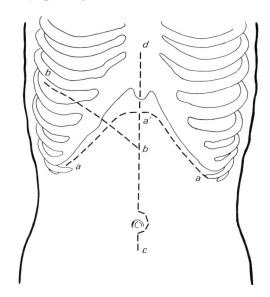

Fig. 16.2. Incisions available for hepatic surgery.

The incision depends on the indication for operation and the site of the lesion. Most elective operations can be managed through a high subcostal incision (*a–a′–a*), which can be extended to right or left depending on the lobe which is to be excised. A thoracic extension (*b–b*) may be necessary for lesions which are very large or lie posteriorly, when early access to the hepatic vein is required.

Laparotomy for blunt abdominal trauma is usually carried out through a midline incision (*a′–c*). Although this incision permits access to other intra-abdominal injuries, it is often inadequate for dealing with hepatic trauma. Early control of the hepatic vein(s) may be required and this can only be accomplished by extending the incision into the right chest. Thoracotomy can be rapidly performed by splitting the lower sternum (*a′–d*) and dividing the diaphragm without disturbing either pleural cavity. An alternative is a formal right thoracotomy through the bed of the 7th rib (*b–b*).

Percutaneous Biopsy

Before percutaneous biopsy all patients should be screened for hepatitis B infection, the clotting function should be normal and the blood group known. The usual puncture site is in the midaxillary line in the 8th, 9th or 10th intercostal space; if the liver is appreciably enlarged, a subcostal approach may be employed. The patient lies supine, and the site is infiltrated with local anaesthetic. The biopsy needle is then inserted transpleurally with the patient holding his or her breath in expiration. Many biopsy needles are available, but the Tru-cut needle is probably most popular.

Operative Biopsy

Open liver biopsy is a common diagnostic procedure whenever the liver appears to be abnormal at laparotomy, or a staging operation is undertaken for Hodgkin's disease or other lymphoma. Small samples can be obtained from deep in each lobe by using Tru-cut needles. Digital pressure is applied to the puncture site until any bleeding has stopped. Larger biopsies are obtained by wedge resection of the liver edge (*Fig.* 16.3); either lobe is suitable.

The liver edge to be biopsied is displayed by retraction of the wound. Using a special liver stitch (0 chromic catgut on a curved blunt needle), two sutures are placed to delineate a small wedge of tissue. The sutures are tied snugly to reduce bleeding; excessive tightening of the knots will lead to the sutures cutting through. A V-shaped wedge of tissue is then excised. Any remaining bleeding is controlled either by diathermy or by inserting further sutures to approximate the margins of the V.

CONTROL OF TRAUMATIC HAEMORRHAGE

Over 50 per cent of liver injuries have stopped bleeding by the time of laparotomy, and all that is required is adequate drainage. Bleeding from minor capsular tears or stab wounds can often be arrested by pressure or, if this fails, by simple suture (*Fig.* 16.4); haemostatic agents may also be of value. Deeper lacerations should be explored to remove devitalized tissue; blood vessels are then clipped and tied. No attempt should be made to restore the liver outline with sutures, but omentum can be incorporated into the defect as a pack. These simple techniques are sufficient to deal with over 70 per cent of all liver injuries.

Heavy bleeding can often be controlled by effective packing with gauze rolls. This is not to be recommended as definitive therapy as the infection rate and hence the mortality rate are high. It may, however, suffice to allow the surgeon to gain control or permit the patient to be transferred to a specialist unit. If packing fails or bleeding recurs when the packs are removed, then the hepatic inflow may be occluded (Pringle manoeuvre, *Fig.* 16.5) by placing a soft vascular clamp on the free edge of the lesser omentum. The clamp will occlude both hepatic arterial and portal venous flow and can be maintained for up to 1 hour without untoward sequelae. Venous backbleeding may be a serious problem if the liver is extensively shattered but is usually controllable by pressure. Occasionally hepatic venous flow must be stopped, and this can only be accomplished through the chest. However, recalcitrant bleeding is usually arterial and can often be controlled by hepatic artery ligation. This procedure appears to be safe, but cholecystectomy is advisable if the right hepatic artery is ligated.

Occasionally injuries are very extensive and shatter the liver substance. If the injury is peripheral a resectional débridement is effective; no attempt is made to find the segmental plane. Extensive burst-type injuries are rare, but most commonly affect the right lobe. They require a major resection but rarely a formal lobectomy; again resectional débridement is the treatment of choice.

Injuries to the portal vein can be dealt with by direct suture or, if this is clearly not feasible, by ligation of both ends. Some authors recommend an immediate portocaval shunt if the portal vein is completely ligated, but this is not essential. There is a late incidence of portal vein thrombosis following suture repair. Injuries to the hepatic veins or vena cava are generally fatal. Ligation of the hepatic veins and suture repair of the vena cava should otherwise be attempted. Hepatic lobectomy may be required for access, and intracaval shunts have been described. These are all extreme procedures in a desperately ill patient and are rarely successful.

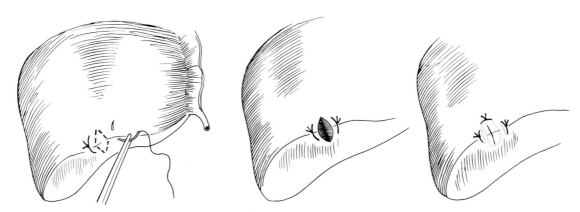

Fig. 16.3. Liver biopsy. After insertion of two catgut sutures a small wedge of liver tissue is removed and the cut edges are approximated.

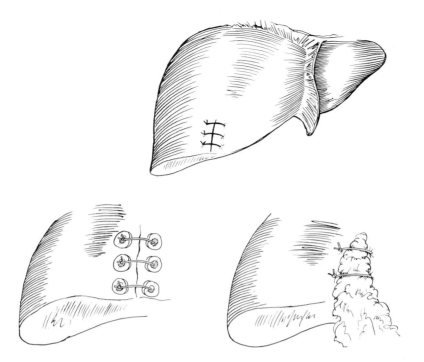

Fig. 16.4. Various techniques employed to control haemorrhage from a simple laceration of the liver.

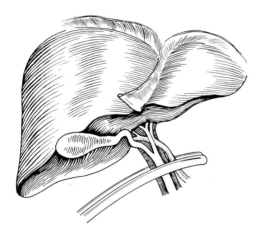

Fig. 16.5. Pringle's manoeuvre. A soft clamp is placed across the free edge of the lesser omentum to occlude vascular inflow to the liver.

PARTIAL HEPATECTOMY

Right Hepatic Lobectomy

Assessment of resectability should commence with full mobilization of the right lobe of the liver from the diaphragm; the falciform and coronary ligaments will need to be divided. The cystic duct and artery are identified and divided, since the gallbladder will be removed with the specimen. The right hepatic duct is then divided, and the common hepatic duct is mobilized and lifted medially to expose the vessels under-neath. The right hepatic artery and right branch of the portal vein are then ligated and divided in that order; the vein is best closed by a running polypropylene suture.

In addition to the main hepatic veins there are usually three pairs of smaller veins which need to be divided (*Fig. 16.6a*). The right lobe of the liver is mobilized upwards and to the left. The inferior vena cava is identified, and the dissection is carried upwards dividing the venous branches as they appear. Superiorly the right hepatic vein will be encountered; this is a short vessel, almost as large as the vena cava. At this stage the vein may be divided or clamped, formal division being delayed until the parenchyma has been divided.

Since inflow and outflow have now been occluded a clear line of demarcation should appear on the liver surface (*Fig. 16.6b*). Glisson's capsule is then divided 1 cm lateral to this median plane, and the parenchyma is divided by finger fracture (*Fig. 16.6c*); some authors recommend the use of a non-crushing clamp to reduce bleeding. As the dissection continues posteriorly the hepatic veins will be encountered and can be suture ligated if this has not already been performed. Bleeding from the raw surface must then be controlled by suture or diathermy; buttressed through-and-through sutures are very effective. Omentum or falciform ligament can be placed over the defect. Several large drains must be placed in the subphrenic space.

An alternative approach is that of *intraparenchy-*

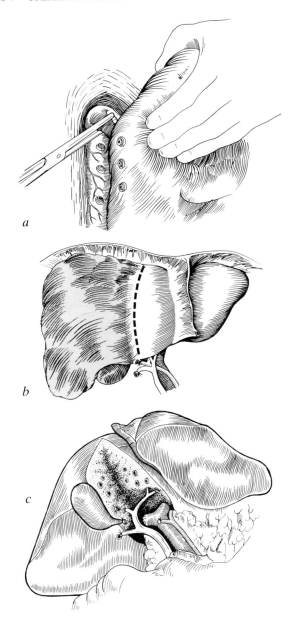

Fig. 16.6. Right hemihepatectomy. *a*, After mobilizing and displacing the liver to the right, three small hepatic veins have been divided between clips and a clamp placed on the right hepatic vein. *b*, The line of parenchymal transection. *c*, After controlling the vascular inflow and outflow to the right lobe, the liver structure is divided between the right and left lobes.

matous dissection. The structures in the porta hepatis are divided as before, but the veins are ligated as they are encountered within the liver substance. Since the median plane passes through the gallbladder bed, this organ must first be mobilized and removed. An incision is then made through Glisson's capsule with the diathermy, heading back from the medial edge of the gallbladder bed towards the vena cava. The liver tissue is then pinched between finger and thumb to divide the soft parenchyma. This tissue

will give way easily until a firm cord is felt. Blood vessels and bile ducts are felt as fibrous cords, which can be clamped, divided and ligated. The finger fracture is carried back until the right hepatic vein is identified, and divided from within the liver.

Extended Right Hepatic Lobectomy

The ability of the liver to regenerate facilitates massive resections of liver tissue. In extended right hepatic lobectomy or trisegmentectomy all the liver to the right of the falciform ligament is removed. Dissection commences as above. The line of incision of Glisson's capsule is then 1 cm to the right of the falciform ligament. The feedback vessels from the umbilical fissue and the median hepatic vein are dealt with by intraparenchymatous ligature to avoid damaging vessels to the left lateral segment. Closure is as previously described.

Left Hepatic Lobectomy

The hilar structures are exposed, and the left branches of artery, bile duct and portal vein are divided. The left triangular ligament is then divided down to the vena cava to expose the left hepatic vein, which is ligated and divided. A line of demarcation should be apparent and the liver tissue is divided 1 cm to the left of this line. The left lateral segment is resected together with the quadrate and caudate lobes.

Left Lateral Segmentectomy

The left lateral segment is fully mobilized, but no hilar dissection is required. The line of division is 1 cm to the left of the falciform ligament. The vascular and biliary structures are divided within the liver substance as they are encountered. The left hepatic vein is divided last; the median hepatic vein should be preserved (*Fig.* 16.7).

INTRAHEPATIC BILIARY-ENTERIC ANASTOMOSIS

Liver Split

Access to the hilar structures of the liver may be accomplished by extrahepatic dissection. However, to enable resection of many cholangiocarcinomas it is necessary to split the liver along the median plane to open the two halves and display the confluence of the ducts. This liver split or hepatotomy is particularly valuable for approaching the right hepatic duct which is completely intrahepatic.

The gallbladder is removed and Glisson's capsule is incised with the diathermy, heading back from the medial edge of the gallbladder bed towards the vena cava. A finger fracture technique is carried out over a distance of 8–10 cm. Careful dissection at the bot-

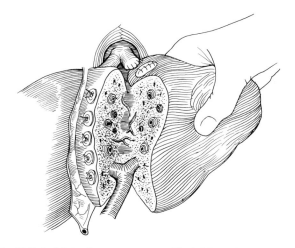

Fig. 16.7. Left lateral segmentectomy. The left branch of the portal vein is exposed in the base of the umbilical fissure. The left hepatic vein has been divided and oversewn.

tom of the liver split should now display the hilar structures completely (*Fig.* 16.8). The origin of the common hepatic duct lies anterior to the hepatic artery and portal vein.

Following resection of a hilar cholangiocarcinoma, reconstruction is achieved by anastomosis of the transected bile ducts to a Roux loop of jejunum. If the intrahepatic ducts are very dilated a mucosa-to-mucosa approximation is feasible. In some cases, however, the bowel will have to be sutured to Glisson's capsule, leaving several ducts on each side to weep into the open bowel. At least one transhepatic stent should be placed through each hepatic lobe and brought to the exterior to drain. If the tumour has extended out into the liver tissue then a central hepatic resection (usually of the quadrate lobe) can be performed prior to the anastomosis.

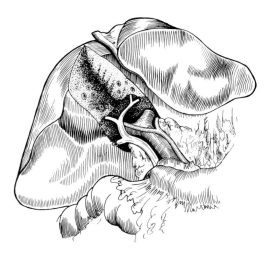

Fig. 16.8. Hepatotomy (liver split). After removal of the gallbladder the liver substance is divided to provide access to the porta hepatis, particularly the origin of the common hepatic duct.

Alternatives to Hilar Dissection

For some patients with obstructive jaundice from a primary or secondary carcinoma at the hilus of the liver, resection is clearly not feasible. These tumours may, however, be slow growing, and biliary decompression provides good palliation. The following are some of the accepted techniques; the choice depends on the site and extent of the tumour.

1. The tip of the right and/or left hepatic lobe is removed to expose a number of transected bile ducts (Longmire's procedure). The large ducts are splinted with small silicon stents, and a Roux loop is anastomosed to the capsule (*Fig.* 16.9*a*).
2. A large right-sided duct can sometimes be identified in the gallbladder bed. Cholecystectomy is performed, and a syringe and needle with intermittent aspiration are used to explore the gallbladder bed. When bile is aspirated the liver tissue is incised to reveal a large tributary of the right hepatic duct. Mucosa-to-mucosa suture is then possible (*Fig.* 16.9*b*).
3. A major duct on the left side can be found by opening the umbilical fissure (*Fig.* 16.9*c*) (segment III bypass). The round ligament is identified and followed down to the liver capsule. The thin bridge of liver tissue at its entry to the umbilical fissure is broken down. The left margin of the round ligament should then identify the duct, which at this point lies just beneath Glisson's capsule; any difficulty in identification can be resolved by needle aspiration. The left hepatic duct (or a major branch) can then be opened over a distance of at least 1 cm before anastomosis to a Roux loop; the liver capsule helps to strengthen this anastomosis. The operation may be termed left intrahepatic cholangiojejunostomy.
4. If 3 is not feasible then a wedge resection of the edge of the left lateral segment will reveal a large duct permitting direct anastomosis (*Fig.* 16.9*d*).

All these anastomoses should be stented by transhepatic tube(s) in the immediate postoperative period.

PALLIATION OF HEPATIC NEOPLASMS

Hepatic Dearterialization

Hepatic neoplasms obtain most of their blood supply from the hepatic artery. Ligation of this vessel will not lead to hepatic necrosis, but it may well shrink the tumour bulk. Although simple the procedure often fails unless a more widespread dissection is performed to ligate all the collateral vessels. Initial results appeared promising but there is no evidence that this procedure prolongs overall survival.

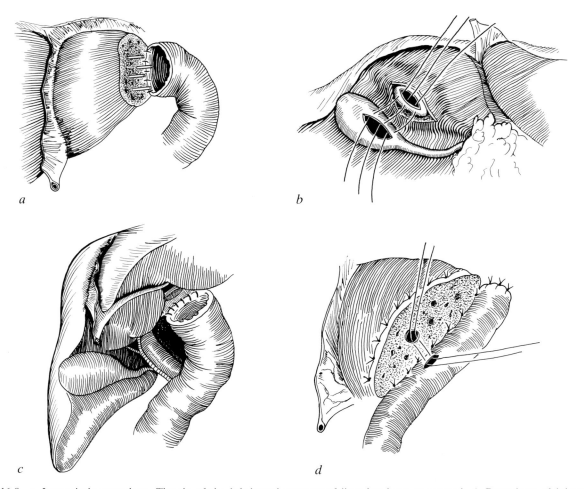

Fig. 16.9. *a*, Longmire's procedure. The tip of the left lateral segment of liver has been amputated. A Roux loop of jejunum is sutured to enclose the raw surface of liver and small tubes are inserted into the transected bile ducts. *b*, Smith's procedure. After mobilization of the gallbladder a dilated branch of the right hepatic duct is exposed in the gallbladder bed. Side-to-side anastomosis is fashioned to the gallbladder. *c*, Segment III bypass. The left hepatic duct is identified in the umbilical fissure and anastomosed to a Roux loop. *d*, A wedge of liver tissue has been removed from the lower edge of the left lateral segment to expose a dilated intrahepatic bile duct, which is anastomosed to a Roux loop of jejunum.

Cytotoxic Infusion

At laparotomy the junction of the hepatic and gastro-duodenal arteries is dissected out and the right gastric artery is ligated. The gastroduodenal artery is ligated distally and a catheter is inserted through a transverse arteriotomy and advanced into the common hepatic artery (*Fig.* 16.10). Each artery is ligated snugly around the catheter (e.g. no. 6 Fr. umbilical catheter or similar). A heparin–saline infusion should be commenced immediately to ensure catheter patency. Post-operatively an arteriogram can be obtained via the hepatic artery catheter to document the size of the lesions and to check that the catheter lies below the bifurcation. Cytotoxic infusion is then commenced. The drug of choice is probably 5-fluorouracil, which is generally well tolerated. These catheters can be retained for weeks or even months. Removal by traction can be safely performed if they are clamped for 48 hours beforehand to permit arterial thrombosis. If the tumour responds, then further oral or intra-

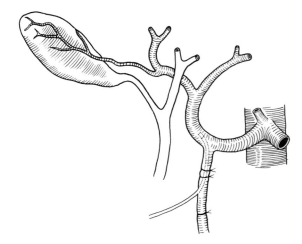

Fig. 16.10. Gastroduodenal artery catheterization for intra-arterial chemotherapy. The gastroduodenal artery is ligated distally, the catheter is inserted via a transverse arteriotomy and advanced into the hepatic artery. It is secured with two ligatures.

venous therapy may be indicated. If arterial infusion is considered necessary after catheter withdrawal, then selective hepatic artery catheterization can be achieved via the femoral artery, provided the artery has not been ligated at operation.

Tumour Embolization

An alternative to mass ligation of the hepatic artery is tumour embolization. This technique can be accomplished by selective hepatic artery cannulation via the transfemoral route. Embolization can shrink the tumour mass and relieve pain, but whether it will prolong survival is uncertain.

Radiation

Normal liver is very sensitive to radiation and only low doses are tolerated. Irradiation has not been shown to improve survival in hepatic neoplasia. The use of intraductal iridium wires to treat cholangiocarcinoma may be more effective, but only preliminary reports are available.

Intubation

An alternative to resection for a hilar cholangiocarcinoma is splintage with a replaceable U-tube. These lesions are often slow growing, and palliation may give as good a mean survival as resection. A choledochotomy is made below the lesion, which is then dilated with Bakes' dilators. The largest dilator is then advanced to a position near the liver capsule and is pushed through. A Silastic tube (usually no. 16 Fr. size) is then impacted or tied to the dilator and is pulled through the liver and the tumour; holes in the tube are aligned to bridge the neoplasm. This tube is brought to the skin surface, and the bile duct is closed around the tube. The two external ends are joined together to complete a loop (*Fig.* 16.11).

External beam radiotherapy may be employed or iridium wire can be placed in the tube. If the U-tube

becomes blocked, it is a simple matter to change it for a new one by a rail-road technique.

PORTO-JEJUNOSTOMY

This procedure is designed to relieve the obstruction of biliary atresia in neonates. The first step is cholecystectomy after an attempt at cholangiography via a cholecystostomy. The common bile duct is identified as a fibrous cord. It is divided at the duodenal border and dissected up to the hilum. The dense fibrous tissue encountered is excised, leaving a defect at the porta hepatis. A Roux loop of jejunum is then fashioned and sutured around the porta. Cholangitis and portal hypertension are the major complications of this procedure. If it fails the alternative is liver transplantation.

LIVER TRANSPLANTATION

Transplantation should be considered for patients with severe parenchymatous liver disease or primary malignancy of the liver. Timing is difficult, and patients with sepsis or bleeding problems are not suitable. In general patients with a slowly progressive downhill course are the most suitable. The indications have already been discussed.

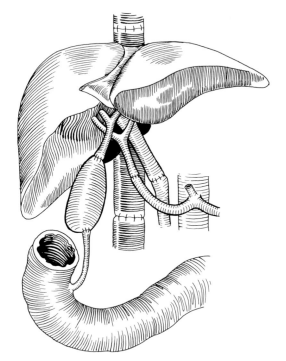

Fig. 16.12. The anatomical position at the completion of liver transplantation. End-to-end anastomoses of hepatic artery and portal vein restore vascular inflow. Venous return is via a segment of donor vena cava which is anastomosed above and below the liver. The donor gallbladder acts as a convenient conduit between donor and recipient bile ducts.

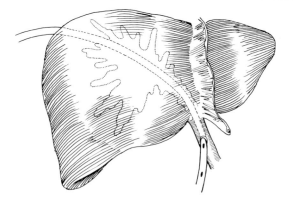

Fig. 16.11. U-tube intubation of the bile duct. The tube is advanced through an incision in the bile duct and passes out through the dome of the liver. Holes in the tube lie on either side of the obstruction.

The most accepted technique is that of orthotopic grafting removing the diseased liver and replacing it with the donor organ. Donor selection is similar to that for renal transplantation but the feasible preservation time is shorter (about 10 hours). Thus two skilled operating teams are required.

The aim of donor procurement is to prevent ischaemic damage to the liver during transfer. The liver is isolated *in situ*, and catheters are placed in the portal vein and hepatic artery. These catheters are perfused with cold Ringer's lactate, and fluid egresses via a vena caval catheter. The liver can then be removed and perfused again before packing in ice for transportation.

While the donor organ is in transit, a second team of surgeons removes the recipient's diseased liver. The completed graft is shown in *Fig.* 16.12. The order of anastomoses is portal vein, inferior vena cava (including hepatic veins), hepatic artery and then the gallbladder as a biliary conduit. Cyclosporin A is used to prevent graft rejection.

Since the 1-year survival rate is now around 50 per cent, this must now be considered an acceptable therapeutic procedure. Better results may be obtainable in children, and certainly in the USA the operation is becoming increasingly common in the younger age group. (*See also* Chapter 60.)

FURTHER READING

Adson M. (1981) Diagnosis and surgical treatment of primary and secondary solid hepatic tumors in the adult. *Surg. Clin. North Am.* **61,** 181–196.

Archampong E. Q. (1977) Amoebic liver disease. *Trop. Doct.* **7,** 161–168.

Barros J. L. (1978) Hydatid disease of the liver. *Am. J. Surg.* **135,** 597–600.

Bismuth H. and Corlette M. B. (1975) Intrahepatic cholangioenteric anastomosis in carcinoma of the hilus of the liver. *Surg. Gynecol. Obstet.* **140,** 170–178.

Blumgart L. H. and Benjamin I. S. (1983) Surgical aspects of liver and biliary cancer. In: Hodgson H. J. F. and Bloom S. R. (eds) *Advances in Gastroenterology.* pp. 251–287. New York, Churchill Livingstone.

Brunt P. W., Losowsky M. S. and Read A. E. (1984) Structure and function of the liver and biliary tract. In: *The Liver and Biliary System.* London, Heinemann, pp. 1–21.

Calne R. Y. (ed) (1982) *Liver Surgery.* Padua, Piccin Medical.

Calne R. Y. and Williams R. (1979) Liver Transplantation. *Curr. Probl. Surg.* **16,** 1–44.

Calne R. Y., Wells F. C. and Forty J. (1982) Twenty-six cases of liver trauma. *Br. J. Surg.* **69,** 365–368.

DeBakey M. E. and Jordan G. L. (1977) Hepatic abscesses, both intra- and extrahepatic. *Surg. Clin. North Am.* **57,** 325–337.

Hays D. M. and Kimura K. (1980) *Biliary Atresia.* London, Harvard University Press.

Healey J. E. and Schroy P. C. (1953) Anatomy of the biliary ducts within the human liver. *Arch. Surg.* **66,** 599–616.

Johnson P. J. (1983) Hepatocellular carcinoma. *Hosp. Update* **9,** 977–991.

Longmire W. P. and Tompkins R. K. (eds) (1981) *Manual of Liver Surgery.* New York, Springer-Verlag.

McPherson S. and Blumgart L. H. (1985) Liver trauma. *Surgery* (Oxford) **1,** 369–373.

Martin E. C., Karlson K. B., Fankuchen E. et al. (1981) Percutaneous drainage in the management of hepatic abscesses. *Surg. Clin. North Am.* **61,** 157–167.

Sanfelippo P. M., Beahrs O. H. and Weiland L. H. (1974) Cystic disease of the liver. *Ann. Surg.* **179,** 922–925.

Starzl T. E., Bell R. H., Beart R. W. et al. (1975) Hepatic trisegmentectomy and other liver resections. *Surg. Gynecol. Obstet.* **141,** 429–437.

Chapter seventeen

The Small Intestine

L. R. Celestin

ANATOMY AND PHYSIOLOGY

General Anatomy

The length in situ of the small intestine is approximately 3 metres, of which the first 25 cm to the duodenojejunal flexure represent the duodenum and the next 100 cm the jejunum, no clear demarcation line separating the latter from the ileum.

Surgical Anatomy

Duodenum

The duodenum is a C-shaped viscus whose two important features are its vascular supply and its peritoneal reflections. The vascular supply lies entirely within the concavity of the C and is derived from the gastroduodenal artery which forks in a Y-fashion astride the head of the pancreas into a posterior and an anterior superior pancreaticoduodenal artery, reuniting below the head of the pancreas to join the superior mesenteric artery. The most important peritoneal reflection of the duodenum lies on the lateral convexity of its vertical portion and its division (or Kocherization) allows posterior access to the head of the pancreas, the bile ducts and their lymph nodes, the inferior vena cava and the superior portion of the right ureter.

The duodenum suffers from a lack of mobility and a restricted vascular supply, both of which limit surgical freedom and lead often to its sacrifice in marked comparison to the jejunum and ileum.

Jejunum and Ileum

The mobility and rich vascular supply of this part of the small intestine makes it of exceptional value in reconstructive gastrointestinal surgery. Equally they make it prone to herniation, volvulus and strangulation.

At laparotomy the omentum usually separates the small intestine from the anterior parietes. Jejunal loops lie in a horizontal fashion to the left of the midline, while ileal loops adopt a vertical lie. This is due to the manner in which the mesentery is suspended from the posterior abdominal wall. After surgery the small bowel should be repositioned in its correct lie as best as possible, and the omental curtain once more pulled down over it. This anatomical lie of the jejunum and ileum is the best landmark in differentiating the two; but in cases of difficulty the dissimilar arterial arcades are of help. The distribution of these arcades is important when a reversed loop is being fashioned.

Physiology

The various juices of gastrointestinal origin add up to some 9 litres, but by the time the ileocaecal valve is reached all but 500–1000 ml have been absorbed. A major function of the small bowel is that of fluid and electrolyte reabsorption, and any condition upsetting this will deeply influence the salt and water homeostasis of the body. Digestion started in the stomach is completed in the small intestine. Stated simply, its function is to convert the polymers of the diet into monomers easily handled by the body. This is done via the digestive influence of enzymes from its exocrine system, which is the target organ of hormones originating from a diffuse complex of endocrine cells in its mucosa, as well as localized endocrine glands of intestinal origin. Digestion and absorption are co-ordinates of the body nutritional patterns and take place at all levels of the intestinal mucosa. Absorption (that is, the net movement into the body from the lumen) differs markedly in the various parts of the small intestine. Per unit length, it is maximal in the duodenum, tapers off in the jejunum, and steps down sharply in the ileum.

The surgical destruction or alteration of any part, or offshoot, of the intestinal tract will bring with it a multitude of problems still beyond biochemical disentanglement. A conservative policy in intestinal surgery reflects good judgement and sensible foresight and must be based on an appreciation of its physiology.

RESECTION OF THE SMALL BOWEL (ENTERECTOMY)

Resection of the small bowel and anastomosis are concurrent in virtually all cases, so that the two techniques are best considered together and are the linchpins of all small bowel surgery.

Indications

Resection is indicated in the following conditions:
1. Congenital lesions, i.e. atresia, stenosis, duplication, ileus.

2. Trauma perforating the bowel or interfering with its blood supply.
3. Strictures from scarring of healed lesions; or in association with active ones as in Crohn's disease and peptic ulceration.
4. Death of bowel from avascularity.
5. Tumours, benign or malignant, affecting the bowel or its mesentery.
6. Complications of obstruction—and less commonly in some cases of intussusception, diverticulitis, fistulas and blind loops.

away, dividing the end arteries and the veins cleanly and tying them. Division is carried out using artery forceps; or by under-running with aneurysm needles. This is the standard procedure for all but cases of malignancy.

2. V-shaped excision, used mostly in malignancy, when the dissection must include the limits of lymphatic spread, divides all arcades until a main branch free from lymph node enlargement is reached. The end arteries of the edges must be seen to pulsate once resection has been completed.

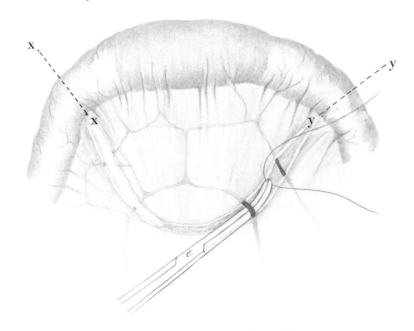

Fig. 17.1. Resection of small intestine.

Principles

In every laparotomy culminating in resection, a firm discipline is imperative:

1. The exposure should be adequate.
2. Exploration must be meticulous and gentle.
3. The area to be resected must be isolated to minimize soiling of the peritoneal cavity and the wound.
4. A perfect anastomosis should be aimed at.
5. All mesenteric gaps must be closed (*see Fig.* 17.11).

The various types of abdominal incisions have already been described elsewhere (*see* Chapter 5), as have the principles of exploration and avoidance of contamination of the operation field. The next concern is prudent resection with sound reconstruction.

Techniques of Resection and Reconstruction

Division of Mesentery

There are two ways of dividing the mesentery:

1. Close to the bowel and parallel to it, about 1 cm

Division of Bowel (Fig. 17.1)

Once the mesenteric vessels have been tied and ligated, the viable edges of the bowel become obvious and division must take place within viable tissue. As a rule this corresponds closely to the mesenteric edge. It continues in the line of the divided mesentery (x–x) if both bowel ends are of the same size; or lies obliquely (y–y) if segments of disproportionate calibres are to be anastomosed, the oblique section providing a larger stoma in the smaller segment, and a longer mesenteric border with a better blood supply.

Crushing clamps are applied to the edges of the loop to be discarded, while soft clamps occlude the segments to be anastomosed. Division is flush with the crushing clamps using either a scalpel or, preferably, a diathermy knife.

Types of Reconstruction (Figs. 17.2, 17.3)

Anastomosis is usually by the 'open' method; the 'closed' method requires care and much experience and its main advantage is the minimal soiling associated with it. Four types of reconstruction are in common use:

1. END CLOSURE

The lumen is closed as a cul-de-sac or stump and is part of any lateral or side anastomosis (*Fig.* 17.2).

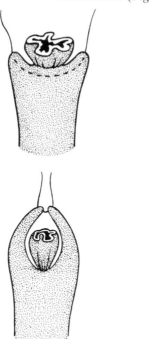

Fig. 17.2. End closure of small bowel by invagination.

2. END-TO-END ANASTOMOSIS

This is a quick but not the safest method. It is customary to practise an oblique cut in both ends to reduce stenosis (*Fig.* 17.3*a, b*). Where a small disparity exists between two loops, accurate apposition is obtained by splitting the less distended loop in its length to bring about an end-to-back anastomosis. Where gross disparity exists, it is better to use a side-to-side anastomosis.

3. END-TO-SIDE ANASTOMOSIS

This is the practice where obstruction causes one loop of bowel to be distended; or in ileocolic anastomosis (*Fig.* 17.3*d*).

4. SIDE-TO-SIDE ANASTOMOSIS

This is the safest method of anastomosis and in many ways the neatest (*Fig.* 17.3*d*).

Principles of Suturing

Before dealing with the practical aspects of suturing, it is essential to understand the principles involved, and appreciate the methods evolved to support these principles. Three golden rules apply to all intestinal suturing: (1) the suture line must be leakproof; (2) the apposed edges must be of viable tissue; (3) the lumen must not be stenosed.

A leakproof anastomosis depends on the manner in which suturing is layered. As a rule four layers are recognized: (*a*) a posterior seromuscular layer;

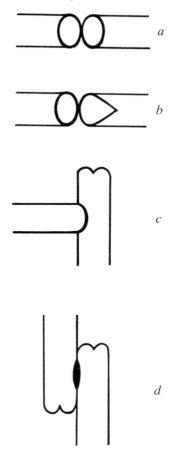

Fig. 17.3. Small intestinal anastomosis. *a*, End-to-end anastomosis. *b*, Tailoring of bowel for end-to-end anastomosis when disparity in size exists. *c*. End-to-side anastomosis. *d*, Side-to-side anastomosis.

(*b*) a posterior all coats; (*c*) an anterior all coats; (*d*) an anterior seromuscular.

In a one-layer closure coats (*b*) + (*c*) only are inserted, while the two-layer closure involves all four coats as described. The three-layer closure has a double posterior and a double anterior seromuscular coat. This latter is uncommonly used, but is highly recommended in Crohn's disease and in constructing reverse loops.

Types of Sutures

Several techniques have been devised to give the best results in the various types of sutures. These techniques are:

1. The 'through-and-through' all coats. Interrupted and continuous; the latter straight or locked.
2. The Connell or 'loop-on-mucosa' stitch.
3. The Lembert—interrupted or continuous.

4. Purse-string.
5. The 'three-bite' stitch.
These are now described in detail.

The Through-and-through all Coats

When interrupted, and in one-layer suturing, unabsorbable material is used (2/0 linen or silk). The stitch goes through all coats in both edges and is inserted from and knotted on the luminal side. The bites take in about 2 mm of the edge and are placed 2 mm apart (*Fig.* 17.4).

thus locking it against the mucosa, before the next stitch is inserted as in a blanket stitch (*Fig.* 17.5).

The Connell Stitch

This is the stitch commonly used for the anterior all-coat suturing. The stitch inverts the edges of the bowel and apposes the serosal surface. It is a continuous stitch.

The first bite starts on the serosal aspect and goes from out in. A loop is then created over the mucosa of the same edge and the next bite is from in out

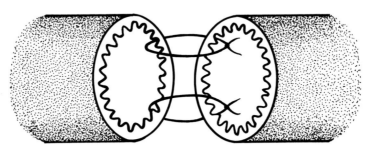

Fig. 17.4. Suture of small intestine. Through-and-through all coats with knots on the luminal side.

The continuous stitch is frequently used in a two-layer anastomosis, 2/0 chromic catgut on an atraumatic needle being the material of choice. Each bite is pulled tight, but as this can purse-string the anastomosis it is best to lock each stitch by passing the catgut loop under the previous through-and-through stitch,

(*Fig.* 17.6). The needle then crosses the gap between the two edges and repeats the same procedure through the other edge. When the suture is pulled the edges are inverted and drawn together. This is both a waterproof and haemostatic suture.

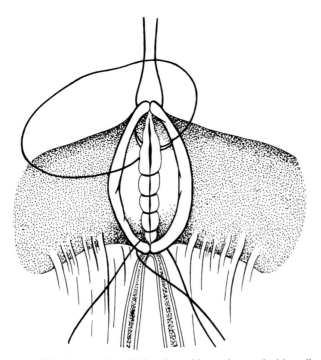

Fig. 17.5. Suture of small intestine with continuous locking all-layers suture.

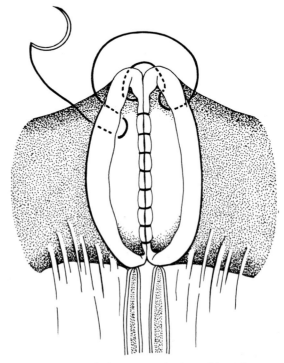

Fig. 17.6. Small intestinal anastomosis. Connell inverting suture.

The Lembert Stitch (*Figs.* 17.7, 17.8)

This is the standard seromuscular stitch of intestinal anastomoses. Silk or linen (2/0) on an atraumatic needle is used. The bite is started about 4 mm from the edge, the needle penetrating the serosa and the muscle to a depth of about 1 mm and coming out

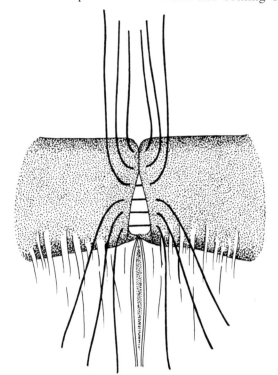

Fig. 17.7. Small intestinal anastomosis. Interrupted Lembert suture.

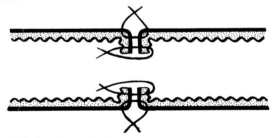

Fig. 17.8. Small intestinal anastomosis using full-thickness interrupted sutures reinforced with inverting Lembert suture.

about 2 mm from the cut edge, to cross the gap to pick up the opposite edge in a similar manner in the reverse order. When pulled together the underlying suture is buried, the serosal surfaces coming together. This is the approximating stitch, releasing tension off the all-coat layer, and providing a seal within 24 hours by endothelial cover. Lembert interrupted sutures are placed 2–3 mm apart.

The Purse-string (*Fig.* 17.9)

This is a series of mattress sutures inserted in a circular fashion around an orifice to be closed or buried.

In a burying purse-string the bowel is crushed with a clamp and tied across the groove so formed with thread or silk. The excess of bowel is trimmed and the stump so left buried by the purse-string. The closing purse-string is to be used only in small openings in the bowel provided it does not constrict them on tightening the stitch.

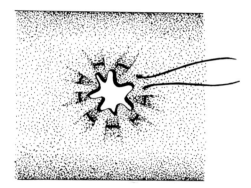

Fig. 17.9. Purse-string suture of small intestinal perforation.

The Three-bite Stitch

This is a very useful stitch for closing awkward corners or approximating more than two edges. It

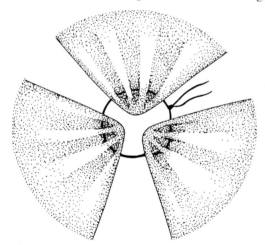

Fig. 17.10. The three-bite stitch is useful for reinforcing closure at awkward corners.

consists of an all-coat stitch taking each corner in turn in a single bite and pulled together to approximate these corners. It can be used to accentuate angles such as the acute one in fashioning a Roux-en-Y loop, or the oblique one at the lesser curve (the 'danger angle' in a Billroth-I anastomosis) (*Fig.* 17.10).

Once the above stitches have been mastered, small bowel surgery should present no difficulties. As a rule it is more practical to carry out the posterior all-coats and the anterior all-coats first, and complete the anastomosis with the seromuscular layers. Special clamps are no longer necessary to approximate the viscera to be anastomosed, all that is required being straight, soft clamps to prevent soiling from the contents of the small bowel.

Viability

The manner in which the mesentery should be divided has already been described. Viable gut is pink and shiny and bleeds on releasing the soft clamp. These features must always be checked before embarking on an anastomosis, otherwise lysis of the bowel wall results with late onset of peritonitis and a high mortality rate.

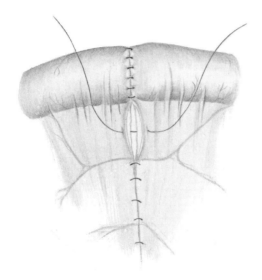

Fig. 17.11. The mesentery must be closed following bowel anastomosis.

Stenosis

Stenosis is avoided by making sure that no anastomosis or closure leads to luminal constriction. The end-to-end anastomosis is most prone to stenosis. Adoption of the oblique cut, as described earlier, will prevent stenosis. When in doubt it is far better to carry out a side-to-side anastomosis. Poor viability of the edges can lead to late stricturing of an anastomosis. This is most commonly encountered in oesophago-jejunal anastomoses.

ENTEROTOMY

This consists in incising the walls of the bowel to have access to its lumen. It has two main indications: (1) *decompression* of a distended bowel and (2) *extraction* of a foreign body or benign tumour.

A third type of enterotomy exists, namely the *traumatic* variety, which is becoming increasingly frequent with road traffic accidents. In decompression, the lumen is opened midway between the duodeno-jejunal flexure and the site of the obstruction to give

maximal reach to the decompressor. Closure is by a purse-string suture.

In extraction, a longitudinal cut is made over the site of the foreign body (gallstone, bezoar, etc.) or tumour, and the enterotomy is then closed *transversely* by layered sutures to avoid stenosing the lumen.

In a traumatic enterotomy, the antimesenteric border may show a ragged tear, often longitudinal. Tears near the mesenteric border tend to be transverse and to give rise to a haematoma within the mesentery.

Technical Details

Decompression

Soft clamps are applied across a loop on either side of the enterotomy site (*Fig.* 17.12), the loop having been milked empty of its contents. Packs then isolate the loop from the abdominal incision.

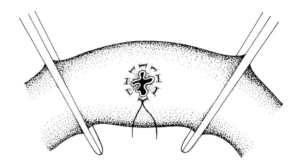

Fig. 17.12. Decompression enterotomy.

A seromuscular purse-string in 2/0 catgut surrounds the chosen site which is then opened with cutting diathermy. The head of the decompressor (*Fig.* 17.13) is slipped inside the lumen and the purse-string firmly tightened over its shaft. The lower clamp is removed and the decompressor advanced some 10–15 cm at a time, suction being *intermittently* applied as more and more loops are telescoped on the decompressor until a satisfactory result has been achieved. The decompressor is then slowly withdrawn and finally swung through 180° to engage the upstream loops that are similarly dealt with. Finally, the instrument is totally withdrawn and the purse-string tied to occlude the enterotomy. The purse-string is oversewn with an interrupted Lembert stitch (2/0 silk or linen) to effect a waterproof closure.

Extraction

The foreign body or benign tumour is easily palpable and as a rule the proximal loop is distended (*Fig.* 17.14).

Soft clamps are placed 8–10 cm away from the lesion, on either side, having emptied the bowel by a milking process. Protective packs are inserted around the surgical field and the bowel incised longitudinally across the foreign body or tumour to well beyond its limits.

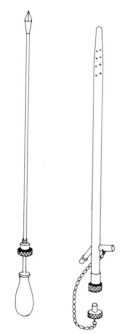

Fig. 17.13. Trocar and cannula used for intestinal decompression.

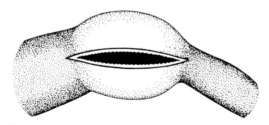

Fig. 17.14. Extraction enterotomy. The longitudinal incision is closed transversely to avoid stricture formation.

Tissue forceps hold the edges of the wound apart and the foreign body should then be extracted without unnecessary force. A benign tumour, if pedunculated, is removed by diathermy. Sessile lesions need resection. A two-layer transverse closure is then carried out. The first layer with catgut using a Connell stitch, and the second by an interrupted Lembert stitch using silk or thread. Should the foreign body, e.g. a gallstone, have possibly damaged the gut at the point of impaction, it should be 'milked' away and extraction enterotomy undertaken through healthy bowel wall.

Traumatic

A longitudinal tear, if less than 4 cm, is trimmed of all ragged edges and closed transversely in two layers. Longer tears, ragged or contused tears and tears with doubtful viability should be excised. Small tears or punctures close together are best dealt with by dividing the bridge between them and converting them into a single larger hole which is then closed transversely. Careful haemostasis of the edges is paramount before any closure. Edges must be trimmed until they bleed as poor viability may lead to fistula formation as a late complication (*Fig.* 17.15).

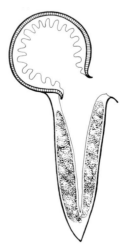

Fig. 17.15. Traumatic enterotomy may be obscured by a mesenteric haematoma.

Transverse tears on the mesenteric border, with mesenteric involvement, require careful assessment. The mesenteric haematoma must be explored and all bleeding points controlled. Once this has been achieved the bowel must be examined for viability. If ischaemia is present a resection is imperative. If the bowel edges are healthy, closure is in two layers, as before, in the transverse lie of the tear.

Duodenal and jejunal tears are not infrequent in road traffic accidents and as the lesion can be in the fixed part of these viscera, resection is often hazardous. A simple solution is to convert the tear into a side-to-side anastomosis with the next mobile distal loop of jejunum.

ENTEROSTOMY

Enterostomies can be conveniently classified as:
1. The high enterostomy—better known as the 'feeding jejunostomy'.
2. The low or terminal enterostomy—universally termed 'ileostomy'.

Jejunostomy

The evolution of fine-gauge nasogastric tubes, of endoscopy and of parenteral nutrition has made the feeding jejunostomy an uncommon operation. However, it still finds a place in:
1. Oesophageal strictures of chemical origin when

both oesophagus and stomach have been severely damaged.

2. Resectable malignant lesions of the stomach in which either a gastrostomy or a gastroenterostomy cannot be fashioned; the patient requiring hyperalimentation in preparation for surgery.
3. In the management of gastroduodenal fistulas.

In fashioning a jejunostomy several guidelines should be followed:

1. The method should be simple and rapid, being easily performed under local anaesthesia.
2. It should be self-closing following removal of the tube.
3. It should be constructed with an anti-reflux mechanism in order to prevent skin digestion.
4. The feeding tube must not obstruct the jejunum.
5. It should be as close to the duodenojejunal flexure as possible to allow maximum absorption by the jejunum (*see* Physiology).

The Witzel jejunostomy or its modifications fulfil these points. It is carried out via a small left paramedian, or better still a left transverse incision. The first jejunal loop which presents itself is brought out and followed proximally until the duodenojejunal flexure prevents any further progress. About 8 cm of the loop are now brought out through the wound. An antimesenteric site is chosen at the distal portion of that loop and held in a silk or thread purse-string. The diathermy knife punctures that site and a no. 20 Fr. gauge Silastic Foley catheter is navigated through it distally. The balloon is inflated with about 10 ml of water and the purse-string tightened around the catheter (*Fig.* 17.16*a*). The catheter and its site

of entry into the bowel are now buried by a continuous Lembert suture using 2/0 catgut, over a distance of 6–8 cm (*Fig.* 17.16*b*). The Lembert stitch is tied, but not cut, and is used to fix that portion of the jejunum to the most medial corner of the abdominal wound, bringing the catheter onto the right of the midline over the skin. The wound is now closed in layers and the jejunostomy is ready for use 24 hours later.

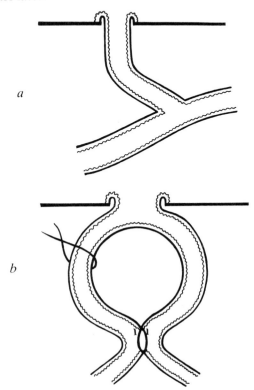

Fig. 17.17. Prevention of reflux in feeding jejunostomy (long term). *a*, Roux-en-Y jejunostomy. *b*, Omega jejunostomy.

If the patient is fit enough an omega jejunostomy or a Roux-en-Y can be constructed, its main indication being a longer term use (*see* Roux loops); otherwise it offers little advantage over the Witzel jejunostomy (*Fig.* 17.17).

Ileostomy (*Fig.* 17.18)
Lateral ileostomies are rarely used and are not described here. The terminal ileostomy takes over an anal function in total colectomy carried out for ulcerative lesions of the colon or polyposis coli, and as such will play a major part in the subsequent life of the patient. It must therefore be constructed with the utmost care, and so sited that appliances can be easily retained during the everyday activities of the patient. The surgeon personally must mark the abdominal wall before the patient comes to the operating theatre. A site is chosen approximately 5 cm below and 5 cm to the right of the umbilicus, and is marked

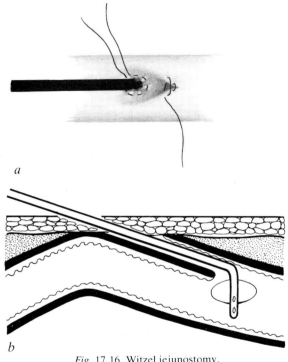

Fig. 17.16. Witzel jejunostomy.

with the patient in the sitting position, to avoid skin creases in the obese and bony protuberances in the slim.

On the operating table a 3 cm circle of skin is removed by lifting the site with toothed forceps and amputating the tented skin so raised. Thereafter using the diathermy needle a hole of the same size is cored until the rectus muscle proper is reached, and split to reveal the posterior rectus sheath or the peritoneum.

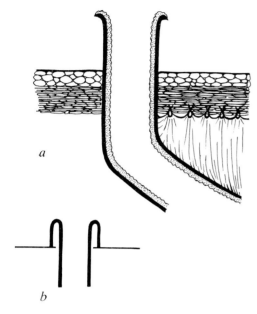

Fig. 17.18. Terminal ileostomy.

After the colon and rectum have been mobilized, the small bowel is prepared as follows:

The last 15–20 cm of small bowel are separated from its mesentery by close division of the vessels, and the mesentery preserved, following which the distal ileum is removed with the colon and rectum, after division with the diathermy knife. The cut edge of the ileum is carefully examined and perfect haemostasis obtained.

The peritoneum at the ileostomy site is opened and tissue forceps used to exteriorize the terminal loop. About 6 cm are brought out. The spared mesentery is then fixed to the anterior parietes with interrupted catgut sutures, and made to curtain across the gap lateral to the ileum to prevent obstruction by intestinal volvulus through that gap. The bowel must not be stitched to the peritoneum as this tends to invite fistula formation.

The exteriorized ileum is then everted using Babcock clamps (*Fig.* 17.18*b*) and maintained in that position by four cardinal stitches between skin and ileum using 4/0 plain catgut on an atraumatic cutting needle. If necessary additional stitches can be inserted. An ileostomy bag (3·8 cm) is applied to the skin immediately.

Stoma care is a subject on its own and a more specialized text should be consulted.

In recent years Koch has devised a 'continent' ileostomy using an ileal reservoir fitting, with an ileal 'valve'. The method has given good results in Koch's hands, but is still being tried by other surgeons and it is too early to give a final account of its indications.

THE ROUX LOOPS

The most important of the Roux techniques is the Roux-en-Y which is an anti-reflux procedure that has evolved from the Roux loop.

A good example of the Roux loop is a simple end-to-side oesophagojejunostomy (*Fig.* 17.19*a*). However, this allows bile and pancreatic juices to reach the oesophagus and cause an oesophagitis.

A simple device to minimize this is the creation of an entero-enterostomy (*Fig.* 17.19*b*) between the loops—the omega loop. However, reflux still takes place but can be prevented by a tie across the afferent loop. This led to the development of the Roux-en-Y.

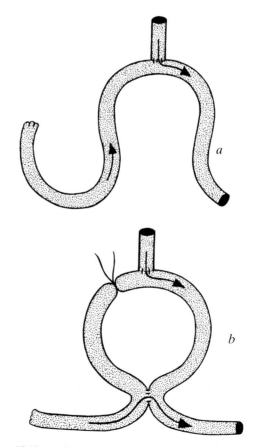

Fig. 17.19. *a*, End-to-side oesophagojejunostomy. This simple loop is useful following total gastrectomy but allows bowel and pancreatic juices to reflux into the oesophagus. *b*, The creation of an entero-enterostomy with stapling or division close to the oesophageal anastomosis will minimize such reflux.

The Roux-en-Y (*Fig.* 17.20)

The jejunal loop is divided 25 cm from the duodeno-jejunal flexure and the distal end anastomosed to the oesophagus. Thirty centimetres further down, the proximal loop is anastomosed end to side into the distal loop, bringing the pancreatico-biliary juices back into the digestive tract, but preventing their reflux into the oesophagus.

A useful method of delaying transit time is to place a 'physiological' obstruction in the path of a peristaltic wave.

This is achieved by isolating a short loop of bowel based on a vascular pedicle, reversing it and replacing

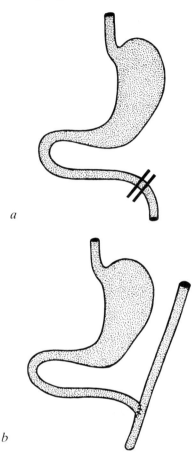

Fig. 17.20. Roux-en-Y anastomosis.

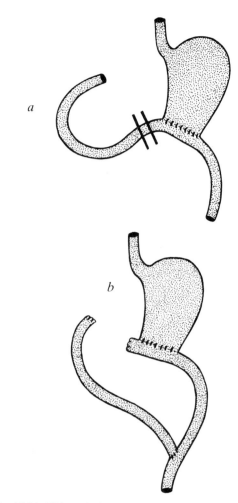

Fig. 17.21. This variation of the Roux-en-Y is used to correct biliary reflux after Polya gastrectomy.

The Roux-en-Y is used:
1. In restoring oesophago-intestinal continuity after total gastrectomy.
2. Preventing biliary regurgitation and biliary vomiting after a Polya gastrectomy (*Fig.* 17.21).
3. Preventing reflux in a feeding jejunostomy (*Fig.* 17.17*a*).
4. Restoring biliary excretion in carcinoma of the head of the pancreas, by a cholecysto-jejunostomy-en-Y.

THE REVERSE LOOP

Conditions occasionally arise when gastrointestinal transit is hurried and gives rise to diarrhoea or to symptoms resulting from the presence of a hyperosmolar solution in the upper intestine.

it in its original position—hence the name 'reverse loop'.

The indications for such a loop are:
1. Post-vagotomy diarrhoea, the loop being mid-ileal.
2. The dumping syndrome, where the loop is upper jejunal and close to the gastric egress.
3. The short bowel syndrome, where the loop is precaecal.
4. The grossly incontinent ileostomy with marked fluid loss, when the loop is in the distal ileum.

The length of the loop is critical and difficult to determine, no exact length being clear. As a rule a 10-cm loop is ineffectual, while a 15-cm loop is likely to give rise to obstructive symptoms and signs. The author has found a 12–13-cm loop useful.

The vascular arches of the relevant bowel loop are carefully studied. Stay sutures then delineate the exact limits of the loop to be reversed after accurate measurement with a sterile steel ruler. Windows are cut fanwise into the mesentery and transverse connections between vessels carefully tied dividing any arch until a single or double vascular supply is left, about which the loop can be twisted a full 180° without occlusion. The loop is then ready for reimplanting. The proximal anastomosis will join together two pieces of bowel with their peristaltic movements meeting head-on and slowing down transit. It is thus an anastomosis of conflict which could disrupt unless carefully fashioned. The inner layer consists of an all-coat one using a continuous locked stitch posteriorly and a Connell stitch anteriorly. Interrupted Lembert sutures, of unabsorbable material, constitute the seromuscular layer; and for greater safety a second similar seromuscular is inserted, thus forming a three-layered anastomosis. It cannot be stressed too much that a leak at this anastomosis is likely to be serious, and therefore great care is imperative. The distal anastomosis is straightforward and in two layers.

During the early postoperative days, more so soon after the return of normal feeding, the patient may suffer colicky abdominal pain. Atropine or Probanthine (probantheline) given regularly will tide the patient over this difficult period.

FISTULAS

Fistulas can be classified as high or low, partial or total. Partial fistula infers that only part of the lumen is involved—the so-called 'lateral fistulas'—and total fistula indicates that the whole lumen is involved, as in the complete breakdown of an anastomosis, when the fistula acts as an ileostomy.

The higher the fistula the greater the problems encountered:

1. A high located fistula causes great loss of fluid and electrolytes.
2. The intestine proximal to the fistula may prove too short for adequate absorption.
3. The effluent has greater digestive power, damaging the skin more severely.
4. Oesophageal, gastric and duodenal fistulas present greater difficulty of excision or bypass.

When obstruction, chronic infection or malignancy does not complicate a fistula, it may close naturally, although this is not often the case. In this situation the most important requirement is adequate alimentation. The patient with a fistula requires hyperalimentation of up to 4000 calories daily with a nitrogen/calorie proportion of 1 g to 200 calories. If intestinal absorption is adequate the enteral route should be used; otherwise it should be supplemented with or even replaced by intravenous feeding.

From a technical point of view fistulas are single or multiple, the latter usually presenting as several lateral holes in matted loops of small bowel emerging through a dehiscence of the anterior parietes.

The majority of fistulas follow sepsis, the breakdown of anastomoses, or accidental damage during surgery.

The Single Fistula

The affected loop may be just beneath the anterior parietes, or lie deep within the abdominal cavity. In the latter instance a full laparotomy is necessary to deal with the fistula.

Methylene blue or a similar dye is injected into the fistula to stain the track and make its recognition easier. An elliptical incision isolates it from the skin, and then by blunt and sharp dissection it is followed through the anterior parietes down to the peritoneum. The involved loop is then freed from any peritoneal adhesion as well as from surrounding loops until it is mobilized sufficiently to be exteriorized without undue traction. Soft clamps occlude the loop on either side of the fistula which is excised with the diathermy needle in a longitudinal plane. The enterotomy is then closed transversely in two layers. Even if excision involves over 50 per cent of the gut perimeter, this remains the method of choice, a posterior wall bridge on the mesenteric border being preferable to enterectomy with end-to-end anastomosis. Resection is justified only when viability is in doubt.

Multiple Fistulas

In multiple fistulas spontaneous resolution is unlikely. The separate closure of each fistula is not practical and resection can be hazardous. Exclusion is the method of choice and has the advantage of simplicity.

The uppermost fistula is explored with a soft sound or catheter to determine the lie of the afferent loop. In a similar manner the efferent loop leading off the lowermost fistula is mapped out (*Fig. 17.22*).

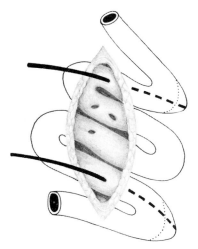

Fig. 17.22. Exploration of multiple intestinal fistulas using sounds.

The abdominal cavity is then opened away from the fistulas over the sites of the tips of the sound, when a clean and free surgical field is obtained. The small bowel is divided on the proximal side of the fistulas on the one hand, and distal to them on the other. The loops bearing the fistulas are then closed by purse-string sutures, while the two free ends are anastomosed to restore intestinal continuity with all the consequent advantages of absorption and fluid preservation. The fistulas become isolated and mucous and may be resected at a later stage and under better conditions (*Fig.* 17.23).

This method of exclusion can also be used in the difficult deep-seated single fistula.

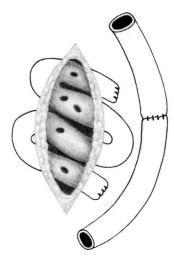

Fig. 17.23. Isolation of fistulous loops of small intestine with restoration of bowel continuity.

TUMOURS

Tumours of the small bowel embrace the varieties of growths that can arise from the various constituent tissues of the intestine.

Benign tumours are commonest but give rise to fewer symptoms than malignant. Of the benign lesions leiomyomas are the most common and like adenomas and haemangiomas may present as bleeding and anaemia. Obstructive symptoms are usually due to intussusception. Carcinoids, by virtue of their humoral secretion, are a group apart and are as common as malignant tumours.

The latter group consists of adenocarcinomas, leiomyosarcomas and the lymphomas, and present with obstruction or bleeding. They are found more frequently in the elderly. Acute presentations require laparotomy and their treatment is discussed later; more chronic cases allow time for investigation of which the small bowel meal and selective mesenteric angiography are the most useful.

Pedunculated benign lesions may be treated by excision through an enterotomy; all other lesions require local or radical enterectomy. Inoperable lesions will require bypass operations. Some tumours, e.g. leiomyosarcomas, may be very vascular and the first step in their excision should be the division of their blood supply with careful haemostasis.

Secondary malignant lesions may be suspected when a previous melanoma has been removed elsewhere in the body. Enterectomy is the treatment of choice, although liver metastases are frequently present.

An unusual lesion causing obstruction by intussusception is the Peutz–Jeghers syndrome in which multiple hamartomatous polyps are present. Great caution should be exercised in limited excisions of the lesions (which are not pre-malignant) rather than by wide multiple enterectomies, or the patient may be left with a short bowel syndrome.

INFLAMMATORY LESIONS

The most important chronic inflammatory lesion is regional enteritis or Crohn's disease. Other lesions are much less common and are due to diverticulitis, granulomas (eosinophilic) and tuberculosis.

Treatment

A period of medical or conservative treatment is always advisable before recourse to surgery which should be indicated only when supportive and medical treatment fails to halt the spread of the condition; or when complications such as protein loss, bleeding, obstruction, fistula formation or perforation occur. On no account should Crohn's disease be explored unless the anaemia, hypoproteinaemia and electrolytic deficiencies have been corrected and the patient is in an anabolic phase. Alimentation, enteral or parenteral or both, must be adequate before embarking on such a major intervention.

The Place of Operative Biopsies

Crohn's disease tends to recur most frequently at the site of a previous anastomosis and it has therefore been suggested that resection should be through a disease-free area. As this cannot be recognized by palpation or macroscopic appearance of the *serosal* surface, either naked-eye examination of the mucosa at surgery or frozen section has been suggested. Neither is very reliable and since minute lesions may be present well away from the main one, the exercise does not seem to be a fruitful one.

A radical approach cannot, therefore, be rationally contemplated and there is more to be gained by conservative surgery preserving as much small bowel as possible. There is a definite place for multiple short enterectomies of skip lesions.

Principles Involved

1. Time must be spent prior to surgery correcting all deficiencies and getting the patient into an anabolic state.

2. In general a bypass, or a bypass with exclusion, should be avoided.

3. All complications are best treated by enterectomy with end-to-end anastomosis.

4. Where fistulas are multiple and loops are bound down by abscess formation avoid the spread of abdominal sepsis by carrying out an exclusion of the fistulas and converting them into mucous fistulas. Once sepsis has diminished, steroids reduced if necessary, and the patient's condition has improved, excision can be undertaken.

The commonest site of Crohn's disease is at the terminal ileum and this is best treated by a limited right hemicolectomy. As recurrence at this anastomosis may lead to early obstruction, as wide a stoma as possible should be aimed at, best achieved by a side-to-side anastomosis at least 5 cm long and preferably in three layers. Loss of the ileocaecal valve, with alteration in the enterohepatic circulation, can lead to postoperative diarrhoea not due to enteritis, and similarly steatorrhoea can be accentuated after surgery. Bile dumping into the colon often responds well to the use of a bile salt-binding resin such as cholestyramine, 12–16 g daily in four divided doses. If steatorrhoea is present dietary fat must be reduced to below 40 g daily. Coarse fibre can be added to the diet at the rate of one level teaspoonful three times a day. More recently loperamide (Imodium) has been tried, the suggested dose being two tablets every morning, plus one after every bowel action.

Crohn's disease of the duodenum and jejunum is uncommon and resection may be hazardous. The main symptoms are those following interference with gastric emptying. It is simpler and safer to undertake gastrojejunostomy to overcome gastric obstruction, and persist with the medical treatment of the duodenitis and the jejunitis with prednisolone or immunosuppression.

ACUTE INTESTINAL OBSTRUCTION

The recognition of obstruction is as important as is the diagnosis of its exact cause.

Early and judicious intervention is the hallmark of the surgery of intestinal obstruction, and a safe approach is to decide on surgical intervention in the first instance, and then proceed to making the patient fit for surgery, altering this policy of intervention only if there are substantial changes leading to a reversal of the initial decision.

Obstruction results from interference with the natural progression of intestinal contents and is of two types, neurogenic and mechanical. In *neurogenic* obstruction the bowel is paralysed and there is little or no peristaltic movement—a state known as 'ileus'.

In *mechanical* obstruction there is an actual obstacle to the peristaltic effort, which increases in an endeavour to overcome the obstruction. At a later stage, either from total decompensation, from loss of viability or from a toxic state, an ileus may set in.

Mechanical obstruction can be simple or strangulated, high or low. Its symptoms, signs and systemic effects are the results of the disturbed physiology of peristalsis, possibly complicated by necrosis and perforation.

Pathophysiology

Interference with peristalsis leads to the damming of secretions and gases proximal to the obstruction, followed very soon by a loss of extracellular fluid into the obstructed loop, thus increasing its contents. This distension is followed by vomiting. The higher the obstruction, the less the distension but the sooner the vomiting, which is small in amounts, frequent and often reflux in nature but leading to a rapid loss of fluid. The lower the obstruction, the greater the distension and the later the vomiting of larger amounts of alkaline contents with, however, a slower loss of fluid. Dehydration and acidosis eventually result. Later, protein is lost into the bowel lumen, increasing the hypovolaemia and interfering with the perfusion of vital organs and the development of shock. Where strangulation exists, whole blood is in addition lost into the bowel lumen and, with the development of gangrene, sepsis sets in, too often with a fatal outcome.

Diagnosis

Interference with peristalsis causes all the following symptoms:

1. *Pain*

A characteristic waxing and waning, termed 'colic', comes on about 4 minutes apart in a high obstruction, and about 8 minutes apart in a low obstruction. With the colicky attacks come typical bowel sounds called 'borborygmi', often heard by the bedside, but usually requiring a stethoscope. The sounds are high pitched, coincide with the pain and die off with a gurgling sound. They should be listened to attentively.

2. *Vomiting*

Pent-up secretions by retrograde peristalsis, and accumulation, find their way back into the stomach and are vomited. There is a tendency to describe such vomit as 'faeculent', a very inaccurate term. True faeculent vomiting is a late sequel of obstruction, being seen several days after its onset and is a sign of impending catastrophe.

3. *Constipation*

Once peristalsis no longer propels intestinal contents into the colon, gas and faeces are no longer passed. However, the contents below a high obstruction may still be passed so that a stool is reported hours after the start of pain.

4. *Diarrhoea*

Associated with obstruction, diarrhoea may be an important guiding symptom. It can occur in a partial obstruction, e.g. Richter's hernia; where an abscess complicates the picture; in intussusception; and very commonly in vascular occlusion.

5. *Past History*

A previous appendicitis, an abdominal or inguinal operation, a history of salpingitis, or a vaginal hysterectomy are all important guides to the most common cause of obstruction, namely bands and adhesions.

Guidelines to the Nature of Obstruction

Every effort must be made to decide whether an obstruction is simple or strangulating. There is no sharp dividing line, but by compounding one's findings a fair judgement can be reached. The following guidelines are useful:

1. *Onset:* A slow, indefinite one favours a simple obstruction. The strangulation is sudden and reflects the sharp interference with vascular supply.
2. *Shock* develops early in the strangulating variety.
3. *Constant pain* in quite sharp distinction to colicky pain suggests a background other than just a simple obstacle, and should be taken very seriously. With constant pain there may also be increased tenderness, but this is not pathognomonic of strangulation. However, its presence should be an indication for laparotomy.
4. *Pulse rate:* Interference with blood supply and the resulting biochemical effects will tend to show a rising pulse rate. A level of 120/minute in a fully rehydrated patient would suggest a major problem requiring early interference.
5. *Temperature, leucocytosis:* Both may be found in either type, but more so in the strangulating variety.
6. *Radiology:* Plain, erect, supine and lateral decubitus scout films should be taken.

Gas shadows may be present and may show a closed loop early in the evolution of signs. Since closed loops are more prone to strangulation, such a finding is most important. A single radiograph, more so an erect one, may not be very contributory if distension is already present, as typical shadows of high and low small bowel will not be seen. However, in a high obstruction, and in mesenteric vascular occlusion, a total lack of gas shadows and fluid levels is seen. Serial films, especially supine, can be useful in showing progression or regression of an obstruction. By and large plain radiology presents its own diagnostic limitations, which only prompt laparotomy will solve.

Management of Obstruction

This is based on two main stages, preoperative and operative.

Preoperative

'Drip and suck' is the description given to this preoperative stage. If little vomiting is present and a scout film shows a fairly empty stomach in the erect film, if the patient's general condition is good and early surgery can be contemplated, it is good practice to pass a nasogastric tube *after* induction of anaesthesia. If Sellick's manoeuvre of oesophageal compression by cricoid pressure is carried out during endotracheal intubation with a cuffed tube, there is little need to fear gastric regurgitation. However, this latter procedure is best handled by a highly skilled anaesthetist. A less skilled anaesthetist would be well advised to pass a nasogastric tube *before* induction. When surgery has to be delayed, or observation is necessary over several hours, or conservative treatment of a subacute obstruction has been elected, nasogastric decompression and replacement therapy are carefully balanced.

FLUID REPLACEMENT

This is not always clearly understood. The danger to life is the obstruction, and its removal will correct metabolic disorders quicker than can non-essential fluid correction. Only when plasma and blood have been lost and a state of shock exists or is impending does one need time to make the patient fit for surgery. As a rule plasma or plasma expanders can be given quickly to restore the circulation, and during surgery electrolytes can be replaced. The production of urine before surgery is a useful guide to the necessity for prolonged fluid replacement. A state of ileus presents a different picture in that it reflects a late stage of obstruction, and here replacement of fluids and electrolytes is required.

If sepsis is suspected antibiotic treatment should be instituted, both aerobes and anaerobes being dealt with.

Operative

Surgery has three main aims: (1) decompression of the bowel, (2) removal of the cause of the obstruction, (3) determining the viability of involved loops.

1. DECOMPRESSION

Most cases will not require aggressive decompression. When ileus has supervened preoperative naso-gastric suction properly carried out would have been sufficient.

Operative decompression is indicated:

a. If the intestinal loops lie fallow and heavy and are thinned out, being then in danger of rupture.

b. If distension interferes with the ease of exploration.

c. If distension is likely to interfere with safe and comfortable abdominal closure. In high obstruction decompression is best done by stripping or milking the bowel contents into the stomach and sucking out via the nasogastric tube. In low obstruction a decompression enterotomy is more easily carried out (*see* Enterotomy, p. 204) until distension has reached a minimum, when the cause of the obstruction can be determined and dealt with.

2. SITE OF OBSTRUCTION (WHEN NOT OBVIOUS)

Inspect the caecum first of all. If it is distended then the obstruction is in the large bowel and the small bowel distension is a secondary phenomenon.

In small bowel obstruction, the caecum is usually collapsed, as is the distal small bowel. Follow these loops proximally until the point of obstruction is reached. Should collapsed small bowel be difficult to follow, exteriorization of the distended loops will facilitate the search.

This may then lead to an internal hernia, a volvulus across a band, adhesions causing hairpin bends, tumours, foreign bodies or an intussusception of a Meckel's diverticulum.

Adhesions between loops should not be separated unless it is to a purpose, for their idle separation can lead to further adhesions. Internal hernias are reduced and unless the neck is tissue that can be safely incised, no more should be done. A volvulus is reduced and the offending band divided. A hairpin bend is straightened by dividing adhesions. Foreign bodies are removed by an enterotomy, while tumours and Meckel's diverticulum are treated by resection. An intussusception is reduced, but if a lesion such as a benign tumour (fibroma, angioma, leiomyoma, etc.) has caused it, the latter is dealt with by resection.

Where strangulation exists and bowel is no longer viable resection is performed. When obstruction cannot be dealt with, be it due to the patient's poor state or to inoperability or inaccessibility, it is wise to do a side-to-side anastomosis astride it and wait for a better day.

3. VIABILITY

Greenish-black gut with no lustre, no palpable pulsating mesenteric vessels or peristalsis is dead gut and must be resected.

Viable gut is usually red, with pulsating vessels, has a sheen and shows peristalsis. However, hypothermia, anoxaemia and shock can cause it to look purple and appear lifeless. On warming it with warm saline and increasing for a short time the anaesthetic oxygen living gut should become bright red to pink with peristalsis, and this should be saved. If there is doubt, resection must be undertaken. This will increase mortality and postoperative morbidity and therefore every effort must be made to prove loss of viability before embarking on resection.

INTESTINAL VASCULAR INSUFFICIENCY

The flow to the midgut is through the superior mesenteric artery which supplies the intestinal arteries arising from its left aspect, and the middle, right and ileocolic arteries on its right. The latter artery is constant and, as will be seen later, is a most useful branch of the superior mesenteric artery. These vessels break up into arcades and terminal arteries to reach the submucosa where they form a rich plexus, from which arise single arterioles to supply individual villi. Plexus and end arterioles constitute the arterial microcirculation of the gut.

The superior mesenteric artery is said to be occluded, partially or totally, in some two-thirds of people past their fifth decade, and its acute angle with the aorta is such that emboli are readily directed into it.

Vascular insufficiency results from any pathological state which reduces the arterial perfusion of the small intestine. The main causes are:

1. *Fall in cardiac output* due to cardiac failure, or the oligaemia of shock and trauma. Myocardial infarction and arrhythmias may aggravate this.

2. *Mechanical obstruction* of the vessels by emboli and thrombi. Embolization is less frequent than was at one time considered.

3. *Damage to the microcirculation* from obstruction interfering with free flow; sensitivity reactions; vasoconstriction by pressor drugs; damage to the mucosa by enzymes such as trypsin, or the endotoxin of organisms such as *Clostridium welchii*, which produces a state of haemorrhagic jejunitis or enterocolitis.

4. *Slowing down of the circulation* from haemoconcentration in dehydration or excessive action of diuretics; from intravascular coagulation and microthrombosis; from venous outlet obstruction as in strangulation and portal hypertension.

Clinical Picture

The onset is sudden with generalized colicky pain and diarrhoea in which blood is present at first in an occult state, and eventually is frank. Vomiting may be a feature. The patient is ill, and in a manner which is out of proportion to the initial signs, which may be disconcertingly few. The abdomen may be soft and not tender and little change may be recorded in the pulse rate, blood pressure and temperature.

As the illness develops the abdomen may become tender, silent and distended and signs of circulatory failure will be recorded. If acute mesenteric insufficiency is suspected a peritoneal tap should be undertaken, and if bloodstained, will suggest the diagnosis.

Serum enzymes and a leucocyte count may be non-contributory in the early stage and a high serum amylase may be present in the absence of pancreatitis.

A scout film will show absence of gas in the early stages, but later a picture of ileus. A rosary of gas bubbles in the portal vein is said to be a preterminal sign.

Selective angiography has been recommended by some authors, but both its execution and its interpretation are difficult, and require expert radiological facilities. If mesenteric occlusion is suspected and other conditions can be excluded, it is more sensible to devote one's time to an exploratory laparotomy than to investigations of doubtful significance.

Management

Causal factors must be dealt with and supportive treatment must precede surgery. Cardiac failure must be treated taking great care that neither digitalization nor the use of diuretics be allowed to aggravate the condition.

Fluid loss and haemoconcentration are treated by replacing both water and electrolytes with Hartmann's solution, and protein with plasma.

Mucosal death takes place early and is associated with bacterial invasion. Antibiotics should be given intravenously using either gentamicin (or a related aminoglycoside) or a cephalosporin.

If intravascular coagulation is suspected the patient should be anticoagulated, and there is a place for routine anticoagulation if surgery is to be delayed and thrombus spread is to be halted. Heparin is given as a continuous intravenous infusion, some 10 000 i.u. 6-hourly, and this can be reversed, should surgery be indicated, by the use of protamine sulphate.

Surgery

It is important to determine whether the obstruction is in a major vessel or is at mucosal level. The vessels are examined, starting at the mesenteric border.

If the intestinal vessels and their arcades are pulsating the ischaemia is probably mucosal in origin. A careful and gentle examination of the bowel wall may detect areas of necrosis. If small they are oversewn, otherwise limited excisions are carried out.

If the vessels are not pulsating they are followed retrograde to the origin of the superior mesenteric artery to determine the site of the block. If the bowel wall has lost all viability arterial reconstruction is a useless exercise, the only hope being resection, but in such a case the prognosis is very poor.

If bowel is viable, then the gut must be revascularized. Direct mobilization and exploration of the superior mesenteric artery can be attempted by the experienced surgeon, but in the majority of cases it is far better to offer the bowel an alternative supply of blood, using the very constant ileocolic artery.

The caecum is mobilized and reflected to the left, exposing the ileocolic artery. Further reflection of the ileocaecal region will expose the bifurcation of the aorta and its common iliac branches. The ileocolic artery having been controlled by light tapes, a generous arteriotomy is carried out. A suitable Fogarty catheter is then passed into this opening and then into the superior mesenteric artery up to its origin and onwards into the aorta to dislodge any emboli and thrombus and perhaps retrieve them. The process is repeated until a free flow is obtained. If this is achieved the superior mesenteric artery will start to pulsate and the bowel will pink up. The arteriotomy may then be repaired. If the procedure fails revascularization of the superior mesenteric artery is carried out by a side-to-side anastomosis between the ileocolic and the right common iliac artery, using 5/0 Prolene. Both common iliacs are palpated for any thrombus that may have escaped and if free the clamps are removed; otherwise the thrombi are removed by small arteriotomies.

The abdomen is closed in one layer and 24 hours later a 'second-look' laparotomy is carried out to assess the success of the revascularization, or to excise any non-viable bowel.

A successful operation may be followed by diarrhoea, blood loss and nutritional dysfunction, but these will settle with time and supportive treatment. An occasional successful result rewards the surgeon for the many failures encountered in the treatment of this condition.

FURTHER READING

Beaton H. L. et al. (1983) Intestinal anastomosis in the neonate. *Surg. Gynecol. Obstet.* **3**, 359–360.
Hamilton J. E. (1967) Reappraisal of open intestinal anastomosis. *Ann. Surg.* **165**, 917.
Jönsson K. et al. (1983) Breaking strength of small intestinal anastomosis. *Am. J. Surg.* **6**, 800–803.
Shackelford R. T. (1981) *Surgery of the Alimentary Tract, Vol. II.* Philadelphia, Saunders.

Chapter eighteen

The Appendix and Colon

H. Ellis

THE APPENDIX

Surgical Anatomy (*Fig.* 18.1)

The appendix originates from the posteromedial aspect of the caecum about 2·5 cm below the ileocaecal valve and varies in length enormously from 1 to 25 cm. Its position is extremely variable and indeed it is said to be the only organ without any anatomy. Most frequently the appendix lies behind the caecum (75 per cent of cases). It is usually quite free, although occasionally it may lie beneath the peritoneal covering of the caecum and, if very long, may actually extend behind the ascending colon with its distal portion lying extraperitoneally against the right kidney. In some 20 per cent of cases the appendix lies just below the caecum or hangs into the pelvis. Less commonly it passes in front of or behind the terminal ileum and occasionally lies in front of the caecum or in the right paracolic gutter.

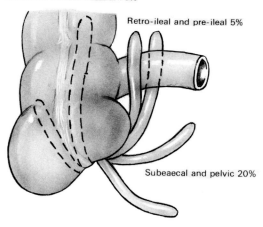

Retrocolic and retrocaecal 75%

Retro-ileal and pre-ileal 5%

Subeaecal and pelvic 20%

Fig. 18.1. Variations in the position of the appendix.

The mesentery of the appendix carries the appendicular branch of the ileocolic artery and descends behind the ileum as a triangular fold (*Fig.* 18.2). The appendicular artery represents the entire vascular supply of the appendix and runs first in the edge of the appendix mesentery and then, more distally, along the wall of the appendix. Thrombosis of branches of this artery in the course of acute infection must inevitably result in gangrene and subsequent perforation. This is in contrast to acute cholecystitis, where the rich collateral vascular supply from the liver bed accounts for the comparative rarity of gangrene of the gallbladder in acute cholecystitis.

Acute Appendicitis

Acute appendicitis is the most common cause of the acute surgical abdomen in this country. The exact incidence is not known because the disease is not notifiable, but probably 125 000 patients are treated annually for acute appendicitis, with some 180 deaths in England and Wales. Its incidence appears to be associated with a Western diet, although the reason for this remains a subject for debate. Although extremely common in Northern Europe, North America, Australia and among the white population of Southern Africa, it is rare in most of Asia, Central Africa and among the Eskimos.

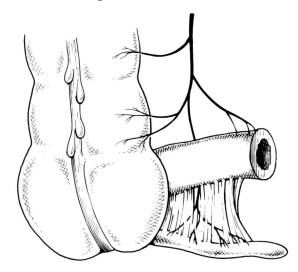

Fig. 18.2. The blood supply of the appendix.

Acute appendicitis is essentially a clinical diagnosis and there is no laboratory or radiological investigation which is diagnostic of the condition. The white count may indeed be raised above 12 000, but in about one-quarter of patients with acute appendicitis the count is normal. The finding of numerous pus cells in the urine on microscopy suggests a urinary tract infection rather than acute appendicitis, but red cells and pus cells may be found if the inflamed appendix involves the adjacent ureter or bladder wall. A plain radiograph of the abdomen may show increased soft tissue density in the right iliac fossa, blurring of the right flank radiolucent line produced by extraperitoneal fat, blurring of the right psoas shadow and occasionally a faecolith in the right iliac fossa. These signs are seen in about 50 per cent of cases of non-perforated acute appendicitis and in some 80 per cent of advanced cases, but may also be seen in about 30 per cent of patients without acute appendicitis who have other causes of acute abdominal pain.

Indications for Operation

In the great majority of cases the treatment of acute appendicitis is urgent appendicectomy—and the sooner the better. There are only four exceptions to this rule:

1. The patient who is desperately ill with advanced peritonitis. Fortunately this is rarely seen in civilized communities nowadays, but here the only hope is to improve the general condition by intravenous fluids, nasogastric suction, broad-spectrum antibiotics and blood transfusion.

2. Where circumstances make operation difficult or impossible, for example at sea or in isolated communities where no surgical facilities are available. Here one has to rely on a conservative regimen and hope that resolution or a local appendix abscess will form.

3. The patient in whom the attack has already resolved. Here, an appendicectomy is advised as an elective procedure and there is no need for urgency.

4. An appendix mass has formed without evidence of general peritonitis (see below).

Operative Technique

If the preoperative diagnosis is one of straightforward uncomplicated acute appendicitis, no specific preoperative steps need be taken apart from those of any routine abdominal operation. However, if the diagnosis is that of perforated appendix with peritonitis, a nasogastric tube is passed, intravenous fluids started and broad-spectrum antibiotic therapy initiated (a third generation cephalosporin or gentamicin, together with metronidazole).

Under the anaesthetic, the abdomen is carefully palpated. Should a mass be felt, the incision can be placed directly over this site. If, however, there is no definite indication of the localization of the appendix, then a routine right iliac fossa skin crease muscle-splitting incision is performed (*Fig.* 18.3). This starts just above and medial to the anterior superior iliac

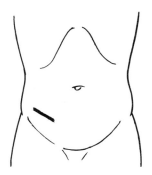

Fig. 18.3. The surface markings of the appendix incision.

spine and is extended medially and slightly downwards. At this level, the rectus abdominis extends two-thirds of the distance from the midline to the anterior superior iliac spine, whereas the oblique abdominal muscles (which are to be split) occupy the lateral one-third (*Fig.* 18.4). Many surgeons in training place the incision far too medially so that it locates

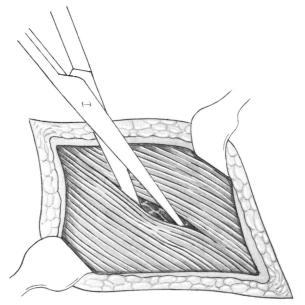

Fig. 18.4. The technique of the muscle-splitting incision for appendicectomy.

over the anterior rectus sheath and not over the oblique muscles. The length of the incision varies according to the build and obesity of the patient. In a very thin subject or a child, a 5-cm incision will suffice. However, in a grossly fat subject, the incision may be three or four times this length for it is preferable to have a rather too long incision than a poor exposure. Once skin and superficial fascia have been divided along the full length of the incision, the external oblique aponeurosis is exposed. This is nicked with the scalpel at its thin medial extremity and then divided along the line of its fibres for the full length of the wound, splitting its muscular part laterally. The external oblique is now retracted, revealing the fibres of the internal oblique muscle, which is fused with the underlying transversus abdominis. These two muscles are to be split together. They are thinnest at the medial extremity of the wound, where they become blended with the lateral edge of the rectus sheath. The tips of the scissors are inserted just at the medial extremity of these muscles adjacent to the rectus sheath. It is a simple matter to penetrate the fibrous expansion, then to insert the tips of the two index fingers into the gap and split the fibres of the muscles along their length (*Fig.* 18.5). Surgical trainees commonly and erroneously attempt to split these muscles at the middle or at the lateral end of the wound, where they are comparatively thick and

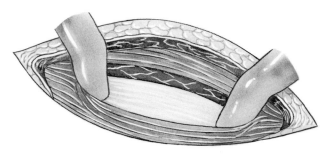

Fig. 18.5. Splitting the internal oblique and transversus muscles.

difficult to divide. The peritoneum, covered by extra-peritoneal fat, is now exposed by retractors. Moistened packs are placed around the wound, the peritoneum held up between two artery forceps and opened with the scalpel, great care being taken to avoid damage to underlying structures.

If difficulty is encountered during subsequent appendicectomy, the surgeon must improve the exposure by extending the incision. This can be undertaken either medially, laterally or occasionally in both directions, the decision naturally depending on the pathology; a difficult retro-ileal appendix needs medial extension, whereas what seems to be an inaccessible retrocolic appendix is mobilized comparatively easily once lateral extension is effected. After lengthening the skin incision, the rectus sheath can be opened widely at the medial end of the wound. Lateral extension is carried out by a combination of splitting and cutting the oblique muscles.

Some surgeons advocate a lower right paramedian incision for appendicectomy, particularly in female patients, or when the diagnosis is in some doubt. There is no doubt, however, that the right iliac fossa incision gives the most direct access to the appendix even in the most difficult cases and this author considers it to be the desirable approach for removal of the appendix. Even when the diagnosis is incorrect in the acute case, a great number of other local pathological conditions can be dealt with through the right iliac fossa incision, especially if it is somewhat extended, and these include ruptured ectopic pregnancy, acute Meckel's diverticulitis and acute caecal diverticulitis. If it is discovered, however, that the cause of the acute abdominal pain is out of reach of the right iliac fossa incision (for example an acute perforated duodenal ulcer or a perforated diverticulitis of the sigmoid colon), then the right iliac fossa incision is left open, an appropriate vertical incision performed, and both are closed at the end of the laparotomy. On the other hand, it may be necessary, having made an inappropriate upper abdominal incision to deal with what was thought to be a perforated peptic ulcer, to carry out a right iliac fossa incision in order to reach the perforated gangrenous appendix!

With the peritoneum opened, the operation of appendicectomy varies in its subsequent steps depending on the pathology and anatomy encountered.

There is usually little difficulty in delivering the early acutely inflamed appendix. The position of the appendix is found by finger palpation and is brought into the wound by drawing the caecum through the abdominal incision, which is a safer manoeuvre than trying to hook out the appendix directly. Occasionally the caecum is extraperitoneal and it is first necessary to mobilize the caecum by dividing its lateral peritoneal attachment to the posterior abdominal wound wall. In cases of difficulty, the appendix is localized by tracing the taeniae coli along the caecum to their junction at the appendix base.

The appendix mesentery may be long, making the operation simple, or the appendix may be closely bound down by congenital adhesions to the caecum and require preliminary mobilization of these strands before the surgeon is able to deal with the vessels in the meso-appendix. The mobilized appendix is grasped and elevated with tissue forceps and the appendicular vessels ligated (*Fig.* 18.6). If running

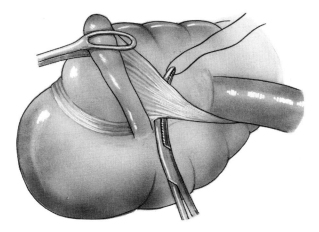

Fig. 18.6. Ligation of the appendicular vessels.

in a narrow pedicle, these may be dealt with by means of a double ligation with thread. When the appendix mesentery is long, it may be safer to clamp and divide the vessels in series, tying each in turn with thread. Should the mesentery be fatty, oedematous or even gangrenous, the ligatures or artery forceps readily cut through the tissues and in this situation transfixion using thread mounted on an atraumatic, curved, non-cutting needle is necessary.

The base of the appendix is now crushed with artery forceps, is ligated with catgut, and the stump surrounded by a purse-string catgut suture which picks up the seromuscular coat of the caecum (*Figs.* 18.7, 18.8). Great care must be taken to avoid pricking blood vessels in the caecal wall (with resultant spreading haematoma), to avoid the bowel lumen and to avoid picking up the edge of the adjacent terminal ileum. The appendix is now removed by dividing its base between the ligated stump and a more

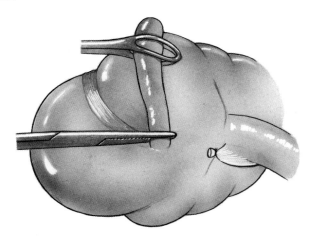

Fig. 18.7. Clamping of the base of the appendix.

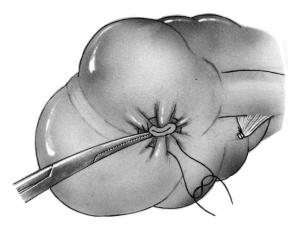

Fig. 18.8. Purse-string invagination of the ligated appendix stump.

distally placed artery forceps, and the purse-string suture is now tied, invaginating the appendix stump. A second purse-string suture invaginates the first and the meso-appendix is now carefully inspected to ensure haemostasis.

If the appendix is gangrenous or perforated this standard procedure may require some modification. The purulent fluid is aspirated, a swab being taken for bacteriological examination. The gangrenous appendix must be mobilized with the greatest care, for it is easy enough to rupture the organ. Once delivered into the wound, the appendix should be wrapped in a small moist swab to prevent further contamination. It may be found that the caecal wall is so oedematous and thickened that invagination is impossible, but fortunately simple ligation of the appendix stump without invagination is perfectly safe. Occasionally the inflamed appendix in the retro-colic position is firmly bound down along the length of the ascending colon and cannot be delivered into the wound. In such circumstances, a retrograde appendicectomy should be performed. The base of the appendix is freed, its base ligated, clamped and divided with invagination of the stump. Using the artery forceps to lift up the divided appendix at its

base, the rest of the appendix mesentery is then serially clipped with artery forceps, divided and tied until the tip has been reached.

Closure

The muscle-splitting incision comes together once relaxation anaesthetic is terminated. The peritoneum is closed with chromic catgut, the transversus and internal oblique muscles are left unsutured and one or two chromic catgut stitches are used to appose the external oblique aponeurosis. The skin is closed with interrupted nylon sutures. A few extra catgut sutures are required where the rectus sheath has been opened or the oblique muscles divided laterally.

Where there is a local abscess, gross infection or difficulty in closing the stump, a corrugated drain is brought out through the lateral extremity of the wound and left for 2 or 3 days.

The Appendix Mass

If a patient has walled off his or her perforated appendix into an appendix mass, there is usually a 4- or 5-day history of abdominal pain, associated with a swinging fever and an elevated pulse rate. Examination reveals a tender mass in the right iliac fossa, which can often also be reached on rectal examination. However, the rest of the abdomen is soft, bowel sounds are present and there is no evidence of a generalized peritonitis. In such cases, the initial treatment is conservative. The patient is put to bed on a fluid diet and careful watch is kept on the general condition, the temperature and pulse and the size of the mass, which is marked out on the abdominal wall with a skin pencil. Antibiotics are not prescribed at this stage because they merely result in a honeycomb of chronic abscess cavities, the so-called 'penicillinoma', although a short course of metronidazole may safely be used. On this regimen, about 80 per cent of appendix masses resolve, but in the remainder the swelling obviously enlarges over the next 1 or 2 days and the swinging fever continues. In such circumstances, the appendix should be drained through a small incision over the apex of the mass with no attempt at appendicectomy (*Fig.* 18.9).

Whether resolution occurs or whether drainage is required, appendicectomy should be recommended after an interval of 3 months which allows the inflammatory condition to settle completely. Unless interval appendicectomy is performed, there is a high risk of a further episode of acute appendicitis.

Postoperative Complications

There is a great difference between the usually rapid recovery which follows removal of an early acutely inflamed appendix and the frequently stormy course of the patient operated on for a gangrenous and perforated appendix. This latter situation still accounts

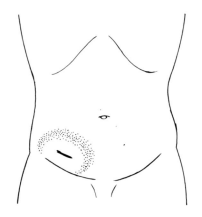

Fig. 18.9. Drainage of an appendix abscess.

for the majority of cases of peritonitis in this country today and with it the invariable associated paralytic ileus.

PARALYTIC ILEUS

Management comprises relief of pain by means of regular doses of morphine, gastric aspiration by means of a nasogastric tube, fluid and electrolyte replacement by intravenous therapy, antibiotic therapy guided, whenever possible, by checking the sensitivity of the responsible organisms, and a careful watch for any localized collection of pus which may require later drainage. Such collections are particularly liable to be found in the subcutaneous space below the incision itself or in the subphrenic spaces or in the pelvis.

Paralytic ileus, if persisting, offers the important differential diagnosis from mechanical obstruction. This decision is vital since the former requires continuation of conservative therapy whereas the latter calls for urgent laparotomy to relieve the small bowel obstruction.

Differential diagnosis is based on the following points: paralytic ileus rarely lasts for more than 3 or 4 days. Persistence of symptoms after this time is always suspicious of mechanical obstruction. An absolutely silent abdomen is diagnostic of paralytic ileus whereas noisy bowel sounds indicate a mechanical cause. The ileus is relatively painless, whereas colicky abdominal pain is present in mechanical obstruction. If symptoms begin after the patient has already passed wind or has had a bowel action, it is very likely that mechanical obstruction has supervened.

The most important and helpful investigation is a plain radiograph of the abdomen. A diffuse distribution of gas throughout the small and large bowel, right down to the rectum, is indicative of paralytic ileus, whereas a localized loop of distended small intestine with fluid levels and without gas shadows in the large bowel is strongly in favour of mechanical obstruction.

SEPTIC COMPLICATIONS

A local wound abscess is a common complication of appendicectomy performed for gangrenous appendicitis. Removal of a suture and gentle probing of the wound release the pus and resolution occurs within a few days. As with the treatment of an abscess anywhere in the body, it is judicious and adequate drainage and not antibiotic therapy that cures the patient rapidly.

Pelvic abscess may follow generalized peritonitis but is particularly common after removal of a perforated appendix. The patient is febrile and toxic, and may complain of diarrhoea with a mucous rectal discharge. Rectal examination reveals a pelvic tender mass which is occasionally large enough to be palpated abdominally.

In the great majority of cases, drainage occurs into the vagina or rectum spontaneously, sometimes assisted by firm pressure by the finger in the rectum. Occasionally, drainage needs to be performed through the rectum or the posterior fornix of the vagina. For this purpose, a pair of sinus forceps is gently passed into the softest part of the mass under a general anaesthetic.

Subphrenic abscess is a much less common complication of peritonitis following acute appendicitis. It is more commonly seen after peritonitis of upper abdominal origin, such as a perforated peptic ulcer or leaking gastrointestinal anastomosis. Pus may collect in either the right or the left subphrenic spaces, lying between the diaphragm and the liver and separated from each other by the falciform ligament, or in the right or left subhepatic spaces below the liver, the right forming Morison's pouch and the left being the lesser sac. About two-thirds of subphrenic abscesses occur on the right side and rarely they may be bilateral.

Subphrenic infection usually follows 10 days to 3 weeks after a general peritonitis, although if antibiotics have been given abscess formation may be disguised and delayed, becoming manifest weeks or even many months after the original episode. There may be no localizing signs and symptoms whatsoever, the patient merely presenting with malaise, loss of weight, anorexia, anaemia and a fever. There may, however, be localizing features of pain in the upper abdomen, the lower chest, or referred to the shoulder, with localized tenderness and signs at the left base.

The white count is raised to the region of 15 000–20 000 ($15 \cdot 0$–$20 \cdot 0 \times 10^9/L$) with a polymorph leucocytosis.

Radiographs of the chest and upper abdomen reveal elevation of the diaphragm on the affected side, a pleural effusion, often accompanied by collapse of the lung base, and a gas and fluid level seen below the diaphragm; the latter occurs in about three-quarters of the cases. Accurate localization may be achieved by ultrasonic scan or computed tomography.

In early cases, where there is no gas or free fluid on radiography, broad-spectrum antibiotic therapy is initiated. If there is a rapid response, the diagnosis is one of spreading cellulitis in the subphrenic space. If resolution fails to occur, or if there is radiological evidence of a localized abscess, surgical drainage is performed. Depending on the localization of the abscess, this is carried out either by a posterior approach through a small incision immediately below the 12th rib, or via an anterior subcostal incision. (*See* Chapter 23.)

Carcinoid Tumour of the Appendix

By far the most common neoplasm of the appendix is the carcinoid tumour, which is found in about 0·1 per cent of all appendices subjected to careful histological examination. Macroscopically, the tumour consists of a yellowish plaque with intact overlying mucosa, which later ulcerates. About three-quarters of the tumours occur at the tip of the appendix and only unusually are they found at the appendix base. Microscopically, the carcinoid is made up of enterochromaffin Kulchitsky cells, which take up silver stains and which arise in the crypts of the intestinal mucosa. Metastatic spread from carcinoid of the appendix is very rare and is practically confined to lesions which are larger than 2 cm in diameter. Such tumours occur only in about 1 per cent of carcinoids of the appendix. The majority of carcinoids are found incidentally on routine histological study of appendices removed during the course of laparotomies for other procedures. Acute appendicitis is not commonly caused by this tumour because of its usual location at the tip of the organ. However, the lumen may be occluded by tumours at the base or in the body of the appendix so that carcinoid may present as a case of acute appendicitis or even an appendix abscess.

If the tumour is discovered at operation, either in dealing with an acutely inflamed appendix or as an incidental finding at laparotomy, the remainder of the small intestine should be carefully examined for other carcinoid tumours, for occasionally these may be multiple. The liver is carefully palpated and the regional lymph nodes examined with care. In the vast majority of cases, the findings will be completely negative, and under such circumstances, particularly if the carcinoid tumour is smaller than 2 cm in diameter, nothing more is required than to carry out appendicectomy. In those rare cases where the tumour is large and/or regional nodes are obviously involved, right hemicolectomy is necessary.

If the diagnosis is not established until the pathological examination of the specimen has taken place, no further procedure need be carried out if this shows that the carcinoid tumour has been completely removed. If the carcinoid involved the base of the appendix and histological examination showed that resection had been incomplete, then there would certainly be a case under these circumstances for re-operation with excision of an adequate cuff of surrounding caecal wall.

The carcinoid syndrome, the results of secretion of serotonin (5-hydroxytryptamine), occurs only in those cases with extensive masses of tumour, usually in the presence of multiple liver deposits, and is very rarely seen in carcinoids originating from the appendix.

COLON

Anatomy

The large intestine is subdivided, for descriptive purposes, into the caecum with the appendix, the ascending colon, hepatic flexure, transverse colon, splenic flexure, descending colon and sigmoid (*Fig.* 18.10).

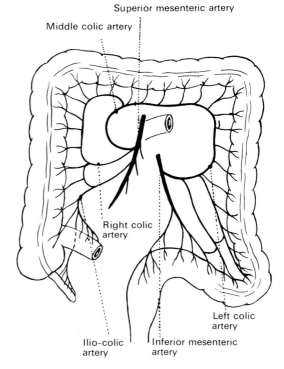

Fig. 18.10. The anatomy of the large bowel and its blood supply.

The large bowel may vary quite considerably in length in different individuals with an average of about 90 cm. At operation the colon is readily identified because of its three flattened bands, the taeniae coli, which begin at the base of the appendix and run the length of the large intestine to end at the rectosigmoid junction. These represent the great bulk of the longitudinal muscle of the large bowel and, because they are shorter than the gut to which they are attached, the colon becomes condensed into its typical sacculated shape. The colon, but not the appendix, caecum or rectum, also bears the characteristic fat-filled peritoneal tags, the appendices epiploicae, which are scattered over its surface and which are especially numerous in the sigmoid loop. The transverse colon is specifically identified by its attachment to the great omentum.

The transverse and sigmoid colon are completely peritonealized. The ascending and descending colon have no mesocolon but adhere directly to the posterior abdominal wall; exceptionally the ascending colon may be wholly or partly peritonealized. The caecum may or may not be completely surrounded by peritoneum (the latter more likely in the female subject), and the appendix, although usually free within its own mesentery, occasionally lies extraperitoneally behind the caecum and ascending colon or adheres to the posterior wall of these structures.

The arterial supply of the colon is derived from branches of the superior and inferior mesenteric arteries. The first branch to the colon from the superior mesenteric artery is the middle colic branch, which originates from the right side of the vessel, enters the transverse mesocolon and divides into its right and left branches; the latter supplies the transverse colon to the region of the splenic flexure and represents the most distal extent of the superior mesenteric blood supply. The right colic artery is relatively small, originates some 5 cm more distally to the middle colic and supplies the ascending colon. The ileocolic artery originates another 5 cm below this and is the only constant branch of these three right-sided colonic vessels. It supplies the terminal ileum, caecum and start of the ascending colon and gives off the appendicular branch to the appendix, the most commonly ligated intra-abdominal artery. The right colic and middle colic arteries are variable and may arise from a common trunk. The right colic artery may originate from the ileocolic artery in about 10 per cent of subjects.

The inferior mesenteric artery arises from the aorta at the level of the 3rd lumbar vertebra and gives off the left colic artery to supply the descending colon, the sigmoid branches, which supply the sigmoid colon, and then descends as the superior haemorrhoidal artery to supply the rectum.

Each branch of the superior and inferior mesenteric artery to the colon anastomoses with its neighbour above and below, so that there is a continuous vascular arcade along the whole length of the large bowel. The anastomosis of this marginal artery (of Drummond) may be small or incomplete between the left branch of the middle colic and the uppermost extent of the left colic in the region of the splenic flexure, and this is the region where ischaemic lesions of the colon are most likely to occur.

The venous drainage of the colon takes place along correspondingly named veins; the inferior mesenteric vein ascends above the point of origin of its artery to enter the splenic vein behind the pancreas. The superior mesenteric vein joins the splenic vein behind the neck of the pancreas to form the portal vein.

Lymph Drainage

The arrangement of the lymph nodes of the intestine is relatively uniform in both small and large bowel (*Fig.* 18.11). Numerous small nodes lie near, or on,

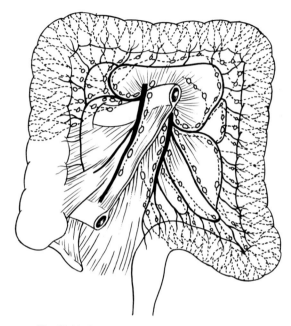

Fig. 18.11. Lymph drainage of the large intestine.

the wall of the intestine and these drain into intermedially placed and rather larger nodes along the vessels of the mesentery and mesocolon. These in turn drain to clumps of lymph nodes situated near the origins of the superior and inferior mesenteric vessels. From these nodes, efferent lymphatics drain into the cisterna chyli.

The lymphatic drainage field of each segment of intestine corresponds fairly accurately to its arterial supply. Thus high ligation of the vessels to the involved segment of gut with removal of a wide surrounding segment of mesocolon will remove the lymph nodes which drain the area; thus division of the middle colic vessels and resection of the wedge of transverse mesocolon would, for example, clear the lymphatic drainage in resection of a growth of the transverse colon.

Diverticula of the Colon

A 'diverticulum' is an abnormal pouch which opens from a hollow organ. In Roman times the word was applied to a wayside house of ill fame and well the diverticula of the colon deserve this name.

Modern Terminology

Until recently, clinicians, radiologists, and pathologists used the term '*diverticulosis*' to imply a colon bearing diverticula in an entirely symptomless patient. '*Diverticulitis*' referred to inflammation of one or more diverticula. Diverticulitis was further subdivided into 'acute' and 'chronic'. The clinical features of the former were easy to define, since these included free perforation and local abscess formation. Those of the latter were considered to be due to long-standing inflammatory changes in the wall of the colon which were manifested clinically by pain, tenderness, constipation and subacute obstruction, while radiologically the barium enema appearances were those of narrowing and distortion of the affected segment of the colon. However, Morson (1963) published detailed studies of specimens of so-called 'chronic diverticulitis', resected by the surgeons at St Mark's Hospital, which showed no evidence at all of chronic inflammation; he applied the term '*diverticular disease*' to denote this situation. The obstructive features in these cases were due to the thickening of the colon musculature together with the further narrowing produced by concertina-like folds of the mucous membrane.

Modern terminology defines three groups of patients (*Fig.* 18.12). The first and very largest comprises subjects with symptomless diverticula; this is termed 'colonic diverticulosis'. The second is made up of those patients presenting with acute inflammation of the diverticulum and its complications, termed 'acute diverticulitis'. The third group is made up of patients with symptomatic disease with no evidence of inflammatory change. The term 'diverticular disease' is a useful description of this state of affairs.

Diverticulosis is entirely symptomless and can only be diagnosed either on routine barium enema examination or discovered at laparotomy or postmortem examination.

Diverticular disease is characterized by lower abdominal discomfort or pain, especially in the left iliac fossa or generalized across the lower abdomen, episodes of severe colic, abdominal distension with belching and often excessive passage of flatus, constipation—which may be complicated by episodes of spurious diarrhoea—and there may be passage of mucus and even of blood per rectum. Not infrequently there are associated dyspeptic symptoms of nausea and heartburn. The patient may even present with acute large bowel obstruction. Clinical examination reveals a tender, thickened sigmoid colon.

Acute diverticultis may present with the features that have been well termed 'left-sided appendicitis', which may settle down over a number of days of conservative treatment or progress to abscess formation, with the development of a paracolic abscess in the left iliac fossa. The acutely inflamed diverticulum may perforate into the general peritoneal cavity rather than forming a local abscess. This, the most serious and acute complication of acute diverticulitis, leads to a general peritonitis, which may be either purulent, from leakage of an enlarging pericolic abscess, or of faecal peritonitis from a wide perforation of a diverticulum. Pericolic inflammation may also lead to perforation into an adjacent organ, particularly the bladder (more commonly in men than women) but also into an adjacent loop of colon, small intestine or vagina. Drainage of a pericolic abscess may lead to a faecal fistula onto the abdominal wall (*Fig.* 18.13).

Haemorrhage may occur either as minor blood loss or as a major sudden bleed. Indeed, severe bright red rectal haemorrhage in the absence of obvious piles is most likely due to diverticula of the colon. The exact pathology of the bleeding is still under debate and in the majority of cases there is no pathological evidence of acute inflammation. Haemorrhage is particularly likely to occur in elderly patients with hypertension and arteriosclerosis, especially in those with diffuse diverticula affecting the whole colon. It may be that haemorrhage in these cases is due to rupture of a tortuous or even aneurysmal

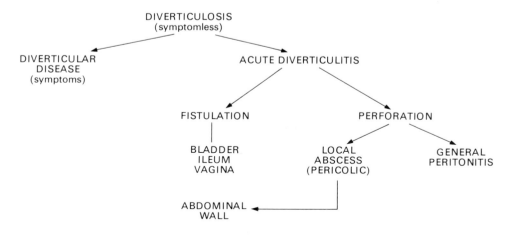

Fig. 18.12. Diverticulosis and its complications.

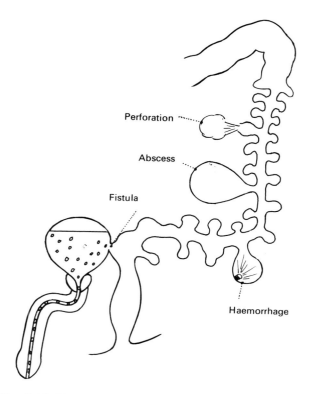

Fig. 18.13. The complications of acute diverticulitis in diagram form.

vessel in relation to a diverticulum or to angiodysplasia.

Acute obstruction may result from diverticular disease alone, or from the associated oedema of pericolic inflammation. Occasionally the obstruction may be due to the adherence of a loop of small intestine to the inflamed segment.

Surgery for Diverticular Disease

The great majority of cases of uncomplicated diverticular disease respond satisfactorily to a high roughage diet containing plenty of fruit, vegetables and bran (Painter, 1975). If medical treatment fails, and the patient's symptoms of subacute obstruction persist, the conventional treatment is resection of the affected segment of colon, with end-to-end anastomosis. Indeed, this remains the standard treatment where there is stricture formation or fistula, and is described later. It may also be needed if, at laparotomy, a clear distinction from carcinoma is not possible. However, recently there has been increasing interest in the procedure first described by Reilly (1970), which is designed to deal with the underlying pathology of thickening of the colonic muscle. He compared the appearance of thickened muscle wall to the pyloric muscle seen in congenital hypertrophic pyloric stenosis and reasoned that an operation similar to Ramstedt's pyloric myotomy might be of benefit when dealing with the thickened colonic wall of diverticular disease. This operation of sigmoid myotomy is valuable in patients with severe diverticular disease without associated inflammatory complications.

Sigmoid Myotomy

SURGICAL TECHNIQUE

Bowel preparation comprises a few days on a fluid diet, emptying the bowel by means of rectal washouts aided by a preliminary dose of magnesium sulphate; metronidazole is given with the premedication. The purpose of this mechanical emptying and attempted sterilization of the large bowel is prophylactic, should there be accidental opening of the lumen of the colon during the operation.

After induction of anaesthesia, a Foley balloon catheter is passed into the bladder and continuous drainage instituted. A lower left paramedian incision is employed. A full laparotomy is performed to ensure that there is no other intra-abdominal pathology. The sigmoid colon is then mobilized by division of its avascular lateral peritoneal attachment. An incision is made along the anti-mesocolic border of the sigmoid colon from the rectosigmoid junction proximally along the full length of the thickened colonic wall; this will usually be found to be from 25 to 40 cm in length. The incision is initially made with the scalpel through serosa and outer muscle wall and is then deepened by means of scissors dissection until the mucous membrane bulges through the divided muscle wall (*Fig.* 18.14). Bleeding is rarely a problem and can be controlled by gauze pressure. Perforation of the mucosa should not occur but, if it does, the hole should be sutured by means of fine catgut and a corrugated drain passed down to the affected area. Routine abdominal closure is carried out and, as might be expected from such a simple procedure, the postoperative course should be uneventful and certainly more benign than can be anticipated following the more extensive procedure of colonic resection.

Sigmoid Resection

In many cases of diverticular disease requiring surgical treatment, the surgeon may feel that a simple sigmoid myotomy would be insufficient to deal with the pathology encountered. For example, when associated diverticulitis has produced severe stricturing of the bowel, protracted pericolic infection, adherence or even fistulization into adjacent viscera, or gross inflammatory disease, sigmoid resection should be undertaken. The left colon is mobilized by division of its lateral peritoneal attachments. The left ureter is identified and carefully preserved. The limits of the gross disease are defined and the levels of resection decided on; there is no need to remove the whole of the colon affected with diverticula since this may greatly increase the extent of resection. Further infec-

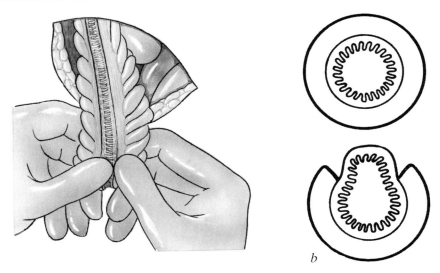

Fig. 18.14. Sigmoid myotomy. *a*, The incision along the thickened sigmoid colon. *b*, The incision is deepened down to the mucosa.

tion in residual diverticula following resection of the main inflammatory mass is very uncommon.

Since the condition is benign, there is no need to carry out wide resection of the mesocolon, which can be divided close to the bowel wall (*Fig.* 18.15). This procedure preserves the vascularity of the cut ends of the colon at the site of anastomosis and ensures that adjacent structures, especially the ureter, are completely safe.

The affected segment of sigmoid loop is removed between Payr crushing clamps, ensuring an adequate blood supply to the cut edges of the colon. Anastomosis is performed using two layers of continuous thread sutures; the outer (serosal) layer may be either interrupted or continuous and the inner layer comprises a simple over-and-over continuous full thickness suture, turning the corner from the posterior to the anterior layer by means of one or two loops on the serosa (*Figs.* 18.16–18.19). The mesocolic defect is closed with a continuous thread suture and the omen-

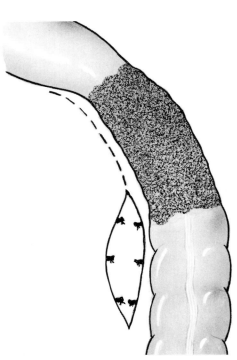

Fig. 18.15. Resection of sigmoid colon for diverticulitis; the mesocolon is divided close against the bowel wall.

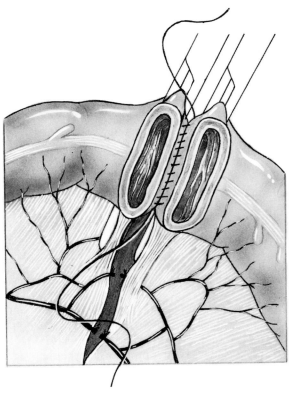

Fig. 18.16. Sigmoid resection for diverticulitis: the first layer of the anastomosis.

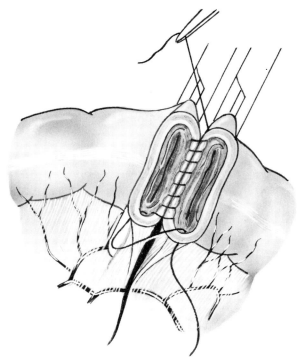

Fig. 18.17. The second layer of the anastomosis.

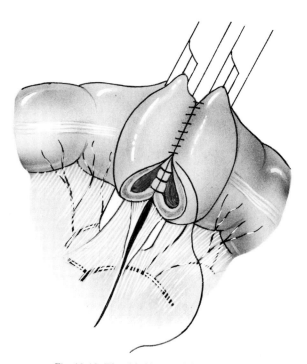

Fig. 18.18. The third layer of the anastomosis.

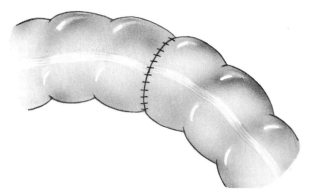

Fig. 18.19. The fourth layer of the anastomosis.

One-layer Anastomotic Technique

Many surgeons favour a one-layer technique for bowel anastomoses. Indeed, I use this myself on occasions although I must express a preference for the two-layer anastomosis for no reason other than habit. Controlled trials have not demonstrated any difference between the two methods as regards leakage rate in colonic anastomosis.

The two ends of colon are held apposed in non-crushing bowel clamps. The posterior layer comprises interrupted simple or vertical mattress sutures of thread placed at intervals of 2 or 3 mm (*Fig.* 18.20*a*). Each corner can be turned by either a continuation of the mattress sutures or by the Connell loop on the mucosal stitch (*Fig.* 18.20*b*). The anterior layer is completed by simple or vertical mattress sutures (*Fig.* 18.20*c*).

If there is any question at all of distal obstruction, a hazardous suture line, or if the anastomosis is performed low down in the pelvis or in the presence of a chronic abscess, the operation should be completed by carrying out a simple loop transverse colostomy performed through a short transverse right upper abdominal incision. The loop of colon is opened for a length of 3 cm and the cut edge of the colon sutured to the lips of the stab incision in the skin by means of a continuous catgut suture (*Fig.* 18.21).

The closure of such a relieving colostomy is carried out 3 or 4 weeks later when the abdominal wound is soundly healed and when the anastomosis has been proved to be intact by means of a limited barium enema examination. If this should reveal any evidence of leakage, however, then colostomy closure should be delayed for a further month.

Surgical Management of the Complications of Diverticulitis

1. *Perforation*

It is not usual for a confident diagnosis of perforated diverticulitis to be made; more often it is simply one of a list of possibilities which are encountered in

tum brought down and wrapped around the anastomotic line. The wound is closed in the routine manner and a corrugated drain passed down to the region of the anastomosis through a lateral stab incision.

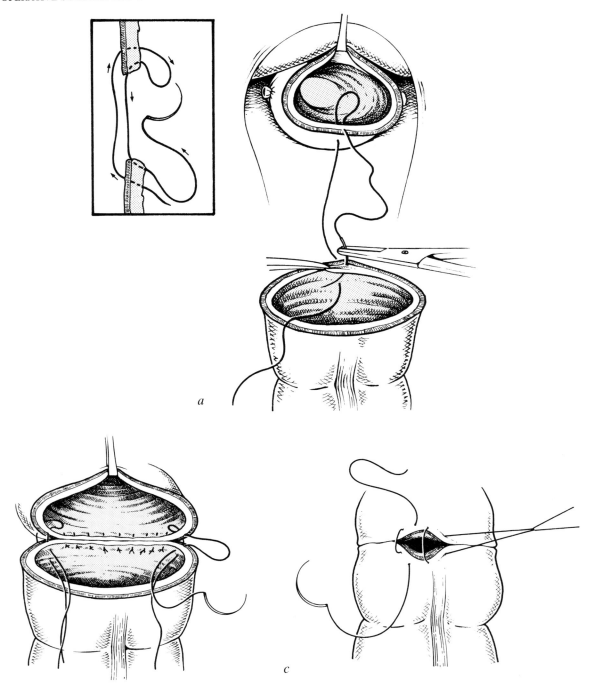

Fig. 18.20. Single-layer colon anastomosis. *a*, Using interrupted vertical mattress sutures of thread placed at intervals of 2 or 3 mm. *b*, Each corner may be turned by a continuation of the mattress sutures or by the Connell loop on the mucosal stitch. *c*, Completion of the anterior layer by simple or vertical mattress sutures.

middle-aged or elderly patients with generalized peritonitis. As a preliminary to laparotomy, a nasogastric tube is passed, intravenous fluid and electrolyte replacement instituted and broad-spectrum antibiotic therapy begun using a cephalosporin or gentamicin, together with metronidazole.

The abdomen should always be palpated under the

anaesthetic. A mass in the sigmoid colon may then be felt which will guide the surgeon to perform a left paramedian incision. If this is not so then the usual routine right paramedian exploratory incision is performed. Pus, faeces or a mixture of the two are encountered on opening the peritoneal cavity and the inflammatory mass in the sigmoid colon is soon

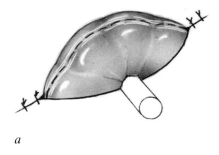

a

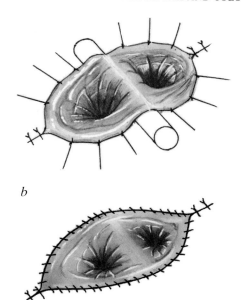

b

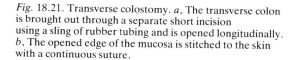

Fig. 18.21. Transverse colostomy. *a*, The transverse colon is brought out through a separate short incision using a sling of rubber tubing and is opened longitudinally. *b*, The opened edge of the mucosa is stitched to the skin with a continuous suture.

revealed. A swab is taken for bacteriological examination. In some instances, no obvious perforation can be detected and under these circumstances we can assume that the perforation has sealed. A transverse colostomy is performed and the abdominal wound closed with drainage. When there is an obvious perforation in the bowel (and this is usually to be found when faecal material is present in the peritoneal cavity) there is some controversy about management. The more conservative approach comprises an attempt to suture the perforation (which usually fails because the stitches cut out from the oedematous colonic wall) or of patching the perforation by means of a pedicled or free omental graft. A transverse colostomy is performed and the area of perforation drained. The more aggressive approach is to resect the affected segment after a preliminary mobilization of the left colon. No primary anastomosis is performed but the ends of the colon brought out as proximal and distal colostomy openings (Hartmann's operation). If the distal stump cannot be brought up to the abdominal wall it should be closed.

The advantage of the conservative procedure is its simplicity and it is to be recommended to the inexperienced surgeon. The disadvantage is that an inflamed infected segment of colon, loaded with faeces and with a poorly closed perforation, persists distal to the colostomy and may produce continued sepsis and fistula formation. The advantage of the more radical resection is removal of the septic colonic segment, but this procedure is safe only in the hands of experienced surgeons.

If the patient survives the initial emergency, later staged resection and closure of the colostomy can be carried out if the conservative method has been used, or closure of the colostomy performed if resection has been effected at the initial operation. It must be pointed out that, in many elderly and feeble patients who have survived this serious emergency, a permanent colostomy may be accepted, and no further procedure is required.

2. Pericolic Abscess

This is more common than free perforation. Treatment is initially conservative. The patient is put to bed on a fluid diet, the extent of the mass marked with a skin pencil on the abdominal wall, with a 4-hourly chart recording the temperature and pulse. Antibiotic therapy should not be prescribed at this stage since it simply leads to a honeycomb of chronic abscesses, the so-called 'penicillinoma'.

If the condition progressively subsides, a subsequent elective resection should be advised after thorough investigation of the patient, which will include sigmoidoscopy and barium enema.

If the mass increases in size, together with continued pyrexia and a rising pulse, then surgical intervention is necessary. The abscess is drained through a small lateral incision over the mass. At the same time, a 'blind' loop transverse colostomy is performed through a small transverse incision in the right upper abdomen in order to defunction and decompress the left colon. Once the whole affair has settled down (usually a question of many weeks or even months) then resection of the affected segment can be performed, followed by closure of the colostomy.

3. Fistula Formation

Fistula formation in the presence of diverticulitis is far from uncommon. As a general surgical principle, it is useless merely to separate the adherent viscus from the diseased segment of colon and to expect that healing will follow. Recurrence of the fistula is almost invariable. In the case of a vesicocolic fistula, it must be decided whether or not the symptoms warrant surgery. If the patient is elderly and frail, he or she may in fact be little inconvenienced by the fistula and is best left alone. In the majority, however, the symptoms demand surgical treatment (*Fig. 18.22*). In the first place it is best to carry out a defunc-

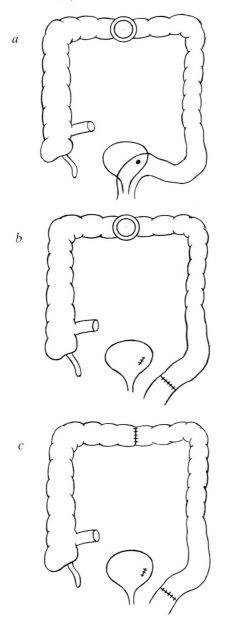

Fig. 18.22. a, Preliminary colostomy. *b*, Resection of sigmoid; closure of fistula. *c*, Closure of colostomy.

tioning transverse colostomy. After some weeks, the inflammatory process will settle down and will enable a much safer second stage to be performed, at which the fistula between colon and bladder is separated, the perforation into the bladder carefully closed with two layers of catgut, the affected segment of colon resected with end-to-end anastomosis and the bladder drained by means of a Foley catheter for 5–7 days. After a delay of some weeks, closure of the colostomy can be carried out.

Occasionally, a feeble, elderly or obese patient with distressing symptoms may require no more than a defunctioning colostomy to relieve the symptoms of the fistula where it is considered that the three-stage procedure outlined above may be too severe a strain.

4. Intestinal Obstruction

Immediate resection is contra-indicated when the diverticular disease is sufficiently far advanced to produce intestinal obstruction. Here, a limited laparotomy is performed, the diagnosis confirmed and a transverse loop colostomy carried out with immediate opening of the colostomy as described above. Resection of the obstructing mass is carried out at a second stage followed by closure of the colostomy after a further period of 3 or 4 weeks.

5. Massive Haemorrhage

Fortunately, the majority of patients with severe haemorrhage associated with diverticula of the colon settle down with conservative treatment in the form of bed rest and blood transfusion. If bleeding continues, surgery becomes obligatory. It is then usually impossible to localize the bleeding site by external examination of the bowel at the time of laparotomy, although a preoperative colonoscopy and/or intestinal arteriogram may give some information about the site of bleeding, if carried out while active haemorrhage is taking place. If there is no clue localizing the site of bleeding, subtotal colectomy with ileorectal anastomosis should be performed. Lesser procedures such as multiple colotomies to determine the source of bleeding are usually unhelpful. If only a partial colectomy is performed it will often be found that further haemorrhage takes place from the residual colon, forcing the surgeon to carry out the more major resection in the much more dangerous situation of a second surgical procedure on a seriously ill patient.

Cancer of the Colon

Carcinoma of the colon, if diagnosed at an early stage, is eminently suitable for surgical resection, with one of the most reasonable prognoses of the common cancers. Here, the principle of the operation is wide resection with adequate removal of the relevant draining lymphatic field and immediate restoration of continuity of the bowel. However, many patients still present with intestinal obstruction and here, except for the relatively unusual obstructing cancers of the right colon, immediate restorative resection is unwise and preliminary colostomy drainage indicated. Other cases may be complicated by invasion of adjacent organs, but here judicious wide resection may still give gratifying results. In others, metastatic deposits may already have spread to the liver and here careful consideration must be given to the possibility of resection for maximum palliation.

Special Investigations

The barium enema examination remains the mainstay of diagnosis of cancers of the caecum and colon. Sigmoidoscopy should never be omitted and enables visualization of growths at the rectosigmoid region with biopsy confirmation of the diagnosis. Even with cancers higher in the bowel, sigmoidoscopy is vitally important to exclude a small second synchronous tumour lower in the bowel or the presence of associated benign polyps. In cases of doubt, fibre-optic colonoscopy may enable a suspicious area to be visualized and biopsy material to be obtained. A routine haemoglobin check is carried out and blood transfusion given preoperatively if anaemia is present. The operation itself will usually be associated with little loss of blood unless this comprises the resection of a large tumour involving adjacent viscera.

Meticulous preoperative bowel preparation is mandatory, as described earlier (p. 223).

Liver function tests and liver scanning are of little value in practical terms. If metastases are clinically undetected, both biochemical tests and scanning have a disappointingly low pick-up rate and even if the tests are positive the abdomen must still be explored in order to assess whether or not palliative resection is worthwhile. Moreover, it would be a disaster if it were to be subsequently found that the abnormal liver tests were due to cirrhosis or that the filling defects on the scan were due to benign cysts or angiomas and that the opportunity of curing a patient of an early cancer had been missed.

Surgical Resection: General Considerations

Certain general principles apply to all resections of carcinoma of the large bowel and can be enumerated before describing the individual operations in more detail.

Preoperative preparation of the bowel is important in order to reduce faecal contamination and bacterial concentration within the lumen. The regimen has already been described under 'Sigmoid myotomy' (p. 223).

A full preliminary laparotomy is mandatory before a final decision is taken as to whether or not resection is possible and, if so, the extent of the operation.

It is wise to palpate the liver for secondary deposits before assessing the primary tumour. The extent of the growth and the possibility of adjacent visceral involvement are assessed. The whole of the large bowel is then carefully examined, since it is not unusual to discover a second primary tumour. At the same time, careful note is made of the state of the large bowel proximal to the growth; the presence of obstruction or of heavy faecal loading of the bowel may indicate that a preliminary colostomy might be necessary before resection is attempted at a second stage. Careful examination of the draining lymph nodes is made in order to determine the presence of clinically obvious lymph node metastases.

When the primary tumour is mobile and there is no clinical evidence of distant spread, curative resection is indicated. A number of scattered liver metastases should not preclude palliative resection, in order to save the patient the miseries of uncontrolled local disease, but if there is extensive hepatic spread, then fine judgement must be used as to whether resection should or should not be attempted. Invasion of adjacent structures again requires careful assessment to determine whether *en bloc* resection is still feasible and this may include anterior or posterior abdominal wall, omentum, stomach, duodenum, small intestine, kidney and pelvic organs. If there is doubt, a trial dissection is always justified for the results of radical surgery in advanced local carcinoma in the absence of evidence of distant dissemination may be surprisingly good (Pittam et al., 1984).

During resection care must be taken to prevent the dissemination and implantation of tumour cells. The growth itself should be wrapped in a gauze pack as soon as possible and packs used to protect the wound edges. Irrigation of the open ends of the bowel at the time of anastomosis should be carried out using a 1 in 500 dilution solution of mercury perchloride or cetrimide.

Position of Patient and Choice of Incision

The positioning of the patient and the choice of incision depend on the site of the cancer and on the build of the patient. Growths of the caecum and of the ascending transverse and descending colon are operated on with the patient supine and horizontal. If the patient is obese, it is advisable to tilt him or her to the opposite side (using either sandbags or a tilting table) in order to allow the small intestine to fall away from the operative site. If the growth is situated in the sigmoid colon, the patient should be tipped into the Trendelenburg (head-down) position which, again, enables the small bowel to be packed away from the operative site as well as assisting with the illumination of the operative area.

The patient should be catheterized when it is anticipated that the operation field will include the pelvis, as in resection of the sigmoid colon, but with tumours situated higher in the large intestine, catheterization is not normally required. An intravenous drip is started as a routine although, under normal circumstances, the transfusion of blood will only rarely be necessary.

An extensive area of the abdomen should be prepared, using iodine in spirit, although a wide range of antiseptics is available. The operative drapes should expose a wide expanse of the abdomen; it may be necessary to extend the incision or to site a colostomy or caecostomy, and inevitably drainage will be required through a separate stab incision. It is a mistake to 'towel up' too narrowly around the proposed line of incision.

For tumours extending from the caecum to mid-transverse colon I prefer a right paramedian incision and use a left paramedian for more distally placed tumours. These incisions give magnificent access, can be extended in either direction and, if necessary, in a grossly fat patient with a lateral adherent tumour, can be extended by means of a transverse limb. Other surgeons employ a transverse or an oblique muscle-cutting incision, but I find that this gives some limitation to full surgical access and is less convenient for the placing of a colostomy or caecostomy, should this be necessary.

Right Hemicolectomy

Right hemicolectomy is indicated for operable carcinomas of the caecum, ascending colon and the hepatic flexure.

A long right paramedian incision is employed and tumour evaluation carried out at full laparotomy as already described. The small bowel is packed off medially. The right colon is freed by incising the lateral peritoneal attachment from the posterior abdominal wall and the right colon mobilized from the posterior abdominal wall to the root of the mesocolon. During this mobilization, the spermatic or ovarian vessels, the ureter and the second part of the duodenum are visualized and carefully preserved from injury.

The hepatic flexure and the right side of the transverse colon must now be mobilized (*Fig.* 18.23). If the tumour is well proximal, this is performed by separating the greater omentum from the right extremity of the transverse colon along what is almost a bloodless plane. If, however, the growth is situated in the hepatic flexure or if the omentum is actually adherent to the tumour, then the adjacent omentum requires detachment and removal with the operative specimen. As soon as possible during mobilization tapes are passed above and below the tumour and firmly ligated to reduce intraluminal dissemination of cancer cells and the tumour itself is wrapped in a gauze pack held by ligatures in order to minimize the handling of its serosal surface.

With the right side of the bowel completely mobilized, the ileocolic and right colic pedicles are tied near their origins using double ligation with thread

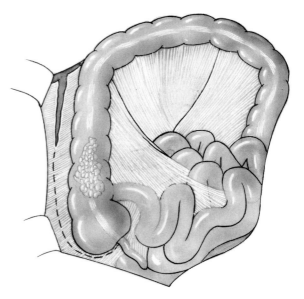

Fig. 18.23. Right hemicolectomy: mobilization of the ascending colon.

and the branches of the middle colic pedicle to the right colon are divided (*Fig.* 18.24). Division of the mesocolon is continued up to the edge of the transverse colon and downwards across the small bowel mesentery to the wall of the terminal ileum. The exact site of division of terminal ileum and transverse colon is chosen with particular attention to the adequacy of the blood supply at the site of the anastomosis and to ensure that at least an 8-cm clearance is obtained beyond the macroscopic edge of the growth. The site of division of the ileum is usually 8–10 cm from the ileocaecal valve.

It is my own practice usually to perform an anastomosis between the end of the ileum and the side of the transverse colon since the colon is much wider

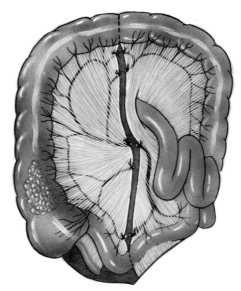

Fig. 18.24. Right hemicolectomy: ligation of vascular pedicle.

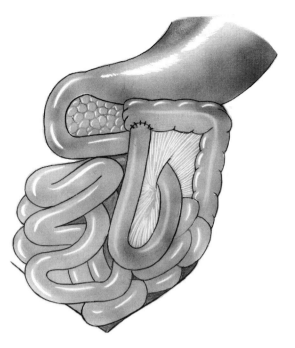

Fig. 18.25. Right hemicolectomy: ileotransverse anastomosis.

be certain that haemostasis is satisfactory. The defect in the mesocolon is closed with a continuous thread suture, care being taken not to prick a blood vessel in either the mesentery or the mesocolon. The remaining omentum is drawn over the anastomotic line and can be tacked over it with one or two interrupted sutures. The abdomen is closed after placing a corrugated drain down to the site of the anastomosis and bringing this out through a separate stab wound.

Resection of Transverse Colon

This is indicated for resection of growths in the transverse colon and comprises removal of the major parts of the transverse colon, its mesocolon and the greater omentum (*Fig.* 18.26).

The stomach is detached from the transverse colon by serial division of the branches of the gastro-epiploic arcade, which are tied with thread and then

than the terminal ileum (*Fig.* 18.25). In some cases there is little disparity in the size of the lumen of small and large bowel and under these circumstances an end-to-end anastomosis can be safely performed. Some surgeons carry out a side-to-side anastomosis having first closed the open end of the ileum and transverse colon. This is time consuming and moreover provides three suture lines, rather than the one of the end-to-end and the two of the end-to-side operations respectively, and I have personally never found any need of, or advantage in, the side-to-side anastomosis.

Having chosen the site of division, the transverse colon is divided between Payr crushing clamps and the ileum divided between non-crushing intestinal clamps. The transverse colon is closed using two layers of 2/0 linen thread. The first is passed loosely through all coats of the colon over the crushing clamp, which is then removed and the suture line pulled tight and tied. The second layer comprises a continuous invaginating layer of the serosal coat. The transverse colon is then picked up in a non-crushing intestinal clamp and apposed to the open end of the terminal ileum. A continuous thread seromuscular suture apposes the peritoneal coats and the colon is then incised longitudinally to a length corresponding to the open lumen of the small intestine. Any faecal material is carefully swabbed away and the open ends of the bowel washed with 1 in 500 perchloride of mercury solution. The inner layer of all-coats 2/0 linen thread is then carried out and the serosal suture then covers the anterior wall. The non-crushing clamps are removed and the anastomosis then checked, both to ensure an adequate lumen and to

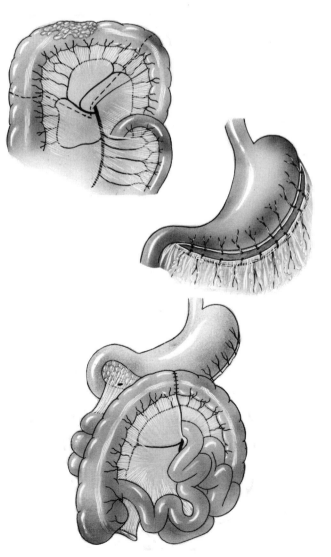

Fig. 18.26. Transverse colectomy: the extent of the resection.

divided between the ligatures. Mobilization continues as far as the hepatic and splenic flexures. The detached transverse colon is held upwards and the middle colic vessels tied at their origins and divided. The transverse mesocolon is incised in an inverted V up to the bowel edge at the selected site of resection. If necessary, with a tumour situated at one or other extremity of the transverse colon, it may be necessary to mobilize the ascending or the descending colon by lateral peritoneal division in order to ensure an anastomosis without tension. Having decided on the level of resection, which must be at least 8 cm from the macroscopic edge of the tumour, the bowel is divided proximally and distally between Payr crushing clamps.

The technique of end-to-end anastomosis in two layers is similar to that described for resection of the sigmoid colon in diverticulitis (*see* p. 223).

Left Colon Resection

Left hemicolectomy is performed for resections of tumours of the descending colon. The left colon is mobilized in a manner similar to the procedure on the right side (*Fig.* 18.27) but is rather more difficult

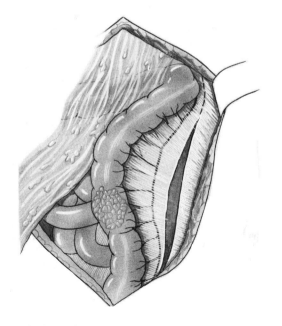

Fig. 18.27. Resection of the left colon: mobilization of the colon.

on account of the higher and more inaccessible position of the splenic flexure. When this is deeply placed in an obese subject, it is better first to mobilize the transverse colon by detaching the greater omentum, to mobilize the descending colon from its lateral peritoneal attachment and then to draw both of these downwards. This enables the splenic flexure to come into view and allows division of the phrenico-colic ligament.

The exact extent of resection depends on the size and site of the tumour, together with the state of the regional lymph nodes. A radical resection of the left colon may necessitate anastomosis between the transverse colon and rectosigmoid. Less extensive resections may require anastomosis of the transverse colon to the sigmoid loop but, in many cases, where there is a relatively small tumour situated in the sigmoid colon itself, resection of the sigmoid loop may suffice with anastomosis of the mobilized descending colon to the rectosigmoid junction. The sigmoid colon itself is readily mobilized by division of its lateral congenital attachments, carefully preserving the genital vessels and the left ureter.

A radical left hemicolectomy will necessitate ligation of the inferior mesenteric pedicle together with the sigmoid branches and the left extremity of the middle colic vessels. A more restricted left hemicolectomy divides the left colic and upper sigmoid vessels and resection of the sigmoid colon itself necessitates only ligation of the sigmoid vessels.

The details of the anastomotic procedure are as described above.

Postoperative Complications

Resection of the colon may be followed by any of the local and general complications which can occur after major abdominal surgery. The important disaster which needs a special note is leakage at the anastomosis. This is especially likely to occur when the blood supply to the cut ends of the bowel is in jeopardy, when the anastomosis has been made under tension, or where the resection has been carried out in the presence of gross distension of the bowel or of heavy faecal loading. No site is immune, but the low anterior resection, performed below the level of the pelvic peritoneal reflection, is at particular risk. It is unusual for a severe degree of leakage to take place distal to a protective colostomy.

Unfortunately, diagnosis is often delayed. Leakage should be suspected in the presence of abdominal pain, distension, toxaemia, a tender swollen reddened wound, a rising temperature and pulse, and abdominal tenderness with guarding and rebound. More often it is only when frank peritonitis is obvious or when there is discharge of faeces through the wound or the drain that the surgeon wakes to the fact that dehiscence of the bowel suture line has occurred.

These cases can be divided into two groups. In the first, there is a minor degree of discharge without any evidence at all of a generalized peritonitis. This may be seen occasionally after closure of a colostomy or where the anastomosis has been protected by a proximal colostomy or caecostomy. Many of these cases are probably accounted for by the rupture of a small abscess at the suture line. Under these circumstances, the patients should be carefully observed, as spontaneous closure of the fistula may be anticipated.

The second group comprise those patients with frank breakdown of the anastomosis with faecal peritonitis. Treatment now needs to be swift if the patient's life is to be saved. Broad-spectrum antibiotic therapy is begun, blood transfusion made available and urgent laparotomy performed. The wound is reopened; no attempt should be made to repair the leakage, but exteriorization of the two ends of the anastomosis must be performed. The contaminated peritoneal cavity is cleared of faecal debris by lavage with saline followed by noxythiolin, povidone iodine or an antibiotic-containing solution.

Obstruction due to Carcinoma

Acute obstruction due to carcinoma of the bowel is a common complication which is much more often seen in association with tumours of the left rather than the right side of the colon. This is partly accounted for by the fluid nature of faeces and the larger lumen of the colon on the right side, the tendency for right-sided tumours to be proliferative compared with the more common constricting growths on the left side and also because the commonest site for cancers in the colon is the sigmoid loop. Dilatation of the colon associated with stretching and occlusion of the blood supply to its wall may result in the development of patches of gangrene which may perforate, producing a generalized peritonitis. This is most frequently seen in the caecum and it is here that gangrene and perforation are most likely to occur. In other instances there may be a stercoral perforation of the colon immediately above the obstruction as the result of pressure necrosis from impacted faeces.

Preoperative radiographs of the abdomen are useful in confirming the diagnosis, and the distribution of the gaseous distension will usually locate the site of the obstruction with a reasonable degree of accuracy.

All patients require a nasogastric tube to empty the distended stomach and fluid and electrolyte replacement by means of an intravenous drip.

In dealing with the acute large bowel obstruction due to neoplasm there are a number of options available. There is the possibility of immediate resection with restoration of continuity of the bowel; the tumour can be resected with exteriorization of the divided ends (the Paul–Mikulicz or Hartmann procedure); a laparotomy with decompression of the bowel by colostomy or caecostomy may be performed and finally a blind decompression may sometimes be indicated.

In general, resection and immediate anastomosis should not be performed in the presence of an obstructed large bowel, which is oedematous and has its blood supply in jeopardy, for there is considerable risk of leakage at the anastomosis under these circumstances. The exception to this general rule is a right hemicolectomy for an obstructing carcinoma of the right colon, for the ileocaecal valve is often competent, the small bowel either not dilated or only moderately affected, and the colon distal to the obstruction is collapsed, with a normal blood supply. In these circumstances right hemicolectomy may be performed but if the patient's general condition is poor or if there is gross obstruction, a caecostomy may be indicated as a preliminary procedure. In some circumstances the obstruction may be due to an extensive and adherent growth in the ascending colon which is of doubtful resectability, and here an anastomosis side to side between the ileum and the transverse colon should be carried out as a definitive palliative procedure.

Resection with exteriorization can be undertaken in mobile segments of the large bowel, that is to say the transverse or sigmoid colon. The divided ends are brought out as a double-barrelled colostomy which can be subsequently closed. These operations may be valuable in the presence of a perforated or gangrenous colon but most surgeons, in circumstances other than these, favour preliminary decompression with subsequent elective resection.

In the majority of cases the obstruction will be found to be situated in the left side of the colon. Laparotomy enables the extent and the site of the tumour to be assessed and then the colon is decompressed by means of a transverse colostomy brought out through a separate incision. The colostomy can be opened immediately, which allows decompression of the distended bowel. In those instances where the growth is in the transverse colon itself, a caecostomy is performed. After 2 or 3 weeks and when the patient's condition has improved, a second-stage resection is carried out and subsequently the colostomy or caecostomy is closed.

In some desperate cases, where the patient's condition is extremely grave, a 'blind' transverse colostomy or caecostomy is performed, if necessary under a local anaesthetic. Study of the preoperative radiographs may localize the distended segment of large bowel. This operation has the disadvantages of the inability to exclude necrosis of the bowel wall and it does not enable an exact diagnosis to be made. It should be regarded only as a last-resort attempt at saving life.

Colostomy

A colostomy is an opening made into the large bowel with a view to diversion of its contents to the exterior. The common sites are transverse colon and sigmoid colon and the following types of colostomy are described:

1. Loop Colostomy

This is usually performed as a temporary vent, for example as a first-stage decompression before proceeding to resection of an obstructing tumour or to provide a temporary 'safety valve' above an anastomosis. It has the advantages of being simple to fashion and easy to close.

2. *Double-barrelled Colostomy*

Here the bowel is divided and each end brought out as a separate stoma through the abdominal wall. This may be part of a Paul–Mikulicz procedure or may be performed when it is essential that no faecal material passes into the distal segment of the bowel, for example where the colostomy is performed above a perforation or a faecal fistula.

3. *End Colostomy*

This is a permanent colostomy in which the divided end of the sigmoid is brought out as a colostomy after abdomino-perineal excision of the rectum or after a Hartmann operation, in which the rectum is excised but the anal stump left *in situ*.

Transverse Colostomy

A transverse colostomy is frequently performed for the relief of intestinal obstruction due to carcinoma or diverticulitis of the sigmoid colon. It may also be required in cases of perforation of a sigmoid diverticulitis, pericolic abscess or vesico-colic fistula and may be utilized in order to protect the anastomosis in a low anterior resection of the rectum.

It may be performed 'blind' in desperate cases of very advanced obstruction, but is more often performed after a preliminary laparotomy.

Although some surgeons advocate bringing out the colostomy through the laparotomy wound itself, this is to be condemned since it will inevitably be followed by serious wound infection and a high risk of dehiscence, and late hernia formation.

The transverse colostomy should be situated at a small transverse incision placed in the right upper quadrant and dividing the right rectus muscle. The length of this incision will depend on the size and degree of obesity of the patient. If the transverse colon is grossly distended and difficult to handle, it may require decompression by means of a trocar attached to the suction pump, closing the site of puncture by means of a purse-string suture. The omentum is separated at the proposed site of colostomy formation from the transverse colon to the right of the main middle colic pedicle. Clearing the omentum in this fashion makes it much easier to bring the transverse colon through the separate incision. A small opening is made through the mesocolon through which is passed a length of rubber tubing. An artery forceps is passed through the transverse colostomy wound, grasps the loop of rubber tubing and is employed to draw the loop of colon through the incision. Gentle traction on the loop maintains the transverse colon in position while the main abdominal incision is closed.

Two procedures which are still used in the construction of a transverse colostomy are now mentioned only to be condemned. The first is the passage of a large glass rod under the colostomy loop which is held in place by attaching a loop of rubber tubing to each end. This is designed to keep the loop of bowel in position, but it merely produces an ugly oedematous colostomy over which it is almost impossible to attach any effective colostomy appliance. The other procedure is to delay opening the colostomy for 1 or 2 days, which simply leaves the patient completely obstructed for a still further period of time. In fact, all that is necessary is to open the colon lumen immediately, using the cutting diathermy, suck away the liquid contents of the bowel with the suction apparatus, and to suture the full thickness of the open bowel to the skin edge using a continuous 2/0 catgut suture (*see Figs.* 18.21*a* and *b*). This has the double advantage of immediately decompressing the bowel and of producing a neat colostomy which is easily accommodated into the modern adherent colostomy appliances. My own preference is a square of Stomahesive with a central opening just larger than the colostomy itself. An adhesive colostomy bag is then applied to the square. Stomahesive completely protects the surrounding skin without any risk of skin sensitization.

In those circumstances where a double-barrelled transverse colostomy (Devine colostomy) is required, the mesocolon is divided to the right of the main middle colic pedicle, tying the vascular arcade at the bowel edge. The transverse colon is divided using De Martel clamps and the proximal and distal limbs brought out through separate transverse incisions on either side of the laparotomy wound. Having then closed to the abdominal incision, the bowel edges are sutured to the skin edges on either side, establishing a terminal colostomy for the proximal loop and a mucous fistula at the distal end of the divided bowel.

Sigmoid Colosotomy

Occasionally a loop colostomy is fashioned in the sigmoid colon in a similar manner to the technique of transverse colostomy. More often, this is fashioned as an end colostomy as part of abdomino-perineal excision of the rectum and is described with this operation (*see* p. 245).

Closure of Colostomy

Formal closure of a colostomy is carried out once the distal anastomosis is soundly healed, and this should be delayed until a check barium enema examination has been carried out. Moreover, the patient should have made a complete recovery from major surgery before this relatively minor operation is undertaken.

The operation can be performed if necessary under local anaesthesia but usually a general anaesthetic is employed. Dissection is facilitated by infiltrating the subcutaneous tissues around the colostomy stoma with a 1 in 250 000 adrenaline solution. An elliptical skin incision is fashioned around the colostomy and dissection carried down to the wall of the colon. A relatively avascular plane is then entered, which enables the colon to be freed from its attachment to the anterior abdominal wall and the peritoneum is opened all around the colostomy loop. The attached rim of skin is now trimmed away with scissors and the stomal wound sutured transversely using a continuous all-coats layer of 2/0 linen thread. The closed loop of colon is returned within the abdominal cavity and the abdominal wall sutured. A corrugated drain is led down to the peritoneal opening.

Recurrent large bowel carcinoma

Recurrence of symptoms after an apparently curative resection of a large bowel tumour will often indicate hopeless recurrent or metastatic disease. However, the following other possibilities should be born in mind (Ellis, 1984):

1. Useful palliation may be achieved by a short circuit or colostomy in the presence of unresectable obstructing recurrent cancer.

2. Occasionally recurrence at the anastomosis or a distant metastasis (including occasionally a solitary deposit in the liver) may be amenable to further potentially curative resection.

3. Metachronous cancer elsewhere in the large bowel may occur in about 5 per cent of long-surviving colonic resections and long-term survival after resection of one or even more such metachronous lesions is well recognized.

4. Occasionally an entirely benign lesion such as a fibrous stricture at the anastomosis or a chronic para-anastomotic abscess may mimic recurrent disease; this happy state of affairs should always be considered.

There has been much interest in the possibility that serial estimations of carcinoembryonic antigen (CEA) might enable detection of early asymptomatic recurrent disease in large bowel cancers, allowing more effective second-look surgery. Wanebo (1981) has pointed out that in four reported series the percentage of positive explorations ranged from 78 to 94 per cent and the incidence of resectable disease from 7 to 72 per cent.

While there is no question that a rising CEA titre following curative resection indicates the probability of recurrent or metastatic disease, it remains to be seen whether second-look surgery based on these estimations will give better results than those obtained by exploring patients with clinical evidence of localized resectable recurrences (Northover, 1985).

Total Colectomy

The most common indication for total removal of the colon (usually combined with excision of the rectum, proctocolectomy) is ulcerative colitis. The operation may also be required for extensive Crohn's disease of the large bowel and for polyposis coli.

In ulcerative colitis the operation is required for two main indications. The first is the emergency situation, that is to say the patient with fulminating colitis, perhaps complicated by perforation, drenching haemorrhage or toxic dilatation of the colon. Under these circumstances, the colon is removed and an ileostomy and a proctostomy performed (see Fig. 18.28). Occasionally severe haemorrhage may necessitate immediate resection of the involved rectum also. At a later date, when the emergency is over and the patient restored to reasonable health, consideration can then be given either to excision of the rectal stump or to performing ileorectal anastomosis between the two exteriorized segments of the bowel. The second group of indications for the operation are elective. These are the patients who have failed to respond to medical therapy or have distressing local or general complications of the disease, including stricture formation, malignant change, gross perianal disease, arthritis and pyoderma gangrenosa. Here the possibility of ileorectal anastomosis may be considered, although the majority of patients will require proctocolectomy and permanent ileostomy.

Investigations and Preparation

In an emergency, little can be achieved by, and time cannot be expended on, elaborate investigations. However, it is important to check for, and to correct, any preoperative anaemia or biochemical disturbances and to remember that many of these patients are on large doses of steroids, so that intravenous hydrocortisone cover will be begun before the operation. Broad-spectrum antibiotics are indicated on account of the very real risk of the patient having either established peritonitis or a rupture of the colon, with considerable peritoneal contamination during the mobilization of the friable bowel. Gentamicin or cephalosporin together with metronidazole is a suitable combination.

In elective cases, the situation is very different. As well as the investigations already described, an attempt must be made preoperatively to delineate the extent of the disease and the presence of local complications in the bowel in addition to attempting to establish the differential diagnosis between ulcerative colitis and Crohn's disease.

Sigmoidoscopy and biopsy are, of course, mandatory. Very severe involvement of the rectum usually precludes any question of its preservation with ileorectal anastomosis.

Fibre-optic colonoscopy will give valuable indication of the extent and severity of the disease and enables any suspicious areas and polypoid lesions to be submitted to biopsy examination.

Barium enema will give information concerning the extent of the disease, the presence of strictures or suspicious areas of malignant change, and often enables a fairly confident differential diagnosis to be made between ulcerative colitis and Crohn's colitis.

A barium meal and follow-through examination are useful in patients with suspected or established Crohn's disease of the large bowel to determine whether or not there is radiological evidence of co-existing small bowel involvement.

Preoperative preparation includes the correction of anaemia, if necessary by blood transfusion, and careful attention must be paid to the general nutrition of the patient, which is often impaired in long-standing cases of colitis. The bowel preparation is similar to that already described above (*see* p. 223) and systemic antibiotics are required because of the risk of operative contamination.

The siting of the ileostomy should be decided on preoperatively. Usually this is fashioned in the right lower quadrant as a tunnel through the rectus muscle. With the patient lying in the supine position, a transverse line is drawn across the abdomen immediately below the umbilicus. Another vertical line is constructed from the pubis to the umbilicus. An ileostomy ring is placed between these two lines (*see Fig.* 18.29) and the centre of this disc represents the site of the ileostomy stoma. If there is extensive scarring at this site, the left lower quadrant may be the position of choice. The patient is sat up and is asked to lean slightly forwards; this is to ensure that the central aperture of the ileostomy appliance will rest at the summit of the fat roll of the lower abdomen. Obesity, emaciation or extensive scarring from previous surgery may make the surgeon alter the situation of the stoma. It is just as well to make the patient acquainted with the ileostomy apparatus and where it will be situated before he or she is submitted to the operation.

General Considerations

Considerable judgement is necessary in the choice of the particular operation to be carried out in each specific case. It has been mentioned that in most emergency situations the life-saving procedure will be total removal of the colon combined with ileostomy and the fashioning of a proctostomy of the proximal end of the divided rectosigmoid through a small separate incision low down in the left iliac fossa. This has the great advantage of removing the vast bulk of the diseased bowel without the need to perform an intra-abdominal suture line. However, in some cases of massive and continued bowel haemorrhage, bleeding may continue from the rectal stump and under these circumstances an immediate emergency proctocolectomy may be indicated.

For the elective operation, the majority of surgeons carry out proctocolectomy and permanent ileostomy as a one-stage operation. The advantages of this procedure over ileorectal anastomosis are that complications are undoubtedly less, there is no possibility of recurrence or reactivation of the disease in the rectal stump nor is there risk of subsequent malignant change in the rectal mucosa. If the indications for surgery are the presence of marked systemic manifestations, only total removal of the diseased bowel will prove effective. Ileorectal anastomosis may be complicated by intestinal fistula formation, stricture formation, recurrence of the complications of the disease and in some cases the very severe associated diarrhoea may prove intolerable to the patient. The great advantage of ileorectal anastomosis, of course, is the preservation of the anal sphincter, and there are many patients who are prepared to put up with all sorts of risks and disadvantages for this one important positive feature. Ileorectal anastomosis should not be considered in those patients where there is already malignant change in the bowel, where the rectum is severely damaged or where the operation is being performed for very severe systemic manifestations, such as joint involvement, iritis, etc. This sphincter-preservation procedure, however, is a worthwhile undertaking particularly in young people who have a reasonable rectal stump both in Crohn's disease and in ulcerative colitis. Long-term results are much better in the colitic than in the patient with colonic Crohn's disease, where rectal recurrence is common.

Operative Procedure

Total colectomy is most efficiently performed through a long left paramedian incision (*Fig.* 18.28).

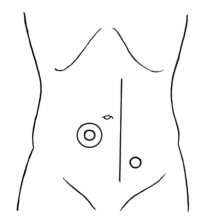

Fig. 18.28. Total colectomy: the abdominal incision and location of the ileostomy. Also shown is the location of a proctostomy, if this is to be used.

The details of the mobilization and removal of the colon are a synthesis of the steps previously described in right-, transverse and left-sided colectomies and need not be repeated in detail. There are, however, two differing features from those resections which are carried out for malignant disease rather than when the total colectomy is performed in cases of colitis uncomplicated by malignant change. First, since the operation is performed for benign disease, there is no need for extensive removal of the meso-colon, and the line of division can be kept very comfortably adjacent to the colon wall. Second, again because the procedure is being performed in a benign situation, the greater omentum should be detached from the transverse colon at an early stage in the operation and carefully preserved attached along the greater curvature of the stomach. At the end of the operation, this enables the greater omentum to be drawn down as a protective sheet under the long abdominal incision and thus act as a useful barrier, preventing the adherence of loops of small bowel to the deep aspect of the abdominal wound.

Removal of the rectum in proctocolectomy again requires no separate description since this is almost identical to abdomino-perineal excision of the rectum for malignant disease. Again, this being a benign condition, the surgeon may stay fairly close to the bowel wall, thus diminishing the risk of impotence and bladder sphincter disturbances.

Ileorectal anastomosis is similar to that of an anterior resection of the rectum (*see* Chapter 19), except that it is the terminal ileum which is brought down to the rectal stump. It is a mistake to try to make the rectal excision too extensive since a small rectal reservoir is associated with intolerable diarrhoea. My own practice is to carry out the anastomosis comfortably at the rectosigmoid junction. The anastomosis should be protected by a temporary loop ileostomy.

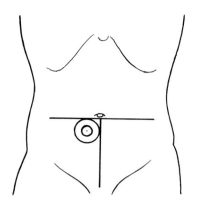

Fig. 18.29. Fashioning the ileostomy wound in the abdominal wall.

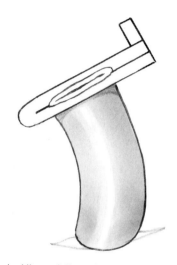

Fig. 18.30. Terminal ileum delivered through the ileostomy orifice.

Ileostomy

The site of the ileostomy will already have been carefully marked out before operation. After total mobilization of the colon and division of its associated mesocolon, the terminal ileum is divided between De Martel crushing clamps and the large bowel is removed. These small clamps are particularly easy to bring through the ileostomy stomal opening. A circular incision about 2·5 cm in diameter is made through the skin at the ileostomy site (*Fig.* 18.29). The rectus sheath is divided in a cruciate manner and the underlying rectus muscle split. The peritoneum is opened and the muscle orifice dilated digitally so that it will admit the index and middle fingers. The clamp holding the divided ileum is then brought out through this orifice for a length of 8 cm beyond the skin edge (*Fig* 18.30). Great care is taken to avoid twisting the bowel during this procedure. The space between the mesentery of the emerging ileum and the abdominal wall is closed by a series of interrupted thread sutures, care being taken to avoid damaging vessels in the mesentery. This procedure has the double advantage of closing a potential internal hernia and of anchoring the terminal ileum in position against the parietal wall of the abdomen. The main abdominal incision is now closed and carefully protected to prevent contamination when the ileostomy is fashioned. The clamp is removed from the cut end of the ileum and the divided edge everted as a cuff over the projecting ileum to produce a mucosal covered nipple about 4 cm in length. The mucosal edge is then carefully sutured to the cut edge of the skin using a continuous running suture of 2/0 chromic catgut (*Fig.* 18.31).

The operation is completed by the application of a suitable ileostomy appliance. The most satisfactory apparatus to use immediately postoperatively is a sheet of Stomahesive with the central orifice cut out exactly to fit the size of the ileostomy. This is applied firmly to the skin and an ileostomy bag is attached to the Stomahesive. This appliance is completely waterproof and non-irritant so that excoriation of the skin, which was once such a problem in the early establishment of the ileostomy, is now rarely seen.

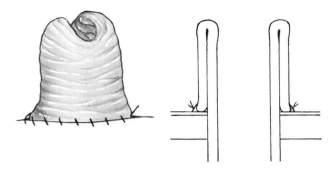

Fig. 18.31. Fashioning of the ileostomy.

Postoperative Complications

The postoperative complications after total colectomy are those seen after any major abdominal operation, but the incidence of postoperative intestinal obstruction due to adhesions is particularly high in most reported series. This is probably because many surgeons remove the whole of the greater omentum and thus, as we have already noted, the small bowel is likely to become tethered to the abdominal wall or pelvic floor closure. If the omentum can be preserved and brought down as a protective layer, the incidence of this complication can be considerably reduced (Ellis, 1982).

The ileostomy itself may be the site of a number of specific complications. Occasionally the blood supply of the terminal ileum is jeopardized and necrosis of the ileostomy ensues. A fistula at the mucocutaneous junction may develop, particularly if deep sutures are used in forming the ileostomy, and these should be avoided. The ileostomy may prolapse or may retract. Under all these circumstances, refashioning of the ileostomy, with careful attention to the technical details described above, is mandatory.

Volvulus

Volvulus of the large bowel occurs most commonly in the sigmoid colon and the caecum. A few cases of volvulus of the transverse colon and of the splenic flexure have been reported. It is a comparatively rare disease in the United Kingdom, Western Europe and North America, but is one of the most common causes of acute intestinal obstruction in Eastern Europe, Russia, Scandinavia, India and Africa.

The twisting of the bowel occurs around its mesocolic axis and results in a closed-loop type of obstruction. This may take either a subacute or recurrent form, or may constitute an acute type if there is tight compression of the blood vessels in the mesocolon. The rotated loop of bowel becomes immensely distended and, if the acute obstruction is not properly relieved, gangrene and perforation supervene with an often fatal peritonitis.

The aetiology of volvulus probably depends on a combination of congenital and acquired factors. There may be an unduly long and mobile mesosigmoid or mesocaecum and it is probable that racial anatomical variation may be at least one factor in the wide geographical variations in the incidence of this condition. Among acquired factors may be adhesions producing narrowing of the base of attachment of a loop of bowel or fixation of its apex to the parietes. A bulky vegetable diet may lead to overloading of the sigmoid colon and certainly the geographical distribution of volvulus corresponds to those populations who live on a mainly bulky vegetarian diet.

Volvulus of the Caecum

This is a misnomer for, in the majority of cases, the adjacent small bowel and ascending colon are involved in the twisted bowel segment.

The patient presents with the features of large bowel obstruction and there is often a history of previous recurrent subacute attacks. The abdomen is grossly distended, but with asymmetry of the abdomen. Gross dilatation of the right side of the colon may produce a tympanitic mass, which may be situated in the right iliac fossa or which may flop over onto the left side of the abdomen.

Radiologically there is gross distension of the caecum, which is often abnormally placed and which may be located in the left upper quadrant of the abdomen and be mistaken for a dilated stomach. A single fluid level is present in the caecum (compared with the usual two large fluid levels in cases of sigmoid volvulus). Distended loops of small intestine are also present.

Treatment comprises urgent operative intervention. The twist has usually taken place in a clockwise direction and if the bowel is viable, gentle detorsion is carried out. The distended loop is then both decompressed and prevented from further volvulus by the fashioning of a temporary caecostomy. Resection is indicated when reduction proves impossible or when the involved segment is obviously gangrenous. The choice lies between a primary right hemicolectomy or exteriorization-resection, which is the wiser procedure in a late case with a seriously ill patient.

Sigmoid Volvulus

In most cases, the twist takes place in an anticlockwise direction. It may present either as an acute episode of sudden complete obstruction, or there may be multiple subacute attacks or occasionally there may be a chronic volvulus. The rapid inflation of the abdomen is a strikingly characteristic feature of volvulus of the sigmoid, and this diagnosis should always be entertained in a case of intestinal obstruction accompanied by massive distension.

Radiological examination of the abdomen usually

reveals a tremendously distended sigmoid loop which may even elevate the diaphragm. The huge gas shadow may be looped on itself, giving the typical 'bent inner-tube sign', and there may be two fluid levels on the erect film, one in the proximal and one in the distal limb of the obstructed sigmoid loop. In late cases there is progressive distension of the distal colon and small intestine with gas and fluid.

Conservative treatment consists of an attempted passage of a soft flatus tube through a sigmoidoscope which is inserted as high as possible into the rectum, with the patient under a general anaesthetic. Gentle manipulation frequently enables the tube to enter into the twisted segment which is followed by a flood of liquid faeces and flatus. If reduction does not take place, the tube should be left *in situ*, to be manipulated into the sigmoid loop at operation.

Operative treatment is required if this conservative method fails or, in advanced cases, with evidence that strangulation or perforation may have taken place. The abdomen is explored through a long left paramedian incision with the rectal tube left in place. The twisted sigmoid loop is reduced and the rectal tube threaded into it in order to facilitate decompression. If reduction is impossible or if gangrene is already present, a Paul–Mikulicz exteriorization is performed, with subsequent closure of the colostomy.

Because of the risk of subsequent retorsion, an elective resection is advised in those patients who have been treated conservatively or by simple untwisting of the volvulus.

REFERENCES

Ellis H. (1982) The causes and prevention of intestinal adhesions. *Br. J. Surg.* **69**, 241–243.

Ellis H. (1984) Second look laparotomy. In: Ellis H. and Schwartz S. (eds.) *Maingot's Abdominal Operations.* New York, Appleton-Century-Crofts.

Morson B. C. (1963) The muscle abnormality in diverticular disease of the sigmoid colon. *Br. J. Radiol.* **36**, 385–392.

Northover J. M. A. (1985) Carcinoembryonic antigen and recurrent colorectal cancer. *Br. J. Surg.* **72**, Supplement S. 44–6.

Painter N. S. (1975) *Diverticular Disease of the Colon: A Deficiency Disease of Western Civilization.* London, Heinemann.

Pittam M R., Thornton H. and Ellis H. (1984) Survival after extended resection for locally advanced carcinomas of the colon and rectum. *Ann. R. Coll. Surg. Engl.* **66**, 81–84.

Reilly M. C. T. (1970) Colonic diverticula: surgical management. *Br. Med. J.* **3**, 570–572.

Wanebo H. J. (1981) Are CEA antigen levels of value in the curative management of colorectal cancer? *Surgery* **89**, 290–294.

Chapter nineteen

The Rectum and Anal Canal

W. S. Shand

SURGICAL ANATOMY AND PHYSIOLOGY

Relations and Structure

The rectosigmoid junction lies approximately at the level of the third sacral vertebra and is a bend of variable acuteness. It was supposed at one time that a sphincter existed at this point but this is now thought not to be the case. The rectum, usually 12 cm in length, first follows the curve of the sacrum downwards and backwards and then downwards and forwards to become the anal canal as it passes through the puborectalis part of the levator ani muscle. At this point the bowel turns through a right angle so that the anal canal, approximately 3·5 cm in length, passes downwards and backwards to the anal orifice.

Each end of the rectum is in the midline but the ampulla between deviates from side to side. This results in folds formed by the circular muscle layer and the mucosa which are best seen at sigmoidoscopy, usually two on the left side with one on the right side between—the rectal valves of Houston.

The upper part of the rectum has a covering of peritoneum that is complete except for a narrow strip posteriorly. As the rectum descends the peritoneal covering becomes reduced so that the middle part has only an anterior covering. The lower part has no peritoneal covering. Approximately at the junction of the middle and lower thirds the peritoneum sweeps forwards onto the bladder in the male and onto the upper end of the vagina and uterus in the female.

On each side of the rectum below the peritoneal reflection there is a collection of fibro-fatty tissue containing the middle rectal blood vessels, the so-called 'lateral ligaments' which tether the rectum to the side walls of the pelvis. Anteriorly the extraperitoneal part of the rectum in the male is related from above downwards to the bladder and ureters, the seminal vesicles and the prostate, and in the female to the posterior vaginal wall, and is covered with a fascial layer, the fascia of Denonvilliers, which runs from the peritoneal reflection above to the urogenital muscular diaphragm below. Posteriorly the rectum is very loosely attached to the front of the sacrum and coccyx which are covered by a thick fascial layer, the fascia of Waldeyer. Between the fascia of Waldeyer and the sacrum lie the middle sacral blood vessels. Inferiorly this fascia sweeps forwards to join the fascia of the rectum at the anorectal junction. The longitudinal and circular muscle layers of the

rectum are complete. The mucosal lining is a glandular columnar epithelium.

The anal canal is related to the coccyx posteriorly, to the ischiorectal fossa on each side, and, anteriorly, in the male to the membranous urethra within the urogenital diaphragm and to the bulb of the urethra, and in the female to the lowest part of the vagina.

The anal canal musculature (*Fig.* 19.1) is extremely important to understand, for inappropriate surgery in this area may lead to incontinence. The external sphincter consists of a cylinder of voluntary striped muscle which is continuous above with the puborectalis part of the levator ani muscle, the whole levator ani muscle and external sphincter forming an inverted cone in which the lower rectum and anal canal lie. The internal sphincter is a downward extension of the involuntary plain circular muscle of the rectum. The longitudinal muscle layer of the rectum also descends as a cylinder but splits to send fibres through the internal and external sphincters to the skin of the lower anal canal (musculus submucosae ani) and to the peri-anal skin (corrugator cutis ani). Of all this musculature much the most important is the puborectalis part of the levator ani muscle which forms a sling around the anorectal junction. Division of this muscle will inevitably lead to incontinence, but the remainder of the external sphincter and internal sphincter muscles can be divided without loss of continence or perhaps with only minor incontinence resulting. The puborectalis muscle together with the internal sphincter at this level is known as the 'anorectal ring'.

The upper half of the canal is lined with columnar epithelium, like the rectum, while the lower half is lined with skin. Halfway down where the two linings meet there is a ring of anal valves, the pectinate (like a cock's comb) or dentate (like a row of teeth) line (*Fig.* 19.1). Above each valve is a pocket known as an 'anal sinus' or 'anal crypt' of Morgagni, into which the duct of an anal gland opens. These glands, up to eight or so in number, lie either in the submucosal layer or in the intersphincteric plane. If they become infected an abscess may result which may ultimately form a fistula-in-ano and they may rarely undergo malignant change, the resulting tumour being an adenocarcinoma.

Blood Supply

The rectum is supplied by the inferior mesenteric artery which, having supplied the sigmoid colon,

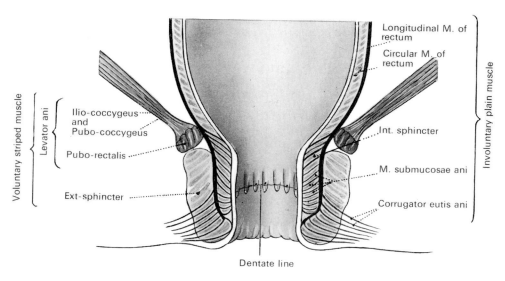

Fig. 19.1. Coronal section through lower rectum and anal canal to show the anatomical features of surgical importance.

becomes the superior rectal or superior haemorrhoidal artery as it crosses the left common iliac artery to enter the true pelvis. At this point it is closely related to the left ureter and to the left testicular or ovarian vessels. It divides at a variable level into right and left branches which may subdivide further as they descend towards the anorectal junction. There is a good marginal communication between the last sigmoid artery and the superior haemorrhoidal artery (Griffiths, 1956). The middle rectal artery, which is variable in size and which may be absent or double, is a branch of the internal iliac artery and reaches the rectum through the lateral ligament on each side. The inferior rectal artery is a branch of the internal pudendal branch of the internal iliac artery and reaches the anal canal by traversing the ischiorectal fossa on each side. All three arteries and their branches supply all layers of the rectum and anal canal, the contribution to each being very variable (Thomson, 1975). Nevertheless, the inferior rectal arteries are always capable of supplying adequately a rectal stump to a point well above the peritoneal reflection, even after division of the middle rectal arteries. The median sacral artery arises from the back of the bifurcation of the aorta. It runs down between Waldeyer's fascia and the sacrum and coccyx and is encountered in excision of the rectum if the coccyx is excised. It supplies a few tiny branches to the back of the rectum.

The venous drainage closely follows the arterial supply. The superior or internal haemorrhoidal venous plexus lying in the submucosal layer of the upper anal canal contributes to three vascular pads or cushions usually found in the left lateral, right posterior and right anterior positions. From it veins drain upwards piercing the layers of the rectal wall to form two main trunks and then a single superior haemorrhoidal or superior rectal vein (part of the portal venous system) which becomes the inferior mesenteric vein as it lies to the left side of the inferior mesenteric artery and which continues upwards to join the splenic vein. The middle rectal vein (part of the systemic venous system) is insignificant. The inferior or external haemorrhoidal venous plexus lying in the subcutaneous layers of the lower anal canal and peri-anal skin drains to inferior haemorrhoidal or inferior rectal veins (also part of the systemic venous system) on each side and thence to the internal iliac veins. The superior and inferior haemorrhoidal plexuses communicate to a variable degree in the subcutaneous and submucosal layers of the anal canal as well as through the sphincter muscles (Thomson, 1975).

Lymph Drainage

Lymph plexuses in the submucosa drain lymph to extramural vessels and nodes and thence in various directions, accompanying the haemorrhoidal blood vessels, upwards to the preaortic nodes via vessels accompanying the superior haemorrhoidal and inferior mesenteric arteries and laterally along vessels accompanying the middle and inferior haemorrhoidal blood vessels to internal iliac lymph nodes on the side walls of the pelvis and thence to para-aortic nodes. In practice the downward spread of rectal carcinoma is very rare and metastasis to superficial inguinal lymph nodes via the external pudendal lymph vessels only occurs if anal or peri-anal skin is involved. Malignant conditions of the anal canal may, of course, metastasize along any of the routes described depending on the exact position of the neoplasm in the canal.

Nerve Supply

The left side of the colon, the rectum and the anal

canal receive a sympathetic nerve supply from the sympathetic chain via the lumbar splanchnic nerves and via the thoracic splanchnic nerves by way of the plexus around the coeliac axis. These fibres converge on the preaortic plexus around the origin of the inferior mesenteric artery and from here they accompany the inferior mesenteric artery and its branches and also form the presacral or hypogastric nerve which descends into the pelvis and divides to send a plexus of nerves to the side wall of the pelvis on each side. From here fibres pass to all the pelvic organs including the rectum and anal canal. A parasympathetic nerve supply comes from the sacral nerves via the pelvic splanchnic nerves (nervi erigentes). These fibres join the sympathetic pelvic plexus to supply the pelvic organs including the rectum and anal canal and passing up the presacral nerve are distributed to the left colon with the sympathetic fibres. Large bowel peristalsis can continue normally in the absence of an extrinsic autonomic nerve supply, but the presence of normal intramuralplexuses is essential. Hence in Hirschsprung's disease, where ganglion cells are absent from a segment of distal large bowel, peristaltic waves fail to pass and functional obstruction results.

It is the hypogastric nerve which may have to be sacrificed in cancer operations of the lower large intestine but which should be very carefully preserved in operations for inflammatory bowel disease. Theoretically division of the sympathetic fibres which are motor to the bladder neck and inhibitory to the bladder wall should cause incontinence of urine, but in practice only slight increase in frequency usually occurs. Sterility in the male may also result, there being normal erection and orgasm but failure of ejaculation. Sympathetic fibres to the anal canal are motor to the internal sphincter but anal reflex mechanisms seem to be unaffected.

Disruption of the autonomic plexus lower in the pelvis may theoretically cause retention of urine and failure of erection owing to division of the parasympathetic element, but in practice there seems to be little permanent effect on the function of the bladder, on sexual function or on anal reflex sphincter mechanisms (the parasympathetic fibres to the anal canal are inhibitory to the internal sphincter), presumably because the plexuses are largely spared unless the lateral ligaments of the rectum are divided very far laterally on the pelvic wall or extensive lymph node dissection is undertaken.

The voluntary muscle of the external sphincter and the levator ani muscle are supplied by the inferior haemorrhoidal branch of the internal pudendal nerve and by the perineal branch of the fourth sacral nerve on each side.

Sensation in the lower anal canal and perianal skin is conveyed by afferent fibres in the inferior haemorrhoidal nerve and this can be abolished by a nerve block in the ischiorectal fossa or in the caudal canal. The much less acute sensation which accompanies injection of internal haemorrhoids, in the upper anal canal for example, is probably conveyed by parasympathetic fibres.

Continence and Defaecation

The reflexes controlling continence and defaecation are complex. From the practical point of view patients who undergo sphincter-saving resections of the lower large bowel retain anal continence. As mentioned above, this may be due to the fact that the autonomic pelvic plexus remains largely undisturbed as do the somatic nerves mediating sensation from the lower anal canal and supplying the voluntary levator ani and external sphincter muscles. Thus the resting tone of the anal internal sphincter which is mediated by its sympathetic supply remains intact as does voluntary control by the external sphincter. Anal sensation may be very important in maintaining continence and this also remains intact. Rectal sensation is probably also an important factor in maintaining continence and this is undoubtedly diminished in such cases, although there is no doubt that most patients retain a degree of 'rectal' sensation, and even patients in whom an ileal reservoir is attached to the upper anal canal may also retain a slight degree of 'rectal' sensation. This would suggest that such sensation is generated to some degree by pressure on surrounding pelvic structures rather than by rectal distension alone (Lane and Parks, 1977).

Defaecation is undoubtedly initiated by a sensation of rectal distension but whether the reflex is completed is of course under strong cortical control. When rectal peristalsis occurs relaxation of voluntary anal control allows defaecation to occur. Even in the absence of all rectal sensation, however, the reflex can be initiated by voluntary straining of abdominal musculature, and thus patients who have had low large bowel resections can always achieve satisfactory evacuation.

INVESTIGATIONS

Investigation of the lower large bowel and anal canal starts with clinical examination of the patient. General examination with reference to the alimentary tract is carried out, abdominal examination being particularly important. The patient is then turned onto his or her left side with the knees drawn up and the pelvis elevated on a pillow (Sims' position). After inspection of the perineum, digital rectal examination is performed. In addition to the large amount of information that can be gleaned by this, it is important to assess whether there is any mechanical contra-indication to the instrumentation which is to follow, for example spasm of the anal sphincters due to a fissure.

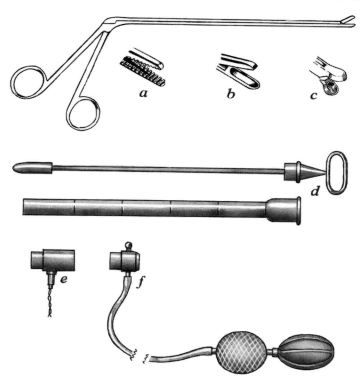

Fig. 19.2. Apparatus for sigmoidoscopy. *a*, Chevalier Jackson grasping forceps with alligator jaws for swabbing. *b*, Paterson's forceps for mucosal biopsy. *c*, Officer's forceps for tumour biopsy. *d*, A 25-cm Lloyd-Davies sigmoidoscope with obturator (1·5-cm diameter). 15-cm, 20-cm and 30-cm versions of wider diameter are available but are usually reserved for use under general anaesthesia. *e*, Light fitting. *f*, Window with bellows. The second bulb is designed to maintain a constant flow of air during insufflation.

Sigmoidoscopy

The apparatus required is shown in *Fig.* 19.2.

This investigation should form part of any examination of the alimentary tract, but it is mandatory in the presence of colorectal and anal symptoms. Bowel preparation is usually not required but massive loading of the lower bowel calls for an enema. Anaesthesia is usually not required but application of a local anaesthetic preparation such as 2 per cent Xylocaine (lignocaine) gel to a tender fissure may be necessary in order to allow the passage of the instrument, and general anaesthesia may be required if spasm or acute angulation in the upper reaches of the rectum cannot be negotiated, or for a child.

The Sims' position is satisfactory but occasionally the knee–elbow position will permit a more satisfactory examination. This is uncomfortable for the patient however. After digital examination the 25-cm sigmoidoscope, with its obturator in place, is lubricated and passed. Once through the anorectal junction (5 cm) the obturator is removed and a light fitting attached. The window with bellows is then attached and the instrument passed under vision with as little air insufflation as possible. Patients should be warned that lower abdominal wind pain may occur, that they may feel a desire to defaecate, and that they may pass wind. The instrument is passed upwards and backwards to the rectosigmoid junction and then downwards and forwards into the sigmoid colon. Swabbing with flat damp cottonwool swabs is carried out when necessary.

If required, a mucosal biopsy is taken with biopsy forceps, as shown in *Fig.* 19.2*b*, but a heavier pair of forceps as shown in *Fig.* 19.2*c* can be used for biopsy of a neoplasm. A biopsy is taken under direct vision having removed the window only. Bleeding is usually not severe and can be controlled by pressure with a swab. As the instrument is withdrawn the patient should be reassured that defaecation is not occurring.

A mucosal biopsy should be gently spread onto a glass cover-slip or onto a piece of blotting paper prior to placing in fixative (10 per cent buffered formaldehyde solution is suitable) while a biopsy specimen from a neoplasm can be dropped directly into the fixative.

Proctoscopy

The apparatus required is shown in *Fig.* 19.3. Proctoscopy is conveniently carried out after sigmoidoscopy with the patient in the same position. Many

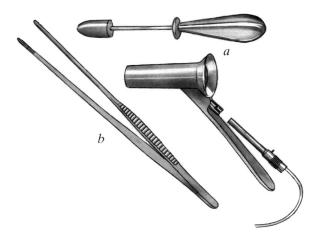

Fig. 19.3. Apparatus for proctoscopy. *a*, St Mark's pattern proctoscope with obturator and light fitting (2·0-cm diameter). *b*, Forceps for swabbing.

different shapes and sizes of proctoscope have been designed and a narrower instrument than the one illustrated may be needed in the presence of anal pathology or for a child.

The proctoscope with obturator and light fitting in place is lubricated and passed, initially upwards and forwards and then upwards and backwards into the lower rectum. The obturator is removed. If desired, an external light source can be used beside the surgeon's right shoulder. Usually little of the rectum can be seen except for an area of the lower anterior wall. As the instrument is withdrawn the anorectal ring closes behind the end of the proctoscope and the presence or absence of internal haemorrhoids in the upper anal canal can be assessed. This is aided by asking the patient to strain down, while reassuring him or her that defaecation is not occurring. The lower anal canal is then examined as the instrument is withdrawn completely.

Barium Enema

A barium enema study adds little to the investigation of the rectum even when the air contrast or Malmo technique is used. Large space-occupying lesions may be seen but these would always be either palpable digitally or visible endoscopically or both. The width of the retrorectal space can be assessed and may be abnormal in certain conditions. Gross dilatation of the bowel such as occurs in Hirschsprung's disease will also be seen. It cannot be over-emphasized, however, that any single examination of the rectum may miss a lesion, and the rectal films of a barium enema study should always be examined with great care.

Colonoscopy

Normally examination with a colonoscope or with a flexible sigmoidoscope has no place in investigation

of the rectum. However, with modern wide-view instruments a small lesion such as a solitary ulcer or even a carcinoma can be picked up during this examination, having been missed digitally, with the rigid sigmoidoscope and on the barium enema examination. It is also possible to obtain a retrograde view of the anorectal region from within. This may be helpful posteriorly where it is not always easy to obtain a satisfactory view by rigid sigmoidoscopy or by proctoscopy.

Computerized Tomography

CT scanning can delineate rectal tumours and can clearly show direct extension of tumour to adjacent structures such as the sacrum or prostate. In practice such scanning is rarely necessary as it adds little to the clinical assessment. It may, however, be extremely helpful in detecting pelvic recurrence of tumour in a patient who has, for example, undergone excision of the rectum.

Sphincter Studies

The anal sphincters and their reflexes can be studied in several ways. Taken together these tests are particularly useful in evaluating cases of incontinence due either to a neurological problem or to muscle weakness or to direct muscle damage for example.

The normal resting tone of the internal sphincter is measured by withdrawing a balloon through the anal canal. The pressure exerted on the balloon is measured together with the additional pressure which the voluntary external sphincter can exert. Rectal sensation is also measured by means of a balloon, the level of awareness and the level when evacuation is inevitable being recorded. With an inflation balloon in the rectum and a recording balloon in the anal canal the relaxation of tone in the internal sphincter as rectal pressure rises, the so-called 'rectosphincteric reflex', can be measured, this being absent in Hirschsprung's disease for example. Electromyographic measurement of resting, contracting and straining action potentials in the puborectalis muscle and in the external sphincter muscles with a needle can also be made. The latency, amplitude and duration of potentials in the external sphincter muscle following stimulation of the perianal skin, the so-called 'anal reflex', are also measured, this being a reflection of pudendal nerve damage. Finally, electromyographic mapping of the sphincter muscles following direct damage can indicate the size and position of the gap between the divided ends of muscle thus aiding their direct suture.

In many cases, however, a good history and a careful digital examination will usually provide as much information as is necessary about the state of the sphincters to decide what local surgery may or may not be required.

SURGERY OF THE RECTUM

Carcinoma of the Rectum

The two procedures most commonly adopted for treatment of carcinoma of the rectum are excision of the rectum and anterior resection (Naunton Morgan, 1965), and several factors influence the decision as to which is used.

The most important factor is the distance of the lower edge of the tumour from the anal margin. Only a rough assessment of this can be made preoperatively by sigmoidoscopic measurement. It has been clearly shown that a 5-cm cuff of rectum below the tumour will achieve complete eradication in all cases (Grinnell, 1954). In many cases, however, a shorter cuff will obviously suffice and it has become common practice to accept less than a 5-cm clearance. Whether this will lead to an unacceptable local recurrence rate in due course remains to be seen. In general, therefore, anterior resection is only possible if the neoplasm is in the upper half of the rectum or at the rectosigmoid junction. For lower tumours excision of the rectum is generally necessary. Sometimes in a slim woman with a wide pelvis an anterior resection is possible for a tumour only 8 cm from the anal margin, while in an obese man with a narrow pelvis anterior resection is impossible for a tumour even as high as 12 cm from the anal margin. With the introduction of the peranal technique of colo-anal anastomosis (anastomosis of the colon to the anal canal just above the dentate line), excision of the rectum can, however, be avoided in a few cases where anterior resection is theoretically possible but technically too difficult. Often a final decision cannot be made until the abdomen is open and the bowel fully mobilized, for in some cases unfolding of the rectum reveals the growth to be much higher than was suspected preoperatively.

The preoperative biopsy of the carcinoma is important, for if the tumour is well differentiated it is well worth trying to achieve restoration of bowel continuity as the chance of local recurrence is low. If the biopsy reveals an undifferentiated tumour, on the other hand, then neither a difficult anterior resection nor a colo-anal anastomosis should be attempted as the chance of local recurrence is high, due to the high incidence of local spread of such lesions in the bowel wall beyond the macroscopic tumour.

Other procedures such as abdomino-perineal pull-through resection, fulguration, trans-sphincteric resection and peranal resection are occasionally appropriate and are briefly described below.

However remote is the possibility of a colostomy the patient must be prepared for this before the operation and ideally should be visited by a stoma-therapist and by a patient who already has an established colostomy. In addition, the site of the colostomy must be assessed and marked with the patient standing and sitting so that it is sited well away from skin creases, the umbilicus, the anterior superior iliac spine and the incision. Also it must be at a level where the patient can see it in order to cope with the changing of the appliance—this is often much higher than one would guess with the patient lying flat in bed or on the operating table.

If there is an element of obstruction, a preliminary defunctioning transverse loop colostomy should be performed. This should be placed in the right hypochondrium to leave the left side of the abdomen free for the subsequent resection. Even in an unobstructed case inadequate preparation of the bowel or a difficult anastomosis may call for a temporary transverse colostomy or for a caecostomy at the time of operation and all patients should therefore be warned of such a possibility.

The most important part of bowel preparation is the mechanical preparation and several methods have been used. A suitable regimen is to start clear fluids on the 3rd preoperative day. On the 2nd preoperative day 10 ml of magnesium sulphate crystals in 60 ml of hot water are given every 2 hours until diarrhoea occurs. On the same evening a phosphate enema is given. On the day before surgery a clear washout is given followed by a Veripaque enema in the evening. Other methods such as giving castor oil by mouth followed by evacuation from below, or flushing through the entire gut with a large volume of electrolyte solution given through a nasogastric tube, have their advocates. Close attention must be paid to fluid and electrolyte disturbance with these latter methods, particularly in the elderly. If there is any suggestion of incipient obstruction, and of course in the presence of frank obstruction, none of these methods is suitable and mechanical preparation should be restricted to evacuation of the bowel from below by enema or washout.

Antibiotic cover is given starting with the premedication and continuing for 48–72 hours postoperatively. A broad-spectrum antibiotic such as an aminoglycoside or a cephalosporin is suitable to cover the majority of large bowel organisms together with metronidazole to cover anaerobic bacteria, including *Bacteroides* species specifically (Keighley, 1983).

1. *Excision of the Rectum*

This operation is performed through the abdomen and through the perineum—abdomino-perineal excision of the rectum. Although it can be performed by one surgeon, the patient being turned between the two stages (Miles, 1908), it is usually done more expeditiously by two surgeons, one at the abdominal incision and one at the perineal working together (Lloyd-Davies, 1939), a synchronous combined approach ('synchronous combined abdomino-perineal excision of the rectum', unfortunately sometimes abbreviated to 'SCAPER').

Under general anaesthetic and with an intravenous infusion running the patient is catheterized and placed in the lithotomy–Trendelenburg or St Mark's

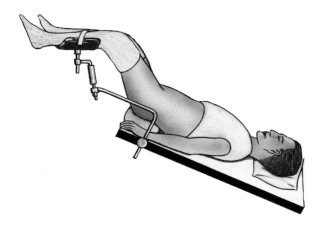

Fig. 19.4. The lithotomy–Trendelenburg or St Mark's position on the operating table for excision of the rectum and anterior resection.

position on the operating table (*Fig.* 19.4). The scrotum is strapped to the right thigh and the anus closed with a purse-string suture.

Through a left (or right) paramedian incision a careful laparotomy is carried out to assess the degree of spread of the neoplasm both locally and distally, the liver being the most important organ to examine. Although a barium enema study will usually have been carried out preoperatively the remainder of the large bowel is carefully examined to exclude synchronous neoplasms. As a result of this examination a decision is made as to whether the resection is to be radical or palliative. In the presence of disseminated disease, unless very extensive, it is generally agreed that removal of the primary neoplasm is desirable even if excision of the rectum is required. This will avoid the problem of obstruction at a later date, together with the pain which local spread of a pelvic neoplasm can cause. If subsequent chemotherapy is to be given in such a case it is better to remove the primary for this is unlikely to respond to such therapy. As already mentioned, a final decision as to whether anterior resection may be possible or not may have to wait until the rectum is fully mobilized.

A self-retaining retractor is inserted. The small bowel loops can either be placed in a bag outside the abdomen or held back by moist packs and a third blade attached to the retractor. The sigmoid colon is then held to the right and the 'white line' marking the junction of the visceral and parietal peritoneum incised. With blunt dissection the spermatic or ovarian vessels and the left ureter are identified and separated from the vascular pedicle of the bowel. The peritoneum on the right side of the sigmoid mesentery is then incised and the vascular pedicle isolated. The inferior mesenteric artery is then divided close to the aorta—the 'high tie', as shown in *Fig.* 19.5 at *a*. The inferior mesenteric vein lying to the left of the artery is divided at the same level. The left colic and sigmoid vessels are divided as shown in *Fig.* 19.5. In some cases, for example in the very old and the very fat,

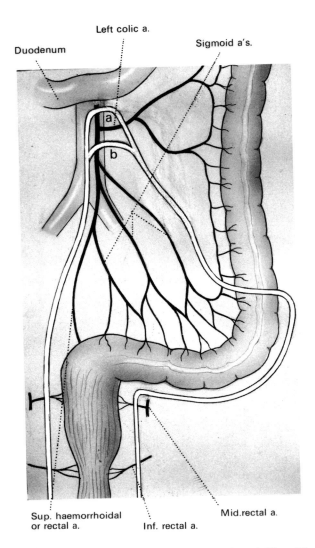

Fig. 19.5. The blood supply of the lower large bowel. The white line shows the area to be resected. *a*, Ligation of the inferior mesenteric artery flush with the aorta, the 'high tie'. *b*, Ligation of the inferior mesenteric artery sparing its left colic branch.

it is prudent to divide the inferior mesenteric artery distal to the origin of the left colic artery as shown in *Fig.* 19.5 at *b*. A good blood supply to the colostomy is thus ensured and the dissection is less difficult. The distance between *a* and *b* is approximately 2 cm so that little in the way of lymphatic drainage is sacrificed.

With the pedicle divided mobilization of the rectum can safely be undertaken (and the pelvic surgeon can start the perineal dissection—*see below*). The peritoneum is incised all the way down on each side of the rectum and the incision joined in front of the deepest part of the peritoneal pouch. The rectum is then lifted forwards and the almost completely avascular presacral plane opened up. In cases where the neoplasm is low and there is no obvious lymphatic spread the presacral nerve can be spared by careful dissection. The abdominal and perineal surgeons meet behind the rectum at this stage. Returning to the front of the rectum, the bladder base and seminal vesicles or vaginal wall are exposed beneath the transverse peritoneal incision using a straight or lipped St Mark's pattern retractor (*Fig.* 19.6*a*). The fascia of Denonvilliers is then exposed and incised, opening up the plane which passes down behind the prostate to its apex. The abdominal and perineal surgeons again meet at this point. The lateral ligament on each

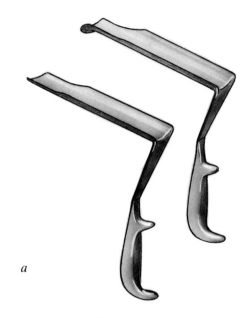

a

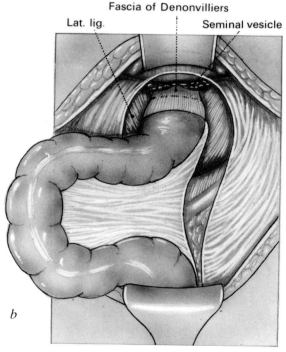

b

Fascia of Denonvilliers

Lat. lig.　　　　　Seminal vesicle

Fig. 19.6. *a*, St Mark's Hospital pattern deep pelvic retractors. *b*, Exposure of the fascia of Denonvilliers.

side is thus defined and divided, the middle rectal vessels being diathermized or ligated (*Fig.* 19.6*b*).

The sigmoid mesentery is now divided, taking care to preserve the blood supply from the left colic branches and the marginal artery. The bowel is divided between crushing clamps at a point that will allow the colostomy to be formed without tension—the point at which the gently stretched sigmoid colon reaches the lower end of the paramedian wound is usually the correct place. A Zachary Cope clamp with three hinged segments is ideal for this step (*Fig.* 19.7). In due course the rectum is withdrawn by the perineal surgeon.

The colostomy site is now prepared. In cases where the rectal tumour is so low that excision of the rectum is inevitable, this step should be undertaken prior to opening the abdomen as this ensures that the incisions in the layers of the abdominal wall are in line when the abdomen is closed. At the previously marked site a circle of skin 2 cm in diameter is removed and a trephine through the whole abdominal wall is made. It is important that the colostomy passes through the rectus muscle as this minimizes the likelihood of paracolostomy hernia. The left paracolic gutter is now exposed with a pair of artery forceps and a non-absorbable purse-string inserted to close the so-called 'lateral space' (*Fig.* 19.8). If a right paramedian incision is used the colostomy can be sited more medially, in which case the 'lateral space' is so large that it need not be closed. Before the pelvic peritoneal floor is closed it is important that the perineal and abdominal surgeons collaborate.

The perineal surgeon proceeds as follows. After applying towels as shown in *Fig.* 19.9, an elliptical incision is made from a point midway between the bulb of the urethra and the anus anteriorly to the point of the coccyx posteriorly. Two pairs of Lane's forceps are applied to the peri-anal ellipse of skin. The fat in the ischiorectal fossa on each side is divided. These incisions are united posteriorly over the tip of the coccyx. A St Mark's perineal retractor is inserted (*Fig.* 19.10*a*). The fibrous attachments of the coccygeus muscles to the tip of the coccyx are divided to expose Waldeyer's fascia. The iliococcygeus muscle is now divided in a forward and lateral direction on each side, the inferior haemorrhoidal vessels being diathermized or ligated. Waldeyer's fascia is now incised with a scalpel exposing the presacral space behind the mesorectum. If desired, the same plane can be reached by excising the distal part of the coccyx, dividing the coccygeus muscles as already described and incising Waldeyer's fascia. This step may give better clearance of low rectal growths but can predispose to coccygeal pain in the postoperative period. The abdominal and perineal surgeons now meet as already described. Anteriorly the subcutaneous fat is divided to expose the superficial transverse perineal muscles and then the deep transverse perineal muscles. The decussating fibres of the external sphincter are divided behind these

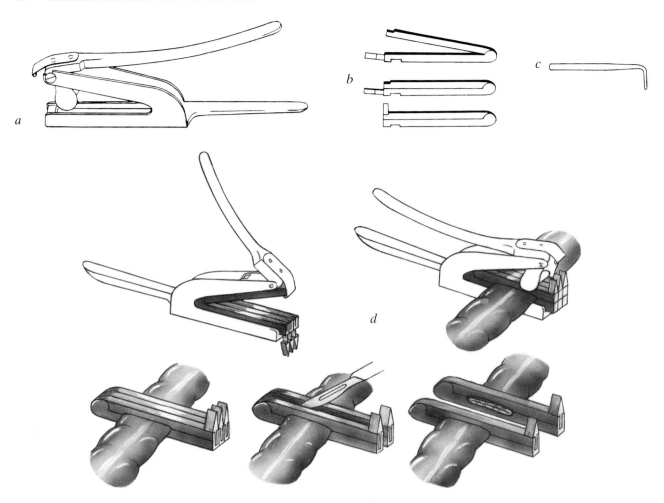

Fig. 19.7. The Zachary Cope intestinal clamp. *a*, The clamp. *b*, Three hinged segments. *c*, Tommy bar for closing and opening segments. *d*, Clamp in use.

pairs of muscles and the plane deepened. At each side the pubococcygeus muscle is now divided followed by the continuation of Waldeyer's and Denonvilliers' fascias. A finger is passed behind the puborectalis muscle on each side to define the plane between the prostate and the rectum. At this point the midline anterior attachment of the rectum to the apex of the prostate and to the membranous urethra

by the recto-urethralis muscle can be gently divided. The abdominal and perineal surgeons meet again in the midline and the puborectalis muscle is divided on each side (*Fig.* 19.10*b*). The lower part of each lateral ligament is now divided and the rectum removed. In the female a strip of posterior vaginal wall is removed with the rectum, contact with the

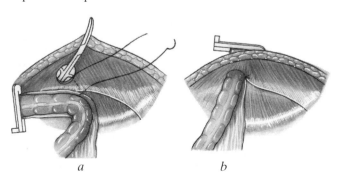

Fig. 19.8. *a*, Exposure of lateral space. *b*, Lateral space closed.

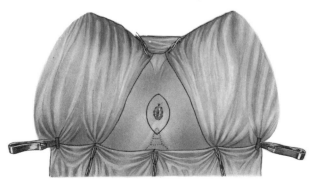

Fig. 19.9. The perineal incision after closure of the anus with a purse-string suture.

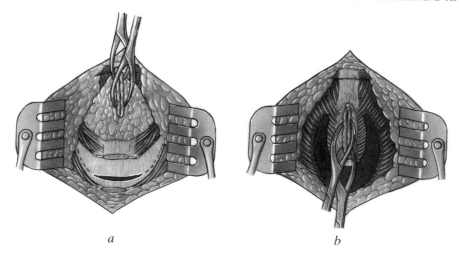

Fig. 19.10. *a*, Incision of Waldeyer's fascia. In this case the tip of the coccyx has been divided.
b, Division of levator ani muscle. The iliococcygeus on each side has been divided leaving the
recto-urethralis muscle and then the puborectalis fibres on each side still to be divided.

abdominal surgeon being made at the posterior fornix.

Both abdominal and perineal surgeons now collaborate to achieve complete haemostasis. The table should be untipped and a check made that the patient's blood pressure is near its normal value. In this way troublesome reactionary haemorrhage can be avoided. The perineal wound is now temporarily closed with tissue-holding forceps and the pelvic cavity filled with a cancericidal agent such as mercuric perchloride (1 in 500) or distilled water for 4 minutes.

If haemostasis is complete the abdominal surgeon closes the peritoneal floor with a continuous catgut suture. The peritoneum over the mesenteric vascular pedicle is closed and the suture is continued laterally to approximate the mesocolon to the peritoneum of the left iliac fossa, the remainder of the lateral space being closed if necessary with a purse-string suture, as already described (*Fig.* 19.11).

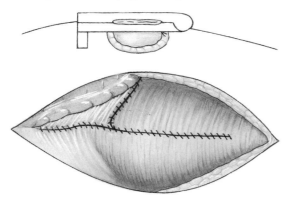

Fig. 19.11. Closure of the peritoneal floor.

The wound is closed in layers without drainage. The colostomy is then fashioned by removing the clamp from the colon, excising the crushed bowel and suturing all layers of the bowel wall to the skin with 12 interrupted 2/0 strength chromic catgut sutures on a tapercut needle. An adhesive colostomy bag is applied.

If pelvic haemostasis is complete the perineal wound can be closed completely in the male with a sump drain through a separate stab incision. Suction is started immediately and continues for approximately 5–7 days. If haemostasis is not adequate the wound is closed with a corrugated drain. The levators are not sutured but the ischiorectal fat can often be approximated with interrupted catgut sutures, thus diminishing the size of the cavity. In the female the edges of the vaginal muscle are oversewn to control troublesome oozing and no attempt is made to reconstitute the vagina. The perineum is closed with a corrugated drain to the pelvic cavity via the reconstituted vaginal orifice. If haemorrhage in the pelvis cannot be controlled the cavity is packed with dry gauze which is removed under anaesthetic after 72 hours. If the pelvic peritoneal floor cannot be closed a plastic bag filled with gauze is placed in the pelvic cavity and this can safely be removed after 4 days without prolapse of bowel.

Postoperative retention of urine may require re-insertion of the catheter on one or more occasions and sometimes prostatic resection is required. Breakdown of the perineal wound requires twice daily irrigation and dressing with an antiseptic solution until healing by secondary intention occurs. The viability of the colostomy must be watched carefully. If the colostomy does not act spontaneously after 5 days or so a suppository or small enema may be required.

The specimen should be taken dry to the histopathology department where it is opened from end to end and pinned out on a board prior to fixation, photography and histological examination.

2. *Anterior Resection*

The preparation for anterior resection should in all respects be the same as for excision of the rectum. Again it is convenient to place the patient in the lithotomy–Trendelenburg or St Mark's position on the operating table for, as already discussed, anterior resection may not in the event be possible and excision of the rectum will have to be carried out.

Following careful laparotomy the sigmoid colon is mobilized and the vascular pedicle divided as for excision of the rectum. The sigmoid mesentery is then divided from this point as far as the point on the bowel wall which will reach to the rectal stump without tension. If necessary the splenic flexure must be mobilized. The rectum is now fully mobilized as described for excision of the rectum. With the lateral ligaments divided the rectal curves are straightened out and a final decision made as to whether anterior resection is in fact possible. The colon is then divided immediately proximal to a Parker–Kerr crushing clamp. The proximal colon is occluded with a non-crushing clamp or if preferred with a ball of cotton-wool in the lumen. The cut edge of the colon and the adjacent lumen are then swabbed out with a cancericidal agent. If the viability of the proximal colon is in doubt mobilization of the splenic flexure and further resection may be required. The mesorectum is now divided at the level of the proposed anastomosis. The vascular pedicle will have divided at this level so that the vessels must be taken on each side and it is convenient to use Parker–Kerr crushing intestinal clamps for this step. The rectum is now clamped transversely with a right-angled crushing rectal clamp at the chosen level below the growth. An assistant now irrigates the rectum per anum with 500 ml of mercuric perchloride (1 in 500) using a rubber catheter passed through a proctoscope. This cleans the rectal stump of any residual faecal matter and destroys loose malignant cells.

Stay sutures are then placed on each side of the rectal stump and the rectum divided below the right-angled clamp. The specimen is removed. A two-layer anastomosis may then be performed as shown in *Fig.* 19.12.

Alternatively a one-layer anastomosis can be performed using a non-absorbable suture such as silk or Ethiflex (*Fig.* 19.13).

A circular stapling device for carrying out colorectal anastomosis following resection of tumours of the middle and upper thirds of the rectum, which was devised in the Soviet Union and perfected in the USA, is now readily available in disposable form. One important advantage over previous devices is that it produces a completely inverted suture line. After resection in the usual way the closed instrument (*Fig.* 19.14*a*) is passed per anum into the rectal stump and on into the pelvic cavity. The instrument is opened and the two bowel ends closed over the device with purse-string sutures (*Fig.* 19.14*b*). When closed

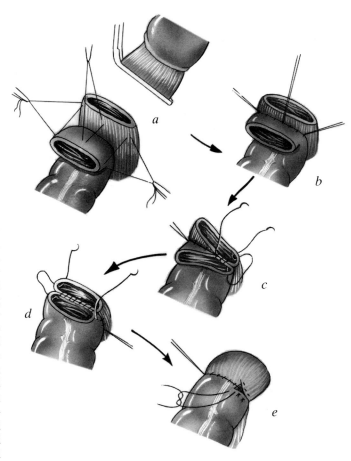

Fig. 19.12. Two-layer anastomosis. *a*, Posterior layer of five, or ideally seven, non-absorbable 3/0 silk Lembert sutures placed as shown and left untied. Stay sutures on each side of rectal stump not shown. *b*, Proximal colon rail-roaded down to the rectum and sutures tied. The central and lateral sutures are held. Stay sutures removed. *c*, All-layer continuous suture started in midline posteriorly using double-ended 2/0 chromic catgut suture. Over-and-over stitch used except at the corners where a Connell or loop on the mucosa stitch negotiates the turn onto the anterior surface. *d*, Connell or over-and-over suture along the front. If used, the cottonwool ball must be removed from the lumen of the proximal colon. *e*, Anterior layer completed with interrupted non-absorbable 3/0 silk seromuscular horizontal mattress Lembert sutures.

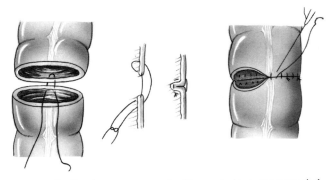

Fig. 19.13. One-layer anastomosis. The posterior sutures are tied on the mucosal surface. The anastomosis is completed anteriorly with horizontal mattress sutures.

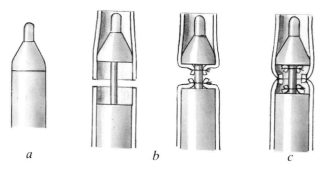

Fig. 19.14. Mechanical stapling device—'the gun'. *a*, Instrument closed. *b*, Bowel ends closed over the open instrument with purse-string sutures. *c*, Anastomosis effected with clips, bowel ends resected by the circular knife and the instrument opened to release the anastomosis.

and fired the device effects the anastomosis with a double row of metal clips. At the same time a circular knife cuts the bowel ends within the circle of clips. The device is opened again to release the anastomosis (*Fig.* 19.14*c*) and withdrawn. Integrity of the anastomosis can be tested by filling the pelvis with saline and insufflating the rectum gently with air. Any defect is made good with additional seromuscular sutures. It is doubtful whether this device allows a lower anastomosis to be carried out than can be achieved by conventional hand-sewn techniques, but it may in some instances allow an easier anastomosis and is undoubtedly an important addition to the armamentarium of the colo-rectal surgeon.

The peritoneum is closed over the mesenteric vascular pedicle and the suture continued towards the pelvis closing the gap between the mesocolon and the parietal peritoneum on its right side. The abdomen is now closed with stab drainage to the anastomosis (a length of Paul's tubing inside a similar length of wider Paul's tubing is satisfactory). The anal sphincters are gently dilated to allow easy passage of flatus.

The complication of anastomotic breakdown and subsequent pelvic infection is best avoided by meticulous attention to haemostasis and avoidance of tension at the anastomosis. A covering transverse colostomy (or caecostomy) should be performed if there is any doubt about the adequacy of the procedure. If dehiscence of the anastomosis occurs it usually heals spontaneously, but if more extensive a transverse colostomy should be raised until healing occurs.

3. *Peranal Anastomosis* (Parks, 1977)

In general, carcinomas of the upper third of the rectum are treated by anterior resection while those of the lower third are treated by excision of the rectum. Middle-third tumours may be treated by either technique depending on the various criteria already described. However, a few of these cases may be suitable for resection followed by colo-anal anastomosis.

The tumour must be mobile, without evidence of palpable mesorectal lymphatic spread and the histology must not be anaplastic.

Preparation is as for the two procedures already described. The splenic flexure is mobilized. The rectum is fully mobilized as far as the anal canal and resected as for anterior resection. A Parks retractor (*Fig.* 19.15*a*) is now inserted into the anorectal stump

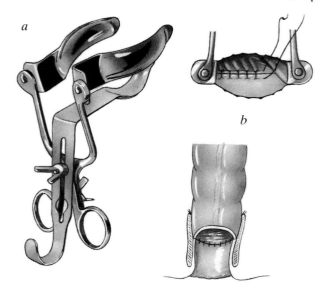

Fig. 19.15. Peranal anastomosis. *a*, Parks anal retractor with detachable third blade. *b*, The colon anastomosed to the anal canal just above the dentate line.

and the mucosa removed in strips from just above the dentate line upwards, after submucosal infiltration of normal saline containing adrenaline (1 in 300 000). The colon is then brought down into the muscular cuff and after insertion of the retractor into the colon itself, it is anastomosed to the divided mucosal edge using interrupted non-absorbable sutures which include the anal mucosa, internal sphincter fibres and the whole thickness of the colon wall (*Fig.* 19.15*b*).

Suction drainage to the potential space between the colon and the rectal cuff is inserted. The anastomosis should be covered with a transverse colostomy. The tendency to stenosis can be resisted by daily dilatation for a short period by the patient with a St Mark's anal dilator for a period of a few weeks.

4. *Abdomino-perineal Pull-through Resection*

This technique for tumours of the middle and upper rectum is not generally used in the United Kingdom as it offers no advantages over the three techniques already described and carries the distinct disadvantage of temporary if not permanent disruption of sphincter function. Preparation of the patient and mobilization of the rectum are identical to those already described. An obturator is then passed into

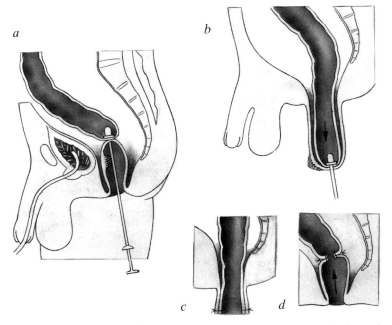

Fig. 19.16. Abdomino-perineal pull-through resection. *a*, Rectum tied round an obturator above the carcinoma. *b*, Rectum intussuscepted to the outside. *c*, Rectum resected. *d*, Anastomosis completed and stump returned to pelvis.

the rectum and the bowel tied round it (*Fig.* 19.16*a*). The rectum is then intussuscepted to the outside and resected (*Fig.* 19.16*b*,*c*). Immediate anastomosis in two layers can be carried out with subsequent reduction of the stump to the pelvis (*Fig.* 19.16*d*), or alternatively the second stage can be delayed for 10 days or so.

5. *Fulguration*

There is a limited place for fulguration of lower rectal neoplasms but this must not be used at the expense of the ultimate prognosis. It should perhaps be reserved for very early tumours and in patients who are medically unfit to undergo routine resection. The neoplasm is removed with a clear margin of the normal tissue using a diathermy needle. Regular re-examination is required to look for and to treat any residual tumour.

6. *Trans-sphincteric Resection* (*see* p. 253)

7. *Peranal Resection* (*see* p. 254)

Hartmann's Operation

In this operation the upper rectum and sigmoid colon are resected, the rectal stump being closed and a terminal colostomy formed. It is indicated in a few cases of carcinoma of the mid- or upper rectum where local spread of malignant tissue would make anterior resection unwise or where the patient is medically unfit to undergo an abdomino-perineal resection. It is also indicated in patients with diverticular disease in whom gross inflammatory changes in the pelvis make primary anastomosis dangerous.

The preparation of the patient is as already described for resections, although this procedure can safely be performed in the emergency situation when bowel preparation has not been possible, for example when obstruction has occurred. The lithotomy–Trendelenburg or St Mark's position is used. The degree of mobilization of the bowel is dictated by the pathology. The rectal stump is washed out and closed with catgut in two layers. If possible the pelvic peritoneum is closed over the rectal stump. The colostomy is made in the left iliac fossa.

Continuity of the bowel can always be re-established at a later date if the general condition of the patient allows or when pelvic inflammation has settled.

Conservative Excision of the Rectum for Inflammatory Bowel Disease

In patients undergoing proctocolectomy for ulcerative colitis without malignant change or for Crohn's colitis or in patients who have primarily undergone subtotal colectomy, usually for ulcerative colitis in a toxic phase, in whom the rectum is not suitable for ileorectal anastomosis, a much less extensive procedure can be carried out than is required for malignant disease of the rectum.

The patient is prepared in the usual way and under

general anaesthetic is placed in the lithotomy–Trendelenburg position on the operating table. Through a left paramedian incision the bowel is mobilized above. The dissection in the pelvis should be kept very close to the rectum. Posteriorly, the superior rectal vessels are preserved and the dissection is kept close to the rectal wall. This is a very vascular plane and numerous branches of the rectal vessels have to be ligated or diathermied. This preserves as much of the mesorectal fat as possible. The lateral ligaments are divided close to the rectum and anteriorly the dissection continues down through the recto-vesical pouch, through the fascia of Denonvilliers to the plane behind the prostate or vagina.

The perineal surgeon closes the anus with a stitch and makes a small elliptical incision around the anus over the intersphincteric groove. The dissection is carried up in the intersphincteric plane to meet the abdominal surgeon above the level of the external sphincter posteriorly and laterally. Anteriorly decussating fibres of the external sphincter which are attached to the recto-urethralis muscle must be divided to reach the abdominal surgeon in the plane behind the prostate. In the female the vaginal wall is kept intact.

This rather tedious dissection leaves a very small pelvic cavity. The pelvic peritoneum is closed from above and the pelvic wound closed with sump drainage, the external sphincter muscle being closed completely. In these cases the perineal wound heals well, the sump drain usually being ready for removal at 5 days and the sutures at 10 days. Antibiotic cover is essential.

Perineal Crohn's disease may call for a more extensive perineal dissection and any pelvic inflammation may call for open rather than closed drainage.

The Trans-sphincteric Approach to the Rectum
(York Mason, 1974)

With a suitable proximal defunctioning colostomy the rectum can be exposed by an incision starting at the anal margin in the midline posteriorly and lying to one side of the coccyx and sacrum. The external anal sphincter is then divided followed by the lower part of the levator ani muscle and a few fibres of the gluteus maximus muscle. This exposes the rectum. A complete tube of rectum can be removed with subsequent anastomosis (*Fig.* 19.17*a*). If necessary the muscle coat of the rectum and anal canal (internal

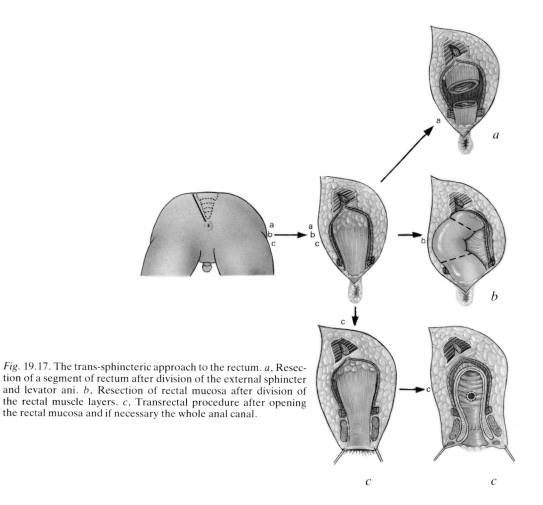

Fig. 19.17. The trans-sphincteric approach to the rectum. *a*, Resection of a segment of rectum after division of the external sphincter and levator ani. *b*, Resection of rectal mucosa after division of the rectal muscle layers. *c*, Transrectal procedure after opening the rectal mucosa and if necessary the whole anal canal.

sphincter) can be divided and the mucosal lining of the rectum and anal canal exposed. Submucosal resection of extensive benign lesions such as rectal adenoma can then be carried out. If necessary a complete tube of mucosa can be removed with subsequent mucosal anastomosis (*Fig.* 19.17*b*). Alternatively the rectum can be opened and a transrectal full-thickness resection carried out (*Fig.* 19.17*c*). This approach can also be used for repair of a rectoprostatic or a rectovaginal fistula.

The Kraske Approach to the Rectum

The rectum can also be approached through a midline incision over the sacrum, coccyx and anococcygeal raphe. The muscular and ligamentous attachments to the coccyx are divided. The anococcygeal raphe is divided in the midline from coccyx to external sphincter and the coccyx removed. The fifth and, if necessary, the fourth sacral vertebrae can also be removed. Waldeyer's fascia is now exposed and when divided in the midline access to the whole rectum is achieved. Procedures such as described in the previous section can now be carried out. The technique offers little advantage over the trans-sphincteric approach, except perhaps in the removal of an extensive retro-rectal lesion such as a teratoma or dermoid cyst. The divided sacrum can cause discomfort postoperatively when the patient is sitting.

The Peranal Approach to the Rectum

1. *Rectal Polyp*

These should all be removed for histological examination. Barium enema and sigmoidoscopy are essential prior to this to exclude other pathology and to detect other polyps. The bowel is prepared with a disposable phosphate enema. General anaesthesia is usually employed but local anaesthesia to allow adequate relaxation of the anal sphincters can be used. The patient is placed in the left lateral position.

Through an operating sigmoidoscope (*Fig.* 19.18*a*–*e*) the stalk of the polyp is encircled with a diathermy snare and with a low-intensity cutting current the whole lesion is removed for histological examination (*Fig.* 19.18*f*). Any bleeding can easily be arrested with a diathermy coagulation button. In the lower rectum some polyps can be delivered to the outside so that the stalk can be ligated and the polyp excised.

2. *Sessile Rectal Adenoma* (Parks, 1966)

Preparation is as described for the removal of a rectal polyp. The lithotomy, left lateral or prone position is used according to the site of the lesion. With a Parks anal retractor in place the submucosal layer is infiltrated with normal saline containing adrenaline (1 in 300 000). The lesion is excised with a small cuff

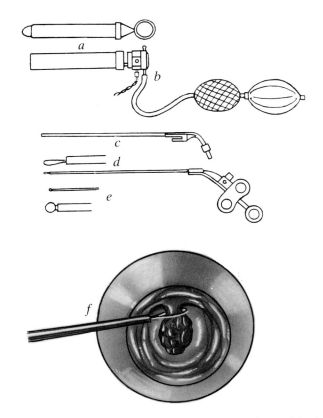

Fig. 19.18. Peranal diathermy snare of a rectal polyp. *a*, Lloyd-Davies operating sigmoidoscope with obturator—15 or 20 cm in length. *b*, Light fitting with window and bellows. *c*, Sucker. *d*, Diathermy snare. *e*, Diathermy buttons. *f*, Stalk of polyp encircled by snare.

of normal mucosa (*Fig.* 19.19*a*). The underlying muscle is left bare but epithelialization rapidly covers the defect. Tumours as high as 20 cm can be brought down by intussusception and removed. It is possible to remove three-quarters of the circumference of the rectal mucosa in this way and still achieve satisfactory healing without stenosis. In the case of circumferential lesions, however, the mucosal defect must be closed. This can be done by imbricating the muscle wall with non-absorbable sutures (*Fig.* 19.19*b*) and then closing the mucosa with catgut sutures (*Fig.* 19.19*c*). A trans-sphincteric approach as already described can also be used and, if very extensive, resection with colo-anal anastomosis is appropriate.

3. *Rectal Carcinoma*

Very small rectal carcinomas may be removed per anum using an anal retractor. Full-thickness resection of the anal wall is required and the defect closed using a single layer of non-absorbable sutures. The indications for such a procedure are rare as there must be no extrarectal extension of the tumour, which is very difficult to assess clinically and impossible to assess histologically as no lymph nodes are removed, and lesions of high-grade malignancy must

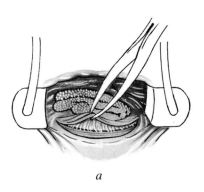
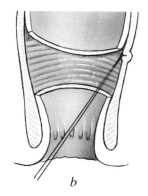
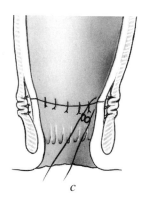

Fig. 19.19. Peranal resection of sessile rectal adenoma. *a*, Excision of mucosa with lesion after submucosal infiltration. *b*, Imbrication of muscle wall after circumferential mucosal resection. *c*, Suture of mucosa.

be excluded. In a very old patient or a medically unfit patient or in someone who adamantly refuses to have a colostomy, such a procedure may be justified.

The Soave–Denda Operation

This operation is used for extensive benign conditions of the rectal mucosa such as haemangioma or circumferential adenoma or for Hirschsprung's disease where it is unnecessary to disturb the pelvic nerve plexuses. After the usual investigation and preparation a laparotomy is performed through a left paramedian incision. The upper rectum is divided (*Fig.* 19.20*a*) and as much of the proximal segment of rec-

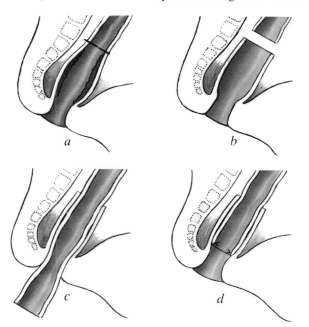

Fig. 19.20. The Soave operation with the Denda modification. *a*, Division of the upper rectum. *b*, The mucosa of the distal rectum is removed. *c*, The colon is brought down within the rectal muscular cuff and left protruding from the anus until adherence is complete—Soave operation. *d*, The colon can be brought down within the rectal cuff and sutured to the anal canal mucosa just above the dentate line—Denda modification.

tum and sigmoid colon resected as is necessary to remove pathology. The mucosa of the distal rectum is then removed (*Fig.* 19.20*b*) from above and from below (using an anal retractor) following submucosal infiltration with normal saline containing adrenaline (1 in 300 000). The proximal colon is brought down into the muscular cuff of the rectum. The colon is loosely tacked to the anal verge and left protruding from the anus (*Fig.* 19.20*c*). Three weeks later when adherence is complete the protruding colon is excised (the Soave operation). Alternatively the colon is sutured to the cut mucosal edge just above the dentate line in the anal canal (*Fig.* 19.20*d*) at the first operation (the Denda modification of the Soave operation). A suction drain is placed in the plane between the colon and the rectal colostomy and antibiotic cover is given.

Complete Rectal Prolapse

Many operations have been devised to treat this extremely distressing condition which is associated in a large percentage of cases with grossly abnormal bowel function and/or faecal incontinence. Of all these the one producing the best results is the Ivalon or polyvinyl alcohol sponge repair (Wells and Naunton Morgan, 1962), and only this is described in detail. The principle of the repair is that the reaction that the Ivalon excites retains the rectum in the pelvis and so prevents intussusception and therefore prolapse.

After a full investigation to exclude other pathology which may initiate intussusception, and therefore prolapse, the bowel is prepared mechanically with aperients and washouts. Antibiotic cover is essential. With the patient prone and the bladder empty a left paramedian incision is made. After laparotomy and packing of the bowel into the upper abdomen, the lower sigmoid colon and rectum are mobilized by incising the peritoneum on each side of the pelvic mesocolon. These incisions are continued down beside the rectum and joined in front of the rectum in the rectovaginal pouch. The presacral space is opened up as far as the anorectal junction and the lateral ligaments divided. Anteriorly only a little dissection is required to expose the vaginal vault or seminal vesicles as the pouch is always deep due to the hernial sac. Meticulous haemostasis is essential. A piece of Ivalon sponge is then cut as shown in *Fig.* 19.21*a*, the exact size depending on the ana-

uncommon and if caught in the sphincters in the upper anal canal may give very distressing discomfort or pain. This can often be relieved by one or two submucosal injections of 5 per cent phenol, as for internal haemorrhoids.

Circumferential mucosal prolapse must be dis-

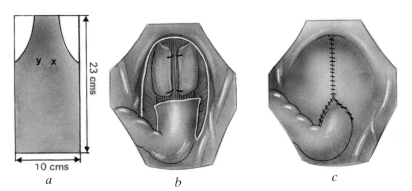

Fig. 19.21. Ivalon sponge repair of complete rectal prolapse. *a*, Ivalon sponge sheet cut to size. *b*, Ivalon sponge in place. *c*, Peritoneal floor closed.

tomy of each patient. A non-absorbable suture is now put through the Ivalon sheet at x. It is then passed through the fascia in front of the sacrococcygeal junction and returned through the Ivalon sheet at y. The sheet is then moulded to the curve of the sacrum and coccyx with the 'tail' lying on the pubococcygeal muscles, and the suture is tied. The rectum now falls back into the sacrococcygeal curve and the Ivalon is wrapped round three-quarters of the circumference of the rectum. It is loosely tacked to the rectal wall with non-absorbable sutures at all four corners (*Fig.* 19.21*b*). The mesorectum is then fixed to the lumbosacral disc in the midline with one non-absorbable suture. The pelvic peritoneum is reconstituted so that the sponge is completely extraperitonealized (*Fig.* 19.21*c*). The abdomen is closed without drainage.

Careful attention to bowel function is essential. A hydrophilic aperient such as Metamucil (ispaghula) in a dose of 15 ml at night is very effective, and this may have to be continued indefinitely. Frequent rectal examination is essential to ensure that impaction does not occur and the daily use of a glycerin suppository may be helpful. If troublesome incontinence continues due to weakness of the anal sphincters a post-anal repair (*see* p. 269) may ultimately be necessary.

Another satisfactory procedure is the Ripstein operation. This consists of placing a wide band of non-absorbable material as a sling around the rectum to retain it in the hollow of the sacrum. Less dissection is required than for the Ivalon repair but in all other respects operative details and management are the same (*Fig.* 19.22).

Mucosal Prolapse

A degree of anterior rectal mucosal prolapse is not

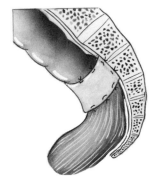

Fig. 19.22. Ripstein operation for complete rectal prolapse.

tinguished from complete rectal prolapse. In those cases in whom there is no incontinence ligation and excision of the redundant mucosa, as for internal haemorrhoids, is very satisfactory, the preoperative and postoperative management being exactly the same.

If incontinence remains a troublesome symptom a Thiersch procedure (*see* p. 269) may be needed or in a few cases post-anal repair may be indicated.

Rectocele, Enterocele and Pelvic Floor Descent

Descent of the pelvic floor in the female may consist of uterine prolapse, prolapse of the bladder into the anterior vaginal wall (cystocele), prolapse of the urethra in the anterior vaginal wall (urethrocele), prolapse of the intestine into the pouch of Douglas (enterocele), prolapse of the rectum into the posterior vaginal wall (rectocele), and weakness of the urogenital hiatus, or any combination of these. A chapter on rectal surgery would be incomplete without mentioning the latter three conditions which may present as a palpable swelling at the introitus, with difficulty in achieving rectal evacuation without digital pressure on the posterior vaginal wall.

The operation that deals with this situation is posterior colpoperineorrhaphy, with or without vaginal hysterectomy if appropriate. The posterior vaginal wall is opened vertically and the perineal body divided. The sac of the pouch of Douglas hernia, if present, is identified, ligated and excised. If the uterus is removed the uterosacral ligaments are approximated. The anterior rectal wall is now invaginated with a continuous vertical suture. The pubococcygeus muscles are then approximated in front of the rectum and inferiorly the puborectalis muscles are approximated in front of the upper anal canal. Anterior plication of the anal sphincters can then be carried out if appropriate and the perineal body reconstituted. The vaginal wall is finally closed vertically to complete the operation.

Rectovaginal Fistula

Preliminary preparation for surgery may include examination under anaesthetic, sigmoidoscopy (and if necessary colonoscopy), radiography, and biopsy of the rectum and of the fistula track, in order to determine, first, to which part of the bowel the fistula connects and, second, whether there is any underlying pathology such as Crohn's disease or malignancy which may affect the management. In a few cases of inflammatory bowel disease the fistula will close with medical treatment.

A traumatic fistula of obstetric origin can usually be dealt with by a conservative repair in which the anatomical layers, rectal mucosa, muscle layer, vaginal mucosa, are identified and closed separately using either a vaginal or an abdominal approach. Alternatively the fistula can be converted into a third-degree perineal laceration with repair of the resulting defect in layers and reconstitution of the perineal body. A covering colostomy is not essential unless a urinary fistula is also present. In these cases a colostomy is essential and the urinary fistula should be dealt with before the rectal fistula as a separate procedure. In some cases the fistula can be approached through the anus using a Parks retractor, and occasionally a York Mason trans-sphincteric approach is appropriate.

A very high rectovaginal fistula due to obstetric trauma or a fistula associated with inflammatory bowel disease usually requires a bowel resection with restoration of continuity and possibly a hysterectomy. This is occasionally suitable for a fistula associated with malignant disease. It will also be suitable for an irradiation fistula if normal bowel is present on each side of the affected area. Occasionally restoration of continuity may not be possible and excision of the rectum with colostomy is the only alternative.

Adult Megacolon: Full-thickness Rectal Biopsy

Adult megacolon may be due to adult Hirschsprung's disease or to intractable constipation which has required long-standing use of laxatives to which the bowel has become unresponsive. It is important to distinguish between these two conditions and although X-ray studies and sphincter studies may be helpful a full-thickness rectal biopsy is conclusive.

The bowel must be mechanically clear and this may take many days in the face of long-standing constipation. With the patient under general anaesthetic and in the lithotomy position an anal retractor is inserted. A stay suture is placed through the full thickness of the rectal wall just above the ano-rectal ring in the left lateral quadrant and is tied, leaving the needle attached. A second suture is placed 3 cm proximal to the first and this also is tied. The bowel wall is then incised just proximal to the first stitch and a strip of bowel wall 3 mm wide is removed between the two sutures. The edges of the defect are then oversewn using the first stay suture, which is tied to the second suture at the upper end of the wound.

Cases of adult Hirschsprung's disease will require a Duhamel procedure. For the rest a subtotal colectomy with caeco-rectal or ascending colo-rectal anastomosis may be indicated in those cases with a thin dilated large bowel. In a few cases the large bowel is hypertrophied indicating a probable sphincter problem, and in these a colostomy is probably indicated as local procedures on the sphincters, such as sphincterotomy, rarely help.

Hirschsprung's Disease (*see* Chapter 58)

Cases presenting in the first few months of life should be given a defunctioning colostomy, usually a right transverse colostomy, as the primary treatment. For cases presenting in later life a period of rectal irrigation may prepare the bowel sufficiently prior to the definitive procedure, at which time it is usually wise to add a covering colostomy. Three principal procedures are used. In each, frozen section examination of a piece of bowel wall must confirm that the colon to be brought down for anastomosis is normal.

1. *Swenson's Operation*

In this procedure the aganglionic segment of rectum is resected and an abdomino-anal pull-through anastomosis in two layers is performed (*Fig.* 19.23a).

2. *Duhamel's Operation*

In this procedure the rectum is preserved and a retro-rectal peranal pull-through performed. The spur can be dealt with by a stapler or by intestinal crushing clamps (*Fig.* 19.23b). The potential rectal pouch (marked X) can be avoided by leaving the rectal

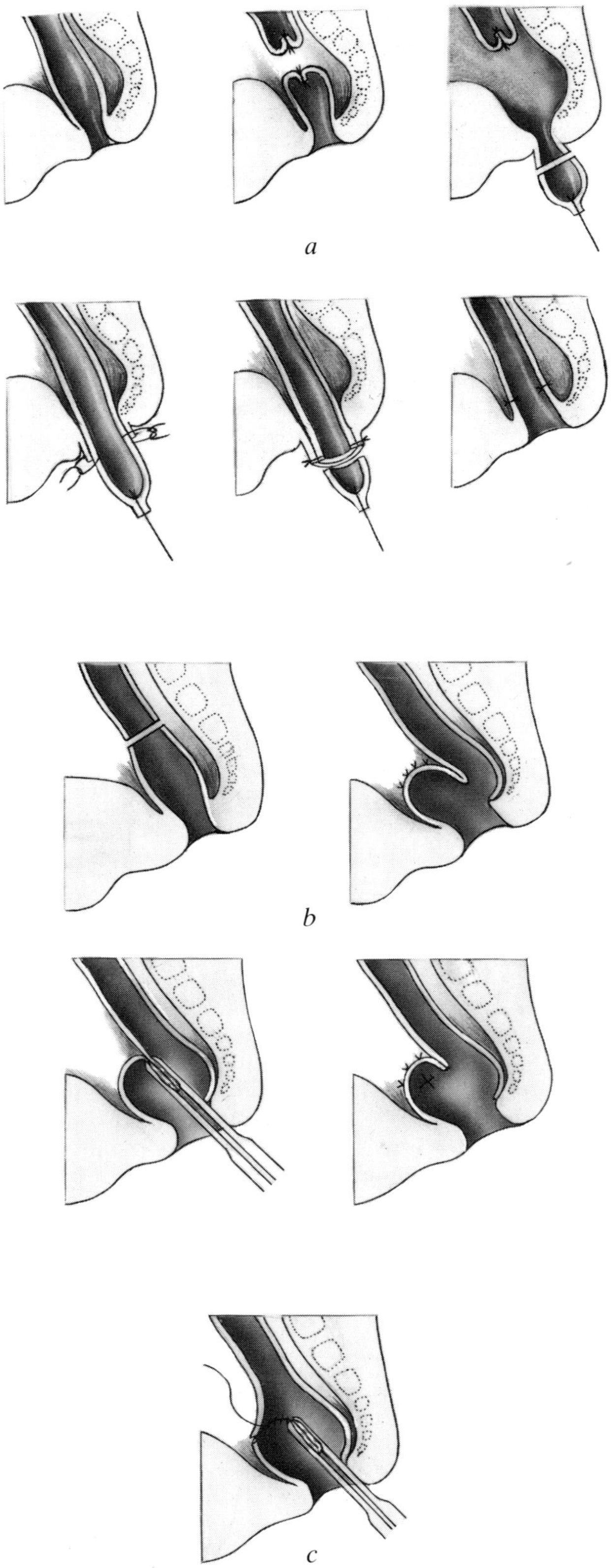

Fig. 19.23. Hirschsprung's disease. *a*, Swenson's operation. *b*, *c*, Duhamel's operation.

stump open, opening the colon at the same level and suturing the anterior colic wall to the anterior rectal wall (*Fig.* 19.23*c*).

3. *The Soave–Denda Operation*
This is described earlier in this chapter (p. 255).

SURGERY OF THE ANAL CANAL

Internal Haemorrhoids

1. *Conservative Treatment*
The single most important prophylactic treatment is the avoidance of straining at stool and this can best be achieved by the addition of bulk to the diet in the form of natural bran in order to achieve a satisfactory stool consistency.

Application of ointments and creams and insertion of suppositories rarely produce anything but temporary relief of anal discomfort or irritation and do nothing for bleeding.

A. INJECTION
The symptom of bleeding resulting from first-degree internal haemorrhoids can in the majority of cases be kept under control by injection treatment (Gabriel and Milligan, 1939). Some patients with second-degree internal haemorrhoids can achieve similar relief and injection therapy is often worth trying in these cases, perhaps in combination with banding (*see below*). Third-degree haemorrhoids will not be helped, and indeed troublesome prolapse and thrombosis may be caused by injection. Pregnancy is no contra-indication to injection treatment, although other conservative measures are perhaps better in early pregnancy as a mother with an abnormal baby might always wonder whether the injection had been responsible.

After general examination and sigmoidoscopy to exclude other pathology such as colitis or neoplasm, proctoscopy is performed to establish the diagnosis. Occasionally a barium enema will be necessary to exclude absolutely colonic pathology. Bowel preparation and anaesthesia are unnecessary. No assistant is required. The proctoscope is repassed and it is convenient to insert a cottonwool swab into the lower rectum to hold back any faecal material and to put the rectal wall slightly on the stretch. A 10-ml Gabriel syringe with a bayonet-locking guarded needle is used. The solution for injection is 5 per cent phenol in almond oil with 0·5 per cent menthol added. The menthol helps to dissolve the phenol crystals during preparation and is said to reduce the discomfort of the injection. The needle is inserted into the submucosal layer just above each haemorrhoid and approximately 3 ml injected (*Fig.* 19.24). No more than 10 ml

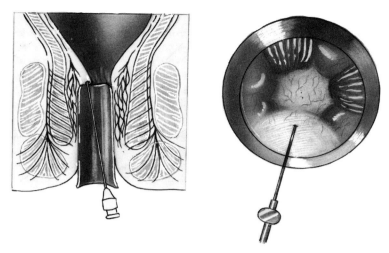

Fig. 19.24. Injection of internal haemorrhoids.

should be used. Ideally the mucosa should balloon up as the injection proceeds. If it is too superficial the mucosa goes quite white and the injection must be discontinued or an ulcer will result which may lead to secondary haemorrhage. The needle can be inserted too deeply in which case no ballooning will be seen and it is possible to inject into the prostate in which case haematuria or haematospermia may result. In that case a broad-spectrum antibiotic must be administered immediately. Occasionally, following an otherwise satisfactory injection, a submucous abscess occurs or, rarely, an oleogranuloma.

During the injection the patient will either feel nothing or at most a feeling of distension. The rectal swab is then removed and a clean swab inserted at the level of the injection site before withdrawing the proctoscope. If the injection site bleeds a swab should be placed at the ano-rectal junction and the proctoscope removed. After a few minutes bleeding will have stopped in the majority of cases. If bleeding persists local application of a swab soaked in adrenaline (1 in 1000) will be effective. Very rarely packing as for secondary haemorrhage after haemorrhoidectomy is required. Ideally the patient should avoid defaecation until the following day. Patients should be warned that they may see the cottonwool swab, that they may notice more bleeding than usual at defaecation for a day or two and that they may be aware of leakage of mucus for a few days.

A second injection can be given if the haemorrhoids are sizeable but this should not be done for 6 weeks in order to allow the first injection to have a full effect and also to avoid mucosal ulceration.

B. BARRON BAND LIGATION (Barron, 1963)

Occasionally a second-degree internal haemorrhoid, a residual secondary haemorrhoid after haemorrhoidectomy or a recurrent haemorrhoid is suitable for banding. The procedure can be carried out follow-

ing the routine examination described above, without bowel preparation or anaesthetic.

A proctoscope is passed and held by an assistant. The instrument for banding is shown in *Fig.* 19.25*a*.

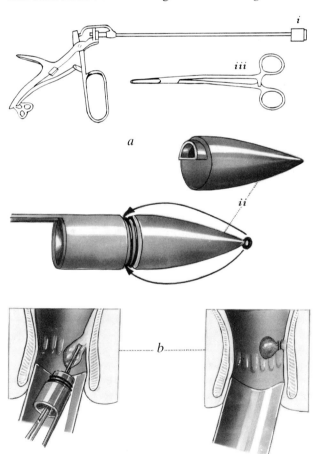

Fig. 19.25. Barron band ligation of internal haemorrhoids. *a*, The instrument. i, Double cylinder. ii, Cone for mounting the rubber bands. iii, Grasping forceps. *b*, The firing of the instrument and the end result.

It consists of a double metal cylinder (*i*) onto one of which two rubber bands are mounted using a detachable cone (*ii*). Once loaded, the haemorrhoid to be banded is grasped near its base with forceps (*iii*) through the double cylinders. The instrument is then fired and this places the bands in position as shown in *Fig. 19.25b*.

Oral analgesia may be required. Sloughing occurs between 4 and 10 days and may be accompanied by bleeding. Rarely this is severe and requires hospitalization and packing as for secondary haemorrhage after haemorrhoidectomy. It is wise only to band one to two haemorrhoids at any one session and to wait at least 3 weeks before contemplating further banding.

C. MAXIMAL ANAL DILATATION—LORD'S PROCEDURE
(Lord, 1972)

As already mentioned, straining at stool undoubtedly predisposes to the formation of internal haemorrhoids. The condition can be helped by the addition of bulk to the diet but another factor may be constriction of the anal canal and this may be helped by gentle dilatation of the canal. This conservative measure may be particularly useful in a very young patient or in pregnancy. Bowel preparation is unnecessary. A general anaesthetic is required.

With the patient in the left lateral position the surgeon inserts the index finger of each hand into the anal canal and with gentle stretching in a lateral direction he or she may be able to insert six or even eight fingers. This must be done with the greatest care and it is best to do too little rather than too much. After the dilatation a foam rubber sponge can be inserted for an hour to reduce the risk of haematoma.

Postoperatively a special dilator 3·8 cm in diameter may be passed daily for 2 weeks or so and then less frequently for a further period to prevent constriction recurring.

Incontinence of flatus may occur for a time, but more serious incontinence can be avoided by gentleness. Mucosal prolapse may occur but usually resolves spontaneously. If it persists a further procedure may be necessary.

2. *Surgical Treatment*

A. HAEMORRHOIDECTOMY—LIGATION AND EXCISION (ST MARK'S OR MILLIGAN–MORGAN TECHNIQUE)

This operation (Milligan et al., 1937) is indicated for internal haemorrhoids that are large and therefore prolapse and also if conservative measures have failed. The presence of a skin tag, fissure or superficial fistula is an additional indication. Pregnancy is not a contra-indication but palliative treatment is best until the pregnancy is over as the situation will then improve and surgery may be avoided. With modern anaesthetic techniques, old age is not a contra-indication. Prolapsed thrombosed internal haemorrhoids can be removed by the technique to be described, within 48 hours of the event, but thereafter there is a danger of portal pyaemia and a conservative regimen of bed rest and local application of cold lead lotion should be adopted. Other causes of symptoms must be excluded prior to surgery. This entails general examination and sigmoidoscopy and, if indicated, a barium enema. It is particularly important to exclude a colonic or rectal neoplasm. Haemorrhoidectomy should not be carried out in the presence of dysenteric infection, or any form of colitis, as the wounds will prove difficult to heal and a flare-up of the colitis may ensue. Copious reassurance is required that this need not be the painful procedure that it is sometimes made out to be.

The patient is admitted on the day before operation and a phosphate enema given. The peri-anal skin is shaved, but it may be necessary to complete the shave on the operating table. If very constipated a rectal washout with tube and funnel can be given 2 hours prior to surgery the following day, but care must be taken that all fluid is removed from the rectum.

General anaesthesia is usually employed but a caudal or spinal anaesthetic in the elderly is satisfactory. The patient is placed in the lithotomy position with slight headdown tilt, the lower end of the table removed and the buttocks positioned well over the end of the table. In the male the scrotum should be elevated with a thick rubber tube or with strapping. The peri-anal skin is cleaned with cetrimide and the anal canal and lower rectum swabbed out digitally with cottonwool soaked in cetrimide until all traces of faecal material have been removed. It is convenient to start towelling with leggings. A large towel is then placed across the buttocks below the anal orifice and fixed to the leg supports with pole clips. The lower abdomen is covered with a further towel and a towel-covered Mayo table is positioned in front of the seated surgeon. This routine is suitable for all anal surgery. If necessary shaving is completed with a scalpel.

The operation starts with an inferior haemorrhoidal nerve block. This allows a much lighter general anaesthetic to be given and reduces postoperative discomfort to a remarkable degree. Lignocaine 1 per cent with adrenaline (1 in 200 000) is used, provided there is no cardiac contra-indication to the use of adrenaline. The skin behind the anus is swabbed with Hibitane (chlorhexidine) in spirit. With a finger in the anal canal a no. 19 Fr. gauge 50-mm needle on a 20-ml syringe is inserted in the midline and passed in turn into each ischiorectal fossa where 7 ml of solution are injected. Three Dunhill artery forceps are now placed on the peri-anal skin in the left lateral, right posterior and right anterior positions, corresponding to the usual sites of the primary internal haemorrhoids. Traction on these brings the internal haemorrhoids into view and three more Dunhill forceps are placed near the apex of each haemorrhoidal

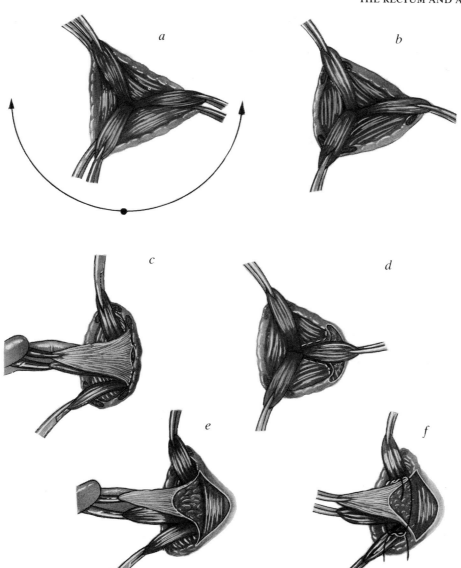

Fig. 19.26. Ligation and excision of internal haemorrhoids (St Mark's or Milligan–Morgan technique). *a*, Site of inferior haemorrhoidal nerve block and the 'triangle of exposure'. *b*, A cut on each side of the haemorrhoidal mass at the anal margin. *c*, Cut outside the haemorrhoidal mass. *d*, Mucosal incision on each side of each haemorrhoidal mass. *e*, Dissection of the haemorrhoidal mass off the internal sphincter. *f*, Ligation of the pedicle.

mass. Secondary haemorrhoids can be clipped with a further Dunhill forceps and included with the nearest primary mass for dissection. Traction on all six forceps reveals the 'triangle of exposure' between the three haemorrhoidal pedicles (*Fig.* 19.26*a*). By holding each pair of Dunhill forceps apart in turn the mucocutaneous junction is put on the stretch and 2 ml of the above local anaesthetic solution are injected subcutaneously using a no. 25 Fr. gauge 16-mm needle. This step cuts down troublesome minor haemorrhage very significantly and it is therefore worth waiting for a few minutes for it to take effect.

The dissection now starts using blunt scissors, sur-geon's straight scissors being suitable. It is very important throughout to make sure that muco-cutaneous 'bridges' are maintained between each area of dissection. A cut on each side of the haemorrhoid/skin tag mass at the anal margin marks the limit of the sideways dissection of each haemor-rhoid. When learning the technique this can be done to all three haemorrhoid/skin tag masses at this stage, thus marking the base of each 'bridge' at the start (*Fig.* 19.26*b*). The two forceps on the left lateral haemorrhoid/skin tag mass are now held in the left hand with the index finger of the left hand in the anal canal and a cut is made outside the mass midway between the two cuts already made (*Fig.* 19.26*c*). These three cuts are then joined along the dotted line in the illustration. In order to be certain that the 'bridges' are maintained the haemorrhoid/skin tag mass is then held laterally and with narrow-bladed scissors (McIndoe scissors are suitable) the mucosa on each side of the mass in the anal canal is divided as far as its apex (*Fig.* 19.26*d*). The dissection must go no higher than this as stenosis may result. The index finger of the left hand is then reinserted into the anal canal and with blunt scissors the dissection of the haemorrhoid/skin tag mass from the whitish circumferential fibres of the internal sphincter continues to the apex of the haemorrhoid (*Fig.* 19.26*e*). The pedicle of the haemorrhoid/skin tag mass is then transfixed and ligated with '0' (No. 4) strength chromic catgut (*Fig.* 19.26*f*). This process is repeated for each haemorrhoid in turn and the haemorrhoidal masses excised leaving a good cuff of tissue and a 2-cm length of ligature. Any residual veins beneath the bridge edges are removed by filleting, residual tags of skin trimmed from the edges of the external wounds and bleeding points diathermied. A small piece of Paul's tubing is then inserted into the rectum and taped to one buttock. This gives warning of reactionary haemorrhage into the rectum and is removed after 24 hours. Flat dressings of gauze soaked in cetrimide, Eusol (1 in 8) or Hibitane (1 in 2000) are applied with a wool pad and a T-bandage.

The patient is started on an aperient such as Mil-Par (magnesium hydroxide) in a dose of 15 ml three times a day, until the first bowel action is achieved. Thereafter a bulk-forming laxative is used and should be continued in diminishing dosage until the anal canal is healed and an easy daily bowel action with a formed motion is achieved. The author uses Normacol (sterculia) granules and Senokot granules in a dose of 10 ml of each twice daily at the start. Senokot can usually be discontinued after a few days and the Normacol dosage reduced, but this usually has to be continued for a week or two after discharge from hospital. In due course natural bran may be all that is required to maintain a satisfactory bowel action.

After 48 hours the patient starts a twice daily regimen of hot baths and redressing. Flat dressings of Eusol (1 in 8), Hibitane (1 in 2000) or Milton (sodium hypochlorite) (1 in 40) are applied with a wool pad

and kept in place with a T-bandage or Netelast 'pants'. Adequate analgesia should be given as necessary. At the 6th day an index finger is passed to ensure that stenosis is not occurring. If the canal feels a little tight the patient should be shown how to pass a no. 2 St Mark's pattern anal dilator. This should be done twice daily until the first outpatient visit 4 weeks after operation, at which time a finger should again be passed (but not a proctoscope) to assess progress. The anal canal will always feel somewhat 'stiff' at this time. Further follow-up is not necessary unless a further period of dilatation is thought to be desirable.

Complications include retention of urine which may require catheterization, reactionary haemorrhage from an external wound, which is usually slight and responds to local application of a swab soaked in adrenaline (1 in 1000), haemorrhage from a slipped ligature on a pedicle which requires religation under general anaesthesia, and the formation of a fistula due to the edges of a wound falling together, which must be laid open. The most serious complication, however, is secondary haemorrhage which usually occurs at about the 8th postoperative day and which usually requires pressure to control it. This is achieved by passing a large rubber tube wrapped in gauze into the rectum and anal canal via a large proctoscope. A broad-spectrum antibiotic is given for 5 days and the pack is gently removed after 48 hours.

B. CLOSED HAEMORRHOIDECTOMY

This technique, not widely practised in the United Kingdom, aims to preserve as much of the lining of the anal canal as possible. Healing by first intention is usually achieved and postoperative pain is said to be minimal.

Dissection of each haemorrhoid/skin tag mass starts at the anal margin (*Fig.* 19.27*a*) and as narrow a strip as possible of skin and mucosa is removed together with underlying haemorrhoidal tissue until the internal sphincter is exposed (*Fig.* 19.27*b*). Further haemorrhoidal tissue is removed from beneath the edges of the wound (*Fig.* 19.27*b*) and the wound is closed with a continuous catgut suture (*Fig.* 19.27*c*).

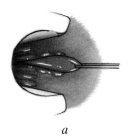
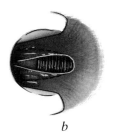
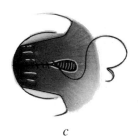

a   *b*   *c*

Fig. 19.27. Closed haemorrhoidectomy.

C. HAEMORRHOIDECTOMY—LIGATION AND EXCISION
(PARKS' TECHNIQUE)

This technique (Parks, 1956) aims to remove haemorrhoidal tissue, restore sensitive prolapsed anal skin to the lower anal canal and remove an equivalent amount of mucus-secreting columnar epithelium from the upper anal canal and lower rectum.

A Parks anal retractor is used (*Fig.* 19.28). Normal

be used to freeze haemorrhoidal tissue. Patients with a lax anus can receive treatment on an outpatient basis, perhaps with intravenous diazepam, while those with spasm require dilatation under a general anaesthetic prior to treatment. No bowel preparation is necessary. With the patient in the left lateral position the anus is lubricated with KY Jelly (good conductor) and a proctoscope is passed. The cryoprobe

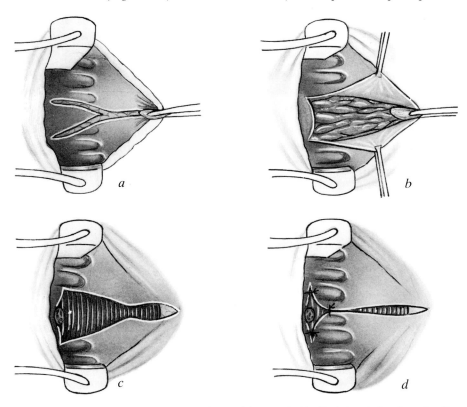

Fig. 19.28. Ligation and excision of internal haemorrhoids (Parks' technique). *a*, Small amount of tissue at skin edge raised. *b*, Dissection of haemorrhoidal mass. *c*, Dissection completed. *d*, Anal mucosa advanced up the canal and sutured.

saline containing adrenaline (1 in 300 000) is injected subcutaneously and submucosally at the site of each haemorrhoidal complex in turn. The dissection starts at the anal margin and as little anal skin as possible is removed (*Fig.* 19.28*a*). As the dissection proceeds flaps of anal skin and mucosa are raised (*Fig.* 19.28*b*). The small piece of anal skin and underlying haemorrhoidal tissue is dissected from the internal sphincter, ligated and excised (*Fig.* 19.28*c*). The two flaps of anal skin and mucosa are then advanced up the canal and sutured as shown in *Fig.* 19.28*d* using '0' strength chromic catgut. The stitches should include internal sphincter muscle fibres to fix the flaps more securely. Postoperative pain is less than in the standard ligation and excision operation and anal stenosis is rare.

D. CRYOSURGERY (Goligher, 1976)

A liquid nitrogen or nitrous oxide closed probe can

is applied to the apex of each haemorrhoidal mass in turn. Freezing takes 2–3 minutes. A nitrous oxide probe will stick to the tissue and will only separate when rewarming occurs. It is important to ensure that the haemorrhoidal mass remains mobile over the internal sphincter during the whole procedure.

Oedema and discharge will require the wearing of a pad and frequent hot baths, but no other treatment. Pain requires oral analgesics only. Healing is complete in 3 weeks. Secondary haemorrhage and sepsis have been reported. Stenosis is rare.

SUMMARY

As far as conservative management is concerned there is no doubt that injection and banding are the most effective forms of treatment. Manual dilatation can be useful in a few cases. With regard to operative treatment the standard operation of ligation and excision (St Mark's or Milligan–Morgan) is by far the most widely practised and produces excellent results. The Parks method is a difficult technique to learn and initially is a more bloody and a more time-consuming procedure. It produces excellent results, however, and in the right hands is a very acceptable alternative to standard ligation and excision. Closed haemorrhoidectomy is theoretically attractive but is a difficult technique and has no real advantages over the previous two methods. Cryosurgery is not widely used in the UK as it is felt to be unpredictable, the postoperative oedema and discharge can be troublesome and residual tags of skin often call for a further procedure. Infra-red coagulation is a newer technique, not fully evaluated as yet, which seems to have no obvious advantages over established procedures.

Anal Skin Tags

Skin tags alone rarely give symptoms but if hygiene is difficult pruritus may be troublesome. Often they occur in association with other conditions, especially internal haemorrhoids, and may be removed in the treatment of these conditions. Small tags can be removed as an outpatient procedure under local anaesthetic. No sutures are required and a simple dry dressing only is needed for a few days. Larger tags will require general anaesthesia for their removal.

Fibrous Anal Polyp (Hypertrophied Anal Papilla)

Rarely one or more fibrous polyps may develop at the dentate line midway up the anal canal and if prolapse occurs they are noticed by the patient. They may occur with other conditions, for example with a fissure-in-ano, and may be treated with that condition. If they occur alone they should be ligated and excised under general anaesthetic using a Dunhill artery forceps and '0' strength chromic catgut.

Peri-anal Haematoma (Thrombosed External Haemorrhoid)

Thrombosis in an external haemorrhoidal vein is usually an acutely painful condition associated with the appearance of a tender bluish swelling of variable size, from which clot may begin to extrude spontaneously.

If very painful and comparatively small the whole area can be excised under local anaesthetic. A Hibitane-soaked dressing is applied for 24 hours and thereafter frequent hot baths and dry dressing are all that is necessary. A gentle aperient is advisable. Relief of pain by incision of the lesion and evacuation of the clot can be dramatic, but a troublesome oedematous tag usually results.

If a large area is involved conservative treatment with bed rest, oral analgesics and frequent applications of cold lead lotion is advisable until the acute episode has settled. Resolution is usually complete in 2–3 weeks. A complete proctological examination is then essential to exclude other pathology.

Fissure-in-ano

Simple anal fissure occurs in the lower half of the anal canal, in the midline posteriorly in 75 per cent of cases, in the midline anteriorly in 15 per cent of cases and at both sites in the remaining 10 per cent of cases. It is associated with spasm of the anal sphincters.

Inspection of the anus will usually reveal the lower end of the fissure even in the presence of marked spasm. Digital examination is usually possible if 2 per cent lignocaine lubricant is used and if great care is taken. Sigmoidoscopy or proctoscopy may not be possible initially. A fissure that is not in the midline, is extensive and irregular, or which is multiple, is suspicious of other pathology such as inflammatory bowel disease which must be investigated appropriately, syphilis which must be diagnosed by dark-ground illumination of a smear, or neoplasm which must be biopsied.

As a fissure passes from the acute to the chronic stage several changes may occur (*Fig. 19.29a–f*). Initially the vertical muscle fibres of the musculus submucosae ani are seen (*a*) but as the fissure deepens the horizontal fibres of the internal sphincter are seen (*b*). A sentinel tag of skin may then develop at the lower end of the fissure (*c*) together with a hypertrophied anal papilla on the dentate line at the upper end (*d*). Undermining of the edges may lead to abscess formation (*e*) and finally a subcutaneous fistula may develop at the lower end (*f*).

Stages (*a*) and (*b*) can be treated conservatively by the passage of a St Mark's pattern dilator (*g*), no. 2 in the series of three being ideal. This is passed by the patient twice daily using 2 per cent lignocaine gel as a lubricant, and is kept in place for a period of 1–2 minutes. Patients must do this themselves in the clinic to reassure themselves and the surgeon that it can be done. This should be continued for 6 weeks and a bulk-forming laxative taken in addition. For the remainder, and for those cases in whom conservative management does not succeed, lateral subcutaneous internal sphincterotomy is indicated (Hawley, 1969).

This procedure can be performed under local anaesthetic on an outpatient basis, but the author prefers to admit the patient on the day before surgery when a phosphate enema is given, and to use a general anaesthetic. With the patient in the lithotomy position a bivalve speculum is passed (Eisenhammer). When opened, the lower fibres of the internal sphincter can be felt as a tight band between the blades of the instrument (*h*). Lignocaine 1 per cent with adrenaline (1 in 200 000) is then infiltrated between the sphincter and the mucosa of the lower anal canal and into the intersphincteric plane. The

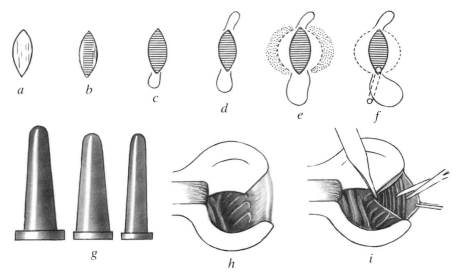

Fig. 19.29. Fissure-in-ano. *a*, Vertical fibres of musculus submucosae ani exposed. *b*, Horizontal fibres of internal sphincter exposed. *c*, Sentinel tag of skin develops. *d*, Anal papilla develops. *e*, Undermining and abscess formation. *f*, Subcutaneous fistula develops. *g*, St Mark's pattern anal dilator—three sizes. *h*, Bivalve speculum inserted into anal canal. *i*, The internal sphincter exposed.

speculum is removed and a circumferential incision made in the lateral position just outside the external anal ring (*i*). The speculum is reinserted and the wound edges held apart with tissue-holding forceps. The white lower fibres of the internal sphincter can then be seen and these are divided up to the level of the dentate line.

The wound is closed with absorbable sutures. Any sentinel skin tag or anal papilla is removed from the fissure. Undermined edges are trimmed and a fistula if present is laid open. The temptation to carry out the sphincterotomy in the base of the fissure should be resisted as a dorsal wound may not heal well. A flat dressing is applied. A gentle aperient is given and the patient may leave hospital when comfortable, ideally after the first bowel action.

Peri-anal and Ischiorectal Abscess

Infection in this area may localize as a small but obvious abscess adjacent to the anal orifice or spread through the ischiorectal fossa on one or both sides to form a large abscess which may initially be difficult to diagnose. Final assessment includes sigmoid-oscopy and proctoscopy but this may be very painful and may have to be deferred until the patient is under a general anaesthetic in the lithotomy position.

If the presence of an abscess is confirmed an incision is made over the most fluctuant part. A swab of the pus is sent for bacteriological culture. The cavity is explored digitally to assess its extent and to break down loculi. Instruments should never be used for fear of penetrating the levator ani muscle, thus causing a supralevator extension of infection. The wound edges are trimmed to allow free drainage and the corner of a gauze dressing soaked in Eusol

(1 in 8) or Hibitane (1 in 2000) inserted to keep the wound open—it should not be packed. The dressing is changed at 24 hours and thereafter the patient has a twice daily bath with reapplication of the dressing.

Although infection, in a sebaceous cyst for example, can occur in this area, such infection is usually associated with a fistula-in-ano but the track to the anal canal is totally obscured by oedema in the acute stage. At 10 days a further examination under anaesthetic may reveal the internal opening in the canal and the track can then be laid open. Any further trimming of wound edges can be done at this stage. Persistent discharge or recurrent abscess invariably means that a fistula is still present.

Fistula-in-ano

A fistula-in-ano will not heal spontaneously and apart from causing recurrent abscess may in very rare cases become malignant. Inflammatory bowel disease and large bowel neoplasia must be excluded by sigmoid-oscopy and proctoscopy and if necessary by barium studies prior to surgery. The nomenclature associated with this condition is difficult and several classifica-tions of fistula-in-ano exist (Hawley, 1975; Parks et al., 1976). To describe a fistula as 'simple', if it con-sists of a radial track running from an external open-ing to an internal opening in the anal canal, and all others as 'complex' is insufficient. To describe a fis-tula as 'low' when it arises from an anal gland regard-less of whether it tracks above the levator muscle, and 'high' only if it has an opening in the bowel above the levator muscle, is helpful, although many sur-geons would regard any extension above the levator muscle as being a 'high' extension, but this again is insufficient. What is required from the practical point of view is an accurate understanding of the anatomy of the anal canal musculature together with a clear appreciation of the relationship of the fistula track and its openings to these muscles. Several complicated situations can arise which are very difficult to deal with but which are fortunately very rare. Only the more common situations are dealt with in this chapter and only nomenclature about which there is no debate is used.

A fistula nearly always arises from an infected anal gland (*Fig. 19.30a*) and in 80 per cent of cases the

rarely upwards through the levator muscle where again it may track circumferentially (*Fig. 19.30g*). Very rarely such a track may enter the rectum (*Fig. 19.30h*).

In cases of inflammatory bowel disease a fistula may pass from the rectum or more proximal diseased bowel to the outside directly (*Fig. 19.30i*), there being no connection with the anal canal. This is an extrasphincteric fistula cured by dealing with the proximal disease. Very rarely such a track may pass down in the intersphincteric plane (not shown).

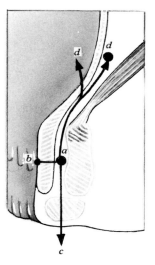
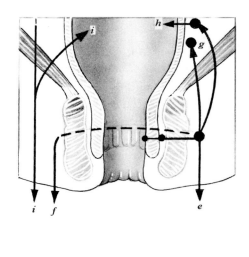

Fig. 19.30. Fistula-in-ano. *a*, Anal gland. *b*, Opening of gland into a crypt. *c*, Low intersphincteric fistula. *d*, High intersphincteric fistula. *e*, Trans-sphincteric fistula with opening directly to the outside. *f*, Trans-sphincteric fistula with circumferential extension. *g*, Trans-sphincteric fistula with supra-levator extension. *h*, Trans-sphincteric fistula opening into the rectum. *i*, Extrasphincteric fistula.

gland involved is in the midline posteriorly. The duct of each gland opens into a crypt at the dentate line (*Fig. 19.30b*) and this becomes the internal opening of the fistula. The glands themselves are in the intersphincteric plane and a resulting abscess can extend in one of several directions. If it extends downwards to the peri-anal skin, the most common situation, it is a low intersphincteric fistula (*Fig. 19.30c*). If it extends upwards and opens into the rectum it is a high intersphincteric fistula (*Fig. 19.30d*). Extension upwards and downwards and circumferentially in this plane can of course all occur in the same fistula. Very rarely the track of such a fistula may pass up in the intersphincteric plane to the supralevator space and thence down through the levator muscle to the ischiorectal fossa and so to the outside. This is a suprasphincteric fistula (not shown) and calls for very careful management (Parks et al., 1976). If infection spreads through the external sphincter the fistula becomes trans-sphincteric and the track may thence pass directly to the outside (*Fig. 19.30e*), or spread circumferentially outside the external sphincter beneath the levator muscle and thence to the outside (*Fig. 19.30f*), occasionally by several openings, or

The patient is admitted the day before surgery and given a phosphate enema. A rectal washout is given 3 hours before operation. A light general anaesthetic is given so that the tone in the puborectalis part of the external sphincter is not lost and the patient put in the lithotomy position.

Instruments

A set of H. E. Lockhart-Mummery directors is required (*Fig. 19.31a*). There are four instruments in the set and they are characterized by a groove running the whole length of the instrument down which a scalpel blade can be passed. A malleable silver probe-ended director, together with a set of Anel's fine malleable silver probes, may also be helpful.

Intersphincteric Fistula

A low intersphincteric fistula is the type most commonly encountered. With one finger in the anal canal a director is gently passed from the external opening. Under light anaesthesia the anorectal ring can be

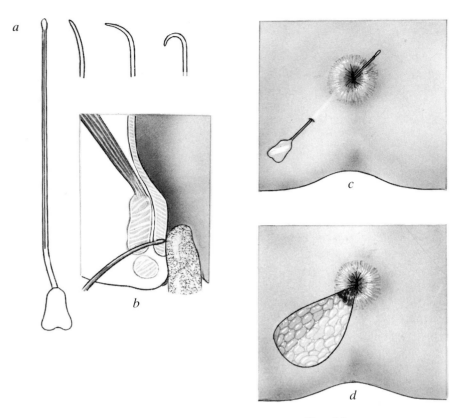

Fig. 19.31. Fistula-in-ano. *a*, Set of H.E. Lockhart-Mummery directors.
Low intersphincteric fistula-in-ano. *b*, Probing of fistula. *c*, Director passed to the outside. *d*, Track laid open.

clearly felt above the track containing the director (*Fig.* 19.31*b*). The point of the director is then brought to the outside (*Fig.* 19.31*c*). The track is laid open by cutting along the groove on the director with a scalpel. The track is curetted and the tissue sent for histological examination. A gentle search is made for communicating tracks which are laid open if found. The main track is then extended outwards for a short distance and the whole wound trimmed to make a triangular wound which is as shallow as possible (*Fig.* 19.31*d*). If there is an upward extension in the intersphincteric plane without an opening into the rectum, it will usually drain satisfactorily when the lower part is laid open as just described.

A flat gauze dressing soaked in Eusol (1 in 8) or Hibitane (1 in 2000) is tucked into the anal canal to reach the apex of the triangular wound. A wool pad is applied and a T-bandage. The inner dressing is kept moist with Eusol, Hibitane or Milton and is soaked off in a hot bath at 48 hours and thereafter reapplied twice daily after a hot bath. Two people are required to do the dressing in order to ensure that it reaches the apex of the wound in the canal each time. A gentle laxative is given.

If the abscess in the intersphincteric plane tracks upwards only, then it calls for different management.

With an anal rectractor in place a director is passed up the track in a cranial direction from the opening in the anal canal to the rectal opening if there is one. If there is no rectal opening one is made artificially with the director and the track laid open with a cutting diathermy needle. No dressing is required.

Trans-sphincteric Fistula

Sometimes such a fistula can be laid open as already described for a low intersphincteric fistula. Often, however, when the director is passed into the external opening of this fistula it passes parallel to the anal canal to the apex of the ischiorectal fossa of one side rather than to the internal opening in the anal canal (*Fig.* 19.32*a*) and great care must then be taken not to push it through the levator muscle or, worse still, on into the rectum. The ischiorectal part of the fistula is laid open first by passing the director forwards and then backwards (*Fig.* 19.32*b–d*). If the track passes to the other ischiorectal fossa this too must be laid open (*Fig.* 19.32*e*). Search is then made for the internal opening which is often in the midline posteriorly and this too is laid open provided it is below the anorectal ring.

Dressings are applied and changed as for the low

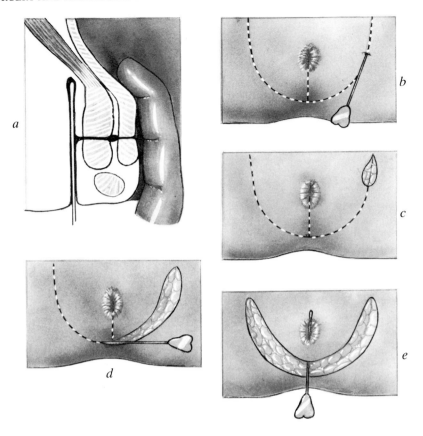

Fig. 19.32. Trans-sphincteric fistula-in-ano. *a*, Probing of fistula. *b*, *c*, *d*, Ischio-rectal part of fistula laid open. *e*, Track to internal opening probed and laid open.

intersphincteric fistula but initially a general anaesthetic may be required for the dressing if the wound is extensive. Weekly revision, under general anaesthetic if necessary, is needed throughout the healing process and if any missed tracks become apparent (a bead of pus in otherwise healthy granulations) they must be laid open. Active sphincter exercises are encouraged and a gentle laxative given.

Extension of such a fistula through the levator muscle to the supralevator space will close satisfactorily provided adequate drainage is established and if there is an opening into the rectum this should be closed with monofilament wire. Of prime importance in the management of these more difficult and fortunately rare fistulas is the integrity of the puborectalis muscle. In such difficult cases a covering sigmoid colostomy may be necessary.

Malignant Neoplasms of the Anal Canal

The three common malignant conditions of the anal canal are adenocarcinoma arising in the lower rectum or anal glands, squamous cell carcinoma of the anoderm and malignant melanoma.

Adenocarcinoma should be treated by abdominoperineal excision of the rectum with wide clearance of the perineal and ischiorectal tissues. Because of the lymphatic drainage of the peri-anal skin close attention must be paid to the inguinal glands. Excision biopsy and frozen section examination of a superficial node may be called for, if necessary followed by a block dissection of nodes.

Squamous cell carcinoma may require excision of the rectum, but wide local excision may be feasible if the upper part of the sphincter mechanism is uninvolved as this is a comparatively less aggressive tumour. Interstitial radiotherapy with or without external beam irradiation may also give adequate control of such tumours, the treatment being covered by a defunctioning colostomy. External beam irradiation may also be used to treat metastatic inguinal lymphadenopathy.

Malignant melanoma may also require excision of the rectum but, because of the very poor prognosis, local excision, if possible, is perhaps a more sensible and humane procedure.

Anorectal Incontinence

This distressing symptom can occur as a result of sphincter damage, for example after fistula operation or after difficult childbirth or by trauma. It is best treated by direct repair of the sphincters. It can also occur in association with complete rectal prolapse and, thirdly, in a group of patients who have minimal prolapse but who have weakness of the pelvic floor muscles, including the sphincters, for other reasons, for example due to nerve damage during a difficult labour. In the latter two groups postanal repair of the sphincters may be appropriate. Sphincter studies which may be helpful in the evaluation of these difficult cases have already been described (p. 244).

a. Repair of Injured Sphincters

When divided the ends of the sphincter muscles spring apart and the gap between them becomes filled with fibrous scar tissue. A large circumferential incision around the anus is made centred on the site of maximal damage as determined by electromyographic studies. The scar tissue is carefully excised and the muscle ends identified. The mucosal lining of the anal canal is separated from the muscle layers and repaired with continuous chromic catgut (*Fig. 19.33a*). The muscle ends are then overlapped and loosely sutured with monofilament wire (*Fig. 19.33b*). The free edge of the anal canal mucosa is sutured to the muscle and the wound left open to granulate. A covering colostomy is essential.

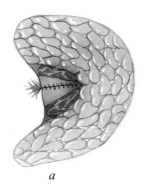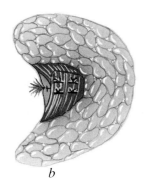

a   *b*

Fig. 19.33. Repair of injured sphincters. *a*, Mucosa of anal canal repaired. *b*, Sphincter ends overlapped and sutured.

b. Postanal Repair (Parks, 1975)

The aim of this repair is to plicate the sphincter muscle cylinder from within (in order to preserve its nerve and blood supply) and so re-form the right-angled anorectal angle which is invariably lost in these patients, the puborectalis part of the levator ani being the most important factor in this respect.

The patient is placed in the lithotomy position and a solution of normal saline with adrenaline (1 in 300 000) infiltrated into the postanal tissues. A V-shaped incision is made 6 cm behind the anus and the anterior flap of skin elevated as far as the anal margin (*Fig. 19.34a*). The plane between the white internal sphincter muscle and the reddish external sphincter is then opened up round half the circumference of the anal canal and lower rectum, Waldeyer's fascia being divided (*Fig. 19.34b*). Two or three sutures of braided nylon are then inserted loosely to approximate the two sides of the iliococcygeus part of the levator ani (*Fig. 19.34c*). Below this similar sutures are placed in the pubococcygeus part of the levator ani, with a third layer in the puborectalis and a final layer in the lower part of the external sphincter muscle.

The anterior flap of skin is taken up into the anal canal by this procedure and the wound is therefore closed as a Y with suction drainage (*Fig. 19.34d*). Magnesium sulphate is given for 10 days to achieve diarrhoea and so avoid any straining whatsoever. Thereafter a hydrophilic laxative is used regularly and glycerin suppositories inserted every morning to achieve an easy bowel action.

c. Thiersch's Operation

This procedure is helpful in a few elderly people with mucosal prolapse or with poor anal tone after repair of complete rectal prolapse as already described in the section on surgery of the rectum (p. 256). The bowel must be completely evacuated. General, spinal or epidural anaesthesia is suitable and the lithotomy position is used. Two small incisions are made, one in front of and one behind the anal orifice. A curved Doyen needle is passed from one incision well out into the ischiorectal fossa outside the sphincters to the other incision. Monofilament nylon (or wire) is then threaded and the needle withdrawn. This is repeated on the other side using the same nylon, thus encircling the anal canal. If nylon is used it can be passed around the anus two or three times. It is then tied while a no. 18 Hegar dilator is held in the anal canal. The small wounds are closed with absorbable sutures.

Impaction is common after this procedure and must be guarded against with paraffin emulsion in the early postoperative period and a bulk laxative with or without suppositories subsequently.

Anal and Peri-anal Warts (Condylomata Acuminata)

These must be distinguished from condylomata lata of syphilis. A full proctological examination is essential as they may occur in the anal canal and more rarely in the lower rectum. The external genitalia must be examined also for if all warts are not treated recurrence is inevitable.

If confined to the peri-anal skin, small numbers of warts can be treated with 25 per cent podophyllum in tincture of benzoin compound. This is touched onto the warts twice weekly until all have gone. Care must be taken not to touch the normal skin as it tends to burn and it is advisable for the patient to have a bath 4 hours after each application.

More extensive peri-anal warts or warts in the anal canal call for excision under general anaesthesia. A

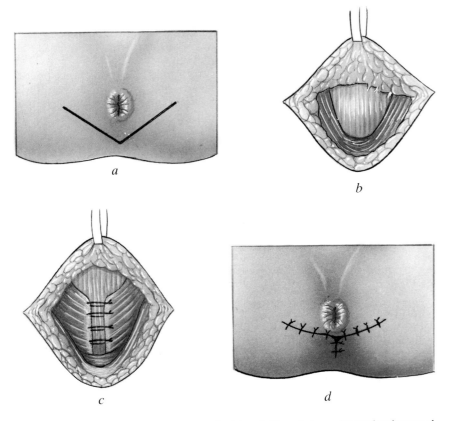

Fig. 19.34. Postanal repair of sphincters. *a*, Incision. *b*, Plane between internal and external sphincters opened up. *c*, Loose repair of levator ani and external sphincter. *d*, Closure of incision.

phosphate enema is given. With the patient in the lithotomy position the affected area is infiltrated with normal saline containing adrenaline (1 in 300 000). This elevates the warts on a balloon of skin or mucosa and they can then be cut off with fine-pointed scissors preserving as much normal skin as possible. Diathermy excision tends to destroy slender skin bridges and thus healing takes longer.

Extensive removal in the anal canal calls for the use of an anal dilator postoperatively until healing is complete. If very extensive, the operation may have to be done in stages to avoid anal stenosis. Close follow-up is essential as recurrence is common, but any such recurrences can usually be treated successfully with podophyllum.

Imperforate Anus (*see* Chapter 58)

In half of these infants the abnormal opening of the bowel lies below the level of the levator ani muscle so that incontinence is not a problem. In the male the opening is in the perineum anterior to the normal siting of the anus and may connect with the outside via a small track running forwards onto the scrotum. In the female the opening may be in the perineum anterior to the normal siting of the anus or in the lower vagina. In a few cases dilatation is all that is necessary. However, in the majority a simple episiotomy in a posterior direction in the midline is required as a primary procedure and may prove sufficient. If the opening is grossly displaced, however, the lower end of the bowel can be mobilized and moved back within the lowermost fibres of the external sphincter, which must be divided and then resutured in front of the bowel. This second procedure is done when the child is older and continent.

In the remaining half there is usually a fistulous connection with the bladder, urethra or vagina and the lower bowel may end above the levator ani. Much more extensive surgery is required to correct these cases. A defunctioning sigmoid colostomy is raised as a primary procedure until the infant is larger. Investigation is made for genito-urinary and skeletal anomalies. The definitive repair operation starts with separation of the pubo-rectalis sling from the urethra through a perineal incision. Anterior to this incision the external sphincter muscle (usually intact and normally sited) is exposed through a small incision which will become the new anus. From this incision a clamp is passed through the external sphincter and anterior to the pubo-rectalis sling. The child is then turned and the colostomy mobilized. The distal bowel is resected from the colostomy to the level of the bladder and the mucosa of the remaining rectum is filleted out and tied off at the level of the fistulous opening into the genito-urinary system. The clamp from below is then passed through the wall of the blind rectal stump to grasp the colon which was previously the proximal colostomy stoma. The colon is drawn through to the perineum where it is sutured to the skin, so becoming the new anal orifice.

REFERENCES

Barron J. (1963) Office ligation of internal haemorrhoids. *Am. J. Surg.* **105**, 563–570.

Gabriel W. B. and Milligan E. T. C. (1939) Haemorrhoids. *Br. Med. J.* **2**, 412.

Goligher J. C. (1976) Cryosurgery for haemorrhoids. *Dis. Colon Rectum* **19**, 213–218.

Griffiths J. D. (1956) Surgical anatomy of the blood supply of the distal colon. *Ann. R. Coll. Surg. Engl.* **19**, 241–256.

Grinnell R. S. (1954) Distal intramural spread of carcinoma of the rectum and rectosigmoid. *Surg. Gynecol. Obstet.* **99**, 421–430.

Hawley P. R. (1969) The treatment of chronic fissure-in-ano: a trial of methods. *Br. J. Surg.* **56**, 915–918.

Hawley P. R. (1975) Anorectal fistula. *Clin. Gastroenterol.* **4**, 635–649.

Keighley M. R. B. (1983) Perioperative antibiotics. *Br. Med. J.* **286**, 1844–1846.

Lane R. H. S. and Parks A. G. (1977) Function of the anal sphincters following colo-anal anastomosis. *Br. J. Surg.* **64**, 596–599.

Lloyd-Davies O. V. (1939) Lithotomy–Trendelenburg position for resection of rectum and lower pelvic colon. *Lancet* **ii**, 74–76.

Lord P. H. (1972) A new approach to haemorrhoids. *Prog. Surg.* **10**, 109–124.

Miles W. E. (1908) A method of performing abdomino-perineal excision for carcinoma of the rectum and of the terminal portion of the pelvic colon. *Lancet* **ii**, 1812–1813.

Milligan E. T. C., Naunton Morgan C., Jones L. E. et al. (1937) Surgical anatomy of the anal canal, and the operative treatment of haemorrhoids. *Lancet* **ii**, 1119–1124.

Naunton Morgan C. (1965) Carcinoma of the rectum. *Ann. R. Coll. Surg.* **36**, 73–99.

Parks A. G. (1956) The surgical treatment of haemorrhoids. *Br. J. Surg.* **43**, 337–351.

Parks A. G. (1966) Benign tumours of the rectum. In: Rob C., Smith R. and Naunton Morgan C. (eds) *Clinical Surgery. Vol 10, Abdomen and Rectum and Anus*. London, Butterworths, pp. 541–548.

Parks A. G. (1975) Anorectal incontinence. *Proc. R. Soc. Med.* **68**, 681–690.

Parks A. G. (1977) A technique of colo-anal anastomosis. In: Rob C. and Smith R. (eds) *Operative Surgery: Colon, Rectum and Anus*. London, Butterworths, pp. 164–167.

Parks A. G., Gordon P. H. and Hardcastle J. D. (1976) A classification of fistula-in-ano. *Br. J. Surg.* **63**, 1–12.

Thomson W. H. F. (1975) The nature of haemorrhoids. *Br. J. Surg.* **62**, 542–552.

Wells C. and Naunton Morgan C. (1962) Polyvinyl alcohol sponge prosthesis: the use of Ivalon sponge. *Proc. R. Soc. Med.* **55**, 1083–1085.

York Mason A. (1974) Trans-sphincteric surgery of the rectum. *Prog. Surg.* **13**, 66–97.

FURTHER READING

Gabriel W. R. (1963) *The Principles and Practice of Rectal Surgery*, 5th ed., London, H. K. Lewis.

Goligher J. C. (1984) *Surgery of the Anus, Rectum and Colon*, 5th ed. London, Baillière Tindall.

Todd I. P. and Fielding L. P. (eds) (1983) *Rob and Smith's Operative Surgery, Alimentary Tract and Abdominal Wall*. Part 3: *Colon, Rectum and Anus*, 4th ed. London, Butterworths.

Chapter twenty

The Biliary System

C. M. Davidson

Operating on the biliary tract for calculous disease is one of the commonest laparotomies in the Western world. Over 40 000 cholecystectomies are performed in England and Wales each year and about 750 000 in the United States of America. Unfortunately, operations for complications of cholecystectomy, principally biliary stricture, still occupy a significant place in biliary tract surgery.

SURGICAL ANATOMY

An understanding of the basic embryology (Hamilton et al., 1945) in the development of the gallbladder and pancreas helps to explain the many possible anomalies in this region which the surgeon may encounter. During the early stages of the formation of the duodenum, a small hepatic bud arises as early as 27 days at the junction of the foregut and midgut. The hepatic bud divides into a larger cranial portion, which forms the liver, and a smaller caudal portion, which is closely associated with the ventral pancreas and forms the gallbladder and cystic duct. The single hollow stalk of attachment of these two parts to the duodenum forms the bile duct. Initially, like the hepatic bud, the bile duct is attached to the ventral aspect of the duodenum, but by the 7-mm stage growth changes and the rotation to the right of the duodenum brings its attachment to the dorsal aspect of the duodenum. At about the 12-mm stage the two pancreatic primordia fuse to form a single organ in which the ventral pancreas forms the lower part of the head and the remainder of the pancreas (tail, body and upper part of head) is derived from the dorsal pancreas. The main duct is formed distally by the dorsal component and usually opens with the bile duct. The proximal part of the original dorsal pancreatic duct may persist as the accessory duct.

Variations in the arrangement of the ducts and the blood vessels have been exhaustively studied. A knowledge of the most frequent variations is of the greatest importance to the surgeon (Graham et al., 1928) (*Fig.* 20.1).

The arrangement of the arteries around the gallbladder is as variable as that of the ducts. The cystic artery most frequently arises from the right hepatic artery and passes behind the duct but may pass anteriorly. The hepatic artery itself may twist in front of and to the right of the common hepatic duct and the cystic artery may arise from the left hepatic artery. An accessory cystic artery is not an uncommon finding (*Fig.* 20.2).

The gallbladder (Gray, 1946) is a pear-shaped sac adherent to the visceral surface of the liver. The normal organ has a thin wall and presents a glistening appearance. There is little or no fat beneath the peritoneum and there are no adhesions between the gallbladder and the adjacent viscera. It is described as having a fundus, body and neck. The neck frequently shows an asymmetrical dilatation close to the exit of the cystic duct and in this way a pouch is formed (Hartmann's pouch). The mucosa is composed of tall columnar cells set on a vascular stroma. Underlying the mucosa is a muscle layer covered by peritoneum except where it is in contact with the liver. The blood supply is from the cystic artery which is an end artery, and the venous drainage is through the cystic vein to the right branch of the portal vein and through direct venous channels with the liver. The lymphatic drainage is via the cystic duct gland which lies close to the cystic artery. The nerve supply is vagal and sympathetic.

GALLSTONES

The solubility of cholesterol in bile is limited and depends on the presence of conjugated bile salts and phospholipids. Bile salts are water soluble, whereas both lecithin (which constitutes 90 per cent of phospholipids in bile) and cholesterol are insoluble in aqueous systems. However, bile salts are capable of dissolving both lecithin and cholesterol. The bile of stone formers is supersaturated with cholesterol, and this is also true of non-stone formers following a period of starvation or overnight fasting. On eating, however, bile salt secretion is increased and the bile becomes unsaturated. The bile salt pool circulates 5–15 times in 24 hours. In diseased states such as ileitis, where there is loss of bile salts due to defective reabsorption, the enterohepatic circulation is deficient and the incidence of stones is increased. Besides cholesterol stones, it is also possible to form pigment stones. These are small black stones formed when excess unconjugated bile pigment is excreted in the bile. The excess free pigment may result from increased haemoglobin breakdown and possibly chemical alteration of conjugated bile in the gut or gallbladder. These stones can form in the ducts and in the pure variety are called 'mulberry calculi', although they are usually yellow and crumbly.

Recently there has been increasing interest in altering the physicochemical composition of bile to effect dissolution of gallstones. It has been shown that by

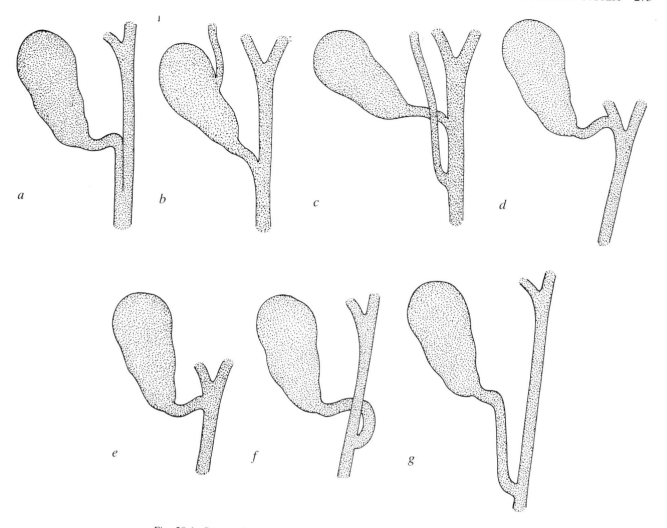

Fig. 20.1. Some of the more common variations of cystic duct anatomy.

giving chenodeoxycholic acid orally, there is an increase in the bile salt pool and a fall in the bile cholesterol content of the bile, which results in dissolution of certain cholesterol stones. However, such treatment is time consuming, expensive and does not alter the underlying abnormality responsible for stone formation. Thus recurrence of stones on cessation of therapy is likely, and furthermore the consequences of such treatment are uncertain. The increased bile salt pool may result in increased cholesterol absorption. In addition, reduced endogenous bile salt synthesis eliminates a major pathway for cholesterol excretion and consequently hypercholesterolaemia may result. There is also the theoretical possibility that a chenodeoxycholic acid-rich bile salt pool would result in bacteria in the bowel producing more hepatotoxic lithocholic acid.

The prevalence of gallstone disease in the general population is unknown as many patients with gallstones are asymptomatic. The incidence is considerably greater than the number of operations performed. In a prospective study (Lund, 1960) of 562 patients with asymptomatic gallstones for 5–20 years it was found that 50 per cent of the women and 30 per cent of the men developed symptoms within 5 years and 2·5 per cent had died during that period from biliary tract disease.

With more advanced diagnostic facilities, antibiotics, and improved anaesthesia and resuscitation techniques, surgery should usually be advised for gallstones provided there is no contra-indication such as asymptomatic stones in the elderly. The hospital mortality is well below 1 per cent for elective cholecystectomies, although the mortality and morbidity are higher in surgery for acute cholecystitis (Flemma et al., 1967) because the bile is usually infected and also because the disease occurs more frequently in older patients with concomitant pathology. Exploration of the common bile duct also increases mortality and morbidity. In the presence of free perforation of the gallbladder the perioperative mortality may rise to as high as 30 per cent (Godfrey et al., 1984).

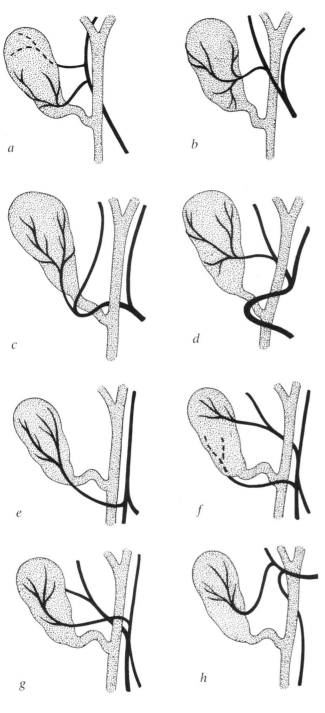

Fig. 20.2. Although the arrangement of the cystic artery is constant in the majority of patients, these variations may cause problems.

Gallstones are more than twice as common in women than in men and the age of presentation seems to be getting younger. It has been shown that emptying of the gallbladder is delayed in the third trimester of pregnancy and women on the contraceptive pill are twice as likely to develop gallstones as those not on the pill, possibly related to an oestrogen effect resulting in lithogenic bile. A genetic factor has also been demonstrated which shows that those with gene A have a 17 per cent increased likelihood of gallstones compared with the general population. Certain surgical procedures such as gastrectomy and vagotomy with pyloroplasty predispose to gallstone formation, possibly by reducing cholecystokinin release.

CHOLECYSTITIS

Cholecystitis is traditionally classified as 'acute' and 'chronic', but most surgeons will find that the histology report is often at variance with the clinical findings. Indeed, it may be impossible to distinguish a normal gallbladder at operation from one which shows chronic cholecystitis on histology. Many surgeons refer to 'clinically acute' or 'clinically elective' biliary tract surgery and there is continuing debate on the place of emergency surgery in biliary tract disease. It is, however, generally agreed that emergency biliary surgery should only be performed by a fully trained surgeon experienced in this field, and it should be undertaken within 48 hours of the onset of the attack.

Chronic Cholecystitis and Cholelithiasis

The symptoms of chronic cholecystitis, postprandial flatulence, epigastric distension and pain after fatty or starchy foods may be due to a diseased gallbladder with or without stones. It must be remembered, however, that similar symptoms may be present in peptic ulcer disease and reflux oesophagitis. It is essential, therefore, to demonstrate pathology of the gallbladder or ducts radiologically, before ascribing the dyspepsia to biliary tract disorder, and to realize that cholecystectomy may not cure dyspepsia. If stones are present the patient may experience so-called 'biliary colic', which is rarely a true colic but a constant pain in the right upper quadrant which reaches a peak and then eases off over a period which can vary from 15 minutes to several hours. A history of jaundice with pale stools and dark urine or the alteration in stool and urine colour alone is a useful aid to diagnosis. Transient jaundice may occur without a stone in the common duct; indeed a stone is found in only about one-third of such cases. Such symptoms may also suggest the passage of a stone through the ampulla. If fever and rigors occur then choledocholithiasis is likely.

Acute Cholecystitis

Acute cholecystitis is the most frequent complication of gallstones and may progress to a mucocele, 'empyema', perforation, gangrene, fistula formation or ascending cholangitis. The incidence of this condition in the population is difficult to determine; many cases do not reach hospital and the definition in hospital reporting varies. Reports in the literature indicate that the disease accounts for between 5·3 per cent (Lahey Clinic) and 20·8 per cent (Massachusetts General Hospital) of all cases operated on for biliary tract disease. In 95 per cent of cases the obstruction of the cystic duct is due to a calculus, but other causes, such as fibrosis, torsion or biliary mud, may be found. As the gallbladder becomes swollen and distended, the blood vessels and lymphatic channels become compressed, thus leading to ischaemic necrosis, gangrene and perforation. The bile is infected in 50 per cent of cases of acute cholecystitis compared with 25 per cent in elective cases. The most common organism is *Escherichia coli* followed by *Streptococcus faecalis* and *Staphylococcus aureus*. Rarely, emphysematous cholecystitis may occur due to organisms such as *Clostridium* and gas-forming coliforms. It is not uncommon for a point of necrosis of the gallbladder wall to be sealed by the omentum which, when dislodged at the time of surgery, allows bile to spill. In these cases a bile-stained transudate may be found in the peritoneal cavity, but this fluid is not the result of perforation. Perforation, however, does occur but is uncommon and is associated with a high mortality. At operation it may be associated with a pericholecystic abscess, subphrenic collection of infected bile or generalized peritonitis. 'Empyema' of the gallbladder is a misnomer and true empyema is uncommon although it is lethal in the elderly. It is a term handed down for a condition in which the gallbladder is distended with creamy material consisting of mucus, cholesterol and calcium carbonate. On occasions acute cholecystitis may follow other surgical procedures, burns or trauma and this may be due to thicker bile and gallbladder stasis following starvation, fever, dehydration and narcotics. Common duct calculi are present in less than half of these patients although some series have reported a higher incidence of choledochotomy being required in acute cases.

There has been much debate concerning surgical treatment of acute cholecystitis but with the advent of antibiotics and improved diagnostic facilities, urgent surgery is now fashionable. There is no doubt, however, that these patients should be operated on by an experienced surgeon, because the mortality and morbidity from reported series are greater than in the elective cholecystectomy. Cholecystostomy is the safer procedure when an inexperienced surgeon encounters an unexpected acutely inflamed gallbladder and in these circumstances it would be the treatment of choice. In view of the higher incidence of infective organisms in the acute case, perioperative antibiotics are indicated (Haw and Gunn, 1973). This is especially so in patients who are at risk of developing wound sepsis such as patients over 50 years of age, those with jaundice, the obese and those who have been shown to have a non-functioning gallbladder.

Emphysematous cholecystitis is a specific form of acute cholecystitis caused by gas-forming organisms, usually of the clostridial group. The gas is trapped in the gallbladder wall and is seen on a plain radiograph of the abdomen. It is surprising that this is not seen more often because of the frequency of *Clostridia* in bile culture, and this may be due to the low virulence of the organisms. The condition occurs more commonly in males than females, who are not infrequently diabetic, and it is therefore important to exclude diabetes in these cases and to look for the condition in diabetic patients with acute cholecystitis, particularly if they appear more toxic than one would expect.

Acalculous cholecystitis does occur but is uncommon and clinically difficult to diagnose. Success in the management of these cases varies greatly in the reported series. In a review of over 29 000 gallbladders removed in the Mayo Clinic, 9·6 per cent showed chronic cholecystitis with no calculi present. The aetiology of this condition is uncertain but there is fairly good evidence that bacterial and viral infections may be a contributing factor in certain circumstances which produce inflammatory changes of the gallbladder. Fifteen per cent of cases in one review gave a history of hepatitis in acalculous cholecystitis. Histological changes due to reflux, vascular abnormalities and even allergic factors have been implicated in the aetiology of this condition. The clinical presentation is similar to that of calculous gallbladdder disease. Diagnosis is difficult but faint gallbladder opacification on repeated oral cholecystogram should raise suspicion. Other suspicious features are poor contraction after a fatty meal and a small gallbladder volume. Cholecystokinin and cholecystography have been used to try to reproduce the pain experienced but reports vary on their effectiveness. When the diagnosis is considered, every effort should be made to exclude peptic ulcer disease, reflux oesophagitis and the irritable bowel syndromes. If, after repeated gallbladder investigations, dieting and regularization of bowel habit, the syndrome persists, then cholecystectomy is indicated.

CHOLEDOCHOLITHIASIS

Common duct stones arise most commonly in the gallbladder and pass into the duct although this has recently been challenged. Primary common duct stones, however, do occur with a very wide range of reported incidence. Stones formed in the common bile duct may form around foreign bodies such as a ligature or a parasite. Inflammation of the duct wall and bacterial contamination frequently accompany choledocholithiasis giving rise to a varying degree of ascending cholangitis. The duct is usually dilated and the tissues surrounding it adherent, probably secondary to the inflammation, and the gallbladder when present usually contains stones. The frequency of choledocholithiasis increases with age but this does not exclude the possibility in the young. Approximately 15–20 per cent of all patients undergoing cholecystectomy have common duct stones. Despite recent advances in biliary instrumentation and radiology, rates of retained stone have been reported at between 5 per cent and 35 per cent. On the other hand, it is also claimed that the incidence of unnecessary exploration of the common duct may be as high as 30–50 per cent. The previously stated indications for choledochotomy—small stones in the gallbladder, history of jaundice and a dilated common bile duct—are not satisfactory. A raised bilirubin at the time of surgery and a measured common bile duct greater than 10 mm are, however, reliable indicators (Reiss et al., 1984).

Instrumentation alone has a 20 per cent failure rate (Shore and Shore, 1970) for retained stones and intraoperative radiology a 7 per cent one (Way et al., 1972). Choledochoscopy, however, reduces the incidence in most series to 2 per cent. There is now substantial evidence that all cases of choledochotomy should have biliary endoscopy (Kapper et al., 1982).

STRICTURES OF THE BILE DUCT

Surgical trauma is the most common cause of bile duct stricture. Stricture at the lower end of the common duct is usually associated with false passages made during a forceful dilatation of the sphincter of Oddi and subsequent fibrosis. These are usually discovered when operating on recurrent common duct stones and are best repaired by a transduodenal sphincteroplasty or alternatively a choledochoduodenostomy. Failure to identify the local anatomy, operating with inadequate exposure and operating on the acutely inflamed gallbladder when identification of the anatomy is extremely difficult, are liable to be associated with common duct damage.

It has also been suggested that with increased use of choledochoscopy the possibility of stricture due to damage of common bile duct blood supply is possible, and therefore delicate handling with this procedure is essential.

Lord Smith (1978) has recently reviewed his extensive experience in dealing with such strictures and points out the increased frequency of this complication in the hands of inexperienced surgeons. He also mentions that such cases are all too frequently not considered to be difficult cholecystectomies at the time. Damage to a main bile duct may be recognized at the time of the surgery, in the immediate postoperative period with the progressive onset of jaundice, or after discharge home when the stricture results in further duct calculi, rigors, fever and jaundice. A large amount of bile drainage following cholecystectomy should be a cause for concern and even if the drainage should suddenly stop the possibility of a retained stone should be considered. If the injury is recognized at the time of surgery, end-to-end anastomosis should be performed with 3/0 chromic catgut interrupted sutures and the duct splinted with a T-tube brought out through a separate opening in the common bile duct, preferably below the repair.

It is unfortunately a fact that further stricture following this procedure is not uncommon and therefore a reason for choledocho-enterostomy to be preferred. When the stricture is in the common bile duct, this is not a difficult surgical procedure but it is essential that good mucosal approximation is achieved without tension. The stoma must be wide to reduce the incidence of stenosis and to prevent accumulation of intestinal contents within the duct system. The intestinal loop (Roux-en-Y) selected must have a good blood supply and should not be under tension. Common hepatic duct strictures are more difficult to manage and restenosis is more frequent. In this situation a mucosal tube and transhepatic splinting will give the best long-term result.

POST-CHOLECYSTECTOMY SYNDROME

It is difficult to define this syndrome but it is clear that continuing symptoms are less common in the older patient, in those who have had a long history of biliary tract disorder and in severe pathology in the gallbladder. The results of cholecystectomy depend on the accuracy of the preoperative diagnosis and in the absence of biliary colic pain in the initial history, a thorough appraisal must be carried out if the incidence of post-cholecystectomy syndrome is to be reduced. If symptoms are assessed following cholecystectomy it is well to remember that should a stone have been overlooked for one reason or another at the initial operation in the common bile duct, patients frequently have further trouble within 1 year, whereas recurrent stones do not often present one with problems during the first year. It is also well recognized that if jaundice or acute cholecystitis is present at the first operation, stenosis of the sphincter of Oddi or sclerosing cholangitis must be considered a possibility, and some authors suggest that 55 per cent of cases of post-cholecystectomy syndrome are due to fibrosis at the sphincter resulting from a previously impacted stone or traumatic bouginage at the time of exploration. It can be stated, therefore, that in patients in whom symptoms persist following cholecystectomy, a normal ERCP (endoscopic retrograde cholangiopancreatogram) indicates that the symptoms are due to some other pathology. It has been suggested that symptoms may be produced from a cystic duct remnant, but this is rare.

DIAGNOSIS OF BILIARY TRACT DISEASE

When biliary tract disease is suspected from the history it is essential to obtain radiological confirmation before advising treatment. This is a rapidly changing exercise in the department of radiology.

1. A straight radiograph may suggest stones in the right upper quadrant or demonstrate air in the biliary passages suggesting a biliary intestinal fistula. Only 15 per cent of gallstones are radio-opaque.

2. Ultrasonic scanning is now the first-choice investigation but if negative should be followed by an oral cholecystogram. Ultrasound is non-invasive and involves no radiation but unfortunately may be unsuccessful because of gas in the colon. It demonstrates stones and dilated ducts and pancreatic neoplasms.

3. Oral cholecystography involves the absorption, excretion and concentration of contrast material by the gallbladder. In 95 per cent of cases the presence or absence of gallbladder disease will be demonstrated, provided the tablets are taken, there is no small bowel malabsorption, liver disease or biliary intestinal fistula. Non-visualization of the gallbladder, suggesting cystic duct obstruction, from gallstones or cholecystitis, should be confirmed by a repeat double-dose oral cholecystogram because up to two-thirds of studies may prove to be normal on repeat examination. Non-opacification on two examinations is diagnostic of disease.

4. Endoscopic retrograde cholangiopancreatography (ERCP) is becoming available in most centres and has added a new dimension in the diagnosis and treatment of biliary and pancreatic disease.

5. Percutaneous fine-needle transhepatic cholangiography complements ERCP by outlining the proximal ductal system and it is employed if obstructive jaundice is suspected. It is successful in 95 per cent of cases with dilated ducts. The procedure should be covered by an antibiotic and if obstruction is demonstrated, laparotomy may be carried out on the same day.

6. Intravenous cholangiography does not depend on the concentrating function of the gallbladder for opacification; the bile is already radio-opaque when it is excreted by the liver.

7. Liver function tests should be undertaken routinely and will help in many cases to distinguish obstructive from hepatocellular jaundice. Abnormal prothrombin levels should be corrected before surgery using vitamin K.

8. Radiography of the chest is essential before operation as one of the most common postoperative complications is atelectasis.

OPERATIVE PRINCIPLES

Position of the Operating Table

It is essential to position the patient accurately on the cassette changer tabletop so that the tip of the 9th right costal cartilage is opposite the centre of the grid. It is also important to place a wedge of foam or a sandbag under the lower left ribs so that the common bile duct will not be superimposed on the lumbar spine in the operative cholangiogram pictures.

Incisions

The incisions most commonly used for cholecystectomy and surgical exploration of the bile ducts are:
1. Kocher's right subcostal incision.
2. A midline incision.
3. A right paramedian incision.
4. A right upper quadrant transverse incision.

The transverse incision which is placed in the natural fold is very satisfactory and is situated halfway between the umbilicus and the xiphoid process. It extends from the midline across the rectus muscle and when necessary is extended into the external oblique muscle. It provides good exposure, and may be extended across the epigastrium or when necessary in a vertical direction either up or down. It heals well and the incidence of incisional hernia is extremely low.

Abdominal Drainage

Drainage of the peritoneal cavity following biliary tract surgery to remove collections of bile and blood is essential. A Redivac drain should be placed posterior and lateral to the right lobe of the liver and if no drainage occurs this should be flushed with 5–10 ml of sterile saline and a revacuumed bottle applied. The drain may usually be removed on the 3rd postoperative day when drainage has ceased.

Wound Closure

Closure of the wound should be in two layers, preferably with an absorbable suture because of the incidence of wound infection in these procedures.

CHOLECYSTECTOMY

Many techniques are described for cholecystectomy but of paramount importance in all cases are good exposure, good assistance, good light and a complete display of the anatomy before structures are divided or ligated. Anatomical variance occurs in at least 10 per cent of cases and this adds to the hazards and to the demands on the surgeon. The main dangers of this operation are partial or complete division of the common duct and this preventable complication occurs in approximately 0·02 per cent of cases in the United Kingdom. Ideally, two assistants are required but failing this there are many self-retaining retractors which can be used. The majority of surgeons performing cholecystectomy stand on the patient's right-hand side, but some prefer to stand on the left side. All surgeons should try each side because when two assistants are not available it can be an advantage to operate from the left side using one's own left hand to displace the duodenum and expose the cystic duct and common duct.

Through a transverse incision the right hand is introduced over the right lobe of the liver to allow entry of air which allows the liver to descend for better exposure. A full laparotomy is then performed with special reference to the oesophageal hiatus, the duodenum to exclude an ulcer, the terminal ileum to exclude ileitis, and the sigmoid colon to exclude diverticulitis. The remaining viscera should be palpated also to exclude unexpected pathology. A pair of angled sponge-holding forceps is then placed on the fundus of the gallbladder. Sometimes the gallbladder is too distended to be grasped and requires to be emptied by means of a trocar and cannula being inserted through the purse-string suture in the fundus in order to prevent contamination. It may also be found that a small fibrotic gallbladder full of stones is difficult to grasp and in these circumstances the straight forceps can normally grasp the wall of the gallbladder. Frequently, before the gallbladder can be clearly displayed adhesions between the omentum, the colon and the duodenum require division and this is best done by the assistant putting each structure under tension to allow division of the adhesions close to the gallbladder. The hepaticocolic ligament is then divided and the peritoneal reflection of the duodenum incised while the duodenum is held under tension by the assistant.

Two packs are then inserted, one to hold the large bowel down and in the right paracolic gutter and the second placed carefully over the duodenum and held by the assistant. The assistant's left hand should have the fingers extended so that the index finger lies medial to the common duct while the remaining fingers are flexed at the interphalangeal joints over the duodenum, thus putting the free edge of the lesser omentum under tension. A swab should now be placed in the hepatorenal pouch to absorb any blood or soiling which results from the dissection. A short broad Deaver retractor should now be placed on the medial side of the gallbladder to retract the liver and it is wise to place a long swab under the retractor to prevent tearing of the liver. Forceps are placed on Hartmann's pouch so that the cystic duct and the free edge of the lesser omentum are put under tension. The peritoneum overlying the free edge of the lesser omentum is now incised with care to dissect the cystic duct, common bile duct, hepatic duct and cystic artery. Having incised the peritoneum, blunt dissection may be used by means of a pledget, and gentle stroking across the ducts will usually displace the fat and allow exposure of the duct system. Care, however, must be taken to avoid damage to small vessels which may bleed and obscure the anatomy. Small fibrous strands will be encountered which are probably lymphatic channels and autonomic nerves, some of which may need division.

After the common bile duct and common hepatic duct have been adequately displayed, attention is focused on the cystic artery which is carefully identified and confirmed by digital palpation. The cystic artery is traced onto the surface of the gallbladder. It is frequently necessary to incise the peritoneum up towards the gallbladder in order to display Calot's triangle adequately, and it is essential to define the gap between what is considered to be the common hepatic duct and the gallbladder (*Figs.* 20.3, 20.4).

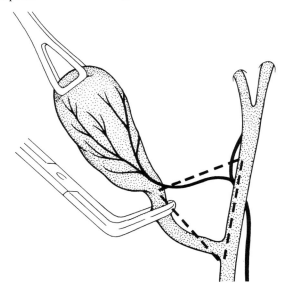

Fig. 20.3. Calot's triangle.

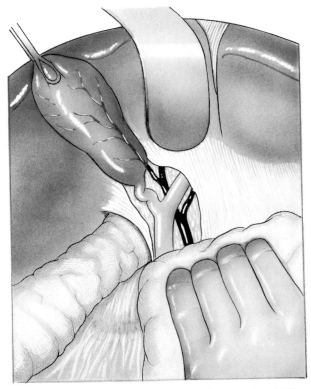

Fig. 20.4. Exposure of the gallbladder and its associated biliary ducts and vessels.

The cystic gland is often a very good guide to the cystic artery and there is also a fairly tough layer of parietal peritoneum posterior to the cystic duct which is incised with care. Right-angled forceps are used to pass a ligature round the cystic artery and subsequently a similar ligature may be passed round the cystic duct (*Figs.* 20.5, 20.6). Either catgut or Dexon should be used for the cystic duct and a non-absorbable suture for the artery. The right hepatic artery not infrequently runs close to the neck of the gallbladder but can be seen to turn back towards the

porta hepatis. Any large vessel in this region should be treated with caution (*Fig.* 20.7). Having clearly defined the cystic duct, cystic artery and the junction of the cystic duct to the common bile duct (*Fig.* 20.8), the ligature on the cystic duct is tied at the neck of the gallbladder leaving adequate space for the cholangiogram catheter to be placed in the cystic duct

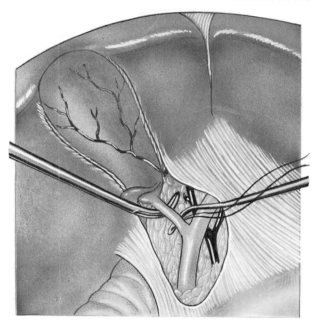

Fig. 20.5. Following identification and division of the cystic artery, a ligature is passed around the cystic duct.

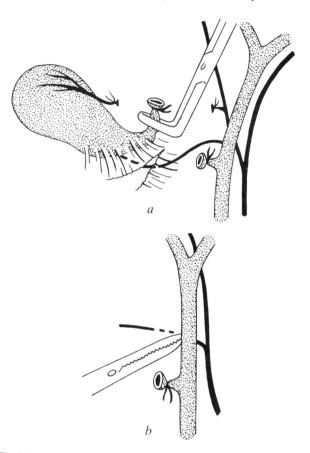

Fig. 20.7. An accessory cystic artery may be divided during dissection of the gallbladder and blind application of haemostats in this situation is dangerous.

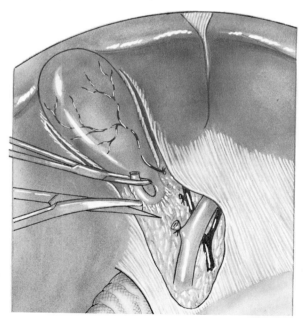

Fig. 20.6. Ligation and division of the cystic duct.

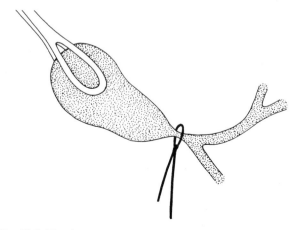

Fig. 20.8. Traction on the gallbladder may tent up and angulate the common bile duct.

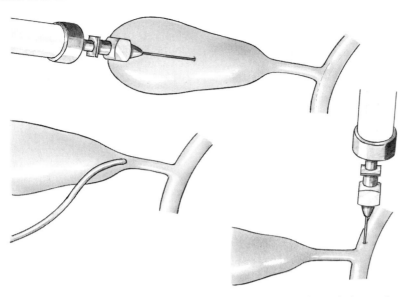

Fig. 20.9. Operative cholangiography may be undertaken through the gallbladder, the cystic duct or the common bile duct.

(*Fig.* 20.9). The operative cholangiogram can also be performed by inserting a needle in the gallbladder or common bile duct, which can be useful when the anatomy is difficult to determine.

After the cholangiogram has been performed a second ligature is passed round the cystic duct and is ligated close to, but not flush with, the common duct, as this may cause narrowing either at the time of ligation or subsequently due to tissue reaction. If one chooses to clamp the cystic duct before ligation, it is essential that the clamp is removed after the first knot has been applied so that the tissues are not fixed by the clamp, which can mislead one into believing that the knot is secure. The cystic artery is then ligated and divided. Should bleeding occur pressure should be applied by means of the left index finger and thumb in the foramen of Winslow which will compress the hepatic artery and thus control haemorrhage, allowing accurate application of an artery forceps to the bleeding point. It is unwise to use diathermy in this region because the depth of the burn cannot be estimated and damage to the ductal system is therefore possible.

The gallbladder is now dissected free leaving a good cuff of peritoneum if possible to be sutured over the gallbladder bed (*Fig.* 20.10). During removal of the gallbladder, diathermy to the gallbladder bed should be used for small bleeding points and any accessory biliary ducts should if possible be ligated. If freeing the gallbladder has been difficult and bleeding areas of liver tissue have been created, a Sloan–Robertson coagulation sucker can be a great help. Suturing the peritoneum over the gallbladder bed is not essential but preferable as this will improve haemostasis, reduce bile leakage from small biliary radicles in the gallbladder bed and reduce the likelihood of other viscera becoming adherent to a raw gallbladder surface.

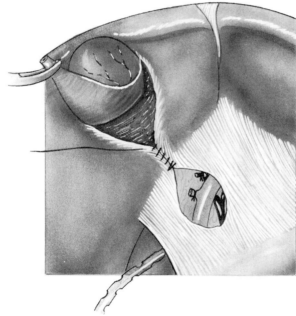

Fig. 20.10. The peritoneum is closed over the gallbladder bed.

Retrograde Cholecystectomy (*Fig.* 20.11)

When difficulty is encountered in defining the anatomy of the biliary tree or if the surgeon has any doubt in his mind concerning the cystic duct or cystic artery, the safer method of removing the gallbladder from the fundus should be used. In this method a tissue forceps is applied to the fundus of the gallbladder and the peritoneum between the gallbladder and the liver incised with a knife or diathermy. A plane can be found deep to the peritoneum, and using dissecting scissors the peritoneum is gradually undermined and incised on the medial and lateral side of

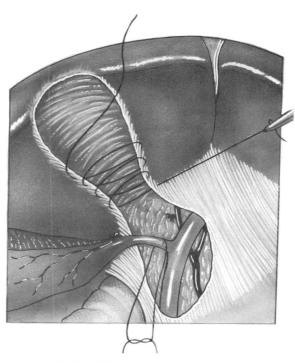

Fig. 20.11. Retrograde cholecystectomy.

the gallbladder. This may be facilitated by the use of a dissecting pledget. The vessels are coagulated as they are encountered. As one reaches the triangle between the gallbladder and common hepatic duct, the cystic artery becomes obvious and should be ligated and divided.

The cystic duct is readily identified at its junction with the common bile duct. The cystic duct is then ligated close to the neck of the gallbladder and the operative cholangiogram performed as previously described. The gallbladder bed is closed using a 2/0 chromic catgut suture. Haemostasis is checked, and palpation of the common duct carried out if there is any doubt on the findings of the cholangiogram. The swab is removed from Morison's pouch and a Redivac drain is placed on the posterolateral aspect of the right lobe of the liver and brought out through a separate stab wound. The wound is closed, the omentum having previously been placed over the duodenum towards the gallbladder bed. The wound should be closed with two layers of Dexon and either a subcutaneous closing stitch or interrupted Prolene to the wound. Unless there is swelling of the wound or haematoma the sutures are removed on the 6th or 7th postoperative day.

Complications

The commonest complication following cholecystectomy is pulmonary atelectasis, and should the patient have a fever in the first 4 days postoperatively a chest radiograph should be taken and appropriate physiotherapy given.

If the radiograph is normal and the patient continues to be febrile, a subhepatic collection should be suspected and radiological screening of the diaphragm could be helpful. If no drainage occurs through the Redivac drain in the immediate postoperative period, 5–10 ml of sterile water should be injected into the Redivac drain and a revacuumed bottle applied. If excessive bile leakage occurs from the drain this may be due to either a divided accessory duct, not noted by the surgeon, or a slipped ligature on the cystic duct. If bile drainage continues and the patient's general condition deteriorates, a further laparotomy should be performed. A leaking cystic duct may be found and if so a further ligature applied. If no obvious cause can be discovered for the bile leakage and a subhepatic collection of bile is present, it is wise to decompress the biliary tree by means of a T-tube in the common duct.

If jaundice occurs postoperatively, it may be due to: (1) a retained stone in the common duct; (2) a damaged main duct; (3) anaesthetic agent; (4) blood transfusion. (3) and (4) should be excluded by laboratory tests, but to exclude (1) and (2) endoscopic retrograde catheterization of the duct should be undertaken. Failing this, and if jaundice deepens, a transhepatic cholangiogram can be done and appropriate treatment instituted.

CHOLECYSTOSTOMY

Cholecystostomy rather than cholecystectomy should be performed only in special circumstances, either on account of the general condition of the patient or as the result of the unexpected finding of acute cholecystitis by an inexperienced surgeon. It is not an operation without difficulty because the obstructing stone may be impossible to dislodge in which case mucous fistula persists.

Technique

The abdominal cavity and the wound edges are protected by means of packs. The gallbladder is then held with the surgeon's right hand while a trocar and cannula is inserted into the fundus. The trocar is then withdrawn allowing emptying of the gallbladder, following which the cannula is withdrawn slowly and a light bowel clamp applied. The opening in the fundus is enlarged and held open by means of Babcock's tissue forceps. The bowel clamp is removed and any remaining content within the gallbladder is sucked out. Palpation at this stage will usually demonstrate stones at the neck of the gallbladder, many of which can be milked out or removed by means of the Desjardin forceps. Small stones are best removed by using a dry swab on the index finger which is rotated in the gallbladder, thus collecting grit and small stones.

A purse-string suture is inserted around the opening in the fundus of the gallbladder and a Foley catheter previously introduced through a stab wound is placed in the gallbladder and the purse-string tightened and tied. The Foley catheter balloon is then inflated with 5–10 ml of water. A second purse-string seromuscular suture is then inserted in order to inkwell the fundus of the gallbladder as a further protection against leakage. After tying the second purse-string, the long ends should be brought out through the stab wound alongside the Foley catheter which helps to anchor the gallbladder to the deep surface of the wound. The wound is closed after placing a Redivac drain below the right lobe of the liver. The Foley catheter should be left on open drainage until the 5th day, when a cholangiogram should be performed. If the radiograph shows a patent cystic duct with no obstruction then the Foley catheter may be removed on the 8th day. If, however, obstruction to the cystic duct is demonstrated then the gallbladder Foley catheter should be left on open drainage until a secondary procedure may be carried out and the gallbladder removed.

CHOLEDOCHOTOMY

Exploration of the common bile duct may be a primary or secondary procedure. It is indicated as a primary procedure when a dilated common duct is demonstrated radiologically either by a transhepatic cholangiogram, an intraoperative cholangiogram or ERCP. The radiograph may show intraductal stones or obstruction due to a stricture or tumour. The duct may be explored at two levels—supraduodenal and transduodenal.

The *supraduodenal approach* is commonest and demands full mobilization of the duodenal loop and a clear demonstration of the duct in the free edge of the lesser omentum. Routine operative cholangiography has reduced the frequency with which exploration of the common duct has resulted in negative findings. The first step (if not already carried out prior to cholecystectomy) should be division of the hepatico-colic ligament, which allows the hepatic flexure of the transverse colon to be displaced downwards and held by a moist pack. The peritoneum is then incised lateral to the duodenum while the assistant holds the duodenum with a moist swab under tension with two hands. The peritoneum should be incised right up to and round the junction of the second and third parts. It is then possible by blunt dissection, using the left hand, to free the duodenal loop and head of the pancreas until the inferior vena cava is exposed. The peritoneal fold passing from the superior border of the first part of the duodenum should also be divided to complete the mobilization.

The common duct may now be palpated in its entirety between the fingers and thumb of the left hand. The common duct gland is probably enlarged in these cases and acts as a guide to the common duct. Using flexed fingers behind the head of the pancreas, the duodenal loop should be palpated by the thumb and thus the ampulla can be detected as a nipple-like structure on the medial side of the loop, usually more distal than expected. Stones may or may not be palpable but the groove on the posterior aspect of the pancreatic head may be readily defined. Either supporting the supraduodenal portion of the common duct with the left hand or following insertion of two closely placed stay sutures of fine catgut in the common duct, the latter is incised vertically close to the duodenum (*Fig. 20.12*). As a guide, the vertical incision should be twice the diameter of the common

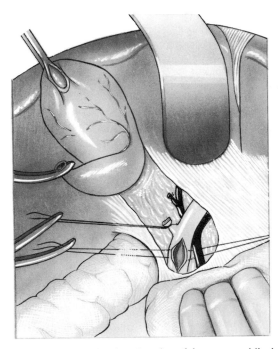

Fig. 20.12. Supraduodenal exploration of the common bile duct.

duct. It is also prudent to place a swab in the hepatorenal pouch close to the free edge of the lesser omentum to absorb the bile which leaks when the duct is opened. The swab also tends to hold small stones, which may be extruded. A swab for bacteriological examination of the bile should be taken at this stage. The nature of the bile should be noted, because if there is a preponderance of sludge not only does this suggest stasis but it influences the surgeon in an older patient to consider a transduodenal sphincteroplasty or a choledochoduodenostomy to prevent recurrent trouble.

A Fogarty catheter is now passed down the common duct through the ampulla into the duodenum. The balloon is then inflated and the catheter withdrawn, allowing accurate location of the ampulla. The balloon should now be deflated to allow passage through the ampulla and immediately reinflated to a pressure which just allows withdrawal and this pushes out intraductal stones. Compression of the duct proximal to the opening to prevent stones going back up can be achieved by use of a bulldog clamp. The proximal ducts are explored in a similar fashion. Saline irrigation using a Rochester syringe can then be carried out, flushing the ducts. This manoeuvre should be repeated for the distal common bile duct. Gentle probing of the ducts may now be carried out using Desjardin forceps. The forceps should be passed up the left and right hepatic ducts and any major stone will be discovered as resistance is transmitted through the instrument or debris is retained in the jaws of the instrument following withdrawal. If a stone is palpated it should be delivered into the forceps or milked up to the opening in the duct. The choledochoscope, either the rigid or flexible one, should then be used. It is first inserted distally and a good view of the ampulla should be obtained and then proximally into the right and left hepatic ducts. A Dormia basket is required to remove stones which cannot be withdrawn with a Fogarty balloon or Desjardin forceps. A Bakes dilator should only be used if stenosis or visualization has not been obtained with the endoscope and should be passed down the common duct with extreme gentleness and without force and the ampulla is passed over the dilator. Any force using a dilator may produce a false passage and a possible stricture later, but when the dilator passes cleanly through the ampulla the tip should shine through the opposing duodenal wall (*Fig.* 20.13). The ampulla is then palpated carefully over the dilator, any thickening or irregularity indicating the need for transduodenal exploration and biopsy. If the dilator, however, cannot be passed with ease and the cholangiogram shows a hold-up, transduodenal exploration should be carried out. If a choledochoscope is available this should be passed proximally and distally after exploration. If this is not available, the duct should be checked by means of a cholangiogram using a small Foley catheter technique.

The catheter is inserted proximally through the choledochotomy and the balloon inflated, following which the duct is irrigated with at least 20 ml of saline to reduce the likelihood of introducing air bubbles. Six ml of contrast are injected and the film taken, but the amount of contrast must be judged by the size of the ducts, remembering that overfilling or underfilling can equally give false positives. With great care and in order to prevent any stone being displaced from the lower end of the duct, the balloon is deflated and the catheter placed in the distal component and a further radiograph taken. If there is any doubt regarding clearance of the duct, a choledochoduodenostomy should be performed. Following choledochotomy the duct may either be closed primarily or drained by means of a T-tube. When closing a choledochotomy over a T-tube interrupted sutures of 3/0 catgut should be used in the proximal portion of the duct leaving the vertical limb close to the duodenum. A continuous suture for this procedure may

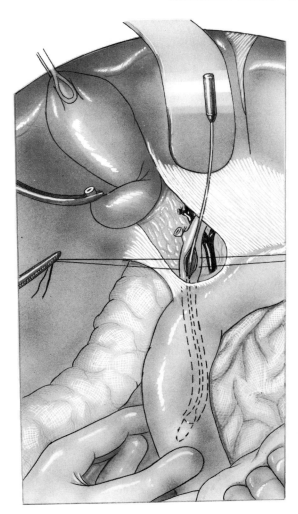

Fig. 20.13. Passage of Bakes dilator through the common bile duct to the ampulla.

be disrupted when removing the T-tube. If the duct, however, is closed primarily then a continuous suture is preferable.

TRANSDUODENAL CHOLEDOCHOLITHOTOMY, SPHINCTEROTOMY AND SPHINCTEROPLASTY

It is occasionally impossible to pass a dilator or catheter down the common bile duct and through the ampulla onwards into the duodenum. This difficulty may be caused by the immovable impaction of a stone in the ampulla of Vater or a fibrous stricture of the sphincter of Oddi, and sphincterotomy is occasionally indicated when the common bile duct is widely dilated down to its termination. When gallstones are associated with recurrent pancreatitis it is advisable to undertake transduodenal sphincterotomy or sphincteroplasty.

Technique

After adequate exposure of the common bile duct, a vertical incision is made in its anterior wall, following which a 3- or 4-mm Bakes dilating sound or a no. 8 Fr. gauge catheter is passed downwards to the obstructed ampulla. The olive-shaped tip of the dilator is then projected forwards towards the anterior wall of the second portion of the duodenum where it may be palpated tenting the duodenal wall. A vertical incision is then made through the anterior wall of the duodenum over the point where the dilator is palpable. The edges of the open duodenum are carefully retracted with light tissue forceps, exposing the tip of the dilator or an impacted ampullary stone. The ampulla may be cautiously dilated from below, following which an impacted stone can be removed with Desjardin forceps, and following this graduated dilators can be readily passed from above through the sphincter and into the duodenum.

At this stage it is advisable to flush the common bile duct from above using saline which will hopefully wash away fine biliary stones and detritus. When sphincterotomy is undertaken, a pair of fine forceps is passed from below into the ampulla and the tips of these are separated, following which the ampulla and anterior wall of the common duct are incised for 8–10 mm over a grooved director using either the diathermy or scalpel (*Fig.* 20.14). Once the incision in the ampulla is started and the orifice opened, extension of the incision may be facilitated by the introduction from either below or above of a Bakes dilator. The incision to divide the sphincter of Oddi is best undertaken in the 10 o'clock position. Following completion of this manoeuvre the emergence of the main pancreatic duct should be identified and a fine probe gently passed.

Most surgeons now convert the sphincterotomy into a sphincteroplasty by suturing the mucosal edges of the cut ampulla back to the duodenal mucosa, thus avoiding later restricture. (For a full description of sphincteroplasty *see* Chapter 14.) The incision in the duodenum is closed transversely in two layers and the common bile duct is almost invariably drained using a T-tube.

PRIMARY CLOSURE OF COMMON BILE DUCT OR DRAINAGE?

Primary closure of the common duct is permissible in certain cases but should be considered only by a surgeon experienced in this field. When primary closure is carried out it is by a continuous suture of 3/0 catgut, starting just above the opening and finishing just below it, small bites being taken which are closely placed. Primary closure certainly allows greater postoperative mobility and a reduced wound infection rate. However, for most patients it is safer for the common duct to be drained either by a straight catheter or a T-tube. It has been suggested that when a T-tube is removed some leakage of bile occurs and certainly a spike of fever and pain in the right upper quadrant for 24 hours after the T-tube is removed is not uncommon. In order to facilitate removal of the T-tube, the horizontal limb (which lies vertically in the duct) should be converted into a gutter and a 'V' cut out opposite the vertical component. The T-tube should be inserted with the aid of a right-angled forceps and should be tested by an upward and downward movement holding the vertical limb to ensure that no kinking within the duct has taken place. The duct should then be closed above with interrupted 3/0 chromic catgut (*Fig.* 20.15). The vertical limb should be brought out through a separate stab wound in a lateral position in case there is a retained stone and removal is required using the image intensifier at a later date, for if the vertical

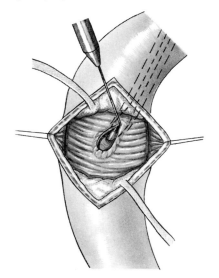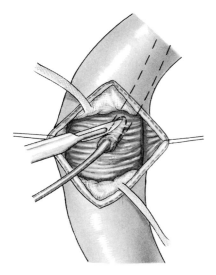

Fig. 20.14. Transduodenal sphincterotomy may be undertaken using the diathermy or scalpel.

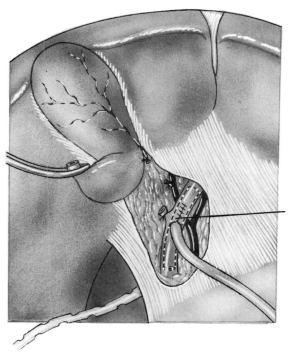

Fig. 20.15. The common bile duct is sutured snugly over the T-tube.

limb is not lateral visualization is obscured. It should be sutured to the skin by a bootlace technique. The gallbladder, if not previously removed, should now be removed and the wound closed after placing a Redivac drain in a posterolateral position to the right lobe of the liver.

CHOLEDOCHODUODENOSTOMY (*Fig.* 20.16)

The duodenum is the most suitable viscus for biliary intestinal anastomosis when it is used for recurrent

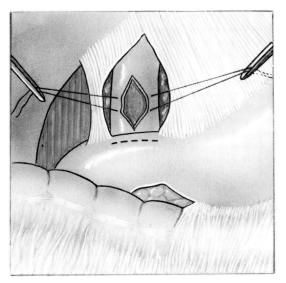

Fig. 20.16. Choledochoduodenostomy.

stones in the common duct. It should, however, be employed with discretion as it may leave a sump which can only be drained by means of overflow and therefore may give rise to continued symptoms of pain and fever (sump syndrome). When employed the stoma should be 2·5 cm in diameter to allow easy to-and-fro drainage. A long vertical incision in the common duct should be made close to the duodenum and an incision on the superior aspect of the duodenum in the line of the bowel should be made of similar length. The seromuscular layer should be incised first so that the length of the cut can be defined and the mucosa is opened and will immediately evert. Two lateral seromuscular sutures between the duodenum and the common duct should be placed as anchors and held as stays, preferably using non-absorbable material. The anastomosis should be completed by means of a continuous 2/0 chromic catgut suture using a separate length for each side and starting at the point nearest to the duodenum. A one-layer anastomosis is sufficient and great care should be exercised to prevent inadvertent approximation of the anterior and posterior walls of the stoma. The abdomen should be closed after carefully placing a Redivac drain below and behind the right lobe of the liver.

CHOLEDOCHOJEJUNOSTOMY

The use of jejunum to drain an obstructed common duct is preferable when a high anastomosis is desired, and the incision and exposure are as described for cholecystectomy. When it has been decided that a palliative bypass operative procedure is the treatment of choice, and in the absence of a gallbladder, a loop of jejunum is selected. The duodenojejunal junction should be identified and a site for anastomosis not less than 12 cm from this point should be selected. When selection has been made the site should be approximated to the porta hepatis to ensure that it is long enough and lies at the site without tension. The site is then marked by using either a seromuscular stitch or a tissue forceps. The bowel is then divided using a soft bowel clamp on the proximal end and a crushing clamp distally. The loop should be held up by the assistant to allow the surgeon to view the vascular arcades by transillumination. It will be necessary to divide two or three of the vascular arcades, taking care to maintain the integrity of the blood supply to both limbs. It is essential to ensure that the mesentery is not under tension when placed at the porta hepatis. The vessels should be ligated using an aneurysm needle technique rather than clamping, for should the clamp slip or should the assistant remove it prematurely a spreading mesenteric haematoma will occur and place that portion of intestine in jeopardy. The vertical limb (Roux-en-Y) anastomosis may be ante- or retrocolic, whichever seems to lie best, and the open end should be closed in the manner described below.

The crushing clamp is held by the assistant and a similar clamp laid on top while an over-and-over suture of 2/0 chromic catgut is inserted. The free end should be held in forceps by the assistant. When the through-and-through suture is complete, a moist swab is placed over the forceps and held by the surgeon's left hand while the top forceps is removed and the free ends of catgut lifted up, while the crushing clamp is removed. This technique prevents intestinal spillage and gives good haemostasis. The suture is then returned as a seromuscular stitch and tied to the free end. A choledochojejunostomy may be side to side or end of common duct to side of jejunum, using a 3/0 chromic catgut as a continuous suture. When the anastomosis is complete, the intestinal limb should be attached to the liver capsule with interrupted seromuscular sutures of non-absorbable material. The Roux-en-Y is completed by end to side, a two-layer anastomosis 12 cm distal to the choledochojejunostomy. The distance is important because this limits reflux into the common duct. The abdomen is closed after placing a suction drain behind and lateral to the right lobe of the liver.

CHOLECYSTENTEROSTOMY

Anastomosis between the gallbladder and the jejunum is a useful palliative procedure in obstructive jaundice. It may also be used as an initial procedure in the deeply jaundiced patient who has an operable carcinoma of the common duct or ampulla but whose liver function is impaired and whose albumin is very low. At the time of laparotomy multiple lymph node biopsies should be performed, especially the suprapancreatic and coeliac group of glands, the histology of which will assist in deciding any further definitive treatment.

Technique

Laparotomy and exposure are as previously described for cholecystectomy. A liver biopsy should be performed and after positioning the packs around the gallbladder it is decompressed by means of a trocar and cannula which reduces spillage. A swab for bacteriology is taken and cultured for both aerobes and anaerobes. A loop of jejunum is selected and after placing a soft bowel clamp across the jejunum a posterior layer of interrupted non-absorbable seromuscular sutures is placed before opening the bowel. The stoma should be wide enough to allow free to-and-fro movement of biliary intestinal content. The inner layer of continuous 2/0 chromic catgut should be inserted in an over-and-over fashion for haemostasis, care being taken at the corners where a loop on the mucosa stitch can be helpful to invert the mucosa. The anastomosis is completed with an anterior layer of interrupted non-absorbable sutures. Side-to-side anastomosis of the vertical limbs of the loop is advocated by some surgeons but it is not necessary if the cholecystenterostomy is wide. The abdomen is closed after placing a Redivac drain behind and lateral to the right lobe of liver.

OPERATIONS FOR RETAINED OR RECURRENT STONES IN COMMON BILE DUCT

It may be possible to remove retained stones via the track of the T-tube, the latter having been exchanged for a simple tube through which a Dormia basket may be passed and the stone removed under X-ray control (*Fig.* 20.17) (Geenen et al., 1984). Alternatively an endoscopic sphincterotomy may be performed (*Fig.* 20.18). The immediate effect of endoscopic sphincterotomy on biliary and sphincter of Oddi motility is to decrease the pressure gradient that normally exists between the common bile duct and duodenum and to abolish the normal sphincter of Oddi phasic contractions (Escourrou et al., 1984).

In experienced hands this is the treatment of choice for retained stones, acute pancreatitis with common duct stones, papillary stenosis and the 'sump syndrome' sometimes seen after choledochoduodenostomy.

Endoscopic Retrograde Cholangiopancreatography (ERCP)

This was introduced about 10 years ago and the asso-

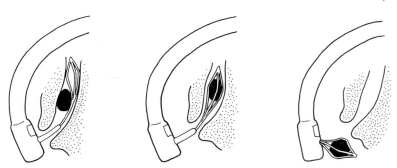

Fig. 20.17. Transendoscopic removal of common duct stone using Dormia basket inserted via the duodenoscope.

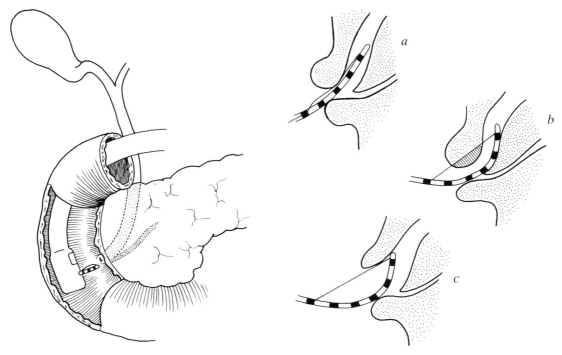

Fig. 20.18. Endoscopic sphincterotomy using the hot wire technique.

ciated radiological and histological information which may be obtained from this examination, together with the performance of specific surgical procedures, has provided a great advance. In addition to the diagnostic advantages of this method, operative endoscopic procedures have been developed to remove stones and to deal with strictures at the lower end of the common bile duct and to establish biliary and pancreatic drainage.

ERCP must be performed with facilities for constant radiological screening and requires the services of a skilled radiologist. Following cannulation, the biliary tree can be outlined with radio-opaque dyes and a pancreatogram can be performed with great ease.

Endoscopic Sphincterotomy

Endoscopic sphincterotomy is performed routinely in most major hospitals and although the procedure was originally confined to elderly patients with retained or recurrent stones following cholecystectomy, it is now clear that a considerable proportion of those undergoing endoscopic removal of stones from the common bile duct have not undergone removal of the gallbladder as most of these patients were frail and future cholecystectomy was not contemplated.

Once the presence of a stone has been confirmed in the common bile duct the papillotome is inserted into the papilla. This instrument is a wire encased in a plastic tube and once its position is confirmed in the common bile duct the wire is tightened and

the roof of the papilla is cut using an electrical current (*see Fig.* 20.18). Following sphincterotomy, spontaneous passage of the stone is common but in many cases introduction of a Dormia basket or balloon catheter is necessary. It is, however, less easy to remove a large stone from above a tight stricture of the common bile duct although a variety of instruments to break up the stone are being developed.

An inflammatory or malignant stricture at the lower end of the duct may be divided with the papillotome and a prosthetic stent may be inserted if surgery appears to be impossible. Furthermore, high common duct strictures can also be passed with a tube and some strictures may be dilated from below with balloon catheters.

Complications of ERCP

The incidence of cholangitis and acute pancreatitis is low and generally regarded as in the region of about 1 per cent. The mortality of ERCP without an additional therapeutic procedure is extremely low and death is almost invariably unrelated to the procedure but to pre-existing serious diseases. However, the incidence of complications associated with therapeutic procedures is greater than that following simple diagnostic ERCP and it is generally considered that the mortality of endoscopic sphincterotomy is 1–2 per cent. Other complications include cholangitis, pancreatitis and severe haemorrhage, in some patients requiring transfusion and laparotomy.

Despite these risks, the diagnostic advantages of this recently introduced investigation, together with the ability to undertake procedures on the sphincter or within the common bile duct, represent a very great advance in this field.

BILIARY FISTULAS AND INJURIES TO THE DUCTS

Biliary fistulas, although uncommon, are a real problem following biliary surgery. A fistula may be difficult to diagnose as it may discharge intermittently. It is not uncommon to have some bile drainage following cholecystectomy and this probably arises from small accessory ducts in the gallbladder bed, and this normally stops within 48 hours. If bile drainage continues, it is likely that an accessory duct has been divided. It is unusual, however, to require operative treatment for this condition, as usually it dries up and ceases. If, however, discharge is associated with fever and malaise, re-exploration should be considered. At reoperation any bile collection is sucked out and an omental patch sutured over the gallbladder bed. During re-exploration the cystic duct stump is carefully checked to see if a ligature has slipped. This accident usually occurs on about the 4th or 5th postoperative day and it is sudden in onset with the patient complaining of pain in the right upper quadrant; it is accompanied by some degree of shock. If no obvious cause can be found a transhepatic cholangiogram should be done to exclude a posterior tear of the duct. If bile drainage through the fistula continues in the absence of general toxic signs, and the stools are normal in colour, then a 'wait-and-see' policy may be adopted. Like many other fistulas, these usually cease to drain within 3 weeks. If, however, diminished drainage is accompanied by deepening jaundice, fever and pale stools, re-exploration is mandatory.

Before a second operation is performed, it is helpful to undertake either a percutaneous transhepatic cholangiogram or an endoscopic retrograde catheterization of the common duct to demonstrate the leak. If a straightforward cholecystectomy is followed by a deepening jaundice, light stools and dark urine, a presumptive diagnosis of stricture may be made. Traumatic rupture of the bile ducts may follow closed trauma or penetrating injuries, and may occur in the absence of injury to the liver. The clinical picture is one of shock followed by recovery but persistent pain in the right upper quadrant and progressive abdominal distension, fever and jaundice. Peritoneal lavage demonstrates the presence of bile in the peritoneal cavity.

SECONDARY OPERATIONS ON THE COMMON BILE DUCT

Secondary procedures on the biliary tree are tedious and hazardous in any surgeon's hands. The main technical difficulty is adhesions which have obliterated the anatomical planes and fixed the various viscera to the neighbouring structures. Entry into the peritoneal cavity may be facilitated by lengthening the previous incision or using an alternative incision, thus avoiding parietal adhesions. After entering the peritoneal cavity parietal adhesions to the back of the previous incision are carefully divided and the free edge of the liver identified. The first and safest step should then be to separate the structures from the right lobe of the liver starting as far lateral as possible and working medially, the assistant keeping the infrahepatic structures under tension. The colon, duodenum and omentum are often densely adherent to the gallbladder bed. Even in the most experienced hands, small tears in the intestine may occur which must be sutured immediately with atraumatic 2/0 chromic catgut. Tears are not serious when seen and repaired but when unnoticed they can be disastrous.

If cholecystectomy has previously been performed there is no real guide to the common duct other than an anatomical knowledge of where it should be. If the opening into the lesser sac is patent, which is unlikely, a finger in the foramen and palpation of the hepatic artery will help in identifying the duct, but one usually requires to use an exploring syringe and needle. In cases of extreme difficulty it may be necessary to open the second part of the duodenum, and following identification of the ampulla of Vater, retrograde catheterization will assist identification of the common bile duct. Haemostasis is essential throughout this procedure and enthusiastic use of diathermy should be deprecated. Should the portal vein be opened during dissection, primary suture using 5/0 Prolene should be carried out and similarly a lateral tear in the hepatic artery should be sutured. When the common duct has been identified an on-table cholangiogram using the needle technique in the common duct should be carried out. This should demonstrate the underlying pathology and the appropriate surgical procedure should be performed.

HEPATICOJEJUNOSTOMY (*Figs.* 20.19, 20.20)

Anastomosis between the proximal hepatic ducts and the jejunum may be necessary in cases of stricture, either benign or malignant, or in the reconstruction following a pancreaticoduodenectomy. It is now generally accepted that when these patients develop symptoms suggestive of cholangitis, this is due to stenosis of the anastomosis and not to intestinal content reflux. The anastomosis should be as wide as possible and it should be without tension, and it is also important to ensure that the bile duct lining is in complete apposition to the jejunal mucosa. Jejunal anastomosis ensures a wide and secure anastomosis conforming to all three requisites and thus minimizes the complication of stenosis. It is technically very difficult on many occasions to perform an accurate anastomosis at a high level in the porta hepatis. The anastomosis is splinted by means of an intrahepatic

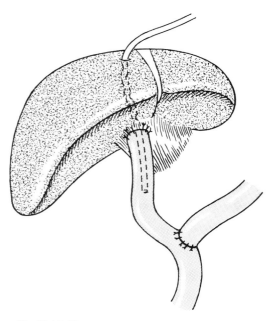

Fig. 20.19. Hepaticojejunostomy using a Roux loop.

which should protrude some 10 cm beyond the anastomosis. Prior to pulling the tube through, several lateral holes should be cut for the intrahepatic portion and the transhepatic tube should be brought out through a separate stab wound (*Fig.* 20.20).

Postoperatively the transhepatic tube should be on continuous low suction for 4–5 days and then discontinued. At that time close observation of the suction drain should be made so that if bile drainage is persistent suction of the transhepatic tube should be reinstituted. A tube cholangiogram is performed on the 10th postoperative day to check that there is no leakage from the anastomosis. If this is confirmed the tube is spigoted off during the day and allowed to drain freely at night, being washed out with sterile water once daily. The transhepatic tube should be left *in situ* for 6–12 months before it is removed, and a check cholangiogram should be undertaken before its withdrawal.

tube through the anastomosis; this is not milked out by the normal bowel peristalsis. After the hepatic duct has been found and opened, it should be irrigated to remove small stones and biliary mud and then by means of a right-angled Desjardin forceps the transhepatic route can be fashioned. The forceps is introduced into the hepatic duct and then into the right hepatic duct and by gentle manipulation into a subdivision of the duct, which usually allows the forceps to be palpated easily through the surface of the liver. Following a small incision on the surface of the liver, the forceps may be pushed through to protrude from the liver surface. A large latex rubber tube is then pulled down through the liver and ducts to the anastomosis. A Roux loop is then fashioned some 20–25 cm in length and brought up to the porta hepatis. The open end of the loop is closed and sutured to the capsule of the liver and a separate opening for the anastomosis made on the anterior surface (*Fig.* 20.19). The anastomosis is fashioned with interrupted 3/0 catgut over the latex rubber tube

TUMOURS OF THE GALLBLADDER AND EXTRAHEPATIC BILE DUCTS

Carcinoma of the Gallbladder

This commonly arises in association with cholelithiasis. The clinical presentation is not very dissimilar to that of cholelithiasis but loss of weight is noted in over 60 per cent of these patients. Anorexia, nausea and vomiting are usually seen in these patients, over 50 per cent of whom give a history suggesting gallstones. The most prominent physical finding in these patients is a palpable mass in the gallbladder area. Histologically a differentiated adenocarcinoma is the most common finding. The spread of tumour may be direct into the liver or by lymphatics. The treatment of carcinoma of the gallbladder is surgical provided that surgery is possible at the time the tumour is recognized. The prognosis in gallbladder carcinoma is poor and it is usually considered that the patient lives for 6 months or less after the symptoms of the disease become manifest.

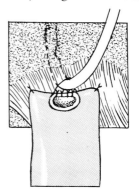
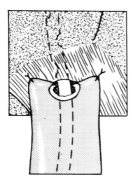
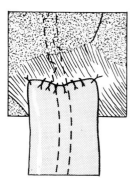

Fig. 20.20. Hepaticojejunostomy: details of anastomosis over the transhepatic tube.

Carcinoma of the Extrahepatic Bile Ducts

These tumours occur at an earlier age than does gall-bladder carcinoma, and there is a 3:2 male:female ratio in bile duct carcinoma. The symptoms of carcinoma of the extrahepatic bile duct are primarily the result of obstruction. Progressive and unremitting jaundice usually occurs within 4 months before admission to hospital. Pain occurs in some patients and as a rule is intermittent and colicky. Weight loss is frequent and usually accompanied by anorexia, nausea and vomiting. Often the carcinomas are small and difficult to palpate. This is particularly true of carcinomas occurring near the junction of the hepatic ducts, but it may be true of any carcinoma along the bile passages. Operative cholangiography, percutaneous cholangiography and choledochoscopy have greatly helped in the diagnosis of these patients but the results of surgical treatment of these carcinomas are poor. The commonest site is at the confluence of the extrahepatic bile ducts. Treatment is surgical, by resection or intubation where possible, but there have been some reports of a favourable response to radiotherapy in a small percentage of cases. It is now possible following ERCP to obtain a biopsy and in some cases dilatation of the stricture followed by the introduction of a stent may be the best way of palliation. Malignant mesodermal tumours are rare and usually occur in children. They present as biliary obstruction, grow rapidly and are rapidly fatal.

Intraduodenal Bile Duct Carcinoma

Malignant epithelial tumours of the duct at this site are usually well-differentiated adenocarcinomas. There is no sex difference in the incidence of these tumours which usually occur in the sixth decade. They usually occur at the junction of the mucosa of the common bile duct with that of the papilla. Because of their site they present early with jaundice, pain, weight loss, chills and fever. Jaundice has usually been present for only a few weeks before admission to hospital. Infiltration of carcinoma along the major ducts is usually limited but, when present, it occurs both in the periductal lymphatic system and in the mucosa. Carcinomas of the intraduodenal bile duct are most often slow-growing, well-differentiated tumours that produce obstruction of the duct and jaundice before they have spread widely. For this reason, they are often amenable to surgical treatment. Radical surgery by pancreaticoduodenectomy is the treatment of choice. Both systemic and intra-arterial chemotherapy have had little success in the management of cholangiocarcinoma.

REFERENCES

Burnstein M. J., Ilson R. G., Petrunka C. N. et al. (1983) Evidence for a potent nucleating factor in the gallbladder bile of patients with cholesterol gallstones. *Gastroenterology* **85**(4), 801–807.

Escourrou J., Cordova J. A., Lazorthes F. et al. (1984) Early and late complications after endoscopic sphincterotomy for biliary lithiasis with and without the gall bladder 'in situ'. *Gut* **25**(6), 598–602.

Flemma R. J., Lewis M. F., Osterhout S. et al. (1967) Bacteriologic studies of biliary tract infection. *Ann. Surg.* **166**, 563–572.

Geenen J. E., Toouli J., Hogan W. J. et al. (1984) Endoscopic sphincterotomy: follow-up evaluation of effects on the sphincter of Oddi. *Gastroenterology* **87**, 754–758.

Godfrey P. J., Bates T., Harrison M. et al. (1984) Gall stones and mortality: a study of all gall stone related deaths in a single health district. *Gut* **25**, 1029–1033.

Gollish S. H., Burnstein M. J., Ilson R. G. et al. (1983) Nucleation of cholesterol monohydrate crystals from hepatic and gall-bladder bile of patients with cholesterol gall stones. *Gut* **24**(9), 836–844.

Graham Cole W. H. et al. (1928) *Disease of the Gall Bladder and Bile Ducts: A Book for Practitioners and Students.* Philadelphia, Lea & Febiger.

Gray H. (1946) *Gray's Anatomy, Descriptive and Applied*, 29th ed. Edited by T. B. Johnston and J. Whillis. London, Longman.

Hamilton W. J., Boyd J. D. and Mossmann H. W. (1945) *Human Embryology: Prenatal Development of Form and Function.* Cambridge, Heffer.

Haw C. S. and Gunn A. A. (1973) The significance of infection in biliary disease. *J. R. Coll. Surg. Edinb.* **18**, 209–212.

Kapper S. K., Adams M. B. and Wilson S. D. (1982) Intraoperative biliary endoscopy: mandatory for all common duct operations? *Arch Surg.* **117**, 603–607.

Lord Smith (1978) Injuries of the liver, biliary tree and pancreas. The Sir Ernest Finch Memorial Lecture. *Br. J. Surg.* **65**, 673–677.

Lund J. (1960) Surgical indications in cholelithiasis: prophylactic cholecystectomy elucidated on the basis of long-term follow up on 526 nonoperated cases. *Ann. Surg.* **151**, 153–162.

Reiss R., Deutsch A. A., Nudelman I. et al. (1984) Statistical value of various clinical parameters in predicting the presence of choledochal stones. *Surg. Gynecol. Obstet.* **159**, 273–276.

Shore J. M. and Shore E. (1970) Operative biliary endoscopy: experience with the flexible choledochoscope in 100 consecutive choledocholithotomies. *Ann. Surg.* **171**, 269–278.

Way L. W., Admirand W. H. and Dunphy J. E. (1972) Management of choledocholithiasis. *Ann. Surg.* **176**, 347–359.

Chapter twenty-one

Hiatal Hernia

D. B. Skinner

Proper surgical management of hiatal hernia and gastro-oesophageal reflux is based on principles and understanding learned only recently. Hiatal hernia was not diagnosed in a living human being prior to the introduction of oesophageal radiography early in this century. Until the mid-century, hiatal hernia was thought to be an anatomical problem similar to hernias elsewhere in the body, and the usual surgical treatment emphasized obliteration of the hernia sac and suturing of the diaphragmatic crura to narrow the oesophageal hiatus. In 1951 Allison's description of gastro-oesophageal reflux and reflux oesophagitis established this as the disease causing the symptoms of heartburn and regurgitation and the complications of stricture and bleeding. Subsequently, Hiebert and Belsey (1961) convincingly demonstrated that patients could have abnormal oesophageal reflux causing complications in the absence of a hiatal hernia, and it became gradually appreciated that most patients with hiatal hernia did not have abnormal gastro-oesophageal reflux and did not require treatment.

Now it is generally accepted that hiatal hernia and gastro-oesophageal reflux are different conditions which commonly occur together, but may occur independently. A large number, estimated at 10 per cent of the adult population, of North Americans and Europeans are known to have a hiatal hernia, but very few of these people are troubled by the symptoms or complications of reflux. On the other hand, approximately 80 per cent of those with pathological degrees of reflux causing symptoms and complications have an associated hiatal hernia, but 20 per cent do not. It is the frequent entry and prolonged presence in the oesophagus of acid peptic secretions, and occasionally pancreatico-biliary secretions which cause the symptoms of heartburn and regurgitation and the complications of reflux.

TYPES OF HIATAL HERNIA

The very common type I, axial or sliding hiatal hernia by itself generally causes no symptoms or complications unless associated with abnormal reflux. Accordingly, the type I hiatal hernia should not be considered to be a disease, and does not require any type of medical or surgical treatment. The rarer type II, para-oesophageal or rolling hiatal hernia presents a different problem (*Fig.* 21.1). In this instance the herniation of stomach is into a free peritoneal sac extending into the thorax. Since abdominal pressure is consistently higher than thoracic pressure this sac will naturally tend to enlarge until the entire stomach

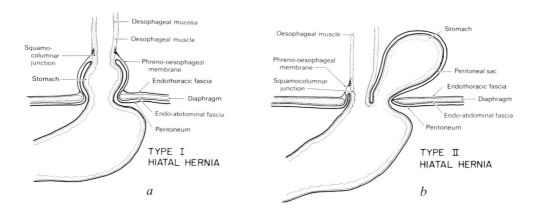

Fig. 21.1. The anatomical abnormalities for a type I sliding or axial hiatal hernia (*a*) and a type II rolling or para-oesophageal hiatal hernia (*b*). In the type I defect the phreno-oesophageal membrane remains intact but is displaced in a cephalad direction. This membrane is formed by the fusion of the endo-abdominal and endothoracic fascia coming off the diaphragm. Normally it inserts 3–4 cm above the junction of tubular oesophagus with gastric pouch. The insertion of the membrane is into the submucosa of the oesophagus. If insertion of the membrane occurs at a normal level, the hiatal hernia pouch remains intra-abdominal, as does the lower oesophagus, so no reflux may occur.

In the type II hiatal hernia there is a defect in the phreno-oesophageal membrane permitting a true peritoneal sac to enter the thoracic cavity. The junction of oesophagus and stomach remains at a normal location and is fixed by the insertion of the remainder of the intact phreno-oesophageal membrane.

is in an intrathoracic location. Even though such hernias may be asymptomatic, they are potentially lethal because of the high incidence of gastric obstruction, volvulus, infarction, bleeding and intrathoracic gastric dilatation. For this reason, the large type II para-oesophageal hernias should be repaired surgically when they are encountered even if they are asymptomatic. This type is the only variety for which surgical repair of hiatal hernia is always indicated.

The diagnosis of hiatal hernia is generally made by radiography. Since the common type I hiatal hernia is not always a disease and may not require therapy, the diagnostic problem is documentation of gastro-oesophageal reflux. For this purpose, radiography is much less effective than in diagnosing hiatal hernia. Only about 40 per cent of those patients who eventually are proved to have abnormal degrees of reflux are shown to have reflux demonstrated spontaneously during radiographic studies including ciné barium swallow techniques.

OESOPHAGEAL FUNCTION TESTS

To make the diagnosis of abnormal gastro-oesophageal reflux, oesophageal function tests are frequently required. Several of these tests are widely employed, and are generally done at the same sitting.

Manometry

The first of these tests to be introduced was oesophageal manometry. Observations of oesophageal peristalsis dated back many years, but modern oesophageal manometry was developed in a systematic fashion by Code and associates at the Mayo Clinic in the mid-1950s (Fyke et al., 1956). The technique was refined (Winans and Harris, 1967) to provide more quantitative data by using infused catheters.

To perform oesophageal manometry a triple lumen fluid-filled catheter with orifices spaced 5 cm apart is introduced like a nasogastric tube into the stomach. The catheter channels are connected through pressure transducers to a recorder. Alternatively, miniaturized electronic transducers may be used in place of the open-tipped water-perfused catheters. The train of catheters or transducers is slowly withdrawn from the stomach into the oesophagus. Normally each pressure detector passes from the stomach characterized by baseline pressure slightly higher than atmospheric, through a zone of high pressure between the stomach and oesophagus, and finally into the less than atmospheric pressure environment of the oesophagus (*Fig.* 21.2). The high-pressure zone usually measures between 3 and 4 cm in length. One-half to three-quarters of this high-pressure zone is located within the abdominal environment as indi-

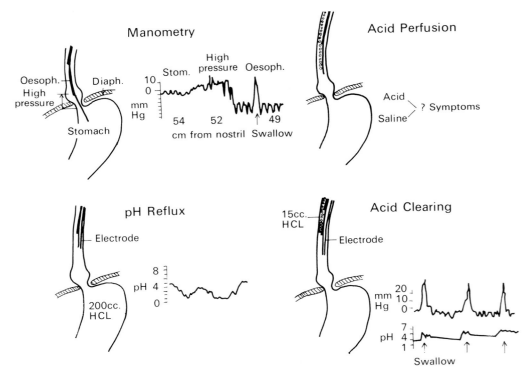

Fig. 21.2. Diagram of commonly used oesophageal function tests. Manometry is performed with triple-lumen catheter to record pressures across the gastro-oesophageal junction. The pH reflux test detects drops in pH 5 cm above the gastro-oesophageal junction after placement of an acid load in the stomach. The acid clearing test determines the ability of the oesophagus to empty 15 ml of 0·1-N HCl from the mid-oesophagus. Normally this occurs with swallowing. The acid perfusion test correlates the presence of the patient's own symptoms with the perfusion of acid or saline into the mid-oesophagus.
(Reproduced by kind permission from D. B. Skinner and D. J. Booth (1970). *Annals of Surgery*, vol. 172, p. 627.)

cated by positive-pressure deflections with respiration. The functional level of the diaphragm is determined as the place where respiratory pressure deflections reverse as the thorax is entered. The high-pressure zone is believed to represent the distal oesophageal segment which extends several centimetres within the abdominal cavity before the gastric pouch is entered (*see Fig. 21.1*). There is a statistical correlation between the magnitude of the high-pressure zone and the presence or absence of gastro-oesophageal reflux in a population of patients and normal subjects. However, the overlap in pressures recorded in patients with or without abnormal reflux is too great to employ manometry as a diagnostic measurement of reflux in an individual patient.

Besides assessing and locating the distal oesophageal high-pressure zone, manometry provides other valuable information. Findings diagnostic for achalasia, scleroderma or oesophageal spasm may be observed in patients with symptoms of oesophageal disease which might otherwise be confused with some manifestations of reflux. The principal function of manometry is the exclusion or diagnosis of other motor disorders which may accompany or be confused with an incompetent cardia and gastro-oesophageal reflux.

pH Reflux Tests

Oesophageal pH studies are another commonly used test of oesophageal function, and are routinely employed in conjunction with oesophageal manometry. A long gastrointestinal pH electrode is passed like a nasogastric tube into the stomach. As this electrode is slowly withdrawn a sharp rise in pH is noted over a 1-cm distance corresponding to the level of the distal oesophageal high-pressure zone. Such a sharp rise in pH is seen in approximately 80 per cent of normal people. Patients with an incompetent cardia frequently have a gradual and prolonged rise in pH. Unfortunately this may occur in normal individuals if acid and mucous material from the stomach are coated on the pH electrode. Although this pH electrode withdrawal technique is the first pH test for reflux described (Tuttle and Grossman, 1958), it is not widely used because of the high rate of false positive examinations.

A standard acid reflux test developed in the mid-1960s places the pH electrode 5 cm above the top of the high-pressure zone and after an acid load is placed in the stomach (Kantrowitz et al., 1969). Patients are asked to perform a series of respiratory and postural manoeuvres to challenge the cardia while pH is being recorded in the oesophagus. During a standard acid reflux test, patients perform coughing, deep breathing, Valsalva manoeuvre and Müller manoeuvre, in the supine, right side down, left side down and head down positions. After each bout of reflux, time is allowed for pH to return to above 4 before the test is resumed. More than two drops in pH during the performance of these manoeuvres is determined to be abnormal when compared to healthy controls (Skinner and Booth, 1970). This test is performed in conjunction with oesophageal manometry and provides a rapid and effective screening test for patients with abnormal reflux. It is more accurate than manometry alone or the Tuttle test for the diagnosis of abnormal reflux. Because the test is of limited duration and imposes severe stresses on the cardia, it still carries a small incidence of false positive and false negative results.

Acid Clearing

It requires two abnormalities for reflux oesophagitis to develop. A patient must have frequent episodes of gastro-oesophageal reflux, and, in addition, must have some disorder of normal oesophageal clearing which permits the regurgitated gastric contents to have prolonged contact with the squamous epithelium. It is normal for everyone to have reflux on occasion, particularly after meals. Regurgitated gastric contents are cleared from the oesophagus only by coordinated peristalsis. A disorder in oesophageal clearing permits refluxed contents to remain in the oesophagus. Animal studies demonstrate that it requires approximately 45 min for acid perfused into the oesophageal lumen to penetrate the squamous epithelium and cause a drop in pH which may be a trigger for an inflammatory reaction. A test of acid clearing is used routinely in conjunction with the standard acid reflux test. After the reflux test is completed and shown to be abnormal, a 15-ml bolus of 0·1-N hydrochloric acid is placed in the mid-oesophagus. Distal oesophageal pH is monitored while the patient is asked to swallow at 30-sec intervals. Normal individuals without reflux oesophagitis clear this bolus of acid from the oesophagus in 10 swallows or less. Those with oesophagitis are likely to have a marked prolongation of clearing, or to have repeated drops in pH during the test as further reflux occurs. This test is useful as a screening method to identify those at greatest risk for having oesophagitis.

Acid Perfusion

The symptoms of epigastric pain and heartburn are non-specific, and may be caused by a variety of other conditions including coronary heart disease, other oesophageal diseases, gastritis, gastric ulcer or duodenal ulcer, pancreatitis or biliary tract disease. For this reason the acid perfusion test is often performed when symptoms are atypical to determine if the patient's symptoms may be provoked by infusion of acid into the oesophagus. The test is generally conducted at the end of the battery of oesophageal function tests. The infusion catheters are left in the mid-oesophagus and 0·1-N HCl or normal saline are alternately perfused for 10-min intervals into the oesophagus without the patient being informed as to which substance is being infused. If the patient's spontaneous symptoms are elicited by acid and relieved by saline, it can be stated that the symptoms are acid induced and of oesophageal origin. When coupled with the documentation of abnormal reflux, the presumption of reflux causing symptoms may be made. With the use of oesophageal manometry, standard acid reflux test, acid clearing test, and the acid perfusion test, the functional disorders of the oesophagus, including gastro-oesophageal reflux, may be diagnosed in a high proportion of patients with studies which are simple to perform and can be used on an outpatient basis. These tests provide the most commonly and effectively employed methods for diagnosing abnormal gastro-oesophageal reflux.

Prolonged Oesophageal pH Monitoring

Continuous oesophageal pH monitoring over 24 hours or longer provides additional insight into the disordered pathophysiology of reflux, and is of great value in the diagnosis of the atypical or difficult patient. The technique employed is that described by Johnson and DeMeester (1974) in which the long gastrointestinal pH electrode is left in position 5 cm above the high-pressure zone. The grounding circuit is completed by strapping KCL ground electrode embedded in conductive paste and wrapped with Saran Wrap on the patient's forearm. This allows a long-term satisfactory contact. Commercially available systems have the earth electrode incorporated in the catheter assembly. The long electrode is connected to a portable pH meter and recorder so that the patient may be up and around in the hospital or at home during the time of observation. The subject is instructed to note changes in position, symptoms or other activities so that correlations may be made between activities and intraoesophageal pH. The patient is maintained on a diet adjusted to eliminate low pH foods. A portion of the test is performed while the patient is in the sitting or upright position, and the other half of the test is performed while the patient is lying flat in bed overnight. From the tracing obtained over a 24-hour period it is possible to calculate the proportion of time in the upright position or supine position in which oesophageal pH is less than 4, the total number of reflux episodes in each position, the number of episodes longer than 5 minutes, the longest episode of low pH and the total time during which pH is abnormally low. A scoring system is devised to take each of these factors into account.

Studies in normal healthy individuals demonstrate that everyone has some reflux usually after meals. This generally occurs in the upright position, and the bouts of reflux are limited in number and of short duration. Individuals with pathological reflux demon-

strate three patterns (DeMeester et al, 1976). Most commonly seen is the patient who has multiple and prolonged bouts of reflux in both the upright and supine positions. These individuals tend to be both symptomatic and subject to oesophagitis. Another smaller group of patients has reflux only in the supine position. Since this reflux generally occurs while the patient is asleep at night, the individual may be unaware of the reflux. Swallowing occurs rarely at night, so the duration of contact of the regurgitated substances and the oesophageal mucosa may be prolonged. These prolonged bouts of reflux are correlated with an increased incidence of oesophagitis. If this occurs only while the patient is asleep, he or she may not be aware of reflux until the onset of dysphagia occurs. This may explain an earlier observation that 20 per cent of patients seen with oesophageal strictures do not request medical help for their symptoms prior to the onset of dysphagia.

The third subset of abnormal reflux is that which occurs only in the upright position. These patients reflux frequently with any change of activity or body position during the daytime while they are up and around. They are often highly symptomatic, but protect themselves against complications of reflux by swallowing air, antacids or food. They complain frequently of belching as well as heartburn, and are often overweight. If these patients have no supine reflux, the chance of oesophagitis is small since the acid is cleared by the swallowing manoeuvres which the patient employs. Most of these individuals acquire the habit of aerophagia which may be difficult to correct after a successful anti-reflux repair. These patients may be more subject to abdominal distension and the gas bloat syndrome after anti-reflux surgery, but have a small risk of oesophagitis. Accordingly, it seems inadvisable to operate on such patients, and great efforts are made to treat them medically unless frank oesophagitis develops.

The 24-hour continuous pH monitoring studies are especially useful in diagnosing those patients in whom reflux causes pulmonary symptoms, and those individuals in whom an alkaline component to reflux is present. Respiratory symptoms are common in North America and Europe. It is well known that chronic or acute aspiration of gastric contents into the lung may lead to respiratory disease. The frequency of respiratory symptoms in patients with reflux is as high as 60 per cent. However, it is often difficult to demonstrate a direct cause-and-effect relationship between reflux and respiratory complaints. By continuous pH monitoring it is possible to identify those patients in whom bouts of reflux regularly precede the onset of coughing and respiratory symptoms. This occurs in less than 10 per cent of patients with abnormal reflux. In others the coughing itself is a cause of abnormal reflux. When respiratory symptoms are prominent and are considered as a possible indication for anti-reflux surgery, the use of continuous pH monitoring will determine whether this is a justifiable indication for surgery in an effort to relieve the respiratory disease (Pellegrini et al., 1979).

It has been known for some time that acid-reducing gastric operations such as pyloroplasty and vagotomy or antrectomy with or without vagotomy do not relieve, and may aggravate, symptomatic reflux and oesophagitis. Careful analysis of 24-hour pH recordings demonstrates a small group of patients in whom the pH intermittently rises above 7 to the range of 7·6 which is equivalent to the alkalinity of pancreatic and biliary secretions. This may occur with or without acid reflux depending on the amount of acid production by the stomach. Based on such studies, patients are identified with oesophageal strictures in spite of achlorhydria, and in whom the alkaline regurgitation is frequent and the probable cause of the oesophagitis and stricture.

When the symptoms are atypical and radiographic studies do not convincingly demonstrate spontaneous reflux, the oesophageal function tests serve as the standard for diagnosis of functional disorders including an incompetent cardia and gastro-oesophageal reflux. In difficult or unusual cases, continuous pH monitoring in the oesophagus provides additional valuable information. Once the diagnosis of abnormal gastro-oesophageal reflux is established by one of these methods, further investigation for the presence of complications is indicated.

DIAGNOSIS OF OESOPHAGITIS

Oesophagitis is the most common complication of reflux and the precursor to stricture and bleeding. Since oesophagitis is a pathological diagnosis it requires direct observation of the condition of the lower oesophagus, most frequently by endoscopy. For routine diagnostic work the flexible fibre-optic oesophagogastroscope is commonly employed. Based on the appearance of the distal oesophagus, oesophagitis may be graded from O to IV. Grade I oesophagitis is recorded when erythema of the oesophagus near the gastro-oesophageal junction is seen but there are no frank ulcerations. A biopsy of the mucosa may show hyperplasia of the basal epithelial layers of the squamous epithelium and close proximity of the rete pegs and vascular bundles to the surface giving the red appearance. However, no inflammatory cells are seen and this should not be considered as true oesophagitis. Grade II oesophagitis is noted when there is a break in the mucosa with frank ulceration. This is a visual diagnosis made by the endoscopist and does not require microscopic confirmation. Oesophagitis progresses to grade III when the ulcerations are confluent and accompanied by fibrosis and rigidity of the wall. When a frank stricture develops so that the oesophagoscope cannot be passed, grade IV oesophagitis is recorded. The degree of oesophagitis is an important determinant when considering indications for surgery.

ANTI-REFLUX SURGERY

Indications

After completion of the work-up, including barium swallow, oesophageal function studies when indicated, and endoscopy, and a general evaluation of the patient's health, consideration of treatment is undertaken. Surgery is reserved for those patients with the complications of reflux including ulcerative oesophagitis, stricture, bleeding documented to come from oesophagitis, Barrett's oesophagus and documented repeated bouts of aspiration causing lung disease. All other patients with uncomplicated reflux should be treated medically in an effort to relieve their symptoms. Only if symptoms are clearly known to be caused by reflux, and cannot be relieved by rigorous medical treatment over approximately 6 months, should a patient with uncomplicated reflux be considered for surgical treatment. Even in these circumstances the pure upright refluxer who has the habit of aerophagia is probably not a surgical candidate because of the high incidence of symptomatic gas bloat syndrome after operation. As indicated above, only the large type II para-oesophageal hiatal hernia is an indication for surgery based on the diagnosis of hiatal hernia. The rationale for recommending surgery when ulcerative oesophagitis is present is that recurring bouts of ulcerative oesophagitis may lead to fibrosis and stricture which are much more difficult to treat, and have less chance of being cured. Ulcerative oesophagitis may progress to frank stricture formation in a remarkably short time, so that surgical treatment is generally advisable when oesophagitis reaches this degree of mucosal damage.

Principles

Once a decision to operate is reached, the operation to be performed should be an anti-reflux repair rather than simply an obliteration of the hiatal hernia sac and narrowing of the oesophageal hiatus. A number of anti-reflux repairs have been advocated in recent years. Allison (1951) initially described a repair which he hoped would prevent reflux by reattaching the phreno-oesophageal membrane to the margins of the hiatus. This did not succeed in correcting reflux in many patients, and Allison eventually acknowledged this after long-term follow-up of his cases (1973). The Allison repair is not now recommended for anti-reflux surgery.

There are a number of effective anti-reflux operations under evaluation. Each of these recognizes similar principles. For an anti-reflux operation to be successful, it should restore the normal or somewhat exaggerated length of intra-abdominal oesophagus. Evidence compiled in recent years indicates that it is the intra-abdominal segment of narrow-diameter swallowing tube entering the large-diameter gastric pouch within a common pressure chamber of abdomen which accounts for the normal control of reflux.

When described in this way, it is obvious that the Law of Laplace governing wall tension of tubes applies. This causes the smaller-diameter swallowing tube to remain closed and requires a greater force to distend its lumen than is the case for the larger-diameter stomach.

If the intra-abdominal segment of oesophagus is lost so that the swallowing tube is in the less than atmospheric pressure environment of the thorax as it enters into the gastric pouch, then it will tend to have a larger diameter and be a less effective barrier to reflux when challenged by increased gastric pressure. The evidence for this mechanism is documented by a number of experimental and clinical observations (DeMeester et al., 1979; Skinner, 1985). A true anatomical sphincter in the distal oesophagus of human beings has never been convincingly demonstrated, and current evidence indicates that a sphincter muscle per se is not present or necessary in the distal oesophagus to prevent reflux. Rather the anatomical location of the intra-abdominal oesophagus and its geometric relation with the gastric pouch is critical in preventing reflux. Each of the successful anti-reflux repairs emphasizes the restoration of the intra-abdominal segment of the oesophagus and restricts the diameter of the lumen by a partial or full plication of stomach around the intra-abdominal oesophageal segment.

Selection of Approach

In Europe and North America, the anti-reflux repairs developed independently by Nissen (1961) and by Belsey (Skinner and Belsey, 1967) both in 1955, are most widely used. The repair described by Hill (1967) of Seattle has many advocates in North and South America, and a repair described by Guarner of Mexico City recognizes similar principles (Guarner et al., 1975). The Belsey Mark IV operation can only be performed through a thoracotomy incision. The Nissen fundoplication may be performed transthoracically or transabdominally. The Hill posterior gastropexy and calibration of the cardia are performed through an abdominal approach, and the Guarner operation is similarly done transabdominally. Unfortunately the choice of operation is often governed more by the experience and credentials of the surgeon rather than by the needs of the patient. When a surgeon is familiar and comfortable with anti-reflux operations being done either transthoracically or transabdominally, indications for one approach or the other are recognized. A common cause of failure of anti-reflux surgery is insufficient reduction of enough length of intra-abdominal oesophagus or reduction of it under too much tension. The transthoracic approach allows more oesophagus to be completely mobilized which facilitates establishment of the intra-abdominal segment of swallowing tube. For this reason the transthoracic approach is preferred in patients with severe oesophagitis or in patients who have recurrences following previous efforts at anti-reflux surgery. The transthoracic approach offers advantages in the obese patient in whom exposure of the cardia through an abdominal incision may be unduly difficult. The abdominal approach is highly satisfactory for the first time anti-reflux operations in thin patients, and is clearly the procedure of choice when other intra-abdominal disease requires correction at the same time.

Because the Belsey Mark IV operation and Nissen fundoplication are probably most widely used, and because of space constraints in this chapter, only these two repairs will be described in detail. The interested reader is encouraged to investigate the techniques and attributes of the Hill and Guarner repairs by using the cited references.

Mark IV Anti-reflux Repair

The Belsey Mark IV operation was so named because it represented the fourth modification or variation employed by its developer, Ronald Belsey of Bristol, England. Finding that the original Allison repair did not succeed in preventing reflux, Belsey instituted a series of modifications until the Mark IV operation proved to be a successful anti-reflux procedure. These modifications proceeded between approximately 1949 and 1955.

The operation is performed through a left 6th interspace thoracotomy. The 6th interspace is chosen both because a higher thoracotomy seems to cause less postoperative pain and discomfort due to less rib motion, and because this repair is used when extensive mobilization of the oesophagus up to the aortic arch is desired. It is essential to avoid undue stretching, breaking of ribs, or damage to the chest wall during the performance of this operation, so as to minimize post-thoracotomy discomfort.

After the thorax is opened the pulmonary ligament is divided, ligating a small vessel at its free margin. An incision in the pleura is made just anterior to the aorta. The oesophagus is dissected from its bed ligating two or three direct branches from the aorta to the oesophagus. Because of the extensive submucosal collateral circulation of the oesophagus these vessels may be ligated without fear of causing ischaemia. As the oesophagus is elevated from its bed the adherent right pleural surface is dissected free bluntly to prevent opening of the right thorax with accumulation of blood in the downside chest during the remainder of the procedure. Anteriorly the oesophagus is dissected free from the pericardium from which some of the oesophageal muscle fibres arise. Eventually the entire oesophagus with its adjacent vagus nerve branches should be completely freed from the rest of the mediastinum up to the level of the aortic arch (*Fig.* 21.3).

The reflection of the greater peritoneal sac onto the anterior surface of the oesophagus is incised by pulling up on the oesophagus and cutting directly into

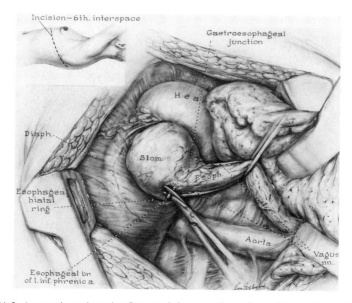

Fig. 21.3. A transthoracic anti-reflux repair is generally performed through the left 6th intercostal interspace. The oesophagus is mobilized up to the arch of the aorta to enable reduction of the intra-abdominal segment of oesophagus. All attachments to the hiatus are divided. In this figure the ascending branch of the left inferior phrenic artery is being divided.

(*Figs.* 21.3–21.7 are reproduced by kind permission from Belsey R. H. R. and Skinner D. B. (1972) Surgical treatment: Thoracic approach. Chapter 11 in: Skinner D. B., Belsey R. H. R., Hendrix T. R. et al. (eds) *Gastroesophageal Reflux and Hiatal Hernia*. Boston, Little, Brown.)

the tissues at the anterior margin of the oesophageal hiatus. After the pleura is divided the next layer is the phreno-oesophageal membrane which represents a fusion of the endo-abdominal and endothoracic fascia. This membrane inserts into the submucosa of the oesophagus several centimetres above the oesophago-gastric junction. After incising the phreno-oesophageal membrane, retroperitoneal fat is encountered. Deep to this lies the peritoneal reflection which is opened. The cardia is completely freed from its attachments to the diaphragm by incising the phreno-oesophageal membrane circumferentially. An ascending branch of the left inferior phrenic artery is encountered laterally close to the left vagus nerve. This artery is ligated and divided but the nerve is carefully preserved. Medially the hepatic branch of the vagus nerve should be preserved. Just posterior to this lies the ascending, communicating branch of the left gastric artery (Belsey's artery) which is ligated and divided. Once this is done the lesser peritoneal sac reflection off the intra-abdominal oesophagus is easily identified and entered. The dissection is completed preserving the two main vagus nerve trunks and their branches. At the end of this dissection it should be possible to pass a right-angle clamp or the operator's fingertip completely around the free edge of the hiatal muscle.

The fibro-fatty tissue remaining on the anterior and lateral oesophageal wall is excised so that the fundoplication of stomach serosa will be against bare oesophageal muscle to encourage adhesion (*Fig.* 21.4).

Several vessels are usually encountered in this fat pad. It is important to dissect this tissue from a cephalad direction distally. Otherwise the dissection is likely to follow the phreno-oesophageal membrane into the submucosal layer of the oesophagus.

The pleura overlying the junction of diaphragm and pericardium is incised medially. The pericardium is bluntly elevated off the right portion of the diaphragm so that the tendinous origin of the diaphragm may be identified. By pulling the diaphragm forward with a tenaculum, the tendinous right pillar of the diaphragm is identified. A spoon bowl may be introduced posteriorly into the hiatus to protect the liver while large needles bearing 2/0 silk sutures are passed through the right and left margins of the oesophageal hiatus to narrow it posteriorly (*Fig.* 21.5). The number of sutures required to obliterate the posterior hiatus from its vertebral origin anteriorly varies with the size of the hiatal hernia, but three such sutures is an average number. These sutures are laid in place but not tied until the fundoplication is completed. Up to this point, the dissection is the same whether a Belsey or Nissen type of fundoplication is subsequently employed.

If the Mark IV operation is chosen, a first row of three 2/0 silk sutures is placed. Laterally the first stitch passes from fundus of stomach to the oesophageal muscle 2 cm above the gastro-oesophageal junction just adjacent to the left vagus nerve. The suture is reversed and passed back through the oesophagus catching both transverse and longitudinal muscle

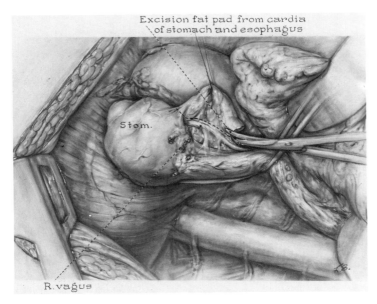

Fig. 21.4. After full mobilization of the oesophagus the hiatal hernia sac and redundant fibro-fatty tissue on the cardia are excised to permit close apposition of the fundus of the stomach to the oesophagus when the fundoplication is performed. The vagus nerves are preserved.

fibres by a slightly oblique direction of the stitch. The stitch then passes through the fundus of the stomach. The mattress suture is tied to begin the approximation of the gastric fundus to the distal oesophagus. A similar stitch is placed anteriorly, and the third suture in this row is placed medially adjacent

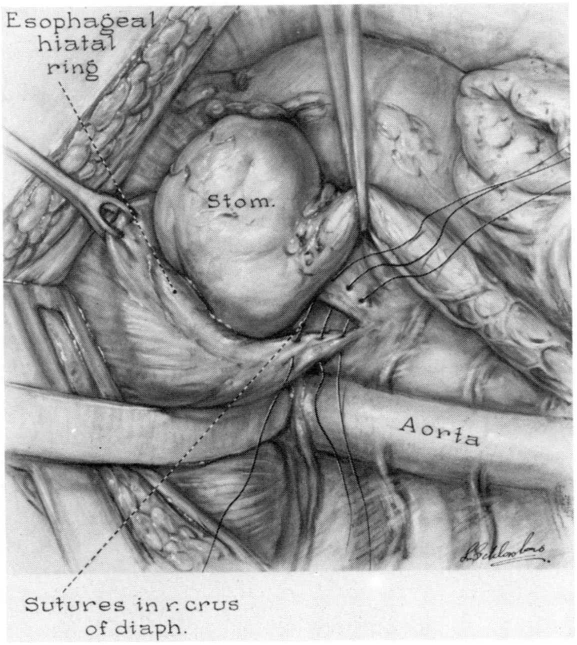

Fig. 21.5. After full mobilization of the gastro-oesophageal junction the repair is started by narrowing the hiatus posteriorly. Up to this point the steps in the transthoracic anti-reflux operation are the same for either a Belsey Mark IV or Nissen fundoplication procedure.

to the right vagus nerve. This brings approximately 2 cm of distal oesophagus within the gastric wrap.

A second row of sutures is placed passing initially through the diaphragm, then fundus of stomach and oesophagus and reversing back through the three structures in reverse order (*Fig.* 21.6). The suture passing through the diaphragm is placed into the bowl of a spoon inserted beneath the diaphragm to protect the intra-abdominal organs. The diaphragm suture should catch the edge of the central tendon of the diaphragm rather than the muscular layers of the margins of the hiatus since the muscles do not hold sutures well. The first stitch is again placed laterally through the diaphragm, fundus of stomach and oesophagus 4 cm above the gastro-oesophageal junction. The stitch is then reversed and passes back obliquely through the oesophagus, stomach and diaphragm. The two additional sutures are placed anteriorly and medially. These sutures are held until all three are inserted.

The gastro-oesophageal junction is placed manually beneath the diaphragm where it should remain without tension prior to the sutures being tied (*Fig.* 21.7). When it is seen that the repair is satisfactory, the sutures are pulled up individually to avoid sawing through the oesophageal muscle. Sutures are tied without tension so that they do not cut through the fragile muscle of the oesophagus. When the fundoplication is completed in this fashion, the posterior sutures in the diaphragmatic crura are ligated also avoiding strangulation of the muscle. A chest tube is inserted, and the chest is closed in layers avoiding overtight suturing which increases post-thoracotomy discomfort.

A nasogastric tube is not routinely used but may

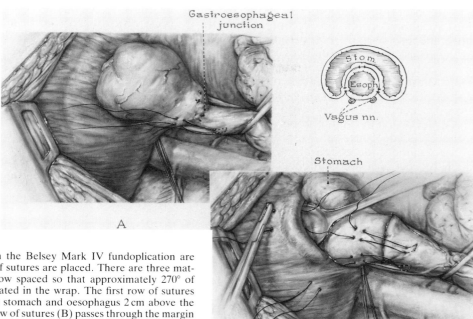

Fig. 21.6. The steps in the Belsey Mark IV fundoplication are illustrated. Two rows of sutures are placed. There are three mattress sutures in each row spaced so that approximately 270° of oesophagus is incorporated in the wrap. The first row of sutures (A) passes through the stomach and oesophagus 2 cm above the junction. The second row of sutures (B) passes through the margin of the tendinous portion of the diaphragm, stomach and oesophagus 4 cm above the junction. The suture is reversed back through the same structures. The spoon retractor prevents injury to intra-abdominal organs.

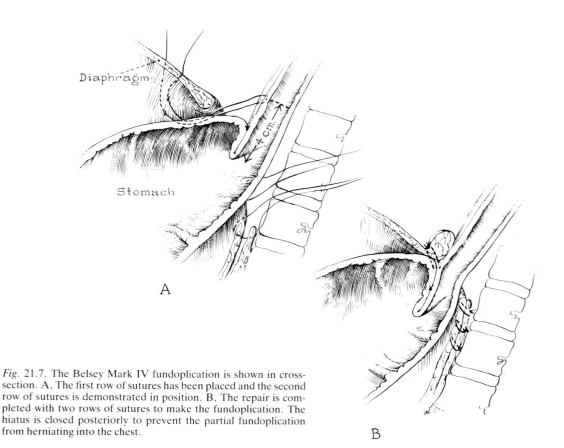

Fig. 21.7. The Belsey Mark IV fundoplication is shown in cross-section. A, The first row of sutures has been placed and the second row of sutures is demonstrated in position. B, The repair is completed with two rows of sutures to make the fundoplication. The hiatus is closed posteriorly to prevent the partial fundoplication from herniating into the chest.

need to be inserted postoperatively if the patient develops abdominal distension. Preoperative, intra-operative and also 48-hour postoperative antibiotics are given because of the possibility of a needle entering the oesophagus and contaminating the mediastinum. The chest tube is removed when drainage has decreased to less than 200 ml in 24 hours. Liquids are given by mouth as soon as bowel sounds return which is generally on the 2nd postoperative day. The patient receives a barium swallow study prior to discharge to document the effectiveness of the repair. On discharge patients are cautioned to chew their food well, eat slowly, and to avoid a large bolus or sticky foods for several weeks after surgery.

Nissen Fundoplication Anti-reflux Repair

The Nissen fundoplication may be performed either transthoracically or abdominally. When done through the thorax, the incision and dissection are identical to those used for the Mark IV repair and described above. After complete mobilization of the intrathoracic oesophagus and cardia from the diaphragm and removal of the para-oesophageal fibro-fatty tissues, the posterior sutures are placed to narrow the hiatus and again left untied until the fundoplication is finished.

To facilitate a loose and easy complete wrap of stomach around the oesophagus, the two or three highest short gastric arteries from the spleen to stomach are divided by drawing them up into the hiatus and individually ligating and dividing them (*Fig.* 21.8). The posterior fundus is passed behind the oesophagus and the anterior fundus is passed medially so that the suture line is placed on the medial

or right aspect of the oesophagus. This causes the least distortion of the stomach. The first suture is passed between the posterior fundus of stomach, muscle of the gastro-oesophageal junction, and anterior aspect of the fundus just at the cardia. The vagus nerves are left adjacent to the oesophageal wall. These sutures should be placed far out on the fundus of the stomach on each side so that a substantial amount of gastric fundus is folded into the wrap to ensure that it will not be too tight. Normally three or four additional such sutures are placed progressing in a cephalad direction until 4 cm of distal oesophagus has been included in the fundoplication (*Fig.* 21.9).

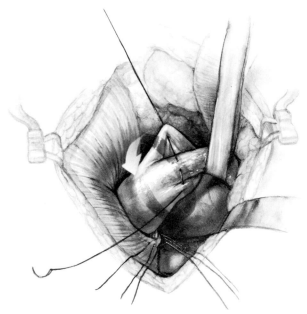

Fig. 21.9. After the posterior sutures are placed in the hiatus the fundoplication is performed. The lateral fundus is wrapped posteriorly behind the oesophagus. A series of sutures is placed through anterior and posterior stomach and oesophagus on the medial aspect of the oesophagus.

At this point it is important to ascertain that the wrap is not too tight. The operator's finger should slide easily through the tunnel caused by the full fundoplication, or a no. 60 Fr. gauge bougie may be passed by mouth by the anaesthesiologist and be shown to enter easily into the stomach without tearing the sutures of the fundoplication. Once this is done the fundoplication is placed beneath the diaphragm where it should remain without tension. The posterior sutures are tied to complete the repair (*Fig.* 21.10). Chest closure is similar to that described for the Mark IV operation.

When performed transabdominally, the Nissen operation may be done through several incisions. Some surgeons prefer a midline incision, others choose a left paramedian incision. Some employ a bilateral subcostal incision. The author generally prefers a right subcostal incision extended across the midline to the left costal margin just missing the tip

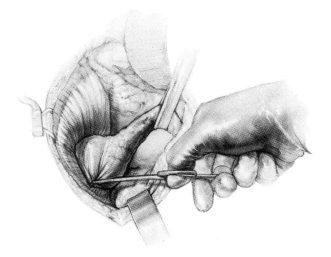

Fig. 21.8. If a transthoracic Nissen fundoplication is selected, the highest short gastric vessels are divided as they are drawn up into the hiatus. The dissection of the oesophagus and cardia is the same as for the Mark IV repair.

(*Figs.* 21.8–21.10 are reproduced by kind permission from Skinner D. B. (1976) in: *Surgical Techniques Illustrated*, Vol. 1, No. 2, pp. 33–41. Boston, Little, Brown & Co.)

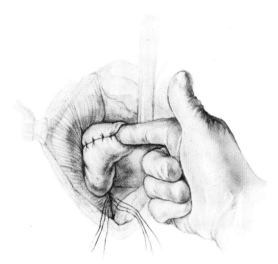

of the xiphoid cartilage. After thorough abdominal exploration, the left lobe of the liver is taken down by dividing the triangular ligament. Frequently a small vessel is encountered in the free margin of this ligament which should be ligated. Care is taken to avoid injury to the nearby phrenic vessels. The triangular ligament is divided past the midline avoiding the junction of phrenic and hepatic veins. The stomach is pulled down to reduce the hiatal hernia sac and expose the intra-abdominal segment of oesophagus. A transverse incision is made through the peritoneum overlying the abdominal segment of oesophagus. This incision should be carried the full width of the hiatus. It is carried slightly down onto the gastrohepatic omentum, taking care not to divide the hepatic branch of the vagus nerve which passes in this layer of tissue. To the left this incision is carried out onto the crus of the diaphragm. The operator's finger is inserted in the groove between the exposed oesophagus and left crus of the diaphragm. By dissecting bluntly in a straight posterior direction, the aortic pulse is palpated. The operator's finger should use the aorta as a guide and slide off the aorta onto the vertebral column and then back up medially to encompass both the oesophagus and its adjacent vagus nerves. When the blunt dissection is carried out in this manner there is little danger of injury to the oesophagus itself which may occur if the dissection is carried too close to the oesophageal wall. After the oesophagus and adjacent nerves are encircled a tape is placed around them to provide subsequent traction.

The reflection of the peritoneum from the gastro-oesophageal junction over to the spleen is incised and the highest short gastric vessels are exposed. Two or three of these are dissected, ligated and divided

to provide mobility to the fundus. When this is completed the posterior fundus should easily pass behind the oesophagus without putting undue tension on the remaining short gastric vessels. The lower oesophagus is dissected bluntly from the mediastinum to be certain that at least 4 cm of distal oesophagus can be delivered into the abdomen. When this is accomplished the oesophagus is drawn down and retracted to the left to expose the decussation of the diaphragmatic crura. With the operator's finger protecting the coeliac axis, a large needle bearing a 1/0 silk suture is passed through both crura being certain to include endo-abdominal fascia in each bite (*Fig.* 21.11). Usually three or four such sutures are placed

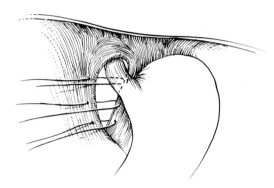

in a cephalad direction to narrow the oesophageal hiatus so that it will accept only one of the operator's fingers without being too tight. The diaphragmatic sutures are tied at this time.

The mobilized fundus is passed posteriorly behind the oesophagus and grasped with a non-crushing clamp such as the Lockwood clamp. A portion of the anterior fundus near the greater curvature is rolled over the anterior aspect of the oesophagus. The first suture of the fundoplication is inserted from the anterior fundus through the muscle of the oesophagus at the gastro-oesophageal junction and through the posterior fundus. These sutures are placed widely out onto the fundus to roll a good amount of gastric wall into the tunnel around the oesophagus to prevent the repair from being too tight. As with the thoracic approach, four or five such sutures are placed until a measured 4-cm length of intra-abdominal oesophagus is completely wrapped by gastric fundus (*Fig.* 21.12). The vagus nerves are left within the wrap. When this is achieved, a no. 60 Fr. gauge bougie or operator's finger are passed through the tunnel to be sure that it is loose and will not obstruct the lower oesophagus. After careful inspection for haemostasis, the wound is

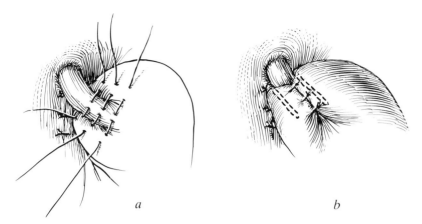

a　　　　　　　　　　*b*

Fig. 21.12. To complete the transabdominal Nissen fundoplication a series of sutures is placed through the anterior and posterior stomach and oesophagus. The fundus is brought posteriorly behind the oesophagus. Approximately 4 cm of intra-abdominal oesophagus should be included in the fundoplication. It should be loose enough to accept the operator's finger.

closed with great care, as ventral hernia is one of the known complications of this approach.

When done transabdominally, great care must be taken to be certain that enough lower oesophagus is mobilized to prevent the repair from being performed on the upper stomach. If the repair is done too low or if the oesophageal sutures do not hold and the repair slides down onto the stomach, a portion of the stomach above the wrap is partially obstructed and leads to severe reflux as a complication of the operation. This is the so-called 'slipped Nissen' effect.

As with the Mark IV operation, preoperative, intraoperative and postoperative antibiotics are used for approximately 48 hours in case one of the sutures has been placed too deeply in the oesophageal wall. With the full fundoplication postoperative intubation of the stomach may be more difficult, so a nasogastric tube is routinely left in the stomach until bowel sounds have returned and feeding can then be started. A barium swallow is routinely obtained before the patient's discharge from the hospital to ascertain that a proper repair has been achieved without complication.

Postoperative Results

A properly performed Mark IV operation or fundoplication should demonstrate the intra-abdominal segment of oesophagus on the postoperative barium swallow. If this is not seen, the patient does not have a successful anti-reflux repair. When a 4-cm segment of intra-abdominal oesophagus is restored, early postoperative standard acid reflux tests or 24-hour pH monitoring demonstrate that both of these repairs are highly effective in restoring competency to the cardia. Both repairs generally cause a rise in magnitude of the distal oesophageal high-pressure zone (Skinner and DeMeester, 1976). The Nissen fundoplication causes a slightly higher and more consistent rise which is probably caused by the fact that a full

fundoplication rather than partial fundoplication around the oesophagus is done. Both repairs as well as the Hill and Guarner repairs are highly effective in relieving the patient's symptoms and complications of reflux. Which of the repairs will prove to be most effective in the long run remains to be determined as long-term randomized follow-up studies of the several repairs by the same team of surgeons are not yet completed and reported.

In a 10-year follow-up study, the success rate in patients followed for more than 10 years after the Belsey Mark IV operation is 85 per cent with all symptomatic patients undergoing oesophagoscopy, and all patients being followed with barium swallow examinations during the follow-up period (Orringer et al., 1972). Comparable 10-year follow-up studies are not yet available for the other types of repairs but should be reported in the near future.

Recurrences may develop at any time following operation even up to 10 years after the repair, so short-term reports of success with anti-reflux surgery are not very meaningful. At present these several repairs all employ the same principles and are known to be effective in preventing reflux in the early months and years after operation. Which repair will prove to be best depends not only on long-term success in eliminating recurrences of hiatal hernia and reflux, but also on which repair has the least incidence of side-effects such as persisting dysphagia and the gas bloat syndrome. When a satisfactory anti-reflux repair can be achieved at the initial operation, it can be expected that at least 85 per cent of patients will have successful long-term control of their symptoms and complications of reflux.

REFLUX STRICTURE

Management of the patient with a stricture of the oesophagus caused by reflux is much more difficult. This may require oesophageal resection and replacement, as described in Chapter 9. A variety of methods short of resection are described. When a stricture is formed, the overall experience is that any repair short of resection and reconstruction has approximately a 70 per cent success rate at best in eliminating postoperative dysphagia and recurrence of reflux and the hiatal hernia. At present our policy is to invest substantial time in the preoperative preparation of patients with strictures prior to their first anti-reflux operation. The preoperative preparation includes intensive antacid therapy over a number of days in the hospital, and daily dilatation until a no. 40 Fr. gauge dilator can be passed easily for several consecutive days prior to surgery. When this is achieved it is usually possible to continue dilating the stricture to a no. 60 Fr. at the time of operation. Repairs for stricture should be performed transthoracically to allow extensive mobilization of the oesophagus in an effort to restore the intra-abdominal segment of oesophagus. In nearly all cases this can be accomplished. However, some patients continue to require dilatations after a Mark IV or fundoplication procedure for stricture, and the recurrence rate is higher in these patients.

Reflux-induced strictures consist of both an element of inflammation, oedema and muscle spasm, as well as fibrosis of the oesophageal wall. The spasm and oedema may be eliminated by intensive preoperative preparation, but the fibrosis may not be reversible. When the latter is severe, it may be difficult or impossible to reduce the swallowing tube to an intra-abdominal location. Several alternatives other than resection are available, and are employed at the first anti-reflux operation. When reoperation is necessary for recurrence after treatment of a stricture, resection and reconstruction as described elsewhere are preferable.

The three most commonly used operations short of resection include a Nissen fundoplication left in the thorax, an extension of the swallowing tube by a gastroplasty (Collis, 1957) coupled with a Nissen or Belsey reconstruction, or the Thal gastric patch procedure (Thal et al., 1965) coupled with a fundoplication left in the thorax. Because the Nissen fundoplication is a 360° wrap, it is effective mechanically even if left in the chest (Safaie-Shiraze et al., 1974). However, this operation has several disadvantages in that the incidence of progressive enlargement of the iatrogenic hiatal hernia is high. The intrathoracic gastric pouch seems to be subject to gastric ulceration, bleeding and perforation as has been observed in several series. For this reason, treating the strictured shortened oesophagus by intrathoracic fundoplication alone is currently not widely practised. When this is done, the stomach must be carefully sutured to the margins of the hiatus in an effort to prevent

further herniation, and the hiatus must be left widely open to prevent congestion and obstruction of the gastric pouch.

A more widely favoured alternative is the Collis gastroplasty manoeuvre (*Fig.* 21.13). In this procedure the swallowing tube is lengthened by fashioning a tube of lesser curvature of the stomach as an extension of the oesophagus. This is done by passing a bougie through the stricture into the stomach and fashioning a tube around a no. 40 or larger dilator. The tube may be formed by the use of a stapler or by clamping and oversewing the stomach on both sides of the incision between the fundus and the lesser curvature tube. The remaining exaggerated gastric fundus is used as a plication around the intra-abdominal segment of swallowing tube (Pearson et al., 1978). Either the Mark IV or the Nissen fundoplication may be employed for this manoeuvre. In this fashion a narrow-diameter swallowing tube consisting of stomach is placed beneath the diaphragm to achieve control of reflux. It is important that the diameter of this tube be similar to that of the oesophagus, and that the tube does not flare out as it enters the stomach to avoid an inverted funnel effect which encourages subsequent reflux.

Some surgeons employ the Thal procedure coupled with a fundoplication (Hollenbeck and Woodward, 1975). This is particularly useful when the stricture is very difficult to dilate or when it is split in the course of operation. An incision is made across the stricture which is allowed to gape open. A skin graft is applied to the defect with the adjacent gastric fundus sutured to the margins of the open oesophagus incorporating the skin graft in the suture line. If simply left as a gastric patch across the stricture, free reflux will occur and recurrent oesophagitis and stricture will be the outcome. Accordingly, a full fundoplication of stomach around the lower oesophagus must be employed when this operation is chosen. Both the Collis gastroplasty and Thal procedure with fundoplication have been reported in several series to give approximately 70 per cent relief of dysphagia and long-term control of reflux. Since similar results are achievable with fundoplication alone after intensive preoperative preparation of the patient, we continue to prefer the anti-reflux repair without the Collis or Thal manoeuvre whenever possible.

Until long-term results are reported which clearly establish one repair or another as the best anti-reflux operation, individual surgeons should be encouraged to learn one or more of these procedures, to employ them in carefully selected and fully evaluated patients, and to observe their own postoperative results both by barium swallow studies and postoperative oesophageal function testing to ascertain that they are indeed achieving control of reflux.

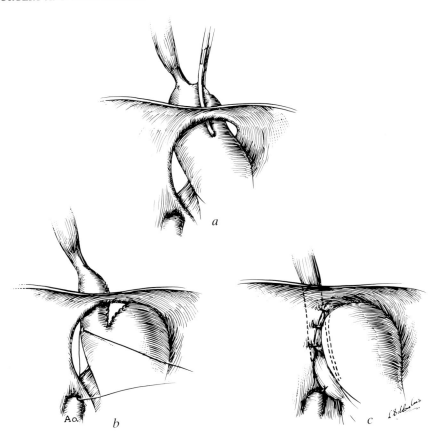

Fig. 21.13. The gastroplasty originally described by Collis is illustrated. A tube is cut from the lesser curvature of the stomach to lengthen the distal swallowing tube. Collis initially described anchoring this to the arcuate ligament. However, a standard Belsey or Nissen fundoplication may be added to complete the anti-reflux repair.

REFERENCES

Allison P. R. (1951) Reflux oesophagitis, sliding hiatal hernia, and the anatomy of repair. *Surg. Gynecol. Obstet.* **92**, 149.

Allison P. (1973) Hiatal hernia. *Ann. Surg.* **178**, 273–276.

Angelchick J. and Cohen R. (1979) A new surgical procedure for the treatment of gastroesophageal reflux and hiatal hernia. *Surg. Gynecol. Obstet.* **148**, 246–248.

Collis J. L. (1957) An operation for hiatus hernia with short oesophagus. *J. Thorac. Cardiovasc. Surg.* **34**, 768.

DeMeester T. R. et al. (1976) Patterns of gastro-oesophageal reflux in health and disease. *Ann. Surg.* **184**, 459–470.

DeMeester T. R. et al. (1979) Clinical and in vitro analysis of determinants of gastroesophageal competence. *Am. J. Surg.* **137**, 39–46.

Fyke F. E., Code C. F. and Schlegel J. F. (1956) The gastro-oesophageal sphincter in healthy human beings. *Gastroenterologia* **86**, 135.

Guarner V., Degollade J. R. and Tore N. M. (1975) A new antireflux procedure at the oesophagogastric junction. *Arch. Surg.* **110**, 101–106.

Hiebert C. A. and Belsey R. (1961) Incompetency of the gastric cardia without radiologic evidence of hiatus hernia. *J. Thorac. Cardiovasc. Surg.* **42**, 352.

Hill L. D. (1967) An effective operation for hiatal hernia: an eight-year appraisal. *Ann. Surg.* **166**, 681.

Hollenbeck J. I. and Woodward E. R. (1975) Treatment of peptic oesophageal stricture with combined fundic patch-fundoplication. *Ann. Surg.* **182**, 472.

Johnson L. F. and DeMeester T. R. (1974) Twenty-four hour pH monitoring of the distal oesophagus: a quantitative measure of gastro-oesophageal reflux. *Am. J. Gastroenterol.* **62**, 325.

Kantrowitz P. A., Corson J. G., Fleischli D. L. et al. (1969) Measurement of gastro-oesophageal reflux. *Gastroenterol.* **56**, 666.

Nissen R. (1961) Gastropexy and 'fundoplication' in surgical treatment of hiatal hernia. *Am. J. Dig. Dis.* **6**, 954.

Orringer M. B., Skinner D. B. and Belsey R. H. R. (1972) Long-term results of the Mark IV operation for hiatal hernia and analyses of recurrences and their treatment. *J. Thorac. Cardiovasc. Surg.* **63**, 25.

Pearson F. G. et al. (1978) Gastroplasty and fundoplication in the management of complex reflux problems. *J. Thorac. Cardiovasc. Surg.* **76**, 665.

Pellegrini C. A. et al. (1979) Gastro-oesophageal reflux and pulmonary aspiration; incidence, functional abnormalities and results of surgical therapy. *Surgery* **36**, 110–119.

Safaie-Shiraze S. et al. (1974) Nissen fundoplication without crural repair. *Arch. Surg.* **108**, 4.

Skinner D. B. (1985) Pathophysiology of gastroesophageal reflux. *Ann. Surg.* **202, 546**.

Skinner D. B. and Belsey R. H. R. (1967) Surgical management of oesophageal reflux and hiatus hernia. *J. Thorac. Cardiovasc. Surg.* **53**, 33.

Skinner D. B. and Booth D. J. (1970) Assessment of distal oesophageal function in patients with hiatal hernia and/or gastro-oesophageal reflux. *Ann. Surg.* **172**, 627.

Skinner D. B. and DeMeester T. R. (1976) Gastro-oesophageal reflux. *Curr. Probl. Surg.* **13**, January.

Thal A. P., Hatafuku T. and Kurtzman R. (1965) New operation for distal oesophageal stricture. *Arch. Surg.* **90**, 464.

Tuttle S. G. and Grossman M. I. (1958) Detection of gastro-oesophageal reflux by simultaneous measurement of intraluminal pressures and pH. *Proc. Soc. Exp. Biol. Med.* **98**, 225.

Weaver R. M. and Temple J. G. (1985) The Angelchick prosthesis for gastroesophageal reflux: symptomatic and objective assessment. *Ann. R. Coll. Surg. Engl.* **67**, 299.

Winans C. S. and Harris L. D. (1967) Quantitation of lower oesophageal sphincter competence. *Gastroenterology* **52**, 779.

Chapter twenty-two

The Diaphragm

K. Jeyasingham

Advances in neonatal surgery, oesophageal surgery and resuscitation have in turn contributed enormously to the operative surgery and management of diaphragmatic pathology. The following specific aspects of diaphragmatic surgery are dealt with in this book:

1. Congenital diaphragmatic hernia (*see* Chapter 58).
2. Surgery of subphrenic suppuration (*see* Chapter 23).
3. Herniation through the oesophageal hiatus (*see* Chapter 21).
4. The anatomy and nerve supply in relation to elective incisions on the diaphragm.
5. Acquired diaphragmatic hernias.
6. Idiopathic unilateral phrenic paralysis and eventration of the diaphragm.
7. Tumours of the diaphragm.
8. Diaphragmatic pacing.

This chapter deals with nos. 4–8.

ANATOMY

The diaphragm is a sheet of muscle and trilobate tendinous aponeurosis, sandwiched between pleura superiorly and peritoneum inferiorly, attached circumferentially to the skeletal structures of the trunk, separating the contents of the thorax from those of the abdomen. Normal anatomical structures passing from one body cavity to the other do so through openings situated in this sheet-like organ, the integrity of which depends greatly on its attachment to the periphery, an intact nerve supply, and on the efficacy with which the openings are filled with the structures traversing them. The strongest parts of the diaphragm are the crural tendons and the trilobate central tendinous aponeurosis. The muscular portion of the diaphragm depends for its strength on the pleural and peritoneal layers, and on an uninterrupted nerve supply from the two phrenic nerves. The left and right crura arise from the anterolateral aspects of the first two and three lumbar vertebrae respectively. Arching between the two crura, at the level of the lower border of the 12th dorsal vertebra, is the median arcuate ligament, posterior to which passes the aorta, and from which also arise some muscle fibres of the diaphragm. The medial and lateral arcuate ligaments, which are but thickened portions of the fascia covering the psoas and quadratus lumborum muscles, give rise to fleshy muscle fibres posterolaterally. The lateral sheet of fleshy musculature arises from the lower six ribs, while anteriorly two slips arise from the posterior surface of the xiphisternum. The muscle fibres all gain insertion into the trilobate aponeurotic central tendon.

Nerve Supply

The right and left phrenic nerves, having travelled the length of the thoracic cavity, on the lateral aspects of the pericardium, reach the diaphragm on its pleural surface, but before doing so they usually send off three or four branches which supply the parietal pleura and pericardium in the vicinity of the central tendon. The right phrenic nerve enters the diaphragm through its central tendon or through the inferior vena caval opening. The left phrenic nerve enters through the muscular part in front of the central tendon, just lateral to the left border of the pericardial sac, and on a more anterior plane than the right. Each main trunk divides, as it traverses the diaphragm, into its main branches, usually three in number (*Fig.* 22.1):

1. An anterior or sternal branch runs medially towards the sternum and ramifies with the corresponding branch of the opposite side.
2. An anterolateral branch which runs laterally, skirting the lateral leaflet of the central tendon.
3. A posterior branch which divides shortly into (*a*) a posterolateral branch coursing behind the lateral leaflet of the central tendon and (*b*) a posteromedial branch that runs towards the crural fibres. Occasionally the posterolateral branch may arise from the main trunk of the phrenic nerve. The portion of crural muscle to the right of the oesophageal hiatus receives its nerve supply from the right posteromedial branch, while that portion which lies to the left of the hiatus is supplied by the left posteromedial branch. The various branches of the phrenic nerve run in the substance of the diaphragmatic musculature, more often on the peritoneal aspect, but can readily be located from the pleural side by identifying the vascular bundles that accompany the nerves.

ELECTIVE INCISIONS IN THE DIAPHRAGM
(*Figs.* 22.2, 22.3)

Diaphragmatic incisions, the majority of which are carried out through a thoracic approach, should be placed in such a manner as to minimize the damage to the branches of the phrenic nerves. However, in the execution of radical procedures for malignant dis-

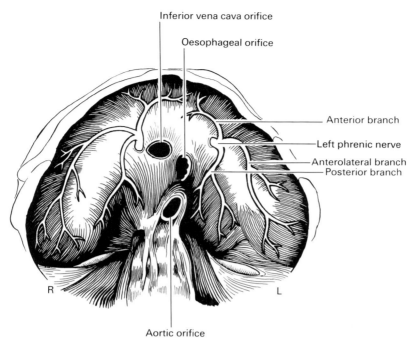

Fig. 22.1. Distribution of the branches of the phrenic nerves in relation to the anatomy of the diaphragm, as viewed from below.

ease, these considerations have to be over-ridden. *Figure* 22.2 illustrates the principal incisions, enumerated in order of frequency of use:

1. Radiate incision from the oesophageal hiatus, preferably stopping short of the anterolateral branch.
2. Radiate incision limited to the aponeurotic area, avoiding damage to any of the branches.
3. Arcuate incision in the aponeurotic central tendon, avoiding damage to the major branches.
4. Anterior costo-abdominal incision in the form of a T, detaching the anterior parts of the diaphragm peripherally and also extending into the anterior abdominal wall through its vertical limb.
5. Posterior peripheral incision, avoiding damage to the major branches of the phrenic nerve, exposing retroperitoneal posterior abdominal wall structures such as the kidneys and suprarenal glands.
6. Circumferential peripheral detachment of the diaphragm to gain access to the major part of the upper abdomen, as for example in hepatic surgery via a right thoraco-abdominal approach.
7. An incision that is rarely employed but one that permits immediate and adequate access to the heart for purposes of resuscitation, should cardiac arrest occur during the course of an upper abdominal operation—the midline incision in the central tendon and fibrous pericardium.
8. Finally, a subxiphoid incision for drainage of the pericardium and for insertion of pacing wires. A vertical anterior abdominal wall incision just below the xiphoid, deepened into the retrosternal space by separating the two slips of origin of the diaphragm from the back of the xiphisternum. The pericardium can then be entered by a sharp incision on its anterior aspect.

A total disregard of the anatomical distribution of the phrenic nerve and its branches during the course of diaphragmatic surgery could lead to immediate as well as long-term postoperative complications that are not altogether insuperable but which are entirely avoidable.

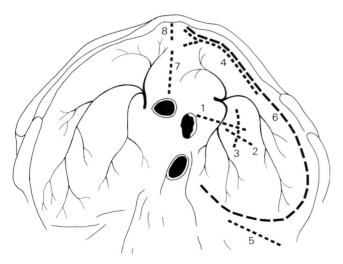

Fig. 22.2. Diaphragmatic incisions.

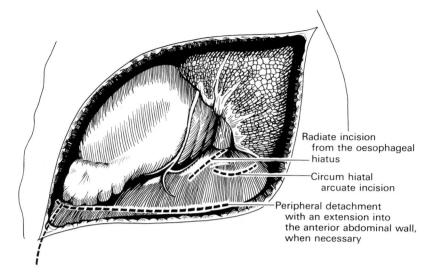

Radiate incision
from the oesophageal
hiatus

Circum hiatal
arcuate incision

Peripheral detachment
with an extension into
the anterior abdominal wall,
when necessary

Fig. 22.3. Diaphragmatic incisions as performed through a left thoracotomy.

CLOSURE OF INCISIONS AND TEARS
(*Fig.* 22.4)

The repair of incisions and tears of the diaphragm demands careful and meticulous approximation of tissues. Where there is no aponeurosis, the strength of the approximated edges depends greatly on the peritoneal and pleural membranes, and less so on the intervening muscle. From the moment the patient recovers from the anaesthetic and muscle relaxants, and begins to breathe on his own, the suture line is subjected to enormous strains, predisposing to disruption. This can occur at any time after the repair, and is encouraged by the following factors:

1. Poor suture technique or suture material.
2. Postoperative abdominal distension.
3. Postoperative pulmonary complications.
4. Impaired nutritional state of the patient before and after surgery.

Attention is paid to the following details of suture technique (*Fig.* 22.4):

a. A non-absorbable suture material is employed.
b. At least two layers of sutures are inserted, one of which is preferably of the interrupted variety.
c. The placement of sutures should be done in such a manner as to avoid interference with the major divisions of the phrenic nerve.
d. Wherever possible, an imbrication or double-breasted suture is preferred to an over-and-over suture.

Interruption of the phrenic nerve by crushing or division in an attempt to rest the diaphragm causes more problems. Similarly, the disadvantages of elective intermittent positive-pressure ventilation for the specific purpose of resting the diaphragm far outweigh the questionable advantages.

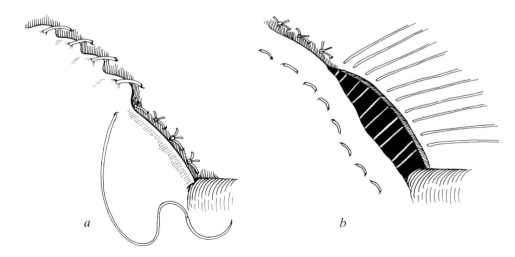

a

b

Fig. 22.4. Two-layer repair of diaphragmatic incision.

TRAUMATIC DIAPHRAGMATIC HERNIA
(Fig. 22.5)

Rupture of the diaphragm usually results from severe blunt trauma to the abdomen and chest. Despite the increasing incidence of high-velocity transportation accidents, the occurrence of traumatic diaphragmatic hernia has in the past not shown a parallel increase. The high immediate fatality rate of such accidents tended to reduce the ultimate number of cases that reached hospital with this specific injury. With the improved mobile resuscitation facilities, the picture is dramatically changing. The diagnosis of diaphragmatic rupture demands an acute awareness of the possibility of this injury. The clinician who first sees trauma patients should always consider this injury. The presence of other serious and life-threatening injuries, while demanding more urgent or immediate attention, should not detract one's thoughts from the possibility of a ruptured diaphragm. At the other end of the spectrum, diaphragmatic rupture has been known to occur even with minimal blunt trauma to the trunk, and the clinician must therefore suspect this injury in any type of blunt trauma to the abdomen or chest.

Penetrating injuries of the diaphragm occur as a result of stab injuries to the chest and abdomen. The site of entry of the weapon may be as high as the axilla and as low as the lumbar region, and yet the diaphragm may suffer injury. The diaphragmatic tears in these cases are not as large as those associated with blunt trauma, and herniation of abdominal viscera does not often occur immediately after injury. Furthermore, herniation rarely occurs unless the tear is larger than 3 cm in length. Gun shots and bullets penetrating the diaphragm in either direction rarely cause herniation. As patients with penetrating injuries of the abdomen and lower chest routinely undergo exploratory surgery, extensive diagnostic tests are not performed. It is, however, the responsibility of the surgeon to inspect the diaphragm and ensure that no tear exists. Such tears are commonly located close to the peripheral attachment of the muscle fibres and are easily missed unless a meticulous inspection of the organ is performed.

Traumatic diaphragmatic hernia occurs after both blunt and penetrating trauma to the diaphragm. In only 40–50 per cent of cases is the diagnosis made at the time of the initial injury. The vast majority (85 per cent) of these patients are males in the 20–30-year age group. In 90 per cent of these patients it is the left dome that is torn. Characteristically the tear is situated in the posterior and central part of the dome and may extend anteromedially to reach the oesophageal hiatus. Circumferential avulsion with immediate prolapse of abdominal viscera occurs in a smaller number. Occasionally a diaphragmatic rupture extends into the lateral pericardial wall, in front of or behind the phrenic nerve. This type of rupture is more likely to be associated with injury to the myocardium and valve cusps. Rarely, the rupture occurs in the pericardial portion of the central tendon and herniation of abdominal viscera occurs into the pericardial sac only. Acute cardiac tamponade and rapid deterioration of the patient may occur.

Surgical Treatment

Once the diagnosis of diaphragmatic rupture and herniation has been made, the treatment is surgical, irrespective of whether the diagnosis has been made at the time of the initial injury, or after an interval of time. The mere fact that the patient may have remained symptom free, is not an adequate reason for postponing surgical intervention, as disastrous complications can occur even in long-standing post-traumatic diaphragmatic hernia. Furthermore, the morbidity and mortality of surgery when a complication such as strangulation or perforation of herniated hollow viscus, has supervened, are considerably increased when compared to the risks of elective surgery.

In the acutely injured patient, the timing of surgical intervention will be determined by the presence and extent of other associated injuries. Where there is clear evidence of intra-abdominal haemorrhage or of injury to small or large bowel, the management of these injuries will undoubtedly take precedence over the repair of the diaphragmatic tear. If, however, there is acute cardiac or respiratory embarrassment produced by the presence of a great bulk of abdominal viscera within the chest, emergency resuscitation by the introduction of an endotracheal tube followed by ventilatory support should be commenced immediately. Once the circulatory state is stabilized, surgery should be undertaken without delay. On the other hand, the presence of extensive and multiple injuries, with the possibility of irreversible intracranial injury, would favour a delay in surgical intervention until a proper assessment of all systems has been achieved.

Surgical Approaches

The ideal approach for the repair of traumatic diaphragmatic hernia is transthoracic, via an incision made in the 7th interspace. The temptation to make a high incision is great, as radiologically the viscera often reach as far high as the 2nd interspace (*Fig.* 22.5). However, having reduced the viscera into the abdomen, great difficulty can be encountered in repairing a tear in the diaphragm via too high an incision. In those patients where presentation and diagnosis have been delayed, a transthoracic approach is the sensible one, as the herniated organs have had an opportunity to become adherent to their new surroundings, and considerable dissection will be required to free them from the lung and other intrathoracic structures before a reduction can be achieved. In the acutely injured patient with a diag-

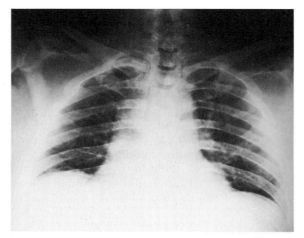

a

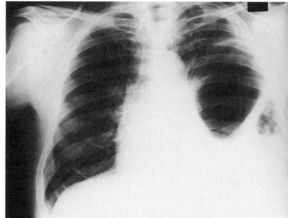

b

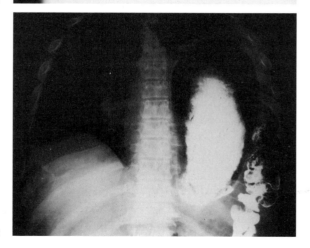

c

Fig. 22.5. *a*, Plain radiograph of chest of an adult male seen in the Accident Department after an upper abdominal and lower chest injury. Note the lack of any features drawing one's attention to the diaphragm. *b*, Chest radiograph of the same patient 10 months later, when he presented with pain in the chest and shortness of breath after meals. Note the dual gas shadows in the left hemithorax, with the lung parenchyma squashed to the apex of the chest. *c*, Contrast study outlines the dual gas shadows seen in *Fig.* 22.5*b* and identifies the stomach and the splenic flexure of colon in the left chest. A misconceived attempt to needle the loculi of gas after the previous plain films could have led to disastrous complications!

nosis of traumatic diaphragmatic hernia, with no evidence of damage to abdominal organs, the transthoracic route should be preferred. However, in the actuely injured patient with diaphragmatic herniation and a suspicion of damage to intra-abdominal organs with or without internal haemorrhage, a thoracoabdominal exploration should be carried out, and the intra-abdominal damage dealt with first, before turning one's attention to the diaphragmatic repair. Occasionally, during the course of a laparotomy for upper abdominal injury, an unsuspected diaphragmatic rupture is encountered by the discerning surgeon. Repair of the tear may then be undertaken from below, provided the herniated organs, if any, are easily reduced. If difficulty is encountered in the reduction of any viscera, a separate anterolateral thoracotomy in the 7th interspace is performed on the side of the tear, without interfering with the costal margin, and reduction and repair are then performed from above. In view of this possibility, among others, a laparotomy undertaken for upper abdominal injury should always be carried out with full skin preparation and draping, exposing the full width of the lower half of the chest and abdomen from one midaxillary line to the other.

Postoperative Management

The postoperative progress of the acutely injured patient in whom a diaphragmatic rupture has been repaired varies significantly from that of a patient who has undergone repair of a traumatic diaphragmatic hernia presenting in a delayed fashion, where surgery almost amounts to an elective procedure. In the former, the main aspects that need consideration are threefold: (1) Other organs may have been injured and would require specialized appropriate management. (2) These patients are prone to prolonged periods of paralytic ileus and will require nasogastric decompression combined with parenteral nutrition for long periods. (3) They are beset with pulmonary complications by virtue of the initial injury, as well as by the direct impairment of diaphragmatic function. High-dependency nursing and close medical supervision are essential in the management of the immediate postoperative period.

In the absence of indications to the contrary, the patient is returned to the postoperative ward, breathing spontaneously, with adequate analgesia. Nasogastric decompression is continued until such time as effective peristalsis has been established. Parenteral nutrition is maintained, special attention being paid to the hypercatabolic state associated with multiple injuries, if any. Intensive physiotherapy to the limbs and chest is continued until such time as the patient is ambulant. Intercostal drainage is discontinued once full expansion of the lungs has been achieved, and no further drainage of blood or air is noted. Once adequate bowel activity has been established, oral feeding is recommended, and parenteral nutrition withdrawn gradually. Radiological monitoring of the state of the pleural cavities and lungs is carried out on a daily basis until the chest drains have been removed, and for several days after, on a bi-weekly basis until the patient leaves hospital.

IATROGENIC DIAPHRAGMATIC HERNIATION

This occurs as a result of dehiscence of the suture line following an elective incision on the diaphragm, or through a reconstructed oesophageal hiatus after oesophago-gastric resection. Although the dehiscence occurs early in the postoperative period, the herniation may not reveal itself for a variable length of time. Apart from the factors that predispose to a diaphragmatic suture dehiscence, one additional factor that promotes herniation of the transverse colon through the reconstructed hiatus is the inadequate mobilization of the greater curvature of the stomach and gastrocolic omentum. When the stomach remnant is pulled up into the chest to be anastomosed to the transected oesophagus, the transverse colon is indirectly pulled up with it, and comes to lie at or near the reconstructed hiatus. The colonic and small bowel distension that follows surgery may, under these conditions, push the colon and omentum into the chest, through the hiatus.

Acute iatrogenic diaphragmatic herniation is a dramatic postoperative complication, requiring urgent surgical attention. Chronic herniation, however, is usually asymptomatic, and may remain undetected for several years. When complications such as incarceration and strangulation supervene, the risks of surgery are high. Elective repair is therefore indicated if the condition is diagnosed even when symptoms are absent. The details of the operative approaches for the two varieties are exactly the same as for the acute and delayed presentations of traumatic diaphragmatic hernia.

POST-SUPPURATIVE DIAPHRAGMATIC HERNIATION

Perforation of the diaphragm as a result of infection above or below the organ is extremely rare. As chronic suppuration is accompanied by dense adhesions, it is often self-limiting. Herniation of abdominal viscera into the chest can, however, occur if a subphrenic abscess should rupture through the diaphragm before such adhesions have formed. When, as happens occasionally in the tropics, an amoebic liver abscess evacuates itself through a fistula into the bronchial tree, after penetrating the diaphragm, the drainage is often complete and if the immediate management of the respiratory tract emergency has been successful, the further management of the patient rarely includes a surgical pro-

cedure. However, if herniation of abdominal viscera occurs as a result of a suppurative rupture of the diaphragm, drainage of both cavities and repair of the diaphragm become unavoidable. Where a subdiaphragmatic focus of suppuration results in an empyema, without herniation, drainage of both collections of pus, above and below the diaphragm, can occasionally be achieved via a catheter placed through a low rib resection and passing through the empyema into the diaphragmatic opening and into the subphrenic collection of pus.

IDIOPATHIC UNILATERAL PHRENIC PALSY AND EVENTRATION OF THE DIAPHRAGM

Phrenic paralysis resulting from an obvious cause such as birth trauma, viral infection, pulmonary and pleural infection, malignant neoplastic infiltration, trauma to the cervical spine, or therapeutic phrenic avulsion is a well-established entity, with very little controversy attached to the condition or to its management. Considerable controversy exists, however, on the phenomenon of an abnormally high position of the intact diaphragm known as 'eventration' and the unilaterally elevated dome of diaphragm which shows frank paradox on deep quick inspiration or sniffing. Although the earlier literature on the subject of eventration attributed this to a failure of muscular development in the diaphragm of the developing fetus, and tended to distinguish it from idiopathic unilateral phrenic paralysis, the current trend is to consider both conditions as one and the same and as being probably acquired. As to whether the diaphragm shows frank paradox, a flicker of a downward movement, or no movement at all during radiological screening, may well depend on the total number of residual functional neuromuscular units present in an elevated diaphragm. The condition may present at any age, from the newborn to old age. It occurs equally in both sexes. Often it is detected as an incidental finding in a routine chest radiograph, but, when it occurs in the neonate, cardiorespiratory failure may lead to death. It is often confused with congenital diaphragmatic herniation or delayed traumatic diaphragmatic hernia.

Diagnosis is made initially on the erect chest radiograph, confirmed on radiological screening for diaphragmatic movement on sniffing. The X-ray appearance of a thin linear line extending the full anteroposterior and lateral diameters of the chest helps to distinguish this condition from a diaphragmatic hernia. A barium meal or barium enema screening may demonstrate the stomach or colon lying beneath the intact diaphragm.

Treatment

In the symptomatic neonate, urgent treatment is imperative. If the infant with an elevated diaphragm is asymptomatic, then close observation of the child is required over the early years of life. In the very elderly, where an elevated dome of diaphragm is picked up as an incidental finding, no surgical treatment is necessary. In young patients with an elevated dome of diaphragm, be they symptomatic or asymptomatic, further objective assessment of pulmonary physiological parameters is warranted. There is increasing evidence to suggest that an improvement in the respiratory function can be achieved by transthoracic plication, or excision and repair of the affected portion of the diaphragm.

A thoracotomy is performed through the 8th or 9th interspace. The lung is retracted and the diaphragm is exposed. The phrenic nerve is identified and the thinned area of diaphragm defined. With careful inspection some functional muscle element can usually be identified along the periphery of the diaphragm. This portion of the diaphragm together with the portion bearing the main branches of the phrenic nerve are conserved. The diaphanous area is then excised and the diaphragmatic edges approximated in a double-breasted (imbricated) fashion. As an alternative, the diaphanous area can be plicated in the manner of a keel repair in order to restore the dome of the diaphragm to its normal level. The entire dome is then reinforced with a sheet of Dacron or Teflon anchored peripherally to the rib cage with interrupted mattress sutures, avoiding the intercostal bundles, and medially to the central tendon of the diaphragm away from the main division of the phrenic nerves.

Short- and long-term assessment of the pulmonary volumes are carried out routinely on these patients, in order to assess the efficacy of the surgical treatment.

TUMOURS OF THE DIAPHRAGM

Apart from the secondary involvement of the diaphragm by tumour invasion or metastases, the diaphragm can rarely be the seat of a primary neoplasm. Benign tumours arise in adipose, fibrous, pleural or neurilemmal tissue. Neurogenic tumours can also be seen involving the diaphragm.

Malignant tumours of the diaphragm are of vascular, neurogenic or striped muscle origin, and present with hypochondrial pain and cough with or without haemoptysis. They are often mistaken for malignant tumours of the lung or liver. Investigation should include ultrasonography, selective angiography of the phrenic, renal and coeliac branches, and computed tomography with contrast injection. Needle biopsy associated with radiological imaging should clinch the diagnosis provided a vascular tumour has been ruled out as a preliminary.

Treatment

Excision of the tumour via a low thoracotomy should be performed wherever feasible. The defect in the diaphragm can then be repaired by direct suture, if it is small. If the defect is large, even if direct approximation is possible, the diaphragm should be supported with an onlay of Teflon or Dacron. Malignant tumours of neurogenic and striped muscle origin should routinely be considered for adjuvant chemotherapy and/or radiotherapy after total surgical excision.

DIAPHRAGMATIC PACING

Recent developments in the field of electronics and the occasional need for physiological diaphragmatic assistance have led to the introduction of phrenic nerve pacing, in an attempt to maintain improved diaphragmatic movements for prolonged periods. Unlike cardiac pacing, where the organ itself is directly stimulated, diaphragmatic pacing has been achieved by stimulating one or both phrenic nerves by the implantation of suitable electrodes in the mediastinal or cervical course of the nerve, 5–10 cm away from the heart. A *train* of impulses lasting 1·20–1·45 seconds (for adults) or 0·5–0·8 second (in infants) is applied at a predetermined *pulse interval* of 50 msec at an *amplitude* of 1800 microamp, later increasing to an optimum of approximately 2500 microamp. The ventilatory *rate*, which is inversely proportional to the duration of the train of impulses, is usually about 12 per minute.

Diaphragmatic pacing may be specifically indicated in the following situations:
1. Sleep apnoea syndrome.
2. Periodic apnoea of neonates.
3. Acute viral encephalitis or transverse myelitis.
4. Acute brainstem lesions of a vascular or neoplastic nature.
5. Traumatic quadriplegia or quadriparesis.

Unfortunately, the clinical usefulness of diaphragmatic pacing has been limited by the duration to which pacing can be effectively continued. In practice, the diaphragmatic response gradually decreases after 20–24 hours. In an attempt to prolong the effective period, pacing can be conducted on a *demand* basis or on an *intermittent* principle. The scope of pacing can conceivably be extended by a judicious deployment of intermittent positive-pressure ventilation alternating with periods of diaphragmatic pacing.

Surgery of Pacing

One of the prerequisites to diaphragmatic pacing is the construction of a tracheostomy. This procedure in itself, by reducing the upper airways' resistance, may prove to be adequate. The phrenic nerve is then exposed via a transverse skin crease incision in the scalene triangle, or alternatively via a parasternal mediastinotomy in the 2nd intercostal space. Uni-

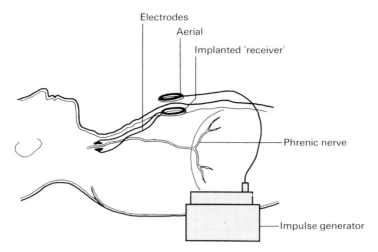

Fig. 22.6. Diaphragmatic or phrenic pacing.

polar or bipolar electrodes (*Fig.* 22.6) are applied around the nerve and the receiver is then tunnelled and positioned under the skin of the front of the chest on the same side. The transmitter 'aerial' attached to the pulse generator is then applied externally to the skin, directly opposite the receiver. The system is now ready for pacing, and should be tested before the patient is returned to the intensive care unit.

FURTHER READING

Brooks J. W. (1978) Blunt traumatic rupture of the diaphragm. *Ann. Thorac. Surg.* **26**, 199–203.
Chin E. F. and Lynn R. B. (1956) Surgery of eventration of the diaphragm. *J. Thorac. Surg.* **32**, 6–14.
Collis J. L., Satchwell L. M. and Abrams L. D. (1954) Nerve supply of the crura of the diaphragm. *Thorax* **9**, 22–25.
Collis J. L., Kelly T. D. and Wiley A. M. (1954) Anatomy of the crura of the diaphragm and surgery of hiatus hernia. *Thorax* **9**, 157–189.
Drewe J. A., Mercer E. C. and Benfield J. R. (1973) Acute diaphragmatic injuries. *Ann. Thorac. Surg.* **16**, 67–78.
Ebert P. A., Gaertner R. A. and Zuidema G. D. (1967) Traumatic diaphragmatic hernia. *Surg. Gynecol. Obstet.* **125**, 59–65.
Glenn W. W. L., Hogan J. F. and Phelps M. L. (1980) Ventilatory support of the quadriplegic patient with respiratory paralysis by diaphragmatic pacing. *Surg. Clin. North Am.* **60**, 1055–1078.
Oakes D. D. (1983) In: Sabiston D. C., Jr and Spencer F. C. (eds) *Gibbons Surgery of the Chest, Vol. II*, 4th ed. Philadelphia, W. B. Saunders, pp. 838–848.
Perera H. and Edwards F. R. (1957) Intra diaphragmatic course of the left phrenic nerve in relation to diaphragmatic incisions. *Lancet* (1957) **ii**, 75–77.
Smith R. A. (1962) Idiopathic paralysis of the diaphragm. *Nederl. Tijdschr. Geneesk.* **106**, 350–351.
Symbas P. N. (1978) Blunt traumatic rupture of the diaphragm. *Ann. Thorac. Surg.* **26**, 193–194.

Chapter twenty-three

Subphrenic Abscess

H. R. S. Harley

ANATOMY

The Intraperitoneal Spaces (*Fig.* 23.1–23.3)

There are five intraperitoneal spaces, namely right suprahepatic and infrahepatic, and left suprahepatic, anterior infrahepatic and posterior infrahepatic.

The right suprahepatic space lies between the diaphragm and right lobe of the liver, limited posteriorly by the superior layers of the coronary and right triangular ligaments and medially by the falciform ligament. The right infrahepatic space is bounded above and in front by the right lobe of the liver and gallbladder, below and behind by the diaphragm, the upper pole of the right kidney, the right suprarenal gland, the second part of the duodenum, a part of the head of the pancreas, the right colic

flexure and the right extremity of the transverse colon and mesocolon.

The left suprahepatic space is large and complicated. It separates the diaphragm from the left lobe of the liver, fundus of stomach and spleen. It is limited medially by the falciform ligament. Posteriorly it is limited medially by the left triangular ligament lateral to which it extends backwards between the diaphragm and spleen and then inwards between the kidney and spleen and the lienorenal ligament.

The left anterior infrahepatic space lies between the left lobe of the liver above and in front and the stomach and lesser omentum below and behind. The left posterior infrahepatic space or lesser sac lies behind the caudate lobe of the liver, the stomach

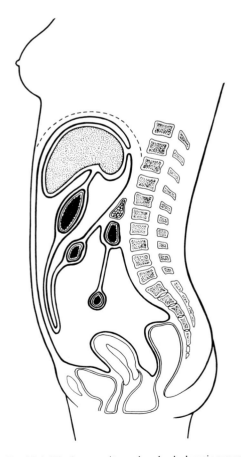

Fig. 23.1. The intraperitoneal and subphrenic spaces.

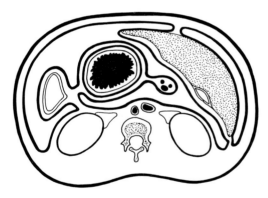

Fig. 23.2. The intraperitoneal and subphrenic spaces.

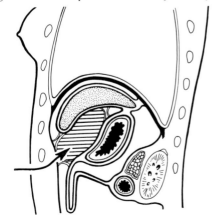

Fig. 23.3. Left anterior infrahepatic abscess. The left posterior infrahepatic space (the lesser sac) lies posteriorly to the stomach.

314

and the lesser omentum and extends downwards for a variable distance into the greater omentum. Behind it are the transverse colon and mesocolon, the neck and body of the pancreas, the upper pole of the left kidney, the left suprarenal gland and a considerable part of the diaphragm.

Communications between the Intraperitoneal Spaces

All the intraperitoneal spaces, except the lesser sac, communicate with each other through a triangular interval bounded above and in front by the free margin of the falciform ligament, below by the transverse colon and behind by the pyloric part of the stomach (Mitchell, 1940). The right infrahepatic space communicates with the two left infrahepatic ones in front of and behind the free margin of the lesser omentum. The opening into the left posterior space is the aditus, bounded above by the caudate process of the liver, below by the first part of the duodenum, in front by the right free margin of the lesser omentum and behind by the inferior vena cava.

The right suprahepatic and infrahepatic spaces communicate around the inferior margin of the right lobe of the liver, but do so freely only posteriorly around the free margin of the right triangular ligament and anteriorly through a quadrangular interval, bounded by the quadrate lobe of the liver above, the transverse colon below, the gallbladder to the right and the free edge of the falciform ligament to the left (Mitchell, 1940). Distension of the infrahepatic space opens up this interval, but elsewhere presses the inferior margin of the right lobe of the liver against the diaphragm and seals off the right suprahepatic space. The left suprahepatic and anterior infrahepatic spaces communicate freely around the inferior margin of the left lobe of the liver, but the left posterior infrahepatic space is closed except at the epiploic foramen.

Infection often remains confined to one intraperitoneal space, but may reach others on the same or the opposite side via the communications discussed above. Extension most commonly occurs between the right-sided spaces.

The Extraperitoneal Spaces

There are two extraperitoneal spaces. The right lies within the coronary and right triangular ligaments between the diaphragm and the bare area of the liver. The left, less well defined, occupies the cellular tissues around the upper pole of the left kidney, the left suprarenal gland, the pancreas and the descending colon.

SITES OF SUBPHRENIC ABSCESSES

The sites of subphrenic abscesses in 217 patients are shown in *Tables* 23.1–23.4

Table 23.1. Site of subphrenic abscess in 217 patients

Site	No.	Percentage
Right	142	65·4
Left	60	27·2
Bilateral	12	5·5
Not known	3	1·9
Total	217	100

Table 23.2. Site of subphrenic abscess in 217 patients

Space	No.	Percentage
Intraperitoneal	199	91·7
Extraperitoneal	14	6·5
Combined	3	1·3
Total	216	100

Table 23.3. Percentages of single and multiple space abscesses

Single space		86·7%
Multiple space		13·3%
Unilateral	7·8%	
Bilateral	5·5%	

Table 23.4. Location of single space intraperitoneal abscesses

Right suprahepatic	87
Left suprahepatic	32
Right infrahepatic	19
Left anterior infrahepatic	9
Left posterior infrahepatic	3
Total	150

SURGICAL MANAGEMENT OF UNCOMPLICATED ABSCESSES

Routes of Drainage

An extraserous route of drainage is mandatory (Harley, 1949, 1955a, 1969, 1974). This means that the incision must not traverse the pleural cavity, even if obliterated, or uninvolved portions of the peritoneal cavity. The parietal peritoneum must be transgressed to reach an intraperitoneal abscess, but transgression must be confined to the adherent zone over the abscess. All abscesses, wherever situated, except those in the lesser sac, can be easily reached extraserously, provided that the whole hand can be inserted through the incision. A transpleural approach, even across adherent pleura, should never be made for three reasons:

1. Pleural complications and mortality rates are increased, even if antibiotics are used.
2. The diaphragm is damaged and immobilized.
3. The infrahepatic spaces cannot be examined. They may be affected with suprahepatic spaces.

The Anterior Extraserous Approach
(*Figs.* 23.4–23.6)

An oblique incision is made 2·5 cm below and parallel with the coastal margin on the side of the abscess, starting over the middle of the rectus muscle and extending well lateral to it. This is deepened through

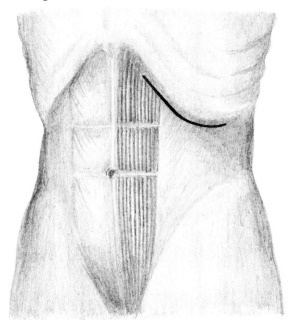

Fig. 23.4. Anterior extraperitoneal approach for drainage of subphrenic abscess.

the three anterolateral abdominal muscles and fascia transversalis, lateral to the unopened rectus sheath. The extraperitoneal alveolar tissue and peritoneum are exposed.

To reach the suprahepatic space on either side the fingers peel the peritoneum off the under surface of the diaphragm. This is easily accomplished, especially when inflammatory oedema is present. When the abscess is reached, as indicated by induration, a finger is plunged through its wall. Pus is evacuated with a sucker, some being kept for bacteriology. The opening into the abscess is then enlarged and any loculi within it are broken down. Thorough exploration of the entire suprahepatic region on either side is possible if the whole hand is inserted through the incision. Suprahepatic abscesses on the right side are located between the diaphragm and the right lobe of the liver, those on the left may be between the diaphragm and the left lobe of the liver, the fundus of the stomach or the spleen.

The right infrahepatic space is explored by passing the fingers upwards and backwards below the right lobe of the liver and above the hepatic flexure and right extremity of the transverse colon. the left anterior infrahepatic space is easily reached by pushing the fingers backwards and upwards below the left lobe of the liver and above the stomach and lesser omentum.

Extraperitoneal abscesses on either side can also be reached by the anterior extraserous route if the incision allows entry of the whole hand.

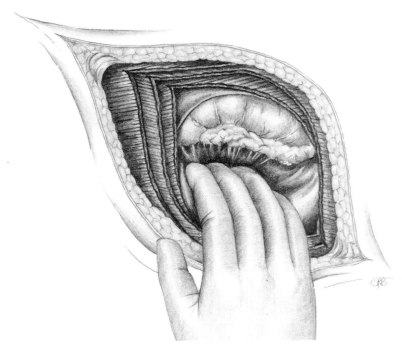

Fig. 23.5. Anterior extraperitoneal approach to subphrenic abscess. The oedematous abscess wall is exposed by blunt dissection.

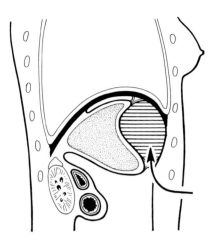

Fig. 23.6. Right anterior subphrenic abscess. Anterior extraperitoneal approach.

The Posterior Extraperitoneal Approach
(*Figs.* 23.7–23.9)

Full details of this approach have been given elsewhere (Harley, 1949, 1969, 1974). The patient is placed as for nephrectomy. The incision starts 2·5 cm from the midline and runs downwards and forwards over or just below the 12th rib, extending beyond its tip far enough to allow insertion of the whole hand. Division of latissimus dorsi and serratus posterior inferior exposes the rib. Its periosteum is divided with diathermy and stripped from the whole length of its upper and lower borders and deep surface. Erector spinae must be retracted backwards to gain access to the posterior end of the rib, and care is required

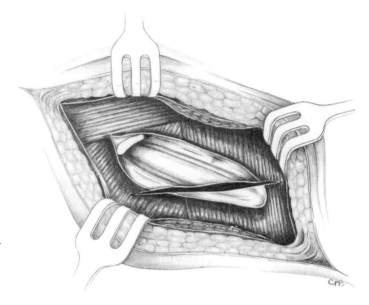

Fig. 23.8. Posterior extraperitoneal approach to subphrenic abscess. The 12th rib has been resected subperiosteally and its bed incised transversely.

to avoid injuring the pleura. After excising the whole rib subperiosteally its bed is incised transversely at the level of the spinous process of the first lumbar vertebra to avoid injuring the pleura. The process must be identified. The incision extends inwards from the periosteum to divide fibres of the serratus posterior and quadratus lumborum muscles, and outwards to sever the muscles of the 11th intercostal space. The exposed attachments of the diaphragm, which may be well or poorly developed, are divided. At the inner end of the incision the subcostal and iliohypogastric nerves must be preserved. Blunt dissection in the paranephric fat reveals the smooth, shiny, thin, fibrous posterior layer of the renal fascia through which the perirenal fat is visible. Blunt

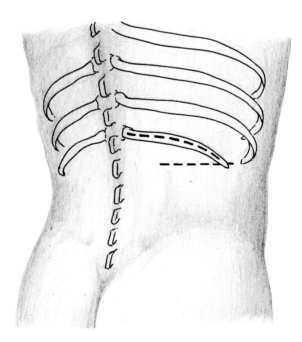

Fig. 23.7. Incision for extraperitoneal approach to posterior subphrenic abscess. The line of the pleura is shown well below the 12th rib.

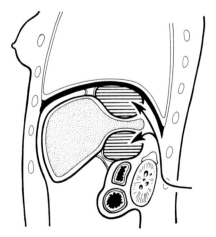

Fig. 23.9. Posterosuperior and posteroinferior subphrenic abscesses. These are readily approached via the posterior extraperitoneal route.

dissection outside the renal fascia exposes the upper pole of the kidney and the suprarenal gland.

The suprahepatic and extraperitoneal spaces on either side are easily explored by passing the fingers upwards under the diaphragm (*Fig.* 23.9). To explore the right infrahepatic space the fingers are pushed forwards and downwards through the junction of the renal and diaphragmatic fascias, above and in front of the kidney and suprarenal gland and below and behind the right lobe of the liver.

Other Approaches

Occasionally a right extraperitoneal abscess extends forwards between the layers of the falciform ligament and is best drained by a midline supra-umbilical incision. Abscesses in the lesser sac usually point anteriorly and are best drained by a laparotomy incision.

Method of Drainage

Subphrenic abscesses are best drained by one or more large, firm rubber tubes with one end doubly bevelled, but with no side-holes, similar to those used for an empyema. The tubes are exteriorized through separate stab wounds. After the anterior extraserous approach an anteriorly placed abscess is drained through a stab below the main incision. A posteriorly located abscess can easily be drained from behind by cutting down the index finger in the extraperitoneal tissues pressing outwards in the loin. A large abscess under the summit of the diaphragm may require tubes placed both anteriorly and posteriorly. The tubes are anchored to the skin by a stitch around a rubber collar encircling the tube at skin level. The wound is closed in layers, with interrupted sutures, and drained by portions of corrugated rubber emerging through one or both extremities. The drainage tubes are attached to water-seal bottles.

Postoperative Management

The patient is kept in bed and given chemotherapy until he or she is apyrexial and ambulation is then encouraged. Suitable supportive treatment and nutrition are administered.

The water-seal bottles attached to the drainage tubes in the operating theatre are connected to wall suction when the patient reaches the recovery room. Suction is maintained until the discharge has decreased to an amount which can be absorbed by one or two dressings per day. Open drainage then becomes preferable, suction is discontinued and the drainage tubes are cut just beyond skin level. Future management of the tubes is controlled by serial sinograms every 7–10 days, made by injecting contrast medium down the tubes. The latter must be left *in*

situ to clarify their relationship to the abscess cavity. Each tube is adjusted so that its tip lies at the bottom of the abscess cavity and is withdrawn only when sinography shows no cavity beyond its end. The tubes are then progressively withdrawn about 2 cm per day.

SURGICAL MANAGEMENT OF COMPLICATED ABSCESSES

Intrathoracic Suppuration

Suppurative complications in the chest developed in 61 (28·1 per cent) of 217 patients studied. These arise largely from the abscess rupturing through the diaphragm into the adherent lower lobe or into the pleural cavity. The former occasions suppurative pneumonitis and a bronchial fistula, the latter an empyema, which may subsequently rupture into the lung to create a bronchopleural fistula.

A subphrenic abscess complicated by suppurative pneumonitis and a bronchial fistula is treated in the same way as an uncomplicated abscess. Its adequate drainage will result in closure of the diaphragmatic perforation and resolution of the suppurative pneumonitis. Delayed surgery for residual bronchiectasis is rarely required.

When intrapleural rupture has occurred the subphrenic abscess and the empyema must each be drained separately by the most appropriate route. Drainage of the former alone will not, unfortunately, cure the empyema.

Abdominal Complications

Other complications, due to the subphrenic abscess or its cause, were present in 99 (45·6 per cent) of 217 patients. These included general peritonitis, intraperitoneal abscesses, rupture into the stomach or intestines, faecal fistulas and liver abscesses, and they all require appropriate treatment.

Liver abscesses occurred in 24 (11·1 per cent) and are a cause of diagnostic and therapeutic difficulty (Harley 1955a, b, 1970, 1974). Liver abscesses may be single (15 cases) or multiple (8 cases). The former may communicate with a subphrenic abscess which has resulted from its rupture through the capsule of the liver, or the two abscesses may be remote from each other. In the former case both abscesses can be drained by the same route, in the latter each must be drained by separate tubes, even if approached through the same incision. Multiple liver abscesses, if few in number and large in size, may also be drained. Multiple small abscesses caused by portal vein thrombosis and suppurative pylephlebitis or suppurative cholangitis must be treated by chemotherapy.

REFERENCES

Harley H. R. S. (1949) Subphrenic abscess. *Thorax* **4**, 1.

Harley H. R. S. (1955a) *Subphrenic Abscess*. Oxford, Blackwell.

Harley H. R. S. (1955b) Suphrenic abscess with particular reference to the spread of infection. *Ann. R. Coll. Surg. Engl.* **17**, 201.

Harley H. R. S. (1969) Suphrenic abscess. In: Rob C. and Smith R. (eds) *Operative Surgery, Vol. 5*, 2nd ed. London, Butterworths, pp. 492–501.

Harley H. R. S. (1970) Radiology in diagnosis and control of surgical treatment of subphrenic and liver abscess. *Proc. R. Soc. Med.* **63**, 319.

Harley H. R. S. (1974) Subphrenic abscess. In: Maingot R. (ed.) *Abdominal Operations, Vol. 2*, 6th ed. New York, Appleton-Century-Crofts, pp. 1430–1465.

Mitchell G. A. G. (1940) The spread of acute intraperitoneal effusions. *Br. J. Surg.* **28**, 291–313.

FURTHER READING

Clairmont P. and Meyer M. (1926) The treatment of appendicitis. *Acta Chir. Scand.* **60**, 55–134.

Nather K. and Ochsner E. W. A. (1923) Retroperitoneal operation for subphrenic abscess. *Surg. Gynecol. Obstet.* **37**, 665–673.

Neck, Face and Jaws

Chapter twenty-four

The Thyroid Gland

N. E. Dudley

THE THYROID

Surgical Anatomy

General Orientations

The thyroid gland is situated in the anterior triangle of the neck, weighs approximately 20 g and consists of two lateral lobes (right and left) which are joined together by a midline isthmus. A small pyramidal lobe (of Lalouette), of varying size, commonly joins the isthmus at its junction with the left lateral lobe by a fibrous band or strand of muscle fibres known as the levator glandulae thyroideae. The lobes measure approximately $5 \times 3 \times 1.5$ cm (slightly larger in women) and extend from the middle of the thyroid cartilage above to the sixth tracheal ring below. Each lobe fills the space between the trachea and oesophagus medially and the carotid sheath laterally. A strong condensation of vascular connective tissue, known as the suspensory ligament of Berry, binds the gland firmly to each side of the cricoid cartilage and it is this ligament, together with the pretracheal fascia splitting to invest the gland, which makes the thyroid move up and down on swallowing. The fascia (false or surgical capsule) sends fibrous septa into the gland substance, dividing it into numerous lobules. These consist of 30–40 follicles which contain colloid and are the main secretory and storage elements.

Development of the Thyroid

The thyroid develops from two distinct embryological structures—the primitive pharynx and the neural crest. A median pharyngeal downgrowth migrates between the tuberculum impar and the second arch component of the tongue and this descends in a caudal direction along a line extending from the foramen caecum at the base of the tongue to the pyramidal lobe of the thyroid. In doing so, the track passes ventral to the hyoid bone and then kinks behind it. The track usually becomes obliterated but occasionally part of it persists giving rise to a thyroglossal cyst or fistula. Rarely the thyroid bud fails to descend but develops *in situ* at the back of the tongue (lingual thyroid). Conversely, it may overshoot the mark and result in a primary mediastinal or retrosternal goitre. The thyroid bud even less commonly may fail to divide into two, resulting in one lateral lobe, usually the left being absent. The parafollicular or C cells scattered between the cuboidal epithelial cells which line the thyroid follicles, are derived from the neural crest. They first migrate to the ultimo-branchial bodies of the fourth and fifth branchial pouches and then to the thyroid. These are the cells which in later life have the potential to undergo hyperplastic and malignant change and result in the calcitonin-producing medullary carcinoma of the thyroid.

Blood Supply

The vascular supply of the gland is impressive and becomes more so in hyperactive thyroid states. The main supply is via two paired arteries and an occasional third to each lobe. The superior thyroid artery, the first branch of the external carotid, runs downward on the inferior constrictor to reach the apex of the lateral lobe where it divides into a large anterior set of branches and a smaller, but equally important, set of posterior branches. Occasionally a branch comes off high on the left to reach and supply the pyramidal lobe fairly near the midline. The inferior thyroid artery is generally much larger than the superior thyroid artery but is less constant, being absent or duplicated on one or other side in 10 per cent of individuals. It arises from the thyrocervical trunk and, passing upwards for a variable distance, loops back down and passes medially behind the carotid sheath to reach the posterolateral aspect of the gland usually at the junction of the middle and lower thirds. Numerous unnamed accessory arteries arise from the oesophagus and trachea but the most frequently encountered is the thyroidea ima (Neubauer's artery), which courses up anteriorly on the trachea to reach the isthmus or one of the lower poles and takes origin from the aorta or brachiocephalic artery. In the absence of the inferior thyroid artery on one side, the thyroidea ima may be the principal source of blood supply to the lobe and is consequently substantial. The named thyroid veins, although three in number like the arteries, do not accompany them and are subject to greater variation. The superior thyroid vein, formed by a confluence of vessels from the upper pole, crosses the common carotid artery high in the neck to drain into the internal jugular. The middle thyroid vein, which overlies the inferior thyroid artery, also ends in the internal jugular vein after crossing the common carotid. The inferior thyroid veins pass down from the isthmus and inferior poles of the lateral lobes to join the internal jugular or brachiocephalic veins in the anterior mediastinum and are intimately associated with the thyrothymic ligaments which expand inferiorly as the lobes of the thymus.

Lymphatic Drainage

The thyroid is no less generously served by lymphatics as it is by arteries and veins. A rich network of lymphatic vessels ramifies throughout the gland and drains primarily into mediastinal nodes inferiorly, tracheo-oesophageal nodes laterally and the midline Delphian nodes superiorly. Dye studies suggest that the majority of the lymph from the thyroid returns to the thoracic duct without reference to the deep cervical lymph node chain or the nodes of the posterior triangle, although these pathways may be used secondarily (*Fig.* 24.1). This factor has implications in the treatment of carcinoma of the thyroid (Crile, 1957).

subclavian artery on the right. It ascends in the tracheo-oesophageal groove and has a variable relationship with the inferior thyroid artery on each side (*Fig.* 24.2). In general the nerve runs deep to the artery but actually passes through or anterior to the branches of the artery as it breaks up close to the gland (Hollingshead, 1952). Occasionally the nerve itself divides early and branches around the artery (10 per cent). In less than 1 per cent of individuals the recurrent laryngeal nerve on the right does not pass down to loop around the subclavian but passes directly from the vagus to the cricothyroid muscle. As it takes the same course as the inferior thyroid artery, it is particularly vulnerable even when this vessel is ligated laterally. Whichever course the nerve takes, it ultimately enters the larynx with the inferior laryngeal artery posterior to the cricothyroid articulation and supplies all the intrinsic muscles of the larynx

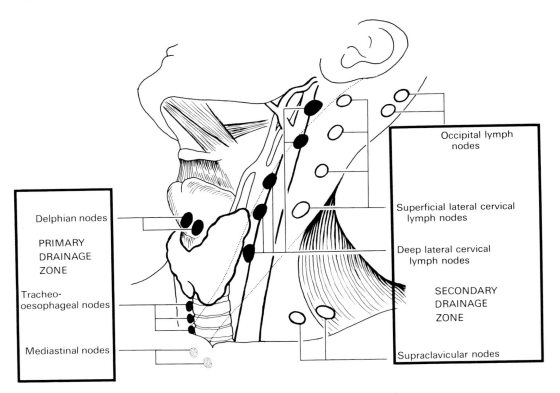

Fig. 24.1. Lymphatic drainage of the thyroid gland.

Important Anatomical Relations

Recurrent Laryngeal Nerves (*Fig.* 24.2)

There are several structures in relation to the gland with which a surgeon must be familiar. The first and most important of these is the recurrent laryngeal nerve, which is a branch of the vagus. The latter, having entered the mediastinum, gives off the recurrent nerve which returns to the neck having looped around the arch of the aorta on the left and the right

together with some sensory supply to the mucosa below the vocal cords. The principal effect of division of this nerve is paralysis of the vocal cord on that side.

The Superior Laryngeal Nerve

This also arises from the vagus (inferior ganglion) and divides at the level of the hyoid bone into a large internal laryngeal nerve and a smaller external laryn-

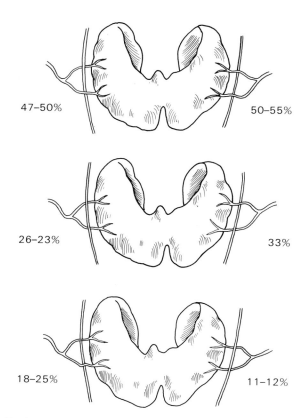

47–50%   50–55%

26–23%   33%

18–25%   11–12%

Fig. 24.2. Variations in relevant positions of inferior thyroid artery and recurrent laryngeal nerve.

geal nerve. The latter runs close to the superior thyroid artery but at a deeper plane, immediately above the superior pole of the thyroid. It terminates as the nerve supply to the cricothyroid muscle which acts as a tensor of the vocal cords on the same side.

The Cervical Sympathetic Chain

This underlies the carotid sheath just medial to the vagus on the prevertebral fascia and is in close proximity to the inferior thyroid artery as it arches around medially.

Indications for Surgery

Thyrotoxicosis

There are three methods of treatment for this condition: anti-thyroid drugs, radio-iodine and surgery. Over a quarter of a century fashions have waxed and waned and the merits of each individual treatment have been argued and frequently overstated. In fact, no one form of treatment is ideal, each having its advantages and disadvantages. These are summarized in *Table* 24.1. In the author's opinion, surgery is clearly most appropriate in the following situations:

1. *Large Toxic Multinodular Goitre*

These glands react in a most labile manner on anti-thyroid drugs and have a notoriously high relapse rate on withdrawal of medication. Radio-iodine often needs to be given repeatedly in high doses and has minimal impact on the size of the gland. Surgery is best carried out sooner rather than later before the airway and cardiovascular system are compromised, the operative procedure indicated being subtotal thyroidectomy.

2. *Toxic Solitary (Autonomous/'hot') Nodule*

Removing such a nodule by surgery is so straightforward that the other methods of treatment need

Table 24.1. Disadvantages of anti-thyroid drugs, radio-active iodine and surgery in the management of hyperthyroidism

Anti-thyroid drugs	'Conservative' [131]I	Surgery
1. Requires compliant and highly motivated patient to cope with variable drug regimen	1. Prospect of radiation therapy may be unacceptable to the patient	1. Prospect of neck surgery may be unacceptable to the patient
2. Needs close clinical and laboratory supervision over 18–24 months	2. Uncertainty about long-term carcinogenic effects of low radiation doses—known to be more oncogenic than high doses	2. Unsuited to patients of advanced age or poor medical status
3. Danger of over-treatment leading to hypothyroidism and thyroid enlargement	3. Uncertainty about teratogenic effects which restricts reproduction for (at least) 2 years post therapy	3. Scar inevitable with possibility of keloid formation
4. Risk of side-effects from drugs—rashes and nausea + potentially dangerous marrow depression	4. Slow response to therapy (3–6 months), especially large multinodular goitres	4. Results are highly operator dependent

5. Poor response with large multinodular goitres	5. Not appropriate for cosmetically unacceptable toxic goitres	5. Small but definite risk of serious complications in skilled hands:
		    Recurrent laryngeal nerve damage <1%
		    Permanent hypoparathyroidism <0·5%

6. Not appropriate for cosmetically unacceptable toxic goitres	6. Cumulative (high) hypothyroidism rate requiring long-term follow-up	6. Modest rate of hypothyroidism
7. High relapse rate		

not be seriously considered, unless the overall medical status of the patient dictates otherwise. Antithyroid drugs would require to be given for life and radio-iodine therapy runs the risk of irradiating surrounding normal tissue with uncertain long-term effects. A further disadvantage is that the nodule usually persists. The operative procedure indicated here is subtotal lobectomy or isthmusectomy depending on the part of the gland containing the nodule.

3. Large Diffuse Toxic Goitre (Graves' Disease)

These are likely to be the most florid cases with the additional problem of cosmetic embarrassment to the patient. There is much to be said for electively operating once toxicity is controlled with anti-thyroid drugs with or without propranolol, although opinion varies in patients with smaller glands. However, in women, especially in their reproductive years, who have relapsed after 12–18 months of a well-monitored course of anti-thyroid drugs or in whom medication has proved impracticable or poorly tolerated, surgery is the first choice providing it is acceptable to the patient and the necessary surgical skills are available. The appropriate operative procedure is subtotal thyroidectomy.

4. Childhood Graves' Disease

In view of the high incidence of benign and malignant nodules in children exposed to radiation (Duffy and Fitzgerald, 1950), radio-iodine is absolutely contra-indicated, and if other anti-thyroid drugs have failed, surgery becomes the treatment of choice. Since hypertrophy of the remnants and recurrent thyrotoxicosis rates are higher in children, surgery needs to be more radical. The extent of the subtotal thyroidectomy performed will rest on the experience and judgement of the surgeon if unacceptably high myxoedema rates are to be avoided. Long-term follow-up is essential.

5. Thyrotoxicosis in Pregnancy

This is a rare combination (0·2 per cent of pregnancies) but can present a difficult management problem. Anti-thyroid drugs given to the mother cross the placenta and may result in hypothyroidism and goitre in the fetus, especially if given in the last trimester. After delivery the same drugs are excreted in the milk but not in sufficient quantities to cause similar effects. Radio-iodine is never given in view of the possible teratogenic effects of irradiation in the first trimester and on the fetal thyroid which is trapping iodine thereafter. If maternal thyrotoxicosis is moderate or severe and especially if the thyrocardiac symptoms exist, heralding possible cardiac failure, subtotal thyroidectomy should electively be undertaken in the middle trimester.

Non-toxic Diffuse or Multinodular Goitre

Benign enlargement of this type occurs for one of three reasons: lack of iodine causing endemic goitre, an inherited enzyme defect within the thyroid preventing iodine trapping or normal metabolism and storage of thyroid hormone causing a dyshormonogenetic goitre, or an acquired defect mutation resulting in a sporadic goitre. Endemic and dyshormonogenetic goitres more usually present in childhood or adolescence, sporadic goitres in adult life. In each instance the gland initially is typically diffuse and soft (colloid goitre) but over several years becomes larger and nodular. This nodularity affects some parts of the gland more than others, often producing retrosternal extensions. Ultimately tracheal deviation and compression occur. In the early stages surgery is usually requested on cosmetic grounds; later to relieve pressure symptoms. The operative procedure indicated is partial thyroidectomy, following which thyroxine replacement is usually required to prevent hypertrophy of the remnants or frank myxoedema.

Non-toxic Solitary Thyroid Nodules

When clinical examinaton, ultrasound and radio-iodine scanning suggest that a nodule is solitary, non-cystic and non-toxic (i.e. isotopically cold or neutral), a tissue diagnosis should be sought to exclude malignancy. This can be done with absolute certainty and comparative safety only by total thyroid lobectomy. In this way the patient is also relieved of what may be a worrying and cosmetically unacceptable lump. Fine needle biopsy (or aspiration biopsy cytology), popularized in Sweden, has reduced surgical exploration rates for thyroid nodules by 24 per cent and has the merit of being quick, painless and convenient, being performed as an outpatient procedure (Hamberger et al., 1985). However, it suffers from the limitations of all biopsy techniques, namely the skill and ability of the operator to obtain a truly representative sample and the experience and accuracy of the cytopathologist reporting the specimen. The only serious limitation of this technique is the failure to differentiate between follicular adenomas and follicular carcinomas which can be done only by studying the overall histological pattern and, in particular, the presence or otherwise of capsular and vascular invasion. Unless the surgeon can depend on a cytology service which has a very low false negative rate, total lobectomy is advocated for all cases especially in children and in males under 40.

Carcinoma of the Thyroid

This is a rare cancer but the incidence appears to be increasing. The indications for and extent of surgery in carcinoma of the thyroid will depend primarily on the histological type, but the age of onset and the mode of presentation will also influence management. These aspects will be considered in relationship to the five main types.

1. *Papillary Carcinoma*

This is by far the commonest carcinoma (60 per cent incidence overall rising to 80 per cent if only children and those under the age of 40 are considered), and women are affected twice as often as men. Occasionally in older patients it occurs in association with follicular lesions when the papillary pattern of behaviour predominates. The typically unencapsulated pale homogeneous primary tumour spreads via the lymphatics, and this is reflected in a 90 per cent incidence of microscopic tumour foci when the whole gland of affected individuals is meticulously examined (Russell et al, 1963). Multiple macroscopic deposits will be evident at operation in 20 per cent of cases and extrathyroid spread to the regional nodes in 50 per cent. These are usually on the same side as the lesion and within the area of primary lymphatic drainage, namely the central group of paratracheal nodes (*see* Surgical Anatomy, p. 324). Where contralateral nodes are involved, or those outside the primary drainage area are affected, widespread disease within the gland itself should be assumed and total thyroidectomy and modified block dissection carried out. There is now little enthusiasm for the classic radical block dissection which confers no improved survival or reduction of recurrences to justify the appreciable mutilation and morbidity. Occasionally, the tumour within the gland is occult, in other words it is impalpable and less than 1·5 cm in size, yet the first evidence of disease is manifested by large deep cervical or posterior triangle nodes. These should be treated in the same way as an overt primary with extrathyroid spread. However, most cases of papillary carcinoma will be diagnosed as a result of frozen section examination of a non-toxic solitary nodule or total lobectomy specimen as already advocated. The problem then arises whether any further treatment is required. Present evidence suggests that only when multiple deposits are seen on the cut surface of the lobe or the pathologist states unequivocally that the tumour is multicentric should the surgeon proceed at once to total thyroidectomy (Wade, 1983). If this information comes to light only subsequently on the paraffin sections, early reoperation and conversion to total thyroidectomy are recommended. If, however, the lesion is unifocal on routine examination, then no benefit is gained by more radical surgery in spite of a known high incidence of microscopic foci on whole gland study already mentioned. This same strategy is advocated for papillary lesions which come to light as an unexpected pathological finding following surgery for thyrotoxicosis or multinodular goitre. Taken overall at follow-up, less than 10 per cent of cases treated by total lobectomy will develop recurrent nodal metastases. Removal of these is aptly described as 'berry picking' for being well encapsulated, they are readily excised and even patients with successive recurrences treated in this way do not appear to have a compromised survival.

2. *Follicular Carcinoma*

This second differentiated tumour accounts for 20 per cent of all thyroid cancers and since the incidence world wide is higher in endemic goitre, would appear to be related to iodine lack and TSH (thyroid-stimulating hormone) drive. Three times as many women as men are affected and the peak age at diagnosis is 45, a decade later than for papillary carcinomas. On microscopic examination the tumour is typically solitary and encapsulated but may very occasionally be multiple and occupy the entire lobe. The degree of malignancy of a follicular carcinoma depends on the extent to which its capsule has been breached and the blood vessels invaded, which can be accurately assessed only by examination of the whole nodule. The tumour characteristically metastasizes by the bloodstream and only rarely via the lymphatics. Presentation, therefore, is typically as a non-toxic solitary nodule with or without evidence of distant spread. Metastases occur in the lungs, bones and occasionally the brain. It is rare for distant metastases to arise without a clinically impressive primary tumour and subsequent management is guided by mode of presentation. Most cases will be discovered on frozen section after total lobectomy as for papillary carcinoma. If the pathologist states unequivocally that the malignant features of capsular and angio invasion are present, total thyroidectomy is the treatment of choice, but if the appearances are not clear-cut, it is better to wait until the definitive paraffin sections are available. These may reveal micro-angio invasion without capsular involvement, in which case suppression of the TSH drive to the gland with T4 0·1–0·2 mg per day for life is all that is required, together with careful follow-up. If, however, overt vascular or capsular invasion is seen, early reoperation is strongly advised converting to total thyroidectomy. The reason for so doing is not only because multifocal deposits may be present in the opposite lobe, but also to remove the main iodine trap. Residual tumour or distant metastases may then be identified by radio-iodine scanning and once detected can be treated with ^{131}I until no further uptake is recorded. Since lymphatic involvement is uncommon (less than 5 per cent cervical nodal involvement) the need for formal nodal dissection is rare, but when it does a modified block dissection suffices.

3. *Anaplastic Carcinoma*

This occurs typically in elderly men and women and accounts for 10–15 per cent of thyroid tumours. It is notable for its speed of growth and extreme malignancy, invasion occurring locally with distant spread via the bloodstream and lymphatics. In the rare case occurring in middle age, total thyroidectomy should be attempted, but for the remainder heroic surgery cannot be justified and, indeed, may do the patient a disservice if it results in implantation of tumour in the surgical incision. The surgeon's role is mainly, therefore, to establish the diagnosis. In view of the bulky nature of most tumours, a good representative biopsy can be obtained with a Tru-cut needle under local anaesthetic. Occasionally, relief of pressure on the trachea can be achieved by removal of the isthmus, but generally local radiotherapy offers the only prospect of worthwhile palliation. The 12-month survival rate is very low and chemotherapy has so far failed to improve this poor prognosis.

4. Malignant Lymphoma

This is a tumour affecting mainly elderly women with a presentation similar to that of anaplastic carcinoma, and it may be difficult to differentiate histologically from the former small cell type. However, the prognosis is vastly better and if the diagnosis can be established on needle biopsy, remarkable regression can be achieved with external radiotherapy and worthwhile 5-year survival obtained. There is no place, therefore, for open surgery if the diagnosis can be estabished clearly by other means.

5. Medullary Thyroid Carcinoma

This rare tumour has attracted great interest since it was first described in 1959 (Hazard et al., 1959) and, clinical awareness having been aroused, it now accounts for 5–10 per cent of cases in reported larger series of carcinoma of the thyroid. It arises from the parafollicular C cells which are distributed throughout the gland but are in highest concentration in the upper poles (Roediger, 1976) and tumours are most likely to be discovered in that location. If the tumour is solitary the disease is likely to be sporadic (80 per cent) (Sizemore et al., 1977) but if multiple the familial form (20 per cent) must be strongly suspected. The latter shows an autosomal dominant pattern of inheritance, men and women being equally affected. Successive generations tend to be diagnosed at a progressively younger age, but this may reflect the improved efficiency of screening. Familial medullary thyroid carcinoma is also associated with tumours of the adrenal medulla (phaeochromocytomas) and with parathyroid hyperplasia—an endocrine triad, recognized as multiple endocrine adenosis (MEA type IIA or Sipple's syndrome). A phenotypically distinct group of patients with medullary thyroid carcinoma and phaeochromocytoma but without parathyroid disease is described—MEA IIB. These patients have characteristic facies, Marfanoid habitus and submucosal neurofibromas of the tongue and lips. In sporadic and familial medullary thyroid carcinoma the C cells produce a near-specific tumour marker—calcitonin—which provides guidance in detection and management. Hypercalcitonaemia is not always present in multiple endocrine adenosis and affected individuals may have a normal basal immunoreactive calcitonin level (ICT). However, the diagnosis of medullary thyroid carcinoma may be assumed if grossly elevated basal calcitonin levels, in the absence of any other malignancy, are recorded. Basal calcitonin levels can be provoked to pathological levels by giving an intravenous injection of pentagastrin ($0.5 \mu g/kg$) plus a calcium infusion sufficient to raise the serum calcium $2.4 mg/100 ml$. When this occurs a small occult tumour or, alternatively, C cell hyperplasia should be suspected, and the latter is recognized and treated as a pre-malignant condition. Surgical management should aim in the first instance to identify familial cases and, having done so, exclude a phaeochromocytoma and hyperparathyroidism, because the dangers of thyroid surgery in the presence of an undiagnosed phaeochromocytoma are considerable. Opinions are divided whether affected patients should be subjected to bilateral adrenalectomy when disease is demonstrable on one side only. Although medullary hyperplasia, or a frank tumour, occurs on both sides in 50 per cent of patients, the morbidity of total adrenalectomy for the other 50 per cent is hard to justify. No such reservations apply to the extent of surgery on the thyroid, which should be total thyroidectomy (Russell et al., 1983) in view of the high incidence of multicentric lesions in familial cases (80 per cent) and in the sporadic variety (30 per cent). Particular attention is paid to the completeness of resection of the upper poles and of the primary lymphatic drainage areas. Dissection of the lymph nodes in the central compartment of the neck extends from the hyoid bone to the innominate vessels, as up to 75 per cent of nodes will be found to contain metastatic disease (Gordon et al., 1973). Lymph nodes in the lateral compartment should be sampled and, if positive, removed in accordance with the modified block dissection technique described for the thyroid. In the author's opinion a patient with medullary thyroid carcinoma revealed later on histology after total lobectomy for a non-toxic solitary nodule need be submitted to total thyroidectomy only if familial disease is subsequently discovered, or elevated basal or provoked calcitonin levels are demonstrated.

6. Secondary Tumours of the Thyroid

Although rare, these most commonly arise from the breast, kidney, ovary or colon. If the primary tumour is under control total thyroidectomy is indicated.

Other Thyroid Conditions

1. Acute Suppurative Thyroiditis

When antibiotics fail to eradicate pyogenic infection, which does rarely affect the thyroid, an abscess may develop requiring drainage by aspiration or open operation.

2. *Hashimoto's Chronic Lymphocytic Thyroiditis*

This is a common cause of enlargement of the thyroid, women being affected 12 times more frequently than men. It is most often seen between the ages of 35 and 55 and onset is rapid over several months. The patient is euthyroid initially but progresses to a hypothyroid state as the lymphocytic infiltration advances throughout the gland. Occasionally there is a toxic phase of variable duration. The goitre is characteristically diffuse and rubbery but may become multinodular and asymmetrical and then shrinks and becomes fibrotic. Symptoms of pressure on the trachea and oesophagus are common and if no response to exogenous thyroxine (0·1–0·2 mg per day) is obtained, removal of the affected lobe or isthmus (partial thyroidectomy) is indicated. Such Hashimoto goitres are relatively avascular and easily separable from the false capsule. The development of malignant lymphoma and primary thyroid neoplasia in a Hashimoto's gland is now considered to be a minimal risk. Antibody levels should discriminate between the two, although high titres for microsomes and thyroglobulin occur in 12 per cent of cases of thyroid carcinoma. The clinical features and radioiodine studies will need to be reviewed and when there is doubt, open or closed biopsy is indicated.

3. *Reidel's Thyroiditis*

This is a very rare disease and some even doubt its existence as a separate entity. It is diagnosed in elderly adults, usually females who complain of pressure symptoms in the neck, weight loss and local pain. The thyroid is woody hard and firmly tethered to the adjacent structures, notably the trachea, which becomes compressed. The clinical signs and symptoms therefore resemble an anaplastic carcinoma or advanced Hashimoto's goitre. The condition may be accompanied by fibrosing mediastinitis, sclerosing cholangitis and retroperitoneal fibrosis. Relief of symptoms may follow division of the thyroid isthmus which is white and brittle, and which can be literally 'snapped off' the trachea with the fingers.

4. *Thyroid Cyst*

The prevalence of cysts of the thyroid increases with age and often reflects a degenerative process in a multinodular goitre. Benign cysts are frequently tense and, due to their location, render the sign of fluctuation hard to elicit. Thyroid ultrasound should reliably identify them as a well-circumscribed echolucent area, but intracystic debris should raise the suspicion of cystic degeneration in a tumour which occurs, notably in papillary carcinomas. Cysts which are smaller than 2 cm in diameter are treated by aspiration, submitting the fluid for cytological examination and the patient to re-examination. Larger cysts are likely to recur when tapped, and may well be cosmetically unacceptable. These carry a risk of sudden airways obstruction due to intracystic haemorrhage, and are, therefore, best dealt with electively by partial thyroidectomy.

Preoperative Preparation

All patients require haemoglobin estimation, chest radiograph, and an ECG, but as intraoperative blood transfusion is only rarely required for any of the procedures to be prescribed, much laboratory time and effort may be saved by blood grouping only.

When the airway is compromised by a retrosternal goitre, thoracic inlet radiological views or tomographs are requested so that the full extent of the problem is appreciated by both surgeon and anaesthetist. The vocal cords are examined routinely by indirect laryngoscopy as a small number of patients have an unsuspected idiopathic unilateral palsy (Neil et al., 1972), the recognition of which is vital if, for example, a total lobectomy is proposed on the contralateral side. Likewise, laryngoscopy is essential if the patient has had previous surgery or has a hoarse voice which might indicate thyroid malignancy or independent laryngeal pathology. Thyrotoxic patients require special preparation prior to surgery and it is essential to establish either a euthyroid state or control the peripheral effects of high circulating levels of thyroxine. The majority of patients referred for surgery are already receiving anti-thyroid drugs but may have unstable thyrotoxicosis. Where toxicity is modest and surgery can be undertaken quickly, the author recommends giving the beta-blocker propranolol in an oral dose of 20–80 mg 6–8-hourly for 10 days preoperatively. Adjustment of the dose is monitored with reference to the patient's sleeping pulse rate which should be brought down below 70 per minute. It is essential to give propranolol on the morning of operation, in other words to maintain the 8-hourly regimen and continue treatment thereafter. The dose of medication is then tapered off over several days in parallel with the anticipated fall in the thyroxin level which has a half-life of 7 days. Some authors (Peden et al., 1982) favour the newer, long-acting beta-blockers which can be given daily, but the same precautions need to be taken pre- and postoperatively. Beta-blockers are contra-indicated in patients with bronchial asthma, sinus bradycardia, second- and third-degree heart block, right heart failure secondary to pulmonary hypertension and congestive heart failure. Patients with severe thyrotoxicosis traditionally receive a 6–8-week course of carbimazole (Neomercazole) 10–15 mg 8-hourly (the timing is critical because of rapid excretion) reducing to a 5 mg 8-hourly maintenance dose once a euthyroid state is achieved. If the patient has an adverse reaction to this drug, propylthiouracil may be given in its place, 100 mg 8-hourly. Extended use of any of the thyourea group of drugs may cause prothrombin deficiency (Naeye and Terrien, 1960), leucopenia and, rarely, bone marrow depression, and a full blood count and prothrombin time are therefore indicated preoperatively for the patients who have been so treated. An alternative to a beta-blocker for these patients in the preoperative phase is Lugol's iodine, 10 drops 8-hourly for 10 days, given in milk to make it more palatable. The mechanism of effect is not well understood, but is thought to diminish hormone output, slow the rate at which stored thyroxine is released and inhibit the organic binding of iodine. There is little evidence that it decreases the vascularity of the thyroid as claimed and may, in fact, increase the bulk, and for these reasons it is not favoured by the author.

Standard Surgical Approach to the Thyroid

The first requirement is to ensure that the patient is comfortably placed and the surgical diathermy indifferent electrode is in firm contact with the buttocks. Good access to the anterior compartment of the neck is best achieved by placing a pillow beneath the shoulders to gently extend the cervical spine. Supporting and stabilizing the head on a padded ring or U-shaped neurosurgical rest are important, for failure to do so, especially in the elderly, may result in severe pain and headaches postoperatively. In patients with short, stocky necks or large goitres, it is helpful to depress the shoulders by gentle traction on the arms in their long axis, securing them to the sides of the body with foam wedges (*Fig. 24.3*). The table is then tilted 15° head up which reduces engorgement in the neck veins and minimizes subsequent bleeding. This manoeuvre may also serve to relieve pressure on the superior vena cava with retrosternal goitres which are compressing the thoracic inlet. A flat board, supported by a pillow, placed horizontally on the upper abdomen and lower chest or a magnetic pad provides a convenient instrument tray (*Fig. 24.3*).

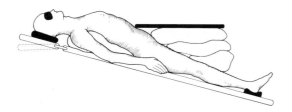

Fig. 24.3. Position of patient for operations on the thyroid gland.

The skin is prepared with chlorhexidine in spirit and the operative area draped. There are several ways of draping the neck. The author favours a four-towel technique with large cottonwool or gauze packs, one on either side of the neck being pushed well down with long-handled forceps into the recess between the head support and the shoulder pillow.

These absorb any blood loss from the lateral extent of the neck incision and provide a good anchor for the towel clips to the side and head drapes. The head towel is reflected forward loosely rather than using a conventional head towel, which prevents ready access to the airway for the anaesthetist in the event of any dislodgement of the endotracheal tube. Although the skin of the head and neck is very vascular, infiltration with 1 in 1000 adrenaline in saline is now rarely practised. Much of the bleeding at the skin edge stops spontaneously and more persistent bleeding vessels are best recognized and coagulated, rather than relying on the vasoconstrictive properties of adrenaline which will lose its effect later and lead to extensive bruising and perhaps a wound haematoma.

Routine operations on the thyroid can be carried out using a Kocher collar incision which is placed in one of the natural skin crease lines (Langer's) approximately two finger-breadths above the sternoclavicular joint (*Fig. 24.4*). This may conveniently

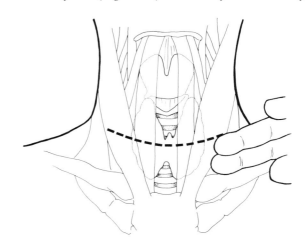

Fig. 24.4. Standard incision for operations on the thyroid gland.

be marked on the skin using a length of silk held taut against the convexity of the neck. Symmetry is important for maturation of collagen in the scar may contract unevenly if the stress lines are unequal, resulting in a poor cosmetic result. It is therefore helpful to check the symmetry by standing at the head end of the table and looking down on the proposed incision directly from above. In view of the risk of keloid formation, the practice of cross-hatching the incision line, using a stylus and ink, or scarifying the skin with a needle is to be avoided. Matching the skin flaps at the end of the operation is rarely a problem for the experienced surgeon. The incision is deepened through the subcutaneous fat and platysma muscle, below which the deep cervical fascia is encountered investing the strap muscles centrally and the sternomastoid muscles laterally. The anterior jugular veins course beneath this fascial layer and, providing the surgeon is careful and keeps to the plane between the platysma and the fascia, blood loss is minimal. Once the layer has been established Babcock or Allis tissue forceps applied to the subdermal layer of each skin flap enable initial, deft scalpel dissection of these using a technique of traction and counter-traction and blunt dissection with a swab on the index finger. Mobilization is extended superiorly to the thyroid notch and inferiorly to the suprasternal notch. The diamond-shaped surgical field is held exposed with a Joll's self-retaining retractor, the wound edges being protected with tetra towels. The deep cervical fascia is then incised vertically in the midline raphe from the prominence of the thyroid cartilage to the suprasternal notch and isthmus of the thyroid. Defining this plane as it extends laterally over the lateral lobes requires care and early recognition of the sternothyroid muscle, which may be thinned to a filmy membrane by compression when the thyroid is enlarged. Difficulties may arise from adherence of these layers due to the inflammation of auto-immune thyroiditis or direct invasion in thyroid malignancy. Exposing the thyroid further requires delivery of each lobe in turn into the wound. In young patients the strap muscles usually present no impediment and the lobe can be freed by sweeping the areolar connections between it and the overlying sternothyroid muscle with the index finger. Alternatively the tissue plane can be gently spread open by widening the jaws of a pair of artery forceps held vertically. Where the strap muscles limit exposure and prevent forward dislocation of the lobe, there should be no hesitation in dividing them. These muscles derive their nerve supply segmentally from the ansa hypoglossi as it loops down from the carotid sheath and it is desirable to preserve this innervation. However, the patient suffers little detectable functional effect even if these muscles are resected as part of a cancer clearance. In practice, a long pair of forceps inserted under the strap muscles at the junction of the upper one-third and lower two-thirds can be brought out at the medial border of the sternomastoid muscle, allowing identification and preservation of the nerve before dividing the muscle with diathermy. Stay stitches to the divided upper and lower muscle flaps are then placed and hitched over the Joll's retractor joints (*Fig.* 24.5).

Specific Thyroid Procedures

Subtotal Thyroidectomy

The aim is to remove sufficient thyroid tissue to abolish toxicity yet preserve a posterior remnant of the gland on each side sufficient to maintain the patient in a euthyroid state. Each lobe will need to be dislocated forward in turn and most surgeons find it preferable to stand on the opposite side of the table to the lobe being delivered. Retraction of the strap muscles is conveniently carried out with a Vaughan–Hudson angled retractor which reduces the risk of

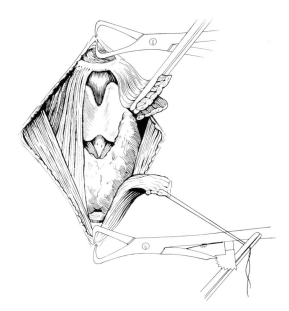

Fig. 24.5. Division and mobilization of strap muscles.

damage to the sympathetic chain. The middle thyroid vein is usually the first structure seen crossing to the gland at its midpoint and this must be ligated and divided before the lobe can be further delivered. This is done with a ligature passed on a small aneurysm needle and then, keeping the gland retracted medially and downwards with a gauze swab, the superior pedicle is defined. It is only after this has been done that the lobe can be fully mobilized. The adherent sternothyroid muscle is conveniently pushed off the surface of the upper pole with a Lahey swab mounted on forceps (beware of fairly constant high unnamed vein running from the pole to the internal jugular) and a thyroid director is then passed between the larynx and the thyroid pedicle. This is a subtle and useful manoeuvre and if damage to the superior laryngeal nerve is to be avoided, the point of the director should be aimed upwards and laterally ensuring by fingertip pressure that the point of the director is passing behind all the upper lobe thyroid tissue but no more (*Fig.* 24.6). Keeping the director in place the pedicle is doubly ligated with a transfixion suture of 2/0 linen passed behind and then anteriorly to secure both branches of the superior thyroid artery. Formal division of the pedicle can often be deferred until the final resection of the lobe is undertaken. The lobe is now grasped with Lahey tenacula and rotated medially. The inferior thyroid artery is identified by opening up the space between the trachea and common carotid artery with blunt forcep dissection and then is under-run cleanly and precisely with a ligature on an aneurysm needle. If this is placed as far laterally as practicable, it is ready for tying in continuity once the recurrent laryngeal nerve and parathyroids have been identified. Gentle traction on this ligature often throws the recurrent laryngeal nerve into prominence as it runs up at an acute

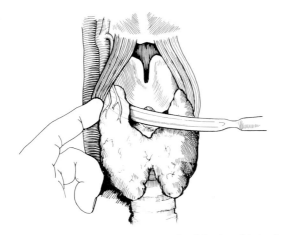

Fig. 24.6. Mobilization of superior pole of the thyroid gland.

angle from the mediastinum to reach the tracheo-oesophageal groove before assuming its intimate relationships with the branches of this artery. When it is not evident, an aberrant course should be suspected, notably lateral or anterior to the trachea or even non-recurrent. The nerve can be confidently identified by its white colour, fine longitudinal surface artery, lack of pulsation and lack of elasticity. Proceeding with the operation at this stage without having identified the nerve is hazardous. The inferior thyroid artery ligature is now tied and the thyroid lobe is freed interiorly by isolating and dividing between ligatures the inferior thyroid veins and thyroidea ima artery where present. During this manoeuvre the recurrent laryngeal nerve should be kept in view and avoided at all times. The inferior parathyroid gland may be seen at this stage, especially if ectopic, lying in the thyro-thymic ligament. This and its blood supply will be preserved if the veins are swept medially and secured close to the gland. In this form of thyroidectomy the parathyroids are not specifically identified and, indeed, attempting to do so may hazard their blood supply. If one is inadvertently excised or devascularized it should be diced into 1-mm cubes and auto-transplanted into the adjacent sternomastoid muscle.

At this stage the surgeon must make the important decision about how much thyroid tissue to leave behind. The empirical formula of resecting seven-eighths and leaving one-eighth of the gland is a useful guideline and results in a gratifying number of euthyroid patients. The merit of this approach is that it requires no modification for varying sizes of gland, but it has the disadvantage that it does not take into account the age of the patient (generally the younger the patient the more radical the resection needs to be) or the presence of thyroid auto-antibodies (which call for less radical excision). Attempts to standardize the size of the thyroid remnant by linear measurement, dental wax stents (Murley and Rigg, 1968) or surgical judgement (Hedley et al., 1972) have been shown to be highly inaccurate so that recommenda-

tions to leave 3 or 4 g of tissue on each side are meaningless. Having decided on the size of the residual thyroid by art or science, and experience, small artery forceps are placed on the posterolateral aspect of the surgical capsule and, generally speaking, injury to the recurrent laryngeal nerve and parathyroids will be avoided if placement is made above the level defined by the anterior surface of the trachea. The gland is then incised with a scalpel blade directed obliquely down towards the trachea (*Fig.* 24.7). The

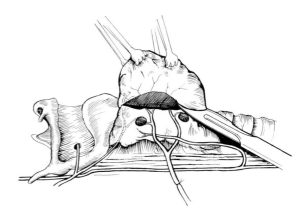

Fig. 24.7. Removal of thyroid lobe by sharp dissection, preserving parathyroid glands.

identical sequence of events is then performed on the opposite side of the neck when some fine adjustment of remnant size will be possible to give an overall one-eighth residue. Both lobes and the isthmus having been freed, the gland now remains attached only by the pyramidal lobe or fibrous remnant of the thyroglossal tract. This requires careful dissection upwards so that no additional thyroid tissue or blood supply is overlooked. The thyroid remnants are then sutured to the pretracheal fascia with continuous chromic catgut in a herringbone fashion, picking up the surgical capsule and rolling the thyroid towards the midline and away from the recurrent laryngeal nerve (*Fig.* 24.8). This is not only haemostatic but

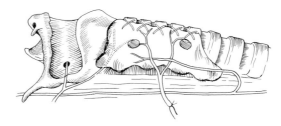

Fig. 24.8. Haemostatic suture of residual thyroid.

if, for any reason, the neck requires further exploration the fibrotic reaction around the thyroid is well away from important structures. The thyroid bed should always be drained on both sides. Where the dead space is modest a Redivac drain is ideal but if the dead space is large or haemostasis has been difficult, a wider-bore drain of the Drayvac type is preferred, and it is exteriorized by a separate small stab incision on each side of the neck. The drains cross in the midline and run for some distance beneath the platysma layer so that superficial as well as deep drainage is provided, avoiding the risk of a subcutaneous seroma. After flexing the head by adjustment of the headrest, the strap muscles are reconstituted with interrupted 2/0 chromic catgut and then approximated with their overlying fascia in the midline with a continuous catgut suture. Finally, the platysma is closed with a running 3/0 plain catgut, picking up the edge of the muscle with evenly matched, very small bites so that the overlying skin is accurately realigned. The skin is closed with (Avlox) clips which produce a better result than routine suturing which tends to tattoo the skin at the needle entry points. After securing the drains with a fine non-slip silk suture a loose thyroid collar crossover type dressing is then applied.

Partial Thyroidectomy

Standard exposure of the thyroid and the subtotal excision technique as described above is performed, leaving as much normal tissue as possible consistent with a modest lateral remnant on each side which will not be evident when the patient swallows. It is inadvisable to leave the isthmus or pyramidal lobe even if apparently normal, for compensatory hypertrophy at that site will be cosmetically unacceptable.

Removal of a Retrosternal Goitre

The surgeon will know of the ectopic site of the gland by preoperative symptoms, examination and investigation, and operating theatre staff will have been alerted to the possibility of an addition sternal splitting approach. In practice, almost all retrosternal goitres can be delivered and removed via a cervical incision which should be placed lower than the conventional Kocher. The anterior chest wall is shaved, skin prepared and draped accordingly and if the airway is severely compromised the services of an experienced anaesthetist are imperative. It is usually safer in these cases to withhold sedative premedication and rely on speedy intubation with the patient awake, having sprayed the vocal cords with local anaesthetic, for inability to intubate a paralysed patient such as this may cause fatal anoxia. Wholly or partially intrathoracic goitres derive their arterial supply from the superior and inferior arteries in the neck and these should be secured in the usual way, and this also applies to superior and middle thyroid venous drainage. Once the upper pole has been freed, an attempt should be made to dissect the retrosternal portion of the lobe with the index finger and gently ease it upwards. Minimal force should be used, otherwise the recurrent laryngeal nerves, which cannot always

be visualized, due to the limited space, may be avulsed or severely stretched. If this manoeuvre fails, the surgeon has one of two choices—intracapsular enucleation or formal splitting of the sternum. The latter is probably only necessary or justified if a retrosternal thyroid malignancy exists or when operating for a recurrent goitre. Intracapsular enucleation of the capsule involves incision of the thyroid transversely just above the sternal notch after which the fibrous septa and colloid nodules within the lobe are broken down with a finger. The contents can then be scooped out with a large Volkmann spoon or a Yanker's sucker. It may then be possible to deliver the capsule to secure the inferior thyroid veins but if there is still concern about the location of the recurrent laryngeal nerve and haemostasis is good, it is best left *in situ*. Two large suction drains are recommended. When sternal split is required an incision is made in the midline down to the periosteum with cutting diathermy from the suprasternal notch downwards for the appropriate distance (*Fig.* 24.9). The

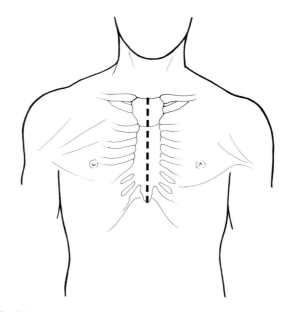

Fig. 24.9. Incision for partial or complete splitting of the sternum to gain access to large retrosternal goitre.

space between the manubrium and the great vessels is gently opened up by finger dissection as far as the digit can reach. Introducing a vertical mechanical saw the manubrium, or sometimes the whole sternum, is divided longitudinally, keeping the saw handle forced upwards at all times. A self-retaining sternal retractor is racked open to spread the divided manubrium or sternum (*Fig.* 24.10). Bleeding from the periosteum is controlled with electrocautery and from the marrow with bone wax. The parietal pleura is freed in the midline and pushed laterally. Removal of the retrosternal goitre proceeds along routine lines and the chest is then closed by accurately reapproximating the sternum using wire sutures. These are passed

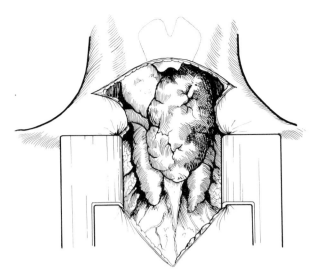

Fig. 24.10. Exposure of retrosternal goitre following splitting of the upper sternum.

through the bone with an awl—the underlying structures being protected by a malleable copper spatula. The wires are held taut with strong forceps, twisted, clipped and the tips of the wire then buried into the periosteum. A retrosternal drain is brought out superiorly and attached to an underwater seal in case a small pneumothorax has been produced. The subcutaneous fat is closed with interrupted catgut sutures and the skin with a running subcuticular nylon one (*see* Chapter 39).

Total Thyroid Lobectomy or Total Thyroidectomy

Thyroid lobectomy is undertaken when the surgeon knows or suspects that the patient has thyroid carcinoma, and if confirmed on frozen section a total lobectomy may in addition be carried out on the other side, completing a total thyroidectomy (*see* Indications for Surgery, p. 326). The approach to the thyroid is standard but the subtotal excision technique described earlier is modified in several important ways. At no stage is the gland grasped with tissue forceps for traction, otherwise a malignant solitary nodule may be ruptured inadvertently with spillage of tumour cells. It must also be assumed that multicentric tumour deposits may exist or capsular invasion be present, hence the need to give a solitary nodule a wide berth by removing the entire lobe, isthmus and a midline portion of the contralateral lobe. However, this ideal should not be pursued to the detriment of the recurrent laryngeal nerve or parathyroids, and where these could be compromised it may be better to leave a little residual thyroid tissue and ablate this later with radio-iodine. The blood supply to each parathyroid is via an end artery arising from the inferior thyroid artery, but it is believed that collaterals to this end artery are picked up on the thyroid capsule from the oesophageal and

tracheal vessels. In this procedure it is better, therefore, not to ligate the inferior thyroid artery in continuity but to trace out each of its terminal branches and individually clip and divide these between mosquito forceps as they enter the false capsule. Concurrently, the recurrent laryngeal nerve will be traced out along its course and it often helps to have this gently retracted laterally on a soft, Silastic sling. As the nerve traverses Berry's ligament to gain the larynx, damage will be avoided by dissecting the nerve free under direct vision, especially when this ligament is divided to free the upper pole. Occasionally, local invasion by thyroid malignancies prevents complete removal, notably on the side of the larynx and oesophagus. In these circumstances the extent of the residual tumour should be marked with small liga-clips to assist the radiotherapist in planning subsequent treatment fields. The safe performance of a standard, total lobectomy should be within the capabilities of most general surgeons but total thyroidectomy is a more demanding procedure and is not for the inexperienced.

Modified Block Dissection for Thyroid Carcinoma

The standard Kocher incision is extended on one or both sides (*Fig.* 24.11) and routine exposure of the

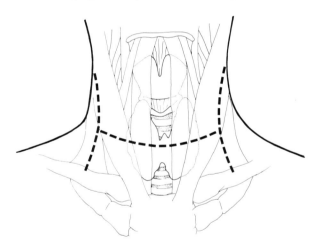

Fig. 24.11. Modification of thyroid incision to include bilateral lymph node dissection.

thyroid gland undertaken. Having raised the skin flaps to their full extent a clearer field may be obtained by suturing the apex of each skin flap to the drapes rather than using two Joll's retractors, which tend to get in the way. Operability is assessed and where there is clear involvement of the strap muscles or sternomastoid on one side, these are resected en bloc with the total thyroidectomy specimen, as described above. The plane between the sternomastoid and strap muscles is opened up and the carotid sheath exposed. Where there is heavy nodal involvement along the internal jugular chain,

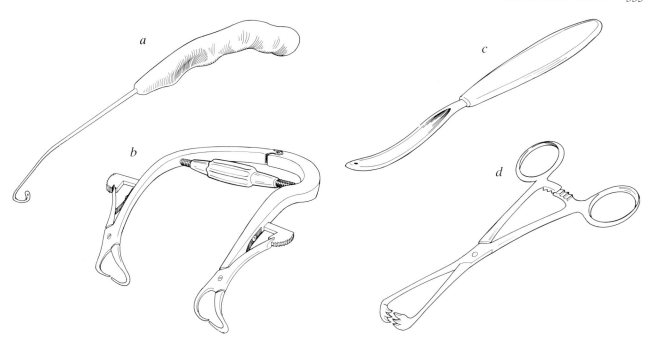

Fig. 24.12. Thyroid instruments favoured by the author. *a*, Small aneurysm needle. *b*, Joll's retractor. *c*, Thyroid director. *d*, Tissue-holding forceps.

extending to the posterior cervical and supraclavicular groups, the author finds it easiest to detach the sternal and clavicular heads of the sternomastoid and rotate this muscle upwards. This provides excellent exposure yet allows preservation of the blood supply (occipital artery) and nerve supply (accessory) so that it may be reattached on completion of the node dissection. Great care is needed when removing the upper and lower deep cervical nodes and their surrounding fat from the surface of the internal jugular vein. Silastic slings placed around the vessel, above and below, provide counter-traction and control the vein wall which, if breached, may result in air embolus as well as serious bleeding. The internal jugular vein may require excision (*see* Chapter 26). Involved supraclavicular and posterior triangle nodes are dissected in continuity with the deep cervical chain and occasionally the posterior belly of the omohyoid muscle may need excision and the transverse cervical and supraclavicular vessels divided. The vagus and phrenic nerves are substantial and easily identified and preserved, but the thoracic duct on the left and the main lymphatic duct on the right are easily damaged. If this occurs, the affected duct should be tied off rather than an attempt made to effect a repair.

Postoperative Care

It is important to recognize promptly any of the possible complications, the management of which will be individually discussed in the next section. The patient is extubated on the operating table. If there has been any concern about the integrity of the recur-

rent laryngeal nerves the anaesthetist is requested to examine the vocal cords. Ideally, the patient is observed in a recovery area close to the theatre until fully conscious, and should reactionary haemorrhage or airway obstruction develop, surgical and anaesthetic help will be readily available. The vital signs, and the appearance of the neck, should be checked half-hourly and then hourly for the first 12 hours and thereafter 4-hourly until the patient is stable. Four-hourly observations of pulse and respiration may be necessary for thyrotoxic patients whose operations have been covered with beta-blockers while the dose is progressively decreased. The suction drains remain for 48 hours but, as always, the moment of withdrawal is variable. Alternate clips are removed at 48 hours and the remainder at 72 hours. Many patients experience some huskiness of the voice due to intubation and this should not cause alarm as this should soon settle. Likewise, soreness of the throat, following vigorous manipulation of a large goitre, is usual and Xylocaine lozenges provide good symptomatic relief. On discharge from hospital, usually on the 3rd or 4th postoperative day, the patient is instructed to gently massage the skin in the region of the incision with lanolin which keeps the scar supple and may prevent adhesion of the platysma to the underlying strap muscles. This latter may cause unsightly puckering of the skin on swallowing.

Postoperative Complications

In competent hands thyroidectomy in all of its forms gives excellent results in the majority of patients.

There are, however, potentially dangerous local and specific complications which can severely compromise the outcome and be life threatening. All are avoidable with sound surgical technique and good preparation (notably of thyrotoxic patients).

Haemorrhage

This is usually reactionary and is a problem in the first 24 hours after surgery. Failure to secure the superior thyroid vessels will result in serious blood loss but slipped ligatures on the inferior and middle thyroid veins may also be dramatic. Bleeding into the dressing alone usually arises from a small skin vessel and placing an extra clip should deal with this. When more profuse haemorrhage occurs the patient should be returned to the operating theatre, where the incision should be opened and the vessel under-run.

Major haemorrhage must be recognized quickly, junior medical and nursing staff being aware of the significance of pallor, respiratory difficulties, stridor and swelling of the wound. No reliance should be placed on drainage to indicate blood loss, as these drains are small calibre and block readily. Immediate action on the ward is to remove the clips or sutures and to open the wound. At the bedside of all patients following thyroidectomy, clip removers, scissors and a pair of artery forceps must always be available. Opening the blades of the artery forceps to distract the skin and then the midline strap muscles will allow evacuation of the clot beneath the deep cervical fascia which should bring immediate relief. The patient is then returned to the operating theatre and under general anaesthesic the bleeding point vessel is identified and ligated. Sometimes a general ooze is seen from the raw surfaces and simply evacuation of the clot and further oversewing of the thyroid remnant achieves haemostasis. There is some evidence that prolonged use of the thyourea group of drugs will sometimes lower the level of prothrombin in plasma (Maeye and Terrien, 1960) and this effect can be reversed by giving vitamin K_1 to promote synthesis in the liver. If, therefore, carbimazole was used in the preoperative preparation of such a patient, vitamin K_1 should be administered, but if the airway obstruction continues, tracheostomy may very rarely have to be considered, particularly if laryngeal oedema has developed.

Recurrent Laryngeal Nerve Damage

This complication is the most publicized and the most feared by patient and surgeon alike, yet the incidence of permanent damage is extremely low in competent hands (less than 0·1 per cent). Injury may be from stretching or crushing (transient) or permanent from ligature or division. Damage is more common when operations are undertaken where the normal anatomy is distorted, for example in multinodular, recurrent or malignant goitres. Unilateral injury may be asymptomatic and go undetected due to compensatory hyperabduction of the uninvolved vocal cord and will be detected only if routine postoperative laryngoscopy is performed. However, most patients suffer postoperatively some loss of power and hoarseness of the voice with a tendency to choke while drinking, especially when tired. If neuropraxia is the underlying pathology recovery can be expected in anything from a few weeks to 6 months, but if the symptoms persist permanent paralysis is likely. Voice improvement in these patients can be achieved by injecting Teflon into the paralysed cord to control the glottic air leak.

Bilateral recurrent nerve paralysis is the most devastating complication in thyroid surgery and is apparent the moment the patient is extubated at the end of the operation. Not only is the patient unable to speak but the unopposed adductor action of the cricothyroid muscles closes the glottis to such an extent that the least exertion results in airway obstruction. When the surgeon is confident that one or both nerves have been identified and preserved, damage due to neuropraxia is a reasonable assumption and reintubation plus hydrocortisone 100 mg t.d.s will tide the patient over the next 48 hours until the oedema settles. If a trial of extubation again fails, tracheostomy is performed and in due course a speaking tube can be inserted.

It is wise to wait for 9 months before accepting the fact of permanent damage, at which stage several surgical approaches are possible. Exploration and resuture of the nerve with grafting as necessary are now feasible with the newer microsurgical techniques, as is anastomosis of the hyperglossal and recurrent nerves. Lateral fixation of one cord by arytenoidectomy to hold the airway open has been practised most widely and there are several subtle modifications of the technique which are outside the scope of this chapter.

Superior Laryngeal Nerve Paresis

The true incidence of this injury is unknown due to lack of any objective test of function until recently. If the patient experiences a change in the voice—loss of pitch and inability to make explosive sounds—damage is likely. Voice analysis using a Visipitch oscilloscope will help to confirm this damage, which may occur in up to 25 per cent of patients (Kark et al., 1984). However, recovery will usually follow for the majority if the nerve has only been stretched. If no improvement is evident after 3 months, it is unlikely to occur. Bilateral damage is said to produce a very flat, hoarse voice which tires easily.

Hypoparathyroidism

If there is any reason to suspect that the parthyroids have been compromised, the serum calcium level should be checked routinely postoperatively and, indeed, there are good arguments for always doing so (Rose, 1963). Hypocalcaemia due to parathyroid deficiency will usually be evident within 1 week of operation and should be suspected if the patient appears unduly agitated, depressed or hyperventilates. Circumoral tingling is generally the first and most sensitive indicator, and paraesthesia in the fingers and toes preceding frank tetany is seen in most profound hypocalcaemia. Tapping over the facial nerve will cause contraction of the facial muscles (Chvostek–Weiss sign) but this phenomenon may be observed in 10–15 per cent of normal individuals (Barnes and Gann, 1974). Carpopedal spasm, provoked by occlusion of the circulation to the arm (Trousseau's sign), indicates severe hypocalcaemia and requires intravenous calcium infusion—10 ml of 10 per cent calcium gluconate (given slowly to avoid cardiac arrest in systole). This may need to be repeated 4–6-hourly. Oral effervescent calcium is commenced at the same time, 4–16 g daily, dose depending on response. If hypocalcaemia persists, vitamin D (calciferol 25 000–100 000 units) as well as 2–3 g oral calcium per day are given until return to a normocalcaemic state. Such patients may lack parathyroid reserve in the future and a challenge, e.g. pregnancy, menopause, etc., will reproduce these signs and symptoms. Other patients, not overtly hypoparathyroid, may suffer vague lethargy and depression or insidiously develop cataracts, mental deterioration and psychosis, a strong argument for establishing that the serum calcium is firmly in the normal range at least once following thyroidectomy.

Hypothyroidism

The ability of the thyroid to produce sufficient thyroxine after thyroidectomy reflects not only the size of the remnant but also the pre-existing pathological processes within the gland. Hypothyroidism is inevitable after total thyroidectomy or malignancy, but less predictable, for example, after a thyroid lobectomy for a benign solitary nodule. Avoiding hypothyroidism is one of the main challenges when operating for thyrotoxicosis. In this instance postoperative function is dictated by several factors:

1. The severity of disease prior to surgery.
2. The age of the patient.
3. The presence of thyroid auto-antibodies.
4. The size of the gland.
5. The surgical judgement which evaluates the foregoing and dictates how much of the gland to remove.

In experienced hands consistent hypothyroidism rates of 10–15 per cent can be achieved while avoiding levels of persistent hyperthyroidism greater than 5 per cent, which would be unacceptable. Formal correction of hypothyroidism should be withheld after total thyroidectomy for malignancy (notably follicular lesions) until a radio-iodine scan has been performed to identify possible distant metastases. Thereafter, tri-iodo-L-thyronine (T3) 50–100 μg per day is given in preference to L-thyroxine (T4) by virtue of its shorter biological half-life of 1 week which enables repeated scans to be performed with minimal delay. Once isotope ablation of residual disease has been achieved conversion to T4 is appropriate. The replacement dose for individual patients varies considerably, the majority only requiring 0·2–0·3 mg a day but some needing three times that amount. Nearly all patients operated on for thyrotoxicosis become biochemically hypothyroid for 2–3 months after surgery and no correction is necessary. The minority who remain or become clinically hypothyroid over the ensuing 2 years require a modest dose of T4 in the order of 0·1–0·2 mg daily. Routine T4 (0·1 mg daily) is recommended for all patients operated on for non-toxic, diffuse or multinodular goitres. Failure to suppress TSH drive can result in recurrent goitre, even if hypothyroidism is subclinical.

Tracheal Collapse

In this condition the trachea has become softened by chondromalacia so that its walls collapse when the goitre is removed, and is rarely seen following removal of a long-standing goitre, especially if retrosternal. In such cases there is likely to be an element of laryngeal oedema and reduced movement of the vocal cords following difficult intubation and delivery of the lobes. Whenever the trachea is noted to be markedly soft and narrow, tracheostomy should probably be performed at the time of thyroidectomy, but this need is most rare.

Thyroid Crisis

Now a very rare event with the improved methods of control of thyrotoxicosis, this state, when fully expressed, is characterized by high fever, tachycardia (atrial fibrillation), extreme restlessness and delirium. Treatment should be given promptly and is based on high doses of anti-thyroid drugs (Neo-Mercazole (carbimazole) 30 mg stat and then 15 mg 8-hourly) plus 1 g of sodium iodide intravenously. The beta-blocker propranolol 2 mg is given slowly intravenously with electrocardiographic control. Fluid replacement, ice pack cooling and sedation may help to abort the crisis.

Cervical Sympathetic Damage

A rare complication resulting from deep, forceful retraction on the carotid sheath producing a Horner's syndrome, notably by the absence of the vascular dilatation component (Smith and Murley, 1965). The myosis and ptosis are frequently permanent.

Wound Complications

Keloid—the laying down of excessive collagen in the

scar—is the most unpredictable wound complication but is said to be more prevalent in negroes, redheads and in pregnancy. Unless the scar can be excised and adapted to conform more readily to Langer's lines, reoperation is unlikely to confer any improvement. Infection is an uncommon complication and when it occurs a foreign body should be suspected—nonabsorbable suture material or, at worst, a stray dissecting swab. Rarely nickel sensitivity from the clips used for the skin closure results in blistering and breakdown.

THE PARATHYROIDS

Surgical Anatomy

There are normally four parathyroid glands in the human, but developmental abnormalities can give rise to a larger or smaller number. Gilmour's much quoted autopsy study of 428 cadavers (Gilmour, 1938) found two glands in 0·2 per cent, three in 6·1 per cent, five in 6 per cent and six in 0·5 per cent, in other words only 87 per cent of cases with the normal complement of four. It is possible that the 6·3 per cent with fewer than four glands were mainly cases of fusion or failed identification. The normal gland weighs 30 mg and measures 3–6 × 2–4 × 0·5–2 mm and is characteristically tan in colour. It is difficult to palpate even when pathological and moves fairly freely within an envelope of surrounding fat.

The upper parathyroids develop from the dorsal endoderm of the fourth pharyngeal pouch, the ventral part of which is fused laterally to the developing thyroid gland on the floor of the primitive pharynx. As a result of this, 92 per cent of the upper parathyroids remain in close contact with the dorsal aspect of the thyroid above the level where the recurrent laryngeal nerve crosses the inferior thyroid artery. The upper parathyroid glands become progressively more dorsally displaced the lower the gland descends, so that in 1·6 per cent they are found between the thyroid and the oesophagus. In 1·5 per cent they lie between the pharynx and oesophagus and in 0·5 per cent of cases, within the carotid sheath (*Fig.* 24.13). It is postulated that pathological enlargement favours dorsal displacement either by the forces of deglutition or negative intrathoracic pressure so that ultimately an upper parathyroid tumour may reach the posterior mediastinum. However, for the most part the upper parathyroid on each side in health and in disease will be found on the posterolateral aspect of the thyroid lobe at or just below the level of the cricoid cartilage. Not infrequently it is tucked behind the upper branches of the inferior thyroid artery as it breaks up to enter the false capsule of the thyroid.

The lower parathyroid gland develops from the dorsal endoderm of the third pharyngeal pouch which also gives rise to the thymus. In contrast to the fourth

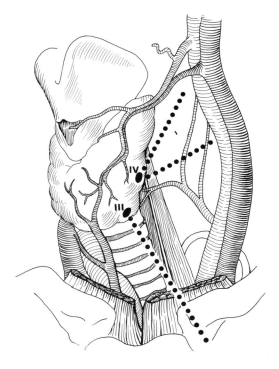

Fig. 24.13. Normal and abnormal position of the parathyroid glands.

pouch, which remains fairly static in position during embryological development, the third leapfrogs over it and descends to the anterior mediastinum. In doing so, it fragments leaving a discrete mass of parathyroid in the neck and a thymus retrosternally. Excessive disruption produces accessory parathyroid and thymic tissue while failure to disrupt at all results in an intrathymic parathyroid. In 20 per cent the parathyroids will actually be within the thymus and this is a bilateral feature in 50 per cent (Proye, 1978). Generally, the lower the parathyroid descends the more likely it is to be intrathymic. Once again, however, the lower parathyroid on each side will normally be found on the posterior aspect of the lateral lobe of the thyroid just below and ventral to the level where the recurrent laryngeal nerve crosses the inferior thyroid artery.

The blood supply to the upper and lower parathyroids is almost exclusively via the inferior thyroid artery; indeed, tracing out the terminal branches of this vessel can aid recognition of the gland. In 5 per cent of cases the upper parathyroids derive their blood supply from the superior thyroid artery in which case the gland is likely to be situated above the upper pole of the thyroid gland itself. Although the ultimate arterial branch of supply to each gland is an end artery, collateral circulation can be observed at a point proximal to the hilum of the parathyroid and is derived from oesophageal, tracheal or superior thyroid arteries.

Preoperative Preparation

In general this is the same as for thyroidectomy patients but the following special recommendations apply. Those primary hyperparathyroid patients with osteitis fibrosa cystica (von Recklinghausen's disease of bone) and most secondary hyperparathyroid patients will require 1-alpha-hydroxycholecalciferol, 2–4 μg/day 2–3 days before operation unless they are grossly hypercalcaemic. This helps to combat the anticipated profound hypocalcaemia due to 'hungry bones' once the pathological parathyroid gland(s) are removed. Grossly hypercalcaemic patients, some of whom may present as emergencies in coma, will require urgent rehydration with phosphate, calcitonin, etc. No preoperative localization studies are advocated unless a previous neck exploration has failed, for most primary operations are successful in competent hands.

Localization studies themselves are costly, not without morbidity and are rarely accurate in the very instances where help is most needed, i.e. small ectopic tumours. However, recent work has demonstrated that venous samples, taken from the subclavian veins, show a raised level of parathormone on the side of the parathyroid tumour. One series (Dennison et al., 1985) reported a high correlation between this higher parathormone level and the side of the parathyroid tumour subsequently confirmed at operation. However, even the most experienced surgeon in the field can have difficulty distinguishing normal and abnormal parathyroids apart from fat lobules, lymph nodes, thymic remnants, thyroid nodules and even bulging inferior constrictor muscles. Indeed, relying on the eye alone has been shown to be only 33·4 per cent accurate (Livesay and Mulder, 1976). There is, therefore, need for some intraoperative help in the identification of parathyroid tissue and the author recommends preoperative infusion of methylene blue (Dudley, 1971) which is selectively taken up by normal and abnormal glands. The intensity of staining is most impressive in stimulated glands, e.g. four-gland hyperplasia in secondary hyperparathyroidism. It is least notable with suppressed parathyroids, i.e. three 'normal' glands in the presence of a large adenoma of the fourth. The dose of methylene blue is calculated on the basis of 5 mg/kg body weight but can be increased to 10 mg/kg in individuals with large muscle bulk who require more dye to achieve comparable results (Rowntree, 1973). The calculated dose is dissolved in 500 ml of dextrose saline, or half that volume as may be indicated in nephrectomized patients, and the infusion started 1 hour prior to surgery. It is essential that the drip rate is adjusted to ensure that the whole dose has been given within 1 hour and by the time the surgical exposure is completed. If given too quickly there is a risk of cardiotoxic effects; if too concentrated, there is a risk of thrombophlebitis in the infused vein. Where the dye is given too slowly, oxidization of the dye to the colourless leucomethyline blue form will occur. The nurses and other medical personnel need to be warned of the cyanotic appearance which the dye gives to the patient, otherwise there is understandable concern and needless alarm.

Indications for Surgery

1. Symptomatic Primary Hyperparathyroidism

The surgeon should have no hesitation in advising prompt exploration of the neck when the biochemical data support this diagnosis. There is good evidence that the incidence of renal stones and infection decreases (McGeown, 1961), osteitis fibrosa cystica improves, subperiosteal resorption resolves and patients with bone and joint pain are dramatically relieved (Kaplan et al., 1976). Where peptic ulceration is present it regresses (Wilder, 1961) and psychological disturbance may well resolve (Aurbach et al., 1973). Hypertension, which is found in 40 per cent of sufferers, is not of itself an indication for surgery and, indeed, deterioration after removal of the parathyroid pathology can occur.

2. Asymptomatic Primary Hyperparathyroidism

Whether to advise surgery or not for patients with mild hyperparathyroidism (serum calcium less than 2·9 μg/ml) and who have no symptoms, is highly controversial. It is an increasing clinical problem, for the widespread use of biochemical screening for conditions unrelated to hyperparathyroidism by multichannel auto-analysers, identifies many patients with unsuspected hypercalcaemia. There is evidence that the incidence of primary hyperparathyroidism in women over the age of 60 is as high as 200 per 100 000 per year (Heath et al., 1980) and if all are to be treated surgically then resources could be overwhelmed. Only limited information is available about the natural history of mild hyperparathyroidism and although 20 per cent of patients in Purnell's series (Purnell et al., 1974) came to surgery, in a 10-year follow-up period not all did so because the patients were being affected adversely. In patients under the age of 50 and in whom follow-up is going to be impractical, sugery is most justified. Whether modest hypercalcaemia, hypercalcuria and raised alkaline phosphatase are reflected in significant renal impairment, osteoporosis, hypertension and decreased survival is unproven. Prospective studies are urgently needed. Meanwhile, the author advises a policy of regular review.

3. Secondary Hyperparathyroidism

This is seen in patients with chronic renal failure and in those being treated by renal dialysis. Occasionally it is seen in cases of long-standing severe intestinal malabsorption. In both, prolonged hypocalcaemia stimulates hyperplasia of the parathyroids with release of high parathormone levels in the peripheral blood. This causes the same pathological bone changes as are seen in primary hyperparathyroidism. Soft tissue calcification, especially in the arteries, and pruritus can also occur. When attempts medically to reverse the hypocalcaemia fail, subtotal parathyroidectomy or total thyroidectomy, cryopreservation and autotransplantation are appropriate.

4. Tertiary Hyperparathyroidism

This is a rare condition seen in patients with long-standing secondary hyperparathyroidism in whom the parathyroid hyperfunction appears to become autonomous, i.e. the hyperplasia and high parathormone levels are attended by inappropriately high serum calcium levels. Again, where medical measures fail, surgery is appropriate as for secondary hyperparathyroidism.

Operative Procedures

1. Routine Approach

The surgical approach to the parathyroids is identical to that described for the thyroid and no modifications are required (*see* p. 330). However, meticulous haemostasis is even more crucial, especially at the stage of freeing the thyroid from the strap muscles laterally and opening up the space between the gland and the carotid sheath. When blood extravasates it stains the surrounding connective tissues, including the parathyroids themselves, so that identification is made much more difficult. Quite simply, there is no substitute for patient, careful dissection, which must not be compromised by considerations of time. Where present, the middle thyroid vein is divided in order to allow full mobilization of the lateral lobes medially and forwards. It is preferable to keep the lobe retracted with a gauze swab on the finger, rather than use a transfixion suture or grasping with tissue forceps, both of which can lead to bleeding. The inferior thyroid artery and recurrent laryngeal nerve are next identified and soft, Silastic vascular slings are then placed around them. This is an important step, not only in the prevention of nerve damage, but also to localize the parathyroids which largely derive their blood supply from the inferior thyroid artery. Additionally, the parathyroids, unless ectopic, have an intimate anatomical relationship with both nerve and artery (*see* Surgical Anatomy, p. 338). Identification of the parathyroids may well, of course, be made much easier if stained deeply with methylene blue. Even normal and suppressed glands have a subtle, pale-greenish tinge which helps their recognition. Several other factors aid the surgeon in identifying the parathyroids:

a. The gentlest compression of the parathyroid gland between non-toothed forceps will cause it to 'blush' due to the richness of its blood supply causing subcapsular haemorrhage.

b. Compared with lymph nodes, thyroid nodules and fat globules, parathyroids are so soft as to be impalpable and also very mobile within their fatty envelope.

c. The cut surface of a parathyroid is homogeneous, shiny and vascular, contrasting with lymph nodes which have a visible cortex, are duller and relatively avascular.

d. There is usually a definite sharp edge to the parathyroid adjacent to its vascular pedicle once it has been freed from the surrounding fat.

2. Surgery for Primary Hyperparathyroidism

The Routine Case

Statistically, there is a slightly higher probability that the adenoma will be found on the right side of the neck, affecting the lower gland, so this side is usually explored first. The tumour is removed with considerable care since there is a real danger of autotransplantation of parathyroid cells if the capsule is ruptured. Inadvertent or careless spillage of cells may account for some cases of recurrent hypercalcaemia. If the pedicle can be located easily and clipped with mosquito forceps, then the parathyroid can be lifted up by this and dissected clear from the surrounding connective tissues with iris scissors. Prompt frozen section confirmation of the adenoma is sought. Three strategies are then possible:

a. The other three or more parathyroids can be identified visually, surgeons relying on past experience and judgement to satisfy themselves that they are dealing with single gland disease.

b. The other 'normal' gland on the same side of the tumour can be excised and submitted for frozen section (Tibblin strategy) (Tibblin et al., 1982) without exploring the contralateral side at all.

c. A diligent search made for all the parathyroids confirming each with a small snippet biopsy on the sharp edge of each gland, i.e. furthest away from the vascular pedicle to avoid damage to the blood supply at the hilum.

Strategy (*a*) is not recommended and the literature abounds with reports of failed explorations and high recurrent hypercalcaemia rates, demonstrating that in even the most competent hands, 'eyeballing' may be only 30–35 per cent accurate (Wells et al., 1975). Strategy (*b*), more recently advocated, is attractive in so far as it will save time and may reduce the incidence of hypocalcaemia since only one side of the neck is disturbed. If the pathologist reports an unequivocally normal gland in addition to the adenoma, then four-gland disease—hyperplasia—is excluded and the only concern surrounds the remote possibility of one or more adenomas of the contra-lateral parathyroids, a reported incidence of 1–2 per cent. The author favours strategy (c)—hard data about the confirmed presence and histological nature of each parathyroid are established and will be invaluable, especially when later the occasional problem of recurrent hypercalcaemia arises. If the surgeon knows that four parathyroids have been seen and confirmed histologically, a possible fifth parathyroid, probably in the mediastinum, is then most likely. Whichever strategy is adopted, it is imperative that the operative notes include an accurate drawing of the findings showing the precise location of glands removed and those remaining.

The Difficult Case

These fall into two categories: first, where the adenoma cannot readily be located and, second, where there is a dilemma about how much parathyroid to remove. When routine exploration of the normal anatomical sites for the parathyroids fails to reveal the cause for the hypercalcaemia, a methodical dissection of both sides of the neck is undertaken. Abnormal localities for a missing upper parathyroid are looked for first, starting in the vicinity of the upper pole vessels to the thyroid and then the tracheo-oesophageal groove from just below the cricoid cartilage to the posterior mediastinum. This requires careful, bloodless dissection, opening up the space between the trachea and the oesophagus. Care must be taken to avoid damage to the recurrent laryngeal nerve, especially in the mediastinum as it crosses the thyro-thymic ligament. Next, the retro-oesophageal prevertebral space is dissected, remembering that the more cranial and caudal the ectopic site, the more lateral it is likely to be. Next, the carotid sheath is opened and inspected. When the lower parathyroid is missing, or indeed if four normal parathyroids have been identified in a well-documented case of primary hyperparathyroidism, then it is highly probable that the missing fourth or fifth gland will be within the thymus, notably in the anterior horns as they run up towards the lower pole of the thyroid as the thyro-thymic ligaments. Careful inspection of these often identifies the missing parathyroid tumour, even when deeply embedded (if well stained). Routine cervical thymectomy is not advocated for possible fifth-gland disease when one adenoma has already been located but it is recommended when three or four normal glands have been found while a lower parathyroid is still missing. In similar circumstances there is also some justification for performing a 'blind' thyroid lobectomy since up to 7 per cent of missing parathyroid tumours are intrathyroidal. However, careful examination of the thyroid may well reveal suspicious bulging of the false capsule which is well worth uncovering by opening up the clefts between the lobules in the vicinity. Local discoloration, especially if the patient has been prepared with methylene blue, may

again focus the attention of the surgeon to a suspicious area.

The second problem relates to the amount of parathyroid tissue that needs to be removed. Two important basic principles apply: never resect normal glands if the tumour cannot be found and always consider abnormally large glands to be pathological, regardless of the histology. These should be removed in whole or in part, depending on the presence or otherwise of other normal glands. When all four glands are enlarged, due to hyperplasia, a subtotal resection is performed and 30 mg left of the least enlarged gland, i.e. equivalent to the weight of one normal parathyroid. It is important that the remnant is well vascularized and the site is marked with a metal clip or non-degradable suture such as silk. If the viability is dubious or if the gland would be difficult to locate at a future operation, or when the chances of recurrent disease are increased (as in familial hyperparathyroidism, or one of the multiple endocrine adenosis syndromes), then parathyroid transplantation should be considered (see below).

3. Surgery for Secondary Hyperparathyroidism

The operative approach is identical to that described for primary hyperparathyroidism and, generally, there is less difficulty in identifying the parathyroids since all four are uniformly enlarged and hyperplastic. However, occasional asymmetrical hyperplasia is seen and mistakenly reported as multiple adenomas. As a consequence of the patient's renal status, the tissues generally are more friable and oedematous and bleeding is more likely to be due to associated hypertension. The standard approach is to remove three and a half glands and leave a half of one gland in situ with a good vascular supply. This remnant is marked with a metal clip or non-absorbable suture and a recording made of the precise location on a suitable drawing of the operative field for inclusion in the patient's records. Total parathyroidectomy and lifelong support with 1-alpha-cholecalciferol and calcium are inadvisable as these may result in pure osteomalacia in patients with uraemia secondary to chronic renal failure. A viable alternative, popularized by Wells et al. (1975), is to perform a total parathyroidectomy and then autotransplant some of the parathyroid tissue into the forearm. This site is preferred to the sternocleidomastoid as it provides ready access if the secondary hyperparathyroidism persists or recurs and further parathyroid tissue needs to be removed. Once the parathyroids have been removed and confirmed histologically, the tissue is placed in chilled tissue culture medium (Hants' or Waymouth's RPMI 1640 or saline at 4°). The pot containing the medium is placed on an ice bath—a sterile drape over a splash bowl containing crushed ice—and then time allowed for the tissue to become firm. One of the parathyroids is then diced on a flat surface into 1 mm cubes with a scalpel, 50–60 mg of tissue being

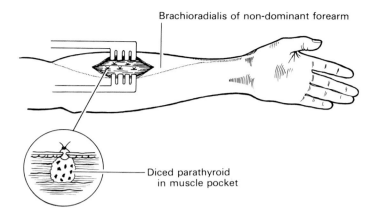

Brachioradialis of non-dominant forearm

Diced parathyroid
in muscle pocket

Fig. 24.14. Transplantation of the diced parathyroid gland into a forearm muscle.

implanted into three or more separate muscle pockets in the brachioradialis of the non-dominant forearm (*Fig.* 24.14). This is a delicate task, requiring fine instruments, and strict attention to haemostasis, otherwise haematoma formation will threaten the viability of the fragments. Each pocket is closed with a fine, easily recognizable, non-absorbable suture, such as Prolene or Tevdek, to prevent extrusion and ready recognition if re-exploration is required. Obviously, if the patient's serum calcium demonstrates only a transient fall there must be concern about a supernumerary gland in the neck or mediastinum which is an argument for delayed autotransplantation. The patient is protected against early or late graft failure by cryopreservation of the remaining excised parathyroid tissue.

Technique
The parathyroids are sliced into $1 \times 1 \times 3$-mm slices and placed in polypropylene vials containing chilled tissue culture medium (80 per cent RPMI 1640) with added glutamine-penicillin-streptomycin and 19 per cent dimethyl sulphoxide (DMSO) and 10 per cent autologous serum. It is important that freezing starts soon after addition of the parathyroid tissue, otherwise the DMSO warms and becomes toxic. The vials are then placed in a freezing chamber and controlled freezing is performed at $-1\,°C/min$, down to $-80\,°C$ for storage in a liquid nitrogen freezer. If hyperparathyroidism develops after grafting, then cryopreserved tissue is thawed in a $37\,°C$ bath until all the crystals have disappeared and then washed straightaway with cold RPMI 1640 culture medium, under strict aseptic conditions. Successful transplantation of cryopreserved parathyroid tissue has been reported after 18 months of cryopreservation (Wells et al., 1977).

4. Surgery after Failed Cervical Exploration for Hyperparathyroidism

This is a challenging situation for both the surgeon and the frequently disillusioned patient. The problem immediately brings into question the validity of the diagnosis of hyperparathyroidism and the experience of the surgeon undertaking the first operation. It is a fact that occasional explorers have a much higher incidence of persistent or recurrent hypercalcaemia but these tend not to be published. The most vigorous appraisal of previous biochemical data, pathology reports and the operative details is the first requirement. Particular enquiry needs to be made into the possibility of previously unsuspected malignancy or sarcoid. Where there is a history of several members of a family with unsuccessful parathyroid operations, the possibility of familial hypocalciuric hypercalcaemia needs to be borne in mind (Marx et al., 1980). This syndrome has been implicated in 9 per cent of patients with failed neck explorations (Marx et al., 1980). Multiple gland disease may be responsible for more than one-third of the rest and efforts must be made to identify individuals affected by familial hyperparathyroid or one of the multiple endocrine adenosis syndromes. Where the general health of the patient and severity of their disease call for reoperation, localization studies are thoroughly appropriate for this particular category of patient, especially if the first exploration was performed by a surgeon experienced in parathyroid surgery. Local facilities and experience of a specific localizing technique will usually dictate which one is used, but selective venous sampling (Dunlop et al., 1980), arteriography (Brennan et al., 1982) and computer-assisted double isotope subtraction scanning, using thallium and technetium (Young et al., 1983), Have proved most helpful. Guided by localization data, surgical attention may be directed back to the neck or into the chest for the first time. Where there is doubt about the completeness of neck exploration, the only course is to re-explore and proceed as for the strategy outlined for a difficult case (p. 341), checking methodically all possible sites. If the mediastinum is to be explored, then this is done by splitting the sternum as for a retrosternal goitre (*see* p. 333).

5. Surgery for Parathyroid Carcinoma

This rare tumour accounts for less than 5 per cent of all cases of hyperparathyroidism (Shantz and Castleman, 1973). Failure to recognize the underlying cause of the disease therefore can, and does, occur with potentially lethal consequences. The surgeon should be alerted to the possibility of the diagnosis preoperatively if the serum calcium is appreciably elevated, i.e. greater than 3·5 mmol/L and especially if levels such as these are recorded in the presence of a palpable mass in the anterior triangle of the neck. It is at operation, however, that an experienced parathyroid surgeon realizes that the parathyroid enlargement responsible for the hypercalcaemia could be malignant. In contrast to a typical adenoma which is soft, deep slate blue (if infused preoperatively with vital dye) and has a delicate capsule, freely dissectable from the local structures, carcinomas are firmer, greyish-white and adherent. Sometimes there is extensive invasion locally. The surgical management recommended is block dissection of the tumour plus all involved soft tissues. Not infrequently an ipsilateral thyroid lobectomy is required to achieve this. Great care must be taken to avoid rupture of the tumour capsule since spillage of cancer cells may lead to local recurrence. All clinically involved lymph nodes should be included in the surgical excision. It is suggested that the strong predilection for local recurrence may be eliminated by postoperative localized external beam radiotherapy (Lilliemoe and Dudley, 1985).

Postoperative Care

This is identical to that described for a patient recovering from routine thyroidectomy with special emphasis on the need to check the serum calcium daily. This is necessary to monitor the anticipated fall to within the normal range, which should be seen within 48 hours with stabilization over a further 48-hour period. Bleeding is rarely a problem, due to the meticulous haemostasis advocated for the procedure so the drains can safely be removed on the 2nd postoperative day. A routine cord check by the anaesthetist on extubation suffices unless particular difficulties have been encountered which might have hazarded the recurrent laryngeal nerve.

Postoperative Complications

Haemorrhage, nerve paresis and the wound complications described for thyroid surgery can all occur and are dealt with accordingly. The main problem after surgery for hyperparathyroidism, however, is failure to achieve normal calcium homeostasis. Persistent hypercalcaemia immediately postoperatively challenges the original diagnosis, the accuracy of the intraoperative histology reporting and may raise the possibility of a pathological (probably ectopic) fifth gland. Patients who are initially normocalcaemic, but become hypercalcaemic again within 6 months, are likely to have had disturbance of blood supply to an abnormal residual gland or glands which has become revascularized and then hormonally active again. An alternative possibility is inadequate excision for four-gland disease. The measures required to investigate all of these hypercalcaemic problems are dealt with earlier (p. 339).

Hypocalcaemia is a much more frequent complication and is encountered in three situations. First, and most commonly, where a large, active adenoma has been removed, the remaining suppressed parathyroids may take several weeks to become fully functional again. Hypocalcaemia in this instance is rarely profound and readily corrected. Second, a prolonged, difficult exploration for ectopic parathyroids with multiple biopsies may inadvertently disturb the blood supply to the normal glands with or without recovery of their function. The third and most predictable cause of postoperative hypocalcaemia is in the 5–10 per cent of patients who have suffered prolonged hyperparathyroid bone disease and have radiological evidence of osteitis. As soon as their parathyroid tumours are removed, switching off the parathyroid drive, demineralized bone rapidly absorbs vast quantities of calcium ('bone hunger'). If this surge of calcium from the systemic circulation to the bones is not anticipated, hypocalcaemia will be profound, the patient exhibiting signs and symptoms of tetany. Some of the patients also have magnesium deficiency requiring replacement. The dietary and systemic measures of providing calcium to correct hypocalcaemia in each of these three situations are discussed earlier (p. 339). In extreme cases 20 ml of 10 per cent calcium gluconate may need to be given hourly via intravenous infusion for 7–10 days and oral l-alpha-hydroxycholecalciferol in doses as high as 8–10 μg/day over several weeks.

REFERENCES

Aurbach G. D., Mallette L. E., Patten B. M. et al. (1973) Hyperparathyroidism: recent studies. *Ann. Intern. Med.* **79**, 566–581.

Barnes H. V. and Gann D. S. (1974) Choosing thyroidectomy in hyperthyroidism. *Surg. Clin. North Am.* **54**, 289.

Brennan M. F., Doppman J. L., Krudy A. G. et al. (1982) Assessment of techniques for parathyroid gland localization in patients undergoing re-operation for hyperparathyroidism. *Surgery* **91**, 6.

Crile G., Jr (1957) The fallacy of the conventional neck dissection for papillary carcinoma of the thyroid. *Ann. Surg.* **145**, 317.

Dennison A., Ball M. and Dudley N. (1985) Preoperative percutaneous localisation of parathyroid tumours; a preliminary report. *Ann. R. Coll. Surg. Engl.* **67**, 276.

Dudley N. E. (1971) Methylene blue for the rapid identification of the parathyroids. *Br. Med. J.* **iii**, 680.

Duffy B. J., Jr and Fitzgerald P. J. (1950) Cancer of the thyroid in children. *J. Clin. Endocrinol. Metab.* **10**, 1296–1308.

Dunlop D. A. B., Papapoulos S. E., Lodge R. W. et al. (1980) Parathyroid venous sampling: anatomic considerations and results in 95 patients with primary hyperparathyroidism. *Br. J. Radiol.* **53**, 183.

Gilmour J. R. (1938) The gross anatomy of the parathyroid glands. *J. Pathol. Bacteriol.* **46**, 133–149.

Gordon P. R. Huves A. G. and Strong E. W. (1973) Medullary carcinoma of the thyroid gland. *Cancer* **31**, 915.

Hamberger B., Gharib H., Melton L. J. et al. (1985) Fine needle aspiration biopsy of thyroid nodules. Impact on thyroid practice and cost of care. *Ann. J. Med.* (in press).

Hazard J. B., Hawk W. A. and Crile G., Jr (1959) Medullary (solid) carcinoma of the thyroid: a clinico-pathological entity. *J. Clin. Endocrinol.* **19**, 153–161.

Heath H., III, Hodgson S. F. and Kennedy M. A. (1980) Primary hyperparathyroidism incidence, morbidity and potential impact in a community. *N. Engl. J. Med.* **302**, 189–193.

Hedley A. J., Michie W., Duncan T. et al. (1972) The effect of remnant size on the outcome of subtotal thyroidectomy for thyrotoxicosis. *Br. J. Surg.* **59**, 559–563.

Hollingshead W. H. (1952) Anatomy of the endocrine glands. *Surg. Clin. North Am.* **32**, 1115–1140.

Kaplan R. A., Snyder W. M. Stewart A. et al. (1976) Metabolic effects of parathyroidectomy in asymptomatic primary hyperparathyroidism. *J. Clin. Endocrinol. Metab.* **42**, 415–426.

Kark A. E., Kissim M. W., Auerbach R. et al. (1984) Voice changes after thyroidectomy: role of the external laryngeal nerve. *Br. med. J.* **289**, 1412–1415.

Lilliemoe K. and Dudley N. E. (1985) Parathyroid carcinoma—pointers to successful management. *Ann. R. Coll. Surg. Engl.* (in press).

Livesay J. J. and Mulder D. G. (1976) Recurrent hyperparathyroidism. *Arch. Surg.* **iii**, 688.

McGeown M. G. (1961) Effect of parathyroidectomy on the incidence of renal calculi. *Lancet* **i**, 586–587.

Marx S. J., Stock J. L. Attie M. F. et al. (1980) Familial hypocalciuric hypercalcaemia: recognition among patients referred after unsuccessful parathyroid exploration. *Ann. Intern. Med.* **92**, 951.

Murley R. S. and Rigg B. M. (1968) Post-operative thyroid function and complications in relation to a measured thyroid remnant. *Br. J. Surg.* **55**, 757–760.

Naeye R. L. and Terrien C. M. (1960) Haemorrhagic state after therapy with propylthiouracil. *Am. J. Clin. Pathol.* **34**, 254–257.

Neil H. B., III, Townsend G. L. and Devine K. D. (1972) Bilateral vocal cord paralysis of undetermined aetiology: clinical course and outcome. *Ann. Otol. Rhinol. Laryngol.* **81**, 514–519.

Peden N. R., Gunn A. and Browning M. C. K. (1982) Nadolol and potassium iodine in combination in the surgical treatment of thyrotoxicosis. *Br. J. Surg.* **69**, 638–641.

Proye C. (1978) Exploration parathyroididienne pour hyperparathyroidie. *J. Chir.* (Paris) **115**, 101.

Purnell D. C., Scholtz D. A., Smith L. H. et al. (1974) Treatment of primary hyperparathyroidism. *Am. J. Med.* **56**, 800–809.

Roediger W. E. W. (1976) Thyroidectomy for non-familial medullary carcinoma. *Br. J. Surg.* **63**, 343–345.

Rose N. (1963) Investigation of post-thyroidectomy patients for hypoparathyroidism. *Lancet* **i**, 124–127.

Rowntree T. (1973) Parathyroid—a personal series. *J. R. Soc. Med.* **73**, 14.

Russell C. F., van Heerden J. A., Sizemore G. W. et al. (1983) The surgical management of medullary thyroid carcinoma. *Ann. Surg.* **197**, 42–48.

Russell W. O., Ibanez M. L., Clark R. L. et al. (1963) Thyroid carcinoma classification. Intraglandular dissection and clinicopathological study based upon whole organ section of 80 glands. *Cancer* **16**, 1425–1460.

Shantz A. and Castleman B. (1973) Parathyroid carcinoma. A study of 70 cases. *Cancer* **31**, 600–605.

Sizemore G. W., Carney J. A. and Heath H., III (1977) Epidemiology of medullary carcinoma of the thyroid gland: a 5 year experience (1971–1976). *Surg. Clin. North Am.* **57**, 633–645.

Smith I. and Murley R. S. (1965) Damage to the cervical sympathetic system during operation on the thyroid gland. *Br. J. Surg.* **52**, 673.

Tibblin S., Bondeson A. G. and Ljungberg O. (1982) Unilateral parathyroidectomy due to single adenoma. *Ann. Surg.* **195**, 245–252.

Wade J. S. H. (1983) The management of malignant thyroid tumours. *Br. J. Surg.* **70**, 253–255.

Wells S. A., Gunnells J. C., Gutman R. A. et al. (1975) Transplantation of the parathyroid glands in man. Clinical indication and results. *Surgery* **78**, 34–44.

Wells S. A., Gunnells J. C., Gutman R. A. et al. (1977) The successful transplantation of frozen parathyroid tissue in man. *Surgery* **81**, 86.

Wilder W. T., Frame B. and Haubrich W. S. (1961) Peptic ulcer in primary hyperparathyroidism: an analysis of 52 cases. *Ann. Intern. Med.* **55,** 885–893.

Young A. E., Grant J. I., Croft D. N. et al. (1983) Location of parathyroid adenomas by thallium-201 and technetium-99^m subtraction scanning. *Br. Med. J.* **286**, 1384.

Chapter twenty-five

The Salivary Glands

R. W. Hiles

THE PAROTID GLAND

Surgical Anatomy (*Figs.* 25.1–25.3)

The surface markings of the boundaries of the parotid gland are the zygomatic arch *above*, the anterior margin of the auricle together with the mastoid process *behind*, and a line drawn from the tip of the mastoid process to the angle of the jaw *below*. *In front*, the gland may extend as far as the anterior border of the masseter muscle, which is readily felt when the teeth are clenched. The line of the parotid duct can be drawn from the lower border of the tragus of the ear towards a point midway between the base of the ala of the nose and the upper limit of the upper lip vermilion. It occupies the middle third of this line and opens on the buccal mucous membrane opposite the second maxillary molar tooth.

The gland is wedged deeply between the mastoid process and the external auditory meatus behind and the posterior border of the mandible in front. The base of this wedge lies outwards and extends forwards over the masseter muscle and constitutes the superficial lobe. The thin edge of the wedge is usually called the deep lobe and extends upwards to reach the glenoid fossa behind the temporomandibular joint. Behind the gland, the mastoid process is sandwiched between the sternomastoid and the deeper digastric muscle. In front the mandible is sandwiched between the masseter outside and the medial pterygoid muscle inside. The accessory portion of the gland lies on the masseter muscle, between the parotid duct and the bone of the zygomatic arch.

The gland is enclosed within a sheath of fascia so that tension and pain are produced when the gland swells. On the surface of the parotid beneath this fascia lymph nodes lie on and in the superficial substance of the gland. Three other structures pass through the gland; the most superficial is the facial nerve with its several divisions and terminal branches. More deeply lies the posterior facial vein and deeper still the external carotid artery. The deepest narrowed edge of the wedge-shaped gland lies against the internal jugular vein. The upper part of this deep portion of the gland is also in contact with the auriculotemporal nerve which gives the gland its secretomotor branch from the otic ganglion.

Blood is supplied to the gland by branches from the external carotid artery and returns via the posterior facial vein. Lymphatic drainage is first to the glands within the parotid and then on to the antero-superior group of the deep cervical lymph glands.

When the gland has been removed, its bed is seen to be made up posteriorly of the posterior belly of

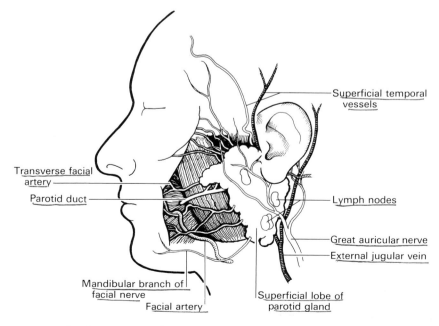

Transverse facial artery

Parotid duct

Mandibular branch of facial nerve

Facial artery

Superficial temporal vessels

Lymph nodes

Great auricular nerve

External jugular vein

Superficial lobe of parotid gland

Fig. 25.1. The superficial lobe of the parotid gland and its relations.

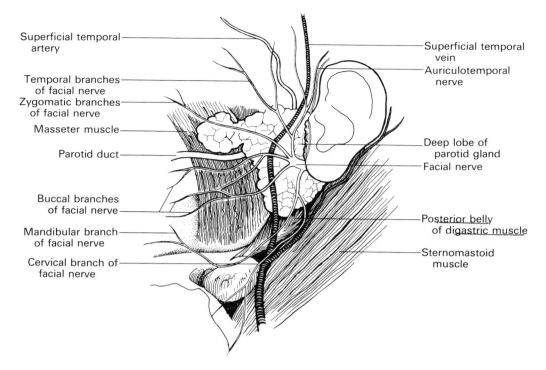

Fig. 25.2. The facial nerve in the parotid gland.

the digastric, the styloid process of the temporal bone and the stylohyoid muscle arising from it. Deep to these is the internal jugular vein passing downwards over the lateral mass of the atlas and being crossed by the accessory nerve. Anteriorly, not quite in touch with the gland, is the internal carotid artery crossed by the tip of the styloid process above and the glossopharyngeal nerve lying on the stylopharyngeus muscle below.

The most important structure in surgery of the parotid gland is the facial nerve. It emerges from the stylomastoid foramen with the digastric muscle origin below and lateral and the root of the styloid process and the tympanomastoid sulcus above and deep. The main trunk of the nerve commonly divides, after a variable distance, into two main divisions and subsequently into branches going to five main areas: temporal, zygomatic, buccal, mandibular and cervical. The mandibular branch is notable in that it emerges from the lower border of the parotid gland passing below the angle of the mandible into the neck. Later it crosses the inferior border of the mandible lying on the facial artery, running upwards into the face again to supply the depressor muscles at the angle of the mouth. There are considerable variations in the pattern of divisions and branches of the nerve, with numerous cross-connections between them. It is best never to take the anatomy of the nerve divisions for granted and to dissect each nerve as if it was the first ever to have been followed.

Special Investigations

Simple radiographs of the parotid area will often reveal calculi but those in the deep lobe are sometimes obscured by the irregular opacities of the skeletal outlines.

Sialography is particularly relevant to the diagnosis of chronic parotitis and duct stenosis, when sialectasis may be evident. It is of little practical value in the differential diagnosis of masses in the parotid area as these almost invariably warrant exploration and resection.

More sophisticated *tests of salivary function* involving the collection, measurement and analysis of salivary fluid from the duct are rarely used in busy surgical practice, although specific findings are documented.

Needle aspiration biopsy is used by some to give a preoperative tumour diagnosis but many consider that, since the commonest parotid tumour (pleomorphic adenoma) shows itself able to seed so readily, this breach of the tumour's integrity is unwise and indeed unnecessary as careful surgical exploration will be necessary anyway in most cases.

Operations

Before any operation on the parotid gland the patient should be warned that the facial nerve is at risk. Also they should be warned that, if adequate tumour treatment demands it, all or part of the nerve may have to be sacrificed.

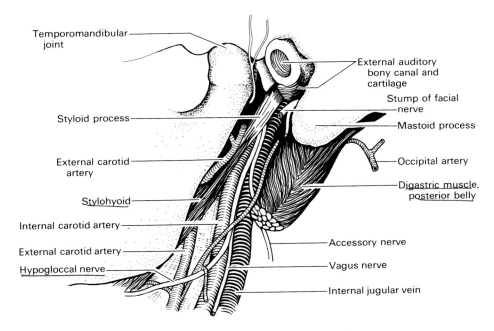

Fig. 25.3. The deep bed of the parotid gland.

Labels in figure:
Temporomandibular joint
Styloid process
External carotid artery
Stylohyoid
Internal carotid artery
External carotid artery
Hypogloccal nerve
External auditory bony canal and cartilage
Stump of facial nerve
Mastoid process
Occipital artery
Digastric muscle, posterior belly
Accessory nerve
Vagus nerve
Internal jugular vein

Incision of Abscess

Acute suppurative parotitis is now quite rare except when patients suffering from other conditions, such as intestinal obstruction or typhoid fever, are allowed to become dehydrated. Prevention is better than cure.

Early infection can be successfully treated with systemic antibiotics but once suppuration is established surgical drainage becomes necessary. If the abscess is already pointing incision is best made directly through the skin at the site of pointing. Once through the skin and the abscess entered and drained, the incision should only be enlarged in a transverse direction so as to minimize the risk of damage to the facial nerve. If no pus is pointing but the gland remains swollen and tender, the parotid is explored through a skin incision as for superficial parotidectomy, the parotid fascia is incised transversely and the gland probed with blunt instruments to release any loculi of pus. The wound is closed loosely with drainage.

Removal of Calculi

Parotid stones are not common and are usually situated deep within the gland. If in the main duct and palpable from the mouth, they can be removed by an approach from the mucosal aspect, slitting open the duct longitudinally. Calculi within the gland are often multiple and if producing symptoms will require parotidectomy. They may occur in association with chronic parotitis.

Exploration of the Gland

Any firm painless mass in the parotid gland is an indication for exploration in the absence of any evidence of systemic disease. Haemangioma, cyst and lipoma all occur occasionally and can usually be diagnosed clinically by compressibility, fluctuance and non-fluctuant softness respectively. Occasionally malignant tumours are found within, or in association with, cysts having a short history. If large and troublesome any of these benign tumours may require formal excision. This can be done using an incision as for superficial parotidectomy and then dissecting out the tumour with due regard to preservation of the integrity of the facial nerve.

Enucleation of Mixed Salivary Tumours

This is mentioned only to be dismissed, as it carries with it a high risk of 'seeding' the operative wound with tumour cells, which may subsequently produce multiple recurrences which are difficult to resect.

Superficial Parotidectomy

This operation is carried out for any firm tumour involving the superficial portion of the gland in the absence of preoperative facial paralysis. Such a tumour usually proves to be pleomorphic adenoma, but less commonly adenolymphoma or early carcinoma is encountered. Rarely, in the course of developing the dissection for superficial parotidectomy, it is discovered that the tumour is a neurilemmoma affecting the facial nerve. Such a tumour is best dissected meticulously from the nerve, if necessary using microsurgical techniques, so as to preserve as much nerve function as possible consistent with total removal of the neurilemmoma. Occasionally pleomorphic adenoma is small, only occupying a small portion of the superficial parotid. In these cases localized resection of the parotid can be performed provided that great care is taken not to breach the integrity of the capsule of the tumour, which would invite recurrence. If in doubt, a formal superficial parotidectomy should be carried out.

Surgical Procedure

Anaesthesia

Parotid surgery should always be performed under general anaesthesia because it is imperative that the patient should be absolutely still and the procedure can be sometimes lengthy.

The anaesthetist is asked not to use any long-acting muscle relaxant which would make it impossible to check on facial nerve function with a nerve stimulator during operation.

It is a great advantage to have a relatively bloodless field which can add to the safety and speed with which the facial nerve can be dissected. This can be achieved with the technique of hypotensive anaesthesia which is safely induced by experienced anaesthetists. Similar operative conditions can be achieved by the infiltration of a solution of adrenaline (1 in 250 000) into the operative area. This should be done by the surgeon at least 5 minutes before beginning the dissection.

Position

The patient is placed supine on the operating table with the head supported by a rubber ring and turned to the contralateral side. Slight head-up tilt of the whole body prevents venous congestion in the operative field. The head is towelled with the whole face exposed so that muscle activity can be observed when the facial nerve is stimulated.

Exposure

The main limb of the incision runs in the preauricular skin crease and is extended upwards above the ear running slightly anteriorly within the temporal scalp. Downwards, the incision is carried around the lobe of the ear to run posteriorly in the postauricular groove for 2–3 cm. The incision is then angled acutely downwards and forwards to form a flap of skin over the mastoid process and then runs approximately two finger-breadths below the angle of the mandible, preferably in a convenient skin crease. Incision should extend at least as far as the anterior border of the sternomastoid (Fig. 25.4).

The skin anterior to this irregularly curved incision is then raised at a level just deep to the subcutaneous fat. Flap edges are held by fine skin hooks and the correct level for developing this flap dissection can often be seen best by tenting the skin towards the

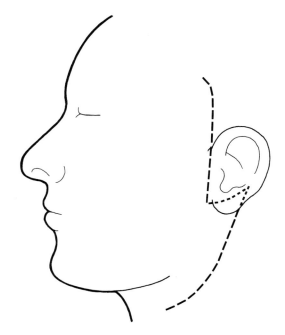

Fig. 25.4. Skin incision to approach the parotid gland.

operator. A thin whitish fornix of air-filled fascia will develop between the subcutaneous fat and a layer of fat of variable thickness which lies on the parotid fascia. Meticulous haemostasis is carried out with the tips of the diathermy forceps so as to keep the operative field unstained with blood. The skin is dissected as far anteriorly as just beyond the anterior border of the masseter, superiorly to just above the zygomatic arch and inferiorly to expose the upper part of the anterior triangle of the neck (*Fig.* 25.5).

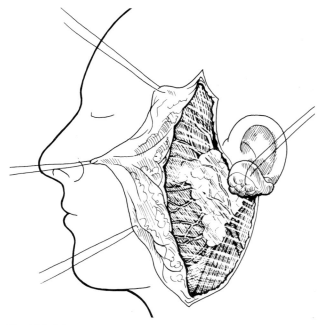

Fig. 25.5. Dissection of the anterior skin flap to reveal the parotid gland.

Dissection

A deeply penetrating natural fascial plane is then opened up running medially between the anterior cartilage of the external auditory meatus and the parotid, in the preauricular groove. This plane will readily open up with blunt dissection. Sharp dissection is then used to extend this plane deep to the ear lobe, inferior to the external auditory meatus and on to the base of the mastoid process. Thence, the deep dissection proceeds downwards along the anterosuperior border of the sternomastoid, thus raising the extreme posterolateral 'corner' of the parotid gland (*Fig.* 25.6). It may be necessary to divide the

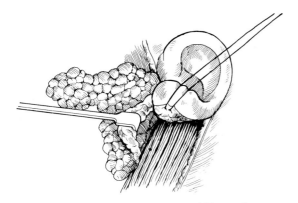

Fig. 25.6. Elevation of the parotid 'corner'.

great auricular sensory nerve. The deeper plane of dissection can be developed with relative safety above and below the mastoid and is then developed with caution in the angle between the cartilage of the external auditory meatus and the anterosuperior aspect of the mastoid process. The small posterior auricular artery is almost invariably encountered, divided and ligated before reaching the vicinity of the main trunk of the facial nerve as it emerges from the stylomastoid foramen (*Fig.* 25.7). Retraction of the parotid gland should be done with great gentleness, otherwise traction forces may be transmitted to the facial nerve and can cause axonal damage.

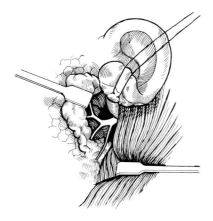

Fig. 25.7. Exposure of the facial nerve.

The nerve is usually covered with a thin fascial sheath which has to be entered before the nerve can be seen clearly. When in the vicinity of where the nerve should be, it often helps to use a nerve stimulator which can detect its position accurately, even before it can be seen. It is necessary to be able to recognize in detail the several distinctive anatomical landmarks in the region of the stylomastoid foramen in order to approach the nerve with careful confidence and not too much anxiety. If the anteroinferior extremity of the conchal cartilage is sought, as it forms the support of the inferior wall of the membranous part of the external auditory canal, it will be seen to form the shape of an arrowhead which points to the nerve. Deep to the tip of this cartilage is the rim of the bony external auditory canal. This rim sits alongside the base of the mastoid process forming a groove between the two which leads downwards in a very short distance to the stylomastoid foramen and the main trunk of the facial nerve emerging from it. If the styloid process can be identified just superior and deep, even merely by touch, this will add confirmation to the supposition that the surgeon is in the right place and looking at the right nerve. The posterior facial vein will be lying deep to the main trunk.

Once the main trunk of the facial nerve has been identified and confirmed by stimulation, the superficial parotid can then be methodically removed as the trunk is traced forwards to its division and branches. Separation of the parotid gland from the nerve can only be achieved with safety by gentle and meticulously accurate dissection. The nerve must not be traumatized by traction or crushing, nor by disturbance of its delicate blood supply which can often be seen running along the epineurium. Small, fine, blunt, curved scissors are used superficial to the nerve by introducing them closed, pushing them gently between the nerve and the superficial parotid in an anterior direction and then gently opening the blades (*Fig.* 25.8). With patience the whole of the nerve can be displayed in this way. Occasionally, fine filaments of nerve, usually cross-connections between the divisions or branches, will be so closely adherent to tumour that it is wiser to sacrifice them, provided they are small. The functional deficit will be barely detectable paresis, postoperatively. As the dissection proceeds anteriorly, the nerve branches become more and more superficial and they often appear to take an abrupt turn laterally as they reach and cross the masseter. It is at this point that they are often most vulnerable to surgical injury, when confidence is running high. Once the anterior border of the masseter has been reached, the plane of the deep dissection can be cautiously joined to that of the subcutaneous dissection, for the superficial parotid and its contained, intact tumour will have been resected (*Figs.* 25.9, 25.10).

Meticulous haemostasis is then secured taking care not to include finer branches of the facial nerve in

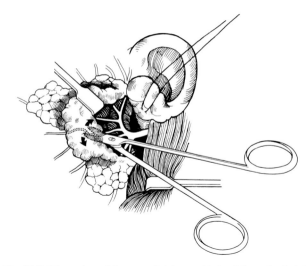

Fig. 25.8. Dissection of the superficial parotid gland from the facial nerve branches without traction.

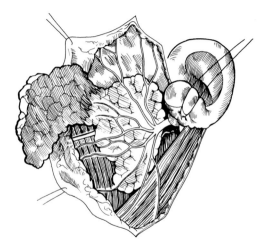

Fig. 25.9. Superficial parotid gland almost resected.

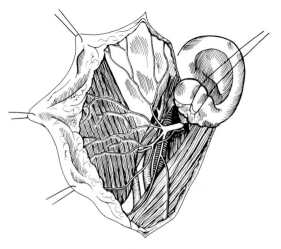

Fig. 25.10. The surgical field after total parotidectomy with preservation of the facial nerve.

ligatures or diathermy points. The wound is drained by a fine perforated plastic tube to a closed suction drainage bottle (*Fig.* 25.11). Skin closure is effected

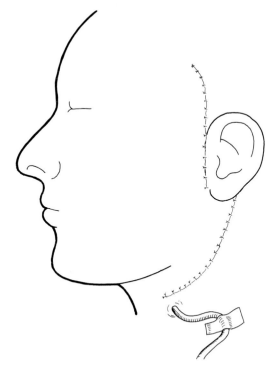

Fig. 25.11. Skin closure with suction drainage of the parotid bed.

with interrupted 6/0 absorbable sutures. If fine, subcutaneous, absorbable sutures are also used, skin sutures can be removed early (after 3 or 4 days) and suture cross-hatch scars of the skin avoided. Suction is maintained until the aspirate is minimal, usually for 2–4 days. The drain is then withdrawn.

Postoperative Complications

1. *Facial Nerve Injury*

2. *Fistulas*

Occasionally salivary fistulas will occur through the scar of the incision but the majority of these close spontaneously. A short course of Pro-Banthine (propantheline) will reduce salivary flow and aid spontaneous closure if used at the first sign of trouble. It is rare for fistulas to persist, but if this happens either the residual parotid is resected or the fistula is dissected out and drained into the mouth.

3. *Auriculotemporal (or gustatory sweating) syndrome (Frey's syndrome)*

This is not uncommon several months after parotidectomy. The patient experiences sweating of the skin over the site of the parotidectomy while eating. It is generally considered to be due to inappropriate innervation of the cutaneous sweat glands by the secretomotor fibres which have regenerated from the divided ends of the auriculotemporal nerve and which previously supplied the resected parotid. Once the syndrome is explained, most patients are able to tolerate it and fortunately the severity of the symptoms tends to diminish over a number of years. Surgical treatment aimed at more central disconnection of the secretomotor fibres is usually reserved for extremely severe cases and is not always of lasting benefit.

Total Parotidectomy with Preservation of the Facial Nerve

Indications
Neoplastic indications for this operation are multiple benign tumours, large benign tumours in the deep portion of the gland and early and low-grade malignant tumours with no or very limited involvement of the facial nerve branches. In the latter case the preservation of the facial nerve is incomplete.

Perhaps the most difficult and hazardous parotidectomy is that required to treat chronic parotitis where the nerve is engulfed in scarred parenchyma.

Surgical Technique
The skin flap is raised as for superficial parotidectomy and the main trunk of the facial nerve identified. If the tumour is large and deep, direct access to the main trunk of the facial nerve may be difficult and it can be easier to find the mandibular branch in the lower part of the operative field in the neck. (This can prove difficult and hazardous for the inexperienced operator.) Once this branch is found it can be traced posteriorly, which will lead to the main inferior division and eventually the main trunk. It is imperative that the nerve be handled extremely gently. Its trunk, divisions and branches all need to be separated from the parotid tissue deep as well as superficial to it and have to be gently retracted from side to side in order to deliver the deep portion of the gland. If there is any danger of reducing the adequate and clean clearance of a malignant tumour by striving to preserve the nerve intact, the nerve or offending part of it is best sacrificed. In order to resect the deep portion of the gland, the posterior facial vein and the external carotid artery have to be ligated at the points at which they leave and enter the gland. Before the gland can be separated anteriorly, the parotid duct is ligated and then divided as it dips behind the buccinator muscle.

Total Parotidectomy with Sacrifice of the Facial Nerve

Indications
Total clearance of the gland together with all its contained and some of its neighbouring structures is indicated when it holds a malignant tumour which is already involving the facial nerve and/or the structures bordering on the gland. Such a malignancy may have arisen in a pre-existing pleomorphic tumour and can be either squamous or adenocarcinoma. Another particularly aggressive tumour is the cylindroma (adenoid cystic carcinoma). More uncommonly an acinic carcinoma is encountered.

Surgical Technique
The positioning, approach and initial dissection are as for superficial parotidectomy. The external carotid artery is divided and ligated above the hypoglossal nerve and digastric muscle as it enters the parotid region. The approach may be complicated by involvement of other structures by the tumour, for instance skin or mandible, which must be removed.

Involved skin must be resected but there may be sufficient skin remaining to allow direct closure. Otherwise, skin flaps will be necessary such as a transposition flap from the neck or, in the male, a scalp flap.

If the mandible is involved, resection of the ascending ramus and angle, together with the attached muscles, may be required. It is sometimes possible to leave the anterior part of the ascending ramus and thus preserve the inferior dental nerves intact. The Gigli saw is passed from the angle of the mandible upwards along the medial aspect of the bone and posterolateral to the inferior dental nerve to reach the sigmoid notch. After section of the bone, the maxillary artery is divided and the condyle of the mandible detached from the glenoid fossa.

If a 5-mm length or more of the proximal stump of the main trunk of the facial nerve can be preserved, immediate nerve reconstruction can be carried out using sensory nerve, such as the great auricular, as a bridge graft. Because of the proximity of the tumour it may not be wise to take the nerve graft from the same side but one can readily be taken from the opposite neck. The graft is taken with an appropriate number of branches from any of the sensory cervical outflow nerve systems (C2 and C3). Nerve suture is carried out with 8/0 or 10/0 nylon, if necessary with the aid of an operating microscope. It is not yet established which technique of nerve suture gives the best regeneration but it has been known for many years that a simple cuff of interrupted fine epineural sutures can give gratifying results. The principle is to effect the most accurate apposition of the nerve ends that is possible while doing the minimum amount of damage to the axons, neurilemmal sheaths and their blood supply.

If cervical lymph node involvement is present or suspected, then total parotidectomy will be performed in continuity with a radical en bloc dissection of the cervical lymph nodes (*see* p. 356). In this case the internal jugular vein will be resected from the deep aspect of the bed of the parotid.

SUBMANDIBULAR GLAND

Surgical Anatomy

As its name suggests, this gland lies under the cover of the body of the mandible. It is cradled by the anterior belly of the digastric muscle in front, the insertion of the stylohyoid below and the stylomandibular ligament behind. Enclosed by deep fascia, it is covered by the skin and platysma and crossed superficially by the anterior facial vein and the mandibular branch of the facial nerve. Similar to the parotid, lymph nodes are found in association with it and a few embedded in it. The facial artery making its way to the face is embedded in a groove, at first in the deep and then in the lateral surface of the gland (*Fig.* 25.12).

The superficial part of the gland lies against the mylohyoid muscle and the nerve and vessels supply-

runs forwards in the floor of the mouth and passes to the opening on the summit of the sublingual papilla at the side of the base of the frenulum of the tongue. Posteriorly, the lingual nerve is above the duct but crosses it laterally at the anterior border of the hyoglossus to pass beneath the duct before turning forwards medially and upwards again into the tongue. The hypoglossal nerve is below the duct. Occasionally, a few small ducts from the sublingual gland, which lies alongside the anterior portion of the duct, open into it. The submandibular ganglion, from which the gland receives its secretomotor fibres, is found attached to the lingual nerve as it approaches the gland and its duct from above (*Fig.* 25.14).

Special Investigations

Simple radiography is the most useful investigation in the case of recurrent submandibular gland enlargement related to meals and will help locate any calculi that may be present. Stones in the duct can often be palpated in the floor of the mouth. Calculi within the glands sometimes have a low mineral content and they are not noticeably radio-opaque.

Sialography is of little value in submandibular disease.

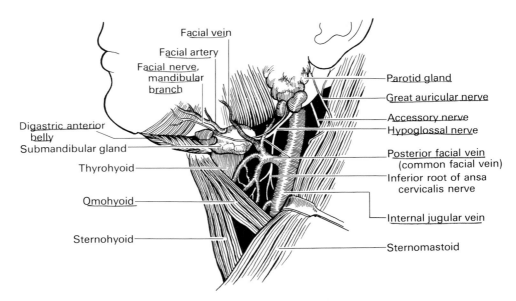

Fig. 25.12. Superficial relationships of the submandibular gland.

ing this muscle. The gland is then hooked around the posterior margin of the muscle so that its deep part rests between the medial aspect of this muscle laterally and the hyoglossus medially. On the hyoglossus its deep relations, in succession from above downwards, are the styloglossus, lingual nerve, submandibular ganglion, the hypoglossal nerve and the deep lingual vein (*Fig.* 25.13).

A 5-cm long duct, which emerges from the hilum of the gland at the posterior border of the mylohyoid,

Operations

Removal of Stone from the Duct (*Fig.* 25.15)

Operative removal of a stone can be carried out under local analgesia or with general anaesthesia. A retraction suture passed below the duct behind and in front of the stone traps it and facilitates longitudinal incision of the duct over it. The stone can then be readily delivered from the floor of the mouth and the open duct is left unsutured.

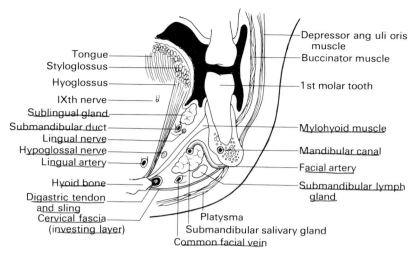

Fig. 25.13. A comprehensive view of the main relationships of the submandibular gland.

Removal of Calculus in the Hilum of the Gland

The whole gland and its duct should be resected in these cases.

Resection of Submandibular Salivary Gland

General anaesthesia is usually employed and the patient is positioned as for parotidectomy. An incision is made almost the whole length of the body of the mandible but some two finger-breadths below it. A convenient skin crease is used for preference (*Fig.* 25.16). Platysma is divided at a low level within the skin wound and elevated with care so as to avoid damaging the mandibular branch of the facial nerve which runs deep to the platysma in the upper part of the operative field. The facial artery and vein are divided and ligated as they reach the lower border of the mandible (at this point the mandibular branch of the facial nerve is particularly vulnerable but should be preserved) (*Fig.* 25.17). The common facial vein is located and divided posterior to the gland. The anterior margin of the sternomastoid muscle is dissected free and the facial artery is ligated again, below the submandibular gland, where it arises from the external carotid artery. The superficial portion of the gland will now be clear and can be dissected from the underlying mylohyoid muscle until the posterior margin of that muscle is reached and the hypo-

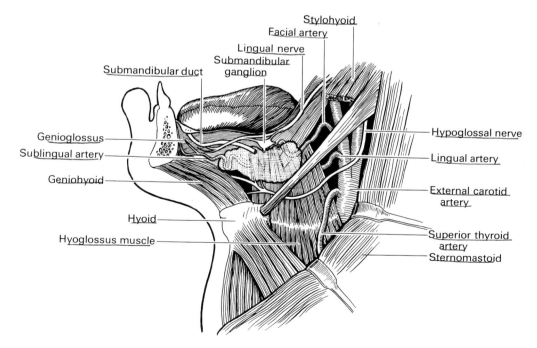

Fig. 25.14. A ghost of the resected submandibular gland showing its deep bed.

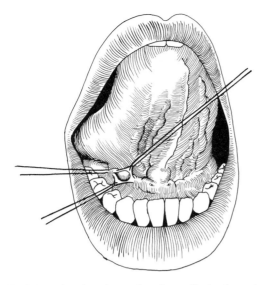

Fig. 25.15. Securing the release of a submandibular duct calculus.

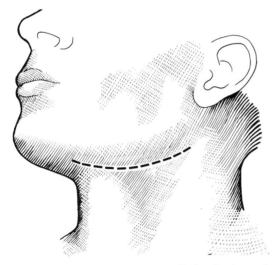

Fig. 25.16. Skin incision for submandibular gland resection.

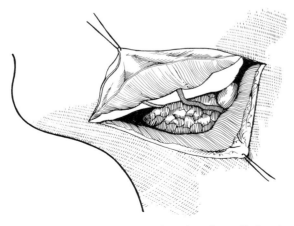

Fig. 25.17. The superficial approach to the submandibular gland. The mandibular branch of the facial nerve is preserved on the back of the platysma muscle sheet.

glossal nerve is preserved below the gland. The muscle border is then retracted and the deep part of the gland delivered by careful dissection to separate it from the lingual nerve above. The submandibular ganglion is then divided from the lingual nerve. Careful, complete haemostasis is achieved on the plexus of sublingual vessels in that area. The gland now remains attached only by its duct which is divided and ligated well forward in the floor of the mouth (*Fig.* 25.18).

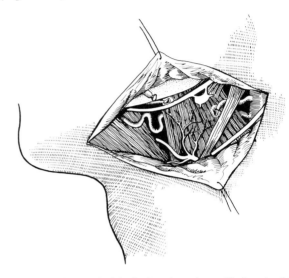

Fig. 25.18. The surgical bed after the submandibular gland has been resected.

The wound is closed with fine absorbable sutures to the platysma, taking care not to entrap the already carefully preserved mandibular branch of the facial nerves. A small corrugated or closed suction drain is inserted into the deep bed from which the gland has been removed. The skin is closed with 6/0 non-absorbable sutures. The drain can usually be removed in 24–48 hours.

Gland Resection for Tumour

Neoplasm occurs in the mandibular gland only one-tenth as frequently as in the parotid. Tumours can be benign (pleomorphic adenoma) or malignant. Pleomorphic adenoma and low-grade malignancy restricted to the gland are treated by resection as described for recurrent sialoadenitis and calculi within the glands.

Radical Resection for Aggressive Malignancy

In order to establish the diagnosis, an excision biopsy of the *total* gland may be necessary, with frozen section histology. If the aggressive nature of the tumour is evident by its short history and fixity, formal radical resection can be carried out *ab initio*, as the diagnosis is obvious. Local recurrence after the rare poorly differentiated tumours is common, distressing and difficult to treat, particularly if less than a radical operation has been performed. Full radical resection will often mean resection of the hemimandible on the affected side, full clearance of both submandibular triangles and an en bloc excision of the ipsilateral cervical lymph nodes. If involvement of the mucosa of the floor of the mouth is extensive, plastic surgical repair of the lining may be required using a forehead flap of skin based on the superficial temporal vessels. If neck skin is also involved and requires resection,

fresh cover may be required. Transposition neck flap is sometimes feasible but often a deltopectoral axial pattern skin flap or a myocutaneous pectoralis major flap will be necessary. A more sophisticated repair by composite free flap of iliac crest bone and groin skin can be used in suitable cases after radical clearance of tumour. Such a free flap is raised on the deep circumflex iliac artery and vein which is then divided and anastomosed, by microvascular technique, into a convenient neck artery of compatible size.

Chapter twenty-six

Block Dissection of the Glands of the Neck

R. T. Routledge

Surgical ablation of the lymph nodes and the lymphatic network remains the most effective method of controlling lymphatic metastases from primary tumours of the head and neck, despite recent claims of 'neck node control' by radiotherapy. The incidence of recurrent tumour after a skilfully performed radical neck dissection is extremely low and most recurrent problems in dealing with tumours of the head and neck relate to inadequate clearance of the primary.

INDICATIONS

The question is often posed, 'At what stage, when dealing with head and neck malignancies, should a neck node clearance be carried out?' We have learned, over the years, to be somewhat more selective and have concluded that bigger and better operations do not necessarily bring larger rewards. No self-respecting surgeon will embark on mutilating surgery without good justification for its use and the day of the so-called 'prophylactic neck dissection' has, hopefully, disappeared. There are always those who can produce the series of cases who have undergone neck dissection when clinically there has been no evidence of secondary involvement of nodes, and in which careful microscopical studies have shown in a small percentage of cases malignant cells in lymph glands. But we recognize that not all such malignant cell inclusions necessarily prosper and that the body is capable of dealing with many of them; and we have no evidence that removal of affected nodes at this early stage gives better results than neck dissection carried out when a node is first discovered. It is certain that if a policy of 'prophylactic neck dissection' is carried out, very many patients will be subjected to mutilating surgery who might never have needed it.

With some few exceptions it is sound policy to institute a careful follow-up of all patients treated for a primary malignant growth of the head and neck, with a particularly rigorous search for any possible involvement of neck nodes at 3-monthly intervals, and to proceed to neck dissection if nodes are palpable or if, indeed, there is any doubt that involved nodes are present in the neck. No policy, however, should be adhered to invariably and there could be occasions when it would seem politic to carry out a neck dissection at the same time as ablation of the primary growth, even though neck nodes are not clinically involved. In those cases in which reconstruction following ablative surgery of the primary involves introducing tissue employed in the reconstruction into the neck it is safer to clear the neck first. Potentially infiltrated tissue is being opened up and tissue introduced which may mask nodes which later become enlarged so that they would have been palpated but for the bulk of material introduced beneath the neck skin. This applies particularly in cases where pectoralis major myocutaneous flaps are routed on a muscle pedicle beneath the skin of the neck or where a sternomastoid-clavicle myo-osseous repair of an ablated mandible is carried out.

On occasions the biological behaviour of the primary, usually of posterior tongue or upper pharynx, is so disturbingly aggressive that wisdom dictates that early lymphatic spread is inevitable and an en bloc clearance of primary and neck nodes is advisable. Similarly, patients who present late in the course of their disease with an uncontrolled primary growth probably merit neck dissection, even though nodes are not clinically palpable.

Having said all this, it remains a fact that the majority of patients with primary tumours of the head and neck will have a neck clearance only if and when nodes become clinically evident.

There is no indication for needle biopsy of suspect nodes. If there exists that much doubt concerning a node, it is better to take the decision to carry out a formal neck clearance.

The term 'block dissection of neck' covers a number of related procedures which may be summarized as follows:

1. Radical
2. Suprahyoid.
3. Supra-omohyoid.
4. Function-preserving.
5. Bilateral.

1. RADICAL DISSECTION

This is the standard full clearance of neck nodes, the most usually employed procedure and one which forms the basis of all types of neck clearance.

Preoperative Considerations

It goes without saying that a full standard preoperative preparation of the patient is mandatory. Age, per se, is no contra-indication to operation. There will be times when no amount of preoperative therapy will get a patient as fit as one would have desired, but in such cases it must be remembered that this is an emergency procedure. Without it the affected gland may become uncontrollable and risks may have to be taken in order to spare the patient a miserable death from eventual fungating neck growth.

Anaesthesia

Standard general anaesthesia via an endotracheal tube suffices for most cases. In certain ear, nose and throat procedures a preliminary tracheostomy is prepared and anaesthesia is continued via this route. Similarly, major lower jaw resections involving excision of the entire symphyseal region so disturb tongue fixation that a preliminary tracheostomy becomes essential. In those cases where it is safe to employ it, hypotensive anaesthesia controls bleeding and speeds the operation. In other cases simple head-up tilt and maintenance of an unobstructed airway produce effective control of bleeding and enable the surgeon to carry out the operation in the manner of a strict anatomical dissection which, in effect, it is.

The patient lies flat on his or her back with the neck extended and the chin turned towards the opposite side. Skin towels are conveniently fixed by suturing them, in places, to the skin and are arranged to provide access to the whole neck, the lower face and upper chest.

Incisions

Numerous patterns of incision have been employed since Crile described linked double horizontal incisions which were standard for many years. In essence, incisions must provide unobstructed access to the entire operative field and ideally should be placed, so far as is possible, within normal skin crease lines. Two forms of incision will be described which adequately provide for most eventualities.

The McFee incision is mostly commonly employed (*Fig.* 26.1). This is an unlinked, double horizontal pattern which raises a wide strap of skin to expose the whole of one side of the neck and submandibular region. The upper component extends from just beyond the midline in the symphyseal region at the level of the lower border of the mandible, downwards and backwards in a deep curve to the posterior border of the mastoid process. Taking this incision beyond the midline medially facilitates thorough clearance of the submental glands, an important group and one that is often missed. The lower incision extends from the midline at the suprasternal notch along the line of the clavicle to beyond the anterior border of the trapezius.

This is the safest and most elegant of all the incisions described for the operation of block dissection of the neck. Being an unlinked combination of two parallel, horizontal neck incisions there are no awkward 'T' junctions, which commonly lead to delayed healing, and no vertical component to lead to postoperative webbing of the scar. In those cases who

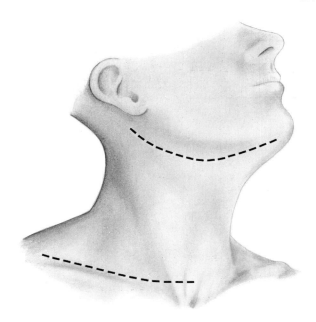

Fig. 26.1. McFee unlinked double horizontal incisions for block dissection of the neck.

have received preoperative radiotherapy, with consequent diminution in vitality of the treated soft tissues, it is by far the safest pattern of incision to use. Breakdown is uncommon and the final cosmetic result could not be improved.

It is, however, not so suitable for function-preserving neck dissections, and an alternative pattern is recommended and is described later (p. 361).

Procedure

Lower Dissection

When the horizontal incisions have been made, down to platysma, the upper skin flap is raised in full length to a level above the lower border of the mandible. This flap may then be conveniently anchored out of the way by means of a temporary suture fixed to the head towel.

The whole of the neck skin, bounded by the two horizontal incisions, is then raised by sharp dissection in the form of a wide strap extending from the midline anteriorly to beyond the anterior border of the trapezius posteriorly. It is essential that the whole of the anterior border of the trapezius is displayed, so that it can, during the course of the dissection, be stripped of its fatty-fascial investment. There is a posterior group of deep cervical nodes which is contained in this tissue and which it is important to remove with the main specimen.

There remains controversy as to what should be the fate of the platysma; whether this muscle should be taken with the specimen or left on the skin flaps in the belief that the flaps will be protected from necrosis. It is difficult to see what protection to a skin flap can be provided by denervated devascularized muscle. Skin flaps, properly designed and handled, should not necrose and in order to adhere to the monobloc principle the authors feels that it is essential that the platysma be removed with the contents of the neck (*Fig.* 26.2).

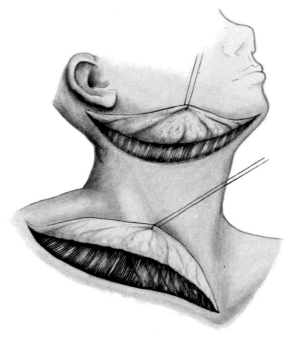

Fig. 26.2. The platysma muscle is separated from the skin flaps.

Elevation of the skin strap displays the platysma, a well-defined muscle sheet except for the posterior and inferior margins where it tends to tail off. This muscle sheet is divided along its entire length in the midline and inferiorly, ligating and dividing the external jugular vein low down. Retraction in an upward direction, by means of a tissue forceps gripping the lower border of the muscle, will begin to display the deeper structures at the root of the neck. The medial, intermediate and lateral supraclavicular nerves will be seen fanning out across the clavicle and these are divided.

The insertion of the sternomastoid into the clavicle and the upper border of the sternum is clearly displayed and then divided (*Fig.* 26.3). Tissue forceps grasp the thick, divided muscle and retract upwards to expose part of the lower belly and the tendon of the omohyoid. This muscle is divided below its intermediate tendon and is lifted upwards by an artery forceps gripping the tendon. Immediately deep is the internal jugular vein. About a 2 cm length of this vein, just above the clavicle, is carefully cleaned so that it can safely and easily be ligatured and divided. There is, quite constantly, at the level of the clavicle, a fairly large tributary running medially and it is good practice to display this clearly, so that the lowest ligature may be placed just above the junction. This

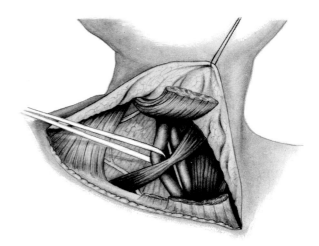

Fig. 26.3. The sternomastoid muscle is divided almost at its insertion and the internal jugular vein mobilized.

avoids accidental damage to the tributary and consequent bleeding in a particularly inaccessible area. Two ligatures are tied above and below the point of division of the vein and it is wise to secure the lower stump with a transfixation tie.

Careful finger dissection deep to the vein will free it for 1 or 2 cm from the carotid sheath and the vagus nerve, which must be identified and preserved.

Attention now focuses on the areolar content of the root of the neck. Working from medial to lateral, a combination of sharp and finger dissection will allow the fatty pad to be swept outwards and upwards off the scalene muscles and the brachial plexus. The phrenic nerve running obliquely across the face of the scalenus anterior will come into view and the transverse cervical vessels will be encountered in the fatty tissue. They can usually be cleared of fat but a constant branch running vertically upwards towards the levator scapulae will need to be ligated and divided. Sharp dissection continues up the anterior border of the trapezius, dividing the accessory nerve as it enters the muscle, having emerged from the sternomastoid at the junction of its middle and lower thirds, and is extended as far as access from the lower skin incision will allow, and then the medial portion of the operative site is cleared, again as far as access from the lower incision permits. The internal jugular vein together with the carotid sheath is easily stripped from the common carotid artery and vagus nerve (*Fig.* 26.4).

At this stage in the dissection the skin strap is retracted downwards and the dissection specimen is passed under it and upwards, to appear in the upper wound and the dissection can then be completed from this access point.

Middle Dissection

Special care must be taken at this stage to avoid damage to the phrenic nerve. This nerve arises mainly

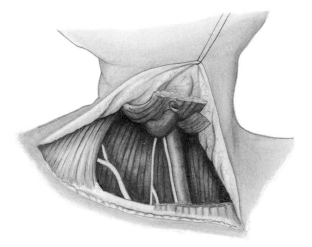

Fig. 26.4. The internal jugular vein is ligated and divided at its lower end and the dissection specimen is cleaned and passed under and above the skin flap.

from C4 but has connections from C5 and C3 as well. As freeing of the internal jugular vein proceeds, deep to it can be seen the cervical plexus with the individual nerves emerging from between the scalenus anterior and the scalenus medius, and it is all too easy, if care is not exercised, to lift forwards the upper end of the phrenic nerve, by retraction on the overlying vein, and damage it as the cervical nerves are cut. The author makes it a rule to divide the cervical nerves well forward of the roots of the phrenic nerve and to avoid heavy retraction on the specimen at this stage, so that distortion of the underlying structures is minimized.

Broadly speaking the internal jugular vein is the key to the operation. Dissection proceeds in its plane, separating it and the carotid sheath from the carotid artery and vagus nerve and extending posteriorly to the anterior border of the trapezius and anteriorly to denude the strap muscles up to the midline, so that the neck contents are removed in one and the same plane. Large thyroid venous tributaries are divided between ligatures.

The first major arterial branch to be encountered is the superior thyroid artery as it turns over and runs for a short distance parallel to the carotid artery. With primary tumours of the oral cavity it can be left intact, though it will need to be sacrificed with primary growths of the larynx and thyroid. The carotid bifurcation can be seen at about the level of the hyoid and at this stage the cervical fascia may be boldly incised from the attachment of the intermediate tendon of the digastric to the greater horn of the hyoid, along the line of the anterior belly of the digastric as far as its insertion into the symphysis. Posteriorly the fascial incision is continued up to the mastoid process and these two manoeuvres then permit rapid advance of the dissection into the submandibular triangle. The internal jugular vein and carotid

sheath are stripped upwards until the origin of the occipital artery is visualized (*Fig.* 26.5). The hypoglossal nerve hooks round at this point to cross the

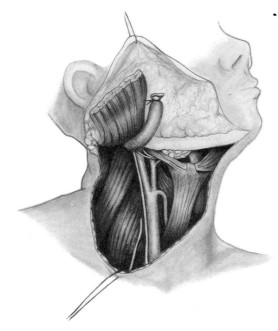

Fig. 26.5. The dissection is completed into the submandibular triangle and the internal jugular vein is dissected up until the origin of the occipital artery is visualized.

internal and external carotid arteries, and it should always be secured at this stage so that it may be protected in the rest of its course towards the tongue. It will be necessary, now, formally to divide between ligatures the large lingual tributary of the internal jugular vein. It is often duplicated and easily damaged, to cause considerable bleeding which can be difficult to secure.

If, at this point, the carotid artery and vagus nerve are displaced forwards the sympathetic trunk, with the superior and middle ganglia, are clearly seen lying parallel and deep to the vessels. Aimless dissection from behind forwards, in the middle part of the neck, could damage the trunk. The capsule of the submandibular salivary gland is freed from its attachments to the digastric muscle and a tissue forceps grasping the lower pole of the gland lifts it upwards and outwards to expose the gland bed comprising the mylohyoid and hyoglossus muscles.

Upper (Submandibular) Dissection

Periosteum is divided along the lower border of the anterior part of the mandible and the fibro-fatty contents of the submental triangle are swept away from before backwards from the muscle bed. At the anterior border of the masseter the facial artery and anterior facial vein are divided between ligatures. Traction on this superoanterior corner of the specimen will now expose, in full, the muscle bed of the submandibular gland, crossed diagonally by the hypoglossal nerve. Upward traction shows the facial artery entering the posterior part of the gland accompanied by the common facial vein. The vessels are divided and ligated (*Fig*. 26.6). Downward traction

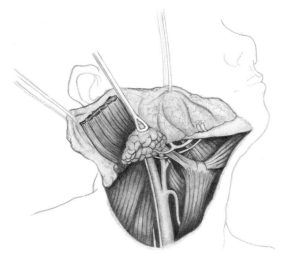

Fig. 26.6. The facial artery and the facial vein are exposed and divided following dissection of the fibro-fatty contents and the submental triangle.

pulls a U loop of lingual nerve into the operative field. The lingual nerve is attached to the deep lobe of the submandibular gland and the origin of the submandibular duct by means of its branches to the submandibular ganglion, which supplies the gland. The ganglion is usually quite obvious and, as it is divided from the deep lobe, the lingual nerve tracks back into place, deep to the ramus of the mandible. The submandibular duct is ligated as close to the oral mucosa as possible, and divided, and the whole contents of the submandibular triangle are then free.

In the posterosuperior angle of the field the lower pole of the parotid gland is transected. It contains a large venous trunk, the posterior facial vein, which is divided between ligatures. The upper attachment of the sternomastoid is cut through to expose the posterior belly of the digastric. Deep to this lies the upper end of the internal jugular vein and the accessory nerve, and from these the whole of the specimen is now suspended. The nerve is closely applied to the vein and is separated and divided. The jugular vein is divided between ligatures and the upper end is further secured by a transfixation tie. The specimen is now free (*Fig*. 26.7).

Complete haemostasis is secured, and the wounds are then closed in layers with suction drainage.

Postoperative Management

Postoperative therapy is determined by the extent of any other ablative procedure, which may be car-

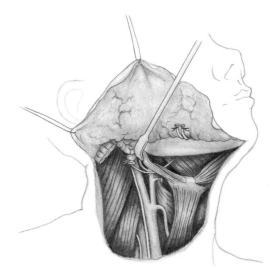

Fig. 26.7. The lower pole of the parotid gland is transected, the upper attachment of the sternomastoid is divided and the jugular vein is ligated and divided as high as possible.

ried out together with the neck dissection, such as a jaw or laryngeal resection. No special postoperative care is required following a straightforward block dissection of neck. The operation can be fairly swiftly concluded and, in many cases, without blood transfusion. Morbidity is not marked and patients are usually ambulant by the day after operation. Suction usually continues for 48–72 hours, and sutures are removed at 7 days.

Complications

The incidence of serious complications is low. Using a McFee incision even minor wound breakdown is uncommon, and frank skin necrosis is almost never seen.

Wound breakdown with carotid blowout is always quoted as a complication, yet the author has only encountered this on two occasions and in both very heavy irradiation had been followed by ill-planned incisions. If there is very real doubt that heavy irradiation may have lowered soft tissue viability to a point where skin necrosis is inevitable after added surgical trauma, before closing the wounds the levator scapulae can be freed and turned over medially as a hinged flap in order to provide muscle cover to the denuded carotid.

If, in spite of everything, there is a major skin breakdown, so as to threaten exposure of the carotid, swift action to replace non-viable skin using a convenient deltopectoral or pectoralis major flap will save the day.

On occasions dissections at the root of the neck may damage the thoracic duct. Even if the duct is visualized during the dissection it can be difficult to secure between ligatures, as it so easily tears. Division of the thoracic duct leads to a discharge of milky fluid from the wound, which is mostly of nuisance value. Such fistulas always close spontaneously in time, though they may give trouble for several weeks. No special treatment is indicated.

Postoperative Sequelae

It cannot be denied that sacrifice of the accessory nerve does pose problems for the patient in the way of a paralysed trapezius, often with complaints of continuing discomfort in the neck and shoulder. The surprising feature is that so few patients have difficulty in adjusting to this disability, which will, of course, be permanent. Very often I have been intrigued to find, 6 months after a radical neck dissection, a surprisingly powerful shoulder shrug against resistance. This can be due to only two factors. First, that the levator scapulae compensates in large measure for the lost trapezius action. Second, that there is an additional motor supply to the trapezius, which is not routinely damaged in a neck dissection.

Further investigation revealed that it is possible to identify a nerve trunk of not inconsiderable size, posteriorly in the lower third of the neck, which arises from the cervical plexus and joins the accessory nerve within the substance of the sternomastoid muscle at a point about 2 cm from its posterior border. Routinely, now, when performing a radical neck clearance, the author dissects out this cervical branch and divides the accessory nerve proximal to the junction. Careful postoperative assessment has demonstrated that in all cases some trapezius function is preserved and patients have made no complaint of shoulder weakness or stiffness, or of the constant dragging ache which so commonly follows trapezius paralysis. The minimal added dissection required in no way compromises the radical nature of the operation as, for most of its course, the cervical component runs in the plane of the scalene muscles deep to the block of tissue to be excised and, having carefully sectioned the accessory nerve, the sternomastoid muscle can be elevated and removed as previously described.

Excision of the mandibular branch of the facial nerve, as it loops down into the neck and then ascends to cross the facial vessels as they overlie the mandible at the anterior border of the masseter, leads to paralysis of half the lower lip with a very obviously asymmetrical appearance, particularly when the face is in animation. It has to be accepted, though, that this is a small price to pay to ensure a complete clearance. A small lymph node is constantly encountered just at the point where the nerve crosses the facial vessels, and any attempt to dissect out the nerve must jeopardize a total clearance.

2. SUPRAHYOID CLEARANCE

The suprahyoid clearance is a poor substitute for a radical neck dissection and I believe that it has no place in the treatment of head and neck cancer. It was said to be indicated in an unfit patient in whom lymphatic involvement was limited to mobile nodes confined to the submandibular triangle, or in cases of bilateral node involvement where a full block dissection was carried out on the most heavily involved side, and a suprahyoid clearance on the least affected side, in order to avoid the complications of a bilateral radical neck dissection.

The suprahyoid dissection, as such, is little more than a clearance of the submandibular triangle and removes the gland and its duct, the fascial investments of the triangle and only the extreme upper part of the carotid sheath, and fascial coverings of the jugular vein. It must be considered to be a pale, inadequate imitation of a radical neck node clearance and cannot be justified on any grounds.

3. SUPRA-OMOHYOID CLEARANCE

This extended operation does have rather more indication and can be considered in grossly unfit patients whose glandular involvement is limited to a single, mobile node in the submandibular triangle, or in cases with bilateral, palpable nodes in whom, on one side, there is only one mobile node in the submandibular triangle.

Only one incision is required, corresponding to the upper horizontal incision of the radical operation. The upper flap is raised and retracted as already described in the radical neck dissection, and the lower skin edge is undermined and retracted downwards so that dissection can begin at a point well below the carotid bifurcation. It is not usual to transect the sternomastoid which can be retracted posteriorly to obtain a good view of the middle of the neck. The internal jugular vein is divided between ligatures just above the superior thyroid tributary, and the carotid sheath is stripped from this level upwards. The remainder of the dissection proceeds as already described for radical dissection (p. 356), save that the upper end of the sternomastoid remains attached to its origin on the mastoid process, and because of this the internal jugular vein has to be ligated at its upper end, lower down than can be attained in a radical block dissection.

It is to be noted that this procedure does not permit clearance of the nodes at the root of the neck, nor along the anterior border of the trapezius.

It does not match up to the standards required of curative surgery for malignant conditions, in that a deliberately incomplete procedure is being carried out and the field is seriously jeopardized if glands, which are left behind, become involved, so that further surgery of the neck has to be undertaken.

4. FUNCTION-PRESERVING NECK DISSECTION

The 'function-preserving' neck dissection is an interesting concept and is a valuable procedure so long as fairly limited indications are adhered to. Described by Bocca for the treatment of lymphatic spread from primary laryngeal growths, it has been applied to other malignant head and neck conditions, notably to patients with primary growths of the oral mucosa.

As originally envisaged, the procedure was carried out as prophylactic clearance so that it can, with justifiction, be employed in patients with aggressive tumours or late tumours in whom no nodes are palpable but where experience dictates that an elective neck dissection is indicated. It is probably safe also to advise such a procedure in patients in whom a single, small, mobile node is noted in the submandibular triangle. Any suspicion of multiple nodes or of fixation of nodes to deeper structures, or overlying muscles, should rule out this more limited clearance.

Paradoxically, though the dissection is less radical it is a more difficult procedure to carry out, because so many structures have to be identified and preserved and because, to an extent, surgical access is more restricted. For these reasons the McFee approach tends to be too limiting and an alternative incision is recommended. It consists of a horizontal and a vertical component (*Fig. 26.8*). The horizontal

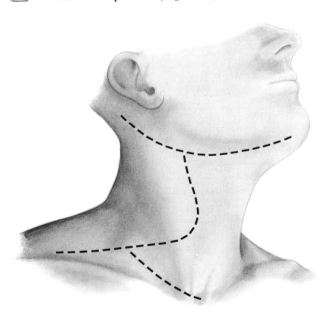

Fig. 26.8. Incisions for 'function-preserving' block dissection of the neck.

limb corresponds exactly to the usual long submandibular incision, which is the upper component of the McFee procedure. From the midpoint of this limb an incision extends in lazy S form to the midpoint of the clavicle. Three skin flaps are thus outlined and are raised to expose a wide triangle of neck. If required, greater access to the root of the neck may be achieved by incorporating an additional horizontal component to the vertical neck incision at the level of the clavicle. Bocca describes a thorough clearance

of all fascial and aponeurotic investments from the line of the posterior border of the sternomastoid to the midline, preserving the sternomastoid muscle, the accessory nerve, the internal jugular vein and the submandibular salivary gland.

It is claimed that the procedure from a cancer 'cure' standpoint is as effective as other methods, yet avoids all the major disabilities associated with these methods. The concept has gained in popularity over the past year or two, but it should be emphasized that its main indication is in those cases in whom no lymph nodes are palpable—that is to say as a prophylactic procedure, an attitude to treatment which is by no means accepted by the majority of head and neck surgeons. It would seem to the author that a great danger of this method is that attempts may be made to apply it to totally unsuitable cases and that a full radical neck dissection, with preservation of trapezius function, as already described, provides safer management from the cancerological viewpoint, with little increase in postoperative disability. Its chief value may lie in the management of patients with bilateral node involvement, where a radical neck dissection can be performed on one side, and a function-preserving clearance, which leaves the internal jugular vein intact, on the other.

5. BILATERAL NECK DISSECTION

The prognosis for any patient suffering from primary malignancy of the head and neck, who presents with bilateral cervical node involvement, must necessarily be grave. This does not mean that the case is lost and that energetic salvage attempts should not be instituted. Many such patients have been saved and, indeed, cured by an aggressive policy.

A bilateral, radical block dissection of the neck performed at one operation carries postoperative hazards so severe and a mortality rate so high as to preclude its justification in any case. The dangers stem from the removal on both sides of the internal jugular vein. This vein provides almost all the drainage from the head and neck and sudden simultaneous bilateral interruption causes severe congestion of all the territory drained. The risks of irreversible brain damage, due to venous stasis, are high, particularly so as we are dealing with patients in the older age groups whose cerebral reserve, in any event, is probably low. If a period of not less than 3 months can be allowed to elapse between the two block dissections, morbidity and mortality are greatly reduced, probably as a result of vertebral vein hypertrophy following ligation of the internal jugular vein on one side.

A standard radical clearance can therefore be performed on both sides of the neck, so long as the two procedures can be separated by not less than 3 months. Such a policy can be applied to those cases in whom glands appear on the other side of the neck after one side has already been cleared.

Often, however, on clinical examination glands are palpable bilaterally and the need arises for simultaneous attack on both sides of the neck. It is advised that a radical operation be carried out on the most affected side or on the side of the primary if both gland groups are equally involved, and some form of internal jugular vein-preserving clearance on the other side—either a function-preserving operation or supra-omohyoid clearance as described earlier (p. 361).

Chapter twenty-seven

Maxillofacial Surgery

J. W. Ross

INFECTION

Acute Alveolar Abscess

This arises within the bone of either jaw and is usually due to a tooth with dead pulp or nerve. It can also arise between the gum and a tooth and often will have been preceded by chronic inflammation of the area. Other pathological conditions in the jaws may produce abscesses, such as cysts, buried teeth or fractures. If a tooth is involved, it becomes very tender to pressure. The infection may resolve, discharge into the mouth or penetrate into the soft tissues, and whether the latter produces cellulitis or an abscess depends on the infecting organism and the patient's resistance. Extension into the various potential spaces around the jaws can result in external swelling, trismus and danger to the airway when sublingual, submandibular and pharyngeal spaces are involved (*Figs.* 27.1, 27.2).

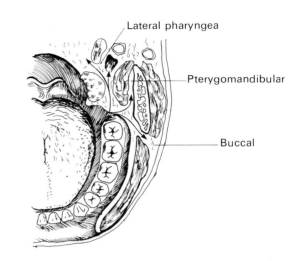

Fig. 27.2. Possible pathways of infection arising from infection around wisdom tooth. (Transverse section.)

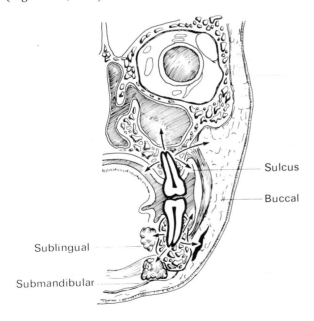

Fig. 27.1. Possible pathways of infection arising from an apical abscess. The proximity of the maxillary sinus is clearly shown. (Coronal section.)

Pus formation, which may be detected by fluctuation or pointing, should be relieved as soon as possible by incision and drainage, either intra-orally or extra-orally at dependent points. The best place for incision can often be located by asking the patient to indicate the most painful spot with one finger. Intubation of the patient is sometimes needed for operation but can be difficult and dangerous when there is poor mouth opening or potential airway obstruction. Forced opening of the mouth or manipulation with a laryngoscope may cause premature bursting of an abscess intra-orally which could result in inhalation of pus and airway restriction.

External incision should extend to the subcutaneous level and continue with sinus forceps to avoid damage to important underlying structures, such as the facial nerve. The sinus forceps should be inserted closed until the pus is reached and then withdrawn open to ensure free drainage. A careful check should be made that all loculi have been entered and a finger is effective for this purpose.

An essential part of the operation is the drainage but removal of the cause is usually carried out under the same anaesthetic.

It is uncommon to insert drains into intra-oral wounds but this is usually necessary for external drainage. A corrugated rubber drain, trimmed at a 45° angle but with the point removed to avoid vessel erosion, is inserted to the depth of the cavity. Multiple drains are used if there is more than one loculus.

The drain is usually retained for 48 hours only but, if pus is draining freely at that time, it may be kept in place or shortened and removed later. After 4 days, retention of the drain may induce discharge by acting as a foreign body.

Complications

Actinomycosis

If there has been surgery in the mouth or fracture of the mandible some few weeks before the acute episode, or there is an unusual amount of induration associated with the swelling, the first sample of pus should be taken in a tube rather than on a swab for investigation in the laboratory for actinomycosis. This is a chronic condition but may produce an acute abscess. Colonies of the bacterium (*Actinomyces israelii*) may be seen as 'sulphur' granules in the pus which may be crushed and examined under the microscope revealing a typical pattern of radiating filaments or 'ray fungus'. If actinomycosis is diagnosed, prolonged antibiotic treatment is indicated, usually with penicillin.

Facial Sinus

Rarely, an alveolar abscess will track to the skin surface and discharge, producing a chronic discharging sinus which may be some distance from the tooth. These sinuses are commonly misdiagnosed and a dental opinion should always be obtained when there is uncertainty about the diagnosis.

Treatment is removal of the cause and excision of the sinus tract, if the sinus is not of recent origin.

Cavernous Sinus Thrombosis

Although rare, cavernous sinus thrombosis is a serious complication of infection in and around the jaws. Spread is presumed to take place by infected thrombi in the pterygoid plexus or anterior facial vein which connects with the cavernous sinus. The patient will develop rigors and a high swinging temperature with oedema around the eyes and exophthalmos. Involvement of the nerves in the sinus results in ophthalmoplegia on the affected side.

Treatment is by anticoagulants and antibiotics and again removal of the cause and drainage where required. The patient should be under neurosurgical care.

Sterile Abscess

This condition is becoming more common and is sometimes known as 'antibioma'. It is due to treating abscesses with antibiotics but without drainage, and occurs when the antibiotic sterilizes the pus, leaving a fluctuant abscess which, when incised, does not grow an organism.

Clinically, the patient presents with a fluctuant swelling and is afebrile. Incision and drainage are indicated.

Osteomyelitis

Occasionally, infection in or around the jaws can result in extension through the medulla. When acute, the patient has a high temperature, severe pain, loosening of teeth, lymphadenitis, swelling of the face and eventually multiple discharging sinuses within the mouth and on the face. Pus may discharge around the teeth.

In the lower jaw, involvement of the mandibular nerve may produce anaesthesia of its distribution.

The condition is predisposed by systemic and local factors causing lowered resistance, including diabetes, agranulocytosis, hypogammaglobulinaemia, typhoid, marble bone disease, Paget's disease, radiotherapy and, of course, fractures.

The mandible is more commonly affected and this is thought to be because of its denser bone and poor collateral circulation. However, in infants the condition occurs more commonly in the maxilla and is believed to be haematogenously spread or due to local trauma. Metastatic osteomyelitis may spread to or from the mandible.

It is considered that an important factor in the spread of osteomyelitis may be the stripping of the periosteum from the bone by the pus, thus depriving it of its blood supply. As the infection spreads, pieces of bone become isolated from their blood supply and die. These sequestra may be seen on radiography and are related to the areas of bone destruction.

As with the treatment of acute alveolar abscess, pus is collected as soon as possible for identification of the organisms and a sensitivity test.

Although the organism is usually *Staph. aureus*, a wide variety of organisms has been associated with the condition.

Surgical drainage and sequestrectomy are carried out under general anaesthesia, care being taken not to strip healthy periosteum from the bone.

Control of the disease process has to be exercised mostly on clinical evidence as the radiographic appearance lags some 10–20 days behind the clinical state.

Weakening of the mandible can advance to the stage where fracture readily occurs and care must be taken to continue antibiotic treatment until the condition is completely under control. Inadequate treatment may lead to chronic osteomyelitis which is most difficult to treat.

There is good evidence that some cases of chronic osteomyelitis of the mandible are associated with the 'incompetent leucocyte syndrome'.

MAXILLOFACIAL INJURIES

Most fractures of the facial skeleton are due to road traffic injuries. Maxillofacial injuries commonly occur in association with injuries to other parts of the body and the most important of these is the head injury, which occurs in approximately one-third of the cases. Impact to the head is transmitted not only to the brain but to the cervical spine and a careful check must be made for injuries in this region. A general examination of the patient must be carried out and one should suspect other injuries if the patient is in shock as this generally does not occur with facial injuries in isolation.

As the facial skeleton consists of thin bones with certain reinforced buttresses, it collapses in a relatively easy manner when the body is projected on to a stationary object. The face therefore acts as a shock absorber and lessens trauma to the brain.

Severe injuries are common in the driver and front seat passenger, and fragmentation of the windscreen may cause permanent disfigurement and disabilities, such as blindness and facial palsy, a condition which is seen less frequently since the legislation on the wearing of seat belts was introduced.

External haemorrhage is rarely a problem with maxillofacial injuries and the correct treatment is reduction of the fractures and suturing of the lacerations as soon as possible.

The most likely cause of problems in these cases, particularly where there is unconsciousness, is the airway. Careful pharyngeal toilet with suction should be carried out wherever possible and with swabs and forceps where suction is not available. The hazards include blood, vomit, broken teeth, dentures, oedema and falling back of the tongue where the anterior part of the mandible and the attachment of the tongue are separated from the rest of the jaw.

With fractures of the maxilla, there will be swelling of the palate and spasm of the pterygoid muscles which tend to draw the maxilla downwards and backwards, thus aggravating the compromised airway. Therefore, the face-down position is most important and, where necessary, the tongue should be held forward together with the maxilla, if this is displaced, to free the airway until intubation.

It is a good working rule that patients with severe facial injuries in combination with a head injury should have a tracheostomy performed at the earliest opportunity, to protect the airway and also facilitate future treatment by removing the endotracheal tube from the areas of injury. The chest should always be radiographed for missing tooth fragments and dentures.

The fractured maxilla may be displaced by the pull of muscles, which also occurs in the mandible when the muscles of mastication cause upward rotation of a ramus fragment where the fracture is anterior to the attachments of medial pterygoid and masseter muscles.

When fractures of the mandible are bilateral, inframandibular muscles will cause downward and backward displacement of the symphysis.

Fractures of the Mandible

Fractures of the mandible occur in any situation but the common sites are the subcondylar, the angle, the body, the canine and symphysis regions. Those frac-

tures of the jaw which involve teeth are inevitably compound to the mouth and, where the teeth are grossly involved, or are themselves damaged in the root, they should be removed or they will tend to retard healing.

Fractures of the Maxilla (*Fig.* 27.3)

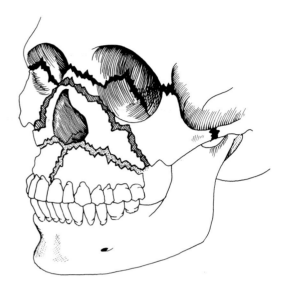

Fig. 27.3. Le Fort I, II and III fractures with split palate.

As the bones of the maxilla are thin, they do not tend to fracture along simple lines but tend to comminute and collapse. Le Fort carried out experiments on cadavers and showed that there were three main levels of maxillary fracture.

The first and lowest is the Le Fort I, which is a horizontal fracture passing above the floors of the antra and nose, through the septum and lateral walls of the nose, zygomatic buttresses and pterygoid plates.

A Le Fort II fracture is the so-called 'middle-third' or 'pyramidal' fracture which ascends from zygomatic buttresses through the infraorbital margins and high into the nasal cavity.

A Le Fort III fracture is at a higher level and involves the roof of both orbits and, as the zygomas are below the level of the fracture, the face as a whole is separated from the skull. The latter is a rare fracture but a possible complication of both the Le Fort II and III fractures is involvement of the base of the skull in the region of the cribriform plate, causing a dural tear and consequent leakage of cerebrospinal fluid. There is a danger of infection passing from the nose and becoming established within the cranium, causing meningitis.

These patients, whether they show cerebrospinal fluid leak or not, are treated prophylactically with antibiotics.

About 20 per cent of maxillary fractures include

a split of the palate which is sometimes severe enough to cause rupture of the oral mucosa but usually results only in a widening of the maxillary arch, It is important that this fracture is recognized if correct reduction is to be achieved,

Fractures of the Nose

The nasal bones may be fractured and displaced in any direction but are usually pushed backwards. If the blow is severe enough, the ethmoids are collapsed and the medial walls of the orbits and canthal ligaments shifted laterally, producing a condition known as 'telecanthus'. The lateral cartilages of the nose may be displaced and one side over-ride the other and the cartilaginous septum may be displaced from its groove in the vomer and curved to one side or the other,

Fractures of the Zygoma

One or both zygomas are commonly fractured in combination with a fractured maxilla and may be depressed, producing a flattened cheek prominence. The main fractures occur at the zygomatic buttress, infraorbital margin, involving the infraorbital canal and at the zygomaticofrontal and zygomaticotemporal sutures, or some other place on the arch.

Fracture and displacement of the zygoma can, of course, occur in isolation, and fracture of the zygomatic arch with depression is commonly seen, This depression consists of a triple fracture with the apex of the two fragments pushed medially, which is usually the direction of the trauma. However, downward displacement rarely takes place because of the strength of the investing temporal fascia,

Blowout Fracture

Since this injury was first described there has been much debate about its cause. It was originally believed that a blowout fracture of the orbital floor was caused by compression all around the rim of the orbit from an injury, such as a ball striking the orbit. It is now considered that a blow to the inferior orbital rim is sufficient to cause this type of fracture in the orbital floor without the rim itself fracturing,

Characteristically, the blowout fracture of the orbit shows radiographically that some of the contents of the orbit have dropped through into the antrum and will appear as a 'teardrop'. Confirmation of this is by tomography, which may show a trapdoor deformity of the thin bones of the orbital floor. It was said that trapping of the inferior rectus or inferior oblique muscles was the cause of the diplopia which often results from this injury.

However, recent work has shown that the eye is held in position in the orbit by radial fibrous bands and it is believed now that it is the trapping of the fibrous bands which produces the immobility of the eye,

Whatever the cause of injury in these cases, the eye itself may have sustained trauma and careful inspection should be made by an ophthalmic surgeon,

Treatment of Maxillofacial Injuries

Fractures of the mandible, where most of the teeth are present, are treated by interdental or eyelet wiring (Fig. 27.4, 27.5). This consists essentially of passing a wire loop around two teeth, twisting to tighten into the concavities of the teeth at the gum margin. This leaves an eyelet protruding and the process is continued with other pairs of teeth in both jaws until sufficient eyelets have been applied to allow the

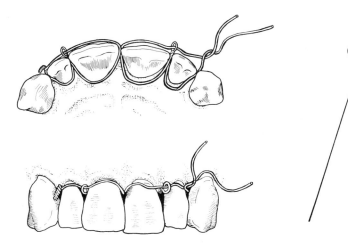

Two stages of eylet wiring

Eyelet wires
0·4 mm soft stainless steel

Fig. 27.4. Eyelet wiring of teeth for immobilization of fractured jaw.

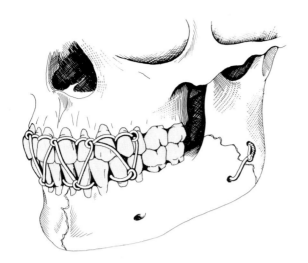

Fig. 27.5. Eyelet wiring of a fractured symphysis; interosseous wiring of angle fracture.

eyelets themselves to be joined from upper to lower jaw, fixing the jaws together. This can be carried out under local anaesthesia but general anaesthesia is commonly used.

Consideration of the airway must be given at all times and the patient's stomach must be empty before the jaws are fixed together. The patient is returned to the ward with wire cutters so that, in an emergency, the fixation can be cut to open the jaws. Since the teeth have been brought together in their correct occlusion, the attached bone will be reduced into its correct position but problems arise where there are few or no natural teeth.

When without teeth and with dentures, fixation of the jaws is achieved by wiring the jaw fragments into the dentures using circumferential wires and then wiring the dentures together, producing reduction of the fractures.

These methods will stabilize those fractures which have teeth attached to them or which can be included in dentures. However, fractures behind this region may require separate fixation by direct bone wiring, either from the mouth or through the skin. The choice will depend on the position, extent and displacement of the fracture.

One simple wire loop is usually sufficient to fix this proximal fragment because the anterior part of the jaw has already been fixed.

Where there are no teeth and dentures have been lost or broken, it is necessary to construct facsimiles of the dentures without teeth and wire these into position as one would have done with the dentures. The lower four incisors are usually removed from the dentures to facilitate feeding but, with the acrylic splint, provision is made anteriorly for a feeding gap.

With unilateral fracture in the subcondylar region, patients can often achieve their correct bite with effort and take a soft diet. When they are unable to bite correctly, as with marked displacement of the fracture, the jaws are wired together for 10–14 days. With bilateral subcondylar fractures, jaw fixation is necessary for 4 weeks at least or shortening of the ascending rami may develop.

Reduction and fixation of the fractured maxilla are invariably carried out under general anaesthesia and, because the bite relationship is important in achieving correct reduction, the anaesthetic is administered via a nasal tube.

If there are fractured zygomas it may be necessary to elevate these to allow for disimpaction of the maxilla, and these movements are carried out with care to avoid penetration of sharp bone fragments into the orbits.

When the palate is split reduction is necessary, which requires compressing the posterior ends of the arch of the teeth together with either finger pressure or a special instrument. It will be clear that when reduction has been achieved the upper and lower teeth will match and bite together accurately.

When the maxilla has been set in the correct position, judged in a lateral and anteroposterior plane by the matching of the bite, it is necessary to displace it upwards into the correct position to re-establish facial height. This is a matter of judgement as overcorrection can be achieved where there is comminution, and if the face is too long, healing will be delayed because of the lack of bone contact. Interdental wiring may be applied between the teeth to fix the bite when it is then necessary to hold the face height until healing takes place. There are a number of methods available for this, of which the most common is four-screw fixation, comprising a screw on each side of the mandible, anterior to and below the mental foramen. There are special self-tapping bone screws which are inserted with a hand drill through a small incision in the skin. Two screws are applied to the supraorbital region in the same way and the face height assessed. Vertical bars and joints are used to lock the upper and lower set of pins together. It is then necessary to join the screws horizontally to brace this apparatus, sometimes known as the 'box frame' (Fig. 27.6).

With the combined injury of mandible and maxilla, it is essential that a platform be formed to allow reduction of the maxilla into the correct position. It may therefore be necessary to insert intraosseous wire across the fracture lines in the mandible to render it 'intact', and a suitable basis on which to build the rest of the face.

Before the application of external fixation, it is necessary to deal with the zygomas and naso-ethmoidal complex.

Zygomatic fractures will usually respond to the Gillies approach from the temple, when Bristow's elevator is inserted through a small incision above the hairline between the temporal fascia and the temporal muscle, passed easily down under the zygomatic arch or zygomatic body and pressure is applied outwards to elevate the fragments.

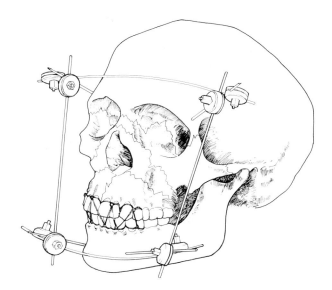

Fig. 27.6. Screw fixation of fractured maxilla using 'box frame'.

Care must be taken to avoid inward pressure on the temporal bone. This method leaves a scar which cannot be seen when the hair grows. If the zygoma proves unstable, it may be necessary to carry out open reduction of the fractures with wiring.

Fractures of the nose are treated by manipulating the lateral cartilages and nasal bones with Walsham's forceps; the outer blade is covered with rubber tubing to protect the skin. The septum is repositioned if displaced and the nasal bones brought forward using Asch forceps. A problem arises when the ethmoids have been compressed as it is necessary to apply strong pressure with thumb and forefinger far back on the medial walls of the orbits while bringing the septum and nasal bones forward with the forceps. This squeezing-in action helps to restore the medial canthi to their correct position but, if the canthi are completely free from the skeleton, it may be necessary to make small incisions to pick up their ends and wire them together across the nose. If these are still attached to bone and if it is possible to collect them with the rest of the nasal fragments, they may be controlled using thin lead plates on each side, which are wired across the nose and maintained for 10 days.

The problem of soft tissue injury should be considered before extubation, and after fracture fixation. Even in the most severe facial injuries, there is usually no loss of tissue but, in cases where tissue has been lost, e.g. a piece of lip, initial treatment is to suture the mucosa to the skin accepting the defect temporarily and later carrying out a secondary plastic surgical repair.

The patient is carefully extubated and the pack removed before the jaw fixation is finally tightened. The pharynx is sucked out through the mouth and via the nose and, if there is no tracheostomy, it is wise to leave an endotracheal or nasopharyngeal tube in position to maintain the airway until such time as this can safely be removed.

Postoperative Care

The patient should be returned to the ward with wire cutters where the jaws are wired together, and when there is external fixation of the box-frame type it will be necessary to send a spanner back to the ward with the patient. All staff dealing with the patient postoperatively should know exactly which procedures are required to open the mouth and should appreciate that the patient may still have food in the stomach and may therefore vomit.

The patient takes a purely fluid diet after the operation, but if there is any doubt about the patient's ability to do this, an i.v. line is left in place and a nasogastric tube should be inserted before the patient leaves the operating theatre.

It is important that all patients have thorough oral hygiene to keep the mouth scrupulously clean, and regular checks of the fixation should be carried out, particularly in the restless patient; loosening of wires can occur and there may be disturbance of external fixation.

The average time for union of fractures is 3 weeks for the maxilla and 4 weeks for the mandible.

SURGERY OF THE TEMPOROMANDIBULAR JOINT

Indications for temporomandibular joint surgery include:
1. Ankylosis.
2. Dislocation—recurrent or long standing.
3. Arthrosis—not responding to conservative methods.
4. Osteoarthritis with pain.
5. Jaw deformities, e.g. condylar hyperplasia.
6. Fractures.

The preauricular incision is the most common approach to the temporomandibular joint. The upper end of the incision should be about 3 cm in length, angled forward at about 45°. Its posterior end should be at the groove where the helix joins the scalp. The incision then continues in the groove anterior to the helix and tragus and ends anterior to the lobe attachment.

The incision is therefore above the main trunk of the facial nerve but care must be taken to avoid the upper branches crossing the zygomatic arch superficial to the periosteum.

Dissection is carried out anterior to the external auditory meatus cartilage and the temporal part of the incision deepened until the temporal fascia is reached. This is incised exposing the temporal muscle and subperiosteal dissection is carried out along the zygomatic arch. This will expose the joint capsule and its thickened lateral ligament. Incision of the cap-

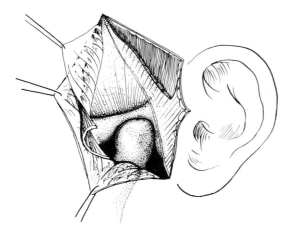

Fig. 27.7. Preauricular approach to temporomandibular joint.

sule from above and posteriorly will expose the condyle (*Fig.* 27.7).

1. Ankylosis

In severe cases of bony or fibrous ankylosis of the joint, dissection is extended well along the arch to expose the affected area. The aim of the operation is to produce a gap between the mandible and the skull to allow free movement. This gap may be left open or filled with a foreign material, such as Silastic, to prevent reattachment.

Costochondral grafting is used when a space maintainer or functional hinge is required. This will require augmentation of the preauricular incision with a submandibular approach as the rib will be wired to the ramus and the cartilage inserted into the fossa at the base of the skull, which is prepared to receive it if necessary.

2. Dislocation

Cases of long-standing dislocation of the mandibular condyle are rare and even fewer require open reduction. However, chronic recurrent dislocation is more common and occurs unilaterally or bilaterally. Reduction is usually possible without general anaesthetic, local anaesthetic or sedation and, as it becomes more frequent, reduction becomes easier and can quite often be achieved by the patient.

Its occurrence is nevertheless an inconvenience and many operations have been devised in the past to prevent it. These range from plication of the capsule of the joint to removal of the articular eminence, and have met with varying degrees of success. Dautrey's operation has proved to be very successful (*Fig.* 27.8).

3. Arthrosis

This is a very common affliction of the temporoman-

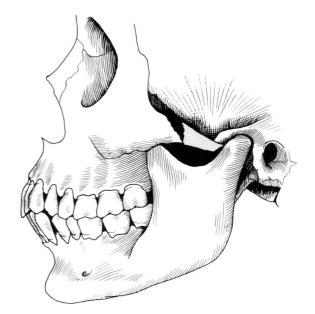

Fig. 27.8. Dautrey's procedure for recurrent dislocation of the temporomandibular joint. The zygomatic arch is transected and the posterior end is depressed to prevent forward movement of the condyle.

dibular joint, particularly in young females. It is believed to arise from a disturbance of the complex neuromuscular control of the joint. This painful disturbance is often associated with anxiety and tension, but after conservative methods have been fully explored surgery may be necessary.

Some success is claimed with condylotomy, which can be carried out as a blind procedure using a Gigli saw, or as an open procedure via a preauricular incision, or through the mouth.

It has become apparent due to improved diagnostic methods, e.g. video-arthrography, that some of the problems are due to disc detachment or perforations and these can be repaired surgically.

4. Osteoarthritis

Severe pain may occur in the proliferative phase of this disease and surgery is often the only way to deal satisfactorily with the problem. The aim is the removal of the irregular part of the condylar head undertaken as a high condylectomy, or so-called 'shave'.

5. Condylar Hyperplasia

Unilateral growth of the condyle may occur after normal skeletal growth has ceased, and may be associated with deformity of the condyle. In these patients, removal of the condyle (condylectomy) is indicated.

6. Fracture

Gross displacement of the fractured condyle in children may have serious growth consequences and occasionally open reduction is required. The preauricular incision is used often with a submandibular incision to allow manipulation of the fragment or fragments into position.

TREATMENT OF ORAL MALIGNANCY

The commonest form of oral malignancy is the squamous carcinoma, 50 per cent of which involve the tongue. Leucoplakia is said to predispose to malignancy but only 4 per cent of these white patches become malignant. Leucoplakia, when it arises in the floor of the mouth, produces a higher incidence of malignancy, thought to be due to pooling of carcinogens or possibly to the endodermal origin of the floor of the mouth.

Tumours are usually classified on the S.T.N.M. classification:

S—Site.
T—Extent of primary tumour.
N—Involvement of regional lymph nodes.
M—Presence of distant metastases.

Each category is graded and the grades are combined to ascribe a staging to the tumour. Some sites are known to have a poorer prognosis than others, e.g. those situated towards the posterior of the mouth in the oropharynx or posterior tongue.

The extent of the primary is obviously important in the prognosis as well as being an important consideration in the mutilating effect of any surgery.

Involvement of the regional lymph nodes implies serious spread of the disease and the presence of distant metastases a bad prognosis. The rate of growth of a tumour is a most important prognostic index.

Preoperative Considerations

A careful examination of the mouth should be carried out, particularly down the sides of the tongue and back in the floor of the mouth, using spatulas or dental mirrors. The patient should be asked to lift the tongue into the palate so that the root of the tongue, sides of the tongue and floor of the mouth can be examined anteriorly. The examiner will then be able to assess the full extent of the tumour already seen and may possibly detect other primaries.

Fixation of the tongue is an ominous sign.

Pre-malignant Lesions

Localized pre-malignant lesions are generally excised but can be treated by cryosurgery. The more extensive pre-malignant lesions which can involve much of the mucosa inside the mouth, producing the so-called 'hot mouth', may eventually result in multiple primary tumours. Serial excision with skin grafting has been carried out in these cases, although some authorities advocate the use of radio-active yttrium, which has a very low penetration.

Methods of Treatment

Choice of treatment for oral cancer is as follows:
1. Surgery.
2. Radiotherapy.
3. Cytotoxic drugs.
4. Combinations of these treatments.

The choice of treatment will depend on the stage of the disease, the biological activity of the tumour, the general fitness of the patient and the question of whether any treatment has already been attempted and been unsuccessful. The commonest combination therapy is to carry out excision of the tumour and follow this by radiotherapy. Cytotoxic drugs can be administered by intra-arterial perfusion but are more usually given systemically. Lymphomas and sarcomas are rarely treated by surgery.

Surgical Treatment of Tumours

The tumour is excised with a margin of surrounding normal tissue to an extent which depends on the location and histology of the tumour but is usually about 2 cm. Allowance must be made for special situations where the tumour is known to spread preferentially, such as into the mandibular canal and greater palatine canal. These excisions may mean loss of large portions of upper or lower jaw and, if there is lymph gland involvement, block dissection is performed in continuity with the tumour.

CARCINOMA OF THE LIPS

Small carcinomas involving the vermilion of the lip can be excised by wedge excision allowing 1 cm on each side of the tumour and closed directly with little deformity. If this excision of the tumour would result in the loss of more than one-third of the length of the lip the defect can be filled by a cross-lip flap, i.e. swinging a flap from the other lip on a pedicle to help fill the defect. Larger excisions than this will need more complicated flaps to restore the sphincter to a reasonable aesthetic and functional size.

CARCINOMA OF THE MANDIBLE

In the mandible, where excision of the tumour has resulted in loss of the body or angle on one side, it is preferred to disarticulate the condyle and coronoid process in continuity if immediate reconstruction is not contemplated. Otherwise, the proximal fragment will flex and will cause extreme discomfort if the upper natural teeth are present or will rub on the upper denture.

If the excision terminates anteriorly between the canine region and the centre line of the mandible, it is possible to leave the patient without any reconstruction, apart from that necessary to restore lost soft tissue. The importation of a pedicle or flap to provide soft tissue cover helps to prevent the swing of the mandible to the operated side and also serves partly to fill in the defect caused by the loss of bone.

Many patients can wear lower dentures on edentulous remaining fragments of lower jaws provided that they extend across the midline to the excised site, and most, when faced with the proposition of reconstruction, invariably prefer to accept the situation and wear a new reduced lower denture.

Because the tongue tends to fall backwards without anterior support, postoperative nursing and feeding can be difficult should it be necessary to excise the symphysis. The airway may be so at risk that tracheostomy is necessary, and feeding will be by nasogastric tube inserted at operation, in combination with an intravenous infusion. Fortunately, symphysis tumours are quite rare but, for the above reasons, an attempt is made to reconstruct the anterior mandible even if this is only on a temporary basis, e.g. by a titanium implant allowing the tongue to be sutured forward and stabilized.

When the tumour is confined to the floor of the mouth or alveolus and is superficial in a reasonably deep mandible, it is permissible to cut out a block of mandible with the tumour, leaving a lower border strut intact. This also enables one to stabilize the tongue, but the same rules of excision apply as far as the safety margin is concerned and it is not therefore always possible to leave a deep strut. The patient must take care postoperatively as fracture may readily occur.

CARCINOMA OF THE TONGUE

The tongue may be involved primarily in a tumour or by extension. This may necessitate excision of a small part of the tongue which may be closed directly or a large part may need removal, care being taken to give a good margin around the tumour. This may cause difficulty in swallowing and speaking, but most patients adapt quickly to the smaller tongue.

If the excision is large, the tongue tip can often be rotated and sutured to cover a raw area anteriorly and large superficial defects can be covered with quilt grafts. A split-skin graft is applied to the raw area and sutured to it around the edges and to the bed of the graft. The grafted skin is then perforated in a number of places to allow free escape of blood.

CARCINOMA OF THE MAXILLA

Malignant tumours of the maxillary alveolus invariably require removal of a section of the maxilla and quite frequently this entails a hemimaxillectomy and includes the removal of varying amounts of soft tissue from the cheek. The hemimaxillectomy includes the lateral nasal wall but it is often possible to leave the septum intact and attached to the remaining part of the maxilla, although there should be no hesitation in removing whatever structures may be involved in the tumour. Superiorly, the excision usually stops at a level which leaves the infraorbital rim intact. If, at operation, it is found that the tumour involves the roof of the antrum or the infraorbital rim, this is excised and, if the orbit is involved, enucleation of the eye may be required.

Only rarely does the tumour involve the overlying skin and this is more common with alveolar tumours than with those originating within the antrum, which may themselves present on the alveolus. When skin is involved, it is excised with the usual normal margin.

Occasionally, maxillary tumours extend from the orbit or nasal cavity into the ethmoidal air cells or into the base of the skull. On these occasions it is usual to carry out the operation in cooperation with a neurosurgeon, but spread to this extent implies a very poor prognosis. Enucleation of the eye is usually followed by excision of the edges of the eyelids which are sutured together and the defect is eventually covered by a prosthesis attached to spectacles. Defects in the skin can often be covered by locally mobilized flaps when small but larger defects will need imported skin from other sites.

Although it is possible to carry out a limited hemimaxillectomy without incision of the skin, in those cases where the operation is likely to be more extensive a Ferguson incision is used. This passes upwards through the vermilion of the lip and philtrum and around the ala of the nose in the crease at the lateral margin towards the medial canthus and from there laterally under the eyelid as far as is necessary to achieve access. After excision is complete, the maxillary defect is filled with either plastic foam or a gutta percha mould covered with a split-skin graft. The plastic foam is held in place by sutures and the mould by some form of dental appliance which is made before the operation and which can be supported by a frontal bar and external screws or by bilateral circumzygomatic wiring, if the zygomatic arch on the affected side is intact.

Complications

These include salivary fistulas, breakdown of wounds with exposure of bone grafts and implants, and necrosis of flaps or pedicles. The early postoperative complication, once the airway has been ensured, is bleeding, the source of which is sometimes difficult to detect and can be rapidly fatal.

When the histological report is received after the operation, it may reveal that excision is incomplete. A decision is then made whether further surgery will be carried out or whether the patient will have radiotherapy or cytotoxic therapy. This will depend on the type of tumour and the surgeon's impression of the extent and spread of the tumour gained at operation and discussion with the oncologist.

JAW RECONSTRUCTION

Defects and deformities of the jaws occur in the following circumstances:

1. Excision for malignancy.
2. Excision of large benign tumours and cysts.
3. Severe accidents including missile injuries.
4. Osteomyelitis and osteoradionecrosis.
5. Congenital anomalies.

The aim of treatment is to restore mastication, deglutition without leak into the nose, speech and appearance.

1. After Excision for Malignancy

In the maxilla, restoration of function and appearance is usually achieved by fitting a prosthesis known as an 'obturator' (*Fig.* 27.9). A rapidly constructed

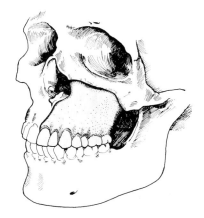

Fig. 27.9. Obturator replacing resected maxilla.

temporary obturator is inserted 7–10 days postoperatively when the plastic foam or mould is removed. This is replaced by an appliance, hollow for lightness, which can be of an elastic material to allow insertion into undercuts to improve retention.

Defects in the maxilla can be repaired by the use of rib grafts covered by nasal and oral mucosal flaps but this is rarely necessary as obturators are well tolerated.

In the mandible, reconstruction is complicated by the inevitable loss of soft tissue which may be extensive and will certainly include the periosteum. Lost soft tissue may be replaced by flaps.

When it is necessary to maintain space between the bone ends or to establish postoperative stability of the tongue, foreign material may be used until such time as bone grafting can be safely undertaken. It is not common practice to carry out primary bone grafting in malignant cases, because of the difficulty in achieving adequate soft tissue coverage, and also on account of the possibility of recurrence of tumour. The presence of hidden metastases must also be considered.

Many materials have been used as implants between the bone ends. These include stainless steel strip, titanium bars and Kirschner wires. The importance of symphysis replacement has been mentioned in the postoperative forward fixation of the tongue

and any of these materials may be used for this. All except the Kirschner wires are attached to the fragments by screws of the same metal.

Unfortunately, many of these cases suffer perforation of mucosa or skin postoperatively in relation to the implant, or wound breakdown, in spite of prophylactic antibiotics and double suturing of the mucosa. In the mouth, this is considered to be due to the movements of the mucosa over the implant, possible impairment of blood supply and contracture of scar tissue.

However, exposure is not always a disaster as loss of the implant can be deferred until the patient is over the dangerous postoperative phase, when fibrosis will tend to hold the tongue forward as well as retaining some separation of the fragments. When it is decided eventually to replace the implant by bone, grafting can be carried out in a variety of ways.

Figure 27.10 shows grafting of the symphysis using

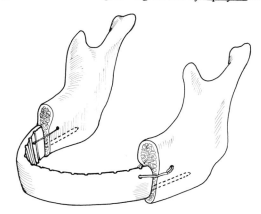

Fig. 27.10. Replacement of symphysis and parts of lower jaw using rib autograft. The rib is notched on its inner surface to allow bending without fracture.

a rib that has been notched on its inner surface to allow it to bend without breaking after skewering it with a Kirschner wire of about 2 mm diameter. The ends of the wire are inserted at least 2·5 cm into the medulla of the mandibular remnants. The ramus and gaps in the body can be replaced by iliac crest or rib grafts, which are wired into place.

Clinical experience suggests that chip and medulla grafts have a higher resistance to infection than solid pieces of bone and, to this end, grafting of these into a mesh trough has been used in the mandible. The trough can be made of titanium or Dacron and is attached by screws to the cut end of the mandible. Suitable medulla can be excavated from the iliac crest via a small incision.

Following radiotherapy, the blood supply to the soft tissues is impaired, and this will have an adverse influence on the survival of the bone graft. This difficulty may be overcome by the removal of a piece of iliac crest or rib with its arterial supply and venous drainage, followed by microvascular anastomosis of these to suitable vessels in the neck. Although these operations are necessarily prolonged, the results are promising. Myocutaneous flaps with rib attached and based on pectoralis major are also used to reconstruct both jaws.

More recently, split clavicle including part of the sternal articulation and skin has been used to replace parts of the mandible, including the condyle. The microvascular anastomosis is based on the acromio-thoracic axis.

2. After Excision of Benign Lesions

Immediate reconstruction is carried out, which avoids the difficult dissection often encountered in secondary grafting.

A great advantage of benign tumour excision is that periosteum may be retained, maintaining some osteogenic potential. Iliac crest or rib grafting is used.

3. After Traumatic Loss

In general, immediate grafting is avoided owing to wound contamination and soft tissue loss, and is postponed until the wound is cleanly healed and adequate soft tissue is available for cover, either by importation from other regions as pedicles or flaps or locally from advancement or rotation.

In the meantime, the space for the graft must be maintained without insertion of foreign material in the wound.

When teeth are present, the upper and lower jaws are fixed together with wires or splints and external fixation is used to hold the bone fragments. This con-

sists of bone screws inserted into the bone at each side of the gap and joined by external bars and joints, and is used without joining the jaws in edentulous cases.

4. After Osteomyelitis and Osteoradionecrosis

Bone grafting may be required after oesteomyelitis once infection has been controlled and healing is complete. Periosteum is often present and the above techniques are used (*see Figs.* 27.13, 27.14).

Following bone loss due to osteoradionecrosis, bone grafting is avoided, as healing is unlikely on account of poor blood supply, both in the bone and soft tissue, and the likelihood of chronic infection. The main problem is that the bone affected by radiation, and which should be excised, cannot be defined. These cases are rare but the use of bone grafts with their own blood supply must improve the prognosis.

A new technique after excision in these circumstances is to fill the defect at the angle and ramus with a rotated temporal muscle flap which has the advantage of bulk and its own blood supply.

5. Congenital Anomalies (*Figs.* 27.11–27.15)

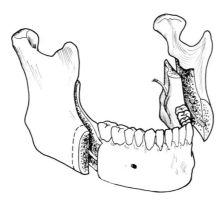

Fig. 27.11. Sagittal split of the mandible may be used for correction of prognathism or retrognathism as there is a large area of bone contact between the fragments.

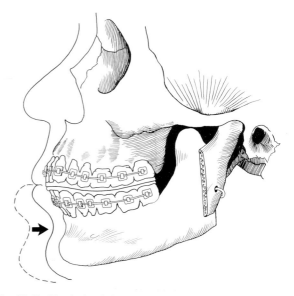

Fig. 27.12. Vertical subsigmoid osteotomy for prognathism can be performed intra-orally or extra-orally. Intra-oral operation avoids potential damage to the facial nerve.

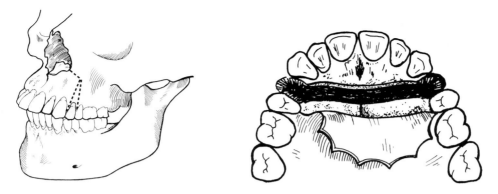

Figs. 27.13, 27.14. Osteotomies can be performed on the maxilla at any level up to and including the base of skull in extreme deformity, e.g. Crouzon's disease. Minor local deformities are corrected by segmental osteotomies, e.g. anterior maxillary osteotomy.

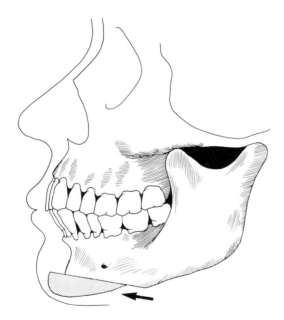

Fig. 27.15. A retruded chin, with teeth in a normal bite, can be corrected by genioplasty carried out intra-orally. For protruding chins the movement is backwards.

FURTHER READING

Cawson R. A., McCracken A. W. and Marcus P. B. (1982) *Pathologic Mechanisms in Human Disease*. St Louis, C. V. Mosby.

Epker B. N. and Wolford L. M. (1980) *Dentofacial Deformities. Surgical-Orthodontic Correction*. St Louis, C. V. Mosby.

Jones J. H. and Mason D. K. (1980) *Oral Manifestations of Systemic Disease*. Philadelphia, W. B. Saunders.

Rowe N. L. and Williams J. Ll. (1985) *Maxillofacial Injuries*. Edinburgh, Churchill Livingstone.

Shafer W. G., Hine M. K. and Levy B. M. (1983) *Textbook of Oral Pathology*. Philadelphia, W. B. Saunders.

Breast, Skin Grafting and Lymphoedema

Chapter twenty-eight

Principles of Skin Cover

J. Lendrum

The importance of the skin's integrity cannot be over-emphasized. Whenever breached, its function of maintaining the *milieu intérieur* is impaired. Control of body fluid and heat is lost; protection from toxic fluids, rays and solids is lost; colonization by micro-organisms is inevitable and invasion likely. The skin's sensory and expressive roles may be destroyed.

Subsequent scar contracture may destroy the function of the structures, particularly joints, which skin clothes. The patient's body image and acceptability in society may be altered, making him or her a psychiatric cripple.

The principles of skin cover are to restore form and function as rapidly as possible, leaving as inconspicuous scars as possible, without creating further avoidable damage.

The priority of skin cover must follow only maintaining the airway and control of bleeding, for without an intact skin envelope all deep structures are at risk of continuing damage, and elaborate surgery on brain, bowel or bone will have been wasted.

To heal and function skin must be live and cover live tissue. The diagnosis of dead, dying or irrevocably damaged skin and the recognition of impending or potential risks to its blood supply are therefore fundamental to its handling.

The assessment of skin viability is often difficult and can only be made from experience. The successful handling of skin can be learned, but not taught, and depends on gentleness, sympathy and imagination. The colour and feel will guide the surgeon who may persuade but never compel skin.

BASIC PRINCIPLES OF SKIN HANDLING

Gentleness is the key to success. Skin should be handled as little as possible. The major enemies are tension and haematoma.

1. *The Patient*
Patients should be as fit as possible. Diabetes, anaemia and malnutrition should be corrected. Arteriosclerosis, particularly in the legs, delays healing.

2. *The Operation Site*
This must be anaesthetic and well illuminated.

3. *The Surgeon*
The surgeon must be comfortable and relaxed.

4. *Colourless Antiseptic*
Skin preparation is essential. Dyes obscure colour and make vitality impossible to assess.

5. *Instruments*
These need be few and simple. Suction should be available. Knives should be sharp. Hooks should be used to move skin. Holding in the fingers, crushing in heavy dissecting or ratchet forceps must be avoided.

6. *Retraction*
This must be done cautiously. Bruising, crushing and kinking under forceful retraction will damage skin. Continuous rubbing with instruments and sutures will burn it as effectively as hot compresses or careless diathermy.

7. *Skin Edges and Raw Surfaces*
These must be kept moist. Desiccated tissue dies.

8. *Stop All Bleeding before Closure*
Haematoma becomes colonized by bacteria and will form an abscess. Haemostasis must be accurate and delicate so that no damage is done to other tissue.

Where bleeding cannot be stopped completely, wounds should either be drained, left open or temporarily covered by a dressing.

The commonest cause of postoperative wound sepsis is inadequate operative haemostasis and is usually an avoidable technical disaster.

9. *Remove All Dead and Foreign Material*
Avascular fat, muscle and bone necrose to form abscesses.

10. *Avoid All 'Dead' Spaces*
Wounds should be closed in layers, taking care not to leave gaps which will inevitably fill with exudate or blood and form abscesses.

The minimum amount of buried suture material should be used to achieve this. Each suture acts as a potential nidus for infection. Heavy, tightly tied sutures strangulate tissue.

Where subcutaneous fat does not survive between

the skin and the deep fascia or periosteum the scar will adhere to the deep layer and produce a tender, puckered, obvious, depressed scar.

11. *Bony Ridges and Depressions*

These should be smoothed down or padded over with soft tissue. Skin stretched tight over a ridge will necrose.

12. *Skin Edges*

These must come together easily *without tension*: The ultra-structure of dermis permits a certain limited amount of stretch and no more. Attempts to force skin beyond this inbuilt limit are fatal.

Judgement of the amount of extension possible can be learnt only by experience and is critical. Hauling on skin with thicker and thicker stitches, placed further and further from the edge ending with 'deep tension sutures', shows a lack of understanding of skin physiology and a lack of judgement which ends at best in a hideous scar, but more often in wound breakdown.

If sutures cheese wire through, thicker ones will not relieve the tension. If the skin feels tight as it is closed postoperative oedema will make it tighter still. If skin blanches as it is moved its circulation has stopped and no amount of hyperbaric oxygen will keep it alive.

There is always an alternative method of closure which should and must be used.

13. *Dressings*

These should protect the wound from shearing, pressure and rubbing. The old concept of the 'pressure' dressing has been shown to exert either no pressure or so much that venous return is prevented, thereby causing necrosis. The idea has been abandoned. Wound immobilization postoperatively for a few days relieves pain, reduces bleeding and reduces the risk of external forces disrupting the wound. This may be achieved by a soft, bulky gauze pad, firmly bandaged in place, which protects the patient and his or her relatives from an unsightly wound. This type of dressing may be used to absorb exudate from a wound, but it must be thick enough to remain dry on its outer surface and stable enough to remain in apposition with the wound. A wet or displaced dressing will militate against healing and must be removed.

Skin itself is the best wound dressing and often needs no additional cover. Micro-organisms will not invade a well-closed wound from outside, but will always disrupt a badly closed wound from within.

14. *Sutures*

These should never be tied tightly. The area enclosed in a tight suture will necrose. Postoperative oedema makes tight sutures tighter still, and the stitch will cut through the skin.

Sutures should be removed as soon as possible; no later than 48 hours from the eyelids, 4 days from the rest of the face and 7 days elsewhere. If the wound then opens, it was not correctly closed in the first place.

Non-absorbable sutures should not be used on the pinna or genitalia: their removal from these sites causes agony. Absorbable materials such as catgut and Dexon should not be used as percutaneous sutures.

The methods of covering skin defects are:
1. Direct approximation.
2. Transplantation.

DIRECT APPROXIMATION

Indications

1. Surgical incisions.
2. Clean lacerations.
3. Small areas of skin excision/loss.

Method

Plan the incision or excision to lie in or parallel to a natural skin crease where tension is least and scarring least conspicuous (*Fig.* 28.1). There is never any indication for vertical incisions in the neck. (N.B. Abdominal striae run across the lines of minimal tension.)

Draw on the skin a plan of the proposed incision, checking the line of skin crease and the available skin that can be removed by gently pinching it up between finger and thumb.

The amount that may be excised will depend on:
1. *The Site.* Beware the presternal, infraclavicular and deltoid regions, which almost invariably produce hypertrophic scars. Thick skin of the palms, sole and back are least extensible.
2. *Local Anatomical Landmarks.* Landmarks such as the mouth, eye or nose will limit what can be removed without distortion.
3. *The Age of the Patient.* The patient's age is proportional to what may be excised. Infants' skin is not extensible. Increasing age diminishes tension and produces folds of stretched skin which permit large areas to be sacrificed. Cut the skin with a sharp knife. Avoid stretching and tearing. Cut perpendicular to the surface. Bevelled edges heal with a heaped up conspicuous scar.

Stop all bleeding.

Check tension before suturing by the feel and colour of the skin on drawing it together with hooks. If it feels tight a little more gain may be made by cautiously undermining the adjacent skin, but beware, especially in the leg, that this does not destroy the blood supply (*Fig.* 28.2).

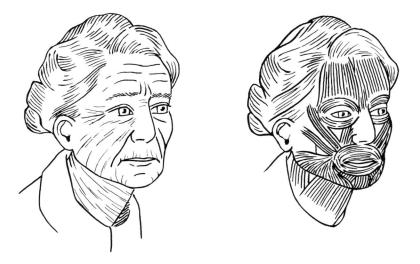

Fig. 28.1. The lines of facial wrinkles which correspond to the elective site of scar direction when compared with the underlying muscles.

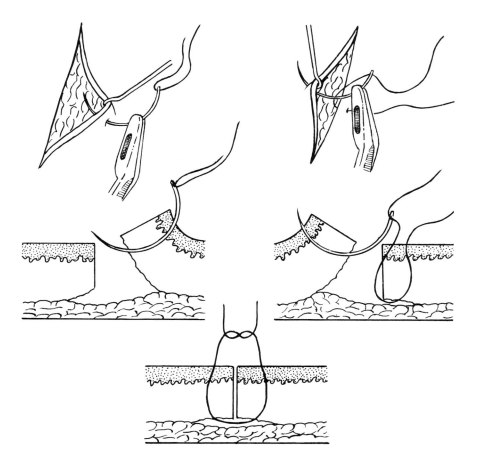

Fig. 28.2. Suturing with eversion of the skin edges. Note that the skin is lifted with a hook and not crushed with dissecting forceps.

Check that local landmarks are not distorted, for example by pulling a lip or eyelid into ectropion.

Edge-to-edge skin apposition must be exact. Fine sutures should be used on curved cutting needles: 3/0 is the strongest needed; the maximum on the face is 5/0 and on the eyelids 6/0.

Types of Direct Closure

The defect must be converted into either a fusiform or wedge shape.

FUSIFORM

This is usually incorrectly known as 'elliptical'. The length-to-breadth ratio should be as great as possible to avoid pleats at the apices known as 'dog ears'. A length at least four times the breadth is usually necessary. The two sides must be of equal length (*Figs.* 28.3, 28.4).

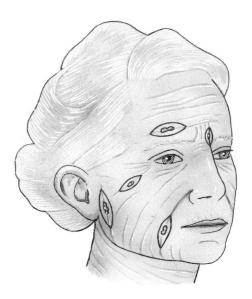

Fig. 28.3. 'Elliptical' facial incisions and excisions. Lines of election.

WEDGE

Where skin of the margin of lip, eyelid, nostril or pinna is to be removed this may be done by excising a wedge of the full thickness of the structure.

Up to one-quarter of the length of the free margin of these may be sacrificed with a good structural and functional reconstruction by careful closure of each separate layer (*Figs.* 28.5, 28.6).

Contra-indications

1. Where tension would result.
2. Where displacement, distortion or destruction of anatomical landmarks would result.
3. Where the resulting scar would cross a natural skin crease.

TRANSPLANTATION

Definition

Movement of live tissue from one site to another where it can produce a lineage of live cells.

Types of Transplantation

1. Grafts.
2. Flaps.

Indications

Wherever skin loss is too wide for the area to be closed directly.

SKIN GRAFTS

Definition

Skin removed from one site, with complete division of its vascular connections, transplanted to another site where it revascularizes by capillary anastomosis. Skin grafts are classified according to:

1. Their donor–recipient relationship.
2. Their thickness.

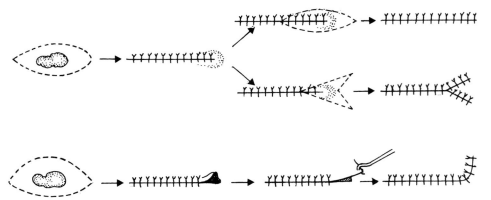

Fig. 28.4. Alternative methods of excising the 'dog ear' produced by a short ellipse.

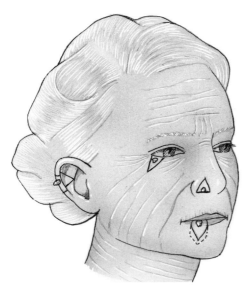

Fig. 28.5. Wedge excision through the full thickness of the pinna, eyelid, nostril and lip.

TYPES OF GRAFT CLASSIFIED BY DONOR–RECIPIENT RELATIONSHIP

1. *Autograft:* Tissue transferred from one part of an individual to another part of the same individual.

2. *Isograft:* Tissue transferred from one individual to another of identical genetic constitution (identical twins).

These two categories are the only ones which can provide permanent skin cover.

3. *Homograft* (American equivalent: allograft): Tissue transferred from one individual to another of the same species who is not genetically identical.

Homografts even of close genetic similarity are rejected after a very variable unpredictable time, ranging from days to months. Their use is restricted to the temporary cover of large raw areas resulting from burns, while awaiting healing of the donor site before recropping.

4. *Heterograft* (American equivalent: xenograft): Tissue transferred from an individual of one species to one of a different species.

Freeze-dried pigskin, often used as a skin substitute dressing in extensive burns, is incorrectly named a 'graft' as it is dead and does not 'take'.

Take: Of a graft, this means its biological reattachment to its recipient area and consequent normal physiological behaviour.

TYPES OF FREE SKIN GRAFT CLASSIFIED ACCORDING TO THICKNESS (*Fig.* 28.7)

1. *Split-skin Grafts* (partial-thickness or Thiersch grafts).

2. *Full-thickness Grafts* (whole-thickness or Wolfe grafts).

3. *Composite Grafts.*

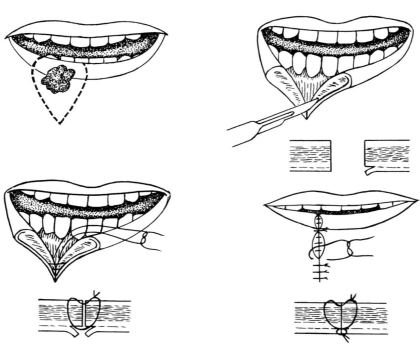

Fig. 28.6. Two-layer closure of wedge excision defect of the lip.

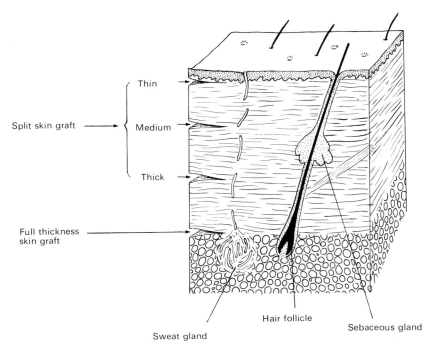

Fig. 28.7. Thickness of skin grafts. Split-skin graft.

1. Split-skin Grafts

These consist of epidermis and the subjacent dermis, the thickness of which may be thin, intermediate or thick according to the depth of dermis included.

Indications

Split-skin grafts are used for free skin grafting where skin or mucosal defects too large to be closed directly have a base (graft bed) which has a vascular supply sufficient to support the graft.

Free grafts begin to necrose and autolyse when detached from their donor site. If they revascularize before this happens they will survive and regenerate. The recipient graft bed must therefore be capable of producing granulations.

It is, however, unnecessary and usually inadvisable to wait for granulations to form before applying a graft. Delay allows the exudate from the raw surface to be converted to fibrin through which capillaries cannot penetrate. Massive bacterial colonization of the raw surface also prevents take.

Contra-indications

1. Where the raw area has an avascular bed formed by:
    a. Bare cortical bone deprived of its periosteum (medullary bone readily accepts grafts).
    b. Bare cartilage deprived of its perichondrium.
    c. Bare tendon deprived of its paratenon or sheath.
    d. Open joints or other fistulas.
    e. Prostheses and foreign bodies.
2. On major arteries, veins and nerves which are not only unable to support grafts, but which need padding between themselves and the skin.
3. Where it is planned to do subsequent surgery. Skin grafts cannot be lifted as flaps without necrosing.
4. On irradiated tissue.
5. As a substitute for conjunctiva. Desquamating skin, especially if hairy, abrades, ulcerates, and causes vascularization and consequent corneal opacity.

Principles of Split-skin Grafting

1. The patient should be as fit as possible.
2. The thinner the graft the more rapidly does the critical basal cell layer revascularize so that the more certain is successful take. Thin grafts therefore take on areas where the blood supply is least good, such as fat and fibrous tissue, or where there is some bacterial contamination.

Thin graft donor sites heal more rapidly with less scarring. However, thin grafts have disadvantages when compared with thick ones:
    a. Contracture is inversely proportional to graft thickness.
    b. Thin grafts are more likely to change colour than thick ones. Mottled areas of de-, hypo- and hyperpigmentation alternate within the same sheet of graft to a greater extent in thin than in thick grafts.
    c. Graft skin consistency is less like the normal.

Thin grafts tend to remain shiny and stiff for longer.

d. They are less robust and stand less wear and tear. They are more prone to breakdown and ulceration after trivial trauma.

e. Hair regeneration is less common and sparser with thinner grafts.

For these reasons the thickest graft which will take on the recipient area should always be used.

Thin grafts should be used only:

a. In the emergency cover of burns.

b. For temporary repair, following trauma, and for covering the raw surfaces of open flaps.

c. On chronic ulcers the beds of which cannot be excised completely.

d. Where the defect is not over or near a joint.

e. Where the graft is not easily seen.

Thick grafts should be used:

a. For the release of contractures.

b. Over or near joints.

c. On the face, hands and feet.

d. When the donor site can be hidden.

Wherever possible a single sheet of skin should cover the whole defect. Where there are joints in a graft hypertrophic scars result.

Mesh Grafts

Multiple parallel rows of offset slits cut in a graft permit its expansion in both planes by up to six times its original dimensions. When stretched a lattice work of holes appears, so that it resembles a string vest. The holes epithelialize within a few days by growth from the edges of the strings. These grafts are useful for:

1. Grafting areas larger than the available donor sites (i.e. burns over 30–40 per cent of the body surface area).

2. Grafting uneven surfaces, especially small radius convexities such as the scrotum or concavities such as the defect following maxillectomy or orbital exenteration where sheet grafts would pleat.

DISADVANTAGES

1. Until epithelialization is complete the recipient area is still open.

2. They contract more than do sheets.

3. The 'string vest' appearance remains as a permanent cosmetic deformity.

Donor Site (Figs. 28.8–28.11)

Almost any area may be used as a source of donor skin. In extensive burns whatever is undamaged may be used to repair what is. Where there is a choice:

1. Like should replace like if possible. Each area of skin is unique and only identical with the same area on the opposite side of the body.

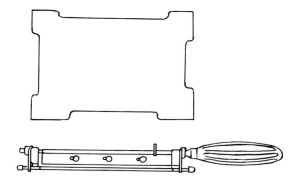

Fig. 28.8. Gabarro board. Skin graft knife.

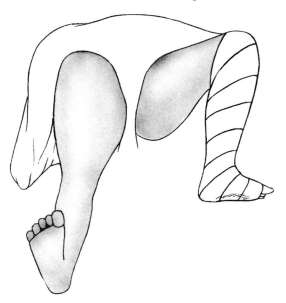

Fig. 28.9. Taking a skin graft. Position of patient.

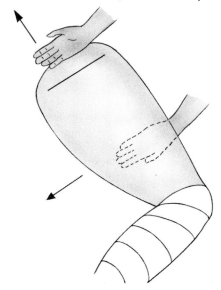

Fig. 28.10. Taking a skin graft. Position of assistant. The left hand is flattening the thigh by lifting and pushing in the direction of the lower arrow. The right hand is tensing the skin by pulling in the direction of the upper arrow.

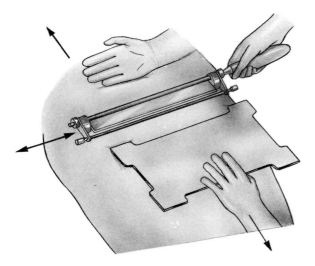

Fig. 28.11. Taking a split-skin graft. Continued tension and stretching of the thigh in the direction of the arrows by the assistant is imperative, while the action of the surgeon is at right angles to this.

2. Broad, smooth, flat or convex surfaces are easiest to shave.
3. Take the nearest colour match. (The postauricular sulcus and upper medial aspect of the arm are best for the face.)
4. Take the graft from an area which is normally hidden. Shaving off a layer of skin leaves permanent scarring: the thinner the graft the less conspicuous this will be.

In young girls the first choice must be the buttock. The front of the chest should be avoided.

The face, hands, feet and genitalia are always the last resort. When grafting a defect resulting from excision of a malignant neoplasm the same limb should never be used as a donor site. The donor site is a large raw wound which should be protected until healed by an occlusive dressing.

The healing time of the donor site is proportional to the thickness of graft taken from it. A thin graft donor site should heal within 7 days and a thick one within 3 weeks by coalescence of epithelium spreading from hair follicles, sebaceous and sweat glands in the base.

A thin graft donor site will leave barely detectable discoloration, whereas a thick one will always remain shiny, mottled and noticeable and is best treated by covering with a thin graft.

Skin Storage

Split-skin grafts may be stored in airtight containers suitably labelled with the patient's name and date of operation:

1. For up to 3 weeks at 4 °C wrapped in a gauze well wrung out of normal saline.
2. For up to 6 months at −196 °C wrapped in a glycerol gauze, the container being bathed in liquid nitrogen.

The Recipient Area

The success of a graft is proportional to the care with which the recipient area is prepared. Ideally, this should be a clean, vascular (but not bleeding), smooth, flat, raw surface.

Fluid or solid between graft and bed will prevent take.

Haematoma and *exudate* are the most common causes of graft failure and must be prevented by meticulous haemostasis. Patient pressure on a raw bleeding surface is an investment which will save time, trouble and regrafting later.

Foreign bodies should be removed. Old scar tissue and exuberant, proud, oedematous, gelatinous, grey or yellow granulations must be excised, for example from chronic ulcers. This process is called 'débridement'. Irradiated tissues must be excised.

Avascular structures should be covered by vascular ones. Bare limb bone can be covered by transposing a muscle belly over it. The outer table of the skull may be sacrificed to graft the diploë. Major vessels and nerves should be covered by vascular soft tissue. Open joints or fistulas should be closed.

The base should be levelled to permit the graft to adapt accurately to its surface. Hollows fill with exudate through which capillaries cannot grow.

The wound should be free from beta-haemolytic streptococci, even small numbers of which destroy grafts. Small numbers of other pathogens do not prevent graft take, but heavy infestation by *Staphylococcus* and *Pseudomonas* may.

A single sheet of skin graft should be applied to the defect whenever possible, making sure that there are no pleats or overlaps, especially at the graft edge. When two or more sheets are needed to cover a single defect they should be butt jointed accurately. Whenever there is skin overlap both layers and the surrounding graft will die.

When a graft is put on to deep fascia the skin at the perimeter should be sewn both to the graft and the deep fascia, so that there is no shearing between them.

Check that no haematoma is present under the graft after its application. This is visible through all but the thickest grafts and must be removed before dressing.

Graft Dressing

More grafts are lost because of bad dressings than are saved by good ones. Dressings therefore should be avoided whenever possible and made simple and secure when they are used.

The objective is fixation of the graft to its bed, so that capillary anastomosis can take place without mechanical interference. This is a natural process which does not require a cover, but does need protection from shearing, sliding or rubbing forces moving the graft on its bed and protection from pressure which prevents capillary blood flow.

The 'pressure dressing' should be regarded as a means of preventing pressure necrosis of the graft rather than a means of squashing the graft home.

AIMS OF DRESSINGS

1. To immobilize the graft in relation to its bed.
2. To protect the graft from pressure.
3. To protect the patient and those around him or her from the unsightly appearance of the patch.

INDICATIONS FOR USE

1. When treating outpatients.
2. When treating an elderly or arthritic patient who must be kept mobile with a graft on the leg.
3. When grafting concavities, such as the orbit, maxilla or mouth.
4. When grafting over paratenon or tendon sheath.
5. When using mesh grafts.
6. When a double surface or a full circumferential area on trunk or limb makes it necessary partially to bear weight on the graft.

METHOD

The graft edge should be sutured accurately to the perimeter of the defect without overlap. The sutures should pass through a covering single layer of tulle gras and overlying piece of polyurethane foam sponge cut accurately to fit the defect. These sutures should be tied radially over the foam.

Where grafts are used over or near joints these should be immobilized by appropriate splints.

The dressings should be removed as soon as possible for inspection. Haematoma or seroma which have lifted small areas of graft (less than 1 cm diameter) should be expressed by nicking the graft and pressing it back to its bed. Larger areas should be removed and replaced by stored skin.

CONTRA-INDICATIONS

1. On the neck.
2. On the trunk, especially the back.
3. Where a previous graft has failed.

EXPOSED GRAFTING

Grafts not covered by dressings may be watched and haematoma and seroma expressed before they cause skin necrosis.

It is not necessary to suture the graft to its bed.

Immobilization of the area is mandatory. Infants need immobilization of all limbs.

The graft must be protected from accidental knocks and rubbing. Great ingenuity is required to devise protection by cages, splints or cradles.

Delayed Grafting

Grafts applied to unconscious patients are often disturbed as the patient regains consciousness. Changes of blood pressure and violent movements may cause bleeding under the graft.

To obviate these risks it is preferable to store the graft and wait for 48 hours before applying the graft to the defect. At operation the recipient area is prepared for grafting, but covered instead by a dressing of tulle gras and saline- or eusol-soaked gauze.

The dressing can be removed painlessly 48 hours later, blood and serum washed off with a gentle saline douche and the skin graft applied as a dressing and left exposed.

Extensive burns and areas of skin loss where the débridement cannot be guaranteed should not be grafted primarily.

It is better to give a second general anaesthetic at 48 hours and if necessary complete the débridement before applying the grafts.

Postoperative Care

Grafts should be protected from mechanical injury and underlying fluid aspirated or expressed whenever necessary until take is assured at 8 or 10 days. By then grafts are sufficiently adherent to withstand washing and gentle handling. A graft which moves on its bed at this time has failed to take and should be replaced (remember the fault lies with the bed and not the graft).

The graft subsequently scales, crusts at the edges and becomes shiny. It does not secrete sebum. It remains insensitive and therefore liable to damage from unnoticed trauma over the next few months. It should therefore be gently but thoroughly washed and greased by massage with lanolin or ung. aquosum for at least 6 months until supple, sensitive and matt surfaced.

Grafts should be protected by clothing or barrier creams from bright sunlight for at least 12 months.

Cosmetics may be used to disguise the graft as soon as it has completely healed.

Excess scar tissue forms under grafts and their edges hypertrophy unless continuously compressed for 6 months after they have taken.

As soon as take is assured and healing complete a two-way stretch compression garment should be worn to minimize this risk. To be effective it must be worn 23 hours a day.

Graft contracture continues for at least 3 months and cannot be prevented by splints. Early mobilization and compression may prevent joint stiffness, but are not always successful.

Causes of Graft Loss
1. Fluid between the graft and bed. Common. Usually due to bleeding.
2. External mechanical force.
   a. Inadequate immobilization.
   b. Poor dressing. Common. Usually due to carelessness.
3. Necrotic or avascular tissue in the graft bed. Common. Usually due to inexperienced surgery.
4. Poor general health of the patient. Usually due to diabetes or anaemia.
5. Infection. Rare. Usually due to beta-haemolytic streptococci.

Antibiotics are only indicated if beta-haemolytic streptococci are grown from the wound or an infection elsewhere merits appropriate treatment. Neither systemic nor topical antibiotics will induce graft survival if anything prevents capillary anastomosis between bed and graft.

Graft Inadequacies
Failure to restore form and function may result from:
1. Graft loss.
2. Graft contracture. This flattens normal contours, bridging concavities and grooving convexities. Joint movement is limited particularly in the neck and over joint flexures.
3. Junctional scars hypertrophy and add to the contour distortion. They are inelastic. Grafts commonly wrinkle adding to the contour problem.
4. The colour seldom perfectly matches the surrounds and is often mottled.
5. Hair may be inappropriately transferred and causes problems in mucosal replacement. On the scalp, free grafts do not grow sufficient hair to match normal scalp.
6. Fragility of the grafts. Thinner than normal dermis and less subcutaneous padding make grafts less robust than normal skin. In early months they lack sensation and are therefore at greater risk of injury, especially on soles, palms and shins. Protective sensation usually returns within 2 years.

2. Full-thickness Grafts

These require perfect apposition to a perfect bed for survival. Their use is therefore limited to replacement of small areas on the face and hand where the recipient area blood supply is excellent; where contracture would be disastrous, and where their excellent cosmetic and wear properties are required.

Donor Sites
The postauricular sulcus is the best match for the face. An area of skin adequate to cover an eyelid can be removed from behind one ear and the secondary defect closed by direct suture. Larger areas of less good colour match and consistency for facial reconstruction can be taken from the supraclavicular fossa, with direct closure of the donor site. This area should be avoided in girls.

Small areas can be taken from groin, elbow and wrist flexures for use on the hand with direct closure of the donor site.

On the rare occasion when large grafts are needed the secondary defect must itself be grafted by split skin.

Principles of Use
Full-thickness grafts should never be used in the emergency cover of injuries. All subcutaneous fat must be removed from the grafts. They must be made to fit the defect exactly in shape and size and must be sutured under their original tension. They must be efficiently immobilized and applied under a tie-over dressing. They cannot be stored nor can their application be delayed. They will not take on granulations.

3. Composite Grafts

These are unreliable and are seldom used. They consist of skin and subcutaneous fat, usually with enclosed cartilage. Their survival depends on very rapid revascularization through their cut edges and they must therefore be very small; 1 cm is a wide composite graft.

Their use is restricted to reconstruction of the nose tip, columella or alar margin by grafts from the pinna and occasionally transfer of a toe tip to a finger or thumb.

They should never be used in the emergency management of trauma. They cannot be used on granulations, stored or delayed.

No sutures should be used to hold them in place. They should be fixed by Micropore tape.

FLAPS

Definition
Tissue transferred from one site in an individual to another site in the same individual while maintaining its vascular supply.

The Pedicle
This is the area by which the blood supply is maintained and is a necessary part of every flap. The term 'pedicle flap' is therefore a tautology. The terms 'tube pedicle' and 'tube pedicle flap' are archaic.

The range of flaps used in the cover of skin defects

is vast and continually increasing. Even the classification is altering annually.

Indications for Flap Transfer
1. Where the defect has an inadequate blood supply to support a graft.
2. When a second operation in the area will be required.
3. To cover tendons which have lost their paratenon or sheath.
4. Over divided nerves.
5. For restoring contour.
6. For padding bony prominences.
7. To replace unstable scars or grafts.

Principles of Raising Skin Flaps
The meticulous planning, lifting, transfer and postoperative care of flaps constitute the ultimate challenge to plastic surgeons and are more an art than a science.

Their use should be restricted to those aware of the full range of available methods, with the experience and intuition to choose the most appropriate, the technical skill to achieve transfer safely and who have nurses adequately trained to safeguard the flaps postoperatively. The rewards are great, but the dangers and potential disasters of flap transfer are at least as great.

Planning
The area of the defect is first accurately defined. This may be much larger than apparent, especially if previous scar or graft contracture has dragged surrounding skin into the defect.

The depth of the defect must be gauged and skin, deep tissues and mucosal lining replaced if they have been lost.

The most appropriate flap donor site is chosen, safely to fill the defect with the tissue of nearest functional and cosmetic match. Like should wherever possible replace like. In general the nearer the donor to recipient area the better will be the match.

Local flaps, which move in one stage to an immediately adjacent area, are preferred to distant flaps, of which each stage of transfer adds to their risk and may involve the patient in several weeks of immobilization in uncomfortable positions.

The safety of the flap depends on maintaining its blood supply throughout transfer.

The patient's age and ability to cooperate must be taken into account in planning the most appropriate source and method of transfer.

The flap is designed in reverse; first making a jaconet pattern of the defect and transferring this through each step of the sequence to its donor site. The flap should be designed slightly larger than the defect if more than one stage of transfer is involved to allow for shrinkage and trimming. In transferring the pattern each stage must be checked to ensure that there is no tension or kinking, and that there is no pressure on the flap. Any of these hazards may occlude the venous return from the flap and cause its necrosis.

Types of Flap

The Rhomboid Flap (Fig. 28.12)
This is an elegant example of the local flap. It usually has a *random* pattern blood supply (lacking an anatomically distinct arteriovenous system) and is very safe because the ratio of its length to breadth is nearly equal. If a named artery and vein run in its subcutaneous tissue it is an *axial* flap.

The main use is on the face and the trunk. *The defect* must first be converted into a parallelogram, the sides and short axis of which are equal and the acute angles of which are 60°.

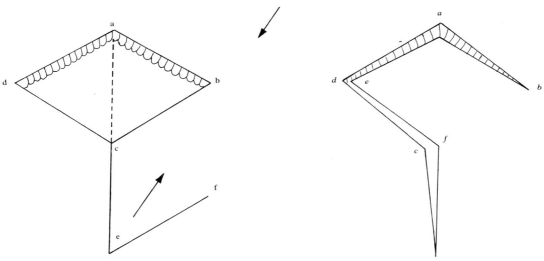

Fig. 28.12. The rhomboid transposition flap. The arrows in the left-hand diagram are in the line of the skin crease.

The donor site is the adjacent area of skin which most readily can be spared. There are four possible areas for each rhomboid. The line of the short axis of the rhomboid (a–c) is extended on to the adjacent skin for an equal distance (c–e) and a second line (e–f) drawn from its end equal in length to, and parallel with, one side of the defect (c–b), so that the angle between the two lines enclosing the flap is 60°.

The incision is made along this line into the subcutaneous fat, which is raised with the skin and transposed through 60° to fill the defect. This involves direct approximation of points c–f, which should therefore lie in the plane of maximum skin extensibility (at right angles to the creases). The feasibility of this closure should be checked in the planning by pinching up the skin between these two points.

Latissimus Dorsi Flap

Originally described in 1896 to reconstruct the ablated breast, it is a historical tragedy that this flap has only recently gained the popularity that it deserves. It consists of the latissimus dorsi muscle with some, all or more than its overlying skin and is classified as a 'musculocutaneous compound flap' as it consists of more than one type of tissue.

Most areas of skin receive their blood supply from vessels that leave the muscle to traverse the deep fascia and supply the immediately overlying skin. Latissimus dorsi occupies a large area of the back, and the skin over and immediately around it can survive solely on these radiating vessels. The blood supply to the muscle comes mainly from the thoracodorsal artery, which is the terminal branch of the subscapular artery, with a corresponding venous drainage. Thus a huge area of skin, measuring up to 30×15 cm, may be moved on a pedicle lying in the axilla.

USE OF THE LATISSIMUS FLAP (*Fig.* 28.13)

1. As a *local* flap to reconstruct the chest wall and breast. This is a *transposition* flap which retains a skin pedicle in addition to its thoracodorsal vessels.
2. As a *distant* flap on the:

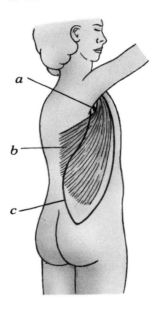

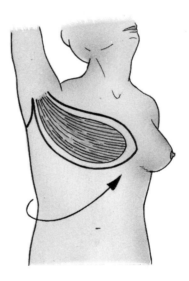

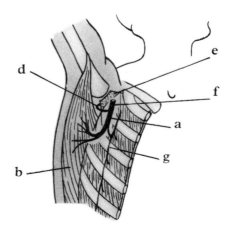

Fig. 28.13. The compound myocutaneous latissimus dorsi flap. *a*, Thoracodorsal neurovascular bundle. *b*, Latissimus dorsi muscle. *c*, Outline of skin flap. *d*, Circumflex scapular vessels. *e*, Scapula. *f*, Subscapular vessels. *g*, Lateral thoracic vessels.

a. Upper limb.

b. Neck (including the mucosal lining of the oesophagus and pharynx).

c. Face (for cheek lining or skin cover).

d. Head.

The required area of skin is detached entirely from its surroundings, and only its muscle attachment on its vascular pedicle is left. The flap is tunnelled under the intervening skin to reach its new destination. It is then known as an 'island flap'.

3. As a *free* flap. Skin and muscle are detached as an 'island' of which the artery and vein (which have diameters of about 2 mm) are also divided and anastomosed under the operating microscope to suitable vessels adjacent to the recipient areas, which may be anywhere on the body but are most commonly in the leg.

OPERATIVE TECHNIQUE

The defect is first outlined and a pattern transferred to the skin overlying the muscle. When used as a transposition or island flap the pattern is used to check that the proposed pedicle is long enough easily to reach the recipient area.

The skin and subcutaneous fat are incised directly down to muscle and the cut edge of the flap sutured temporarily to the muscle to prevent shearing damage during the remaining dissection. These sutures are removed before suturing the skin to the recipient area.

The lateral border of the muscle is identified and lifted. The origins are divided from their inferior and medial attachments to the iliac crest, the lumbar fascia and the thoracic vertebrae. The muscle is turned upwards from the underlying deep muscles of the back, dividing two posterior rami of the lumbar segmental vessels in the process. Care must be taken at the inferior angle of the scapula to avoid raising serratus anterior with the latissimus muscle. The neurovascular bundle appears deep to the latissimus near the lateral border of the scapula, and its branches to serratus anterior are divided. If more mobility of the flap is needed the insertion of the latissimus to the humerus may be divided. If, as is usual, the bulk of the muscle is greater than required, its motor nerve, the thoracodorsal, may be divided to induce atrophy without prejudicing the blood supply to the overlying skin.

Both muscle and skin are sutured into their new positions. Usually the donor site can be closed by direct suture, but if a wide flap has been raised from a thin patient the secondary defect should be grafted with split skin rather than close the wound with tension. Suction drains should be inserted at the lower end of the donor site and retained until dry.

The loss of function resulting from this musculocutaneous transfer is surprisingly small. Forced adduction of the arm is probably taken over by teres major.

MANAGEMENT OF WOUNDS INFLICTED OUTSIDE THE OPERATING THEATRE

This depends on the type and site. Such wounds should all be treated with suspicion and a careful eye for the unexpected. The surgeon should aim to repair the wound with full skin closure by the most rapid means, even where this means temporary loss of form or function. Reconstruction should never be attempted at the time of initial repair; it must always be planned, timed and executed under ideal conditions on a fit patient.

Avoid making the damage worse. Attend first to the airway and the blood loss. Conserve all viable tissue. Excise all dead tissue and foreign bodies.

1. *Abrasions*

Tattooed dirt should be scrubbed out with a wire suede brush and hydrogen peroxide. Superficial dermal damage should be covered by a non-adherent bulky dressing. If there is complete dermal destruction or friction burning a skin graft dressing should be applied.

2. *Clean Lacerations*

Explore the full extent of the wound and repair:

1. Damaged deep structures such as tendons and nerves.

2. The wound in layers.

3. The skin after trimming dead or bevelled edges—if these can be done within the first few hours of injury. If not, await resolution of oedema before repair.

3. *Crush Injuries*

Caused by blunt impact, these injuries produce skin and subcutaneous fat necrosis which may not be immediately obvious. Complex patterns of tissue disruption may be difficult to piece together. These wounds are usually ragged, untidy and dirty. Simplify them as much as possible. Cut back skin and subcutaneous fat to bleeding tissue. Convert a stellate to a circular or elliptical shape. Remove all haematoma and foreign bodies. Cover with a temporary graft or perform delayed primary suture (q.v.).

4. *Avulsion Injuries*

These are injuries in which a tangential impact tears up a flap of skin. They must be treated with the utmost care. Successful healing is a tribute to surgical judgement.

Gently lift the flap, clean the whole bed and stop all bleeding. Further management depends on the site of injury:

a. *Head, Face, Neck and Hand:* Err on the side of conservation. Flaps of dubious viability should be laid back on their site of origin without sutures. Trim the minimum skin from the flap margins.

b. *On the Arm, Trunk and Genitalia:* It is preferable to excise the whole flap and replace by an immediate graft.

c. *On the Leg:* It is mandatory to excise the whole flap and replace by an immediate graft.

A major cause of morbidity is the mismanagement of the trivial avulsion flap injury of the skin of the shin in the elderly and in patients on long-term corticosteroid treatment. The anatomy of the blood supply to the skin of the shin precludes flaps surviving and they must always be replaced by grafts.

5. *Projectile Injuries*

The management depends on the type and velocity of the missile.

a. *Shotgun Pellets:* These should be removed unless they have penetrated deeply and a search for them would inflict worse damage.

b. *Shrapnel and Low-Velocity Bullet Wound:* The wound tracks should be laid open and drained. The missile should only be removed if it can be found without extending the damage. Skin entry and exit wounds should be excised and packed loosely open and, if extensive, grafted secondarily.

c. *The Modern High-Velocity Bullets:* These bullets leave tiny entry and often as tiny exit wounds, but expend their enormous kinetic energy in the deep tissues which are therefore torn up and disrupted for a wide distance round the track.

All fascial planes traversed by these bullets must be opened widely, and no attempt made to close anything except major vessels. Only in this way can oedema be prevented from occluding the circulation to the part and making damage worse. Delayed primary closure is essential.

Loss of Full Thickness

Lips, eyelids and noses should be closed as a wedge if possible, but loss of more than one-quarter of the free border should be closed by loose approximation of skin to mucosa. Reconstruction should only be started when healing is complete.

Burns

Nice judgement is required to determine the depth of dead tissue which should be excised and grafted. This should be done as soon as the decision is made:

1. That the depth of injury is greater than will heal under a dressing within 10 days.
2. That the patient's general condition and particularly fluid balance are stable.

Delayed Primary Closure

Make haste slowly is the rule for all dirty and untidy wounds. As soon as possible after injury:

1. Lay the wound open widely to allow drainage, to relieve compression, to promote blood circulation, to explore and to remove all dead, damaged and foreign material.
2. Stop as much bleeding as possible.
3. Close open joints and cover major vessels and nerves with local soft tissue. Cover exposed brain by dura or a fascial patch.
4. Loosely pack the wound with well-padded gauze, firmly bandaged.
5. Splint fractures comfortably.

After 48 hours reanaesthetize the patient and remove all the packing. Check and if necessary complete the débridement. Close the skin, usually best done with a thin split-skin graft.

Correct primary or delayed primary treatment of skin loss usually obviates the need for subsequent scar revision. The majority of scars and areas of skin loss sent to plastic surgeons for revision result from inept initial management. If these simple guidelines are followed patients will be saved from delayed healing, disfigurement and demoralizing additional surgery.

FURTHER READING

Converse J. M. (1977) *Reconstructive Plastic Surgery, Vol. 1*, 2nd ed. Philadelphia, W. B. Saunders Co.

Dowden R. V. and McCraw J. B. (1981) Myocutaneous flaps. In: Jackson I. T. (ed.) *Recent Advances in Plastic Surgery*, Edinburgh, Churchill Livingstone, pp. 29–44.

Gillies H. D. (1920) *Plastic Surgery of the Face*. London, Hodder and Stoughton.

Grabb W. G. and Smith J. W. (1973) *Plastic Surgery*, 2nd ed. Boston, Little Brown & Co.

Hunt T. K. and Dunphy J. E. (1979) *Fundamentals of Wound Management*. New York, Appleton-Century-Crofts.

McGregor I. A. (1980) *Fundamental Techniques of Plastic Surgery*. Edinburgh, Churchill Livingstone.

Chapter twenty-nine

Management of Lymphoedema

G. W. Taylor

Chronic lymphoedema as a sequel of lymphatic insufficiency can occur in many anatomical areas but it is in the limbs, and particularly the lower limb, that surgical treatment is most frequently indicated.

ANATOMICAL CONSIDERATIONS

Lower Limb

The lower limb is served by a superficial and deep system of lymph trunks. The superficial system parallels the long and short saphenous veins but, unlike the veins, the trunks become more numerous as they ascend the limb. Lymph from the lateral side of the foot and heel follow the short saphenous vein and pierce the deep fascia in the popliteal fascia to join the popliteal lymph node. Lymph from the remainder of the limb is collected into trunks which accompany the long saphenous vein and end in the inguinal lymph nodes. In a normal lymphangiogram between 6 and 12 trunks may be seen at this level. The deep system of lymphatic trunks follows the course of the deep veins and terminates in the deep inguinal lymph nodes.

Unlike the venous system, there is no communication between the deep and superficial system of lymphatics apart from the terminations in the popliteal and inguinal lymph nodes. The lymph trunks are small in diameter (1–2 mm) and are valved at frequent intervals and rely on the massaging effect of muscular movement to promote lymph flow in a proximal direction.

Function of Lymphatics

In the limb the lymphatics subserve two main functions. They remove excess tissue fluid and also scavenge from the tissue space substances of large molecular size. In lymphatic insufficiency, therefore, not only is there failure to remove fluid from the interstitial space but there is accumulation of the small quantity of plasma protein that normally leaks through the blood capillary wall. This concentration of extravascular protein produces an abnormal interstitial osmotic force which leads to further water retention and clinical oedema.

The high protein content of the oedema fluid is responsible for secondary changes of fibrosis that occur in chronic lymphoedema and for the common complication of recurrent cellulitis. In long-standing lymphoedema the subcutaneous tissue and covering skin become permanently stretched and the normal intrinsic tissue tension is lost. Restoration of this latter factor is an important consideration in surgical treatment.

SURGICAL TREATMENT OF LYMPHOEDEMA

The multiplicity of operations that has been tried in lymphoedema emphasizes the difficulty of obtaining surgical cure and to date there is no completely satisfactory surgical solution. Operations may be classified as 'restorative' where an attempt is made to restore normal lymphatic function, 'excisional' where the bulk of the oedematous tissue is excised, or a combination of these two aims. In order to establish a rational basis for the use of these methods, the aetiological factors in the patient under consideration must be clearly understood. The lymphatic fault in lymphoedema may be of congenital origin as in primary lymphoedema or secondary to acquired disease involving the lymphatic system.

In the context of surgical treatment primary and secondary lymphoedema differ fundamentally. In primary lymphoedema the congenital malformation of the lymphatic system usually involves the whole limb and both lymph trunks and lymph nodes may be abnormal. The common abnormality in severe primary lymphoedema is hypoplasia of the lymph trunks in which lymphangiography demonstrates a solitary subcutaneous lymph trunk often draining into scanty maldeveloped inguinal lymph nodes. By contrast, in secondary lymphoedema the abnormality is usually a localized obstruction at the root of a limb and the lymphatic system distal and proximal are grossly normal. Most of the so-called 'restorative' operations rely on construction of a lymphatic bridge across the root of the swollen limb. It can be seen, therefore, that such procedures have a rational basis only in secondary lymphoedema where a localized fault exists, and will fail in the presence of the more extensive defects of primary lymphoedema. Choice of operation must depend on an accurate diagnosis of the underlying lymphatic pathology and lymphangiography is an essential investigation if restorative procedures are under consideration.

Indications for Operation

Surgical treatment of lymphoedema should only be considered when non-operative measures have failed to control the situation or where neglect of treatment at the outset has resulted in permanent gross swelling. The less severe degree of lymphoedema of whatever aetiology can be controlled by a conservative regimen and such measures as night elevation of the foot of the bed, the wearing of elastic stockings by day, and the intermittent use of diuretics will often bring worthwhile improvement and will halt the progression of the swelling.

In the severe varieties of lymphoedema these measures may fail and the swelling becomes burdensome by virtue of the increased weight of the oedematous tissue, and clothing will require alteration to encompass the abnormal limb. Thus limitation of normal activities is the main indication for operation. Women often request operation because they are disturbed by the appearance of even a mild degree of lymphoedema. Cosmetic indications alone should rarely be the basis for surgical treatment because operation, although successful in reducing the size of the limb, usually leaves an inelegant and extensive scar. Recurrent cellulitis due to invasion of the swollen tissues by the *Streptococcus* or other bacteria is a common and troublesome complication of lymphoedema. If such inflammatory episodes occur frequently and are not controlled adequately by prophylactic antibiotic therapy then surgical excision of the oedematous areas will be necessary.

Restorative Operations

Many ingenious techniques for restoring or rerouting lymph flow have been tried but none has produced consistent benefit. Lymphangioplasty using buried strands or tubes, first reported by Sampson Handley in 1908, continues to be revived with differing materials and techniques but without long-term success. Bridging procedures using a pedicle containing lymphatic trunks could eventually restore lymph flow if used across a localized area of lymphatic obstruction as might occur in secondary lymphoedema. Gillies and Fraser in 1935 described an operation in which a skin and subcutaneous pedicle was transplanted from the arm, across the groin to an oedematous leg. This procedure has never gained substantial acceptance and has largely been abandoned.

In 1968 Lanzara reported the use of pedicle grafts of the greater omentum into the base of the limb but this operation too has not stood the test of time. Professor J. B. Kinmonth (1972) has reported an ingenious variation of this theme. His procedure uses a pedicle of isolated small bowel, laid open and denuded of its mucosal layer, to bridge localized lymphatic obstruction in the groin. Functional lymphatic connection across this intestinal bridge has been demonstrated by lymphangiography and evaluation of its clinical efficacy is being continued.

The creation of lymphovenous shunts proximal to an area of lymphatic obstruction is an attractive concept and was first introduced into clinical practice by Nielubowicz and Olszewski in 1968. Their method involved horizontal transection of a lymph node proximal to the level of obstruction and implantation of the raw lymph node surface into a neighbouring vein. Unfortunately, consistent benefit has not followed the use of this procedure and it is likely that lymph transfer through the transected node is obliterated by fibrosis. With the development of microvascular surgery direct anastomosis of lymphatic trunk to vein is possible and has been used in lymphoedematous limbs by B. McC. O'Brien (1976). Multiple lymph trunks proximal to an obstructive site are visualized following a distal injection of patent blue dye and are then anastomosed end to end to suitably sized venous radicles. Measurable improvement in the oedematous limb has occurred after this procedure, but long-term evaluation is not yet available.

Excisional Procedures

In chronic lymphoedema the main site of lymph stasis is the subcutaneous layer and excisional procedures achieve their effect by radical excision of this tissue. In Homans' operation the subcutaneous tissue is excised beneath thin but viable skin flaps, while in the Charles operation both skin and subcutaneous tissue are excised en bloc and skin cover provided by free split-thickness skin grafts. The Charles operation is successful in producing a light leg with little tendency to swell but has two serious disadvantages. The cosmetic result is often poor because the resulting leg is almost literally only skin and bone, and more seriously a significant proportion of patients suffer late change in the grafted area which becomes nodular, hypertrophied and the site of intractable weeping eczema. The Charles operation, therefore, should only be done in the rare cases of 'tropical elephantitis' in which the local skin has become grossly hyperkeratotic and damaged by recurrent infection.

The less radical Homans' operation, however, produces worthwhile reduction in the oedematous area and is applicable to most cases of primary or secondary lymphoedema.

Homans' Operation

It is important that the patient should be rested for several days before operation with long periods of elevation of the oedematous limb. The skin of the limb should be washed daily with Chlorhexidine (Hibitane) solution and interdigital tinea pedis eradicated.

Homans' operation is performed in stages, the number of which are dependent on the severity of the oedema. For a moderate degree of swelling it may be sufficient to reduce the medial side of the leg only. In more severe cases a second stage on the lateral side may be done after an interval of 2–3 months and in gross lymphoedema a third, posteriorly based excision may be required.

The patient lies supine on the operating table. The excisional part of the operation is done under a bloodless field and if the thigh is not involved an inflatable tourniquet is used. If the thigh is to be included in the operative field a sterile Esmarch bandage can be applied to the root of the limb after completing the skin preparation.

INCISIONS

These are marked out with sterile ink (*Fig.* 29.1) and are similar for either the medial or lateral side of in the region of the lateral popliteal nerve in a lateral dissection and medially the posterior tibial neurovascular bundle lies just beneath the deep fascia behind the medial malleolus. Perforating vessels are ligated and divided at the level of the deep fascia, and any obvious bleeding points are dealt with at this stage. Hot packs are then applied to the wound and the tourniquet is released. Firm pressure is maintained for 5 minutes, and the packs are then removed. Careful haemostasis is then carried out with ligation of any visible vessels and diathermy coagulation of minor bleeding points. When the wound is dry the now redundant skin flaps can then be manipulated

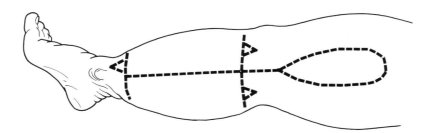

Fig. 29.1. Incisions for Homans' operation. The anterior and posterior flaps are approximately equal. One or more triangular dart excisions may be necessary at the proximal and distal transverse incisions.

the limb. If the thigh is to be included in the reduction, an ellipse of skin is marked for excision extending from the upper third to the level of the knee joint. From here a straight mid-medial or lateral incision is carried distally to join a transverse incision at a level just below the malleoli. A similar transverse incision is made at the level of the tibial tuberosity. The length of the transverse incisions determines the circumferential extent of the excisional procedure and thus the ultimate size of the skin flaps. It is advisable not to be too ambitious in this respect and the exposure should be something less than half the circumference of the limb. The thigh ellipse is excised first and includes the subcutaneous tissue to the level of the deep fascia. Only minimal mobilization of skin flaps should be done in this area. The posterior flap of the leg component is then developed to its full extent. In cutting the skin flaps a balance must be struck between keeping them sufficiently thin to avoid recurrence of the oedema and leaving enough subcutaneous tissue to ensure an adequate blood supply. They should thicken gradually towards their base. At the ankle the transverse incision should be undermined distally in order to facilitate excision of the bulge below the level of the malleoli. Excision of the subcutaneous layer is then done, starting proximally, and by sharp dissection keeping to the plane of the deep fascia which is left intact.

The long saphenous vein is usually excised with the specimen on the medial side and it is impracticable to spare cutaneous nerves. Care should be taken in order to gauge the extent of their excision so as to produce a 'snug' fit to the deep fascial layer. Equal increments are excised from each flap and it is best to start the excision and approximation (with interrupted sutures) proximally and proceed a few centimetres at a time. It is surprisingly easy to excise too much skin if this is done in one manoeuvre.

As the closure proceeds multiple suction drains of the Redivac type are laid under the flaps. Usually between four and six of such drains are needed. It will then be found that because of the loss of the excised subcutaneous pad the proximal and distal transverse incisions will be over-length (to the same degree as the excised portions of the skin flaps). This must be corrected by V-shaped excisions proximally and distally. The placement of the V is not critical but it should be kept away from the line of the main longitudinal suture line. After massive excisions more than one V excision may be required. The limb is then cleaned with Savlon solution, dried and covered with a copious gauze and wool dressing. A crêpe bandage is applied snugly but not too firmly over this. The patient is kept in bed with the limb elevated until the sutures are removed on the 10th postoperative day. Graduated ambulation is then encouraged with the limb supported by an elastic bandage. At this stage the limb is fitted with an elastic stocking which should be worn permanently. In severe oedema a second stage on the opposite aspect of the limb can be done after an interval of 2–3 months.

POSTOPERATIVE COMPLICATIONS

The most frequent complication is necrosis of a portion of one or both flaps. This usually results in an area where the flap has been fashioned too thinly or is over-long. Small patches of necrosis will heal by secondary intention but larger areas should be excised and skin grafted.

Homans' Operation in Other Areas

The principle of the operation is the same and local flaps can be raised to suit the particular anatomical circumstance. The dorsum of the foot is best dealt with by a midline incision with equal medial and lateral flaps extending to the base of the toes (*Fig.* 29.2). Post-mastectomy oedema of the upper limb

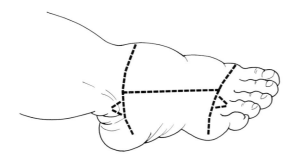

Fig. 29.2. Incisions for Homans' operation on dorsum of foot.

can be sufficiently massive to warrant operative reduction. The upper arm is often the most troublesome area in that armholes in dresses and coats will not accommodate its girth. In the arm a posterior midline incision is used meeting transverse extensions at axillary and elbow level. The forearm can be dealt with at a second stage with an incision running longitudinally on the anteromedial aspect to join transverse extensions at wrist and elbow. If there is gross forearm swelling a third stage may be added with the incision placed on the posterolateral aspect. The dorsum of the hand can be dealt with in the same fashion as the dorsum of the foot.

Combined Restorative and Excisional Operations

The Kondoleon operation was the first to combine an excisional procedure with an attempt to deviate lymphatic flow, by excision of a strip of deep fascia. In 1962, Thompson described an operation with the same objective. In Thompson's operation lymph from the skin and superficial tissues was theoretically enabled to drain into the deep lymphatic system by burying an abraded skin flap into the deep compartment of the leg. This was combined with a major excisional procedure much on the lines of the Homans' operation already described. The evidence that lymph transfer occurs after this operation is conflicting and in our hands the long-term outcome shows no improvement over the simpler Homans' procedure.

The incisions for Thompson's operation are approximately those for Homans' operation and the flaps are taken back in a similar fashion although the anterior flap is kept shorter (*Fig.* 29.3). After the subcutaneous pad is excised, the soleus muscle is detached from the medial border of the tibia and the shaved edge of the posterior flap is anchored near the posterior tibial neurovascular bundle with interrupted sutures. The free edge of the anterior skin flap is then brought to overlap the buried flap and sutured to the raw dermal area. Multiple suction drains are used and the postoperative management is identical to that in Homans' operation. Complications following Thompson's operation are again largely those of flap necrosis and because of the greater length of the buried compartment the morbidity is higher than in the simpler, purely excisional procedure.

SUMMARY

There is, as yet, no completely satisfactory operation for lymphoedema. It seems unlikely that normal restoration of lymphatic function will ever be achieved by surgical means and the aims of operation should therefore be:

1. To excise the oedematous subcutaneous tissue.
2. To restore tissue tension in the affected area.

These objectives can largely be met by simple excisional procedures of the Homans type.

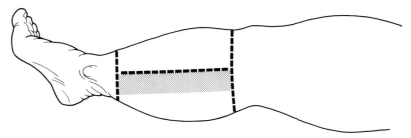

Fig. 29.3. Incisions for Thompson's operation. The hatched area of the posterior flap is shaved with the dermatome.

REFERENCES

Gillies H. and Fraser F. R. (1935) Treatment of lymphoedema by plastic operation: preliminary report. *Br. Med. J.* **1**, 96–98.

Kinmonth J. B. (1972) *The Lymphatics.* London, Arnold.

Lanzara A. (1968) Surgical treatment of lymphoedema by omental transplantation. *J. Cardiovasc. Surg. (Torino),* p. 122. Special number for XVIIth Congress of the European Society of Cardiovascular Surgery.

Nielubowicz J. and Olszewski W. (1968) Surgical lymphatico-venous shunts in patients with secondary lymphoedema. *Br. J. Surg.* **55**, 440.

O'Brien B.McC. (1976) Replantation and reconstructive microvascular surgery. *Ann. R. Coll. Surg. Engl.* **58**, 171.

Thompson N. (1962) Surgical treatment of chronic lymphoedema of the lower limb. *Br. Med. J.* **2**, 1566.

Chapter thirty

The Breast

A. J. Webb

In dealing with breast surgery the major consideration is for female breast disease; a small section on diseases affecting the male breast is placed at the end of the chapter. Benign and malignant breast lesions are an important and worrying aspect of general surgical practice. They cause great anxiety for the patient and her family and it behoves the surgeon to make a precise diagnosis and deal with the problem in an efficient, compassionate and informed manner. Breast carcinoma is a continuing scourge; epidemiological studies would suggest that the numbers will increase. In the USA during 1976, 88 000 new cases presented of which around 30–40 per cent might be cured, i.e. achieve a 15-year disease-free survival. For England and Wales during 1974, breast cancer accounted for 4 per cent of all female deaths—for the 35–54-years age group it caused 1 in every 6 deaths. There exist interesting differences in the age-adjusted incidence of breast cancer between countries. Hawaii shows a high incidence at 80/100 000 women, Oxford, England is 54/100 000 and Osaka, Japan 12/100 000 women. There are, in addition, inexplicable variations in incidence between social classes (Henderson et al., 1984).

There are many poorly understood factors in the presentation, behaviour and management of breast cancer and much research effort is expended to elucidate them. It remains a perplexing and capricious disease which demands a team effort comprising radiotherapist, oncologist, surgeon and others.

CLINICAL EXAMINATION

For an organ as accessible as the breast one might assume that clinical examination would be precise. This is not so. Clinical errors are a frequent event in clinical practice even among experienced surgeons, and more so among general practitioners. Forrest (1974) states his accuracy rate at 80 per cent and this level is confirmed by other studies. Carelessness in examination is seldom the reason for mistakes; the physical form of female breast tissue accounts for much of the difficulty. Small cancers can present within a large breast and the signs are masked by breast tissue and fat. Buried cysts are often referred to outpatient clinics as an 'undoubted malignancy' because the smooth cyst outline is obscured. Areas of lumpiness or breast thickening are often difficult to assess.

This does not absolve the surgeon from performing a careful clinical examination. Although there are many good descriptions and illustrations available in the literature (Handley, 1964; Widow, 1968; Thomas and Boulter, 1984), it is worth while emphasizing certain aspects. Inspection is essential, preferably with the patient sitting up and arms braced on the hips. Contraction of the pectoral muscle will reveal any deep tethering or skin attachment and elevation of the arms above the head will confirm. Sometimes it is valuable to palpate the breasts as they lie away from the chest wall. But the best position is the patient lying on her back and the hands placed on the head or behind the neck. Careful reinspection, especially of the nipple area, should precede palpation. Feel the breast with the flat of the slightly flexed fingers (*Fig.* 30.1). It is sensible to use the dominant

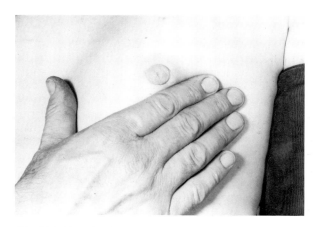

Fig. 30.1. Examination of the breast using the flat of the hand.

hand but a certain element of ambidexterity can be rewarding and is not bad practice. A finger-and-thumb feel is sometimes needed to elucidate a deeply placed feature or to gently express discharge from the nipple. Often the patient will be successful in expressing discharge in order that smears can be made. Delicate finger-and-thumb palpation is essential to assess thickening of the lactiferous ducts. Provided the examiner is thoroughly familiar with the surface characteristics of natural breast tissue there is much to be said for examining with a light soapy lathering of the breast skin: alternatively 0·5 per cent Hibitane (chlorhexidine) in spirit is equally effective. Haagensen (1971) preferred talcum powder for a similar purpose. Skin friction is diminished and the palpatory features are significantly enhanced. Cysts in particular are far easier to identify by this simple trick.

Axillary examination is even more unreliable than breast palpation. There is at least a 30 per cent error either way in feeling the axillary contents. Provided the axillary fascia is relaxed by the position of the arm, and the examiner's fingers pass gently high into the axilla, sweeping its contents against the medial axillary wall, then there is some chance of a useful yield. It is easy to neglect the axillary tail and the pectoral nodes lying close to it. The supra- and infra-clavicular regions must be carefully palpated.

Mammography used in the correct circumstances has proved of great value to complement clinical examination. It is probable that conventional radiology as opposed to xerography will remain the technique of choice in Great Britain. But xerography, if available, is especially valuable for the radiography of biopsy specimens (Dodd, 1970; Frischbier and Lohbeck, 1977). For screening purposes, a single mediolateral oblique film as opposed to lateral and superoinferior projections has been developed and awaits evaluation (Tabàr and Dean, 1984).

BREAST ABSCESS

Three types of abscess occur. First, infection at the areola in a tubercle of Montgomery. This presents like a boil and is incised directly the presence of pus is clinically detected. Occasionally it may present as a chronic folliculitis. Second, and much more extensive, there is inflammation connected with the nipple or elsewhere in the breast due to mammary duct ectasia. This important lesion may be subacute in its presentation and varies in degree depending on how much of the breast tissue is involved. Rarely a four-quadrant swelling develops accompanied by erythema and *peau d'orange*, completely mimicking an inflammatory carcinoma in form and timing. A precise diagnosis is essential and for this purpose fine-needle aspiration cytology from several sites is invaluable. Surgery is not immediately indicated and the process usually improves slowly with antibiotics. Surgical drainage can then be more precisely directed. Unfortunately repeated procedures are often necessary and the whole process may take weeks to settle. The more usual subareolar presentation of actasia is of inflammation confined to the nipple area forming an abscess which points at the areola. This should be drained by a direct circumareolar incision. A para-areolar fistula may follow and later definitive duct dissection will be required for the underlying duct disease (Hadfield, 1968). Third, intramammary abscesses occur associated with lactation, be it due to secondary infection following milk retention or a florid tissue reaction following duct rupture. The process begins as a congested area of the breast due to nipple oedema from a fissure or a creamy plug in the duct orifice. Local treatment with heat, expres-

sion of the milk and a systemic antibiotic may be effective. The infant continues to feed from the opposite side. If after 4 days an area of induration with oedema and erythema persists then incision is required. Preliminary aspiration with an 18-gauge needle to confirm the presence of pus is optional. A peri-areolar skin incision is made and with a long artery forceps gentle penetration into the indurated breast tissue usually leads to pus. The entry is widened and a finger inserted to break down all the loculi and allow free drainage. A second, dependent counter-incision is necessary if the cavity is large and both incisions should be kept open for a few days.

Occasionally, a deep chronic abscess deriving from an infected cyst, localized ectasia or lactational abscess overtreated with antibiotics presents as a hard lump. The unusual lesion, breast granuloma, may also present in this manner and can be accompanied by erythema nodosum (Koelmeyer and MacCormick, 1976). The physical signs can be worrying due to local skin adhesion and oedema. Needle biopsy will reveal the true nature of such a mass and excision biopsy usually provides the swiftest and most permanent relief.

BIOPSY OF THE BREAST

Biopsy is the removal of tissue or cellular material from an organ during life for the purposes of pathological examination. Following clinical examination it is the essential sequel to establish a definitive diagnosis. It is the classic and widely held view that such proof must be histological, whereas a minority opinion would accept cytological evidence. The history of biopsy in general and breast biopsy in particular forms a critical chapter in the development of modern surgery since 1850. Controversy abounds regarding the most convenient, safe and accurate method of biopsy (Burn, 1973; Editorial, 1977; Rilke, 1984). Needle biopsy and surgical procedures are the two contenders and they are now considered.

1. Needle biopsy embraces three differing techniques.

a. Fine-needle (18–23 gauge size) aspiration biopsy incorporating some form of constant suction obtains a yield for cytological examination and enjoys scattered but increasing popularity in Europe, the USA and Great Britain (Grubb, 1981).

Its accuracy in skilled hands is undeniable and too often its detractors have failed to employ the technique correctly (Magarey and Watson, 1976; Davies et al., 1977). It possesses many advantages, being supremely convenient, atraumatic, swift to report and economical. Very small (0·5 cm diameter) breast lumps, regional lymph nodes and soft tissue deposits are all suitable for this technique (Webb, 1982).

b. Large-needle (Tru-cut style) biopsy employs a small trocar and cutting cannula principle to remove a core of tissue from the breast for histology (Roberts et al., 1975; Davies et al., 1977; Baum, 1981). The procedure necessitates a small skin incision under local anaesthesia and is reported to be rather inaccurate for lumps less than 2 cm in diameter.

c. Drill biopsy (Burn et al., 1968) aims for a similar tissue yield by an ingenious high-speed pneumatic drill apparatus (Morrison and Deeley, 1955). Like large-needle biopsy, this procedure is a compromise to obtain histological material yet avoiding surgical incision or excision. In skilled hands the results are very good but it is more cumbersome, traumatic, technically involved and expensive than fine-needle biopsy.

2. Incision biopsy has received the support of eminent surgeons in the past (Haagensen, 1971) but is currently regarded as an inferior technique only to be considered if the lesion is greater than 5 cm in diameter. For clinical cancer opinions differ as to whether incision really involves minimal trauma to obtain a representative sample as it directly exposes and enters malignant tissue. For possible benign dysplastic lesions incision is the rule; there seems to be no sense in wide excision of an area of fibrocystic dysplasia when the aim of the intervention is to sample the area in doubt for histological proof of its innocence or otherwise. The same principle applies to mammary ectasia and excision of the major duct system. One is establishing the diagnosis by sampling; the diseased ducts may well extend throughout the whole breast.

3. Excision biopsy is a favourite operation for the removal of fibroadenomas, small cysts and uncertain lumps less than 5 cm in diameter (Hughes, 1982). For benign lumps, diagnosis and treatment are achieved, while for carcinoma some surgeons favour marginal local excision and macroscopy with frozen section prior to mastectomy or axillary node biopsy. A minority favour wide excision biopsy or segmental resection for certain low-grade breast cancers already identified by needle biopsy. Medially placed neoplasms may be treated in this way. It is advisable to limit this surgical approach to tumours ≤2 cm diameter; adequate axillary node biopsy is obligatory. Others favour excision biopsy and paraffin section so that the patient may decide in the light of her diagnosis what surgical operation she desires. With actively spreading high-grade cancers such an excision will run the risk of transgressing involved lymphatic fields, and cells could implant during mastectomy. The approach is very controversial.

There is undoubtedly an increasing tendency among British surgeons to use less invasive breast biopsy procedures. All the needle methods mentioned here are in current use. Fine-needle biopsy suffers from unreasonable prejudice and a relative lack of trained cytologists. With large-needle and drill biopsy not all histopathologists are at ease examining small tissue fragments. Fine-needle biopsy is the least traumatic (Webb, 1970, 1975; Coleman, 1982; Melcher et al., 1984) and is safely applicable to other relevant sites, e.g. lymph nodes, hepatic, skeletal and soft tissue deposits.

Each biopsy procedure is now described in further detail.

Fine-needle Biopsy

The lump or lumpiness is steadied with the fingers of the left hand and a disposable no. 1 (21-gauge) needle, with a 20-ml syringe attached, is gently inserted after cleansing the skin. Constant suction is produced either by a syringe pistol or more simply by the 'braced-thumb' trick (*Fig.* 30.2). The needle

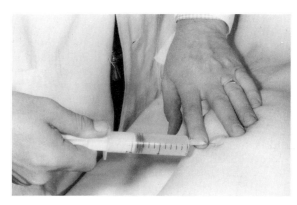

Fig. 30.2. Fine-needle aspiration biopsy of a lump in the breast which is steadied by the fingers of the left hand. The braced-thumb method of constant suction is shown.

is moved delicately through the lesion in several directions sucking tissue juice and cells into the bore of the needle and syringe stem. Suction is reduced before withdrawing the needle. The needle is detached and the contents carefully blown onto slides and spread into smears. Rapid air drying is essential, followed by fixation in methanol (5 min). Giemsa staining gives uniformly reliable results, but wet fixation and Papanicolaou staining are performed by some cytologists. The procedure should be repeated at a different site if required. The total biopsy from puncture to microscopy and diagnosis can be achieved well within 30 min.

Large-needle and Drill Biopsies (Baum, 1981; Hughes, 1982)

Cutting edge cannulas and trocars, together with drill biopsies, demand a very similar procedure. Most cases are performed on an outpatient basis. Common to both styles is the insertion of local anaesthetic and a 3–5-mm skin incision to allow entry into the breast tissue. The large needle is inserted into the lesion which is steadied in the standard manner. The needle is thrust into the breast mass and rotated to obtain a core of tissue. Syringe suction is applied to withdraw the specimen. The drill biopsy needle attached to the apparatus is inserted through the skin and the drill speed adjusted to obtain a cut core. The needle is detached and syringe suction applied to withdraw as for large-needle biopsy. With both methods the syringe contains 2 ml of 3·8 per cent sodium citrate solution to protect the tissue. The biopsy specimen is gently extruded on to a watch glass and carefully transferred to fixative. The standard and variable laboratory processing time for paraffin sections applies but frozen sections may be feasible if necessary.

Excision Biopsy

For small, superficially placed lesions in selected patients, sedation and local anaesthesia are acceptable and widespread office practice in the USA, but for the vast majority general anaesthesia is preferred although this can be arranged on an outpatient, daystay basis. The patient is towelled with the arm abducted on a board or adducted. This depends on the site of the lesion, its probable nature and the size of the breast. Ideally para-areolar, circumferential skin crease or marginal (Galliard–Thomas) incisions are made for cosmetic and aesthetic reasons provided that there is no likelihood of malignancy (*Fig.* 30.3). After skin incision the breast (large

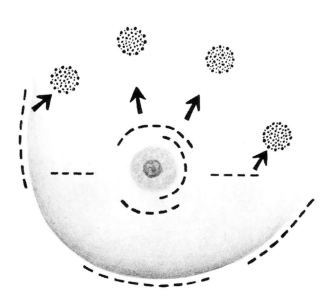

Fig. 30.3. Excision biopsy. Para-areolar, circumferential skin crease or marginal (Galliard–Thomas) incisions are made for cosmetic and aesthetic reasons.

lobule) fat is reflected to reveal the breast tissue proper. The lesion is relocated and this may be difficult as all breast lumps become less obvious once the skin is incised. The breast tissue is held with Poirier or Allis tissue forceps; for a very mobile lump fixation with a no. 1 needle is recommended. Using

sharp dissection the breast is incised and the lesion exposed. Three alternatives are then possible.

1. For fibroadenoma, the lump is totally excised with a narrow (1–2 mm thick) margin of breast tissue. Because of their extreme mobility fibroadenomas do carry the risk of being incised at surgical excision unless a precise technique is followed.
2. For an area of fibrous dysplasia a sample is excised, preferably in a coronal rather than a radial segmental direction. It is sometimes possible to 'shape' the residual edges of dysplastic breasts after excision to improve cosmesis.
3. If careful palpation reveals suspicious induration then of course this should be cut away *in toto*.

If cysts are found during biopsy they can be aspirated or emptied by incision. Painstaking haemostasis is essential following biopsy. Obvious major vessels on the surface are ligated with 3/0 silk or catgut; smaller mammary bleeding points are coagulated with diathermy. To facilitate this, the edges of breast tissue are held up with tissue or artery forceps and small rectractors to expose the depths of the biopsy space. Drainage is a matter of judgement. Large cavities are best drained using thin corrugated rubber brought out through a small separate stab incision. The drain is tethered with a silk suture and a 3/0 silk 'pull-out' suture tied after removal of the drain adds neatness. Breast tissue should never be sutured after excision. The fat may be loosely sutured before skin closure to avoid an unsightly hollow. Skin suture by fine silk or nylon gives tidy results, but if a thick corium dermis is present then a subcuticular 4/0 plain catgut, polyglycolic or monofilamentous suture gives excellent results.

If doubt exists as to whether the lesion is malignant the biopsy incision must then lie within the bounds and line of a possible subsequent mastectomy or further local excision.

Incision Biopsy

This style of biopsy may be considered for a possible malignant mass greater than 5 cm in diameter. The aim is to obtain a representative sliver of tissue for frozen section and macroscopical diagnosis. Some surgeons are content to perceive the characteristic feel of the scalpel blade cutting into scirrhous cancer and thereafter proceed to mastectomy. Incision biopsy is an unsatisfactory procedure. The incision should avoid obvious subcutaneous veins and be as small as is feasible, cutting directly through skin, fat and breast tissue. It is important that the depth of the incision should reach the cancer. Diathermy haemostasis is ideal and the skin should be closed with a tight inverting suture, hopefully to prevent contamination during the mastectomy. Some surgeons prefer to insert a swab soaked in a cancerocide such as cetrimide before skin closure.

ADAIR'S OPERATION is excision of the major duct system or lactiferous sinuses, 'macrodochectomy'.

This simple and usually effective operation was initially described by Adair and Urban and was popularized in Great Britain by the reports of Hadfield (1960, 1968). The indications for it are troublesome mammary duct ectasia, para-areolar fistula, which is a complication of ectasia, and intraduct papilloma. Inverted nipples can also be corrected by this procedure. Some surgeons prefer the operation of microdochectomy for possible intraduct papilloma, having localized and cannulated the offending duct. Others prefer to remove all the ducts in the light of sound evidence that more than one duct is commonly involved.

Mammary duct ectasia is a prevalent and perplexing disease; its incidence is probably underestimated and it frequently passes unrecognized. The aetiological basis of the underlying abnormality is poorly understood and some surgeons prefer the term 'periductal mastitis' (Thomas et al., 1982; Dixon et al., 1983). In its milder forms the clinical presentation may be as follows:

1. Pain in the nipple and surrounding breast.
2. Discharge from the papilla; varying in amount and character.
3. Small tender areas in the sub- and para-areolar region.
4. Progressive retraction of the nipple(s).
5. Mild, self-resolving episodes of subareolar inflammation.
6. A discrete breast lump.

Confirmation of the diagnosis can usually be made on clinical grounds, supplemented by mammography, fine-needle aspiration biopsy of any masses and microscopy of the nipple discharge. The indication for surgery depends on the severity of the symptoms and the presence of a discrete lump. Para-areolar fistula following abscess formation demands intervention, whereas intermittent nipple discharge seldom requires it unless atypical cells are found by cytology or the discharge is persistent and a nuisance.

Technique (*Fig.* 30.4)

The nipple is stretched to expand the area and small skin scratches are made in three places to ensure precise suturing. Usually an inferior hemicircumferential skin incision is made at the precise junction between areola and breast skin proper. The areola is elevated by skin hooks or tissue forceps. Very careful scalpel dissection is begun towards the papilla remaining between the ducts and smooth muscle corium of the areola. Thickened ducts are easy to see and are

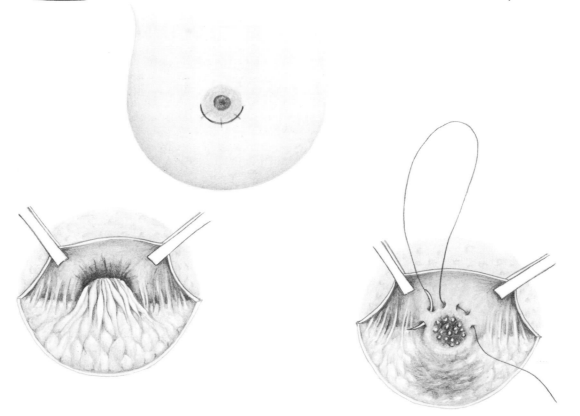

Fig. 30.4. Adair's operation. Excision of the major duct system or lactiferous sinuses through a peri-areolar skin incision.

detached from the papilla by sharp dissection. The duct cluster is held with an artery forceps. Once the papilla has been cleared the ducts are incised at their emergence from the breast tissue. If necessary, and it often is so, thickened breast or a subareolar mass of uncertain nature is excised. Where possible the ducts are ligated with fine silk or underpinned as they emerge from the breast stroma. Gentle bimanual pressure on the breast will usually reveal large abnormal ducts by the issuing discharge. This stage of the operation can be technically difficult and it may be possible only to diathermize the orifices of ducts lying in dysplastic breast. Fine ligature and diathermy haemostasis having been achieved, a purse-string suture of 4/0 plain catgut is inserted behind the papilla to lightly protrude it.

Drainage may be necessary using a thin corrugated rubber strip brought out through a separate stab site. Skin closure is by two layers of 4/0 silk sutures or by subcuticular material. The vascularity of the mammillary skin may be impaired if the dissection is excessive or carried too close to the corium of the areola; delicate dissection is required.

The operation is usually successful but not invariably so. Para-areolar fistula with extensive scarring, periductal inflammation and squamous metaplasia of the ducts may recur. In some cases, despite great care, nipple vascularity is prejudiced and skin is lost. Reoperation becomes necessary with unavoidable segmental resection of breast tissue containing an obviously diseased ductal tree. Rarely simple mastectomy offers the only cure.

MICRODOCHECTOMY

A bloodstained nipple discharge is uncommon and happens less frequently than patients will allege. It is often caused by an intraduct papilloma and thickened ducts may be felt. A distinct mass and a bloody discharge are far more suggestive of intraduct and invasive carcinoma. Cytology of the discharge is essential and will confirm the presence of erythrocytes together with clumps of benign and often atypical papillary epithelium. Carcinoma cells are distinctive and easy to identify. Mammography is helpful to show evidence of carcinoma. Ductograms are sometimes diagnostic. If the offending duct can be reliably located, then under anaesthesia a lacrimal probe is inserted into it and by a radial incision extending from papilla to areola the duct and papilloma are excised. A no. 15 scalpel blade is ideal for this dissection. Subcuticular 4/0 plain catgut or 4/0 interrupted silk sutures will give an excellent cosmetic result.

CARCINOMA OF THE BREAST

The Surgical Alternatives

Once the diagnosis of carcinoma has been established by some form of biopsy then there is a choice of procedures. There are five operations currently favoured.

1. Limited excision with only enough surrounding tissue to allow a clear margin together with axillary dissection of variable extent; otherwise known as 'lumpectomy' or 'tumourectomy' (Harris et al., 1981).
2. Segmental mastectomy or quadrantectomy involving a wide removal of the cancer (Veronesi et al., 1981). Through one incision, it may be possible to dissect the axilla also—or a separate approach is dictated depending on the site of the primary. In the Veronesi procedure, pectoralis minor is removed together with the apical and central axillary contents.
3. Simple or total mastectomy where axillary nodes remain.
4. Extended simple or total mastectomy where axillary node biopsy is added.
5. Subradical or Patey mastectomy where complete axillary dissection is attempted with removal of the breast and pectoralis minor. Pectoralis major is preserved.
6. Radical mastectomy where the breast, pectoral muscles and axillary contents are removed en bloc.

1. Lumpectomy
2. Segmental Mastectomy and Axillary Dissection

These procedures are followed by radiotherapy. The techniques are controversial and require a very precise surgical skill. Some 10-year surgical results in respect of sizeable series have been published (Brady and Bedwinek, 1984). For a variety of reasons an attempt to construct a controlled, randomized trial comparing them with extended local mastectomy and irradiation for both modalities has proved very difficult. They are becoming popular in Great Britain and appear to be within the repertoire of otherwise diehard radical and subradical mastectomists (Handley, 1974). Perhaps they are acceptable practice in the following circumstances:

a. A patient who refuses total mastectomy.
b. An elderly unfit patient with a limited life expectancy from other causes.
c. A small, long-standing breast cancer preferably in a large breast with no mammographic evidence of multiple primary tumours.
d. Biologically favourable, biopsy-proven cancers of acceptable size ($\leqslant 2$ cm diameter).
e. A similar sized cancer lying in the medial quadrants.
f. A cancer that is well distant from the nipple area.

Clinical judgement must be exhibited in all cases. In the proved presence of systemic disease, segmental resection might remain the ideal method of controlling local disease. So often elderly women are unsuited to oestrogen therapy for cardiac reasons.

The patient is towelled as for mastectomy. It is necessary to remove a modest skin ellipse to include also the biopsy site. The skin edges are reflected and a segment of breast including the growth is removed incising 3 cm beyond palpable limits. It may be possible to extend the incision to include the axillary biopsy. Otherwise a separate skin crease incision from the pectoralis major margin to the anterior border of latissimus dorsi is made. Despite precise haemostasis by ligature and diathermy, drainage in some circumstances is wise; a vacuum suction system is best avoided. The 'hollow' induced by the suction is cosmetically ugly and a corrugated drain through a separate stab incision is far better. With long incisions extending to the axilla two suction drains left for 2–3 days only may suffice and leave minimal distortion.

3, 4. Simple and Extended Simple Mastectomy (*Figs* 30.5, 30.6)

These are popular operations and rightly so. The cosmetic and functional results are excellent and the long-term results equal those obtained by more radical procedures. Provided the diagnosis of carcinoma has been confirmed by preliminary needle or excision biopsy the patient can be towelled with the arm abducted. Otherwise preliminary incision or excision biopsy with frozen section is necessary. Following this, the arm is repainted with antiseptic and re-towelled; gowns and gloves are changed. Operating time amounting to at least 30 minutes may be lost thereby. It is necessary to paint the arm, axilla and posterolateral chest most carefully. The chest should lie on a sterile waterproof sheet covered by a towel; a roll of cottonwool wedged into position between chest wall and table preserves sterility there and

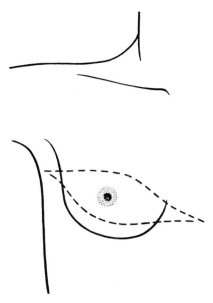

Fig. 30.6. Diagram of mastectomy incision adequate for simple, extended simple and Patey operations.

absorbs oozing from the posterior skin flap. Raising the skin flaps requires special care.

Mammography has confirmed the anatomical fact that two elements comprise the panniculus adiposus overlying the breast, namely the subcutaneous fat proper and the breast fat. The latter is looser and coarsely lobular. When raising the skin flaps, optimal vascularity is preserved by the dissecting between these two layers: scalpel or curved scissor dissection is equally effective, it is a matter for personal preference. Primary healing is anticipated, so a reliable guide to the amount of skin excision with the breast is helpful. The author marks the skin incisions with Bonney's blue dye taking a clearance of around 3 cm from the tumour edges.

First, the upper flap is raised, lifting the skin by hooks or Allis tissue forceps applied to the corium dermis (*Fig.* 30.7). Alternatively, the skin edge may be held in swabs. Elevation of the skin and counter pressure on the breast over a swab reveals the correct tissue plane. Clearance extends to pectoralis major beyond breast tissue to the level of the second costal cartilage, passing laterally to the border of pectoralis major. For simple or total mastectomy the suspensory ligament of the axilla (brachio-pectoral fascia) is not opened but the breast tail, usually with adherent lymph nodes, is detached downwards from serratus anterior. The posterior flap is elevated beginning laterally. Counter traction between breast and skin edge allows dissection to reach the anterior border and lateral surface of latissimus dorsi. The subscapular vessels and nerve to latissimus are sought and preserved.

For extended simple mastectomy, once the lateral half of the anterior flap is raised the axilla may be entered. From above, the breast including the pec-

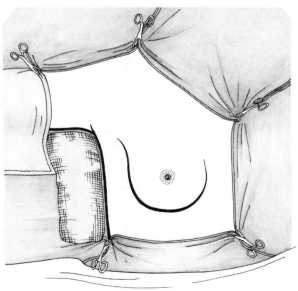

Fig. 30.5. A towelling arrangement suitable for mastectomy. For radical mastectomy the arm should be towelled separately.

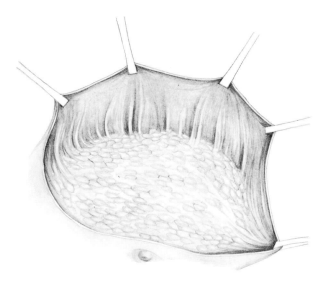

Fig. 30.7. Elevation of the upper mastectomy flap, illustrating the separation between the fatty components of the skin and of the breast.

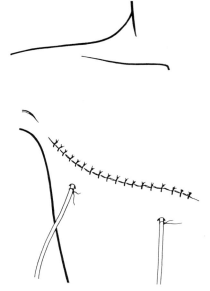

Fig. 30.8. Skin suture and drainage following simple mastectomy.

toral fascia is stripped away from the muscle. The anterior border of pectoralis major is elevated and the suspensory ligament opened to expose the axillary contents. The simplest manoeuvre at this stage is to dissect all the gross axillary contents from the vein downwards to the axillary tail. Alternatively a sample of palpable nodes is taken. The axillary fat and nodes are dissected away by delicate scissor work ligating the central or apical vein of the axilla early on. By pledget and a scissor this tissue mass is detached from the axillary walls and includes any subscapular nodes, but avoiding damage to the neuro-vascular bundle. The lateral thoracic vessels and nerve to serratus anterior are sought and preserved; the intercosto-brachial nerve and lateral cutaneous branch of third dorsal segment are sacrificed. Laterally the axillary tissue is freed from the tendon of latissimus dorsi. Haemostasis is by careful ligature and diathermy to small bleeding points, following which the axillary contents and breast are drawn downwards to meet the already partially detached breast lying over the pectoralis major. The raising of the lower flap is then completed and the breast is removed from above downwards, ligating perforating vessels with 2/0 and 3/0 silk. Care is necessary to avoid leaving a roll of 'breast fat' on both skin flaps.

The skin edges are assessed for apposition and vascularity; trimming may be necessary. Marker sutures are placed along the line of the incision to ensure alignment and two vacuum suction drains are inserted through the lower flap, one to lie medially and the other in the axilla. The wound is then closed with interrupted fine silk sutures (*Fig.* 30.8).

With suction drains, the application of the dressings by Elastoplast or other strapping requires comment, especially as the remaining skin flaps tend to be loose. Skin creases once established and held by suction cannot be rectified and are ugly. The surgeon should perform the dressing, spreading it evenly over the whole wound with the arm lightly abducted. The strapping is added without undue stretching.

The suction drains are removed at 5 days and the sutures at 8 days, provided healing looks adequate. Occasionally there is scabbing and superficial loss at the edge of the upper flap. Some 1 per cent crystal violet paint is applied daily. This simple and inexpensive measure prevents significant secondary infection and ensures that healing proceeds under the scar. Despite drainage, serous fluid may collect beneath the flaps; it is repeatedly aspirated with a fine needle as required. Radiotherapy apart, the scar is ready to accept a prosthesis at 4 weeks from the time of operation.

5. Patey Mastectomy (Subradical Mastectomy) (*Figs* 30.9–30.11)

Some surgeons insist that surgical clearance of the axilla is essential to prevent troublesome nodal recurrence and to clear all local disease, yet they wish to avoid the morbidity associated with radical mastectomy. The operation described by Patey and Dyson (1948) is ideal for them. The towelling preparation differs from that customary for simple mastectomy as the arm is prepared separately in order to allow abduction when the axilla is dissected. Otherwise the skin flaps are raised as for simple mastectomy and the axilla is approached. The ipsilateral assistant then flexes the arm with the elbow held at a right angle. Pectoralis major is retracted and pectoralis minor exposed. This muscle is detached from the coracoid process and turned downwards to expose the apex of the axilla. The fatty and nodal contents are

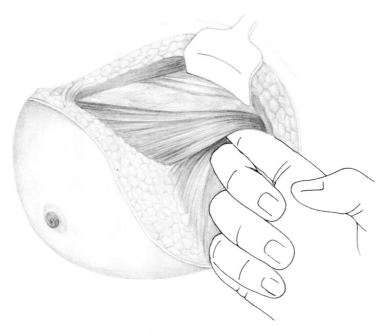

Fig. 30.9. Patey mastectomy. Pectoralis major has been retracted and pectoralis minor defined prior to detachment from the coracoid process.

removed from above and below the axillary vein which necessitates ligating the small veins which drain from the chest wall into the main trunk. It is essential to preserve the lateral pectoral nerve and pectoral branch of the acromio-thoracic artery which pass through the clavi-pectoral fascia to supply pectoralis major. The medial pectoral nerve component to that muscle is sacrificed when the minor is detached. The dissection proceeds downwards towards the central contents which are delicately cleared as for extended local mastectomy, apart from the medial side. Here pectoralis minor is detached from the ribs by cutting

diathermy; any interpectoral nodes are included in the specimen. Alternatively, pectoralis minor is not removed but after axillary dissection is left *in situ* or reattached to its origin. Thereafter the operation proceeds as for local mastectomy.

6. Radical Mastectomy

Despite a large amount of evidence to the contrary, a few surgeons in Great Britain and many in the USA and Australasia still consider that radical mastectomy

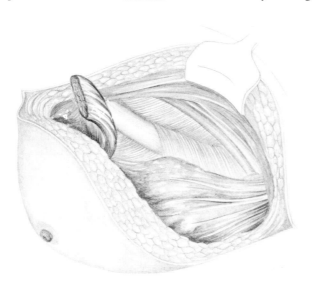

Fig. 30.10. Patey mastectomy. Pectoralis minor, the axilla contents and the breast have been dissected away and drawn downwards.

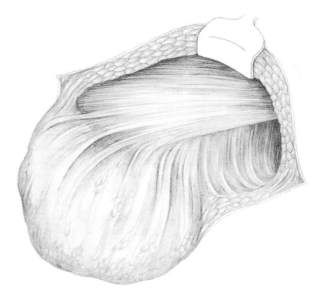

Fig. 30.11. Patey mastectomy. The total specimen is almost fully detached from the pectoralis major.

offers the most effective treatment for stage 1 and 2 carcinoma of the breast. The approach to T1b and T2b tumours in the absence of detectable distant metastases is problematical. Such cases are few but a significant number of surgeons would opt for radical mastectomy in such a presentation. Similarly, local recurrence after simple mastectomy or local excision and irradiation might be suitable. The alleged benefit is related to diminished local and axillary recurrence. For technical minutiae the description of Riddell (1954) is unsurpassed.

Ideally the nature of the lesion should be established before radical mastectomy is undertaken, but if not, then an excision or incision biopsy and frozen section are obligatory. The operative field is repainted and retowelled with the arm abducted and pronated on a board. Careful attention must be paid to the painting and towelling of the posterolateral aspect of the chest and brachioscapular area. The arm is then firmly attached to the board.

The incision varies with the position of the carcinoma. For centrally placed lesions a transverse or oblique approach is possible but for most cases a more vertical oblique direction is correct. The incision should be planned before surgery and the growth included in a skin ellipse adequate to provide 2–3 cm clearance each side and yet allow for primary skin closure. With a large tumour in a small breast, skin grafting is necessary and the ipsilateral thigh is prepared accordingly. The vertical oblique incision begins at the tip of the coracoid process and follows as far as possible the line of a brassière shoulder strap—then encompassing the growth and finishing close to the xiphoid process.

The lateral flap is first elevated down to the anterior border of latissimus dorsi; extending up to its tendon of insertion and below the full length of the rectus sheath. The outer third of the medial flap is next raised to the clavicle above and sternum medially down to the first perforating artery. The interval between the clavicular and sternal heads of pectoralis major is entered and the muscle separated by careful digital dissection. At the lateral end the bilaminar tendon of insertion is divided close to the humerus. Pectoralis major is turned downwards; the lateral and medial pectoral nerves are divided and pectoralis minor exposed. The acromio-thoracic vessels are ligated as they perforate the clavi-pectoral fascia. This layer is incised and pectoralis minor is elevated from the axillary vein, divided at its insertion and turned downwards. Division of the suspensory ligament of the axilla in the line of the axillary vein exposes the axilla and its contents. Starting laterally and proceeding towards the thoracic inlet, the veins draining from the axillary contents and chest wall into the main vein are secured, allowing fat and nodes to be drawn downwards. The fascial and fatty attachment of axillary contents to the lateral skin flap and latissimus is now divided. Finally, the fascial layers overlying subscapularis and serratus are incised and

lifted digitally from the muscles to enclose the axillary contents.

At the angle between the scapula and chest wall, these fascial layers are divided by scissors from above downwards. The axillary contents with the fascia are cleaned downwards, dividing the intercosto-brachial nerve and lateral intercostal vessels as necessary. It is important to preserve the nerves to latissimus and serratus anterior. Pectoralis minor is detached from its origin and with the major is lifted upwards and medially, taking the breast with it until the perforating vessels of the internal mammary artery are reached. These vessels are clipped and ligated. In thin subjects the intercostal muscles and anterior intercostal membrane are very tenuous where the vessels emerge. Pectoralis major is excised from the sternum. The breast and attached muscle are then laid back over the chest and the remainder of the medial skin flap is elevated. The breast with attached muscles and axillary contents are finally removed by sharp dissection. Depending on the size of the vessels, absolute haemostasis is achieved by ligature or diathermy. Skin trimming may be necessary. Two suction (Redivac) drains are inserted through the lateral flap at the axillary and sternal ends: skin closure is by fine interrupted silk sutures.

Should grafting be required, the gap is closed as far as possible and a split graft is taken from the thigh to match the defect. The graft is laid on petroleum jelly gauze over a board and trimmed to approximate size; spare portions are saved in a sterile jar and refrigerated in case of graft failure. The graft is sutured to the edges with interrupted 3/0 silk sutures which are left long to tie over plastic sponge or flavine wool. Postoperative wound management is as has been previously described.

Postoperative Care

Limited arm and shoulder movements are allowed from the start but it seems sensible to restrict abduction movements until around 14 days postoperatively, by which time most of the serum collections will have resolved. The patient should be warned of the possibility of lymphatic vessel thromboses in the axilla and arm. These are manifested by tight, painful wire-like strands extending even as far as the cubital fossa; arm movements should continue and the process will resolve.

When the wound has healed, or after radiotherapy has been completed and the skin recovered, a light dusting powder to the chest wall is soothing and a mammary prosthesis can be inserted inside the brassière. Until that time, improvisation with cottonwool suffices.

REGIONAL NODE BIOPSY

To assess the spread of breast cancer and prescribe surgical and other measures accordingly, some surgeons favour biopsy of the apical, axillary and internal mammary nodes (Blamey et al., 1979).

The argument is reasonable: if the apical axillary nodes are involved then cure is unlikely, even more so if the internal mammary nodes contain tumour. Also, that if both sites are invaded then this simple biopsy evidence is as reliable a predictor of widespread micrometastases as skeletal and liver isotopic scanning.

The principle and practice of this type of biopsy do remain controversial, and many surgeons are happier assuming the presence of disseminated disease if a certain number—the favourite number at present is four—of axillary nodes contain tumour. The dilemma is as yet unsolved. These biopsy procedures should, however, lie within the repertoire of a surgeon interested in breast cancer as they may become increasingly important.

Isolated Axillary Biopsy

This applies when the mammary incision for segmental excision or lumpectomy cannot be conveniently extended. A skin crease incision is made to extend from the palpable borders of the pectoralis major and latissimus dorsi. The axillary space is opened through the suspensory ligament and wide exposure developed by gentle blunt dissection and retraction. A generous representative sample of the central contents and palpable nodes is effected. The exposure tends to be modest; obsessive haemostasis and drainage are advisable.

Internal Mammary Node Biopsy

It is probably wise to confine biopsy to the second and third interspaces, through a short vertical or transverse incision. Pectoralis major is detached from the sternal edge and perforating vessels are ligated. For a distance of 4 cm lateral to the sternal edge, the intercostal muscle and anterior intercostal membrane are incised to expose the internal mammary vessels. Fatty and nodal tissue is isolated by delicate pledget dissection, taking care to avoid puncturing the pleura. The nodes may be as diminutive as 2–3 mm diameter. Haemostasis accomplished, the pectoral is reattached with interrupted 3/0 or 4/0 silk sutures, and the skin likewise.

Apical Axillary Node Biopsy

A short incision of around 6–8 cm in length is made below and parallel to the middle third of the clavicle. The pectoral is detached subperiosteally from the clavicle and retracted downwards. The clavi-pectoral fascia is divided and the axillary vein identified. The space between the axillary vein and the upper chest wall is cleaned. One expects to find fibro-fatty tissue, including some apical nodes.

RECONSTRUCTIVE SURGERY

Subcutaneous Mastectomy with Insertion of Prosthesis or Reconstructive Prosthetic Mammoplasty following Mastectomy

Like many aspects of breast surgery this fairly recent addition to the surgeon's repertoire is controversial both in technique and application. Cronin and Gerow (1964) reported on the reliability and suitability of Silastic gel mammary prostheses, both for augmentation mammoplasty and replacement. Williams (1972) wrote that during the previous 9-year period Dow-Corning Corporation sold over 50 000 Silastic prostheses: since then interest in reconstructive breast surgery has increased (Georgiade, 1977). Adjacent editorial articles by Freeman (1972) and Weiner (1972) counselled caution and enthusiasm respectively. The issues involved are fundamental and may be itemized as follows:

1. There are no long-term studies of subcutaneous mastectomy with prosthetic inserts.

2. In North America there is an increasing tendency to offer mastectomy and prosthetic replacement for non-malignant lesions or symptoms, e.g. mastodynia, recurrent breast cysts, multiple biopsies for dysplasia, atypical epitheliosis, a strong family history of breast cancer.

In Great Britain this unorthodoxy is under consideration but at present receives modest support. The procedure may be acceptable for atypical and preferably bilateral intraduct cellular proliferation. So infrequently is breast cancer discovered 'early' that a more aggressive approach to the presumed premalignant state demands serious consideration (Weiner, 1972).

3. Troublesome complications may arise following prosthetic insertion, the sole aim of which is to retain a cosmetic effect. The prosthesis does not bounce naturally with movement; nipple sensation is significantly altered and may be lost. Skin healing may fail and the prosthesis becomes exposed. The cosmetic effect may be marred by a firm subcutaneous reaction producing skin wrinkling. It is essential that the patient and, if appropriate, her husband are fully aware of these risks. Considering the very heavy bill for drugs and appliances an additional load from widespread use of expensive Silastic prostheses demands careful assessment. For malignancy, a total mastectomy with a well-fitting prosthesis serves superbly well for most women. It is common experience that most cope psychologically with their physical loss.

Operative Details

A selection of sterile Silastic prostheses should be available in the theatre together with a scale to weigh excised breast tissue. General anaesthesia without intentional hypotension is required, but a 20–30° head-up tilt is useful. The towelling arrangement includes elevation to paint the back and lie the patient on a sterile towel. Both breasts are exposed and the towels are sutured in place; the opposite side is covered initially, to be exposed later for comparison.

A submammary incision is ideal but a reasonable alternative is an oblique approach behind the anterior axillary fold. Previous biopsy scars may dictate another incision such as subareolar or lateral radial. By firm retraction over swabs, the skin edges are separated and it is critical to the success of the procedure to enter the correct plane. The separation lies between the breast fat and subcutaneous fat. The latter contains a network of veins, and the fat is finely lobular; it varies in thickness according to build. Delicate elevation of the skin edges by skin hooks or Allis tissue forceps is performed, followed later by appropriate retractors. When the nipple is reached, the ducts are divided, leaving a thick corium layer to preserve vascularity and hopefully eventual sensation. It is sensible to mobilize an edge of the breast and elevate it from the pectoral fascia. Thereby the breast tissue can be turned deep side out and dissection simplified. The major arterial supply to the breast skin enters on the medial and lateral side, so it is prudent to dissect very carefully there in order to ligate the arterial branch entering the breast while preserving the skin vessel.

Careful and patient retraction will enable the breast to be removed and preferably a biopsy of low axillary (pectoral) nodes also. Total haemostasis is achieved by fine 3/0 silk ligatures or very precise fine diathermy coagulation. The incision is held open by retractors, and the gel-filled, round, patchless prosthesis is slipped into the vacated space and checked for size; the opposite breast is exposed and comparison made. If necessary, the prosthesis is replaced to fit. The skin is then closed in two layers. A deep subcutaneous layer of 2/0 or 3/0 chromic catgut is carefully placed followed by subcuticular or fine interrupted skin sutures according to preference. The wound is sealed with mastiche or Nobecutane (resin wound dressing, Astia), followed by some form of supportive dressing. A cotton brassière is applied over the dressing.

Variations in Technique

It is important to mention these; they are interesting and instructive. Watts (1977), who has assembled a wide experience of subcutaneous mastectomy, requires careful resterilization of the prosthesis, despite assurance from the manufacturer. Also a 'no touch' technique is used throughout the mastectomy, in particular for insertion of the prosthesis, when new gloves are taken. He avoids both drainage and antibiotics. Others employ a far less rigid technique seemingly content to handle both skin and prosthesis. In one large American series (Williams, 1972) local steroid (triamcinolone acetate) and antibiotic (cephaloridine) are injected into the space. Suction drainage

is widely used. Insertion of the prosthesis following subcutaneous mastectomy may be immediate or delayed for 3–6 months. Immediate insertion carries a greater risk of complications especially where the skin is thin and biopsy scars are present. Delayed insertion allows skin vascularity to reach an optimal state but sadly the cosmetic result tends to suffer. Some surgeons routinely excise and resuture previous biopsy scars at the time of mastectomy.

Postoperative Management

Certain details are very important. A soft lateral pad of sterile cottonwool is inserted inside the brassière cup to prevent the prosthesis from sliding laterally into the axilla. Arm and shoulder movements are restricted for 2 weeks. Occasionally a collection of serous fluid requires careful aspiration.

Complications

If a significant haematoma develops, it is sensible to evacuate it at around 48 hours. Skin loss of minor degree can be excised down to the prosthesis and resutured. Gross exposure of the prosthesis necessitates its removal with resuturing or grafting. Skin loss may not be immediate but may take many weeks to develop. Later complications have already been mentioned. They include rupture of the prosthesis, its dislocation into the axilla and the formation of a firm or even hard fibrous capsule. The latter may respond to firm massage but, as with the others mentioned here, reoperation and a new prosthesis may be required.

A modification in the insertion of Silastic mammary prostheses has recently appeared. To overcome the very troublesome complication of capsule formation some surgeons insert the prosthesis deep to the pectoralis major. The route is either by splitting the muscle centrally; by incising serratus anterior laterally and tunnelling behind pectoralis. Alternatively the sternocostal origin of pectoralis is detached and the prosthesis slipped upwards. A modest-sized (200–250 ml) prosthesis may be inserted, but the procedure is controversial and awaits further evaluation. An additional modification is to use tissue expansion incorporating a prosthesis which is progressively inflated over a period of weeks with saline injections (Radovan, 1982).

The principal use of this novel technique is to expand a subcutaneous space for insertion of a prosthesis where, due to the previous mastectomy, skin is short.

Additional Techniques and Aspects of Breast Reconstruction

The present position has been well reviewed by Hughes (1984) but there is much controversy in the philosophy and practice of this branch of breast surgery. First, if less radical procedures for selected breast cancers are successful, then the need for reconstruction will be less than if mastectomy is the rule. Although breast cancer is a very unpredictable disease it would appear reasonable to incorporate some prognostication and withhold reconstruction for at least 2 years. This would exclude the group in whom early recurrence develops.

The overwhelming reason for reconstruction is to relieve the psychological distress consequent on mastectomy in many women. Whereas some 20–30 per cent of women suffer a significant psychological reaction to mastectomy (Maguire, 1984), the reaction is much improved by 1 year afterwards (Dean et al., 1983). The results of reconstruction are generally rather discouraging so there would appear to be sound reasons for delaying it beyond 2 years. The majority of women adjust very quickly to a tidy mastectomy and a neatly fitted external prosthesis.

Two further questions are perhaps best reserved for either plastic surgeons or general surgeons with a dominating interest in breast cancer and also a belief in reconstruction. The procedures are the latissimus dorsi flap and the rectus abdominis flap—both rather complex techniques. Details are provided in publications by Bostwick et al. (1978), Webster and Hughes (1983) and Nash and Hurst (1983).

Subcutaneous mammary prostheses have been attended by rather modest results (Dean et al., 1983; Ward and Edwards, 1983) and have not gained great acceptance. It remains to be seen if 'flap' techniques are more successful. The indications for their use need to be very precisely defined.

PLASTIC SURGERY PROCEDURES IN RELATION TO THE BREAST

The most dramatic of these is mammoplasty but this is a difficult and unpredictable technique even in skilled and experienced hands (McKissock, 1972). A variety of procedures is currently employed, which probably means that the perfect operation is elusive. The operation should not be undertaken by a general surgeon. Nevertheless, he may feel competent to excise resistant locally recurrent breast carcinoma or an area of radionecrosis. To close a chest wall defect, a simple split-skin graft or a rotation flap with grafting of the exposed area is employed (Dudley, 1977). This is not a difficult technique; it demands clean excision even down to and through the muscle layer if necessary and the construction of an adequate rotation flap. The need for this operation arises very infrequently and it should only be performed if there is no evidence of distant metastases. Otherwise, hormonal measures or chemotherapy are the logical approach.

Augmentation Mammoplasty

This commonly performed operation, which employs a Silastic silicone gel prosthesis, is considered for hypoplastic breasts or where, following childbirth and lactation, the breasts undergo a degree of atrophy and ptosis. The indication is a relative one and is purely concerned with cosmesis. The stress and unhappiness which some women allege in these circumstances should be carefully evaluated by the surgeon. The technique is not difficult and in the absence of available plastic surgical expertise could reasonably be acquired and practised by a general surgeon concerned with breast disease.

Operative Details

Under general anaesthesia an incision is made just above the inframammary crease in order to preserve a small fringe of breast tissue attached to the chest wall close to the lower skin edge. The incision is deepened to the pectoral fascia and the breast is lifted away from the fascia by blunt swab or digital dissection. Unlike subcutaneous mastectomy, the dissection is easy and there is little risk to blood supply. After a suitable bed is fashioned and haemostasis secured, a round, correctly sized, low-profile Silastic prosthesis is eased in and manipulated into place. According to Williams (1972) a safe size is 225 ml and a volume of 315 ml should never be exceeded.

The skin is closed in two layers, the first by 2/0 plain or chromic catgut making use of the fringe of breast and fatty subcutaneous tissue to produce a ledge which will prevent the prosthesis from slipping downwards. Skin closure is according to the preference of the operator.

An alternative approach relies on an oblique axillary incision hidden by the anterior axillary fold. The breast is dissected away from pectoralis major as with the inferior approach, and to reach the lower quadrants of the breast a thick blunt metal sound has been advocated. The prosthesis is inserted as previously described and the use of topical steroids and antibiotics is favoured by some surgeons.

The complications match those which may follow subcutaneous mastectomy. For 608 patchless Silastic prosthetic augmentations Williams (1972) reported infection in 3, exposure due to skin loss in 6 and ptosis of the prosthesis in 14.

MANAGEMENT OF THE BREAST CANCER PATIENT

The early 1970s were associated with new concepts in relation to breast cancer and its management. Diagnosis was improved by the adoption of low-dose mammography and the recognition that the identification of a cancerous lump by some form of needle biopsy in the clinic led to more enlightened investigations. The concept of micrometastases and the faltering importance of radical local surgery were easily accepted by most surgeons. The implications and irregular availability of cellular hormone receptors were and are more difficult. Adjuvant chemotherapy and hormonal treatment for high-risk groups enforced on all the importance of an oncological team to sustain long-term treatment for all cases.

The recognition of early metastases and the near-total eclipse of radical surgery led to greater emphasis on rehabilitation and an as yet unfulfilled and unsubstantiated requirement for breast reconstruction.

The formulation and execution of controlled clinical trials for breast cancer treatment may have created more problems than provided solutions. Some are of much greater potential than others. Hopefully the maturation of important studies within the next 10–15 years will be rewarding.

It is difficult within a few pages to appraise a problem which taxes modern oncology to its limit and concerning which so much is written. Apart from understanding up-to-date and substantial scientific fact one needs a basic philosophical approach to this killing disease. It is sensible to begin by relating certain dilemmas in basic knowledge apropos breast cancer—it is understandable that so many disagreements still exist. Over the past 40 years there has been no improvement in the survival rate from breast cancer (Bonnadonna et al., 1976), although disease-free intervals may have been increased. Figures differ for survival, but they suggest that at 10 years 30–50 per cent of all cases are alive. Forrest (1974) reported that for stage 1 and 2 only, the 15-year survival rate was around 30 per cent, and these figures were confirmed by other British workers. Unhappily, epidemiological studies have yielded little because the 'high-risk factors', e.g. family history, previous breast carcinoma, previous biopsies for mammary dysplasia, are not strong enough to construct study groups.

Mammographic measurements, animal studies and cell kinetics enable calculations to be made for a 1 cm diameter breast cancer: Silvestrini (1984). It contains numerous cells and a doubling time of 100 days for the primary is a reasonable assumption. Extrapolation shows that the lesion began at least some 8 years before discovery at 1 cm and was capable of metastasis in its preclinical stage. This casts some doubt on the value of screening, as the time gained may not be effective enough to be valuable. Perhaps cancers discovered during screening are of a slower growing type with lesser metastatic potential. The question is unanswered (Baum, 1981, 1982).

Breast cancer is an extremely capricious and unpredictable disease. It has even been suggested that it is several different diseases (Baker, 1977). Certainly each case is cytomorphologically unique. Although statistics show trends within a large group of cases there are differing forms of tumour–host behaviour. In very few reports is management 'tailored' to the clinico-pathological state. We are still unable to reliably predict how a particular patient will progress.

Dormancy in breast cancer is a well-recognized clinical phenomenon: it must mean either a slower tumour doubling time or, more likely, an effective tissue resistance. The latter must surely be an immunological host response. Yet attempts to identify and harness this response have proved largely fruitless. Similarly, quantitative and qualitative understanding of the cellular heterogeneity of breast cancers is not yet possible.

The logistics of clinical and mammographic screening show that it might succeed in so-called 'high-risk' women. Wholesale screening is expensive and the yield of latent cancers is barely worth it. The idea that a breast cancer is but the local manifestation of an already generalized disease process has gained acceptance—for some very grudgingly—but with a hope that in 20 per cent of cases the disease is truly local (Gazet et al., 1978). The problem is detection of metastases. Scanning techniques for bone and liver are very approximate and expensive. Several studies have revealed that in breast cancer follow-up clinical examination supplemented by chest radiographs at regular intervals, together with measurements of the serum alkaline phosphatase and gamma-glutamyl transferase, will discover 90–96 per cent of metastatic presentations (Perez et al., 1983). Nodal spread is most easily determined from the axilla and the number of nodes involved there is a predictor of micrometastases elsewhere. Micronodular deposits may be present in posterior intercostal and mediastinal lymph nodes—unseen and unsampled. Perhaps these nodes account for metastatic spread in pathologically node-negative cases.

In the past, the importance of specific local surgery has been overemphasized. In Great Britain total mastectomy with axillary clearance or adequate biopsy (4 lower pectoral lymph nodes) has found widespread favour. American and European monographs (Heuson et al., 1976) still refer to radical and super-radical mastectomy—procedures shown to be of no benefit over total mastectomy. A useful review of the more important clinical trials in respect of local treatment for breast cancer is provided by Veronesi (1984). It is indeed surprising that radical mastectomy still finds a place. The chemotherapists have also entered the field (Bonnadonna et al., 1976) to persuade surgeons to remove all local tumour (primary and nodes). This does not necessitate a radical mastectomy, however, at most a Patey procedure will suffice.

Lumpectomy or segmental mastectomy followed by radiotherapy are perhaps illogical procedures in the face of sound evidence that many breast cancers are multicentric. It is also common knowledge for any surgeon and radiotherapist experienced in the field that some breast cancers fail to respond to radiotherapy. Controlled trials are in progress but may fail to resolve the problem as the study groups are biologically heterogeneous. Yet in certain circumstances the procedure is an attractive one for tumours less than 2 cm in diameter. It is more suitable for low-grade cancers where mammography reveals a single lesion. Peripheral small cancers are ideally suitable, especially if the patient is in poor health. The procedure carries a risk of local recurrence that is greater than that following mastectomy.

Primarily involved or recurrent axillary metastatic nodes are best managed by axillary clearance and not by radiotherapy. Radiotherapy maintains its strong place in the management of breast cancer. First, it is invaluable for osseous deposits, especially for pain relief. Second, soft tissue and skin recurrence following surgery may respond very adequately to local radiotherapy.

The role of postoperative irradiation is now less certain. It is contra-indicated for node-negative, Mo cases (the TNM international classification), but where nodes are involved it is frequently given. It delays local recurrence but has no beneficial effect on survival. Hormonal treatment has for long been popular in the therapy of metastatic breast cancer because of its minimal side-effects. Perhaps 30–40 per cent of all cases showed some response but where treatment was effective 20 per cent of all cases remitted for at least 1 year—some with long-term free periods. It is currently suggested that cytoplasmic oestrogen receptors (ER) are important as predictors (McGuire et al., 1975). If present, then 60 per cent of ER-positive patients will show a response; if not, then the treatment has negligible effect. This investigation is a refined assay performed on frozen tumour tissue in but a few laboratories. Not many metastatic cases will yield tumour material and ER status is ideally estimated at the time of mastectomy. The result is held for future application. Work on progesterone and other receptors is in progress and could be of equal importance as many postmenopausal patients respond well to norethisterone acetate (SH 420). The significance of receptors is not yet fully understood and a simpler method of recognizing their presence would be a great advance.

The whole subject of receptor assay and significance is both important and complex. The reader is referred to an authoritative chapter by Scholl and Lippman (1984) for a detailed review. In clinical management three other factors require consideration. Not every centre managing breast cancer has access to receptor assays and the likely status of a tumour can in any case be largely predicted from its differentiation. Finally, the addition of an alleged anti-oestrogenic substance—tamoxifen—to the therapeutic field has complicated management. It might be expected that ER + status would predict the cases likely to respond to tamoxifen. There are significant exceptions to this which could mean that tamoxifen, which is a most acceptable drug because of its efficacy and lack of side-effects, may function other than as an anti-oestrogen.

Many surgeons and oncologists use tamoxifen as a first line of therapy—reverting to chemotherapy if no response is detected. The operation which has stood the test of time is oophorectomy for the pre-

menopausal woman. Adrenalectomy has been superseded by the adrenal suppressant aminoglutethimide supplemented by steroids.

The case most likely to respond to these measures will be at least 2 years premenopausal; having shown a long free interval (> 2 years) between mastectomy and first recurrence, and where the metastatic manifestation is either skeletal, soft tissue or pleural. Cerebral, hepatic and other abdominal metastases are unresponsive to hormonal measures.

In postmenopausal women who have shown some response to tamoxifen but relapsed, then a trial of progestagens is well worth while.

The indications for surgical hormone ablation are modified.

Chemotherapy and breast cancer are a modern dilemma both for advanced metastatic disease and in an adjuvant role. The position has been summarized and appraised by Powles et al. (1978), Turner (1978) and Bonnadonna and Valagussa (1984). There is disagreement on the application of chemotherapy. Chemotherapy should only be administered in a skilled unit run by radiotherapists or physician oncologists. There are dangerous side-effects from chemotherapy. One of its major disadvantages is that unnecessary deaths may follow inexpert practice. For advanced disease, single drug regimens such as thiotepa or chlorambucil may induce a response; simplicity if effective obviously carries advantages. Combination therapy is more popular, however; cyclophosphamide, methotrexate and 5-fluorouracil (CMF), also vincristine, adriamycin and prednisone (CAP), are commonly administered. Treatment regimens and dosage vary. The response rate for CMF is reported as 70 per cent, with complete remission (total disappearance of clinical disease) at 30 per cent. The response lasts for up to 1 year with longer free intervals following complete remission. Useful prolongation of active life may result. Turner (1978) obtained excellent response rates in the 1950s using Durabolin (nandrolone phenylpropionate) combined with thiotepa. There seems little point in extending combination therapies beyond three drugs and the aim would be a single drug regimen. Chemotherapy in advanced disease demands sympathetic skill for its humane administration.

The place of adjuvant chemotherapy is as yet unsolved but may yet be revealed from trials already in progress. After several years involving trials of adjuvant chemotherapy there is very major disagreement, for instance between British and American oncologists. The controversies relate to the morbidity of the treatment, its ability to prolong survival and cost. The principle is basic. Chemotherapy kills most efficiently any small tumour deposits up to 1 mm in diameter by first-order reaction kinetics. Based on axillary (and no other) nodal metastases, Fisher et al. (1968) proposed that where four or more nodes were involved by tumour that without adjuvant therapy the 5-year relapse rate was 80 per cent with a survival rate of 31 per cent. Metastases extant at the time of mastectomy must explain these figures, hence improvement could only be obtained by some early systemic 'cancer kill' therapy. The adjuvant therapy trials of Fisher et al. (1968) and Bonnadonna et al. (1976) for stage 2 breast cancer reveal a dramatic initial delay in the appearance of metastases of sixfold over the control group. The benefit is not sustained, however, and by 33 months the difference reduces to twofold. Premenopausal patients benefit more than postmenopausal. Several authorities suggest that this effect is hormonal—ovarian and adrenal —induced by the chemotherapy. Also that the benefit derives from chemotherapy delaying the development of micronodular disease rather than true micrometastases. The current trend in chemotherapy is to stratify more precisely groups likely to respond. Predictability is important in the assessment of trials and at present we cannot predict. At 5 years without chemotherapy, some 46 per cent of stage 2 patients will be alive. It is generally agreed that once distant metastases develop the patient cannot be cured by any known means. The best that can be attained is tolerable survival until perhaps some other cause of death supervenes.

Even now, methods of determining metastatic disease are gross, rendering each case assessment very imprecise. The discovery of a reliable tumour marker for serum estimation in early as opposed to late cases is urgently required but sadly elusive. Of considerable interest and importance are the different response rates for chemotherapy depending on disease site. With combination chemotherapy, lymph node, soft tissue, skin and lung deposits show a 50 per cent response rate; bony secondaries are refractory, whereas they respond far better to hormonal measures. Thiotepa alone or in combination with testosterone or Durabolin did affect osseous metastases. There is as yet no explanation for this.

Taking all of these factors into account, a reasonable plan of management for breast cancer is shown in *Figs* 30.12–30.14.

FUTURE DEVELOPMENTS

In respect of breast surgery there is no shortage of questions which need to be answered (Baum, 1982; Veronesi, 1984).

Properly constructed trials based on comparable prognostic groups should be established to decide whether local excision and axillary sampling or extended local mastectomy, both followed by radiotherapy for positive nodes, are comparable procedures. The ethics of such a trial present difficulties but the question has never yet been properly answered. Similarly the margin of local excision for a breast cancer amounting to either lumpectomy (minimal clearance) or segmental removal (2–3 cm) requires solution. Veronesi (1984) has drawn atten-

tion to the relevance of the tumour size/breast size ratio. At present it appears that only tumours of up to 2 cm diameter (radiologically measured) should be offered for local excision.

The implication of multicentricity in breast cancers is becoming increasingly well studied but the implication is uncertain.

The extent of axillary dissection varies much between surgeons. There is room for a trial to compare axillary clearance with minimal sampling followed by irradiation. There is good evidence that internal mammary node biopsy is inappropriate. Further study is required to settle the matter.

For a contemporary volume on current aspects of breast cancer the reader is referred to that edited by Bonnadonna (1984). The incorporated bibliography is exhaustive.

DISEASES OF THE MALE BREAST

The commonest lesion encountered in general surgical practice will be gynaecomastia. There are many possible aetiological factors and these are discussed in a monograph by Hall (1959). Idiopathic gynaecomastia in young and middle-aged men is often unilateral and socially embarrassing. Bilateral gynaecomastia may develop also and an underlying cause should be sought; usually none is found. The exclusion of a drug factor, cirrhosis of liver, testicular trophoblastic teratoma and Klinefelter's syndrome having been achieved, simple surgical excision is effective treatment.

A submammary as opposed to a subareolar incision is preferable. An adequate subcutaneous fatty layer should be preserved or the cosmetic result may be sunken and ugly. If the breast is excessively large, the opinion of a plastic surgeon should be considered.

Occasionally bilateral gynaecomastia related to the administration of spironolactone may be troublesome in the nature of cyst and abscess formation. Following simple drainage of infection, mastectomy should in due course be performed.

Carcinoma of the male breast is a rare disease, accounting for 0·7 per cent of all male cancers and 1 per cent of all primary breast cancers (Holleb, 1970). Pathologically the majority (62 per cent) are infiltrating duct cancers. It presents at a median age of around 58–60 years. The patient often delays reporting and advanced disease is the rule; up to one-third of cases are inoperable when first seen. The diagnosis must always be suspected in unilateral gynaecomastia and needle biopsy is an invaluable simple means of diagnosis.

Excision biopsy with frozen section is the alternative means of confirmation. The majority of cases have undeniable clinical signs of malignancy. If the nipple is extensively invaded by tumour or the growth is tethered to pectoralis major then a radical mastectomy is advisable. With lesser involvement extended local or Patey mastectomy will suffice. Axillary clear-

PLAN FOR INVESTIGATION OF BREAST LUMP AND LUMPINESS

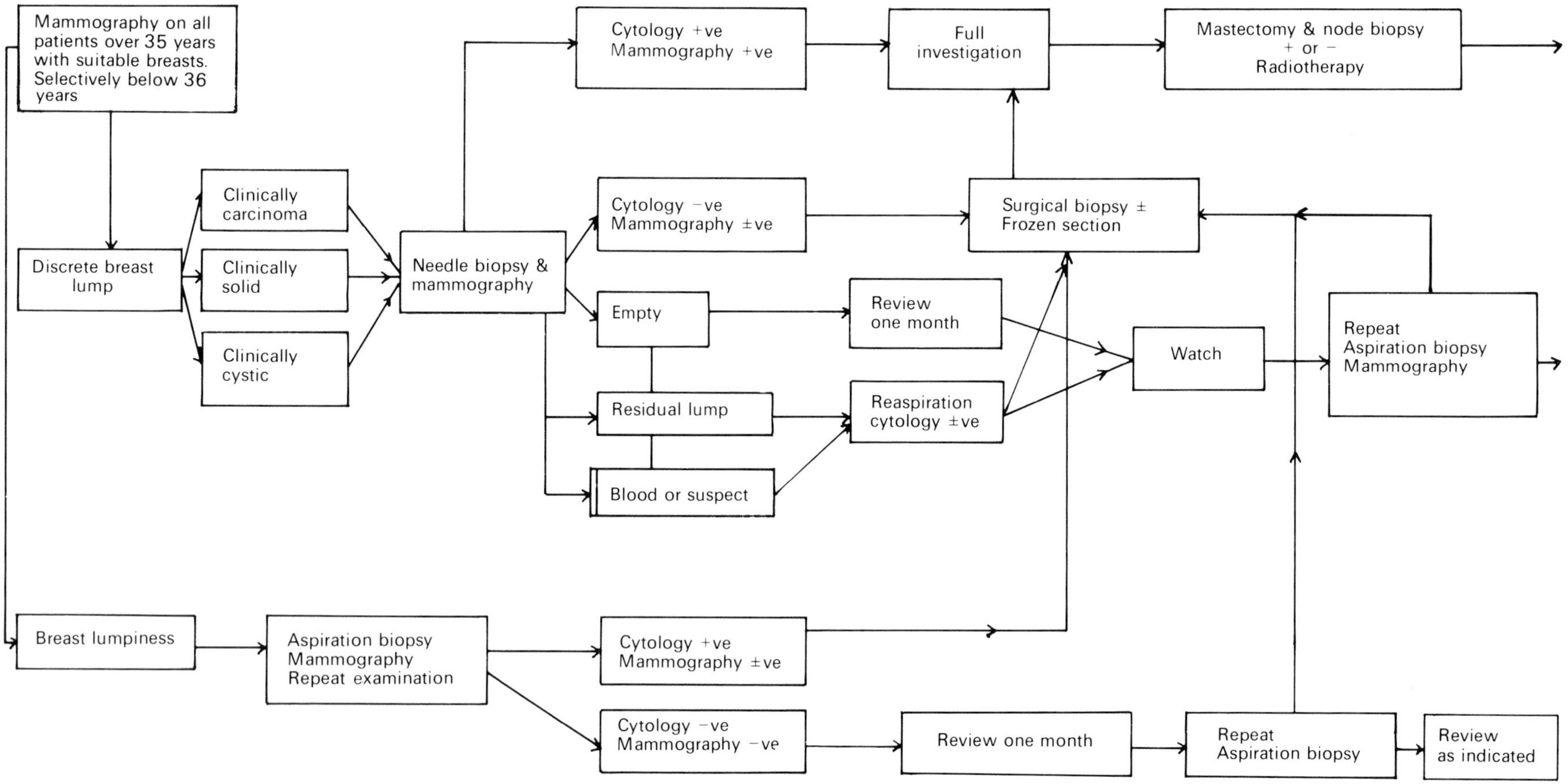

Fig. 30.12

A SCHEME FOR THE MANAGEMENT OF
PRIMARY BREAST CANCER

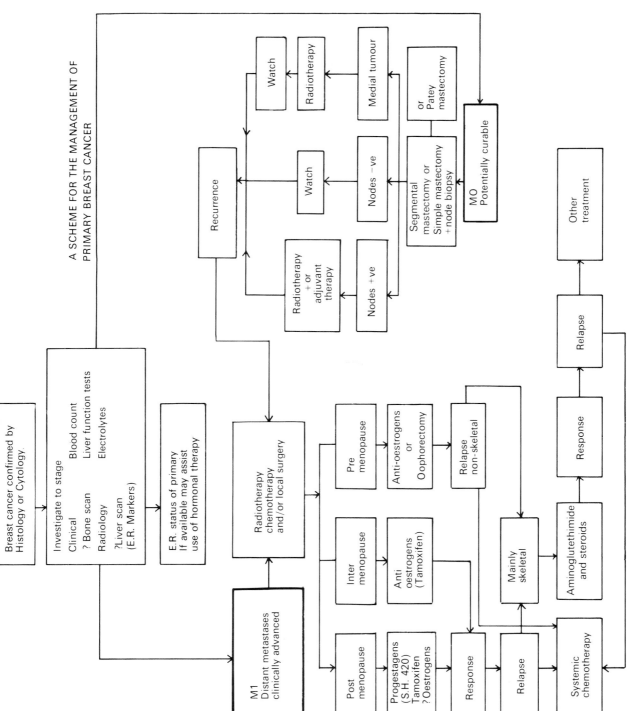

Fig. 30.13

INVESTIGATION AND MANAGEMENT OF NIPPLE DISCHARGE—SPONTANEOUS OR EXPRESSIBLE

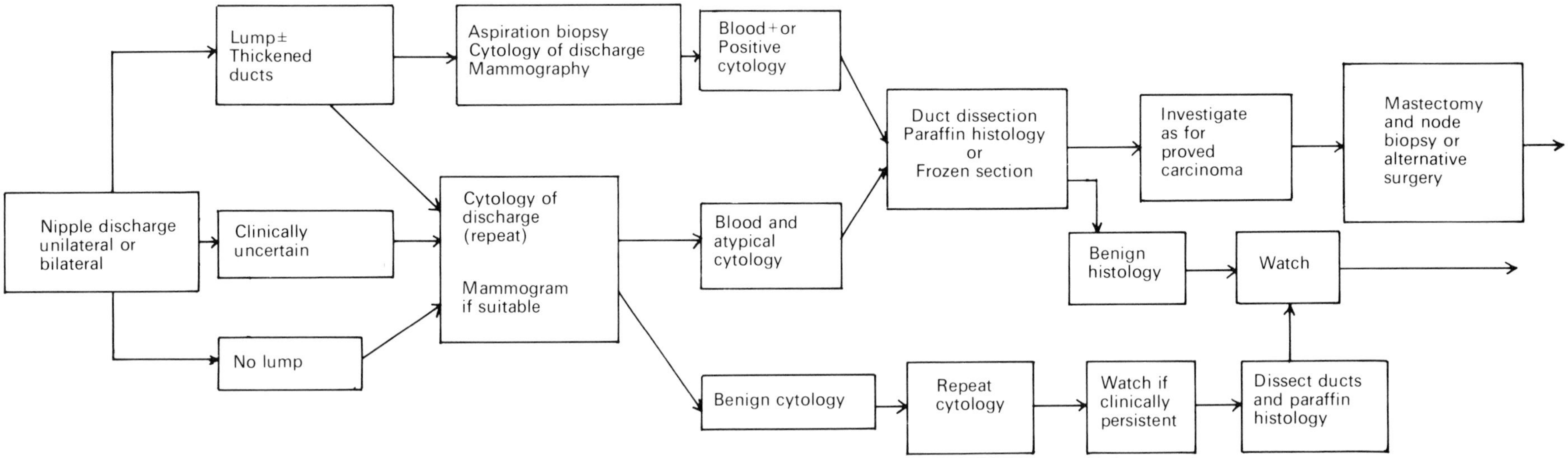

Fig. 30.14

ance and wide skin incision with skin grafting offer the best chance of controlling local disease. If nodes are involved by tumour it is customary to prescribe postoperative irradiation.

Inoperable and metastatic male breast cancer is resistant to treatment. A 45 per cent response rate has been reported following bilateral orchidectomy.

There are reports of beneficial effect from adrenalectomy. Drug therapy with oestrogens, androgens and steroids has been universally disappointing.

There is no confirmed aetiological cause for male breast cancer and no explanation for its left-sided predilection. For the matched pathological stages the survival rates equal those for females.

REFERENCES

Baker R. Robinson (ed.) (1977) *Current Trends in the Management of Breast Cancer*. London, Baillière Tindall.

Baum M. (1981) *Breast Cancer, The Facts*. Oxford, Oxford Medical Publications.

Baum M. (1982) Will breast self examination save lives? Editorial. *Br. Med. J. (Clin. Res.)* **284**, 142.

Blamey R. W., Davies C. J., Elston C. W. et al. (1979) Prognostic factors in breast cancer—the formation of a prognostic index. *Clin. Oncol.* **5**, 227.

Bonnadona G. (1984) *Cancer Investigation and Management. Vol. 1. Breast Cancer: Diagnosis and Management*. Chichester and New York, Wiley.

Bonnadonna G. and Valagussa P. (1984) Combined modality approach. In: Bonnadonna G. (ed.) *Breast Cancer: Diagnosis and Management*. Chichester and New York, Wiley, p. 281.

Bonnadonna G., Valagussa P. and Veronesi U. (1976) Results of ongoing clinical trials with adjuvant chemotherapy in operable breast cancer. In: Heuson J. C., Mattheiem W. H. and Rozencweig M. (eds) *Breast Cancer: Trends in Research and Treatment*. European Organization for Research on Treatment of Cancer Monographs. New York, Raven Press, p. 239.

Bostwick J., Vasconex L. O. and Jurkiewicz M. J. (1978) Breast reconstruction after radical mastectomy. *Plast. Reconstr. Surg.* **61**, 682.

Brady L. W. and Bedwinek J. M. (1984) The changing role of radiotherapy. In: Bonnadonna G. (ed.) *Breast Cancer: Diagnosis and Management*. Chichester and New York, Wiley, p. 205.

Burn J. I. (1973) Biopsy. In: Taylor S. (ed.) *Recent Advances in Surgery*, Ch. 18. Edinburgh, Churchill Livingstone, p. 442.

Burn J. I., Deeley T. J. and Malaker K. (1968) Drill biopsy and the dissemination of cancer. *Br. J. Surg.* **55**, 628.

Coleman D. V. (1982) Fine needle aspiration of solid tumours. In: Dudley H. and Pories W. (eds) *Rob and Smith's Operative Surgery*, 4th ed. London, Butterworths, p. 254.

Cronin T. D. and Gerow F. J. (1964) Augmentation mammoplasty: a new 'natural feel' prosthesis. *Transactions of the International Society of Plastic Surgeons, 3rd Congress, 1963*. Amsterdam, Excerpta Medica, p. 41.

Davies C. J., Elston C. W., Cotton R. E. et al. (1977). Preoperative diagnosis in carcinoma of the breast. *Br. J. Surg.* **64**, 326.

Dean C., Chetty U. and Forrest A. P. M. (1983) Effects of immediate breast reconstruction on psychosocial morbidity after mastectomy. *Lancet* **ii**, 459.

Dixon J. M., Anderson T. J., Lumsden A. B. et al. (1983) Mammary duct ectasia. *Br. J. Surg.* **70**, 601.

Dodd G. (1970) Mammography and thermography in the diagnosis of breast cancer. In: *Breast Cancer: Early and Late*. Proceedings of the 13th Annual Clinical Conference on Cancer, Houston, Texas, 1968. Chicago, Year Book Medical Publishers, p. 77.

Dudley H. (1977) In: Dudley H., Rob C. and Smith Sir R. (eds) *Operative Surgery*, 3rd Ed. *General Principles, Breast and Hernia*. London, Butterworths, p. 113.

Editorial (1977) Pinning down the diagnosis in breast cancer. *Br. Med. J.* **2**, 282.

Fisher B., Ravdin R. G., Ausman R. K. et al. (1968) Surgical adjuvant chemotherapy in cancer of the breast: results of a decade of cooperative investigation. *Ann. Surg.* **168**, 337.

Forrest A. P. M. (1974) Primary cancer of the breast—indications for therapy. In: Atkins Sir H. (ed.) *The Treatment of Breast Cancer*. Lancaster, MTP, p. 9

Freeman B. S. (1972) Whither subcutaneous mastectomy? *Plast. Reconstr. Surg.* **49**, 654.

Frischbier H. J. and Lohbeck H. U. (1977) *Früh Diagnostik des Mammakarzinoms*. Stuttgart, Thieme.

Gazet J.-C., Ford H. T. and Powles T. J. (1978) Surgical management of breast cancer. In: Joslin C. A. (ed.) *Aspects of Cancer Management: Carcinoma of the Breast*. Proceedings of a Symposium held at the University of York, 13 April 1977. Tunbridge Wells, Medical Congresses and Symposia Consultants, p. 7.

Georgiade N. G. (1977) Reconstructive surgery of the breast. In: Sabiston D. C. (ed.) *Davis-Christopher Textbook of Surgery*, 11th ed. Philadelphia, Saunders, p. 666.

Grubb C. (1981) *Colour Atlas of Breast Cytopathology*. England, HM & M.

Haagensen C. D. (1971) *Diseases of the Breast*, 2nd ed. Philadelphia, Saunders.

Hadfield G. J. (1960) Excision of the major duct system for benign disease of the breast. *Br. J. Surg.* **47**, 472.

Hadfield G. J. (1968) Further experience of the operation for excision of the major duct system of the breast. *Br. J. Surg.* **55**, 530.

Hall P. F. (1959) *Gynaecomastia*. Monographs of the Federal Council of the BMA, Australia.

Handley R. S. (1964) Benign breast disease. In: Rob C. and Smith Sir R. (eds) *Clinical Surgery: General Principles and Breast, Vol 1*, Ch. 33. London, Butterworths, p. 349.

Handley R. S. (1974) Techniques of surgical treatment. In: Atkins Sir H. (ed.) *The Treatment of Breast Cancer*. Lancaster, MTP, p. 49.

Harris J. R., Botnick L., Bloomer W. B. et al. (1981) Primary radiation therapy for early breast cancer: the experience at the Joint Centre of Radiation Therapy. *Int. J. Radiat. Oncol. Biol. Phys.* **7**, 1549.

Henderson B. E., Pike M. C. and Ross R. K. (1984) Epidemiology and risk factors. In: Bonnadonna G. (ed.) *Breast Cancer: Diagnosis and Management*. Chichester and New York, Wiley, p. 15.

Heuson J. C., Mattheiem W. H. and Rozencweig M. (ed.) (1976) *Breast Cancer: Trends in Research and Treatment*. European Organization for Research on Treatment of Cancer Monographs. New York, Raven Press.

Holleb A. I. (1970) Cancer of the male breast. In: *Breast Cancer: Early and Late*. Proceedings of the 13th Annual Clinical Conference on Cancer, Houston, Texas, 1968. Chicago, Year Book Medical Publishers, p. 245.

Hughes L. E. (1982) Operations for benign breast disease. In: Dudley H. and Pories W. (eds) *Rob and Smith's Operative Surgery*, 4th ed. London, Butterworths, p. 239.

Hughes L. E. (1984) Breast reconstruction after mastectomy. *Surgery* (Medical Education International Ltd) **1** (7), 165.

Koelmeyer T. D. and MacCormick D. E. M. (1976) Granulomatous mastitis. *Aust. NZ J. Surg.* **46**, 173.

Maguire P. (1984) Psychological reactions to breast cancer and its treatment. In: Bonnadonna G. (ed.) *Breast Cancer: Diagnosis and Management*. Chichester and New York, Wiley, p. 303.

McGuire W. L., Carbone P. P. and Vollmer E. P. (eds) (1975) *Estrogen Receptors in Human Breast Cancer*. New York, Raven Press.

McKissock P. K. (1972) Reduction mammaplasty with a vertical dermal flap. *Plast. Reconstr. Surg.* **49**, 245.

Magarey C. J. and Watson W. J. (1976) The outpatient diagnosis of breast lumps. *Aust. NZ J. Surg.* **46**, 344.

Melcher D., Lineham J. and Smith R. (1984) The breast. In: *Practical Aspiration Cytology*. Edinburgh, Churchill Livingstone, p. 10.

Morrison R. and Deeley T. J. (1955) Drill biopsy: technique using high-speed drill. *J. Fac. Radiol.* **6**, 287.

Nash A. G. and Hurst P. A. E. (1983) Central breast carcinoma treated by simultaneous mastectomy and latissimus dorsi flap reconstruction. *Br. J. Surg.* **70**, 654.

Patey D. H. and Dyson W. H. (1948) The prognosis of carcinoma of the breast in relation to the type of operation performed. *Br. J. Cancer* **2**, 7.

Perez D. J., Powles T. J., Milan J. et al. (1983) Detection of breast carcinoma metastases in bone: relative merits of X-rays and skeletal scintigraphy. *Lancet* **ii**, 613.

Powles T. J., Ford H. T. and Gazet J.-C. (1978) Chemotherapy in advanced disease. In: Joslin C. A. (ed.) *Aspects of Cancer Management: Carcinoma of the Breast*. Proceedings of a Symposium held at the University of York, 13 April 1977. Tunbridge Wells, Medical Congresses and Symposia Consultants, p. 41.

Radovan C. (1982) Breast reconstruction after mastectomy using the temporary expander. *Plast. Rectonstr. Surg.* **69**, 195.

Riddell V. H. (1954) Carcinoma of the breast: a review of the treatment. *Ann. R. Coll. Surg. Engl.* **14**, 215.

Rilke F. (1984) Influence of pathologic factors on management. In: Bonnadonna G. (ed.) *Breast Cancer: Diagnosis and Management*. Chichester and New York, Wiley, p. 50.

Roberts J. G., Preece P. E., Bolton P. M. et al. (1975) The 'Tru-cut' biopsy in breast cancer. *Clin. Oncol.* **1**, 297.

Scholl S. M. and Lippman M. E. (1984) Methods and clinical use of receptor assay. In: Bonnadonna G. (ed.) *Breast Cancer: Diagnosis and Management*. Chichester and New York, Wiley, p. 75.

Silvestrini R. (1984) The cell kinetics of breast cancer. In: Bonnadonna G. (ed.) *Breast Cancer: Diagnosis and Management*. Chichester and New York, Wiley, p. 5.

Tabàr L. and Dean P. B. (1984) Risks and benefits of mammography in population screening for breast cancer. In: Bonnadonna G. (ed.) *Breast Cancer: Diagnosis and Management*. Chichester and New York, Wiley, p. 63.

Thomas B. A. and Boulter P. S. (1984) Clinical examination and investigation of the breast. *Surgery* (Medical Education International Ltd) **1** (4), 86.

Thomas W. G., Williamson R. C. N., Davies J. D. et al. (1982) The clinical syndrome of mammary duct ectasia. *Br. J. Surg.* **69**, 423.

Turner R. L. (1978) The Bradford study: twenty years experience of adjuvant chemotherapy. In: Joslin C. A. (ed.) *Aspects of Cancer Management: Carcinoma of the Breast*. Proceedings of a Symposium held at the University of York, 13 April 1977. Tunbridge Wells, Medical Congresses and Symposia Consultants, p. 47.

Veronesi U. (1984) Current status of primary surgery in the management of breast cancer. In: Bonnadonna G. (ed.) *Breast Cancer: Diagnosis and Management*. Chichester and New York, Wiley, p. 169.

Veronesi U., Saccozzi R., Del Vecchio M. et al. (1981) Comparing radical mastectomy with quadrantectomy, axillary dissection and radiotherapy in patients with small cancers of the breast. *N. Engl. J. Med.* **305**, 6.

Ward D. C. and Edwards M. H. (1983) Early results of subcutaneous mastectomy with immediate silicone prosthetic implant for carcinoma of the breast. *Br. J. Surg.* **70**, 651.

Watts G. T. (1977) In: Dudley H., Rob C. and Smith Sir R. (eds) *Operative Surgery*, 3rd ed. *General Principles, Breast and Hernia*. London, Butterworths, p. 86.

Webb A. J. (1970) The diagnostic cytology of breast carcinoma. *Br. J. Surg.* **57**, 259.

Webb A. J. (1975) A cytological study of mammary disease. *Ann. R. Coll. Surg. Engl.* **56**, 181.

Webb A. J. (1982) Surgical aspects of aspiration biopsy cytology. In: Russell R. C. G. (ed.) *Recent Advances in Surgery*. Edinburgh, Churchill Livingstone.

Webster D. J. T. and Hughes L. E. (1983) The rectus abdominis myocutaneous island flap in breast cancer. *Br. J. Surg.* **70**, 71.

Weiner D. L. (1972) On subcutaneous mastectomy. *Plast. Reconstr. Surg.* **49**, 654.
Widow W. (1968) *Atlas on the Clinical Diagnosis of Mammary Carcinoma*. Berlin, Akademie Verlag.
Williams J. E. (1972) Experiences with a large series of silastic breast implants. *Plast. Reconstr. Surg.* **49**, 253.

FURTHER READING

Atkins Sir H. (ed.) (1974) *The Treatment of Breast Cancer*. Lancaster, MTP.
Breast Cancer: Early and Late. Proceedings of the 13th Annual Clinical Conference on Cancer, Houston, Texas, 1968. Chicago, Year Book Medical Publishers.
Dudley H., Rob C. and Smith Sir R. (eds) (1976–1978) *Operative Surgery*, 3rd ed. *General Principles, Breast and Hernia*. London, Butterworths.
Johnston G. S. and Jones A. E. (1975) *Breast Cancer Diagnosis*. New York, Plenum.
Joslin C. A. (ed.) (1978) *Aspects of Cancer Management: Carcinoma of the Breast*. Proceedings of a Symposium held at the University of York, 13 April 1977. Tunbridge Wells, Medical Congresses and Symposia Consultants.
Voeth J. M. (ed.) (1976) *Frontiers of Radiation Therapy and Oncology, Vol. 2. Breast Cancer*. Basel, Karger.

Chapter thirty-one

Microsurgical Techniques in Reconstructive Surgery

P. L. G. Townsend

The introduction of the operating microscope has facilitated surgery on smaller structures than would be possible without the aid of such magnification.

In hand surgery its value has been established in nerve repair but the main advances have occurred in microvascular work where it is now possible to repair small vessels of diameter 0·5–3 mm. This has enabled replantation of digits to take place and has allowed reconstructive procedures with tissue transfer from one area of the body to another. The blood supply is reconnected, flow restored and living grafts are established.

Microsurgical techniques require training as under the limited field of the microscope, specialized instruments such as fine jeweller's forceps, needle holders and small, non-crushing vascular clamps are manipulated. A bipolar electrocautery is necessary as this allows coagulation between the tips of its fine forceps only. Diamond knives or disposable micro-knives are used for dissecting nerve fasciculi or opening up small vessels to facilitate end-to-side anastomosis. Fine vessel cutters, micro-scissors, micro-irrigation and suction devices and, lastly, a coloured background to provide contrast (blue behind vessels and yellow behind nerves) are all essential.

Microscopes developed for plastic surgery have beam splitters, allowing the surgeon and the assistant to sit opposite each other, which enables them to have an identical operative visual field with stereoscopic vision. The assistant is able to assist the surgeon in, for example, counter-traction or cutting fine sutures and irrigation. A microscope with magnification 25–40 times allows visualization of the connective tissue layer on a nerve 0·1 mm in thickness.

NERVE REPAIR

The results of nerve repair, whether primary or secondary, depend on the ability to bring nerve ends together with minimal tension, carrying out accurate placement of sutures as atraumatically as possible. If after débridement of the ends of the nerve there is a gap, in some situations it may be possible to reroute the nerve, shortening its course as occurs in anterior translocation of the ulnar nerve, but usually a nerve graft is required. The sural nerve is the usual donor site for a nerve graft.

The blood supply to a peripheral nerve is usually via the mesoneurium or suspending mesentery.

Within the nerve trunk itself there is a longitudinal system of vessels which allows nutrition to continue even after some freeing of the surrounding tissue. If after repair the nerve is elongated more than 15 per cent there is evidence that this intraneural flow ceases. Continuous circumferential sutures are not advised as sutures are placed to provide correct alignment and not to provide a watertight seal. It is important during nerve repair to keep the ends moist.

Epineurial Repair (*Fig.* 31.1)

This is the repair of the outer sheath of the divided nerve. Although it may be carried out without magnification, even simple enlargement by the use of

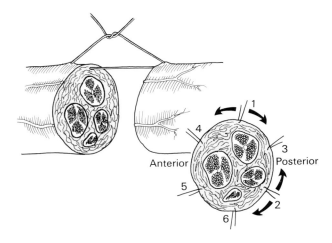

Fig. 31.1. Epineurial nerve repair.

loupes can help to visualize longitudinal vessels which can then be matched. Results are best where the nerves are either purely sensory or purely motor and where the intraneural connective tissue component is small (this can vary from 22 to 80 per cent).

After looking at the longitudinal vessels the epineurium is picked up with jeweller's forceps about 1 cm from the ends, and traction gently decreases the nerve gap. A microsuture (usually 8/0–10/0 Ethicon) is placed through the epineurium about 1 mm from one cut end, starting at the top end or 12 o'clock. This suture passes longitudinally down the axis of the nerve and out of the divided end and then through the equivalent position on the other nerve stump, with the needle bites in the same location in both stumps. The suture is tied relatively loosely and left long to allow rotation of the nerve by traction. A second suture is placed at 120° to the first behind the nerve, and this is also left long. Repair can then be completed and six sutures placed symmetrically may be required. If, after completion, fasciculi are herniating out, further sutures must be placed to prevent a lateral neuroma forming.

Perineurial or Fascicular Repair (*Fig.* 31.2)

The perineurium is the connective tissue condensation around the individual nerve fasciculi, the larger the fasciculus the thicker the layer.

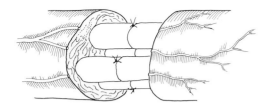

Fig. 31.2. Perineurial or fascicular repair.

With large or mixed nerves where there are a number of fasciculi, accurate alignment of the equivalent ends undoubtedly improves the quality of the result. Within the more distal part of the peripheral nerve, there is less reshuffling of the axons. With more accurate fascicular orientation more peripheral divisions of the nerves should, and usually do, provide the best results following repair. More proximally each fasciculus contains a mixture of components and with even the most accurate reapposition results may be inadequate as it is impossible to align individual axons.

The number of sutures used in fascicular repair must be a balance between accurate alignment and increase in the amount of foreign material introduced.

Perineurial repair is difficult without magnification. Initially, the epineurium is stripped off for about 1 cm as it is believed that this layer is primarily responsible for connective tissue proliferation, and this stripping can be aided by blowing up this outer layer using saline injected via a blunt-ended needle. A cuff of this tissue is resected and allowed to retract, and the fasciculi can then be separated using microscissors and knives. It is best to divide these cleanly at different levels to prevent superimposition of the joins. Sutures (10/0 Ethicon) are placed within the connective tissue layer to prevent damage to the axons. Usually one suture per fasciculus is required but in some mixed nerves, such as the median, which has about 30 fasciculi, only the larger ones may be aligned.

Alternative techniques using epineurial–perineur-

ial sutures can provide the advantages of both methods. The epineurium is picked up accurately, the suture passed more deeply between the fasciculi picking up equivalent ends and not all of these need to be tied since they act as guides.

NERVE GRAFTS

In secondary nerve repair or where there has been a traumatic deficit, or after resection of the ends including neuromas, there may be a deficit which cannot be closed without tension. In this situation a nerve graft is indicated.

In larger nerves, several cables of donor nerve are required, usually from the sural, and these are taken slightly longer than the deficit, to allow for contraction. The epineurium is transected from both ends of the nerve to be repaired. In the nerve graft the epineurium is left intact, partly for placement of sutures but also because the vascular network here needs to pick up a new blood supply from the bed.

Vascularized Nerve Grafts

Long nerve grafts, over 8 cm, and grafts placed in poor vascular beds which are heavily scarred function badly and for this reason techniques are being developed to vascularize nerves using reversed short saphenous vein/sural nerves. This technique is especially indicated where there is an associated vascular deficit such as in the radial or ulnar artery in the forearm.

MICROVASCULAR REPAIR

The technique of learning microvascular anastomosis must be acquired in the laboratory. Although some expertise can be obtained by practising on pieces of rubber glove, silicone tubing or leaves, it is only on blood vessels that the technique may be perfected. Although there is some value in practising on vessels in cadavers or dead animals, it is only in those vessels with blood flow that a real judgement of anastomotic success can be applied. This is usually carried out on animals, such as rats or rabbits, although attempts are being made to substitute the placenta by re-establishing its circulation with blood or fluid.

With nerve repair accurate placement of sutures is required but the only assessment is in the long term, and even then other factors such as infection, haematoma or a poor vascular bed may influence the result.

In microvascular anastomosis poor technique will restrict or terminate blood flow; a single incorrect suture may produce thrombosis at the anastomotic site. The beam splitter enables the assistant to pass judgement on suture placement, tension and numbers required. After removal of the clamps any leaks are immediately apparent.

Microvascular Anastomosis (*Fig.* 31.3)

It is necessary to resect damaged vessels back until they look normal; this pathology may have been due to trauma, irradiation or atherosclerosis. The vessel

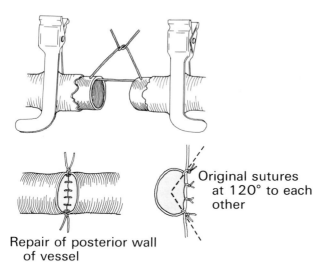

Repair of posterior wall
of vessel

Fig. 31.3. End-to-end anastomosis of small blood vessel using microsurgical techniques.

can then be cleanly resected, either with a vessel cutter or sharp micro-scissors. In the case of the proximal end of the artery, demonstration that a free flow of blood occurs is advisable. If there is vessel disparity, the smaller vessel may be cut obliquely to increase the circumference of the lumen.

The ends of the vessels to be anastomosed are then clamped with non-crushing micro-clamps, which are either individual or special approximating clamps. The adventitia on the outside of the vessels (and which contributes to thrombosis) is cleaned off the ends using micro-scissors and jeweller's forceps. With an artery it is often possible to pull a sleeve of adventitia over the end and then transect it. The adventitia then retracts beyond the media and intima.

The adventitial resection should be for at least 2–3 mm. The vessels often go into spasm and the ends of a micro-dilator can then be inserted into the lumen and allowed to separate without force. The tips of these dilators are machined smooth to minimize intimal damage and should be the only instruments placed on the inside of the vessels. Blood or clots are then washed out using a fine cannula and heparinized saline, and after both vessel ends are so treated they are approximated. Coloured background is placed behind the vessels, to provide contast and to keep blood out of the lumen.

End-to-end Anastomosis

Sutures, usually 9/0 or 10/0 non-absorbable monofilament, are used. The first suture is applied to the posterior wall passing through the media and intima

taking a small bite of the latter. As a separate bite, the suture is then passed through the open end of the other vessel through the intima and then through the equivalent spot on the media. Symmetry is all important. The suture is then tied, more snugly with an artery than with a vein or a nerve. A surgeon's knot is used with the double throw placed squarely so that there is less likelihood of it breaking. The end of this first suture is left long to allow it to be held by forceps.

A second suture is then placed at 120° to the first on the posterior wall. When this is tied the opening on the front of the vessel tends to pout and it is easier to check from the intimal aspect the effect of the sutures placed on the posterior wall. The second suture is also left long so these ends may be grasped and the vessel rotated by the assistant. The repair of the posterior wall is then completed by two or three more sutures depending on the size and type of the vessel. Veins require fewer sutures as the blood pressure is lower.

The long stay sutures are released and inspection again made of the lumen to make sure the initial sutures have not accidentally picked up the anterior wall. A suture is then placed in the front of the vessel at 120° to the first suture and each of the remaining sections then separately sutured. During suturing it is often necessary to irrigate with heparinized saline to remove blood seeping into the vessel ends. Placement of the final sutures may be difficult for when these are tied it may be impossible to visualize the lumen adequately and to ensure that the posterior wall has not been picked up by the needle. A method which avoids this is to pass several sutures through the appropriate layers and divide them, leaving the ends long. A final inspection of the lumen is then carried out with irrigation and these remaining sutures are then tied.

After anastomosis of vein and artery is complete the clamps are removed; venous clamps are usually released before the arterial, and distal before the proximal arterial clamp. Blood should then be seen to cross the anastomosis. Usually there is some seepage of blood in the gaps between the sutures which should stop, but if there is free bleeding further sutures may be necessary.

Should the vessels go into spasm, lignocaine or Praxilene Forte (naftidrofuryl) is squirted on and a warm, moist pack placed over the anastomosis for a few minutes. Assessment of flow can then be made either clinically by obvious perfusion of the replant or flap or by direct vision. The Ackland test is useful. The tips of two micro-forceps are placed beyond the anastomosis occluding the lumen. The forceps downstream are then used to milk the blood out of the lumen so a segment of vessel between the two forceps is collapsed. The forceps adjacent to the anastomosis are then released and blood flow into the collapsed segment indicates a patent anastomosis (*Fig.* 31.4).

The technique for artery and vein anastomosis is

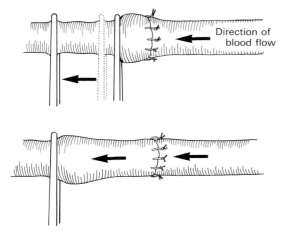

Direction of blood flow

Fig. 31.4. Ackland patency test following microvascular anastomosis.

essentially the same although fewer sutures are required for the vein. Vein walls may be very thin and slightly larger bites may be required, and sutures are tied less tightly. It may be of help with thin-walled veins to float the vessel ends in fluid which helps to separate the walls.

End-to-side Anastomosis

One of the problems of end-to-end anastomosis is the tendency for the vessel to go into spasm occluding the lumen. In a vessel which is partially divided the opening tends to retract which enhances blood flow, a situation well known clinically where a completely transected vessel usually stops bleeding, whereas a vessel which has been nicked tends to bleed profusely.

Advantage is taken of this observation by anastomosing the donor artery in, for example, a free flap into the side of the recipient artery.

The end of the donor vessel and a section of the side of the recipient vessel are prepared by removing adventitia. An appropriate sized stoma comparable to the lumen of the donor artery is made either by a clean longitudinal cut or by picking up the media and intima with forceps and cutting this with curved sharp scissors, although this latter manoeuvre may be difficult. The anastomosis is then carried out, the posterior wall first. It is not usually possible to rotate the vessel by this method so technically this T anastomosis can be more difficult to accomplish although undoubtedly there is an improved patency rate.

REPLANTATION

The first indications for microvascular surgery were for replantation of digits, limbs, scalps or ears although the majority are digital replantations. Amputation may be partial or complete.

In partial amputation the blood supply has been interrupted and necrosis of the end will occur unless this supply is re-established. The connection remaining may be tendon or even a small skin bridge, and the letter may contain valuable veins. If the connection is badly crushed, then débridement may require excision producing a complete amputation.

Complete amputation may be a clean-cut guillotine-type amputation or associated with crushing or avulsion or a combination of these factors.

Treatment of the Severed Part

The amputated part should be placed in an isotonic saline soaked sterile gauze, which may be placed in a plastic bag which is then placed into an outer plastic bag containing ice from a domestic refrigerator. On no account should the digit be allowed to freeze as ice particles will form and the success rate will fall. The bag should not, therefore, be placed in a thermos or insulated box.

If revascularization is achieved within 8 hours' cold ischaemia time, the success rate is as high as 90 per cent, depending on the type of amputation. Particularly successful with guillotine amputations, this success rate falls rapidly after this time. For this reason prior warning to the replantation centre and a two-team approach can improve results. One team identifies the structures on the amputated part and excises traumatized tissue and the other team works in a similar way on the stump.

Indications for Replantation Surgery

Not every patient is suitable for surgery and consideration has to be given to the type and level of the injury. Multiplicity of digital loss, the dominance of the hand, social factors, job requirement, age and the likelihood of long-term use all need careful thought. Absolute indications for replantation are where there is loss of more than one finger, a thumb or whole hand amputation. The presence of severe crushing may be a contra-indication depending on how much shortening is necessary to obtain apposition of undamaged vessels, although vein grafts can reduce the lengths needing resection. Undoubtedly avulsion causes skip lesions in the vessels and reduces the success rate but an attempt at replantation could still be indicated in, for example, complete thumb amputation. Single digit replantations, except in children, are usually unrewarding, often leading to stiff fingers, and the patient ultimately may request the offending digit to be removed.

Clean-cut amputations from distal palm up to distal forearm are very rewarding when replanted. There is relatively little muscle bulk here and, therefore, more tolerance to ischaemia. Repairs are mainly of tendons rather than muscle and return of sensation to fingers and thumb is usually very adequate.

More proximal amputations involve an increasing amount of muscle bulk in the specimen and with it, after circulation has been restored, a definite risk of renal failure with distribution of toxins into the general circulation. In upper arm amputations vessels are large and relatively easy to repair. Nerve repair is, however, disappointing at this level, not only because of the long delay before nerve regeneration reaches the hand but also due to the intermixing of sensory and motor modalities at a higher level. Following replantation at a proximal level on the upper limb some movement of flexion and extension of the elbow may be achieved with some poor protective sensation in the hand, but little else can be expected. In China better functional results have been achieved by shortening the upper arm but this technique is probably unacceptable in the Western world.

Technique

Débridement

The full extent of the injury may only be perceived under magnification. There may be damage at several levels making revascularization, even with the aid of vein grafts, unlikely, and a decision may be made at this late stage not to proceed. Trimming back the vessels until they look normal is essential, and skin-releasing incisions on the side and back may be required to identify arteries and veins.

Bony Fixation

This may be achieved by wires, plates or pins, and may be done after trimming but shortening digits should be restricted to 2 cm.

Tendon and Muscle Repair

Those structures lying deep to the vessels should be repaired, since after the circulation is restored great difficulty may be had in achieving this without damaging the reconstructed vessels. Accurate repair should be carried out in the primary situation as secondary repair is more hazardous.

Nerve Repair

This is usually carried out prior to vessel repair by the techniques described earlier (p. 420).

Restoring Circulation

The more distal the amputation of a digit the more difficult it is to find suitable veins, in which case arterial repair is carried out first, clamps released and veins allowed to dilate up to enable them to be visualized. In amputation of finger tips, arterial anastomosis alone may be sufficient if leeches are used or the patient heparinized. After 48 hours the microcirculation is usually restored.

However, both arteries and veins are usually repaired to prevent congestion, more veins being anastomosed than arteries. Thus if both digital arteries are repaired, the aim should be to reanastomose three veins. If there is a deficit a vein graft, reversed in the case of the artery, needs to be interposed to produce end-to-end anastomosis. In the case of the thumb, opportunity may be taken for a long vein graft to be attached and carried down to anastomose end to side onto the radial artery.

Skin

Suturing should be achieved without tension, allowing for postoperative swelling. Skin grafts may be required or even cross finger flaps from adjacent undamaged fingers.

Postoperative Care

Clinical observation is satisfactory but monitoring may be of help to assess the circulation and to compare, for example, the temperature of the tip of the replanted digit with equivalent tip of a healthy finger. This may give early indication should the circulation become impaired, when re-exploration is indicated. The use of heparin or other anticoagulants may produce more problems than they solve in the form of haematomas but may be useful in fingertip injuries.

DIGITAL RECONSTRUCTION

The techniques used for replantation may be used in reconstruction. In the hand, loss of thumb or digits may be either congenital or traumatic. In traumatic cases, proximal to the site of amputation, the end of the nerves and tendons are all present, as is the case in congenital amputations secondary to amniotic bands. In transverse metatarsal arrest the digits are missing but the equivalent tendons and nerves are absent.

Reconstruction of these digits may be achieved by transferring a toe or toes to replace the missing digits, either to provide a pinch grip between the reconstructed thumb and remaining fingers or between the thumb and reconstructed finger. In the latter case two toes may be taken up to provide a tripod grip.

Dissection of the Toe

The toe, usually the second, is mobilized, together with its metatarsophalangeal joint and metatarsal. The blood supply is usually from the dorsalis pedis and its first dorsal metatarsal artery. This superficial arterial system is connected via a communicating artery with the plantar arch and occasionally it is necessary to anastomose this vessel rather than the dorsalis pedis.

A superficial drainage vein from the dorsum of the foot is mobilized for venous drainage. The plantar nerve branches in the first and second web space are mobilized to provide sensory reconstruction, flexor and extensor tendons to the second toe are traced back as far proximal as possible prior to division.

On the hand the appropriate vessels, nerves and tendons are exposed and in the case of congenital absence equivalent tendons such as the flexor carpi ulnaris may be used. After separation of the vessels and other structures from the foot the second toe, toes or even big toe are transferred to the hand. After fixing the bone in a suitable position the nerves and tendons are repaired. The dorsalis pedis or plantar artery is anastomosed either to the palmar arch or the radial or ulnar artery, the vein is anastomosed to a dorsal vein on the hand. After release of the micro-clamps circulation is restored.

If a big toe is used, to reduce donor skin deficit a wrap around flap has been devised taking the tissue off the tip and lateral aspect of the toe. The donor deficit is then skin grafted. The flap is mobilized with its vessel and nerve supply and is transferred to the hand where the flap is wrapped around a bone graft. As the bone is not vascularized primarily there is an increased tendency for bone absorption.

FREE SKIN FLAP TRANSFERS

Skin grafts will take where there is a vascularized bed. Where there is no such bed, for example following injury where tendons are exposed without para-tendon or bone without periosteum or an exposed joint, alternatives are required to maintain the viability of these structures.

Local flaps may be possible or even distant flaps, bringing the limb up to the flap as in a groin flap to cover the dorsum of the hand, or in a cross-leg flap. In both these cases the flap is still nourished by its attached blood supply.

In certain cases such flaps are difficult or impossible to achieve without multiple stages. In the groin flap mentioned above, the skin and subcutaneous fat of the lateral groin can be mobilized, leaving the flap attached by its arterial supply and venous drainage only. The flap remains viable. These vessels may then be divided and transferred to the lower leg, for example to cover exposed bone in a compound injury. The artery to the 'free flap', either the superficial circumflex iliac or epigastric artery, is then anastomosed under the microscope to a suitable undamaged vessel on the lower leg, either the anterior or posterior tibial artery. A superficial draining vein from the groin flap is anastomosed with an equivalent vein in the leg. After removal of the micro-clamps flow is restored, producing vascularized skin and subcutaneous fat to cover the exposed area.

The advantages of such free flaps are clear. It is possible, for example, to resurface a lower tibia in a compound injury in one stage where earlier, using a tube pedicle, five stages and about 6 months in hospital were required. Early cover of exposed bone may also prevent it drying out and dying.

The free groin flap described above was the first such flap to be used. The disadvantage of this particular flap was the variability of its blood supply, a fairly small calibre artery (range 0·8–3 mm) and a short pedicle.

Latissimus Dorsi Flap

Following development of the groin flap, other sites have been explored to obtain more reliable anatomy, longer pedicles and larger vessels. The latissimus dorsi flap is such a vascularized myocutaneous flap, and flaps from this area are used by translocation to aid breast reconstruction after mastectomy. When dissecting the flap an ellipse of skin is marked out, usually aligned parallel to the direction of the muscle, the anterior edge lying about 3 cm anterior to it. The skin is nourished by the thoracodorsal branch of the subscapular artery and the vessels may be traced proximally into the axilla. Distally the artery and vein run just beneath the free border of the muscle, sending perforating vessels into the overlying skin. Providing this segment of muscle is maintained in the flap, a large portion of skin may be taken with only a relatively small amount of muscle. The advantages of this flap are a long pedicle (about 10 cm) and a large diameter artery (2–3 mm). With a smaller skin flap about 10 cm wide by 15 cm it is possible usually to close the donor defect directly, but if a large flap is required the donor area may require skin grafting. The donor skin ellipse may be orientated horizontally producing a better cosmetic result on closure. The disadvantages of this otherwise very reliable flap are its bulk and the need to sacrifice the nerve supply to the latissimus dorsi.

Other flaps have been developed to provide vascularized skin without sacrificing valuable muscle, such as the scapular flap based on the cutaneous scapular artery originating from the circumflex scapular artery. The skin flap is taken just lateral to the scapula and the vessels are traced through the triangular space.

INNERVATED SKIN FLAP TRANSFERS

The free skin flap transfers outlined above do not regain a significant return of sensation. In certain situations such as loss of skin from the heel or weight-bearing area of the foot, attempts should be made to reinnervate the skin otherwise trophic ulceration will occur. In reconstruction of the hand following extensive injuries a 'sensory' flap will help in regaining use, the nerve supply of the free flap being attached to the divided sensory nerve supplying this area.

Dorsalis Pedis or Dorsal Foot Flap

In this flap the skin on the dorsum of the foot is mobilized, together with the dorsalis pedis artery and a superficial vein. This area is supplied by the terminal branches of the peroneal nerve which may be identified and reanastomosed to the appropriate nerve.

The advantage of this flap includes the possibility of incorporating tendons of the extensor digitorum brevis which are then used to reconstruct, for example, extensor tendons on the dorsum of the hand lost after an abrasion injury. This tendon reconstruction can, therefore, be carried out in one stage using vascularized tendons.

The disadvantage of this flap is the rather precarious blood supply to the skin from the dorsalis pedis vessels which is also a rather poor donor site. A smaller but better innervated flap may be taken from the web space between the big toe and the second toe, the skin being innervated by branches from the medial plantar nerve and terminal branches of the peroneal nerve.

Other innervated flaps are now being developed, such as the lateral arm flap innervated by the lateral cutaneous nerve of the arm or the ulnar artery forearm flap, the latter being innervated by the medial cutaneous nerve of the forearm which runs with the basilic vein.

VASCULARIZED BONE GRAFTS

Where there has been a large segment of bone loss or where extensive resection is required, as in lower jaw malignancies, free non-vascularized segments of bone tend to be absorbed or become infected, and this is especially likely to occur after radiotherapy.

Initial attempts at using vascularized bone were carried out with ribs using the intercostal vessels, but the pedicle is very short and potentially hazardous if the posterior intercostal vessels are used. Vascularized ribs may be raised with the latissimus dorsi flap taking the overlying serratus anterior and arterial supply, which is a branch of the thoracodorsal, so that it is possible to provide skin cover as well as vascularized ribs through a composite latissimus dorsi flap.

Radial Forearm Flap

In lower jaw reconstructions bone and skin are often required, as a thin hairless flap which is pliable and taken with a segment of bone. This may often be provided by the radial forearm flap based on the radial artery. A very long vessel pedicle usually enables vascular anastomosis to be carried out well away from the irradiated area, although only part of the radius can be taken so there is a limit to the amount of mandible which can be reconstructed this way. Prior to surgery it should be demonstrated that the circulation of the hand can be maintained by the ulnar artery. An attempt should be made to restore the original circulation by inserting a long vein graft into the radial artery defect.

Deep Circumflex Iliac Artery Flap (*Fig.* 31.5)

Injuries of the lower leg with skin and bone loss are on the increase, occurring especially following motorcycle accidents. Amputation rates of up to 80 per cent have been reported, indicating the difficulty in reconstruction.

For cases where there is bone loss of less than 12 cm the deep circumflex iliac artery flap is probably the flap of choice, giving good blood supply to the overlying skin in addition to using the whole iliac crest in reconstruction.

Dissection of Deep Circumflex Iliac Artery Flap

The artery (1·5–3 mm in diameter) arises from the external iliac artery and the venae comitans which accompany it usually join to form one draining vein which passes either in front of or behind the external iliac artery to drain into the external iliac vein.

Dissection to find the vessels is through the posterior wall of the inguinal canal beneath the fascia transversalis. The vessels are traced laterally: an ascending branch is given off at a variable distance to the anterior superior iliac spine. This vessel does not provide musculocutaneous perforators. As the anterior superior iliac spine is approached anastomosis with the cruciate anastomosis is noted and carefully tied. The deep circumflex iliac vessels pierce the fascia transversalis and transversus abdominis to run under the internal oblique muscle just beneath the rim of the pelvis. The skin supplied by this artery is centred just above the iliac crest and is nourished by musculocutaneous perforators given off as the artery passes adjacent to the inner lip of the iliac crest.

To reduce the bulk of flap only a cuff of external and internal oblique and transversus muscles are required to protect the vessels. The tensor fascia lata can be divided directly off the lower border of the ilium as there is no contribution to the flap's blood supply from this source.

The size of the bone and skin of the flap depends on the defect being reconstructed. To provide stability afterwards the anterior superior iliac spine and attached inguinal ligament are left behind. The ilium can then be taken as necessary using a power saw. After the composite flap (skin/muscle/bone) (*Fig.* 31.6) has been isolated on its vessels it should be left attached for about 1 hour to allow any vessel spasm to be rectified and for the circulation to re-establish itself. Free bleeding should be noted from the cancellous bone.

In this form of microvascular surgery two teams work simultaneously, one raising the flap, the other

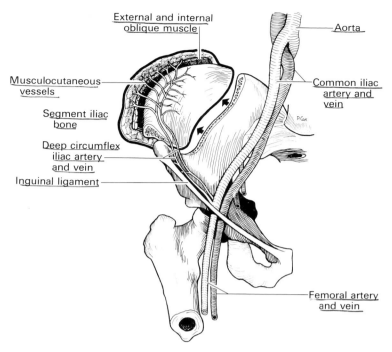

Fig. 31.5. Mobilization and raising of deep circumflex iliac artery flap.

identifying suitable undamaged recipient vessels, usually the anterior or posterior tibial. Bone ends are freshened making certain all devitalized tibia is removed. Bony fixation above and below the defect is provided by external fixators. Normally Hoffmann apparatus is adaptable enough to be positioned to allow access to suitable recipient vessels and to provide visibility for the microvascular anastomosis (*Fig.* 31.6).

Only when these recipient vessels are prepared is the deep circumflex iliac artery flap detached. The bone in the flap is fixed in position and microvascular anastomoses are then carried out, usually end to side for the deep circumflex iliac artery and end to end for the deep circumflex iliac vein, the latter usually to a vena comitans (*Fig.* 31.7). Often a superficial vein is also raised with this flap to anastomose to a superficial vein of the leg which reduces postoperative swelling and makes the flap safer.

In extensively damaged limbs long vein grafts may be required to allow anastomosis to the popliteal artery. In multiple and extensive leg injuries it may be necessary to anastomose the flap vessels to undamaged vessels in the opposite leg (*Fig.* 31.7), the legs being held rigidly together by external fixation. After 5 weeks the vessels may be safely divided and after 6 weeks the skin bridge also. Experience shows that the rate of bony union with full weight bearing is on average 6 months, there being no difference between this, the cross-leg free flap and a flap nourished by vessels on the damaged leg; vascular re-

connection in the former situation occurs via the skin and cancellous bone of the flap to the surrounding equivalent areas and is sufficient to maintain the vascularity of the bone and its capability of behaving like living bone.

Following replacement of a bony defect with vascularized ilium there is an incidence of non-union in one end of the vascularized bone graft. The situation is similar to a double fracture of the tibia which this deep circumflex iliac artery free flap reconstruction clinically reproduces. It is then necessary to freshen up the appropriate end and insert cancellous bone chips. In chronic non-union of the tibia with poor overlying skin the deep circumflex iliac artery flap can be raised taking skin and periosteum only. The ends of the tibia may then be freshened and cancellous bone chips inserted, the area then covered with this vascularized periosteum and skin.

In a successful case of reconstruction of the tibia using vascularized ilium, the living bone graft undergoes remodelling with resorption of the non-stress areas and hypertrophy of the stress lines so that after 2 or 3 years it is often difficult to visualize the original graft.

Following an extended hemimandibulectomy for malignancy the deep circumflex iliac artery flap may be used in reconstruction. The iliac crest is cut to shape and the muscular and tendinous attachments to the iliac crest are then used to reconstruct the temporomandibular joint, and to reattach the temporalis and masseteric muscles.

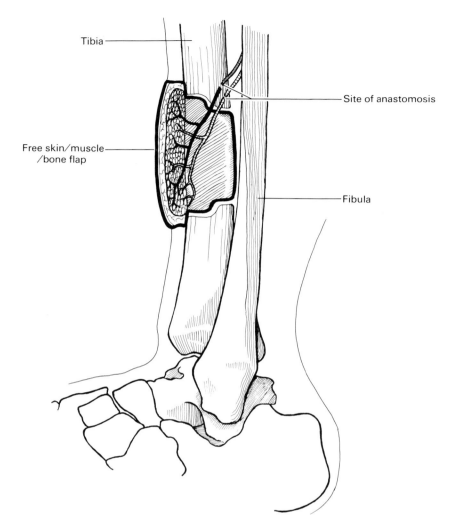

Tibia

Free skin/muscle /bone flap

Site of anastomosis

Fibula

Fig. 31.6. Transplantation of deep circumflex iliac artery flap to bridge tibial defect.

It is possible to use the bone alone in this situation, but the skin in the composite flap may be used to provide cover, especially externally.

Vascularized Fibula

When a bone defect is greater than 12 cm the deep circumflex iliac artery flap is not used for fear of shortening of the limb. This is one of the indications for use of vascularized fibula based on the peroneal artery and veins. Provided about 6 cm of fibula are left at the upper and lower ends, stability is maintained at the ankle and knee joint, and this stability may be enhanced by a screw placed between the lower fibula and tibia.

The nutrient artery to the fibula lies in the middle third so this central segment may be taken alone with the peroneal vessels.

Vascularized shorter segments have been utilized in avascular necrosis of the head of the femur prior to its collapse but a more specific indication is in pseudoarthrosis of the tibia where the fibula may be passed up and down within the shaft of the remaining normal tibia, as ordinary bone grafting techniques in this latter situation have a very high failure rate. Larger segments of fibula have been used in reconstruction of long bone loss in the tibia, femur and humerus. In the forearm where there has been loss of both radius and ulnar bones it has been used to reconstruct a single bone forearm. Unlike the deep circumflex iliac artery flap the fibula does not have the same structural strength and in the lower limb especially some form of extra support is required while the fibula hypertrophies. As indicated previously, this hypertrophy is a function of vascularized bone graft and does not occur with traditional free bone grafts. It is of interest that if the fibular graft fractures, extensive callus is thrown up and this remodelling is often speeded up.

The dissection of the fibula is best carried out by

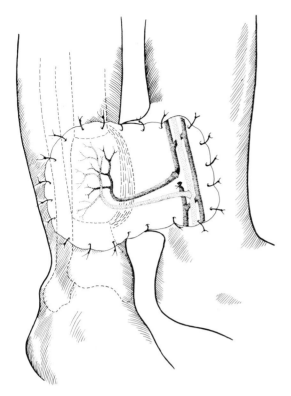

Fig. 31.7. Anastomosis of deep circumflex iliac artery flap to undamaged vessels in opposite leg where there has been extensive leg injury.

a direct lateral incision. There are musculocutaneous branches given off from the peroneal artery, also direct cutaneous branches usually between the soleus and peroneal muscles. It is, therefore, possible to take skin as well as bone if this is wished. Dissection of the fibula at the upper and lower ends is carried out and is divided, usually with a Gigli saw, which allows the isolated segment to be retracted laterally. The interosseous membrane is then identified and carefully released, commencing at the lower end. The peroneal vessels lie just behind this and should be divided and tied at the lower end. The fibula with a small cuff of muscle on the medial side can then be dissected free. The peroneal artery and veins are then traced providing a pedicle of about 5 cm.

If a short segment only of fibula is required this pedicle can be lengthened by subperiosteal dissection of the fibula at the upper end and excess bone removed, maintaining carefully undisturbed the site of the nutrient artery. An extra advantage is that there is now an additional cuff of vascularized periosteum which may be draped around the bone end and may help with final bony union.

The Omentum

It has been known for a considerable time that the omentum may be mobilized by dividing one or other gastro-epiploic vessels and then lengthened by dividing some of the interconnecting vessels but preserving the peripheral arcade. This pedicle flap which is still attached by one of the gastro-epiploic vessels can be brought up subcutaneously on to the chest wall to reconstruct, for example, an area of radionecrosis. Skin grafts can then be applied and these take well on the surface of the omentum.

There are certain areas of the body where such a pedicle flap cannot reach, but the omentum may then be transplanted for microvascular reconstruction. In extensive scalp loss where there is exposed bone denuded of periosteum the area can be covered using omentum, which tends to mould over the area required. Anastomoses can then be carried out between the gastro-epiploic vessels and the superficial temporal vessels although vein grafts may be required to provide anastomosis to the larger facial vessels. The gastro-epiploic artery diameter is a good size, at least 2–3 mm. The veins, however, are very friable and require careful handling.

Another indication for the use of vascularized omentum is in cases of extensive fat atrophy, as in Romberg's disease where the fat on one side of the face may be lost. The omentum may be separated into various fingers and passed subcutaneously onto the forehead, around the eyes and over the cheek and mandible. The omentum is then vascularized.

Previous surgery or history of pelvic inflammation or obesity may make it impossible to use the omentum.

Vascularized Muscles

Using microneurovascular anastomosis it is possible to transfer muscles as free vascularized grafts and expect return of motor function. There are two main indications. Benefit has been achieved after Volkmann's contracture where there has been extensive necrosis and subsequent fibrosis of the flexor muscles of the forearm. The second indication is in the management of facial paralysis.

Both pectoralis major and latissimus dorsi muscles have been used in the forearm to try and re-establish mass flexor movements of the fingers. If the blood supply of the forearm has been partially disrupted this can be repaired at the same time, using in the case of latissimus dorsi the distal end of the thoracodorsal vessels.

In facial paralysis cross-facial nerve grafting has been attempted. Nerve grafts are taken, connecting some of the more distal branches of the normal side which may be sacrificed with minimal functional loss due to interconnection. The graft or grafts are then anastomosed on the paralysed side to the distal ends of the facial nerve. During the long delay before nerve regeneration occurs down these long grafts the facial muscles atrophy and the results have been rather disappointing. This technique may be carried out in two stages, the nerve anastomosis on the paralysed side being carried out after the axons have grown across. To reduce this problem of muscle atrophy, vascularized muscle grafts can be carried out as a secondary procedure using either the extensor digitorum brevis muscle of the foot or the gracilis muscle. The transplanted muscle therefore undergoes earlier reinnervation and does not undergo such excessive degeneration although it seems some allowance should be made for this and a bulkier muscle preferably used.

Vascularized Tendons

As indicated earlier, it is possible to take the dorsalis pedis flap with tendons of extensor digitorum brevis and maintain their blood supply. Results are very encouraging, for example in abrasion injuries to the back of the hand where there is loss of both skin and tendons.

Tendon-like structures such as the external oblique aponeurosis are also used and incorporated in a groin flap. The strip of aponeurosis taken is rolled up to reproduce the tendon, for example the Achilles tendon, in its reconstruction after skin and tendon loss.

Jejunum

In patients with hypopharyngeal carcinoma who have had pharyngolaryngectomy with partial or complete resection of the cervical oesophagus, vascularized jejunum can be considered to restore continuity.

Reconstruction of the upper pharyngeal end is fraught with complications using traditional methods such as mobilizing the stomach or colon and elevating them through the chest or subcutaneously. Anastomotic breakdown often occurs at this upper end at the limit of the vascular supply. To reduce the incidence of this complication, anastomosis may be undertaken between the colonic or gastric vessels, preferably with non-irradiated vessels in the neck. This technique may also be used in reconstruction after excision of the thoracic oesophagus.

In reconstruction using microvascular anastomosis sections of jejunum are taken isolating a single branch of the superior mesenteric artery and vein, as these vessel diameters match well with the superior thyroid artery and external jugular vein. After resection, jejunal oesophageal reanastomosis is carried out in the neck, the lower end first, either with sutures or a stapling gun. By the latter technique the lower anastomosis can be carried out at an intrathoracic level and the upper jejunal anastomosis to the oropharynx is then fairly easily accomplished. After the microvascular anastomoses are carried out peristalsis may return almost at once; it is important to ensure that the jejunum is placed isoperistaltically or there may be constant regurgitation of mucus.

The use of vascularized jejunum allows a single-stage reconstruction and although it requires resection of a section of the bowel, there is far less dissection and morbidity associated with this than with the usual alternatives, and should the vascular anastomoses fail, the consequences are not nearly so catastrophic. However, the success rate world wide is high and as an added bonus it is also possible for the patients to develop oeosophageal speech.

AUTOTRANSPLANTATION OF THE TESTIS
(*Fig.* 31.8)

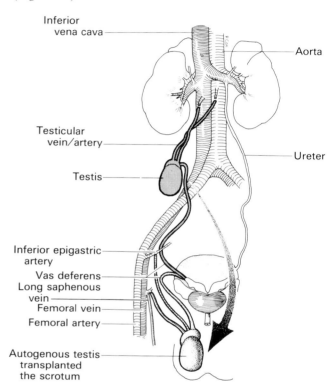

Fig. 31.8. Autotransplantation of the testis.

In up to 5 per cent of cryptorchid testes the testicles are so high that it is necessary to divide the spermatic vessels to allow the testis to be relocated in the scrotum. The blood supply then consists only of collaterals from the vas deferens and cremasteric muscle, with a significant incidence of testicular atrophy. In bilateral cases an attempt should usually be made on one side as it is a relatively simple procedure. If this fails and because of the risk of malignancy, the other testis will be considered for removal. However, the blood supply to the testis can be enhanced by microvascular techniques with prospects of a higher success rate of normal testicular development.

To obtain this renewed blood supply to the testis the testicular vessels are identified close to their origin to achieve as long a pedicle as possible. After division microvascular anastomosis is then carried out. The recipient vessels are usually the inferior epigastric and a superficial vein which have been prepared prior to division of the testicular vessels. This is usually achieved using end-to-side anastomosis for the testicular artery to the inferior epigastric artery and end to end for the testicular vein to a more superficial vein.

Preservation of the stroma of the testis has been demonstrated experimentally using this microvascular anastomosis by the ability to regain spermatogenesis. The operation is, however, best done before 6 years of age. In older patients, even if there is a failure of spermatogenesis, testosterone levels in a successful case can be maintained, thus making it unnecessary for the patients to have testosterone implants indefinitely. In these older patients at a later stage there may still be an increased risk from malignancy and testicular biopsies may be indicated.

CONCLUSIONS

This résumé of microvascular procedures is by no means exhaustive and new indications and methods are being developed. Undoubtedly the long operations and specialized training are very demanding but the operations usually are performed as single-stage techniques reducing hospital stay and allowing earlier mobilization.

The best results are achieved using a team approach and if a flap, for example, develops congestion or becomes ischaemic, then re-exploration of the anastomosis must be carried out at once. This requires some depth of skilled surgical personnel cover and with it the implication that these cases are best undertaken in an appropriate unit.

Urogenital and Adrenal Glands

Chapter thirty-two

The Kidney and Ureter

C. A. C. Charlton

INTRODUCTION

This is an exciting period in the development of the surgery of the kidney and ureter; the change occurring is such that the conventional approach of today's established surgeon is being displaced by the endoscopically trained surgeon.

In the past 5 years, there has occurred a revolution in the surgery of renal and ureteric calculus disease, due to the development of a series of instruments which permits access to the lumen of the upper urinary tract by means of a puncture hole in the loin, or alternatively to the ureter through the urethra; and this, in combination with a variety of stone disintegrating techniques, applied by means of a probe placed in contact with the calculus, is likely to displace the operative approach to stones through conventional incisions by the end of this decade.

Furthermore, it is probable that these modern techniques for stone removal will in turn be superseded by the method of extracorporeal lithotripsy which by the end of the century will be the method of choice for the elimination of stones in the kidney and upper half of the ureter.

Nevertheless, there will always remain the need for the surgeon to approach the kidney and ureter employing the scalpel, and in this chapter the conventional operative approach is described first and so to the development of instrumental surgery and finally, where appropriate, the development of 'non-invasive' surgery.

INCISIONS AND APPROACH TO THE KIDNEY

The surgical approach to the kidneys is conditioned by their position as retroperitoneal structures, with their upper poles protected in part by the lower ribs, and the fact that the artery and vein (occasionally multiple) are situated high up at the back of the abdominal cavity. Surrounding the perinephric fat is Gerota's fascia which resembles a sac with the open end facing inferiorly (towards the bony pelvis).

There are many incisions used for approaching the kidney, and the decision as to which one is employed depends on the pathological process which has determined the need for operation. Since the kidney is a retroperitoneal structure, it is preferable if the surgical procedure remains exclusively located to that compartment, i.e. is extrapleural and extraperitoneal. The advantages of not opening the pleural cavity are that it diminishes the risk of postoperative atelectasis and pneumonia, the development of pleural effusions or pneumothorax, and the possible need for underwater seals and drains. Similarly, opening the peritoneal cavity is more likely to be followed by intestinal ileus, gastric dilatation and the development of peritoneal adhesions than if the surgical manoeuvres are wholly extraperitoneal. Obviously, the need for a nasogastric tube and intravenous feeding is more likely in these circumstances.

However, good access is an important maxim in safe surgery and if it is apparent that the operation would be difficult by confining the operative field to the retroperitoneal space, as might occur with a large upper pole tumour, then there should be no hesitation in opening the pleural and peritoneal cavities.

With these principles in mind, the majority of kidney operations undertaken by the author are by the lumbar route along the line of the 12th rib. If, due to unforeseen circumstances, the access obtained proves unsatisfactory, the incision is extended dorsally into the dorsolumbar approach of Nagamatsu (1950). In the case of large tumours in which it may be expected to find involvement of abdominal viscera (e.g. the spleen or colon) or the diaphragm, or when access to the renal blood vessels from behind can be predicted to be difficult, then a thoraco-abdominal approach along the interspace between the 9th and 10th ribs is employed. Finally, in a selected group, namely thin patients in whom exposure of the renal pelvis is the only consideration, the lumbotomy incision (which is a vertical paravertebral one) is preferred since it does not involve division of the abdominal wall muscles, and so reduces postoperative pain.

Twelfth Rib Resection Incision (*Fig.* 32.1)

Correct positioning of the patient on the operating table is important. The lateral decubitus position is adopted, the patient being so placed that the space between the iliac crest and the 12th rib on the non-operative side is at the level of the 'break' in the table. Two table supports are used along the back of the patient, one at the level of the scapula and the lower one supports the ischial tuberosity. A further support for the forearm of the uppermost arm is positioned, such that the humerus is at right angles to the line of the patient's torso (i.e. the shoulder is flexed to 90°), and the elbow is flexed to 90°. The lower leg is slightly flexed, and the uppermost one

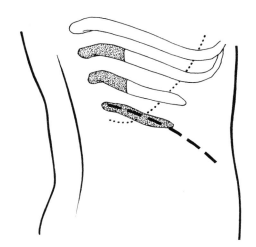

Fig. 32.1. Exposure of kidney via loin incision incorporating resection of the 12th rib. Note the reflexion of the pleura.

is straight. Pillows or Sorbo pads are placed between the knees and ankles of the two limbs.

The table is then tilted laterally towards the surgeon (who is standing facing the patient's back) so causing the patient to lean backwards against the supports which places him or her in a steady and stable position. The table is now 'broken' so that the dip of the patient's waist (on the side to be operated on) is eliminated or straightened out. If the surgeon feels that the patient's position is not stable, a strap encircling the table and the patient's pelvis can be applied at this juncture.

The incision is made along the line of the 12th rib from the angle (i.e. posterior axillary line) to the lateral edge of the rectus sheath. The underlying muscles (i.e. those covering that part of the rib exposed by the incision) are divided. The intercostal muscles attached to the upper border of this part of the rib are detached. Similarly, by keeping the knife blade close to the lower edge of the 12th rib, the attached muscles are divided, avoiding the subcostal blood vessels and nerve. The structures attached to the tip of the rib are also divided, and so the anterior part of the rib (the length of this varies with the length of the 12th rib) is free of any attachments. This protruding portion of the rib is now cut with the costotome. The pleura may now come into view but, with this relatively anteriorly placed incision, should not intrude into the operating field. By introducing a finger into the anterior part of the space made by removing the rib, it is a simple matter to displace the peritoneum anteriorly, by stripping it off the undersurface of the transversus abdominis muscle. Consequently, the external and internal oblique muscles, and the transversus abdominis can be divided without inadvertently opening the peritoneum. At this juncture a self-retaining retractor can be introduced or this can be reserved until the kidney has been mobilized.

Returning to the posterior aspect of the wound, Gerota's fascia is incised for 8 cm or so, as is the underlying perinephric fat. The anterior flap of fat is grasped by a Duval's forceps and the separation of the fat from the kidney capsule is undertaken, preferably with scissors. The capsule should not be breeched since this leads to bleeding.

Subcapsular dissection is to be deprecated, not only because of bleeding, but it also makes access to the renal blood vessels difficult, and, furthermore, in some operations (e.g. partial nephrectomy and nephrolithotomy) the capsule is useful for closing incisions made in the renal cortex. In addition, any subsequent operation on the kidney is made difficult by the absence of the capsule. In the case of reoperation, it may be time consuming, difficult and tedious to aim at preserving the capsule intact, since separation of the perinephric fat and fibrous tissue from the underlying kidney involves sharp dissection, but the surgeon will be rewarded by the resulting decrease in blood loss and improved view which results. When the perinephric tissues are directly adherent to the renal cortex, operating on a kidney subsequently is hazardous, since the dividing line is not apparent and brisk bleeding ensues from incising the renal parenchyma.

Mobilization of the upper pole should also be undertaken with scissors so as to separate the suprarenal from the kidney. This manoeuvre allows the kidney a considerable increase in movement, and it can then be gently retracted downwards into the wound. At this juncture, it is relatively easy to feel the renal artery. In many kidney operations it is desirable to identify the renal artery and dissect it free so that, if at any time bleeding becomes troublesome, a bulldog clamp or digital pressure can be accurately and rapidly applied. By drawing the upper pole of the kidney up towards the surface of the wound, the artery will be found in the angle between the medial aspect of the upper pole and the posterior abdominal wall. Dividing the sympathetic fibres and fascial layers will expose the artery.

Closure of the wound is by interrupted chromic catgut sutures, which pass though all the muscle layers of the abdominal wall, but which are left untied until all the sutures have been placed along the length of the wound. Once all these have been inserted, the 'break' in the table is closed, and the sutures are tied. The fascia overlying the external oblique muscle is closed with a continuous catgut suture.

Dorsolumbar Approach (Nagamatsu) (*Fig. 32.2*)

This approach is used if it is not possible to obtain adequate access to the upper pole of the kidney or the renal blood vessels by the technique described above. It is a relatively simple matter to adapt the 12th rib resection to the osteoblastic flap technique of Nagamatsu by extending the incision backwards along the length of the 12th rib, to the lateral border

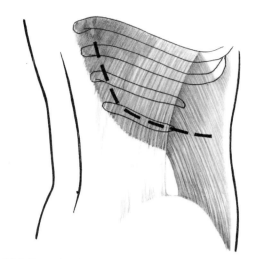

Fig. 32.2. Dorsolumbar approach to the kidney (Nagamatsu).

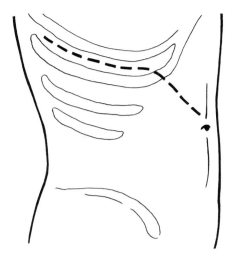

Fig. 32.3. Thoraco-abdominal approach to the right kidney.

of the sacrospinalis group of muscles. The incision is then taken through a right-angle turn to run parallel to the edge of the paravertebral muscles across the 11th and 10th ribs dividing the underlying latissimus dorsi muscle. Some 4 cm of the 10th and 11th ribs are exposed and the muscles attached to the upper and lower borders of these ribs are detached. The remainder of the 12th rib is removed, and some 2 cm of the 10th and 11th ribs are excised with care, so as to preserve the integrity of the pleura. The ligaments tethering the remaining stump of the 12th rib to the transverse process of the first lumbar vertebra (lumbocostal and lateral arcuate) are divided, and the resulting flap is turned up and the large Finochetto retractor can be introduced into the wound. Mobilization of the kidney then proceeds in the manner previously described.

The Thoraco-abdominal Incision

This approach is reserved for extensive malignant disease of the kidney, when it seems likely that the spleen, tail of the pancreas, colon, diaphragm or liver are likely to be involved. The major advantage of such an incision is that with the pleural and peritoneal cavities opened, it is easier to assess the extent of the spread of the tumour, and to remove adjacent involved structures. In addition, for those surgeons who believe in the value of excision of diseased lymph nodes, this incision offers an excellent operative field. Furthermore, rapid access to the aorta or inferior vena cava is possible if troublesome haemorrhage ensues.

The patient is positioned in a semi-recumbent position, with sandbags placed under the scapula and the buttocks so that the patient leans at 25° to the horizontal. The incision extends from the anterior axillary line along the interspace between the 9th and 10th ribs across the costal margin to the level of the umbilicus (*Fig.* 32.3). The intercostal muscles attached to

the upper border of the 10th rib are divided, as are the costal cartilage and the abdominal wall muscles (*Fig.* 32.4). The pleura, peripheral part of the diaphragm and peritoneum are opened in the same line

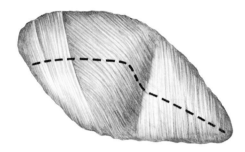

Fig. 32.4. Thoraco-abdominal approach to the right kidney. The skin and subcutaneous fascia have been divided and the abdominal and lateral muscles are incised.

(*Fig.* 32.5), and a large retractor is introduced into the wound. On either side, the colon is mobilized by incising the peritoneum on the lateral aspect. On the right side, the duodenum is reflected medially by Kocher's manoeuvre of incising the posterior layer of the peritoneum along the lateral aspect of the second part of the duodenum. On the left side, the attachments of the splenic flexure of the colon (the

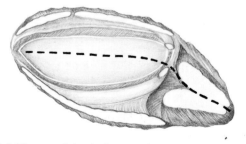

Fig. 32.5. Thoraco-abdominal approach to the kidney. The pleural cavity and the peritoneal cavity have been opened.

phrenico-colic ligaments) are divided. By these manoeuvres, the kidneys and the renal blood vessels are exposed.

The Lumbotomy Incision

The main advantage of this approach is that the large muscles of the abdominal wall (the transversus and oblique muscles) are not cut and so pain in the post-operative period is considerably reduced. However, it has to be admitted that access to the anteromedial aspect of the kidney can be difficult. Consequently the author reserves this incision for simple pyelolitho-tomies.

The patient lies on the non-operative side with the waist at the level of the 'break' in the table. The patient is rolled forwards away from the surgeon, with the lowermost leg flexed at the hip and knee and the uppermost leg stretched out. A sandbag is firmly placed up against the abdomen, so pushing the viscera against the posterior abdominal wall. The shoulder of the uppermost arm is rolled forward and flexed to 90°, as is the elbow. The patient may be secured to the table by encircling the pelvis and table with a strap.

The incision is made along a line 2·5 cm lateral to the edge of the paravertebral muscles extending from the iliac crest to the level of the 12th rib. The underlying latissimus dorsi and serratus posterior inferior are divided in the line of the incision. A 2-cm segment of the 12th rib is removed, as described in the dorsolumbar approach. In the centre of the wound, running in a longitudinal direction, from the 12th rib to the iliac crest, is seen the fused margin of the three layers of lumbar fascia which enclose the sacrospinalis muscle. From the front edge of this conjoint lamellae of lumbar fascia arise the internal oblique and transversus abdominis muscles. Incising the fascia along this line leads directly into the retro-peritoneal space. An opening is made in Gerota's fascia, and the kidney displaced forwards and the posterior surface of the kidney and pelvis exposed by dissecting off the perinephric fat.

A further advantage of the lumbotomy incision is that if it is intended to operate on both kidneys in one session (e.g. bilateral nephrectomy as a prelude to renal transplantation, or for bilateral renal pelvic stones), this is possible by positioning the patient prone, i.e. face down on the table, and breaking it so as to put the patient in the 'jack-knife' position.

RENAL SURGERY FOR CALCULUS DISEASE

One of the main objectives of urological practice is the preservation of renal function, and in the last analysis this is related to the number of surviving nephrons. Nephrons may be damaged or destroyed by infection or obstruction (and of course by malignant disease). Stones which are causing obstruction,

whether to the whole or part of a kidney, will need removing, and so will those which are the cause of recurrent pyelonephritis (i.e. a systemic illness with loin pain). On the other hand, recurring bacteriuria in the absence of pyelonephritis does not necessarily demand the same strict adherence to the principle of elimination of calculous material from the urinary tract.

In planning surgery for stone disease, a guiding principle is that relief of obstruction is a primary requirement. Hence if one kidney is obstructed by a stone at the pelvi-ureteric junction, while the other has a staghorn calculus in the lower half of the kidney which appears to be functioning reasonably well, then a pyelolithotomy on the first kidney should take precedence over surgery for the staghorn calculus.

Prior to any form of renal surgery, an intravenous urogram (IVU) is essential. It will depict the position, shape, size and to some extent the function of the kidneys. An IVU can be used for comparing the function of one kidney with its fellow, but should not be used to assess overall renal function, since such variables as dehydration, size of the bolus of the dye given and its concentration, and technical radiological factors all determine the quality of the pictures which may (if due allowances are not made for these many factors) give a false impression of renal function. Other tests of renal function such as blood urea and serum creatinine with associated electrolyte levels should be done, and a measurement of glomerular filtration rate (by creatinine clearance) is indicated. The haemoglobin level should always be known, and it is advisable to cross-match blood for transfusion purposes. Urine cultures and appropriate treatment are indicated. The various metabolic investigations customary in patients with calculus disease are best undertaken on an outpatient basis, since the urinary calcium levels for an individual leading a normal active life are very different to those obtained in the same patient recumbent in bed and taking a hospital diet.

Pyelolithotomy

Removal of a calculus from the renal pelvis is most commonly undertaken by the lumbar approach, using the 12th rib resection previously described. In a thin patient, in whom there is a reasonable distance (15 cm or so) between the iliac crest and the lower border of the 12th rib (at the lateral edge of the paravertebral muscles), the lumbotomy incision has much to recommend it. This approach has been described earlier in this chapter. Routine mobilization of the kidney is undertaken, so making it possible to lift the kidney 'out' of the wound. It is an advantage to envelop the kidney in a length of Netelast (size B) gauze elastic bandage which provides an atraumatic sling held by the assistant, and prevents bruising from the handling of the kidney which often results from the fingers acting as forceps or tongs in trying to grasp the slippery organ. If the renal pelvis is intrarenal and particularly if it is not dilated, the extended sinus approach of Gil-Vernet (1965) is recommended. A pair of scissors is inserted into the renal sinus and a small curved retractor (the cross-section of which is C shaped) is then so positioned that the blood vessels coursing over the pelvis are lifted free with the renal parenchyma from the renal pelvis proper. This plane is bloodless and leads to the exposure of the intrarenal part of the renal pelvis. The renal pelvis is incised vertically between 4/0 chromic catgut stay sutures and the stone removed. A bougie is passed down the ureter, to ensure that no fragments are occluding the lumen, which would encourage a postoperative urinary fistula. Closure of the pelvis is with interrupted 4/0 chromic catgut sutures. It is advisable to drain the renal fossa.

Nephrolithotomy

Removal of stones from dilated calyces is simply an extension of the pyelolithotomy described above, and it is a simple matter to extract stones through the dilated calyceal necks. If, however, the calyces are of a normal size, the above procedure is often not technically possible; and if there has been previous surgery to the kidney in question, then the renal sinus may be difficult to identify. In these instances, incision of the renal parenchyma (nephrotomy) overlying the appropriate calyx is necessary. This may well result in brisk bleeding, and it is the author's practice to use renal artery occlusion for this type of surgery. The renal artery is dissected out (as previously described) and occluded with a small bulldog clamp (*Fig.* 32.6). The kidney then becomes smaller and softer and it is far easier to feel the stone in a calyx. An incision is made in a radial direction (i.e. in the line of the calyceal necks and major intrarenal blood vessels) and using the blades of the stone forceps, the walls of the nephrotomy are gently parted, when the lining of the collecting system is visualized and incised, and so the calyx entered. In this dry field, the stone can be seen and picked out of the calyx. The renal capsule is closed with 4/0 chromic catgut and the bulldog clamp removed and virtually no bleeding occurs.

If it is envisaged that occlusion of the renal artery will last for more than 10 minutes, i.e. that multiple nephrotomies are necessary, then measures must be taken to protect the kidney from ischaemic damage. The author employs the hypothermic technique developed by Wickham (1968), using the apparatus manufactured by Spembly. Having isolated and clamped the renal artery, two sterilized plastic discs consisting of coiled tubing are applied to each surface of the kidney. The coils are cooled with nitrous oxide gas which is allowed to expand through a system of Joule–Thomson valves. The coils are connected by tubing (which is also sterilized) to the nitrous oxide cylinder, which is readily available in any operating

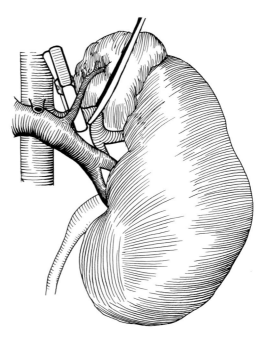

Fig. 32.6. Nephrolithotomy. The renal artery is controlled to reduce bleeding and so improve vision.

theatre. When the temperature of the core of the kidney (measured by a telethermometer supplied by Spembly with the coils) falls to 20 °C, the coils are removed, the calyces opened and the stones removed as described above. To wash out any debris a high pressure flush is employed, using 1-litre bags of sterile normal saline which have been kept in a domestic refrigerator (4 °C). The bags are in a Fenwall bag compressor (used by anaesthetists for rapid blood infusions) and connected to an intravenous drip set. To the end of the tubing, a malleable antral catheter is attached, and by introducing it through the multiple nephrotomies, the calyces are flushed with saline delivered as a forceful stream. To ensure that all the stone fragments have been removed, close-contact radiographs are taken. Localization of the fragments is facilitated by using Cushing silver clip markers fixed to the Netelast gauze. While the radiographs are being developed, it is advisable to recool the kidney if the core temperature has risen above 20 °C. Once all the calculus material has been removed, the nephrotomies are sutured as described above, and a no. 12 Fr. nephrostomy tube placed in the lowermost calyx. The bulldog clamp is then removed, the pyelotomy sutured and the wound drained as before.

A simpler method of preserving renal function with renal ischaemia is by the intravenous injection of 2 g of inosine (Trophycardyl) (Wickham et al., 1979). This latter is a purine nucleotide and its mode of action is not totally understood. It appears that it preserves the integrity of the capsule or envelope of the red cell corpuscle during anoxia, and so prevents the lysis and sludging of red cells which are important factors in the development of acute tubular necrosis. This compound may also be concerned with preserving the brush borders of the renal tubular cell. Two minutes after the intravenous injection (in the antecubital vein), the renal artery is occluded and the removal of calculi is undertaken in a dry field. The period of ischaemia should not exceed 1¼ hours.

Percutaneous Nephrolithotomy

The first stage of this procedure is the establishment of a nephrostomy tract (*Fig.* 32.7). This is done by either a urologist or a radiologist who has developed a special interest in this technique. Initially the tract starts as a needle and is enlarged by dilatation until it is of a size to admit instruments of no. 24 Fr. gauge, whence the urologist gains access to the collecting system, and can either remove the calculus, or disintegrate the stone (lithotrisis) and aspirate the fragments. The lithotrisis is undertaken by electrohydraulic probe and ultrasound probes.

Partial Nephrectomy

The removal of the lower pole of the kidney in calculus disease can only be justified if, after removal of the stone, there remains a thin-walled sump containing a pool of stagnant urine, which readily becomes infected, so providing the conditions necessary for further calculus formation. If the sump is surrounded by a good thickness of renal parenchyma, drainage can be improved and kidney tissue preserved by doing a pyelocalycotomy (*see below*).

In the operation of partial nephrectomy, the kidney must be fully mobilized and the renal artery and its major branches are displayed. The arterial branch supplying that part of the kidney to be removed can be positively identified by injecting methylene blue into the isolated artery and noting the discoloration of the area it supplies. The renal capsule is preserved by incising it along the margin of the kidney and stripping it off that part of the kidney which is to be removed. The identified branch of the renal artery is ligated and divided and the renal parenchyma incised along the line demarcating the discoloured and ischaemic cortex from the normally perfused tissue. If, however, the areas of blood supply of the branches of the renal artery do not match the diseased portion of kidney to be removed, then the author employs the hypothermic technique described in the nephrolithotomy operation. Having arrested the circulation, cooled the kidney and stripped off the renal capsule, the relevant portion of kidney is excised and the larger intrarenal blood vessels (which can be clearly seen in this dry field) are under-run with 4/0 chromic catgut. Defects in the collecting system are repaired with 4/0 chromic catgut and the bulldog clamp is then removed. Any blood vessels which were not secured will now bleed and are now identified and ligated. If bleeding is profuse the clamp can be reapplied while haemostasis is obtained.

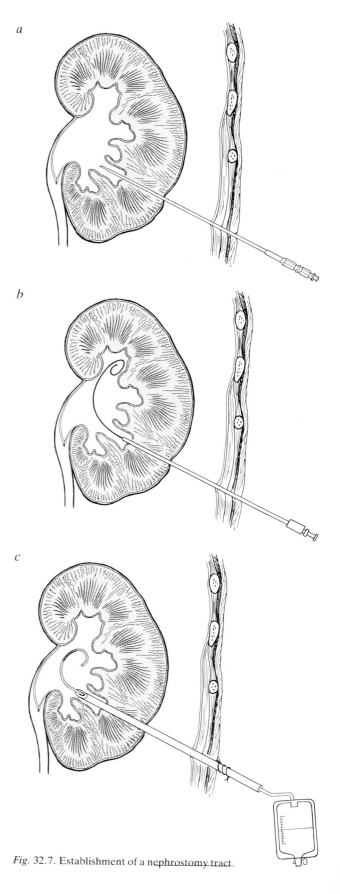

a

b

c

Fig. 32.7. Establishment of a nephrostomy tract.

The exposed renal tissue is covered with the preserved capsule, which is sutured with chromic catgut. Drainage of the renal fossa is advised.

Pyelocalycotomy

Removal of a large amount of calculous material in the lower calyces may be difficult, and it may leave a fair-sized cavity bounded by an adequate thickness or renal parenchyma. To ensure that thereafter there is adequate drainage of urine from the lower pole, a side-to-side anastomosis is made between the opened lower pole calyx and lower major calyx on the one side and the opened upper ureter and lower renal pelvis on the other side so as to form a large continuous cavity.

Initially the lower medial aspect of the renal pelvis is opened between stay sutures. The line of incision along the medial aspect of the lower pole of the kidney is determined by passing a probe through the pyelotomy into the lower calyx which is made to protrude on to the surface. The kidney tissue is cut between the point of the probe and the pyelotomy (*Fig.* 32.8). To avoid the anastomosis being surrounded by renal parenchyma which may lead to an encircling of fibrous tissue with obstruction, the excess kidney tissue is trimmed off. Any bleeding vessels on the incised parenchyma are dealt with by full-thickness calyco-capsular sutures.

A Cummings rat-tailed nephrostomy tube is passed down the ureter before the inferior pyelocalycotomy is anastomosed to the pyelo-ureterotomy, and the larger end of the tube passes through a stab incision in the pelvis to the skin (*Figs.* 32.9, 32.10).

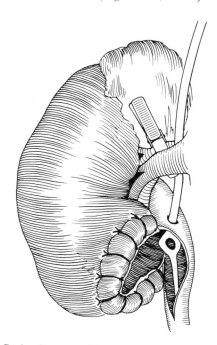

Fig. 32.9. Pyelocalycotomy. Bleeding vessels of the incised kidney substance are dealt with by the use of full-thickness sutures.

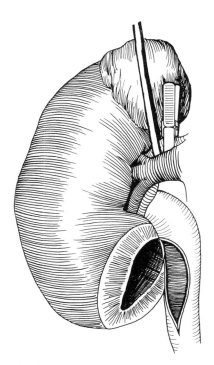

Fig. 32.8. Pyelocalycotomy. The lower medial aspect of the renal pelvis is opened between stay sutures and the line of incision along the medial aspect of the lower pole of the kidney is determined by passing a probe through the pyelotomy into the lower calyx which is then made to protrude on to the surface. The kidney tissue is then cut between the point of the probe and the pyelotomy.

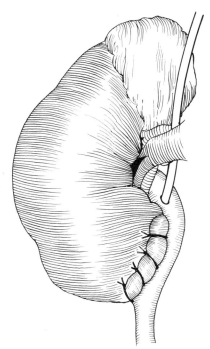

Fig. 32.10. Pyelocalycotomy. A pyelostomy tube is passed down the ureter before the inferior pyelocalycotomy is anastomosed to the pyelo-ureterotomy and the larger end of the pyelostomy tube passes through a stab incision in the pelvis and through the skin.

Lithotripsy

In extracorporeal shock wave lithotripsy (ESWL) a stone can be broken down by focusing shock waves on a kidney stone for about 45 minutes. The procedure involves strapping an anaesthetized patient to a chair placed in a warm water bath. The position of the chair, and so the patient, is adjusted, so that when viewed by two X-ray machines the kidney stone is at the centre of the cross-hairs on both screens. Located at the bottom of the stainless steel water bath are two elliptical-shaped reflector dishes, with an electrode at the focal point of each. These emit shock wave pulses at the same rate as the patient's heart beat (these are synchronized by means of a cardiac monitor) and are focused onto the kidney stone. Over the next couple of days, the stone sediment is voided and if there are any residual calculi which are impacted, or too big to pass spontaneously, then the percutaneous approach is employed, as described above. All stones in the kidney and in the ureter above the level of the pelvic brim are suitable for this extracorporeal shock wave treatment. The intimate relationship of the lower half of the ureter to the bony skeleton is a contra-indication to the use of lithotripsy as a method of stone elimination, but the development of the ureteroscope permits the removal of stones in the lower half, without having to resort to the scalpel. ESWL is at the present time costly and restricted to very few centres.

MANAGEMENT OF UPPER URINARY TRACT OBSTRUCTION

Obstruction to the free drainage of urine leads to impairment of function of the affected part of the kidney, which if maintained may end with irreversible damage, so decreasing the overall renal function.

The diagnosis of upper urinary tract obstruction is commonly made by means of the IVU. A totally non-functioning kidney (e.g. due to arterial occlusion or to very long-standing obstruction with the contralateral kidney having hypertrophied to the extent that the blood urea is normal) will not show any renal opacification despite the injection of large amounts of dye. In the case of a functioning kidney, the dye is first seen as a kidney-shaped shadow due to its distribution through the arterial system which supplies the renal parenchyma. In a kidney with a satisfactory renal blood flow, this opacification will be seen within a minute of injecting the dye, and if the obstruction to urine flow is severe, the dye will continue to accumulate in the renal parenchyma to give a progressively denser shadow. As it emerges from the nephrons into the collecting system, so the calyces and renal pelvis will be seen and the renal shadow will fade. If, due to atrophy of the parenchyma (which may be due to long-standing obstruction) the renal arterial inflow is small, then it may take some hours for enough dye to diffuse through the residual renal

tissue in sufficient quantity to outline this kidney; which is the reason for taking delayed (even up to 1 or 2 days) radiographs in this situation.

It follows from the above that the definition of the level of an obstructive lesion by an IVU depends on the amount of dye which will be excreted by the kidney into the collecting system; and this in turn depends not only on the quantity of dye injected and the taking of delayed radiographs, but also on the quality or potential function of the renal tissue. In most instances, the collecting system and ureter are sufficiently well outlined as to permit accurate localization of the level of the obstruction, but if this is not possible, alternative means of outlining the collecting system are necessary, if correctly planned surgery is to be undertaken. In the majority of cases, a retrograde ureterogram and pyelogram will serve this purpose. This is undertaken using a bulb or Chevassau catheter which plugs the ureteric orifice. Although it is preferable to visualize the ascent of the injected dye using an image intensifier, a satisfactory series of pictures can be obtained by taking the radiographs as the dye is injected. If it is not possible to do a retrograde examination (e.g. the ureter has previously been implanted in the colon or ileum, or access to the ureteric orifice is technically difficult due to a urethral stricture or prostatic projection, etc.) then the radiologists are often able to puncture the dilated renal pelvis through the loin with a long flexible needle, through which is threaded a narrow catheter and dye is injected. The resulting pro- or antegrade ureterogram will clearly define the level of the obstruction and so the correct operation can be planned.

It should be realized that a dilated ureter as seen on the IVU does not necessarily mean obstruction. A ureter which has been damaged by infection, may thereafter be wider and is certainly more distensible than the contralateral ureter. Similarly, certain developmental anomalies lead to a ureter being larger than usual, yet these are not obstructed. If vesicoureteric reflux is marked, then on the IVU a ureter may appear quite dilated. This appearance is further exaggerated if the vesico-ureteric reflux is associated with infection.

Renal Surgery for Obstructive Disease

The pelvi-ureteric junction is probably the commonest site above the level of the bladder neck at which obstruction to urine flow occurs. In the majority of cases, the diagnosis is made on the IVU, there being blunting (to an equal extent) of all the renal papillae, which in the more extreme cases exhibit spherical calyces, a large renal pelvis and a normal ureter.

In the majority, the obstruction is believed to be due to a failure of the transmission of the peristaltic waves from the pelvis passing across the pelvi-ureteric junction and down the ureter so causing the urine to accumulate in a relatively static state. Hydronephrosis may also be due to a stone becoming impacted at the pelvi-ureteric junction, or occasionally due to a polypoid tumour sometimes seen at this site. Hydronephrosis due to stricturing at the pelvi-ureteric junction is seen in tuberculosis, but other stigmas of this disease should also be evident on the IVU. Obstruction of a more temporary nature occurs with a renal papilla or blood clot.

Pyeloplasty

It is the author's opinion that the objectives of a pyeloplasty should be not only to remove the obstruction to urine flow at the pelvi-ureteric junction, but to reduce the volume of the enlarged renal pelvis, so as to permit the rapid 'turnover' of urine in the hydronephrotic kidney and so decrease the liability of urinary infection becoming established in a relatively stagnant pool of urine. The only operation which fulfils these requirements is the Anderson–Hynes dismembered pyeloplasty.

The kidney is approached through the usual 12th rib incision. If complete mobility of the organ is required, the whole of the kidney is freed from the surrounding tissues. In many instances all of the pelvis can be exposed without having to mobilize the upper pole of the kidney. The ureter is identified and the adherent condensed layers of fascia covering the pelvis are dissected off, so that at the time of anastomosis, only the tissues of the pelvis and ureter are sewn together (*Fig. 32.11*). Often the lower pole blood vessels are buried in the peripelvic tissue and these must be completely freed. Although on occasions it may appear that the manoeuvre of separating the lower polar vessels from the pelvis results in relieving the obstructed collecting system, it is difficult to prove whether the same situation persists in a patient who is upright with a significant diuresis. Hence to ensure relief of obstruction, the pelvi-ureteric junction must be reconstructed (*Fig. 32.12*).

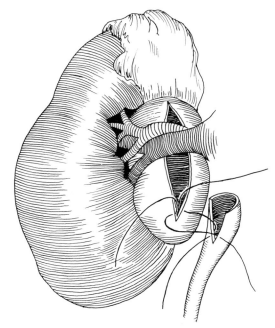

Fig. 32.12. Anderson–Hynes pyeloplasty. Preparation for anastomosis of ureter to lower pelvis.

The redundant portion of the pelvis is excised demarking each end of the incision with 4/0 catgut (on an atraumatic curved cutting needle.) The majority of the gaping renal pelvis is closed with a continuous suture, starting at the superior aspect. The lowermost 2 cm of the pelvis are left open and attached to the spatulated ureter, using once again a continuous suture of 4/0 catgut. This anastomosis is positioned in whichever site it seems best suited, which can be either in front of or behind the lower polar blood vessels (if present) (*Fig.* 32.13). There is no need to use a stent or nephrostomy drainage. A corrugated drain is positioned by the anastomosis.

In the unusual situation of the hydronephrosis being present in a horseshoe kidney, the bridge or isthmus joining the two halves of the kidney must be divided to ensure that there is no further obstruction below the reconstructed pelvi-ureteric junction.

Another advance, which is in its infancy, is the surgery of pelvic hydronephrosis. Access to the lumen of the upper urinary tract, by means of a nephrostomy tract (*see Fig.* 32.7) permits the passage of a urethrotome, and so incision of the mucosal and muscular layers of the pelvi-ureteric junction—a procedure described as pyelolysis.

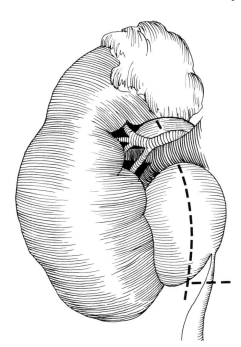

Fig. 32.11. Anderson–Hynes pyeloplasty. Lines of excision.

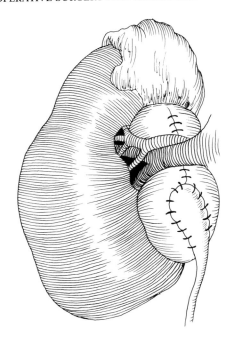

Fig. 32.13. Anderson–Hynes pyeloplasty. Complete anastomosis and repair of pelvis.

Nephrostomy

The function of this operation is to:

1. Ensure urine drainage direct from the kidney so as to bypass an obstruction or protect a recently constructed anastomosis involving the upper urinary tract.
2. Drain from the kidney any blood which may be issuing forth after renal surgery or other trauma.

This is achieved by introducing a catheter or tube into the renal collecting system, and may be part of a more extensive operation or constitute the whole of the operation. In either case a definitive nephrotomy must be made and only then should the catheter be threaded through the renal substance. To ensure that the inner aspect of the nephrotomy is suitably placed, a pyelotomy is necessary. Through the opening in the renal pelvis, a finger is passed into the collecting system and the thickness of the renal cortex overlying an appropriate calyx (i.e. dilated, dependent or easily accessible) can be estimated. The end of a pair of curved nephrolithotomy forceps (e.g. Randall's) is passed through the pyelotomy into the chosen calyx. If the overlying renal cortex is thin, a little pressure on the forceps will ensure its passage through the parenchyma, and so the end of the tube or catheter is grasped and withdrawn into the collecting system. If the thickness of the cortex is substantial, then the nephrotomy is made by cutting down with a scalpel onto the forceps positioned in the appropriate calyx.

One variety of catheter which may be used is a rat-tailed Cummings nephrostomy tube, the tail of

which acts as a splint (no. 8 Fr. gauge) for intubating the upper ureter. This is necessary after doing a ureterotomy, whereby a longitudinal incision is made along a strictured ureter (*Fig.* 32.14) (as occurs in

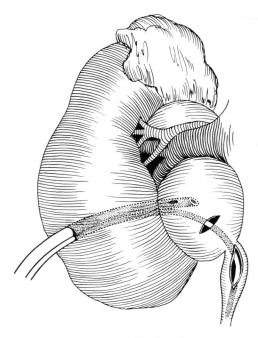

Fig. 32.14. Nephrostomy and intubated ureterostomy.

tuberculosis). Alternatively, if the nephrostomy is being used to drain blood after multiple nephrotomies for stone disease, then a tube (of no. 12–18 Fr. gauge) with a number of openings is necessary. It is rare to envisage long-term catheter drainage from the kidney, but provided the renal pelvis is of an adequate size retaining balloon catheters may be appropriate.

Where possible, the nephrostomy should be sited so that it emerges on the anterolateral aspect of the abdominal wall. This facilitates dressings and care of the tube and also enables the patient to lie on his or her back. Usually a belt with a flange is used to stabilize the position of the catheter.

Ureteric Surgery for Obstructive Disease

As in the case of the kidney, it is preferable if surgical procedure on the ureter are kept in the extraperitoneal space. Naturally this is not possible if an intraperitoneal anastomosis with bowel is necessary, or in dealing with difficult ureterovaginal fistulas; but the incidence of intestinal ileus and peritoneal infection (which may be secondary to the extravasation of infected urine leaking from an anastomosis or ureterotomy) prolongs convalescence and the need for parenteral feeding. In addition, extraperitoneal surgery offers the technical advantages of excluding from the operating field the irritation of obtruding loops of bowel.

The surgical approach to the ureter is conditioned by the nature of the disease process involved. In the case of stone disease, different incisions are used for exposure of the upper, middle and lower thirds of the ureter. In the case of bilateral and advanced retroperitoneal fibrosis, the ureterolysis and biopsy are best undertaken by a transperitoneal surgical exposure.

UPPER THIRD OF THE URETER

The commonest indication for approaching the upper third of the ureter is for removal of a calculus which is causing appreciable urinary obstruction or pain. A stone which lies within 4 cm or so of the pelviureteric junction may, as a result of the dissection, slip back into the renal pelvis, and hence it is the author's practice to use an oblique lumbar incision with the patient on his or her side (see p. 435) so that easy exposure of the kidney is possible if a pyelotomy should prove necessary to recover the stone. Satisfactory exposure of the renal pelvis and upper ureter can also be obtained through the lumbotomy incision (see p. 438). In either case the upper ureter is identified, and an encircling tape placed round the ureter above the level of the stone. In these circumstances there is no need to undertake any dissection in the renal fossa, but if the stone should slip back into the renal pelvis, then this organ will have to be identified and opened to remove the stone.

Once the ureter has been secured and the site of the stone isolated, two stay sutures of 4/0 catgut are placed on the anterior aspect of the ureter overlying the calculus. The ureter is incised longitudinally between the stay sutures. With a blunt (McDonald's) dissector the stone is freed from the adherent ureteric mucosa and removed with stone forceps. Releasing the tape above the ureterotomy should result in a copious flow of urine, which proves that there is no proximal obstruction. To ensure that there is no distal obstruction from a fragment or unidentified lower stone, a ureteric catheter or bougie is passed down the length of the lower ureter. The ureterotomy is closed with a 4/0 catgut suture which passes through the muscle layer of the ureter. A corrugated drain is placed adjacent to the operation site and brought out through the abdominal wall with a stab wound which is separate from the main incision. The muscle layers are closed with interrupted catgut.

MIDDLE THIRD OF THE URETER

The approach to the middle third of the ureter is by means of a muscle-splitting (gridiron) incision of the anterior abdominal wall. The patient lies supine and the incision can be either transversely positioned or in the iliac fossa. If the part of the ureter to be approached is at the mid-lumbar spine level then a transverse incision is used. Laterally it starts at the anterior axillary line, positioned at the midpoint between the tip of the 12th rib and the iliac crest—passing medially to the lateral border of the rectus sheath. The oblique and transverse abdominal muscles are split along the line of their respective fibres, and it is often an advantage to open the anterior and posterior layers of the rectus sheath for 2 cm to allow for an improved exposure. The peritoneum is stripped off the posterior abdominal muscles towards the midline and with the ureter will be found the gonadal vessels. The removal of the stone and subsequent manoeuvres are as described in the previous section.

To isolate the ureter at the level of the bifurcation of the common iliac artery or slightly lower down, an oblique iliac fossa incision is made and the ureter is approached retroperitoneally.

LOWER THIRD OF THE URETER

The pararectal incision immediately overlies the lower part of the ureter, and is made so that it traces the lateral edge of the rectus muscle. The fascia which is immediately lateral to the rectus muscle (formed as a result of the fusion into one layer of the muscles of the abdominal wall) is incised. This exposes the extraperitoneal space from the superior ramus of the pubis to the level of the semilunar line of Douglas (i.e. the lower edge of the posterior rectus sheath). The inferior epigastric blood vessels have to be divided and the peritoneum is stripped medially. If the ureter is not readily identified because of excess fat, it is best to extend the incision superiorly for another 3 cm and carefully separate the peritoneum off the rectus sheath, so that the bifurcation of the common iliac artery can be palpated. The ureter is here identified and traced down into the pelvis.

Mobilization of the ureter to within 3 cm of the bladder is unhindered by any structure until the superior vesical artery and vein are noted to be passing from the lateral wall of the pelvis towards the bladder and are intimately adherent to the ureter. These blood vessels must be divided between Moynihan clamps and securely tied, if access is to be obtained to the lowermost portion of the ureter. Thereafter the muscle fibres of the detrusor will become apparent. Removal of a stone is as previously described.

Drainage of this wound is with a corrugated rubber drain brought out through a stab wound, 5 cm from the lateral edge of the incision. Closure requires one layer of continuous unabsorbable material, since using absorbable material often results in an incisional hernia.

Ureteric Endoscopy

Both rigid and flexible ureteroscopes are available, to be used for diagnostic and therapeutic purposes.

It is not wise to use the instruments if the ureter has been the subject of surgery in the past, since the tethered or scarred ureter invites perforation. The first hurdle to be negotiated is the ureteric orifice, assuming there is no difficulty in visualizing this due to an intervening prostate or other impediment. The intramural ureter should be dilated either with bougies or an inflatable balloon, similar to those used for angioplasty. Having passed through the ureteric orifice, the passage of the instrument is facilitated by injecting fluid along the length of a no. 5 Fr. ureteric catheter which is threaded through the ureteroscope, with its opening at the lens end of the instrument, and so the ureter immediately ahead of the ureteroscope is distended making it easier to visualize the lumen. In addition to examining the interior of the ureter, a number of manoeuvres can be undertaken with the aid of accessories threaded down the ureteroscope. With biopsy forceps and a diathermy electrode, ureteric tumours can be diagnosed and treated. A stone can be retrieved with a wire basket. If the stone is too large, and needs to be reduced in size before attempting its removal, an electrohydraulic or ultrasound probe can be passed up the ureteroscope and the stone partially disintegrated. Alternatively, some upper ureteric stones are best dealt with by pushing them into the renal pelvis and then either submitting them to ESWL (if available) or removing them through a nephrocutaneous tract, as described above.

Considerable care must be exercised when grasping a stone, since it is remarkably easy to injure and perforate the oedematous ureter. In those circumstances it is advisable to thread a double-ended pigtail ureteric splint or stent up the length of the ureter. This often requires X-ray control to be sure that the upper end of the stent is situated in the renal pelvis.

The absence of a ureteroscope entails removal of the ureteric calculus endoscopically using X-ray visualization.

Extraction of a Ureteric Calculus by X-ray Supervision (Fig. 32.15)

A stone which has recently negotiated the upper two-thirds of a ureter should be amenable to removal with a ureteric stone extraction basket. If, however, the stone has been impacted in the lower ureter for weeks or longer, then it may have increased in size to an extent whereby its further passage along the lower ureter and through the ureteric orifice is somewhat optimistic. The intramural ureter is the narrowest part of the ureteric channel, and a stone which is halted at this level may be released with the help of a meatotomy. This latter is best done by incising the meatus with a diathermy electrode, and this manoeuvre alone may be enough to cause the stone to be voided within a few days.

The most commonly used ureteric stone extractor

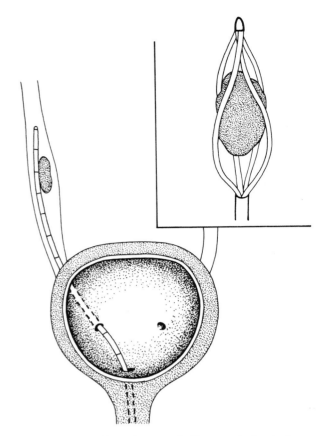

Fig. 32.15. Endoscopic removal of lower ureteric calculus.

is the Dormia basket. Some varieties have a 5-cm bougie guide preceding the basket. Using the operating cystoscope with an Albarran lever, the bougie is lubricated and passed up the ureteric orifice. The catheter of the Dormia is marked with 1-cm rings and so the position of the closed basket from the ureteric orifice can be noted and its relationship to the stone estimated.

In a number of hospitals, an X-ray image intensifier is available for use during the extraction of the ureteric calculus. In these the likelihood of capturing the stone in the wire mesh is obviously considerably increased. The success rate is further enhanced by oscillating movements of the open basket at the level of the stone, which may facilitate engaging the calculus in the basket. The prize is then slowly withdrawn down the ureter and into the bladder.

Ureterolysis

The condition of retroperitoneal fibrosis is becoming more readily diagnosed prior to operation, as a result of the increasing awareness of this disease as a cause of upper urinary tract obstruction. We need not concern ourselves with the symptomatology, but the IVU will show some significant features. The disease may involve one or both ureters, and since the obstruction is extramural, the lower limit of the dilated ureter shows a characteristic tapering or spindle-shaped appearance. There may be other evidence of the cause of the obstruction, e.g. the linear calcification seen in the wall of an aortic aneurysm, which then leaks some blood, and as a result of organization of the haematoma goes on to fibrosis with compression of the ureter.

In so-called 'idiopathic retroperitoneal fibrosis', whereby the disease spreads from the midline laterally, the ureter may occasionally be pulled medially. In this disease and also in that due to spreading carcinoma from the rectum, uterus or prostate, the pelvic portion of the ureter is commonly involved. Retroperitoneal tumours originating in carcinoma of the stomach, pancreas, ovary and breast are other extramural causes of the ureteric obstruction.

It is often necessary to undertake a retrograde ureterogram to define the extent of the ureteric compression, and so plan the correct incision for the operation. A retroperitoneal exposure of the ureter is the best approach if only one ureter is involved, but if both ureters are shown to be obstructed, then a transperitoneal approach may be preferable. The object of the operation is to obtain a biopsy of the material and to free the ureter from the enveloping tissues without making a hole in the ureter. The ureterolysis is best undertaken by identifying the normal ureter below the obstruction, and then by careful dissection establishing the plane which preserves the integrity of the ureter and strips it free from the enveloping tissues. It is important to ensure that the obstruction to the ureter is relieved, which will only occur if the ureter is pared down to the muscle layers. The whole length of the involved ureter must be dealt with in this manner. The vascularity of the ureteric wall is considerably reduced as a result of this periureteric activity, and if the integrity of the mucosa is breached, it may lead to a persistent fistula, despite proximal urinary diversion. In these circumstances, a nephrostomy is to be preferred to the use of a ureterostomy, because of the uncertainty of the nature of the disease process surrounding the ureter (until a histological report becomes available) and subsequent healing.

The exposed ureter should be positioned away from the pathological tissue, and if convenient can be placed in the peritoneal cavity. The biopsy report is important in the further management of these patients. If the patient has bilateral obstruction due to malignant peri-ureteric fibrosis, it is probably inadvisable to undertake proximal urinary diversions. Failure to respond to carcino-chemotherapy will lead to uraemia as a terminal event, which is often preferable to a protracted and miserable terminal illness. If the biopsy shows the obstruction to be due to periureteric fibrosis, corticosteroid therapy is necessary to arrest the disease (the duration of drug therapy is judged by the response to the blood sedimentation rate and degree of ureteric obstruction).

NEPHRECTOMY AND OTHER RENAL OPERATIONS

As previously indicated, the removal of functioning nephrons should not be lightly undertaken. Hence renal surgery should be as conservative as possible, providing this in no way limits the effectiveness of the treatment.

The more common indications for the removal of a kidney vary from malignant disease to that for a severely traumatized organ, or for a kidney virtually destroyed by infection or obstruction (with or without accompanying stone disease). Nephrectomy in vascular disease, e.g. renal hypertension and arteriovenous malformations, should only be considered if other modalities have proved ineffective, i.e. the failure of reconstructive surgery or drug therapy in the case of hypertension.

There are two overriding prerequisites before contemplating nephrectomy. First, a preoperative diagnosis should have been made since exploratory operations of the kidney are a very poor investigative tool (the investigations relevant to a disease process are described on p. 438). Second, the surgeon must be informed of the total renal function and in particular the function of the contralateral kidney. The value of the IVU and blood tests have already been described (p. 438).

Before embarking on a nephrectomy, the haemoglobin level must be known, and blood should have been cross-matched for transfusion purposes. The technique now to be described is that commonly performed by the author when removing the kidney, but when dealing with malignant disease there are some additional features which are mentioned later in this chapter.

The incision and approach to the kidney are determined by the condition of the underlying kidney pathology. The renal artery will be found in the angle between the upper medial border of the kidney and the posterior abdominal wall. It should be traced towards its origin, as far as is possible, to ensure that it is the stem of the artery and not its major branches (which, due to early division, originate close to the aorta) which has been dissected out. Care is taken to ensure that the artery and vein are sufficiently separate to make it possible to put three Moynihan clamps on the artery, without involving the vein in any way. The artery is divided in the space between the clamp nearest to the kidney and that of the adjoining clamp, so that after division there are two clamps on the stump of that part of the renal artery in continuity with the aorta. Using 5 metric (1) chromic catgut, the artery is first ligated behind the furthermost clamp, i.e. the one nearest the aorta, and after removal of that clamp, a second ligature is tied behind the remaining clamp. Finally, the stump of artery attached to the kidney is tied. This procedure is repeated for the renal vein.

Securing and ligating the artery and vein separately

ensure good visualization of the blood vessels. 'Blind' clamping of the renal pedicle may be associated with inadvertently including unwanted structures in the tip of the forceps, On the right side the inferior vena cava is particularly at risk. Furthermore, ligating the major vessels together may lead to the formation of an arteriovenous fistula, Catgut is used in preference to non-absorbable material, to avoid the possibility of sinus formation, which does occur if the wound and renal bed become infected, It is advisable to drain the renal fossa, since there is often some oozing from the smaller blood vessels of the surrounding tissues,

Nephrectomy for Malignancy Disease

The commonest condition for which a nephrectomy is undertaken is a hypernephroma (or carcinoma of the renal tubular epithelium), The diagnosis should be firmly established before embarking on the removal of the kidney. If on the IVU the space-occupying lesion looks more like a renal cyst than a tumour, an ultrasound examination is recommended. If this latter demonstrates that the space-occupying lesion is of a fluid nature, aspiration of this by the radiologist using the image intensifier will often resolve the problem. It is of further help if the fluid obtained is examined by a cytologist for malignant cells. This approach to the treatment of a renal cyst spares the patient an unnecessary kidney exploration.

If, on the other hand, the IVU appearances suggest a renal carcinoma, then arteriography is indicated. The value of this examination is multiple, In the first place, if the characteristic vascular pattern of a hypernephroma is seen, this virtually clinches the diagnosis, and should exclude polycystic disease and the rarer tuberous sclerosis which may look very much like a hypernephroma on the IVU, Other useful information obtained is to depict the number of renal arteries arising from the aorta and may, due to vascular filling, also outline involved lymph nodes. In addition, a free aortic injection may demonstrate the presence of smaller space-occupying lesions in the contralateral kidney (bilateral renal tumours most commonly represent secondary deposits from a carcinoma of the bronchus) and injection of the coeliac axis for tumours of the upper pole of the right kidney help determine whether the liver is involved, since a cross-over circulation may be evident.

Prior to nephrectomy for malignant disease, a chest radiograph is mandatory. Urinary cytology is particularly useful if seeking to establish a diagnosis of a transitional cell carcinoma of the kidney. This information is important, since a nephro-ureterectomy may be indicated,

It should be realized that total nephrectomy is not the only renal operation undertaken for malignant diseases. Transitional cell carcinoma has a multifocal origin, and when this disease is localized to one of the poles of the kidney, it may be justified, particularly in a relatively young individual with similar dis-

ease in the bladder, to limit the renal surgery to a partial nephrectomy (this operation is described in the previous section). It is of course incumbent on the surgeon to examine the ureter (by retrograde ureterography) particularly carefully for evidence of tumour in that organ before planning renal surgery. Partial nephrectomy is also indicated when the tumour occurs in a solitary kidney, or sometimes in bilateral renal tumours,

Nephrectomy is in part being replaced by extensive embolization of the renal artery and its tributaries. In the future it is hoped that the infarcted kidney will be macerated and aspirated by instruments which enter the renal fossa through a loin puncture wound,

Surgery for Renal Trauma

The majority of traumatized kidneys are managed conservatively. Immediate operative interference for an injured kidney is restricted to those cases where continuing significant bleeding persists, or where the IVU shows total absence of function on the side of the injured kidney,

The criteria which indicate continuing significant bleeding from a kidney are a falling blood pressure, rising pulse rate and a progressively enlarging mass in the renal fossa. Haematuria is not a helpful pointer as to the need for surgery, even if it be prolonged for weeks. An IVU is mandatory. It will give valuable information in respect of the number of kidneys and their function. Marked extravasation of dye and urine is not an indication for immediate surgery, although operation may subsequently be required.

Total absence of function on the side of the supposedly injured kidney should be followed by an emergency renal arteriogram. This will give information which is vital to the correct management of the patient. If the angiogram indicates a contusion with thrombosis (or avulsion) of the renal artery, then immediate operation is indicated, and the operator should be prepared to undertake reconstructive arterial surgery. However, complete absence of a kidney on the urogram may be due to a relatively minor injury to a previously poorly functioning kidney, as would be seen in a long-standing pathological condition (e.g. a grossly hydronephrotic kidney) or congenital abnormality (e.g. a hypoplastic kidney). In these cases the treatment of choice is conservative management provided there is no continuing significant bleeding occurring.

Immediate surgery to arrest severe bleeding from a lacerated kidney leads more often than not to nephrectomy. Obviously a more conservative approach is to be preferred, and this may be possible if the damage is localized (as judged by a urogram) to one or other of the poles. Similarly, severe bleeding from a solitary kidney is a fairly desperate situation, and conservative surgery should be attempted. Preferably this requires isolation of the renal pedicle, so as to be able to use bulldog clamps for arresting the haemorrhage. Usually the 12th rib lumbar approach is satisfactory, unless intraperitoneal manoeuvres are also contemplated. Mobilization of the kidney in these circumstances usually means evacuation of clot, and, as indicated above, isolation of the renal artery may be difficult and a pedicle clamp may have to be placed across both the artery and vein for the purposes of controlling the bleeding.

In the less severely injured kidney, soon after the haematuria has ceased, the IVU should be repeated. If there is evidence of persisting extravasation, this may lead to fibrosis with compression of the ureter and/or vascular pedicle. If surgery is delayed until organization of the extravasated blood has occurred, the procedure is difficult. Therefore, operation should not be long delayed, and evacuation and drainage of extravasated fluid and blood are undertaken, with resuturing of torn collecting system and débridement of necrotic tissue with possible extension to partial nephrectomy (as described in the appropriate section).

URETERIC EXCISION, REPAIR AND SUBSTITUTION

Ureterectomy

Removal of a ureter is usually total, and commonly part of a larger operation, namely a nephro-ureterectomy, which may be necessary with tuberculous disease or a transitional-cell carcinoma of the upper urinary tract.

In the case of a carcinoma of the ureter, it may be possible to do a segmental ureterectomy by excising the tumour with a 1-cm margin, and still permit a primary anastomosis. This approach is justified on the grounds that this disease is multifocal in origin, and extirpation of the upper urinary tract for a well-circumscribed lesion of the renal pelvis or ureter may be considered excessive, since recurrent disease can be expected in the bladder or in the contralateral kidney and ureter. Following local removal of a tumour, careful follow-up examinations with urinary cytology, IVU and urethrocystoscopy are mandatory.

Excision of the ureter is also undertaken if a kidney has to be removed due to extensive destruction by tuberculosis, since removal of a kidney alone does not guarantee eradication of the tuberculosis from the residual ureter. To combat active ureteric disease, either the circulating antituberculous drugs must be able to get at the bacillus (which is limited by the blood supply to the ureter) or, alternatively, the drug must come in contact with the ureter by means of its urinary content, and this is only possible if there is a significant degree of vesico-ureteric reflux in the remaining stump.

The operation of nephro-ureterectomy is best undertaken through two incisions. The 12th rib lumbar incision is employed and the routine operation of nephrectomy (see p. 447) is undertaken except that the ureter is not divided. Through the lower regions of the incision, the peritoneum is stripped off the abdominal parietes and the kidney is placed in the iliac fossa. The lumbar incision is closed in the usual manner. The patient is then repositioned and laid supine and retowelled. The incision and approach are as described for the lower third of the ureter. Having dissected the ureter within 3 cm or so of its termination, the superior vesical pedicle is divided which allows the ureter to be followed to the bladder wall. Traction on the ureter makes it possible to put a Moynihan clamp on the tented-up portion of the bladder; and a ligature is applied to the bladder side of the clamp. This clamp is then loosened and repositioned 2 cm up the ureter. The crushed segment is divided and the specimen removed includes a cuff of the bladder.

Primary Ureteric Anastomosis

The ureter may be damaged by trauma, as occurs in penetrating and crushing wounds, or during surgery or by inflammatory and neoplastic disease and other rarer pathological entities. This may result in extravasation of urine, often associated with infection which in turn is followed by upper urinary tract obstruction, intestinal ileus, etc. The defect in the ureter must be repaired or bypassed, if the serious complications of urinary extravasation are to be eliminated.

If the ureter is injured at the time of a surgical procedure, then identification and repair of the defect should be undertaken immediately. Immediate surgery is also recommended following a road traffic accident or other traumatic injuries such as a stab injury. In these circumstances, an IVU should be undertaken before the patient is submitted to surgery, in order to identify the site of the injury and establish the presence of two functioning kidneys.

Factors which determine the type of repair to be undertaken are how recent the injury is, its site and whether there has been any significant loss of ureteric length. If the ureteric injury was not identified at the time of operation, or the defect developed as a complication of other pathology, then it may be wise to first deal with the complications of the ureteric injury, namely infection and fistula formation, by using a proximal urinary diversion, e.g. a nephrostomy. In these circumstances, it will be necessary later to localize the site of the damage by means of an IVU and possibly a retrograde ureterogram.

On those rare occasions that a localized injury occurs to the upper three-quarters of the ureter, local excision of that part of the ureter which may have been devitalized by the inadvertent application of an artery clamp or ligation with a suture is undertaken. The ureteric ends are then spatulated and sutured with interrupted 4/0 catgut material. When healthy ureter is repaired, there is no advantage in intubating the ureter or using a proximal urinary diversion. A corrugated drain is placed down to the site of the ureteric repair.

Uretero-neocystostomy (and Boari Flap) *Figs. 32.16–32.20)*

An end-to-end anastomosis as described above is technically difficult in the lower quarter of the ureter. If the damage to the ureter is within 5 cm of the ureteric orifice, a simple reimplantation of the ureter is done. The bladder is opened and a Leadbetter–Politano type of reimplantation which avoids vesico-ureteric reflux (*see Figs. 32.18–32.19*) is used. If the cut end of the ureter will not reach the intact bladder without tension, then a bladder flap is raised. Construction of a Boari flap implies adequate access to the bladder with ligation of the superior vesical blood vessels on the affected side, so as to be able to mobilize the bladder to a significant extent. The flap is constructed on the superior aspect of the bladder with the base posteriorly. At the level of the hinge flap, the bladder is anchored to the psoas minor muscle at the pelvic brim. The flap is turned up towards the cut end of the ureter and a submucosal re-implantation of this ureter is undertaken, using the tunnel technique as for a Leadbetter–Politano operation. If the anastomosis appears to be under tension, then a ureteric splint is passed up the ureter, and

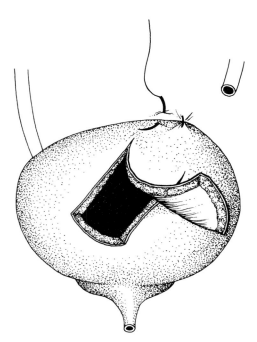

Fig. 32.17. Boari flap. Incision and elevation of flap and psoas hitch sutures.

brought out through the bladder wall and abdominal wall attached to a pointed trocar needle as used with Redivac drains. The bladder flap and cystostomy wound are closed with two continuous layers of catgut. A corrugated drain should be put down to the anastomosis, and urethral catheter drainage maintained for 10 days.

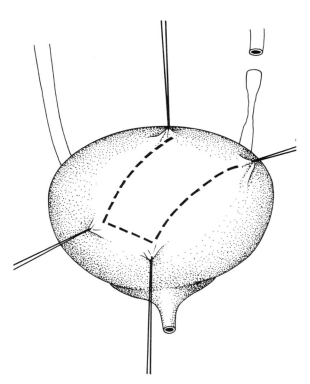

Fig. 32.16. Boari flap for reconstruction of lower ureter. Demarcation of flap.

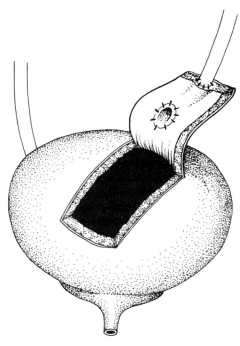

Fig. 32.18. Boari flap. Intramural implantation of ureter.

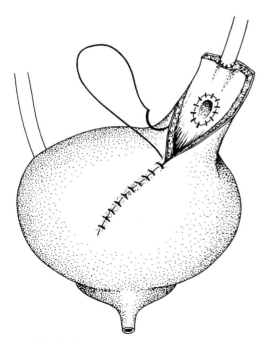

Fig. 32.19. Boari flap. Closure of bladder.

If it is not possible to anastomose the damaged ureter directly to the bladder due to pelvic trauma or disease, or loss of a considerable length of ureter, then the injured ureter should be anastomosed to the contralateral ureter above the level of the pelvic brim—this is known as a transuretero-ureterostomy.

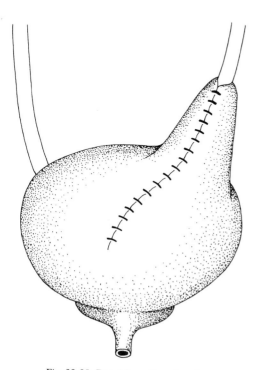

Fig. 32.20. Boari flap. Completed.

Transuretero-ureterostomy (*Figs.* 32.21–32.22)
To undertake an anastomosis of the shortened damaged ureter to the contralateral intact ureter, a

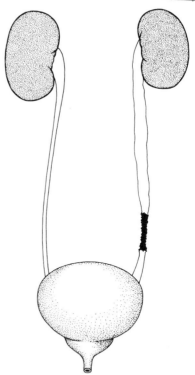

Fig. 32.21. Ureteric stricture following injury.

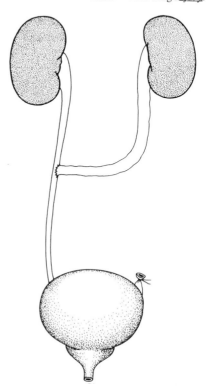

Fig. 32.22. Transuretero-ureterostomy.

paramedian incision is used and the peritoneal cavity is opened. The divided ureter is identified and mobilized retroperitoneally to the mid-lumbar spine level, and a length of 4/0 catgut is attached to the cut end, as a stay suture. The intact ureter is identified at the level where it crosses the common iliac artery, and the peritoneum is incised, the ureter mobilized and isolated between two tapes.

A finger is introduced through the peritoneal opening made over the intact ureter, and passed medially anterior to the aorta and vena cava, but behind the inferior mesenteric blood vessels and mesocolon to emerge at the site where the divided ureter is situated. A pair of artery forceps is now guided along the length of the tunnel created by the exploring finger and the stay suture attached to the cut ureter is grasped and withdrawn across the midline so as to bring it out by the side of the exposed intact ureter. A 4/0 catgut suture is placed either side of the midline of the intact ureter, and a 1·5–2-cm longitudinal incision is made between these two markers. The cut end of the ureter is spatulated by incising it for 1·5 cm.

The anastomosis of the divided ureter to the intact ureter is done with interrupted 4/0 catgut sutures. The peritoneum overlying the incision is not closed, and a corrugated drain is positioned at the site of the anastomosis and brought out through a separate stab incision. The paramedian incision is closed with continuous catgut for the peritoneum and continuous non-absorbable material for the anterior rectus sheath. The peritoneal drain is removed on the 4th postoperative day if there it no urinary leakage occurring. If there is any leakage then it should be left in place for 1 week, by which time a well-established drainage track is formed.

Ureteral Substitution

If a transuretero-ureterostomy is not possible because the contralateral ureter is inaccessible (due to previous surgery or other pathology) or absent (due to previous removal or congenital absence) then the choice lies between a cutaneous ureterostomy or the use of a segment of ileum to re-establish continuity between the ureter and the bladder. A cutaneous ureterostomy in the adult is on the whole an unsatisfactory procedure. In the first place the length of residual ureter is usually short and so the stoma is often situated in the flank, and there is difficulty in conveniently attaching a collecting bag. In a ureter of a normal calibre, the stoma tends to stenose, despite plastic procedures for increasing the lumen and the size of the ureterocutaneous anastomosis.

It is therefore preferable to use a length of bowel to replace the missing part of the ureter, and a segment of ileum is isolated in the same way as described for an ileal conduit. The ureter is implanted into the proximal end of the ileum, some 2 cm from the cut end of the bowel using the nipple technique. To prevent the nipple coming undone, a 4/0 catgut stitch is used to fix the turn-backed flap of ureter on to itself. A splint is secured in position by transfixing (with 4/0 catgut on an atraumatic cutting needle) a suture through both the tube and the ureter at the apex of the nipple. The splint is threaded down the whole length of the ileal segment. The proximal end of the ileum is closed. The bladder is opened between stay sutures. The end of the ureteric splint is attached to a Redivac needle, and this latter is brought from within the bladder through the detrusor and abdominal wall, and the splint is securely fixed onto the anterior surface of the abdomen with a non-absorbable suture. The anastomosis between the bladder and distal end of the ileal segment is done with one layer of interrupted catgut sutures, passing through all layers of gut and bladder. A peritoneal corrugated drain is placed at the site of this lower anastomosis. Urethral catheter drainage is instituted for 14 days. If there is any hint of bladder outflow obstruction, this should have been dealt with prior to the ureteric reconstruction. The splint is removed by gentle traction 10 days after the operation.

REFERENCES

Gardiner R. A., Naunton-Morgan T. C., Whitfield H. N. et al. (1979) The modified lumbotomy versus the oblique loin incision for renal surgery. *Br. J. Urol.* **51**, 256–259.

Gil-Vernet J. (1965) New surgical concepts in removing renal calculi. *Urol. Int.* **20**, 255–288.

Nagamatsu G. R. (1950) Dorso lumbar approach to the kidney and adrenal with osteoplastic flap. *J. Urol.* **63**, 569–571.

Turner-Warwick R. (1965) Lower pole pyelo-calycotomy and retrograde partial nephrectomy and uretero calycostomy. *Br. J. Urol.* **37**, 673–677.

Wickham J. E. A. (1968) A simple method for regional renal hypothermia. *J. Urol.* **99**, 246–247.

Wickham J. E. A., Fernando A. R., Hentry W. F. et al. (1979) I.V. inosine for ischaemic renal surgery. *Br. J. Urol.* **51**, 437–439.

FURTHER READING

Glenn J. (ed.) (1975) *Urologic Surgery*, 2nd ed. New York, Harper & Row.

Wickham J. E. A. (ed.) (1979) *Urinary Calculous Disease*, Edinburgh, Churchill Livingstone.

Wickham J. E. A. and Miller R. A. (eds) (1983) *Percutaneous Renal Surgery*, Edinburgh, Churchill Livingstone.

Williams D. I. (1977) *Operative Surgery: Urology*, 3rd ed. London, Butterworth.

Chapter thirty-three

Functional Assessment of the Lower Urinary Tract

R. C. L. Feneley and J. A. Massey

The routine assessment of micturition disorders often fails to reveal conclusive evidence of their pathogenesis. Furthermore, terms such as 'cystitis' and 'prostatism', based on symptoms alone, can confuse rather than clarify the final diagnosis. Only 50 per cent of women with symptoms suggesting urinary infection have evidence of bacteriuria (Gallagher et al., 1965; Mond et al., 1965), and in a study of male patients with suspected bladder outflow obstruction, 30 per cent had no objective evidence of obstructed micturition (Abrams and Feneley, 1978). Reliable criteria are essential for accurate diagnosis, for selecting appropriate treatment and for monitoring the therapeutic response.

During the past 30 years, urodynamic studies of lower urinary tract function and dysfunction have led to a greater understanding of the pathophysiology of these disorders. Quantitative evaluation of the storage and voiding mechanisms has introduced new criteria in their assessment, which have challenged the validity of traditional concepts. Subjective impressions of prostatic size (Turner-Warwick et al., 1973) or radiological reports of bladder trabeculation and residual urine (Abrams et al., 1976) must now be considered poor indicators of the severity of bladder outflow obstruction. Urodynamic data, however, need to be interpreted as critically as any other specialized clinical report. The subject has generated its own language and both the terminology and the techniques have been precisely defined to allow intelligible communications (International Continence Society 1976, 1977, 1980, 1981). Comprehensive accounts on the subject are available in recent publications (*see* Further Reading).

STORING AND VOIDING FUNCTION AND DYSFUNCTION

The Urinary Diary

Only a minority of individuals have any perception of their total urinary output in 24 hours or the maximum storage capacity of their bladder. A urinary diary, showing the pattern of micturition over a period of 7 days, is a personal record of an individual's frequency and volumes voided, and the value of such a chart cannot be overemphasized. A normal individual passes urine 4–8 times in 24 hours and the volumes usually vary between 250 and 600 ml. These measured volumes give an estimate of the average and the functional bladder capacity of the individual. Diurnal and nocturnal output of urine can be checked for either a reduced output or polyuria. Arousal at night to void urine may be caused by a bladder that has reached the limit of its functional capacity or by wakefulness from other causes that stimulate an increased bladder awareness. In the elderly, an alteration in the normal circadian rhythm can lead to an increased nocturnal output. Small voided volumes may be related to a lifelong pattern of micturition or a habit that has insidiously developed from a change in lifestyle, such as retirement. The bladder capacity may be reduced as a result of structural abnormalities in the bladder wall or by functional disturbances that limit its expansion with or expulsion of urine.

Pressure-flow Measurements

Urine is stored in the lower urinary tract so long as the pressure in the bladder remains lower than the intraluminal pressure in the urethra and voiding empties the bladder completely, if this pressure differential is reversed and sustained throughout micturition. The most comprehensive method of monitoring this dynamic sequence combines pressure-flow measurements from the bladder and urethra with simultaneous radiological display of the lower urinary tract and electromyographic (EMG) recording of pelvic floor activity. This investigation has been called video-urodynamics, which is an abbreviation for synchronous uro-video-cystourethrography (VCU), and the results can be stored on video-tape for 'playback' purposes. Video-urodynamic studies of this type are regularly performed in specialist units, but they are expensive in terms of staff and equipment. The investigation is used selectively for complex problems of incontinence and voiding disorders.

The basic urodynamic investigations provide methods of measuring the urine flow rate, urethral pressures and bladder pressures. Urine flow studies are simple and non-invasive. Intraluminal urethral pressures may be recorded as a static or a dynamic investigation. Recently, synchronous recording of bladder and urethral pressures, termed 'urethro-cystometry', has been facilitated by the development of a dual-sensor microtransducer catheter. Cystometry is used for measuring the pressure–volume relationship of the bladder. Both urethral pressure studies and cystometry have been criticized for being invasive and unphysiological but, with experience and standardization of the techniques, the results can be interpreted to give reliable and repeatable information. The level of the superior edge of the symphysis pubis is taken as the zero reference for the pressure studies, but the results require detailed attention to such factors as the position of the patient, the method of recording the pressure and the rate, temperature and type of medium infused.

DETRUSOR FUNCTION

Filling cystometry can be conveniently performed in the sitting position via a urethral catheter. The filling rate can influence the results, so this is normally specified as a slow fill (up to 10 ml/min), medium fill (up to 100 ml/min) or a rapid fill (over 100 ml/min). During filling the total bladder pressure, termed 'intravesical pressure' (P_{ves}), is usually less than 40 cmH$_2$O. Because the bladder is an intra-abdominal viscus, any rise in abdominal pressure will be directly transmitted to the bladder. Intravesical pressure is thus influenced by posture, obesity, movement or straining. Abdominal pressure (P_{abd}) is conventionally measured via a rectal balloon catheter and electronic subtraction of this from the intravesical pressure is recorded. The resultant pressure is termed 'detrusor pressure' (P_{det}) and this normally remains less than 15 cmH$_2$O throughout filling (*Fig.* 33.1). Bladder function is an ambiguous term, often used to describe the behaviour of the lower urinary tract and, to avoid confusion, the term 'detrusor function' is preferable, as it refers more specifically to the response of the bladder on filling and voiding.

Compliance

During filling, the increasing volume is accommodated with minimal change in pressure and this ratio may be expressed as 'compliance'. Normally detrusor function shows a high degree of compliance; this is related to the passive elastic and active visco-elastic properties of the bladder wall, but the mechanism of the relaxation of the detrusor muscle to stretch is not understood. It is possible to distend the bladder faster than the detrusor can relax and, under such circumstances, the detrusor pressure may increase. Fast-fill cystometry is a provocative test that may simulate reduced compliance. Detrusor hypertrophy is the most common cause of low compliance, although factors such as fibrosis or malignant infiltration of the bladder wall, may produce a similar response (*Fig.* 33.2a).

Contractility

An important feature of normal cystometry is the complete absence of a detrusor contraction during filling. Detrusor contractions are recognized by a transient rise in detrusor pressure during filling and, if these can be demonstrated either spontaneously or on provocation, such as fast filling, movement or coughing, the term 'unstable detrusor' is used (*Fig.* 33.2c). These contractions may be sufficient to produce urinary leakage, presenting clinically as urge incontinence. The patient is normally asked to suppress any attempt to void during the investigation and the ability to do so gives an indication of the individual's detrusor control. If the patient has clinical evidence of a neurological lesion, the term 'detrusor hyperreflexia' should be used to describe these involuntary contractions.

Sensation and Capacity

A sensation of a desire to void is normally experienced by the patient when the bladder has been filled to about 150–200 ml. This first desire to micturate can usually be suppressed, but a much stronger sensation returns when the bladder reaches the limit of

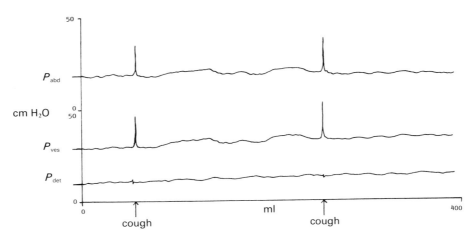

Fig. 33.1. A normal cystometrogram.

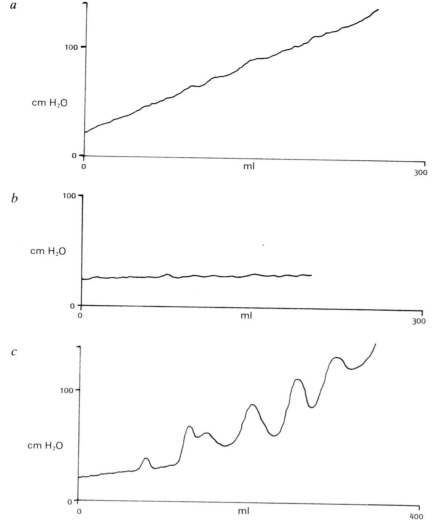

Fig. 33.2. Cystometrograms showing low compliance (*a*), hypersensitivity (*b*) and detrusor instability (*c*).

its cystometric capacity, at about 350–450 ml. Capacity is a term that should always be qualified. The functional bladder capacity has already been mentioned in association with the frequency and volume chart. Maximum cystometric capacity is assessed at the completion of the filling cystometrogram and maximum bladder capacity refers to the measured volume that the bladder will hold under either regional or deep general anaesthesia, usually at the time of a cystoscopic examination. Extreme discomfort may limit the cystometric capacity to 300 ml or less, in which case the bladder is described as hypersensitive (*Fig.* 33.2*b*).

URETHRAL FUNCTION (*Fig.* 33.3)

The storage of urine in the bladder depends not only on the detrusor response, but also on the main-

tenance of an adequate urethral resistance. The sphincter-active zone of the urethra lies between the bladder neck and the pelvic floor. Fluoroscopic studies confirm that the bladder neck normally remains closed throughout filling and, even on provocation by coughing and straining, this proximal sphincter mechanism is competent to withstand the rise in intravesical pressure. Pressure studies of the sphincter-active zone of the urethra have been performed by a variety of techniques, employing fluid perfusion systems, balloon catheters and, more recently, the microtip transducer mounted on a catheter. A static urethral pressure profile is recorded by withdrawing the catheter from the bladder through the urethra and a typical tracing for male and female subjects is obtained. 'Urethral closure pressure' is a term used to describe the pressure differential between the urethral and intravesical pressure ($P_{ura} - P_{ves}$).

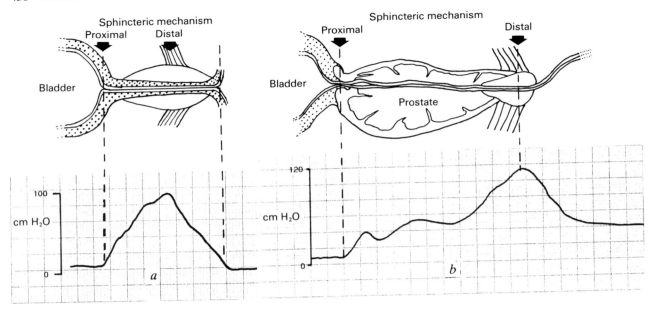

Fig. 33.3. Static urethral pressure profiles in the female (a) and male (b).

The site of the maximum urethral pressure is situated at the level of the external urethral sphincter and pelvic floor and together these constitute the distal sphincter mechanism. Gosling (1979) has described the complex arrangement of the striated musculature at this level. The intramural striated musculature of the urethra appears to be unique. It is supplied by the pelvic parasympathetic nerves and contains only slow-twitch fibres, with no evidence of muscle spindles. The peri-urethral part of the external sphincter is derived from the pubococcygeous component of the pelvic floor muscle and this consists of a mixture of both fast- and slow-twitch fibres, with associated muscle spindles. The peri-urethral muscle is supplied by the pudendal nerve. It would appear that the intramural striated musculature, or rhabdosphincter, is capable of maintaining urethral occlusion for long periods without fatigue and it is presumed that the peri-urethral part responds by contraction to any increase in intra-abdominal pressure. Pressure measurements at this level show that the maximum urethral closure pressure can be increased voluntarily by asking the patient to squeeze the urethra. Enhorning (1961) confirmed that the proximal urethra above the level of the pelvic floor is subjected to the same variations in pressure as any other intra-abdominal viscus. By asking the patient to cough during the measurement of the urethral pressure profile, this hypothesis can be tested. The urethral stress profile demonstrates the maintenance of a positive closure pressure in the normal patient (Fig. 33.4a). Negative closure pressures on coughing are associated with genuine stress incontinence (Fig. 33.4b) and this may confirm clinical observation.

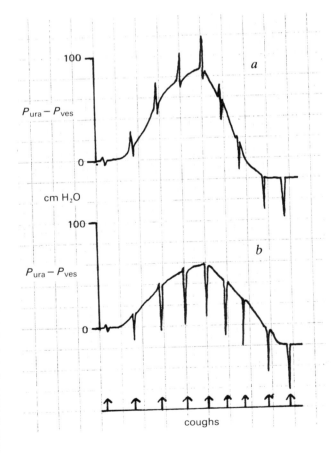

Fig. 33.4. Stress urethral profiles. a, Maintenance of positive closure pressure. b, Negative closure pressure on coughing.

VOIDING STUDIES

The initiation of voiding has been the subject of interest and debate for many years. Video-urodynamic and EMG studies of the pelvic floor have provided a detailed account of the sequence of events. In the majority of studies there is an initial decrease in the maximum urethral pressure at the level of the pelvic floor, associated with a descent of the bladder base and a reduction in EMG activity. This is followed by a rise in the detrusor pressure from active detrusor contraction, opening of the bladder neck and a complete cessation of EMG activity. Urine flow commences and normally the rise in detrusor pressure is sustained until bladder emptying has been completed.

The urine flow tracing normally shows a rapid rise to a maximum flow within 5 seconds of the commencement of voiding (*Fig.* 33.5). Women tend to

trusor pressure (P_{det} iso) and the fluid remaining in the proximal urethra is milked back into the bladder. At the completion of normal bladder emptying, urine flow stops, urethral pressure rises and the detrusor pressure usually returns simultaneously to a low level.

In voiding studies, the two parameters of urine flow rate and detrusor pressure are critical factors. A reduced urine flow rate and a raised detrusor pressure above 100 cmH$_2$O are features of obstructed micturition (*Fig.* 33.6). Interrupted or irregular flow may be due to an unsustained detrusor contraction, which may be associated with outflow tract obstruction or neuropathy. Video-urodynamics demonstrates the complex voiding disorders related to overt or covert neurological conditions, and problems such as detrusor–bladder neck dyssynergia and detrusor–sphincter dyssynergia can be more precisely defined.

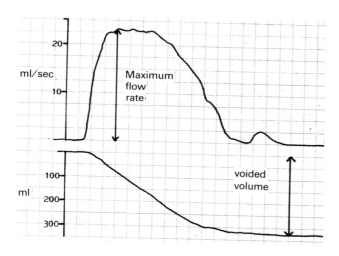

Fig. 33.5. A normal flow trace.

URINE FLOWMETRY

The measurement of the urine flow rate alone is the simplest urodynamic investigation and this can give a reliable indication of the presence or absence of obstruction. The flow rate varies with the volume voided as well as with sex and age and, if the volume voided is less than 150 ml, the measurement is unreliable. A reduced urine flow rate may be associated with a reduced functional capacity and hence it is helpful to check from the frequency and volume chart that the volumes voided are representative of the patient's normal pattern of micturition. Flow studies should be undertaken in privacy and the accuracy of the results can be more reliable if two or three rates are recorded.

void at a faster rate than men, averaging 20–25 ml/sec and with a lower detrusor pressure of 50 cmH$_2$O or less. Some habitually void by relaxation of the urethral sphincter mechanism or by increasing abdominal pressure. In men, the urine flow rate shows greater variation with age, owing to prostatic hypertrophy. Men under 45 years void at rates of around 20–25 ml/sec and this decreases to about 10–15 ml/sec in those over 65 years. Detrusor pressures in men are normally of the order of 70–80 cmH$_2$O. Measurement of the detrusor pressure does not necessarily correspond to the strength of the detrusor contraction. In the presence of a large bladder diverticulum or gross ureteric reflux, the interpretation of the detrusor pressure can be misleading. The strength of detrusor contraction and voluntary control can be estimated by asking the patient to stop voiding during micturition. Contraction of the distal sphincter mechanism is followed by an isometric rise in de-

SUMMARY

Urodynamic studies have exposed the inaccuracy of clinical diagnosis, particularly with regard to the problems of urinary incontinence and outflow obstruction. The preliminary clinical assessment of the patient is based on the history, physical examination, routine urine and blood tests and a plain radiograph of the urinary tract. This initial protocol should identify those patients with significant uropathology, invariably requiring urographic and endoscopic investigations. In the absence of such evidence, the traditional criteria for diagnosis and treatment of micturition disorders were largely empirical. Urodynamic investigations have provided a more scientific approach to the evaluation and management of the patient with lower urinary tract symptoms. Frequency and urgency of micturition, incontinence, hesitancy and a poor stream should be defined in terms of the detrusor and/or urethral dysfunction.

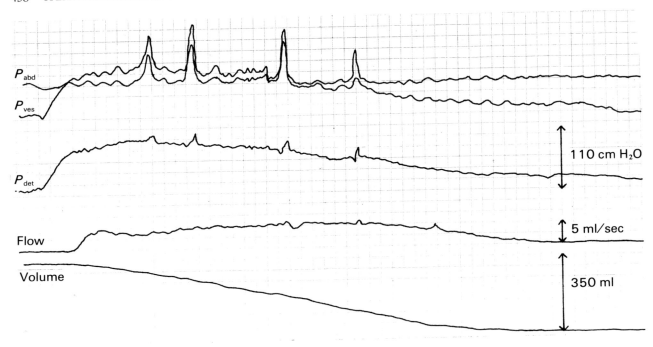

P_{abd}

P_{ves}

P_{det}

110 cm H_2O

Flow

5 ml/sec

Volume

350 ml

Fig. 33.6. An obstructed cystometrogram.

REFERENCES

Abrams P. H. and Feneley R. C. L. (1978) The significance of the symptoms associated with bladder outflow obstruction. *Urol. Int.* **33**, 171.

Abrams P. H., Roylance J. and Feneley R. C. L. (1976) Excretion urography in the investigations of prostatism. *Br. J. Urol.* **48**, 681–684.

Enhorning G. (1961) Simultaneous recording of intravesical and intraurethral pressure. *Acta Chir. Scand.* (Suppl.) **276**, 1–68.

Gallagher D. J., Montgomerie J. L. and North J. D. K. (1965) Acute infections of the urinary tract and the urethral syndrome in general practice. *Br. Med. J.* **i**, 622–626.

Gosling J. A. (1979) The structure of the bladder and urethra in relation to function. *Urol. Clin. North Am.* **6**, 31–38.

International Continence Society (1976) *Report on the Standardisation of Terminology of Lower Urinary Tract Function.* *Br. J. Urol.* **48**, 39–42.

International Continence Society (1977) *Report on the Standardisation of Terminology of Lower Urinary Tract Function.* *Br. J. Urol.* **49**, 207–210.

International Continence Society (1980) *Report on the Standardisation of Terminology of Lower Urinary Tract Function.* *Br. J. Urol.* **52**, 348–350.

International Continence Society (1981) *Reports on the Standardisation of Terminology of Lower Urinary Tract Function.* *Br. J. Urol.* **53**, 333–335.

Mond N. C., Percival A., Williams J. D. et al. (1965) Presentation diagnosis and treatment of urinary tract infections in general practice. *Lancet* **i**, 514–516.

Turner-Warwick R., Whiteside E. G., Arnold E. P. et al. (1973) A urodynamic view of prostatic obstruction and the results of prostatectomy. *Br. J. Urol.* **45**, 631–645.

FURTHER READING

Abrams P., Feneley R. and Torrens M. (1983) *Urodynamics: Clinical Practice in Urology.* Berlin, Heidelberg, New York, Springer-Verlag.

Mundy A. R., Stephenson T. P. and Wein A. J. (1984) *Urodynamics: Principles, Practice and Application.* Edinburgh, Churchill Livingstone.

Turner-Warwick R. and Whiteside C. G. (1979) *The Urologic Clinics of North America* **6**(1). Philadelphia, W. B. Saunders.

Chapter thirty-four

The Bladder and Prostate

J. B. M. Roberts

INTRODUCTION (*Fig.* 34.1)

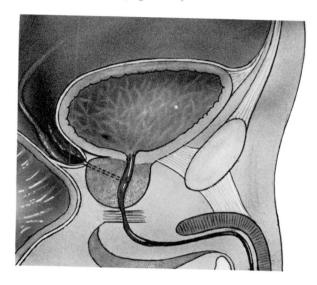

Fig. 34.1. General anatomy of the bladder and prostate.

The surgery of the bladder and prostate as practised in the 1980s involves the use of endoscopic instruments in the majority of cases and open surgical techniques are becoming increasingly rare. Training in these endoscopic manoeuvres is a very different matter from training in open surgery and involves a long clinical apprenticeship and a natural aptitude on the part of the trainee. This aptitude includes both patience and an ability to think in a three-dimensional fashion. This latter ability comes naturally to some and will blossom under supervision, while an unfortunate few will fail to grasp the basic concepts and, though excellent open surgical technicians, will never become competent endoscopic urologists.

Diagnostic ability is again largely a matter of experience. The most raw medical student will recognize the classic bladder tumour on being shown it through the cystoscope, but the borderline between normal and pathological presents perpetual problems to the most experienced endoscopist. An awareness of possibilities allied to a willingness to biopsy when in doubt will, with the backing of expert histological and cytological opinion, minimize mistakes. There is thus no adequate alternative to the carefully supervised clinical apprenticeship in the making of the endoscopic urological surgeon. Nor will the enthusiastic trainee ever regard the chance to see the nor-

mal at cystoscopy as a waste of time for appreciation of the wide range of normality facilitates the recognition of early pathology. Fortunately, modern endoscopic teaching attachments have greatly facilitated the basic teaching of the trainee (*Fig.* 34.2).

BLADDER DRAINAGE

Indications

Tube drainage of the urinary bladder is frequently necessary in surgical practice. It may be required as a temporary measure in cases of acute or chronic retention of urine, during and after surgery in the pelvis where the bladder must be kept empty to gain access to the other pelvic organs, or after surgery on the bladder or prostate. Drainage is necessary in order to drain blood and clots from the bladder, to enable irrigation of the bladder to be performed and to facilitate the healing of bladder incisions by keeping the bladder deflated for 5–7 days. Urinary drainage may also be required in the incontinent or unconscious patient. The urine flow may need to be monitored accurately in cases of oliguria or where a high urine output is expected, as in the treatment of cardiac failure with diuretics.

Permanent tube drainage of the bladder may be required for incontinent patients, those with a small capacity bladder, paraplegics and in the bedridden or terminal patient.

Method

The conventional method of draining the bladder is by a urethral catheter. This must be inserted under strict aseptic conditions and can usually be accomplished using local urethral anaesthesia, which is achieved by instilling 1 per cent lignocaine jelly into the urethra, either direct from its tube or by the use of a plastic syringe without a needle. The local anaesthetic is preferably associated with an antiseptic such as chlorhexidine in order to minimize the risk of introducing infection into the bladder from the infected anterior urethra. Having introduced a quantity of jelly into the anterior urethra, the meatus is then occluded by pressure over the glans and the jelly is massaged back into the posterior urethra. A few minutes are allowed for it to take effect when it should be possible to introduce a well-lubricated catheter without discomfort to the patient. Despite

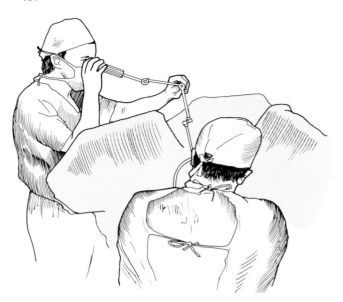

Fig. 34.2. Modern articulated endoscopic teaching attachment.

these precautions, some agitated patients fail to relax adequately and the catheter tip will be held up at the level of the external urethral sphincter. This block can usually be overcome by a combination of reassurance on the part of the operator and deep breathing on the part of the patient which serves largely to distract the patient from the procedure and allows relaxation of the sphincter. The self-retaining Foley balloon catheter is most commonly used and sterility is encouraged by inserting the catheter direct from its sterile plastic container into the urethra without it being touched by hand or instrument. Having introduced the catheter into the anterior urethra, traction on the penis will straighten out the posterior urethra and facilitate the passage of the catheter. The self-retaining balloon is inflated with sterile water or

saline (10–15 ml are usually sufficient) and the catheter connected aseptically to a disposable closed-drainage bag with a non-return valve. The draining tube of the catheter should be fixed to the thigh to prevent repeated traction trauma to the external urethral meatus with the risk of later stenosis. Finally, it cannot be stressed too strongly that having established aseptic catheterization the closed drainage which ensues should be protected as absolutely as possible. Breakage in the closed drainage from the bladder to the collecting bag results in the passage of air bubbles up the column of urine in the catheter and to the bladder, and there is a high risk that these bubbles will be contaminated with the organisms of the hospital ward which are all too frequently antibiotic resistant. Infection is the greatest hazard in bladder and prostatic surgery and the most important step in its prevention is the maintenance of an

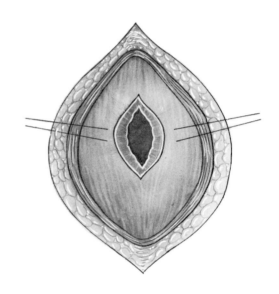

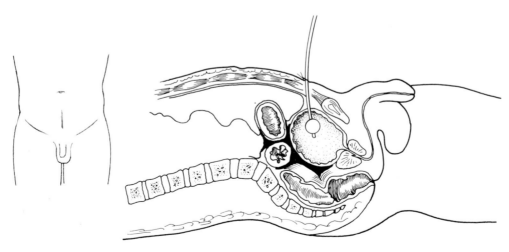

Fig. 34.3. Suprapubic cystotomy and bladder drainage. It is important that the bladder is distended preoperatively.

adequately closed bladder drainage system whenever a catheter is present.

Successful drainage of the bladder may also be achieved by the suprapubic extraperitoneal route, either by a formal operative suprapubic cystostomy or by a percutaneous method using a specially made disposable suprapubic catheter. It is most important that if this route is used the bladder be full and that this be confirmed by needle aspiration of urine before an attempt is made to insert a catheter. Particular care should be taken when there is a previous lower abdominal incision which may have resulted in adhesions fixing loops of small bowel to the dome of the bladder making their perforation a hazard during the catheterization. Suprapubic catheterization is particularly indicated in cases of stricture of the urethra and after failure of the urethral method. Suprapubic catheterization has the advantage of causing less sepsis and, of course, avoids trauma to the urethra. It is also easy to allow a trial of micturition if this is desirable by simply clamping the suprapubic catheter. Again, a strict aseptic technique is used and either method of inserting a suprapubic drain can be achieved under local anaesthetic. The conventional open procedure is achieved through a small suprapubic incision in the midline, incision of the linea alba and then opening of the bladder between stay sutures. A suitable catheter (self-retaining Foley catheter is commonly used) is then inserted and the wound sutured around the catheter. The percutaneous suprapubic catheter is readily inserted under local anaesthetic and a small preliminary skin incision is made with a scalpel blade. This suprapubic catheter can be positioned accurately and has a collar for fixing to the skin and a self retaining balloon which can be inflated via a side arm (*Fig.* 34.3).

Complications

Ascending infection into the bladder can be minimized by the use of a strict aseptic technique and wherever possible it is preferable to perform the catheterization in the operating theatre. The use of an antiseptic lubricant (chlorhexidine and glycerin) is advised. The urine should be cultured repeatedly for evidence of ascending infection and some closed drainage systems now allow for this by inserting a rubber section in the tubing through which a sample can be obtained with a syringe and needle. Regular catheter care is employed for the duration of the catheterization and the patient is encouraged to drink freely in order to ensure good urine flow. Transient bacteraemia may occur during catheterization if the urine is already infected and any instrumentation of the urethra or bladder in the presence of sepsis should be covered by antibiotic as prophylaxis against Gram-negative septicaemia.

Urethral stricture is a particularly troublesome complication of urethral catheterization and the risk

may be minimized by using the smallest catheter compatible with drainage of the bladder.

In long-term drainage of the bladder, phosphatic encrustation on the tip of the catheter will require regular changes of urethral catheter and this complication can be minimized by the use of medical-grade silicone rubber catheters. Using these new catheters it is possible to lengthen the interval between catheter changes.

ENDOSCOPIC INSTRUMENTS (*Fig.* 34.4)

The cystoscope is of course the classic endoscopic instrument used by the urologist, but in the sense of it being an endoscope through which can be assessed only the state of the bladder it has long been superseded by the panendoscope which, with a choice of different telescopes, allows the lower urinary tract to be assessed from the external urethral meatus through the urethra to the bladder. This allows urethral pathology to be accurately visualized and avoids the false passages produced by the blind instrumentation with a cystoscope failing to negotiate an unsuspected stricture (*see Fig.* 34.6).

Both panendoscope and cystoscope consist of a hollow tube which will carry a telescope, a light source and allow two-way passage of fluid from a sterile external source to distend the urethra and bladder.

Panendoscopy (*Fig.* 34.5)

Examination of the urethral and bladder mucosa is readily achieved using a modern irrigating panendoscope with a fibre-optic light source. The procedure is easier to perform under general anaesthesia and this method should always be used for the initial diagnostic cystoscopy for haematuria and when a bladder tumour is suspected. However, under local anaesthesia, achieved by instillation of 1 per cent lignocaine jelly into the urethra, as for catheterization, it can be performed by a skilled operator as an outpatient procedure.

With the patient in the lithotomy position the field is prepared as for an open operation. The assembly and function of the instrument to be used are checked. The panendoscope is passed down the anterior urethra with the penis drawn upwards and during the whole procedure a clear view is obtained of the expanding urethra in front of the instrumental tip. Urethral pathology may be assessed and an obstructing stricture be visualized and dealt with by urethrotomy rather than blindly dilated with the probable production of a false passage. When the tip of the instrument has negotiated the angle at the perineal membrane the outer end of the panendoscope is gently depressed between the patient's legs

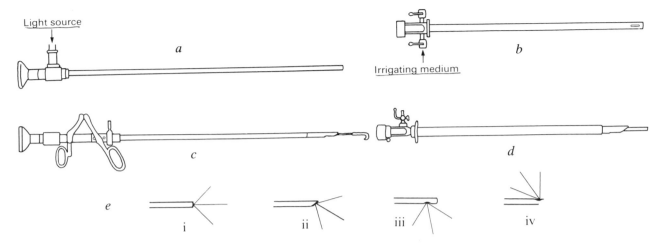

Light source

a

Irrigating medium

b

c

d

e

i   ii   iii   iv

Fig. 34.4. Endoscopic instruments. *a,* Fibre-optic telescope. *b,* Irrigating sheath. *c,* Resectoscope cutting unit. *d,* Resectoscope irrigating sheath. *e,* Telescope types with fields of view: i, 0°; ii, 30°; iii, 70°; iv, 120°.

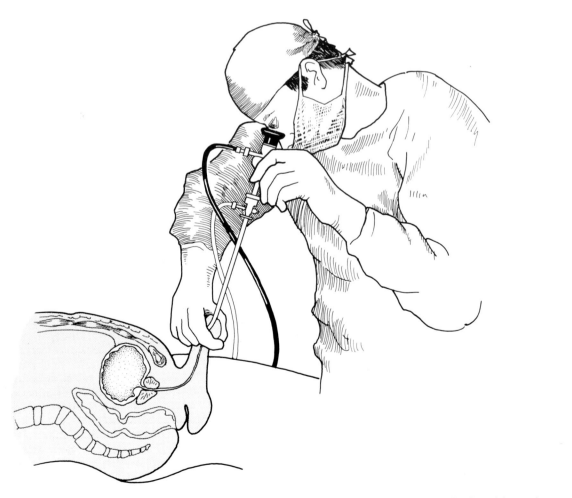

Fig. 34.5. Panendoscopy. The instrument is passed into the bladder under direct vision allowing detailed examination of the urethra.

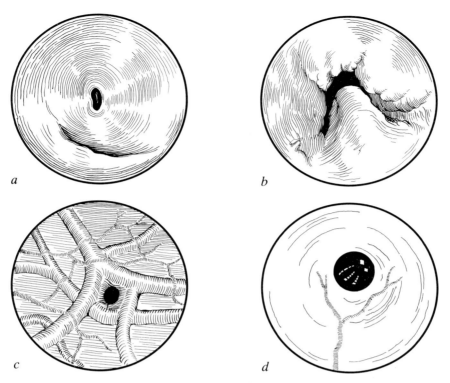

Fig. 34.6. Some typical endoscopic appearances during the passage of the panendoscope into the bladder. *a*, Urethral stricture. *b*, Verumontanum. *c*, Trabeculation with mouth of small diverticulum. *d*, Air bubble in bladder dome.

and the panendoscope should be seen to enter the bladder (*Fig.* 34.6).

In the female the short urethra rarely presents any problem to instrumentation although in postmenopausal patients oestrogen deficiency may produce a stricture and rarely a carcinoma, either of the urethra itself or of gynaecological origin, which may interfere with instrumentation. Routine examination should include an inspection of the urethra, the prostate, the bladder neck and the entire bladder surface. The ureteric orifices should be found and inspected (*Fig.* 34.7) and this apparently simple task requires substantial experience and will often defeat the inexperienced endoscopist. The ureteric orifice has no single classic shape or appearance and this is one of the many features which may vary enormously within the range of normality, hence it is repeated that no student endoscopist should neglect the opportunity to inspect as many normal bladders as is possible in order that the essentially normal should not be mistaken for the diseased.

In the initial stages of the panendoscopy, a 0° or 30° telescope is necessary as the view to be obtained is that directly ahead of the advancing panendoscope. However, once the bladder has been entered a better view is obtained using a 70° instrument which will view laterally while the anterior wall may in some patients not be visualized with other than a 120° telescope which is not commonly found as a part of the urological armamentarium. The bladder mucosa should be inspected for evidence of inflammation which is characterized by increased vascularity, cystic changes or bleeding on distension. The presence of one or more tumours will obviously be a major discovery while trabeculation varying from a fine network under the mucosa to quite coarse sacculation or even diverticulum formation should be assessed. Obviously these signs, which are indicative of either obstruction or bladder dysfunction, should be associated with a careful assessment of the bladder outlet to decide if obstruction is likely to be present and, if so, at what level. When doubt still exists a urodynamic assessment may well be indicated (*see* Chapter 33).

Retrograde catheterization of the ureteric orifice (using a Chevassu catheter) or of the ureter (using a straight ureteric catheter) may be achieved using the catheterizing cystoscope (*Fig.* 34.8). A retrograde ureterogram is performed by the injection of contrast medium into a Chevassu catheter introduced into the ureteric orifice and care must be taken to avoid overdistending the collecting system lest extravasation of the contrast occurs. Radiographs are taken most conveniently using a portable image intensifier. This is not always available and the patient may need to be moved to the radiology department. It must be stressed that with the increasingly impressive standard of excretion urography which is obtained in

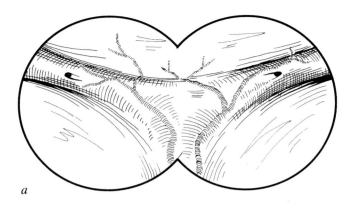

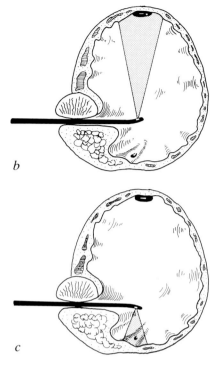

Fig. 34.7. Some typical cystoscopic appearances. *a*, Typical appearance of trigone showing ureteric orifices. *b*, Dome air bubble located with 70° endoscope. *c*, 70° endoscope rotated through 180° to locate the trigone.

modern radiological departments the need for retrograde catheterization to produce X-ray images has reduced enormously and what was once a standard procedure on every urological operating list is now undertaken rarely.

Cystoscopy is indicated in the investigation of bladder infections and of haematuria and may reveal cystitis, bladder tumour, bladder stone, diverticulum or other evidence of bladder neck obstruction such as trabeculation. The presence, position and number of ureteric orifices can be confirmed. The degree of

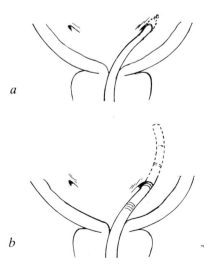

Fig. 34.8. Retrograde catheterization of the ureteric orifice or ureter. *a*, Chevassu catheter which is just introduced into the ureteric orifice. *b*, Straight catheter may be passed well up into the ureter into the renal pelvis.

prostatic enlargement can be assessed by noting the length of the prostatic urethra, the contours of the lateral lobe and projection of the middle lobe into the bladder. The overall size of the prostate can be estimated by simultaneous palpation through the rectum with the cystoscope in place.

BLADDER TUMOURS (*Fig.* 34.9)

Nearly all bladder tumours are transitional cell carcinomas of varying malignancy and truly benign tumours are rare. Squamous cell carcinoma may occur in areas of squamous metaplasia and adenocarcinoma may arise from a urachal remnant or be due to secondary spread. Carcinoma of the bladder arises chiefly from the age of 40 onwards and has a male predominance of 3:1. However, it may occur at much earlier ages; examples in teenagers are well documented. Cytological screening of the urine is carried out on workers exposed to beta-naphthylamines, benzidine, auramine and magenta.

The clinical presentation is classically with painless haematuria, but it may also present with the symptoms of cystitis. Assessment of the patient includes intravenous urography which may demonstrate a bladder tumour (more than 3 cm in diameter), further tumours in the urothelium of the ureter and pelvis of the kidney, and evidence of ureteric obstruction by a tumour of the bladder infiltrating a ureteric orifice. Carcinoma of the bladder is classified by its histological grading and clinical staging. Confirmation of the diagnosis and clinical staging are achieved by cystoscopy, biopsy of a representative portion and bimanual examination of the bladder.

Management of Carcinoma of the Bladder

Transitional cell bladder tumours present a wide range of biological activity varying from the rare and truly benign papilloma to very aggressive, poorly differentiated tumours of high malignancy. Hence, the treatment must be fitted to the particular tumour as demonstrated by endoscopic assessment, palpation under anaesthetic and most essentially biopsy and subsequent histology. All these manoeuvres increase the accuracy of the staging process (*Fig.* 34.9).

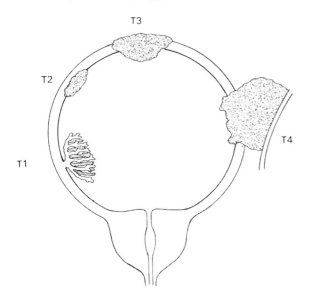

Fig. 34.9. Stages of carcinoma of the bladder with notes on findings at bimanual palpation. T1, Superficial mucosal lesion. Impalpable. T2, Tumour invading muscle wall detectable as a thickening only. T3, The tumour has penetrated the bladder wall. T4, Fixed to the side wall of the pelvis and no longer mobile.

Well-differentiated Superficial Tumours

These are usually managed by transurethral endoscopic resection with diathermy to the exposed tumour base. The bladder should be cleared of tumour at the initial session if possible and the patient warned of the necessity for long-term endoscopic review. Normally the first review should be undertaken at 3–6 months after the initial resection and be performed under general anaesthetic. Later reviews are repeated at increasing intervals until a yearly check is being undertaken if the tumour is obviously controlled. The role of various intravesical cytotoxic agents such as thiotepa and adriamycin has been discussed at great length over recent years, but the results in most series have been disappointing.

It is important in resecting bladder tumours to remove the base completely and extend the resection into bladder muscle, and particularly in the very thin, elderly, female bladder this produces a significant risk of perforation of the bladder. This risk is increased if resection is undertaken when the bladder is partially empty and the resectoscope loop may cut

through a fold of redundant wall related to the tumour, producing a substantial perforation. Should such a perforation occur, prolonged catheter drainage for 1 week should be undertaken unless the breach is extensive when repair and extravesical drainage may be necessary. Prolonged ileus and low-grade peritonitis may ensue from intraperitoneal leakage of urine. Careful haemostasis is essential which can at times be extremely difficult, time consuming and requiring great patience.

The endoscopic appearances of bladder tumours may be very obvious at times, but there are also occasions when a mossy granular appearance is all that will be seen as a guide to areas of activity, while blind biopsy of the four quadrants of the bladder, where the mucosa is apparently normal, will at times produce histological evidence of neoplasia. Such biopsy is desirable in the long-term follow-up of bladder tumours, and is aided by the instillation of methylene blue prior to cystoscopy, areas of neoplasia being stained.

When the bladder surface is diffusely covered with rapidly recurring tumours, it may be treated by the use of prolonged bladder distension under epidural anaesthesia, using an intravesical balloon as has been advocated by Helmstein, which in some cases will produce a most dramatic clearing of the tumour. BCG inoculation, followed by intracavity injection of the BCG, has recently been reported as producing impressive results in the patient with rapidly recurring superficial bladder tumours. Using these various techniques, total cystectomy should rarely be necessary as a means of managing the extensive, well-differentiated, superficial transitional cell carcinoma of the bladder. It is of course important to remember that the nature of the tumour may change and it is not safe to assume that the initial biopsy on discovery of the tumour will act as an infallible guide to the nature of the tumour for the rest of the history of the disease. During long-term follow-up of these tumours, it is important to remember that this is a disease of the whole transitional cell epithelium from the calyces of the kidneys to the distal urethra; the whole of this area has been exposed to an assumed carcinogen and review should, therefore, include excretion urography at intervals of 2–3 years, panendoscopy as well as cystoscopy and cytology when all else appears to be clear. Excretion urography should be undertaken at an earlier interval if the patient experiences recurrent haematuria and the urethra and bladder appear to be clear endoscopically. Equally it is necessary when a positive cytological report remains unexplained by endoscopy.

In the frail and elderly, it may well be wise to minimize endoscopic review which may be more hazardous than the condition being treated. Under these circumstances treatment of symptoms, assisted by cytological review of the urine, may reduce the need for review to 2- or 3-yearly intervals.

Invasive Bladder Tumours

As with all bladder tumours, the first essential is to establish the diagnosis as accurately as possible, which requires bacteriological and radiological screening, followed by endoscopy, biopsy and careful examination under anaesthetic. This will lead to the establishment of the histological nature of the tumour, the grading of the tumour into well or poorly differentiated, and if the biopsy bites are taken well into the bladder muscle this information, together with the examination under anaesthetic, will identify the degree of invasion. It is important to remember that the degree of the spread of the tumour tends to be underestimated rather than exaggerated, and once these facts have been established at the initial endoscopic examination, the surgeon is in a position to commence the treatment which is appropriate to the particular tumour. A small invasive tumour may be completely cleared by an adequate transurethral resection with the resectoscope, and if this is considered to be appropriate it is justifiable to reassess the bladder in 3 months and repeat the biopsy. If the bladder is then tumour free, a watching brief may be maintained. If, however, active tumour is found to be present at this review, various methods of treatment are possible. These include:

1. Radiotherapy in a radical course and unassociated with further surgery.
2. Limited radiotherapy of 4000 rad followed by early total cystectomy and urinary diversion.
3. Total cystectomy and urinary diversion without radiotherapy.
4. If the tumour is very advanced and in the elderly patient, limited radiotherapy in the hope of controlling symptoms, especially haematuria, may be justified.

The results of various regimens of combined chemotherapy are not yet adequately documented. The initial results leave most surgeons depressed and have not been impressive.

Total Cystectomy (Fig. 34.10)

This is a major prolonged procedure with a significant (6–10 per cent) operative mortality. It is rarely indicated in cases of uncontrollable multiple superficial lesions which are beyond the scope of endoscopic diathermy, but is generally indicated for advanced tumours affecting the trigone and for recurrence of tumour or severe haemorrhage after irradiation.

With the patient supine on the operating table and a little Trendelenburg tilt, a long right paramedian or midline incision is made. The peritoneum is opened and the extent of tumour spread beyond the bladder is noted. The peritoneum is then divided circumferentially around the pelvic brim more or less along the line of the external iliac artery and is dissected from this point, proceeding in a plane close to the pelvic wall and this is facilitated by ligation of both internal iliac arteries. This plane is followed

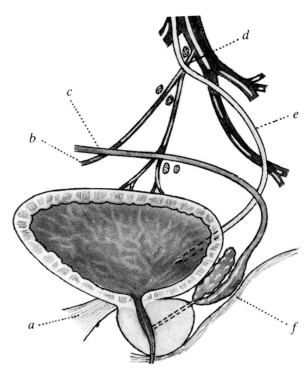

Fig. 34.10. Structures requiring division in total cystectomy. The vas deferens offers a good guide. *a,* Pubo-prostatic ligament. *b,* Obliterated umbilical artery. *c,* Vas deferens. *d,* Anterior division of internal iliac artery. *e,* Ureter. *f,* Denonvilliers' fascia.

towards the apex of the prostate which involves cutting the pubo-prostatic ligaments and ligating a large block of veins running anterior to the prostate. These are very friable and usually it is preferable to control bleeding from them by an adequately placed stitch using either a conventional or a boomerang needle. After this the urethra is divided distal to the prostate and the cystoprostatic mass delivered out of the pelvis dissecting it off the anterior rectal wall. Particularly after radiotherapy it is important to take great care with this dissection as opening the rectum under these circumstances will frequently lead to a faecal fistula despite the most meticulous suturing of the defect at the time of surgery. The prostate and bladder are then delivered abdominally until the initial dissection is encountered. All glands on the lateral wall are removed and identified and great care is taken with haemostasis. If there is evidence of urethral tumour at initial panendoscopy then a urethrectomy should be performed at the same time by dissecting the urethra out from the glans penis to the prostate and then removing it en bloc with the bladder and prostate. A urethrectomy is always performed in the female and most surgeons would remove the uterus and ovaries en bloc with the bladder to minimize the risk of residual disease being left in the pelvis.

When the malignant mass has been removed and haemostasis adequately achieved it is useful to leave a pack in the pelvis and then proceed to urinary diversion, which will be normally by means of an ileal conduit. It is important to remember in choosing the loop of bowel for the conduit that an irradiated loop which has been fixed in the pelvis may have poor healing potential and should therefore be avoided. At the end of the procedure no attempt is made to close the peritoneum. The pelvis is drained both through the wound and usefully through the urethra or the site of the urethra and the wound closed.

Postoperative care involves adequate replacement of blood loss, nasogastric tube suction and intravenous hydration until the often quite significant paralytic ileus has resolved and early mobilization and encouragement which may present some difficulties in the rather frail and elderly patient who is at times exposed to this major surgery. The pelvic drainage can normally be removed after 3–5 days and the patient is frequently ready for discharge in 10–14 days postoperatively despite the magnitude of the surgery and the considerable age of many of the patients.

Partial Cystectomy

Partial cystectomy is a rarely performed operation today, being reserved for tumours of the urachus and perhaps tumours in diverticula. The vast majority of tumours which were so treated previously will now be managed transurethrally.

BLADDER DIVERTICULUM

Most diverticula of the bladder are pulsion diverticula arising as a result of sustained increase in intravesical pressure due to bladder outflow obstruction. There are also rare congenital diverticula unassociated with bladder outflow obstruction, while it is common in severe cases of vesico-ureteric reflux to see a para-ureteric diverticulum whose management is essentially the management of the reflux. A large diverticulum may contain considerable residual urine producing the symptom of double micturition and often producing urinary infection in the stagnant pool of urine which is singularly difficult to eradicate. Stasis of urine within the diverticulum may also be responsible for the occurrence of bladder stone or tumour within the diverticulum, both of which may be difficult to visualize on cystoscopy.

A traction diverticulum of the bladder may be caused by incorporation of the bladder into a femoral or direct inguinal hernia, which may occasionally give rise to urinary symptoms in a patient with a hernia. This is a true diverticulum which is composed of the full thickness of the bladder wall. The extraperitoneal variety places the bladder at serious risk of injury during operations on such hernias, and the bladder may be inadvertently opened during excision of the sac. If this mishap is recognized at the time, the bladder wall should be repaired in two layers and continuous bladder drainage instituted for 5–7 days. If the injury remains unrecognized, a urinary fistula through the herniorrhaphy wound is likely to develop.

The diagnosis of bladder diverticulum may be suspected on clinical grounds or on contrast urography. Diverticulum must be excluded in all cases of prostatic bladder outflow obstruction by cystoscopy prior to surgery. Excision is indicated for large diverticula and for the complications of persistent urinary infection, stone or tumour. As the vast majority of diverticula of the bladder are secondary to bladder outflow obstruction, it is essential that this obstruction should be relieved at the same time as the diverticulum is dealt with otherwise neither the patient's symptoms nor the probable associated infection are likely to be eradicated.

Excision of Bladder Diverticulum

Preliminary cystoscopy confirms the presence and situation of the diverticulum and also enables an adequate assessment of the bladder outlet to be undertaken. Some surgeons prefer to insert a ureteric catheter at this stage while others would carry out the procedure transvesically. It is, however, an essential step in the management of most diverticula whose orifices are near the trigone or on the lateral wall as frequently the ureter is closely related to the diverticulum and may be damaged during the dissection. With the patient in the Trendelenburg position the bladder is exposed extraperitoneally and opened between stay sutures. The orifice of the diverticulum is identified and the diverticulum is packed with gauze; following this an extraperitoneal dissection is undertaken, great care being taken of the ureter which is the more easily identified by the presence of the ureteric catheter. It is useful to open the neck of the diverticulum anteriorly and to insert a retractor or a bladder neck spreader to control the region. In some patients the dissection and excision of the diverticulum are easy, but in others, particularly after long-standing infection, it may be a very difficult procedure. In such cases, if the ureter is significantly at risk then the neck of the diverticulum may be completely divided, the bladder closed and the diverticulum left *in situ* with a drain running down to it for some 10–14 days. Otherwise, diverticulectomy is performed, the bladder is closed with extramucosal catgut sutures and drained per urethram for 5 days.

It cannot be overstated that there is usually associated bladder outflow obstruction which may be dealt with by transvesical prostatectomy at the time of the diverticulectomy or, preferably in the majority of cases, by transurethral resection at the time of the initial cystoscopy prior to diverticulectomy.

BLADDER STONE

A vesical calculus is usually the result of stagnation of urine secondary to obstruction within the bladder or of encrustation on a foreign body within the bladder. The composition of a bladder calculus is usually mixed and so oxalate, urate and cystine may be represented in addition to triple phosphate. When the patient is sitting or standing, the stone lies on the trigone and gives rise to suprapubic discomfort and pain felt at the tip of the penis. The patient complains of frequency of micturition by day and there may be terminal haematuria. On occasion, the stone may interrupt the urine flow, resulting in incomplete emptying of the bladder.

Stones less than 3 cm in diameter may conveniently be dealt with using the cystoscopic lithotrite. The bladder is inspected by cystoscopy. The lithotrite is then inserted and the stone(s) crushed under vision. The debris is evacuated. The patient should be given antibiotics as prophylaxis against Gram-negative septicaemia, if infection is present or suspected.

Larger stones should be removed by open cystotomy and associated bladder neck obstruction or diverticulum can be dealt with at the same time.

PERMANENT URINARY DIVERSION

Diversion of urine with transplantation of the ureters is indicated in total cystectomy, and occasionally for the palliation of ureteric obstruction, for vesicovaginal fistula, the neuropathic bladder (most often due to spina bifida) and in ectopia vesicae. It may also be indicated in patients with a small capacity bladder although this may be enlarged by the operation of caecocystoplasty.

Implantation of both ureters into the sigmoid colon (uretero-sigmoidostomy) has, to a large extent, been replaced by the implantation of the ureters into an ileal conduit. A rectal bladder may also be used by diverting the faecal stream through a terminal sigmoid colostomy and transplanting the ureters into the rectal stump. It is, of course, essential that if this latter procedure is carried out, total continence of the rectal sphincter for fluid be ascertained prior to operation.

Uretero-ileostomy (Ileal Bladder, Ileal Conduit)
(*Figs.* 34.11, 34.12)
Satisfactory long-term diversion of urine can be achieved by using a segment of terminal ileum to conduct the urine from both ureters to the surface of the abdomen where it is conveniently collected in a modern urostomy appliance. The ileal stoma is conventionally sited in the right iliac fossa and the site chosen should be clear of bony points, scars and the umbilicus. The advice of a stomatherapist is invaluable at this stage.

The selection of the most appropriate site should be made preoperatively with the patient up and about the ward, wearing a urostomy appliance to find the most comfortable site, which is then marked on the

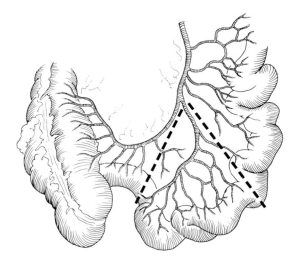

Fig. 34.11. Planning of ileal conduit based on an arteriovenous pedicle.

abdominal skin. With the patient supine and a little Trendelenburg tilt, the abdomen is opened through a paramedian or midline incision. The ureters are identified as they cross the bifurcations of the common iliac arteries, divided and the proximal cut ends are held with stay sutures. Appendicectomy is performed. A length of ileum based on a suitable arcade of vessels is chosen 30–35 cm in length. The ileal segment will protrude through the chosen site on the abdominal wall for some 5 cm so that evagination and suture will produce a spout some 2·5 cm in length (it must be borne in mind that the conduit is not a reservoir and stenosis of the stoma must be guarded against by excision of an adequate disc of skin and careful suture of mucosa to skin without producing

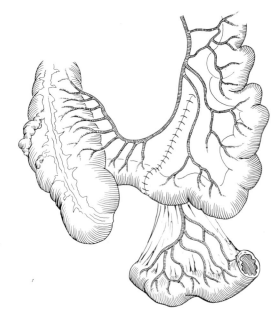

Fig. 34.12. Isolated vascularized ileal loop prior to implantation of ureters.

necrosis of the ileum). The left ureter is brought up through the pelvic mesocolon. Anastomosis of the ureters to the ileum can be achieved in a number of ways, but as the conduit is not a reservoir there should be no necessity for anti-reflux techniques in performing the anastomosis. Anastomosis can be conveniently achieved using the technique described by Wallace. In this technique the ends of both divided ureters are fish-tailed to enlarge them, the two are then sutured together along half the circumference to produce a single joint stoma which is anastomosed to the end of the ileum conduit. The area of the anastomosis is fixed by several interrupted sutures to the posterior wall of the abdominal cavity (*Fig.* 34.13) and the abdomen closed with drainage.

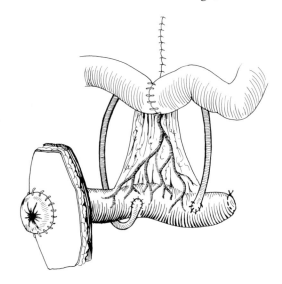

Fig. 34.13. Ileal conduit for urinary diversion. Following resection of the ileal segment the mesentery must be carefully closed.

Opinions are divided whether splintage of the uretero-ileo anastomosis should be undertaken, but certainly it is the preference of the author, although it is important to fix the splints externally so that they do not slip back into the conduit. There should be no tension on the anastomosis and stenosis should be guarded against.

An indwelling Foley catheter is left in the conduit via the stoma for some days to ensure free drainage of urine and to avoid pressure build-up within the ileum. A suitable drainable urostomy appliance may then be used.

Provided that care is taken to ensure an adequate blood supply to the isolated ileal loop and to the ureters by keeping mobilization to a minimum, then problems with healing or stenosis should not occur. The abdominal wall skin is, of course, at risk from ammoniacal dermatitis and the ileal spout is prone to phosphatic encrustation. Hernia, retraction and stenosis of the stoma are all avoidable technical failures. Hyperchloraemic acidosis (*see below*) is

much less likely to occur with an ileal conduit, particularly if free drainage is ensured. However, the use of an excessively long loop of ileum may predispose to the complication.

Ureterocolic Anastomosis (Uretero-sigmoidostomy) (*Fig.* 34.14)

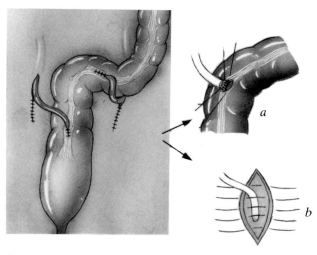

Fig. 34.14. Ureterocolic anastomosis. *a,* End-to-side anastomosis (Cordonnier). *b,* Tunnel insertion (Coffey).

This procedure has, to a large extent, been replaced by the ileal conduit because of the complications which may ensue from anastomosis of the ureters to the colon in continuity. In particular, ascending infection is likely to occur with the production of pyelonephritis and significantly impaired renal function is a contra-indication to this operation. The selective absorption of chloride from the colon is thought to be responsible for the complication of hyperchloraemic acidosis which will require careful long-term observation and regular biochemical monitoring. However, ureterocolic anastomosis can be a useful procedure in those patients who would not tolerate the longer operating time required for the formation of an ileal conduit and in those for whom an abdominal stoma is inappropriate (the elderly, blind or arthritic patient). Total rectal continence must, of course, be confirmed before diverting the urine into the colon.

Bowel preparation by distal washouts and antibiotics unabsorbed by the bowel are necessary to prevent infection. The abdomen is opened through a midline or paramedian incision and the sigmoid colon is exposed by packing off the small bowel. The ureter is divided as low as possible and care is taken to avoid mobilizing the ureter over a distance further than is necessary in order to preserve its blood supply. The proximal cut end of the ureter is held by stay sutures and an appropriate site for anastomosis with the sigmoid colon is chosen to avoid any tension on the ureter. Care must also be taken to avoid angulation or twisting of the ureter which might also embarrass its blood supply. Direct end-to-side anastomosis of the ureter to the colon by the Cordonnier method will usefully guard against stenosis. Mucosa-to-mucosa suturing is employed without undue tension, using interrupted absorbable sutures. To guard against reflux at the anastomosis the Coffey method may be employed, in which a submucous tunnel is fashioned by laying the ureter in a longitudinal incision through all layers but mucosa, the cut end of the ureter entering the colon through a stab hole in the mucosa at the distal end. The ureteric stay suture is then passed through the bowel wall from inside and tied on the serosal surface of the colon. The mucosal tunnel is then fashioned by closing the seromuscular incision over the ureter. The ureter is held in position in this tunnel by picking up its surface with these sutures. Undue tension and constriction of the ureter must be avoided and haemostasis must be meticulous to avoid the occurrence of a haematoma within the wall of the colon which may compress the ureter. Anastomotic leakage and stenosis are the main complications and free drainage into the colon must be ensured. The addition of a sigmoid myotomy to the procedure may help to prevent back pressure effects on the upper urinary tract (*see* Chapter 18).

Postoperatively, regular drainage of urine from the rectum is required and a drainage tube is often left within the rectum immediately postoperatively in order to avoid the accumulation of urine within the rectum. Frequent evacuation of urine from the rectum must be ensured following this procedure and alkalis are indicated if acidosis is a problem. A postoperative intravenous excretory urogram will demonstrate the adequacy of drainage from the ureters.

VESICO-URETERIC REFLUX IN CHILDHOOD

The well-established relationship between recurrent urinary tract infection and vesico-ureteric reflux in the young has led to a variety of operations to correct the reflux. Chronic pyelonephritis and renal scarring are the common sequelae of this combination but as much of the damage is probably produced in the first year of life and before the diagnosis is established the value of such surgery is now under review. The essential element of each of the operations is to reproduce the length of intravesical ureter which is normally present but is lost in these cases. The method used varies from the formal mobilization of the ureter with reimplantation in a long submucosal tunnel (Leadbetter–Politano, Johnson) to operations where the mobilized ureter is pulled through the existing entry point and fixed within the bladder (Cohen).

The reflux requires no correction if merely a transient flicker up the ureter (grade I) at micturating cystography or when reaching up to the kidney without dilatation (grade II) as long as the infection is controlled by antibiotics. When conservative control fails, however, and this is commonly the case when a dilated ureter has been produced (grade III) reimplantation should be considered. There is little convincing evidence that sterile reflux is harmful to the well-developed kidney.

VESICO-COLIC AND VESICOVAGINAL FISTULA

Vesico-colic Fistula

A fistulous communication between the rectosigmoid and the bladder usually results from colonic diverticular disease. Less frequently Crohn's disease affecting the colon or small bowel, carcinoma of the sigmoid colon or carcinoma of the bladder may result in a fistulous communication with the bowel. The clinical results of such a fistula are symptoms of cystitis and, classically, the passage of gas per urethram (pneumaturia) and sometimes faecal material. It may not be possible to demonstrate the communication either by barium enema or by cystography. At cystoscopy, an intense cystitis is found and this often obscures the site of a small communication with the bowel. On bimanual examination, a mass is palpable in the region of the fistula. Such fistulas rarely close spontaneously and require surgical separation of the bowel from the bladder. In view of the dense inflammatory reaction around such a fistula, it is occasionally necessary to perform a defunctioning proximal colostomy. This can result in dramatic resolution of the patient's symptoms and of the inflammation surrounding the fistula so that a subsequent surgical approach to the fistula can be made. The colon and bladder are separated and the defect in the bladder closed followed by catheter drainage for 7–10 days. The diseased bowel is resected and anastomosis performed. The colostomy is closed later if one has been used to cover the resection.

Vesicovaginal Fistula (*Fig.* 34.15)

Vesicovaginal fistula may result from obstetric trauma, irradiation of the cervix, or follow accidental injury to the bladder during gynaecological operations. Those cases which follow childbirth are believed to be caused by pressure necrosis of the bladder wall due to the pressure of the fetal head.

Examination under anaesthetic will reveal leakage of urine into the vagina and the fistula site may be visualized. In view of the difficulty of confirming the fistula site on cystoscopy, help may be obtained by passing a probe through the fistula from the vaginal end. Surgical repair of a low fistula may be achieved by disconnection via the vaginal route, the fistula and its surrounding scar tissue being excised from both the vagina and the bladder wall. If the remaining defect is large, the bladder may need to be mobilized from above in order to achieve satisfactory closure

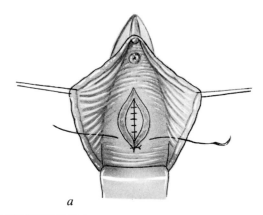

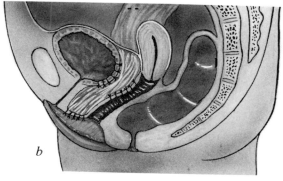

Fig. 34.15. Vesicovaginal fistula. *a*, Closure via the transvaginal route. *b*, Transperitoneal closure utilizing omental pedicle interposition.

without tension. For a high fistula into the vaginal vault, closure may be more conveniently achieved from above by an intraperitoneal operation. Success of such a repair may be facilitated by the interposition of an omental pedicle. This procedure may also be used for fistula recurrence after closure via the vaginal route.

BLADDER OUTFLOW OBSTRUCTION

This is most commonly caused by benign prostatic hyperplasia and prostatic carcinoma. More rarely, the bladder neck may be obstructed by fibrosis or by the ball valve effect of a bladder calculus. Urethral obstruction, due to stricture, congenital valves, etc., is dealt with elsewhere (*see* Chapter 35).

Benign Prostatic Enlargement

The effect of benign enlargement of the prostate is to produce often considerable elongation of the prostatic urethra. In addition, the middle lobe of the prostate may enlarge substantially into the bladder. These changes are compounded by the loss of elastic tissue from the bladder neck and together they inhibit the normal opening of the internal urinary meatus. This results in hypertrophy of the bladder muscle which occurs in irregular bundles throughout the

bladder wall resulting in the cystoscopic appearance of trabeculation. In long-standing cases, there is gradual distension of the bladder due to decompensation of the bladder muscle and the bladder then fails to empty completely. This results in a pool of residual urine within the bladder which predisposes to infection and stone formation. Back-pressure effects on the ureter may result in hydronephrosis and varying degrees of renal failure. If the patient does not present with symptoms resulting from these changes, complete decompensation of the bladder musculature may occur giving rise to retention of urine.

Clinical presentation may therefore be with the symptoms of bladder outflow obstruction which are frequency, urgency and hesitancy, a poor urinary stream and incontinence of urine. Haematuria may occur from congestion of the submucosal veins at the bladder neck. The first presentation may be with retention of urine or indeed with the symptoms of uraemia without complaint of any urinary symptoms.

Management of Bladder Outflow Obstruction

Acute retention of urine is relieved by a urethral or suprapubic catheter. Chronic retention of urine with overflow of small frequent quantities of urine and without pain is best managed by avoiding catheterization in order to avoid the introduction of infection into the bladder. The presence of moderate-to-severe renal failure may, however, necessitate a period of catheter drainage before definitive treatment is entertained. A neurological cause of retention of urine should be sought. The main nerve supply to the bladder is via the nervi erigentes from S2–S4. Retention due to a spinal disc lesion or tumour should therefore produce some perianal anaesthesia and this should be sought. The assessment of the size of the prostate by rectal examination (and by intravenous urography) is often very misleading, especially if the bladder is distended at the time of the examination.

PROSTATECTOMY

Although traditionally known as prostatectomy, the operations generally undertaken on the prostate gland are most accurately regarded as adenomectomies or, in the case of a malignant gland, a subtotal prostatectomy. Indications for operation are essentially outflow obstruction to the bladder of varying degrees; the most absolute presenting in the form of acute urinary retention. The lesser degrees of 'prostatism' present principally as delay in starting, a poor urinary stream and a terminal dribble. Associated symptoms of frequency and urgency of micturition should be regarded with suspicion as they are more likely to be due to bladder instability than obstruction, although in the older male this instability is in itself usually secondary to a primary obstructive pathology.

Essential preoperative investigations must begin with accurate history-taking remembering that in the elderly male the diuretic treatment of cardiac failure may present as nocturnal frequency which is then essentially a diuresis with the passage of large volumes of urine which at times may exceed the diurnal output. This is in contrast with the frequent passage of much smaller volumes commonly seen in the obstructive bladder. Equally, late-onset diabetes commonly masquerades as prostatism with a presentation of either urinary frequency or of a true urinary tract infection, and failure to examine the urine for reducing substances may allow this diagnosis to pass unrecognized. Urinary tract infection is the most common complicating factor in prostatic obstruction hence careful urinary culture and assessment of any infecting organisms are essential. Routine assessment of the blood urea and electrolytes may reveal a uraemic state which is by no means easy to recognize by purely clinical means. Preoperative excretion urography as a routine investigation prior to prostatectomy for outflow symptoms is the subject of some disagreement, but it may well reveal associated abnormalities such as diverticula in the bladder, which will modify the operation to be undertaken, and it is as well to be aware of these facts before proceeding to the operating theatre. A straight radiograph to exclude stone and metastases is certainly the absolute minimum of radiology which is required prior to surgery.

Choice of Operation

There are several anatomical approaches to the prostate, the most commonly utilized in the United Kingdom being the transurethral route. A large number of open prostatectomies, commonly of the retropubic or Millin variety, are still undertaken in non-specialist departments and the choice of operation depends on the general health and build of the patient, the experience of the surgeon and the size of the prostate gland. Most urologists would recognize that each of the three common routes, namely transurethral resection, retropubic prostatectomy and transvesical prostatectomy, has its place in the armamentarium of the urologist. Perineal prostatectomy, which has found substantial favour both in the United States and on the Continent where total prostatectomy is undertaken much more regularly, is very rarely seen in British operating theatres.

Transurethral Resection of the Prostate (*Figs.* 34.16, 34.17)

Once the decision to undertake prostatectomy has been made and the patient taken to the operating theatre, anaesthesia of a variety of forms is available and most urologists would prefer to undertake the operation with some degree of hypotension which may be produced either by inhalational agents or by spinal or epidural anaesthesia. The positioning of the patient is a matter of some controversy concerning the importance of the degree of flexion at the hips resulting in the choice of two types of endoscopic stirrups. Once the patient has been adequately prepared with antiseptic solutions and towels, the procedure is invariably preceded by panendoscopy. The panendoscope (*see Fig.* 34.5) is an end-viewing instrument which allows a clear picture to be obtained of the whole urethra from the external meatus

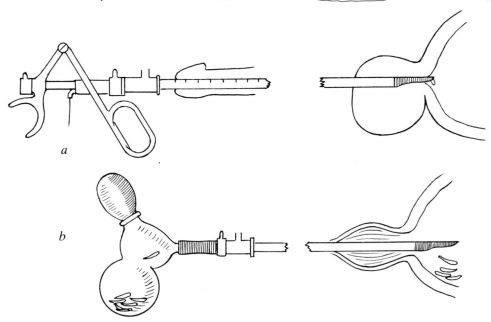

Fig. 34.16. Transurethral resection of the prostate. *a*, Resectoscope in position. *b*, Evacuation of debris with Ellik evacuator.

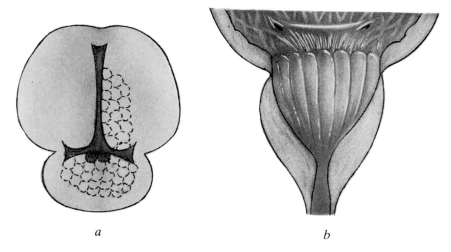

Fig. 34.17. Transurethral resection of the prostate. *a*, Two strips have been cut from the middle lobe. *b*, A common error—leaving too much distal prostate.

through the prostatic cavity into the bladder. The presence of strictures which would be unsuspected by blind instrumentation can be visualized and may be divided by the urethrotome, minimizing the ever present hazard of establishing a false passage. The normal panendoscope is an 18 Charrière instrument and it does not follow that the larger 22 or 24 Charrière resectoscope will pass easily once the panendoscope has been introduced. A careful dilatation with Liston's sounds or, alternatively, a urethrotomy using the Otis urethrotome should therefore be a prelude to the introduction of the resectoscope. Once the panendoscope has been introduced this should be followed by the insertion of further lubricant containing an antiseptic solution, commonly chlorhexidine, because of the risk of introducing infection from the distal urethra into the bladder. The panendoscope is a most necessary instrument for the assessment of the urethra and its effortless passage by the trained urologist should not allow trainees to forget that they are capable of producing substantial urethral damage with false passages which may even penetrate the rectum. Once the urethra has been checked for pathology which would include strictures and transitional cell tumours, the size and nature of the prostate gland are assessed both via the panendoscope and by an associated rectal examination on to the instrument when in position. The *verumontanum* (*see Fig.* 34.6*b*) and external sphincter are assessed and the relationship of the lobes of the prostate to these structures checked. At this stage a decision is finally made concerning the ideal route for prostatectomy and if a gland is particularly large, the patient healthy and not over-obese, a decision may be made to proceed to retropubic prostatectomy rather than carry out the operation by the transurethral route. Whichever decision is finally reached, before proceeding to prostatic surgery a careful and thorough cystoscopic examination is undertaken using a 70° instrument to detect diverticula, stone and especially tumours which will require treatment and will modify the final operative procedure.

Retropubic Prostatectomy (Millin; *Fig.* 34.18)

Preliminary cystoscopy is essential with this method as the bladder is not opened at operation and diverticulum, tumour or stone must be excluded. Under general, epidural or spinal anaesthetic, a vertical midline or Pfannenstiel incision is made. Retropubic extraperitoneal exposure of the prostatic capsule is then achieved and the pre-prostatic veins are secured with suture ligatures. A transverse incision is made in the prostatic capsule just wide enough to allow removal of the enucleated prostate. The plane of enucleation is readily entered by inserting curved scissors and opening the blades in a plane parallel to the capsule. The lateral lobes are freed by digital dissection and the urethral mucosa immediately distal to the prostate is divided with scissors. Both lateral lobes are dislocated out of the capsule and the proximal attachment of the gland is divided. A very large middle prostatic lobe may be removed separately. A wedge is cut from the bladder neck in order to prevent postoperative bladder neck stenosis, having identified the ureteric orifices, and haemostasis secured. The cut edge of the mucosa of the trigone is sutured down into the prostatic cavity. An indwelling urethral catheter is then inserted and the prostatic capsule closed securely to make it watertight. The catheter may be a three-way Foley catheter having an irrigation channel. The suture line in the prostatic capsule is tested by irrigation through the catheter and any clots are evacuated at this stage. A little fluid is left in the bladder to dilute any bleeding which occurs while the wound is closed. The retropubic space is drained.

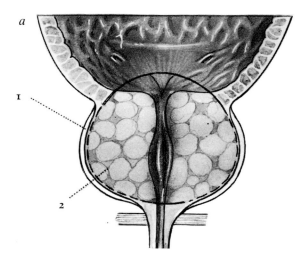

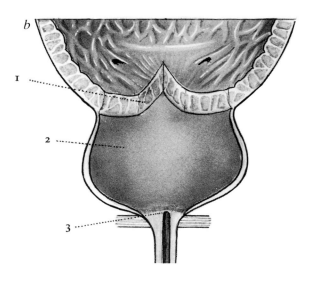

Fig. 34.18. Enucleation of the prostate. *a*, The continuous line indicates scissor dissection and the dotted line finger enucleation of the adenoma. 1, False capsule. 2, Adenoma. *b*, 1, V excised from trigone. 2, Prostate cavity. 3, Cut end of urethra.

A closed irrigation system is then attached to the catheter and irrigation may be by continuous drip or by intermittent irrigation to prevent clot retention within the bladder. A careful check on the volume of irrigating fluid used is important so that the volume of urine flow can be calculated by subtraction from the total. The irrigation is usually necessary for 12–24 hours and the catheter is removed when the urine is macroscopically clear of blood.

The disadvantage of the retropubic approach is that access may be difficult in a fat patient and, in addition, intravesical procedures cannot be performed at the same operation. It is also an unsatisfactory operation for small fibrotic or malignant glands.

Transvesical Prostatectomy (Suprapubic Prostatectomy)

This is indicated when access to the bladder is required in addition to the prostatectomy for removal of a calculus or for excision of a diverticulum.

Through a vertical midline or Pfannenstiel incision, the bladder is exposed retroperitoneally. A vertical midline incision is made in the bladder between stay sutures extending down to the prostatic capsule. By sharp dissection the plane of the false capsule is then entered posteriorly with extension of this plane around both sides to meet anteriorly. Finger enucleation of the prostate completes the dissection. After achieving haemostasis and insertion of a urethral catheter, the bladder wall is closed in two layers and the retropubic space is drained.

In order to allow adequate healing of the bladder incision, the catheter should be retained for 4–5 days. The chief disadvantages of the operation lie in the poor view for haemostasis and the need to open the bladder.

Postoperative Care

Surgery of the prostate gland is dominated by the ever-present risk of infection. This may occur during the operation or at any time postoperatively, particularly when a catheter is *in situ*. The common route of infection is via the lumen of the catheter and this can be prevented by careful *closed drainage* which should not be broken until the catheter is removed. Close cooperation between the clinical department and the microbiologist will allow prompt exhibition of the most appropriate antibiotic when this is required, but hopefully with a sterile urinary tract, careful theatre technique and competent closed drainage postoperatively, the urinary tract will be preserved free from infection in the majority of cases.

Complications

Haemorrhage

Bleeding from the prostatic bed is inevitable after all methods of prostatectomy but is minimized by careful haemostasis. Postoperative irrigation of the bladder is usually necessary unless bleeding is minimal and the use of plastic catheters allows careful suction to be applied to remove clots. Occasionally, return to the operating theatre and removal of clots via the cystoscope is necessary.

Secondary haemorrhage arising from infection within the bladder and prostatic cavity can be severe and result in clot retention.

Perforation of the prostatic capsule may occur as a complication of open prostatectomy or transurethral resection, and the most likely sites for this are at the bladder neck and at the apex of the prostate. If this complication is discovered then drainage of the retropubic space is necessary.

Deep venous thrombosis as detected by ^{131}I fibrinogen uptake has been shown to be considerably less common after transurethral resection (10 per cent) than after open operation (60 per cent).

Infection of the bladder and prostatic cavity is encouraged by preoperative catheterization and when this is undertaken in less than ideal circumstances. If the urine has been infected preoperatively the patient must be given an appropriate antibiotic to prevent Gram-negative septicaemia. Postoperative epididymo-orchitis may occur but few surgeons now perform routine bilateral vasectomy in an attempt to reduce its incidence.

Urinary incontinence following removal of the urethral catheter may occur but is usually temporary and probably results from oedema of the urethral mucosa. This complication is minimized by eradication of infection and avoiding damage to the membranous urethra at the time of operation.

Stricture of the urethra may occur in the prostatic cavity and at the external urinary meatus due to catheter or endoscopic trauma. This is likely to occur particularly after energetic dilatation of the urethra.

Sterility is probable after prostatectomy, even without vasectomy, and is due to retrograde ejaculation.

Recurrent prostatic enlargement is not uncommon after all methods of prostatectomy and, of course, carcinoma may arise in the false capsule. The histological discovery of small foci of carcinoma in an otherwise benign enlargement of the prostate demands no active treatment but careful follow-up of the patient. If carcinoma is unexpectedly found to be extensive in the removed prostate, then hormone therapy may be indicated (see below).

CARCINOMA OF THE PROSTATE

This is the third most common malignancy in men and accounts for 1 in 10 cases of acute retention. Carcinoma may be detected histologically after removal of a clinically benign enlarged prostate or may be found on routine rectal examination. If the carcinoma is producing symptoms then it is likely to have spread locally at the time of presentation. Eighty per cent of patients present with local symptoms of bladder outflow obstruction, urinary incontinence or rectal symptoms. The remainder present with evidence of metastases such as bone pain or a leucoerythroblastic anaemia.

The diagnosis is suspected on rectal examination of the prostate and confirmed histologically by perineal Tru-cut needle biopsy or transrectal Franzen needle aspiration for cytology. The presence of bone metastases may be suggested by marked elevation of the serum acid phosphatase and can be confirmed by isotope scanning using one of the [99]Tc^m-phosphate compounds. These compounds are concentrated in the kidneys and it is essential to maintain a high fluid intake when this procedure has been undertaken. The appearance of metastases on technetium scan may also be used to assess the effect of hormone treatment.

If the carcinoma is causing bladder outflow obstruction, then transurethral resection of the prostate is indicated.

The mainstay of treatment for disseminated carcinoma of the prostate is hormonal and this achieves some response in up to 85 per cent of cases. Subcapsular orchidectomy is preferable on theoretical grounds to the administration of oestrogen as the latter is associated with a very significant morbidity and mortality due to cardiovascular side-effects. However, stiboestrol or ethinyloestradiol treatment is indicated for those patients who refuse orchidectomy.

Supervoltage radiotherapy avoids the complications of hormone therapy but is not without its own side-effects and up to 58 per cent of patients will have histological evidence of active tumour at 1 year after a course of radiotherapy. It has not been shown to have any benefit over hormone therapy.

The choice of treatment should therefore be tailored to the individual patient. Orchidectomy is the first line of treatment, with oestrogen therapy reserved for those who refuse operation. Radiotherapy is particularly useful in the treatment of painful metastases.

LOWER URINARY TRACT TRAUMA

Accidental injury to the bladder requires prompt treatment. The nature of the injury may be deduced from the type of trauma which may be blunt injury, penetrating injury or trauma resulting from operations within the pelvis or instrumentation of the bladder and urethra.

Blunt Injury

A direct blow to the lower abdomen when the bladder is full is likely to result in intraperitoneal rupture whereas a crushing injury to the lower abdomen and pelvis may be expected to produce an extraperitoneal rupture of the bladder or a rupture of the posterior urethra.

Intraperitoneal rupture of the bladder results in leakage of urine into the peritoneal cavity and consequent severe lower abdominal pain which later passes off. There is no desire to micturate and the bladder is impalpable. The presence of lower abdominal peritonitis and the failure to obtain urine on urethral catheterization are indications for urgent excretion urography followed by laparotomy.

Through a lower midline incision, the peritoneum is opened and the small bowel packed off. The injury is usually a small tear on the peritoneal surface of the bladder which should be repaired in two layers.

All urine is removed from the peritoneal cavity and the wound is then closed. A self-retaining catheter is kept in place for 4–5 days.

Extraperitoneal rupture of the bladder is now the commoner injury and is usually associated with fracture of the pelvis. The injury is caused by fragments of bone directly lacerating the bladder or from a tear by traction on the ligamentous attachments to the pelvis. Extraperitoneal rupture occurs in approximately 10 per cent of all cases of fractured pelvis and may be associated with rupture of the urethra.

The clinical picture is of a patient with multiple injuries, often as a result of a road traffic accident or a crushing injury. Deep extravasation of urine into the perivesical tissues occurs over 24 or more hours, and in neglected cases urine tracks into the anterior perineum. This produces a boggy suprapubic swelling which is limited inferiorly by the attachment of Colles' fascia, preventing spread of the swelling onto the thigh or into the posterior perineum. Extraperitoneal rupture of the bladder may be confused with rupture of the membranous urethra but in the case of the latter injury, rectal examination reveals dislocation of the prostate from its normal position and a bogginess around the posterior urethra. If the diagnosis is in doubt, urethrography should be undertaken with aseptic precautions. Immediate laparotomy is performed through a vertical midline incision. The diagnosis is confirmed when the linea alba is divided to reveal extravasated blood and urine. If the injury is high on the anterior wall of the bladder, then direct repair of the defect may be possible. However, if the injury is to the base of the bladder and direct surgical repair is difficult and hazardous, suprapubic drainage of the bladder and separate adequate drainage of the retropubic space are performed. Laceration of the bladder is usually associated with gross contusion of the bladder wall which requires débridement prior to a two-layer closure. Prophylactic broad-spectrum antibiotics are administered from the outset.

Penetrating Injury

Direct injury to the bladder by gunshot or stab wounds is infrequent in civilian practice. The possibility of injury to other pelvic organs must always be considered. Laparotomy and repair of the defect are necessary, combined with an intraperitoneal exploration for other injuries, and penetrating injury to the rectum will require a defunctioning colostomy. Débridement and closure, if possible, of the bladder injury should be followed by suprapubic or urethral catheter drainage with adequate drainage to any extravesical extravasation. Prophylactic antibiotics are mandatory.

Operative and Endoscopic Injury to the Bladder

The bladder and posterior urethra may be damaged by the wilful insertion by the patient of foreign bodies such as hair pins, knitting needles, etc. Injury may also follow surgery to other pelvic organs or result from bladder instrumentation.

The presence of a foreign body within the bladder, once suspected, is readily confirmed at cystoscopy. The patient may not admit to self-instrumentation but may have symptoms of bladder irritation or infection. Fragments of the ruptured balloon of a Foley catheter may produce similar symptoms and most foreign bodies are subject to phosphatic encrustation if they remain *in situ* for long. The smaller foreign bodies are potentially removable via the cystoscope if they can be grasped with the biopsy forceps, but larger foreign bodies or those associated with perforation of the bladder need to be removed by open operation and the bladder repaired.

The bladder and posterior urethra are subject to instrumental trauma following inexperienced vigorous attempts at catheterization, particularly if a catheter introducer is used. The passage of a cystoscope may cause penetration of the posterior urethra during introduction when an attempt is made to traverse the prostatic urethra. The membranous urethra may thereby be perforated and the tip of the cystoscope enter the rectum. The tip of the cystoscope may also be forced through the wall of an undistended bladder, especially when an introducer is used. Damage from the operating resectoscope may occur during treatment of bladder carcinoma or transurethral resection of the prostate. When resecting a large bladder tumour, resection of the base of the tumour involves removal of part of the thickness of the bladder wall. Perforation of the bladder may then readily occur and commonly the perforation is extraperitoneal. Provided that the injury is recognized, then drainage of the retropubic space should be performed immediately and prophylactic antibiotics given. During transurethral resection of the prostate, the prostatic capsule may be inadvertently opened.

If instrumental perforations of the bladder are not recognized at operation, then postoperative extravasation of urine is likely to occur. If this most serious complication is suspected, drainage of the retropubic space should be achieved without delay and prophylactic antibiotics administered.

FURTHER READING

Blandy J. P. (1971) *Transurethral Resection*. London, Pitman Medical.
Blandy J. P. (1984) *Operative Urology*, 2nd ed. Oxford, Blackwell Scientific Publications.
Mitchell J. P. (1972) *The Principles of Transurethral Resection and Haemostasis*. Bristol, John Wright.

Chapter thirty-five

The Penis, Testes and Scrotum

P. J. B. Smith

THE SCROTUM

The scrotum is a musculocutaneous sac containing the testes and the distal ends of the spermatic cords. Beneath the rugose layer of skin is an area of loose connective tissue richly endowed with vascular tissue and containing an attendant layer of muscle known as the 'dartos'. This represents a portion of the subcutaneous muscle that covers many animals, but in man is only represented here in the platysma and in certain facial muscles. In the midline the dartos extends backwards to form a septum which divides the cavity of the scrotum into two parts. Beneath the scrotum lie the fascial tissues that invest the testis and cord. These layers fuse at the triangular ligament and perineum below and above and are continuous with the subcutaneous fascia of the abdominal wall and upper anterior extent of the thigh.

Because of its excellent blood supply and the presence of a cutaneous contractile muscle in the dartos, the scrotum has excellent healing properties. Lacerations heal well and usually require no sutures, the main indication for stitching being to stop bleeding.

Sebaceous cysts are common and, as elsewhere, can be enucleated with minimum dissection. The rarely encountered squamous cell carcinoma is treated by wide excision. Such is the extent of scrotal tissue that primary closure is seldom difficult. These procedures can be done under local anaesthesia, the loose subcutaneous connective tissue being particularly easy to infiltrate with lignocaine. The incisions are closed with 2/0 chromic catgut on a cutting or tapered needle. Non-absorbable stitches are not indicated as they must be removed subsequently, often a more difficult procedure than the original operation. Catgut stitches do produce a local reaction but this disappears since catgut disintegrates in a week or so. Provided the patient bathes daily in saline the discomfort is minimal. The eventual result from either laceration or local sugical excision is excellent and scar formation is never a problem in the scrotum.

By far the most important surgical manoeuvre relating to the scrotum, however, is the formal incision and subsequent closure required for operations involving its contents.

After cleaning the skin with spirit the scrotum is towelled up, particular care being taken to exclude the peri-anal area. The scrotum is then held on stretch and, with one hand holding it behind, a transverse incision made to expose the contents of one or both compartments of the scrotum. The incision is made through all layers including the dartos which is seen

to fall back against the tension of the tissues. Further dissection will now depend on the procedure involved and is discussed individually in detail later.

To close the incision it is important to remember the vascular nature of the tissues for if this is done inadequately a haematoma will occur. With careful closure it should be possible to eliminate the risk of haematoma but as an extra precaution a scrotal hitch-stitch can occasionally be applied. This consists of a nylon stitch through the most dependent part of the scrotum which is then brought up on to the skin of the anterior abdominal wall (*see Fig.* 35.6*b*). On tying this stitch the scrotum is hitched up so as to compress its cavity and discourage any bleeding. The hitch-stitch is removed after 12 hours.

Varicocele (*Fig.* 35.1*a*)

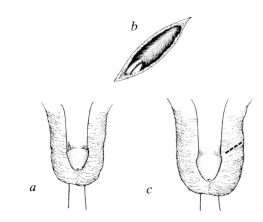

Fig. 35.1. *a*, Varicocele. *b*, Incision for high exposure of varicocele. *c*, Scrotal incision used in low approach for excision of varicocele.

This is a condition of varicosity in the pampiniform plexus and is usually confined to the left side in relation to the drainage of the left testicular vein into the renal vein. If valves are not present there is usually considerable pressure down the vein with subsequent dilatation of the pampiniform plexus. Rarely this situation may arise in association with carcinoma of the left kidney, but there are other more obvious signs present in those circumstances. For practical purposes, a varicosity in isolation is a benign condition and as such there are only two indications for operation—the symptoms produced and any coincident infertility.

A varicosity may produce symptoms due to swelling, local discomfort or cosmetic distress. When associated with male infertility, surgical treatment may improve both sperm count and motility.

The operation consists of ligation of the varicosity, and can be undertaken through either a high or low incision. The high operation is approached through the groin. The testicular veins are identified either in the inguinal canal or above the internal ring in an extraperitoneal plane. The patient under a general anaesthetic is placed on a non-slip mattress. After cleaning the skin and towelling up, an inguinal incision is made. The inguinal canal is opened in the standard fashion with formal incision of skin, superficial fascia, external oblique aponeurosis and external spermatic fascia (*Fig.* 35.1*b*). In the extraperitoneal exposure the abdominal muscles are again incised to expose the deep surface of the internal ring with the cord entering from above. With the cord identified, the dilated veins are now dissected free. Intermittent reverse Trendelenburg tilt may be required to fill the veins for full identification. The vas and testicular artery, often difficult to see, are preserved. All veins seen are divided with the excision of a segment of at least 2 cm to prevent reanastomosis. The incision is closed in layers with catgut to the deep tissues and nylon or clips to the skin. No drain is required.

The low operation approaches the varicosity directly through the scrotum (*Fig.* 35.2). A transverse incision is made through all layers of the scrotum, and the testes and cord delivered through the wound (*Fig.* 35.2*a*). The cord is now carefully dissected through its fascial layers so as to display its contents. Though it may be difficult to see the testicular artery the vas is easily identified and isolated (*Fig.* 35.2*b*). The varicosity is excised, leaving intervals of at least 2 cm between the ligated ends of each vein (*Fig.* 35.2*c*). An intermittent reverse Trendelenburg tilt will help to confirm that all veins involved have been ligated. The scrotum is closed in the manner described above. No drainage is required.

These approaches have their different protagonists but the low approach has certain advantages. First, the varicocele is excised completely, as opposed to the indirect 'defunctioning' of the high operation. Also, with some patients, veins from the back of the symphysis, particularly obturator veins, may contribute to the varicocele. These veins can readily be overlooked in the high procedure, whereas their presence or absence is immaterial to the success of the low operation. Second, with muscle incision and subsequent closure, the high operation is more painful and requires correspondingly longer convalescence.

Finally, in the high operation the varicocele, though collapsed, is still seen to be present and though the veins eventually atrophy, to the patient at least the immediate effect of the operation is not as satisfying as when the varicocele itself is removed.

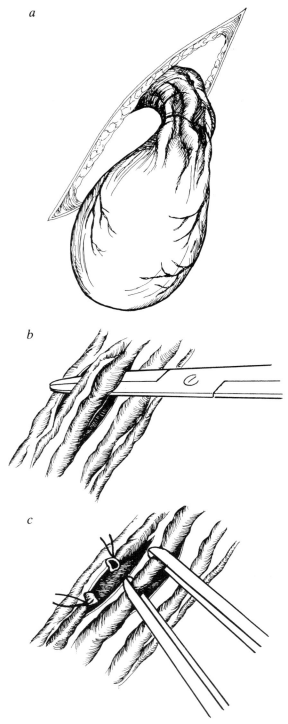

Fig. 35.2. *a*, Delivery of spermatic cord and testis through scrotal incision. *b*, Identification of vas deferens and testicular artery. *c*, Varicocele. Division of veins and removal of varicosities.

Hydrocele

A hydrocele is a cystic swelling of the sac surrounding the testes which persists after closure of the processus vaginalis. It invests the greater part of the testis.

Hydrocele is common in the elderly male where it represents a failure of reabsorption of fluid, possibly associated with degenerative changes of chronic inflammation of the lining of the sac. In the young male it may arise as a reactionary hydrocele due to testicular trauma, infection or, rarely but most important, testicular tumour. Finally, a hydrocele may occur in infants due to failure of the processus vaginalis to fuse; in addition to the cystic swelling this situation also results in an inguino-scrotal hernia in some children.

Surgery for hydrocele is required absolutely to exclude underlying testicular disease in young men, especially tumour, but more commonly to relieve symptoms in the elderly. The symptoms arise as a result of swelling which, as well as causing dragging discomfort, is often most unsightly.

The procedures available may be devided into aspiration of the hydrocele, instillation of sclerosants into the hydrocele, or the excision, plication or eversion of the greater part of the hydrocele sac itself. Aspiration of the hydrocele is the time-honoured method of treatment and at one time involved the use of an impressive array of trocars and cannulas. With the development of modern disposable syringes and needles this elaborate armamentarium can be abandoned. A no. 1 needle connected to a 50-ml Luer–Lock syringe is assembled. The hydrocele is steadied against the scrotum with the left hand, and with the right hand a few ml of 1 per cent lignocaine are infiltrated into the most prominent point of the bulging scrotum, remembering that the testis lies below and behind the hydrocele. On completion of local anaesthetic infiltration and without altering the gentle grip of the left hand, the 50-ml syringe and needle are used to aspirate the hydrocele fluid. This is a simple procedure, taking only a few minutes, and easily accomplished in the outpatient department.

The fluid obtained is traditionally described as 'straw-coloured' but if doubt exists, due to blood staining or cloudiness, it should be sent for cytology and bacteriology (including TB studies).

Where doubt exists beforehand as to the underlying nature of the testes, as in a young man with a short history of testicular swelling, the possibility of reactionary hydrocele due to a tumour should be considered and no attempt made to aspirate in the outpatient department. This situation is described in detail on p. 480. Fortunately, this is a rare occurrence in the management of hydrocele and aspiration is a satisfactory treatment. The main problem is that it is not curative and the hydrocele will re-form, often within weeks, and most patients require more formal surgery to eliminate the hydrocele.

This involves surgery to the wall of the sac itself, either to reduce its size or to open it out so that the fluid can be absorbed through the scrotal tissues. The hydrocele is delivered through a transverse all-layer scrotal incision (Fig. 35.3). Often, with a long-

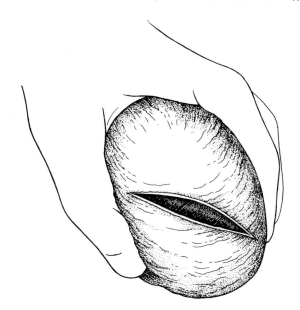

Fig. 35.3. Hydrocele. The scrotum is incised over the tense hydrocele.

standing hydrocele there will be extensive adhesions and increased vascularity in the connective and fascial tissues of the scrotum. These vessels are divided after diathermy or ligation, sufficient only to deliver the hydrocele and testis outside the scrotum. Excessive dissection of the sac and, worst of all, blunt dissection with a gauze swab are to be deprecated. This manoeuvre does not contribute to the operation, and will cause much postoperative oedema with an enhanced risk of secondary infection. Monopolar diathermy can be used safely provided the scrotal contents are kept in close contact with the main body surface during the use of the current. If the testis or cord is pulled up there is a risk, especially in children, of coagulation of vessels in the cord, due to compressed run-off of the current. Bipolar diathermy is, of course, ideal.

Having delivered the hydrocele through the scrotal incision, a scalpel is now inserted into its anterior surface, well away from the testis which is below and behind (*Fig.* 35.4). The fluid is drawn off and the incision in the sac extended with scissors so as to divide it completely in the sagittal plane from the cord above the sinus of the testis below. The testis is now inspected to confirm its benign nature.

Thin-walled hydroceles, seen particularly in children, are treated quickly and effectively by the Jaboulay procedure, in which two halves of the sac are everted and sutured together across the back of the testis (*Fig.* 35.5a). An alternative in children and the usual technique in adults with thin-walled hydroceles is to plicate the sac. A series of 2/0 catgut stitches on a cutting needle is inserted at 1-cm intervals starting in the sinus of the testis and extending radially in a series of loops to pick up small bites of the sac, up to its cut edge. Each stitch is left long until all

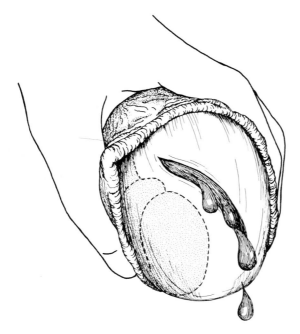

Fig. 35.4. Hydrocele. An incision is made well anterior to the testis.

are inserted and then each is tied separately. This has the effect of bunching up and obliterating the hydrocele wall which is left as a ruff of tissue around the sinus of the testis (*Fig.* 35.5*b*). In experienced hands it is possible to plicate the sac through a small scrotal incision without the need to mobilize or deliver the testis, but the saving in dissection for this is minimal and for most situations the technique described above is satisfactory.

In some, particularly long-standing, hydroceles, however, the sac is thick walled and not suitable for plication. For these patients formal excision is required. Again, this is done, after opening the sac, by cutting each side with scissors so as to leave a small margin of tissue around the testis (*Fig.* 35.5*c*). The sac may extend into the cord and rather more may be left here to obviate the risk of damaging the cord. The problem with excision is that bleeding is prone to occur from the cut surface. Meticulous haemostasis with diathermy and under-running catgut stitches are required to prevent postoperative haematoma formation. On completion of surgery to the hydrocele sac, the testis is returned to the scrotum which is closed in the approved manner. This is one of the few occasions when drainage is required; the exudate of hydrocele fluid produced following surgery may be considerable and particularly if associated with oozing of blood, it can be troublesome. A corrugated rubber drain is effective but carries the risk of retrograde spread of organisms and secondary infection. A suction drain such as Redivac is as effective and much safer (*Fig.* 35.6*a*). Drainage is usually required for 24–48 hours. When both sides of the

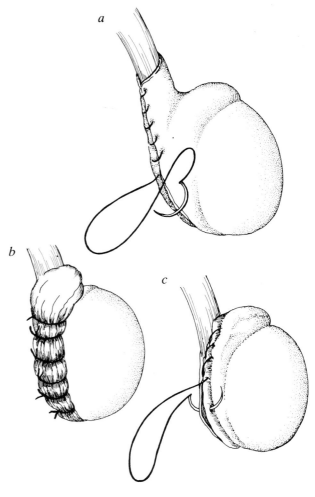

Fig. 35.5. Hydrocele. *a*, The Jaboulay procedure of eversion and posterior suture of the hydrocele. *b*, Obliteration of hydrocele by plication. *c*, Obliteration by excision of redundant tissue and haemostatic suturing.

scrotum are involved, this drain can be laid across the septum.

THE TESTES

Orchidectomy

Indications

Orchidectomy is absolutely indicated for the treatment of malignant tumours of the testis. Occasionally, it may be necessary for advanced cases of torsion of the testis. Some surgeons perform orchidectomy as part of a hernia repair if difficult or recurrent surgical situations have arisen. Though fortunately rare, tumour is an indication for radical orchidectomy. The surgical approach is through the groin, and no attempt should be made to go through the scrotum as there is a real risk of tumour seeding into the scrotal wound. The skin incision is generous so as to

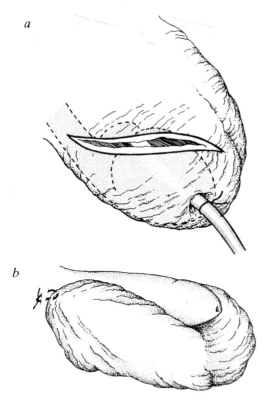

Fig. 35.6. Hydrocele. *a*, Drainage of scrotum using Redivac drain. *b*, Hitch-stitch of scrotum to abdominal wall.

expose the entire length of the inguinal canal. The canal is then opened and on excising the external spermatic fascia, the cord is gently mobilized up to the inguinal ring (*Fig.* 35.7). A compression clamp or constricting loop of a small (no. 8 Fr. gauge) Jacques catheter is now applied to the cord, effectively obstructing both venous and lymphatic circulations, which minimizes the risk of tumour emboli dur-

ing the subsequent handling. By gentle finger and scissors dissection the testis is now delivered up through the neck of the scrotum. Confirmation of the presence of tumour is obtained by palpation and inspection. Any hydrocele fluid should be aspirated before the underlying testis is palpated. In practice there is seldom any doubt about the diagnosis and wedge resection and frozen section techniques have little part to play in the surgery of testicular tumour.

Having decided that the testis contains malignant tumour, and without releasing the proximal compression, the cord is mobilized sufficiently for effective ligation (*Figs.* 35.8, 35.9). Occasionally, the cord may

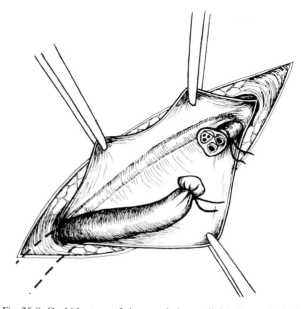

Fig. 35.8. Orchidectomy. It is a good plan to divide the cord within the inguinal canal as early as possible and before delivery of the testis from the scrotum.

be thickened and contain fatty tissue. By division of investing fascia the vas and vessels are dissected free and two separate sets of ligatures are applied, as close as possible to the internal ring, so as to remove the maximum amount of cord tissue. This dissection should also include a careful check to make certain that no hernial sac is involved. The wound is closed in layers with 2/0 catgut and nylon or clips to the skin. No drainage is required.

There is no surgical (as opposed to diagnostic) urgency about orchidectomy for tumour. For at least 24 hours preoperatively, specimens should be collected for serum gonadotrophin and alpha-fetoprotein measurements. These and subsequent lymphogram and scan studies will be important factors in the prognosis and further management.

Surgery alone is rarely recommended and radiotherapy and combination chemotherapy are usually required for the treatment of this tumour.

The same principles of management are required

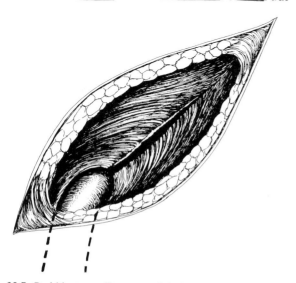

Fig. 35.7. Orchidectomy. Exposure of the inguinal canal and spermatic cord.

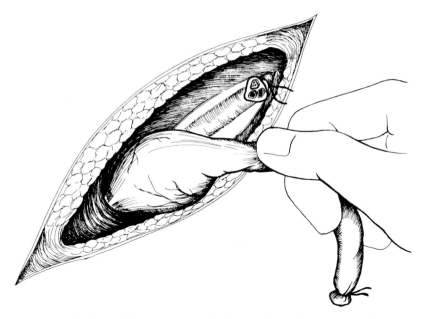

Fig. 35.9. Orchidectomy. Removal of testis following ligation of cord.

for tumours occurring in maldescended testes though obviously the initial mobilization of the cord and testes will vary depending on where the maldescent has finished up. There is certainly statistical evidence to suggest that there is an increased risk of malignancy in undescended testes. This increased incidence is still present even after orchidopexy, if this procedure is deferred until after the age of 5 years.

Subcapsular Orchidectomy

Subcapsular orchidectomy is an operation which removes all functioning testicular tissue, particularly the Leydig cells which produce androgen. This operation is used in the treatment of those prostatic tumours with metastatic disease where oral hormone therapy is not feasible.

Through a transverse scrotal incision both testes are delivered and with a sagittal incision the tunica is divided completely. The soft yellow homogeneous testicular tissue is now expressed by squeezing the testis around a dry gauze swab. Any unremoved testis adherent to the tunica is coagulated. In this way all androgen-producing tissue is removed. The empty shells of the testes are sutured back with chromic catgut and the testicular remnants returned to the scrotum which is closed in the usual manner. No drain is required.

Undescended and Ecotopic Testis

Orchidopexy

This procedure may not influence subsequent spermatogenesis, but the cosmetic and psychological effects of orchidopexy are sufficient to recommend such surgery.

While the operation can be done in the neonatal period, it is best left until the 3rd or 4th year. Care must be taken in diagnosis as some children have retractile testes which, if left alone, will occupy a normal scrotal position in due course. If doubt exists, and careful examination and history usually exclude this, the testes can be examined with the child anaesthetized. If the testis can be persuaded down to the base of the scrotum, the proposed operation can be abandoned. Usually, however, the diagnosis is clear and orchidopexy is indicated.

Under a general anaesthetic and in the supine position, the groin is prepared with spirit and suitable towelling. An incision is made over the inguinal canal, either in an oblique line or transverse crease incision (*Fig.* 35.10). The next step will depend on whether the maldescent has resulted in an ectopic or undescended testis. In the former case the testis usually lies in the superficial inguinal pouch though there are other rare sites in the anterior compartment of the thigh, or even the perineum. An undescended testis lies within the inguinal canal. If under anaesthetic and before incision it is possible to palpate the testis, it is ectopic, and in this situation care must be taken with further dissection of the superficial tissues. The ectopic testis is soon identified beneath the superficial layer of deep fascia, and is best held at this stage by fingers rather than instruments. With the testis on stretch any remaining superficial tissues are dissected free. The testis and its cord are now held by three tissue layers which must be divided to mobilize fully the gland sufficient to place it in the scrotum. These tissues are reily seen after the next step, which is to open the inguinal canal. This

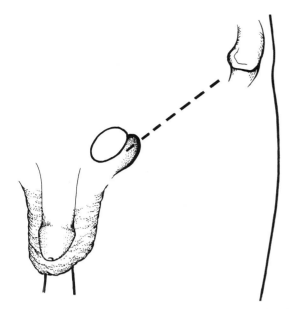

Fig. 35.10. Undescended testis (shown in superficial inguinal pouch). Incision.

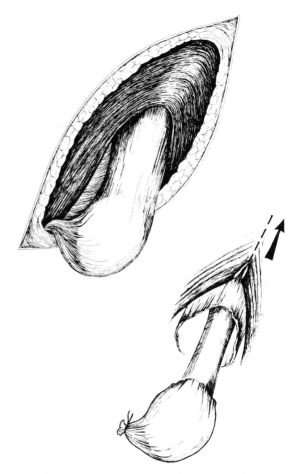

Fig. 35.11. Orchidopexy. Exposure of undescended testis and its investing layers. The investing layers are carefully divided, preserving the cord, following which proximal mobilization of the cord within the inguinal canal will allow the testis to be replaced within the scrotum.

is done by making a small incision with a scalpel in the aponeurosis of the external oblique. This is extended laterally with scissors to reach the fibres of the internal oblique as they sweep upwards across the internal ring. Medial extension of the incision with scissors will open up the external ring and further resection of the same plane will divide the external spermatic fascia, a continuation of the external oblique aponeurosis, the first of three layers. The testis is separated from the external oblique fascia and will already show evidence of increased mobilization (*Fig.* 35.11).

If an undescended testis is present it will be revealed on opening the inguinal canal, in which case there is no external spermatic fascia element. From now on the procedure is the same for both types of maldescent.

The aim of orchidopexy is to mobilize the testis, the limiting factor being its vascular pedicle, which is contained in the cord and which is bound down by the two remaining layers of tissue. The first of these is the internal spermatic fascia and cremasteric muscle, which are parts of the same tissue which derive from the internal oblique muscle. By holding the testis in tension these tissues can be 'chiselled' off the cord using the barely open tips of a pair of fine dissecting scissors. There is surprisingly little bleeding but occasional diathermy coagulation is required. Great care is necessary to prevent coagulation of the cord. This is achieved by either using bipolar diathermy or by avoiding coagulating on a stretched cord, the testis and cord being placed in contact with the body before the current is applied. Division of the cremasteric fascia and muscle exposes the cord which is now further dissected to identify the vas and vascular pedicle. At this stage any hernial

sac present can be detected. Such a sac is common in an undescended testis but rare in the ectopic variety. If present, it is dissected with scissors and ligated at the internal ring. Further mobilization of the cord is obvious at this stage but there is one final tissue layer to be divided in order to obtain the maximum mobilization. This is the layer of deep fascia which invests the testicular vessels as they run through the retroperitoneal space to reach the internal ring. By holding the cord in tension, this tissue is readily seen and divided with scissors. This final manoeuvre is often the critical step in achieving an adequate mobilization of the vessels to enable the testis to lie comfortably in the scrotum. The final stage of this part of the operation is to open the hydrocele sac on the testis and evert the edges. This prevents any risk of hydrocele formation and also encourages subsequent fixation of the testes in the scrotum.

A variety of techniques has been devised to fix the testis after mobilization. Procedures such as the Keetley–Torek or a nylon stitch to the thigh are clumsy and dangerous—they should be avoided. Provided proper mobilization of the cord has been achieved a simple scrotal pouch is all that is required to hold the testis in its proper position. Such a pouch is constructed by first opening up the scrotal canal by finger dissection from above. The index finger is passed through into the scrotal cavity and the scrotal skin stretched over it. A transverse incision is now made at the most prominent point (as low as possible in the scrotum) about 1 cm in length. The incision should only include the skin. With scissors dissection the subcutaneous space is opened up in all directions (*Fig.* 35.12). Small artery forceps are a useful alternative in this part of the procedure. The index finger

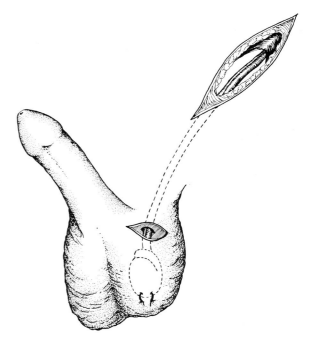

Fig. 35.13. Orchidopexy. Through this opening the testis and the fully mobilized spermatic cord may be drawn into the most dependent part of the scrotum and held in place by sutures.

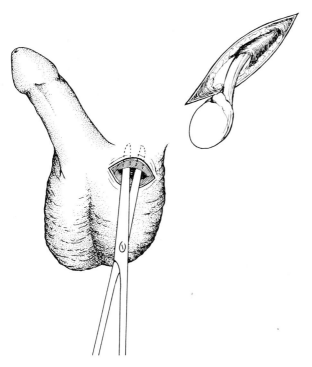

Fig. 35.12. Orchidopexy. Following the creation of a scrotal pouch with the finger, the scrotum is opened.

still in position will now push forward the dartos. This is incised just sufficient to allow an artery forceps to pass through. By simultaneous withdrawal of the finger the forceps are presented through the neck of the scrotum into the inguinal canal where it grasps the base of the testis, which is now drawn into the scrotum and with a certain amount of encouragement squeezed through the incision in the dartos so as to lie in the subcutaneous scrotal pouch (*Fig.* 35.13). The dartos should lie snugly around the cord which should be checked to see that it has not rotated. The scrotal incision is closed with interrupted 2/0 catgut stitches, one of which can pick up a portion of the tunica of the testis to make certain of fixation. The inguinal incision is closed with catgut and either nylon or clips to the skin. No drain is required.

Rarely, and then only with undescended testes, sufficient mobilization may not be achieved, and additional techniques have been suggested. Division of the internal ring by ligation of the inferior epigastric artery has little to offer. Further dissection of the testicular vessels in the extraperitoneal space is likewise unhelpful. Division of the testicular vessels is followed by testicular atrophy. The best procedure in these circumstances is to mobilize the testis as far as possible by dissection of the tissue layers, which will usually help to mobilize the shortest cord so that the testis lies at the neck of the scrotum. The testis and cord are now wrapped in Oxycel and the incision closed. The Oxycel has the effect of preventing adhesions to the testis and cord. Twelve months later the groin is re-explored and the still mobile testis is further dissected to make use of any growth of the cord during this period. It is usually possible to complete the scrotal positioning at this stage. Otherwise, and provided the other testis is normal, orchidectomy is indicated. (*See also* Chapter 31.)

Torsion of Testis

This is a condition of rotation of the testis about its cord producing strangulation. Though it may be congenital or occur in the mature male, torsion most commonly occurs in young boys and adolescents. The onset of pain and swelling in the testes in this age group, particularly if associated with exercise, should suggest torsion, requiring urgent exploration. Manipulation of the testis has been suggested and is worth attempting in the anaesthetic room immediately after induction. Torison is usually anticlockwise so that a reverse movement can sometimes give a vital few minutes of oxygenation. At operation the scrotum is opened through a standard transverse incision and the testes and cord delivered. The incision should include both sides of the scrotum for the reasons stated below. If not already so the testis is now untwisted. Even a dusky, congested testis is worth preserving, though it may have no further spermatogenesis. It can produce hormone activity. The loss of a testis may be psychologically damaging. Only a frankly gangrenous testis which shows no signs of recovery should be excised. This is achieved by simple ligation of the cord at the neck of the scrotum with one suture of 2/0 catgut.

If the testis is preserved, it is vital to fix both it and its companion to prevent repeat torsion. This is the reason both testes are exposed through the initial incision. One or two catgut stitches are placed through the base of each testis and thence to the dartos in the base of the scrotum. These are tied so as to fix the testes. This, plus the local adhesions following surgery, will prevent further torsion. No drain is required.

Finally, a word about testicular prostheses. These are now readily available. The prosthesis has a flange on its lower border which is sutured to the inside of the scrotum. This ensures that it lies correctly. It is impossible to overstate the psychological improvement such a prosthesis can give to a young man unfortunate to lose a testis or, in rare and sad cases, both organs, and who will, in that case, also require androgen therapy.

Epididymal Cyst

The differential diagnosis of epididymal cyst and hydrocele is usually clear. The distinction is that with an epididymal cyst the testis is easily palpated whereas with a hydrocele it is lost within the sac. Further differentiation of epididymal cyst into clear cyst and spermatocele is pointless as both require similar management. As with hydrocele the indications for treatment relate to the appearance and associated discomfort of the cyst. However, the treatment is not the same as the only cure is complete excision of the cyst. Attempts to aspirate or inject sclerosants are unsuccessful. The cyst is usually multilocular and it is impossible to treat all the cysts present. In the same way, plication, though eliminating a large cyst, cannot prevent further small cysts developing.

Excision of the cyst is achieved by careful dissection, under general anaesthesia, following a transverse incision through the scrotal wall. With minimum sharp dissection and, where necessary, careful diathermy coagulation, the testis, cord and cyst are delivered. The epididymal cyst is seen to

be covered with several layers of fascia rich in blood vessels. All of these layers need to be incised, using a scalpel for establishing the plane and scissors to develop it (*Fig.* 35.14*a*).

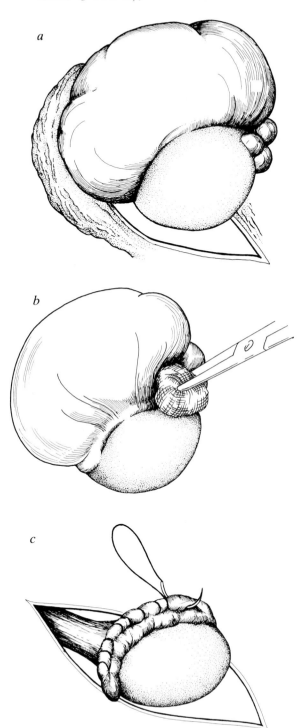

Fig. 35.14. Epididymal cyst. *a*, Delivery following scrotal incision. *b*, Dissection of the cyst from the epididymis and testis. *c*, Following removal of the cyst wall its layers are obliterated using haemostatic suture.

By holding the cyst firmly from behind, these layers are put on tension which facilitates the dissection. If by mischance the cyst is ruptured a forceps such as Duval's or Babcock's should be put across the leak to try and keep the cyst as distended as possible. Eventually a plane is reached in which there are no blood vessels—the outer wall of the epididymal cyst. Using scissors and gentle dissection with a gauze pledgelet, the cyst is mobilized until its base on the epididymis is reached (*Fig.* 35.14*b*). This, though small, is often adherent and may need to be excised, possibly with a small amount of normal epididymal tissue (*Fig.* 35.14*c*). Any bleeding points are coagulated and the scrotum closed (*Fig.* 35.15). No drain is required. The patient will require 48 hours of bedrest postoperatively with 7–10 days' convalescence, and he should be warned of the extensive scrotal oedema which may follow.

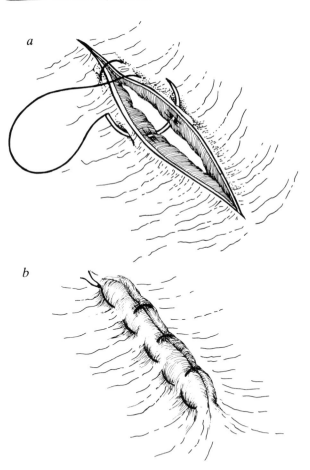

a

b

Fig. 35.15. Closure of the scrotum should be undertaken carefully to ensure haemostasis.

Vasectomy

Vasectomy is ideally performed under a local anaesthetic. Counselling is an essential feature of vasec-

tomy, for as well as detecting the patient's suitability for the operation, he can also be warned of the delayed success of the operation and the need to have two negative sperm counts before he can consider himself sterile.

The operation itself, though simple, and if properly performed very successful, does have a morbidity due to scrotal haematoma and sepsis and, more rarely, sperm granuloma formation. The patient should be warned of these possibilities and reassured that they will settle with conservative treatment. The patient is also to be warned of the rare (1 in 400) instance of spontaneous reanastomosis, usually across a sperm granuloma. Again, he can be reassured that this complication, if it occurs, will be detected at his postoperative sperm test, and further vasectomy performed. Though irrelevant to most patients, it is now possible to state that if there is any change of mind in the future, surgical reanastomosis can certainly be performed with a good (greater than 50 per cent) chance of success.

The essential feature of vasectomy is the division, ligation and repositioning of the vas to prevent reanastomosis. Excision of excessive lengths of vas is meddlesome and may indirectly cause trauma to the ejaculatory ducts and the vesicles making any subsequent attempts at reanastomosis impossible. In the same way dissection of the vas and ligation too close to the epididymis are unnecessary and make subsequent reconstructive surgery difficult. Various additional techniques of banding, clipping and cauterizing the vas have been employed but a simple, careful dissection and ligation will give satisfactory results in the manner now described.

Having bathed and shaved the scrotal tissues the night before, the patient should lie supine on the table. The external genitalia should be cleaned with spirit, the patient being warned in advance of the temporary discomfort associated with this. The genitalia are now towelled up. The testis is held between the finger and thumb of the hand and gently but firmly brought down. Through the tensed scrotum the vas is now detected with the fingers and thumb of the other hand. It is easily palpated as a firm structure and separate from the cord, usually lying medially to the testes. The testis is now released but the finger and thumb remain, presenting 1–2 cm of vas under the scrotum. After skin infiltration with local anaesthetic a 1-cm incision (transverse) is made through the scrotal wall (*Fig.* 35.16*a*). The incision so made is stretched with artery forceps, extending it through any deep connective tissue. The vas is now infiltrated directly with more local anaesthetic in an upward direction, 3–5 ml of 1 per cent lignocaine being infiltrated around the vas about 1–2 cm above the incision. The vas is now seized between the jaws of a pair of tissue forceps.

The tissue forceps and their contained vas are now angled upwards to throw up a loop of vas with its surrounding fascia. This fascia may be extensive and

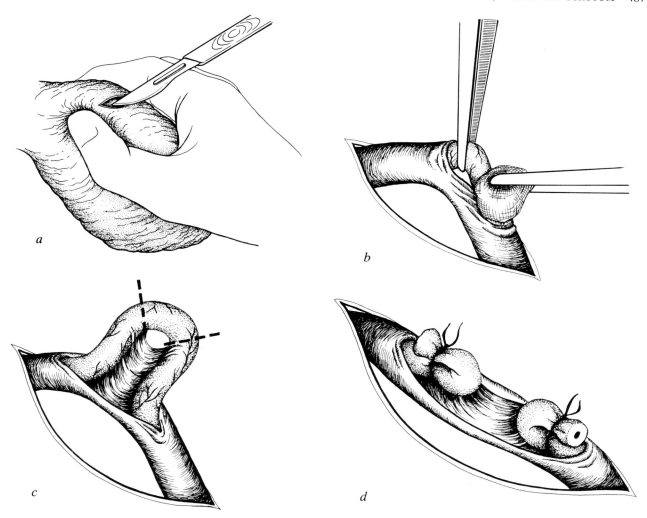

Fig. 35.16. Vasectomy. *a*, The vas is displaced subcutaneously and the scrotal skin is divided over its prominence. *b*, The delivered vas is held with tissue forceps and dissected by sharp and blunt dissection. *c,d*, A short length of vas is removed (*c*) and the ends carefully tied, or folded and tied (*d*).

it is vital to dissect these layers away to reveal an entirely naked vas. This is achieved by vertical incision of tissues along the vas using a scalpel. The fascial layers will fall back as they are divided against the tension, and the pearly white unmistakable appearance of the vas is then evident (*Fig.* 35.16*b*). Any adherent layers of fascia can be gently swept back with a gauze swab. In this way the mesentery of the vas with the terminal branches of its vessels are preserved. Using fine forceps the mesentery is opened and two clips put across the vas so as to isolate 2 cm of tissue. The top of the loop so isolated is excised so as to present two cut ends (*Fig.* 35.16*c*). There is no need to excise any more than a minimum of vas; indeed, it is quite in order to merely slit up the centre of the clamped section of vas.

The cut ends of the vas are ligated with thread, catgut or Dexon (*Fig.* 35.16*d*). The two cut ends of the vas are then returned to the cavity of the scrotum.

The scrotal incision is closed with 2/0 catgut as described previously. No drainage is required.

Both vasa are divided through separate incisions. On completion of the vasectomy the incisions are covered with a gauze dressing and the patient advised to wear two pairs of pants to provide support. The patient should commence with daily salt baths, starting that day, for 7–10 days. He is warned again that the operation is not successful until he has two negative sperm counts, reinforcing the advice given during the preoperative counselling. These sperm tests are done at 14 and 16 weeks postoperatively and occasionally need to be repeated even if only an occasional sperm cell is shown to be present. Although such sperm is likely to have no biological significance it is essential for medicolegal reasons to have two negative sperm counts before declaring the patient sterile.

Ejaculation, either coital or otherwise, should be

encouraged in order that the sperm ducts are emptied. Some patients experience a psychological impotence for a few weeks following the procedure but they are warned of this possibility. No vasectomy procedure is exempt from complications and a proportion of men will complain of pain and local swelling. Most patients, however, are able to return to work in 2 or 3 days but this is by no means invariable and each case requires individual consideration.

Reanastomosis of the vas

The proper care of the vas and its mesentery during vasectomy is essential not only for reasons of good surgical practice but also to give maximum assistance to the surgeon if subsequently a reanastomosis is requested. This technique is simple and carries a high success rate provided the vas is not divided too close to the epididymis and provided only a minimum of vas and mesentery are removed during the original operation. Reanastomosis, though possible under a local anaesthetic, is best performed under general anaesthetic. Both vasa are mobilized through separate scrotal incisions and the area of vasectomy identified. This is readily seen as there is a distinct area of fibrous swelling into which go the proximal and distal ends of each vas. Each segment of vas is carefully dissected, preserving its mesentery down to the scar tissue, and is then divided with scissors to expose a healthy cut surface with a readily identifiable lumen. Microsurgical techniques have been employed for this but are not essential and, for those not used to the operating microscope, may prove to be a positive disadvantage. The two cut ends are now further dissected to ensure comlete freedom and mobilization from the scarred area. The scar itself can be excised but this, though preferable, is not essential.

A 2/0 nylon ligature is now threaded down the lumen of the distal vas for 10 cm or so, in order to confirm its patency. With fine forceps and using 6/0 Dexon, four quadrant stitches are inserted through adjoining parts of both cut ends of the vas. After inserting all four stitches, each is tied. As these stitches are knotted the two ends of the vas are drawn together and after withdrawal of the nylon splint the walls of the vas are brought into opposition. Several interrupted holding stitches are now placed in the surrounding fascia and are used to buttress the anastomosis.

The single, most important feature of reanastomosis is to have an adequate length of well-vascularized vas which again is dependent on the technique of the original vasectomy.

It is the case that where reanastomosis is technically successful, fertility may not necessarily follow, as the sperm in the ejaculate may be of poor quality. Nevertheless, with time there may be an improvement in sperm quality and an optimistic approach can be justified.

THE PENIS

Circumcision

The penis consists of two corpora cavernosa lying either side of a central corpus spongiosum and its contained urethra. The tip of the spongiosum dilates into the glans penis on the surface of which lies the external urethral meatus. Surrounding the corpora is a dense layer of fascia—Buck's fascia. The deep vessels and nerves of the penis lie in the perineal area within the loose area of tissue. Beneath the loosely held skin are several large vessels, particularly the dorsal vein, and underneath within the frenulum to the glans penis. The foreskin or prepuce is the terminal segment of penile skin which connects with the epithelium at the edge of the gland. Removal of this hood of skin is known as circumcision. Ritual circumcision of the newborn is probably one of the oldest and most common operations performed, the technique usually that of simple guillotining of the skin. In children requiring circumcision for symptoms, due to either recurrent balanitis or phimosis (or both), adhesions may be present and proper dissection must take place before excision of the skin. Under general anaesthetic and after cleaning up with aqueous Hibitane (chlorhexidine) the penis is towelled up and the edges of the foreskin seized with the tips of two small forceps at 2 o'clock and 10 o'clock respectively. A fine curved scissors is now passed beneath the foreskin, any phimosis being dilated first. The ends of the scissors are separated to break down any adhesions. The scissors are advanced anteriorly until it is estimated that the coronal sulcus of the skin has been reached. A dorsal incision at 12 o'clock is then made with the scissors to produce a slit in the foreskin down to the level of the coronal sulcus (*Fig.* 35.17*a*). On peeling back the two sides of foreskin, further adhesions between the inner skin layer and glans are seen and divided, using a fine metal probe (*Fig.* 35.17*b*). The small yellowish secretions of smegma are cleaned off and only when the prepuce is fully separated down to the glans is this stage of the operation complete. A clip or skin ink mark is now applied to the ventral surface of the skin to mark the point of the frenulum. This is done with the foreskin relaxed and is essential to ensure a good cosmetic result.

With the two forceps still holding the distal rim of the divided foreskin on stretch and using a sharp curved scissors the 'ears' of foreskin so produced are excised, starting at the tip of the dorsal slit, i.e. at 12 o'clock, and cutting round in an oblique curve to end up at the skin mark on the ventral surface. The foreskin is completely removed without any complicated stitches at the frenulum (*Fig.* 35.17*c*).

Bleeding points, including frenular vessels, are now picked up with fine artery forceps and ligated with 3/0 plain catgut. Bipolar diathermy is acceptable but monopolar diathermy is forbidden due to the risk of deep coagulation of vessels in the base of the penis.

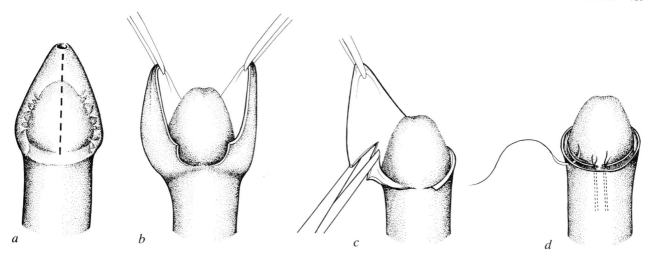

Fig. 35.17. Circumcision. Initial dorsal slit (*a*) followed by separation from the glans (*b*). The foreskin is carefully removed (*c*), leaving a 2–4 mm rim of tissue which is then carefully sutured (*d*).

Occasionally an excess of inner mucosal layer remains and this can be further excised so as to leave a 2–4 mm rim of tissue around the coronal sulcus. This mucosa is now sutured to the skin edge proper with interrupted 3/0 plain catgut on a cutting needle (*Fig.* 35.17*d*).

Special stitching at the frenulum is not necessary but care is required to line up the skin for closure and it is best to insert the 12 o'clock and 6 o'clock stitches first and then fill in the areas on either side, which are attractively presented by traction on these first two stitches. By simple stitching in the area of the frenulum damage to the external meatus can be avoided. The operation site is cleaned with aqueous Hibitane and a simple dressing applied.

The majority of patients can go home the same day, the parents being advised regarding daily saline baths for 10 days and reminded that the catgut stitches fall out at about the same time. A minor analgesic such as Junior Aspirin may be required for 1–2 days postoperatively. Adults having the same operation usually require 24 hours' inpatient stay and 7–10 days' convalescence.

Surgery of the Penis

Carcinoma of the penis is rare but when it does occur it is of the squamous variety and radiotherapy, and occasionally chemotherapy, are the treatment of choice. Extensive radical surgery, with removal of the whole penis and superficial lymph nodes of the groin, does not provide better results and is associated with marked morbidity especially lower limb oedema. In addition, the patient has the problem of a perineal urethrostomy and the psychological trauma of a mutilating procedure.

In some instances of early localized disease, particularly in the elderly, cryosurgery has something to offer. Under general anaesthesia a cryoprobe is applied directly to the lesion and held in position until an ice ball, incorporating the tumour, has formed and this is allowed to slough off over the next few days.

With extensive tumours, partial amputation of the penis can be considered, if necessary followed by radiotherapy to the residual penile shft, inguinal and deep pelvic lymph nodes. Under general anaesthesia and with the patient lying prone a rubber catheter is applied as a tourniquet to the base of the penis. An oblique incision is now made with a dorsal extension so as to provide a flap of penile skin. The incision should be as far down the shaft of the penis as possible to clear the area of tumour, yet at the same time provide an adequate stump of penis for micturition. Superficial vessels, especially the dorsal vein, are ligated with 3/0 catgut and divided. The two corpora are now boldly divided at the line of the skin incision starting dorsally and extending dorsally down on each side, but not through the spongiosum and urethra. The vessels deep in the corpora cavernosa are identified and ligated. If troublesome oozing occurs a figure-of-eight stitch can be placed so as to enclose each of the corpora separately. The spongiosum and urethra are now dissected forwards for at least 1 cm before being divided. This effectively leaves a spout of urethra projecting beyond the cut edges of the corpus. The skin flap previously constructed is now brought down over the raw area and a slit cut in the appropriate space to allow the urethral stump to project through. Excess skin is trimmed from the flap which is sewn with interrupted 3/0 catgut to the cut edge of penile skin.

The urethral stump is left projecting to remodel itself gradually back to the line of skin over the next few weeks. No drain or catheter is required and a simple gauze dressing for the first few hours is more than adequate. This technique tends to provide a better urethral meatus than that obtained by attempting a formal mucosa-to-skin anastomosis.

Meatotomy and Meatoplasty

Meatal stenosis is often symptomless, becoming a problem only when attempting to insert an instrument or a catheter into the urethra. On these occasions a simple meatotomy is all that is required. Under general anaesthesia one blade of a pair of scissors is inserted into the urethra and the scissors then closed so as to divide urethral mucosa and penile skin on the ventral aspect of the penis. The area of stenosis is usually short and one cut is all that is required. The instruments should now pass easily into the urethra. Any bleeding from the urethra usually stops but if troublesome the mucosal edge can be stitched to the skin with 3/0 catgut.

Where a patient is experiencing urinary difficulty due to obstruction, this technique is usually not suitable and a formal meatoplasty is required to clear what is a more extensive area of urethral stenosis. Under a general anaesthetic a flap of skin is raised over the ventral aspect of the penis either in the penile skin or on the inner layer of the retracted foreskin. The skin flap is elevated and the ventral surface of urethra identified. Again, using scissors the urethra is opened from the external meatus downwards so as to divide the whole area of stenosis (*Fig.* 35.18*a*). It is essential to cut through all fibrous tissue and on into healthy urethra (*Fig.* 35.18*b*). When this stage is reached the apex of the flap is sewn down to the apex of the opened urethra. The edges of the flap are sewn to the urethral edges so as to bring this down as a new floor for the distal urethra and its meatus (*Fig* 35.18*c*). The opening of the new meatus is much wider and more ventrally placed but as far as possible should allow for a good, circumscribed

stream of urine. A spraying stream represents too large and too oblique an opening. In an effort to make a more effective meatus the base of the skin flap can be divided to provide a pedicled graft base on the subcutaneous tissue, and this skin can then be sewn in the same manner. In neither technique is a catheter required. The suture material should be 3/0 catgut on a reversed cutting needle. Interrupted stitches are used.

THE URETHRA

Surgery of Urethral Stricture

Extensive stricturing of the urethra can be treated in one of three ways—regular dilatation, urethrotomy or urethroplasty.

Regular dilatation is performed using a variety of curved metal or plastic soft rubber bougies. The metal sounds are shaped to engage the posterior urethra and bladder neck and have olivary tips to reduce the risk of urethral trauma. They are best used for strictures of the posterior urethra. Bougies are less easy to manipulate in the posterior urethra and are to be preferred for strictures of the anterior urethra. The use of any sound requires patience and skill. It also requires proper understanding of the shape and consistency of the urethra.

In most cases sounds are passed on the conscious patient in the supine position. With a meticulous aseptic technique involving aqueous Hibitane skin preparation and full towelling up of the penis, the urethra is filled with a jelly containing lignocaine and Hibitane with each sound fully lubricated with the same material. At the end of the dilatation 10 ml of the same antiseptic jelly are instilled into the urethra and held there for 1–2 minutes, using a penile clamp.

Any sounds procedure is blind and in inexperienced hands can cause serious trauma to the urethra with bleeding and the formation of false passages. While experience will improve technique, dilating a stricture is an unpleasant procedure for the patient.

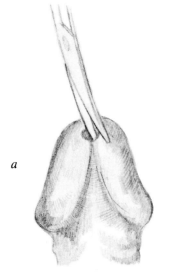
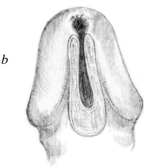
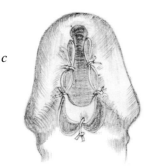

a   *b*   *c*

Fig. 35.18. Meatoplasty. The stricture is opened boldly on its ventral aspect, following which a plastic mucocutaneous repair is undertaken.

It never cures a stricture, the dilatation needing to be repeated at regular intervals with the patient experiencing urinary difficulties between each treatment.

For this reason *urethrotomy* is advised as the initial treatment for strictures, particularly those (and they are now the most common) which arise following urethral instrumentation or prolonged catheter drainage.

The original urethrotomy techniques which involved incising the stricture were blind procedures, but with the development of modern fibre-light optical instruments urethrotomy can now be performed under direct vision.

The optical urethrotome consists of a standard panendoscope using either a 30° or a 0° viewing lens. The scalpel has an anterior and superior cutting edge, mounted into two carrying rods inserted into a Nesbitt action electrotome. The instrument is inserted into the urethra and the stricture visualized. Through a side-arm a small ureteric catheter may be passed through the stricture in order to provide evidence of the direction of the urethra, both through and beyond the stricture. The knife is then extended beyond the panendoscope sheath and the fibres of the stricture are then divided by an upward cutting movement of the blade. The whole instrument is used and the cutting continued until all the fibres of the stricture are divided. It is not difficult to identify the fibres of the stricture and with cutting they can be seen to spring apart. Sometimes the incision needs to be carried deep into the wall of the urethra and bleeding may be encountered, in which case the ureteric catheter can be removed, a diathermy electrode being passed down the side-arm and any bleeding points cauterized. After full incision of the stricture has been performed, the remainder of the urethra, prostate, bladder neck and bladder are inspected. Following the incision of the stricture a fenestrated catheter may be left in place for a period of 1–7 days, the fenestrations in the catheter allowing blood to drain away from the site of the incision.

Properly performed, urethrotomy will give instant and permanent cure from the majority of strictures, eliminating the need for, and the risks of, regular dilatation. The technique, though simple, does require a full understanding of endoscopy.

However, some strictures will not respond to urethrotomy. These are usually dense strictures with marked peri-urethral fibrosis typically seen following urethral trauma, especially that associated with a fractured pelvis. In these situations formal corrective surgery in the form of *urethroplasty* is required.

These operations are of two types, either formal excision of the stricture with direct anastomosis, or skin inlay techniques using scrotal or perineal skin in a one- or two-stage procedure to form a new segment of part of the wall of the strictured area of the urethra. The variations in these techniques and the surgery involved are varied and require great experi-

ence. The more distal the stricture in the urethra, the easier the procedure. Those strictures above the membrane require a retropubic or transpubic approach and are only for those with particular experience working in specialized centres. Strictures below the membrane can be approached through a more accessible perineal exposure.

Excision and Primary Anastomosis

Preliminary urethroscopy is performed to locate the distal end of the stricture, and preoperative ascending and micturating urethrograms should be available to compare with these endoscopic findings. A curved metal sound is now placed in the urethra, its tip lying at the distal end of the stricture. The assistant holds the sound to steady the urethra. A midline incision is made through the perineum and base of the scrotal skin, bleeding vessels are coagulated and the incision deepened with scissors until the urethra is detected (*Fig. 35.19*). The urethra in this position is covered

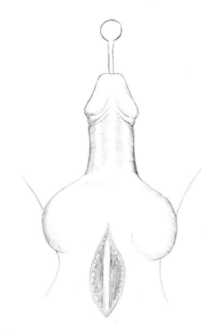

Fig. 35.19. Perineal approach for excision of urethral stricture.

with the bulbospongeosum muscle which is readily identified. The area of normal urethra containing the sound is now dissected further, if necessary dividing the spongeosum muscle. This dissection is completed until the distal point of the strictured urethra can be clearly visualized from the outside. An incision is now made into the distal urethra just beyond the point of stricture. There is sometimes troublesome bleeding from the spongy tissue in the urethra in this area and this may require temporary locking stitching, using a fine nylon stitch. This stitch is removed at the end of the procedure. The site of the strictured opening in the urethra is now seen and a probe passed through across the stricture into the normal proximal segment of urethra. The stricture is now laid open using scissors, one blade being inserted in the urethral lumen across the stricture and the other on the outside. The stricture must be opened across its full length, the incision entering the normal urethra above and below. The area of urethra involved in the stricture is now excised, care being taken on its dorsal surface to avoid bleeding from the corpora cavernosa (*Fig.* 35.20*a*). The cut ends of the urethra

extensive to allow for excision and primary anastomosis, and these may be treated by skin inlay urethroplasty, the details of which are not discussed here.

Rupture of the Urethra

Damage to the urethra may occur as a result of direct injury to the perineum involving the bulb of the an-

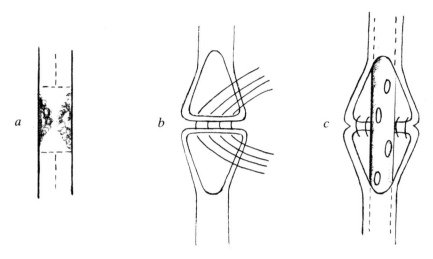

Fig. 35.20. Urethral stricture. The stricture is excised, the healthy urethra is spatulated and carefully sutured on its dorsal aspect only over a fenestrated catheter.

are now mobilized above and below and spatulated (*Fig.* 35.20*b*). With further dissection to mobilize the urethra, both ends of the urethra are brought together and sewn so as to produce an oblique anastomosis incorporating the spatulated segments, using 3/0 Dexon on a tapered cutting needle with interrupted stitches. Holding stitches above and below in the peri-urethral tissues are used to take some of the strain off the anastomosis. A no. 18 Fr gauge catheter is passed having been given some small fenestrations to coincide with the site of the anastomosis (*Fig.* 35.20*c*). These fenestrations drain any local secretions or blood. The bulbocavernosa muscle and its spongy tissue are now enclosed, again using 3/0 Dexon so as to support further the urethral anastomosis on its ventral aspect. The subcutaneous tissue is closed above a Redivac scrotum drain and the skin closed with Dexon. The catheter is removed on the 10th day.

This type of urethroplasty is very effective for small circumscribed strictures, particularly in the bulb. It is, however, difficult for strictures in the membranous urethra or above, particularly those following prostatectomy when there is a marked risk of damage to the remaining sphincter tissue with possible incontinence. In these patients a more specialized technique involving a suprapubic approach and sleeve-type anastomosis is required. Other strictures may be too

terior urethra and indirect trauma to the posterior urethra as a result of the 'shearing' effects associated with fracture of the pelvis or diathesis of the symphysis pubis. While stricture is a common sequel of rupture of the urethra, the severity of the stricture will vary as to whether the injury causes a partial or complete rupture of the urethra.

The passage of blood per urethram with or without retention of urine, following these various types of injury, should suggest the possibility of urethral damage. Incomplete rupture of the urethra will heal spontaneously albeit with the probability of subsequent stricture formation. Such strictures, however, can be dealt with by urethrotomy or simple excision urethroplasty at a later date. Where complete rupture of the urethra has occurred with separation of the urethral ends, a massive impassable stricture occurs, requiring complex repair procedures, possible only in the most skilled hands. If, however, the urethra can be realigned across a catheter the subsequent stricture is less complex and easier to correct. The important management of possible urethral trauma is therefore to recognize complete rupture. The solution lies in suspecting the possibility of urethral trauma following any fracture of the pelvis, diatheses of the symphysis or soft-tissue injury to the perineum. The patient may pass urine spontaneously. If this occurs then there is either no trauma or the urethral tear is incomplete and continuity of its wall is preserved. In this situation no surgical treatment is required, though follow-up for at least 2 years is necessary to detect stricture formation.

If the patient fails to void after 12 hours, an enlarged bladder is both seen and complained of. If no bladder is detected at 12 hours under these conditions, the possibility of either bladder rupture or renal failure with oliguria is likely.

Assuming that a palpable bladder has developed in association with the patient's inability to void, the possibility of complete or partial rupture of the urethra must be considered. The management of such a patient is to proceed to the operating theatre and, in the anaesthetic room before induction is commenced, to attempt to pass a soft latex catheter (no. 16 or 18 Fr gauge for the average adult male) along the urethra into the bladder. This must be done under full aseptic conditions with instillations of Hibitane and lignocaine jelly into the urethra beforehand. The catheterization should be done gently by one skilled in urology. If the catheter passes into the bladder and urine drains, no more need be done, the patient being returned to the ward and the catheter removed in 7–10 days. Again, follow-up is required to detect early stricture formation.

If the catheter will not pass into the bladder easily, no attempt should be made to force it and in particular no use made of a catheter introducer. The possibility of complete rupture must now be considered and, if confirmed, immediate steps taken to realign the severed ends of urethra.

In the supine position, under full aseptic preparation and with the penis exposed and accessible, a lower midline or transverse incision is made to expose the distended bladder.

This is opened between stay stitches, the incision being extended to allow a bladder retractor to be inserted in such a way as to display the internal meatus. A metal (Lister) type sound is now passed down the penile urethra and a gentle attempt made to advance it into the bladder. If the urethral injury is incomplete it may still be possible to do this even after initial failure with a catheter. In that event a nylon ligature is tied to the tip of the sound in the bladder, preferably through a small specially designed eye, which is then withdrawn back across the urethra. The end of the ligature is then untied while its other end is held firmly in the bladder. A catheter is tied on to the distal part of the nylon ligature and by pulling from the bladder end, the catheter is drawn into the bladder. The bladder is closed with 2/0 chromic catgut and the abdominal wound closed in the usual way. The catheter is removed on the 10th day.

If the urethral sound will not pass into the bladder a complete rupture has probably occurred. In this situation an elaborate railroading technique is required to get a catheter to lie across the urethra. A metal sound is inserted through the internal meatus

and advanced along the healthy proximal urethra until it reaches the area of urethral disruption. A sound is now passed down the distal urethra until it too reaches the area of urethral disruption (*Fig. 35.21a*). By simultaneously manipulating the bladder and urethral sounds, it is possible by feel and actual sound to align the two metal ends of the sounds so as to allow one (usually the bladder sound) to be advanced forwards into the other side of the ruptured urethra (*Fig. 35.21b*). Whichever sound is so advanced, be it either bladder or urethra, the tip of that sound is presented at the appropriate meatus. If this is the external meatus a nylon ligature is tied to the specially designed eye of the sound which is then withdrawn into the bladder. The ligature is next tied to a catheter which is pulled across the urethra and up into the bladder (*Fig. 35.21c*). If the urethral sound passes through the internal meatus into the bladder, the ligature is again tied to the tip of the sound which is withdrawn and, once more, by tying the catheter onto the distal end, the catheter can be railroaded back into the bladder. With the catheter lying across the urethra the bladder is closed in the usual way with a suprapubic catheter for drainage purposes.

When the urethral rupture is high, particularly in children, loop stitches of nylon are placed either side of the bladder neck and brought out through the perineum to be stitched to the thigh. These stitches provide traction to the pelvic floor and urethra, and help to bring the ends of the urethra close together around the catheter.

Traction of the catheter may also be applied using a rubber band tied to the end of the catheter and crêpe bandage across the thigh. Such traction should be gentle and only applied for 12 hours as ischaemic damage may be caused to the bladder neck by prolonged firm traction.

In addition, fenestrations should be cut in the catheter prior to its insertion. These drain local secretions and haematoma from the area of ruptured urethra. These fenestrations can subsequently be used to perform an ascending urethrogram via the catheter at about 10 days. Should this show the urethra to have healed the catheter can be removed. Patients with complete rupture will eventually develop a stricture, and panendoscopy at 6–12 weeks is essential to define this and organize further management.

Where complete rupture has occurred but is not detected due to the use of blind suprapubic drainage, the inevitable massive fibrosis makes early urethral reconstruction impossible. At least 12 months should be allowed to elapse before urethroplasty is attempted in order to allow maximum resolution of scar tissue. Such a disaster may be due to inadequately trained surgical personnel or more serious injuries preventing a proper assessment of the urethral injury. In these cases, straightforward suprapubic catheterization is acceptable and preferable to risking the patient's life or worsening the urethral injury.

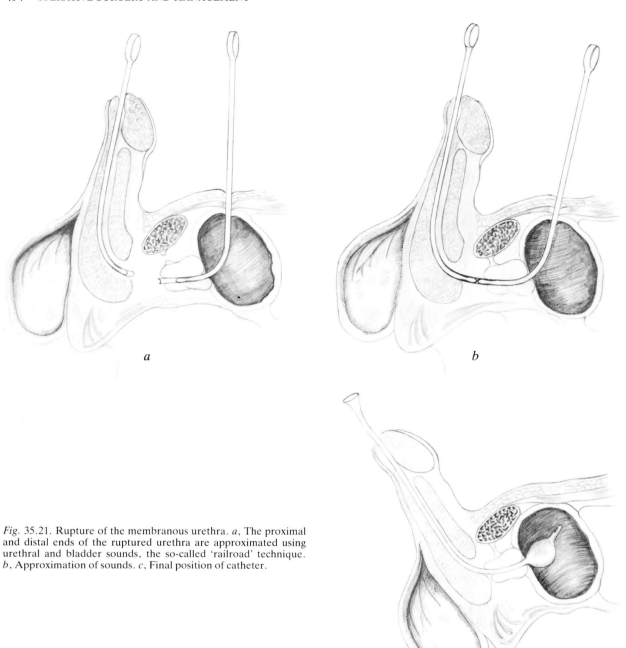

Fig. 35.21. Rupture of the membranous urethra. *a*, The proximal
and distal ends of the ruptured urethra are approximated using
urethral and bladder sounds, the so-called 'railroad' technique.
b, Approximation of sounds. *c*, Final position of catheter.

FURTHER READING

Khezri A. A., Dunn M., Smith P. J. B. et al. (1978) Carcinoma of the penis. *Br. J. Urol.* **50**, 275–279.
Peckham M. (ed.) (1981) *The Management of Testicular Tumours.* London, Edward Arnold.
Smith P. J. B. and Kaisary A. V. (1984) Disorders of the external genitalia in the male. *Gen. Practitioner* **228**, 733–741.
Smith P. J. B., Dunn M. and Roberts J. B. M. (1981) Surgical management of urethral stricture in the male. *Urology* **18**(6), 582.

Chapter thirty-six

The Adrenal Gland

R. N. Baird

The number of adrenalectomy operations performed in the past 10–15 years has fallen, particularly operations for metastatic breast cancer and Cushing's syndrome, because of the development of alternative forms of treatment of comparable efficacy. Nevertheless, adrenocortical adenomas and carcinomas, many of which produce distressing endocrine effects, as well as phaeochromocytomas, may be cured or substantially improved by surgical excision. Patients coming to operation with functioning adrenal tumours undergo time-consuming investigations, often under the care of a specialist physician, so that preoperatively the surgeon is as aware as possible of the location, size and endocrine effects of the growth about to be removed. With good pre-, per- and postoperative management and the appropriate surgical approach the operative mortality should be less than 5 per cent. The long-term results of operations for benign tumours are excellent. Patients with malignant adrenal tumours generally fare badly, and many die of recurrent disease within a year or two.

SURGICAL ANATOMY

The triangular-shaped right adrenal gland lies posterior and lateral to the vena cava and above the kidney. The crescent-shaped left adrenal gland lies medial to the upper pole of the kidney and just lateral to the aorta. The adrenal glands are readily distinguished from the surrounding fat by their chrome yellow colour and firm granular consistency. Their arterial blood supply is inconstant and many small arteries enter the glands, arising from the inferior phrenic artery, the abdominal aorta directly and the renal artery. The single draining adrenal vein on each side is an important surgical feature, especially on the right side where the adrenal vein is short and enters the posterolateral aspect of the vena cava directly. At this point the cava is vulnerable to injury and the right adrenal vein should be dissected with particular care. The left adrenal vein leaves the gland and descends obliquely to enter the left renal vein.

The adrenals are compound glands. The cortex, which produces adrenal steroids, is derived from coelomic mesoderm; the medulla, which produces adrenaline and noradrenaline, is derived from the neural crest ectoderm, and forms part of the neuro-endocrine system of cells known as the 'APUD series'.

CUSHING'S SYNDROME

Clinical Features

The main clinical features of Cushing's syndrome are weakness, obesity—which particularly affects the face (moonface), abdomen and neck (buffalo hump)—hirsutism, acne, purple striae of the abdomen, capillary fragility and skin bruising. Additional features include hypertension, oligomenorrhoea, mild diabetes, mental disturbance and osteoporosis. Middle-aged women are most commonly affected and untreated; the effects of excess cortisol are progressive and often fatal.

Pathophysiology

The cause of excessive cortisol production is usually diffuse hyperplasia of both adrenal glands due to a small ACTH-secreting adenoma of the anterior pituitary, originally described by Harvey Cushing and referred to either as 'Cushing's disease' or 'pituitary-dependent Cushing's syndrome'. Excess ACTH from oat cell carcinoma of the bronchus or thymic tumours may cause adrenal hyperplasia with resulting excess cortisol production, often with marked muscle weakness, hyperpigmentation and oedema not typically seen in Cushing's disease (the ectopic ACTH syndrome). Cushing's syndrome may also be caused by a small functioning adenoma of the adrenal cortex or by an adrenocortical carcinoma, where virilization may be a striking feature.

Investigations

Excess cortisol production, with loss of the normal diurnal variation, is demonstrated as an elevation of plasma cortisol and urinary corticosteroid metabolic products. Pituitary dependence is determined by suppression of urinary and plasma cortisol levels with dexamethasone. Enlargement of the pituitary fossa on skull radiographs and a normal or raised plasma ACTH level favour the diagnosis of pituitary-dependent Cushing's disease. On the other hand, undetectably low plasma ACTH, with a radiological abnormality of one adrenal gland, suggests an autonomous functioning adrenal tumour. Very high ACTH levels raise the suspicion of an ectopic ACTH-producing neoplasm, e.g. from a primary tumour of lung or pancreas.

Pituitary-dependent Cushing's Disease

Patients with mild forms of pituitary-dependent Cushing's disease and bilateral adrenal hyperplasia are usually treated with metyrapone, aminoglutethamide and o,p'-DDD, which block cortisol synthesis in the adrenal gland. In more severe cases excess cortisol secretion can be abolished without the risk of hypopituitarism by bilateral total adrenalectomy. However, the operative mortality, the morbidity, the risk (up to 30 per cent) of an enlarging pituitary tumour (Nelson's syndrome), and the need for life-long replacement therapy mean that operation is reserved for severe cases which fail to respond to medical treatment and for those for whom future fertility is an important consideration. Postoperatively, radiographs of the pituitary fossa and plasma ACTH measurements are obtained at regular intervals.

The pituitary tumour may be treated by radiotherapy, either by external beam or by implant, but there is a risk of hypopituitarism and selective surgical removal of the small functioning pituitary adenoma by the transphenoidal route is now preferred.

UNILATERAL ADRENAL DISEASE

Localization

Only the largest (10 cm or more) adrenal tumours are palpable on abdominal examination. On plain abdominal radiography an adrenal mass may be present above the kidney. The plain film may show adrenal calcification. Other investigations include intravenous urography with tomography, ultrasound and computed tomographic (CT) scanning of the adrenal areas. Arteriography, selective adrenal venography and iodocholesterol isotope scanning may disclose a small functioning adrenal adenoma with typical atrophy of the contralateral adrenal gland. Small (<2·5 cm) tumours are best removed by the anterior (see p. 500) or posterior approach (see p. 499); the lateral thoraco-abdominal approach gives generous access for larger tumours.

Bilateral Nodular Adrenal Hyperplasia

This may be pituitary-dependent or autonomous. If associated with a low plasma ACTH (i.e. autonomous), a bilateral total adrenalectomy may be indicated.

Postoperative Maintenance Following Bilateral Adrenalectomy

The following regimen is suggested, and this is begun as soon as the adrenal(s) have been removed. Hydrocortisone hemisuccinate is given 100 mg 8-hourly i.v., providing a total of 300 mg in the first 24 hours, and in the next 24 hours this is reduced to 50 mg 8-hourly i.v. to give a total of 150 mg for the 2nd day. Thereafter the dose is gradually tapered downwards and converted to oral hydrocortisone, aiming at a daily maintenance dose of 20–30 mg hydrocortisone by 2 weeks postoperatively, with two-thirds given in the morning and 0·1 mg fluorocortisone given once daily. Symptoms suggesting adrenal insufficiency should be treated by increasing steroids; an unexplained fall in blood pressure in the early postoperative period may respond to an extra intravenous dose of 100 mg hydrocortisone. After removal of an adrenal adenoma the remaining suppressed gland will usually resume function in due course, and replacement therapy can be tailed off. Lifelong replacement is necessary after total resections.

PRIMARY ALDOSTERONISM (CONN'S SYNDROME)

Pathophysiology

Aldosterone is released by the outermost layer of cells of the adrenal cortex, the zona glomerulosa, and acts to maintain normal concentrations of sodium and potassium by its action on the distal renal tubule. The main stimulus to aldosterone production is sodium depletion, resulting in a fall in the circulating blood volume, which in turn stimulates the kidney to release renin. Renin causes aldosterone to be secreted via the renin/angiotensin system, and aldosterone acts to restore the circulating blood volume by causing sodium retention. In Conn's syndrome, the autonomous hypersecretion of aldosterone which occurs is not controlled by the renin/angiotensin system and there is excessive sodium retention, causing arterial hypertension and hypokalaemic alkalosis secondary to potassium loss.

Clinical Features

Most patients with Conn's syndrome present with essential hypertension and are found to have persistent hypokalaemia. Occasionally the presenting features are those of hypokalaemia, e.g. polyuria, muscle weakness or tetany. Rarely, carpal spasm is produced by the sphygmomanometer cuff when the blood pressure is being recorded.

Investigations

In patients with persistent hypokalaemia in whom Conn's syndrome is suspected, causes of secondary aldosteronism must be sought. These include malignant hypertension, cirrhosis, nephrotic syndrome and severe cardiac failure. Plasma aldosterone levels and plasma renin activity are measured under standardized conditions. In primary aldosteronism, plasma aldosterone levels are raised but renin activity is suppressed, whereas in secondary forms both levels are raised.

Management

Spironolactone is a competitive antagonist to aldosterone and treatment for 2–3 weeks will correct the metabolic alkalosis and restore the blood pressure towards normal. Bilateral adrenal hyperplasia (diffuse or micronodular) is best treated with spironolactone. Surgical treatment is reserved for patients in whom at least tentative lateralization of a tumour has been achieved. Selective adrenal venous sampling for plasma aldosterone assay, [75]Selenium iodocholesterol imaging (*Fig.* 36.1), ultrasound and CT scanning have successfully lateralized these small tumours, which are seldom of more than 2 cm.

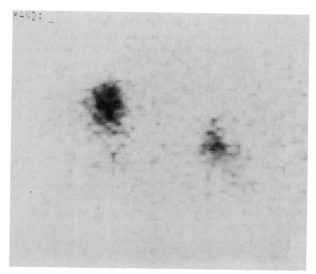

Fig. 36.1. [75]Selenium iodocholesterol scan showing increased uptake from a functioning adrenal tumour (*left*) in Conn's syndrome, compared with normal adrenal (*right*).

Surgical Approach

A solitary tumour (*Fig.* 36.2) is best removed by unilateral adrenalectomy via the posterior approach. In poor surgical risk patients, therapeutic venous infarction of a functioning adrenal adenoma has been

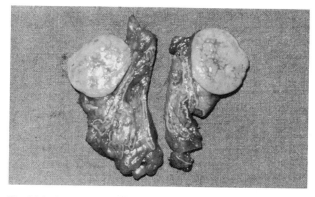

Fig. 36.2. Operative adrenalectomy specimen in Conn's syndrome showing an adrenal adenoma.

described. The adrenal vein is catheterized and sclerosant injected retrogradely into the tumour veins.

VIRILIZING AND FEMINIZING SYNDROMES

The development of masculine features in an adult woman is occasionally due to a functioning benign adrenal tumour, removal of which results in the long-term restoration of the patient's female characteristics. In most instances, however, the adrenal tumour is large and malignant with a poor prognosis following surgical excision. Functioning adrenocortical tumours which cause feminization in males are very rare. These changes towards the opposite sex are much more commonly caused by congenital adrenal hyperplasia (the adrenogenital syndromes), or the exogenous administration of androgens, or by functioning tumours of the ovary, testis or placenta.

ADRENALECTOMY FOR METASTATIC BREAST CANCER

Since the demonstration by Huggins in 1952 of a striking remission of advanced breast cancer after bilateral adrenalectomy, it has become recognized that about one-third of patients with metastatic disease will benefit from operation. A successful response to adrenalectomy is more likely in patients at or beyond the menopause, with a long disease-free interval following primary treatment, a good response to prior ovariectomy, or with metastases located in bone, soft tissue and skin. Secondary growths in the brain, liver and lungs do not respond. The adrenals are removed by the anterior transperitoneal approach (*see* p. 500) and the presence or absence of metastases is noted—a staging laparotomy. Steroid replacement is necessary (*see* p. 496). The benefits of a satisfactory remission have to be set against the response rate, and operative mortality and morbidity of adrenalectomy, compared with comparable treatments such as hypophysectomy, local radiotherapy and chemotherapy. Adrenalectomy is performed less frequently nowadays than in the 1960s, and other palliative treatments are now generally preferred.

Adrenalectomy for metastatic prostatic cancer has produced remission in some patients following orchidectomy and oestrogen therapy, but is not widely used at present.

PHAEOCHROMOCYTOMA

Clinical Features

Patients with catecholamine-secreting tumours of the adrenal medulla characteristically present with symptoms of headache, excessive sweating and palpitations. On examination, the blood pressure is raised, may fluctuate widely and is associated with alternate blanching and flushing of the face. These symptoms and signs are due to the release of excessive amounts of adrenaline and noradrenaline. In the absence of severe paroxysms of hypertension, there may be a variety of features, including tremor, nausea, weakness, dyspnoea and weight loss.

In a few patients the first indication of a phaeochromocytoma is a sudden escalation in blood pressure, when an unsuspected adrenal mass is discovered at laparotomy during routine palpation of the abdominal viscera.

Phaeochromocytomas are particularly hazardous when they occur in children, in pregnancy, and when located extra-adrenally in the wall of the urinary bladder. Rarely, the tumour is familial, as in multiple endocrine neoplasia type II, where there are the associated features of medullary thyroid carcinoma, hyperparathyroidism and submucous neuromas.

Investigations

Confirmation of the diagnosis of a clinically suspected phaeochromocytoma is by finding raised VMA (vanillylmandelic acid) or metadrenaline levels in 24-hour specimens of urine. Urinary free catecholamines and plasma catecholamines may also be measured. If raised levels are found, treatment with adrenergic blocking agents is instituted before further investigations to localize the tumour are undertaken. Two alpha-adrenergic blocking agents are available. Phentolamine is rapid acting and is useful in the acute control of hypertension in intravenous doses of 1–5 mg. Long-term alpha-blockage is achieved using oral phenoxybenzamine in a dose of 20–200 mg daily and takes 5–7 days. Additional treatment with a beta-blocker (propranolol) is given for cardiac dysrhythmias.

Ninety per cent of phaeochromocytomas occur in the adrenal glands. The first localizing investigation is an intravenous urogram with tomography, which characteristically shows displacement of the upper pole of the kidney by an adrenal mass. Ultrasound, CT scanning and ^{131}I-metaiodobenzylguanidine scanning have been used to localize small tumours (less than 2·5 cm). In children, the most common extra-adrenal location of a tumour is on the anterior surface of the aorta, between the inferior mesenteric artery and the aortic bifurcation (the organ of Zuckerkandl). Other rare sites of tumours include the hilum of the kidney, and along the line of the sympathetic chains extending from the abdomen into the neck. Tumours in the bladder cause hypertension on micturition and are diagnosed at cytoscopy, and treated by partial cystectomy.

Operative Management

Alpha-blockade with phenoxybenzamine is given for at least 1 week before operation to control hypertension and to allow the contracted plasma volume to become restored towards normal. Beta-blockade with propranolol may be necessary to slow a persistent tachycardia, but should not be used without prior alpha-blockade because of the risk of precipitating pulmonary oedema.

Premedication is by tranquillizers as opiate narcotics may stimulate catecholamine release. Prior to induction of anaesthesia continuous monitoring of ECG, CVP and arterial pressure is established. Intravenous lignocaine, propranolol, sodium nitroprusside and phentolamine are immediately available to treat dysrhythmias and fluctuations in blood pressure. Prompt replacement of measured blood loss is important and additional fluid replacement amounting to 2–3 L of crystalloid and colloid solutions may be needed to correct the preoperative deficit in plasma volume.

The anterior transabdominal approach is used (*see* p. 500). A generous vertical or transverse incision is made and both adrenals, the renal fossas, paraspinal areas and pelvis are inspected, and the effect of gentle palpation on the blood pressure noted. Multiple tumours present in 10 per cent of adults and one-third of children. Catecholamine release from the tumour is minimized by non-manipulative dissection and early control of the main venous drainage. Phaeochromocytomas are vascular tumours with a generous blood supply. Once the tumour has been removed, the blood pressure falls, and volume replacement and even a noradrenaline infusion may be necessary. If at this stage the arterial pressure does not fall, a further search is made for a second tumour, and any suspicious mass within the abdomen is squeezed gently and the effect on blood pressure noted.

Phaeochromocytoma during Pregnancy

The finding of raised catecholamines in the urine or plasma, or metanephrines or VMA in the urine of a hypertensive pregnant woman strongly suggests an adrenal tumour. If a phaeochromocytoma is diagnosed at any stage during pregnancy it should be removed through a transverse upper abdominal incision because it presents a life-threatening risk to mother and baby. Localizing investigations should not be undertaken because of the radiation risk to the fetus.

Prognosis

The outlook following removal of a benign phaeochromocytoma is excellent, with return of blood pressure towards normal. If hypertension and raised catecholamine levels persist postoperatively, a residual tumour should be sought.

Malignancy is defined as the presence of metastases and occurs in about 10 per cent. The histological features are unhelpful in determining malignancy.

Metastases grow slowly and may not respond to radiotherapy, but alpha-methyl tyrosine, which inhibits catecholamine synthesis, can provide symptomatic relief.

NON-ENDOCRINE TUMOURS OF THE ADRENAL GLAND

The most common non-endocrine adrenal tumour is the neuroblastoma, which occurs only in infancy and childhood. Ganglioneuromas of the adrenal medulla, non-functioning adrenal cysts and adrenocortical carcinomas present as abdominal masses and are removed through a lateral thoraco-abdominal incision.

OPERATIVE TECHNIQUES

Lateral Thoraco-abdominal Approach

The lateral approach is necessary for some large adrenal tumours. The patient is placed in the anterolateral position at about 45°, with sandbags under the shoulder and buttock. The arm is supported across the chest on an armrest and the operating table tilted laterally.

Right Side (*Fig.* 36.3)

On the right side, an approach through the bed of the 9th or 10th rib dividing the diaphragm and partly displacing the liver into the chest, as for a portacaval anastomosis, gives excellent access, particularly for larger tumours. The key to removal of the right adrenal is ligation of the short (0·5 cm) adrenal vein at its confluence with the vena cava. First, the peritoneum at the inferior border of the liver and the lateral edge of the vena cava is incised. The cava is then carefully retracted medially so that the junction of the adrenal vein and the posterolateral surface of the vena cava may be viewed directly prior to ligation or clipping. If the adrenal vein is inadvertently avulsed at this stage blood loss may be substantial and control with a tangentially occluding vascular clamp is more easily achieved if the lateral border of the vena cava has already been mobilized. If access is limited, an Allis clamp may be applied directly to the vena cava to include the torn adrenal vein. Once control has been achieved, the tear is sutured using 5/0 Prolene.

The adrenal is thereafter gradually developed from the retroperitoneal fat by digital dissection.

Left Side

On the left side, an 11th rib approach is better. Following excision of the rib below the pleural reflection and insertion of a Finichietto retractor, the perito-

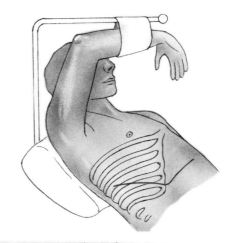

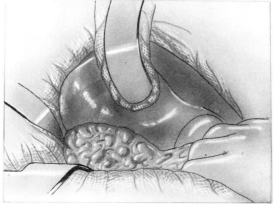

Fig. 36.3. Operative exposure of a large tumour of the right adrenal by a lateral thoraco-abdominal approach through the 9th rib.

neum is swept forwards to reveal the kidney and adrenal. The left adrenal vein is longer (2 cm) than the right and is ligated at its junction with the left renal vein. For larger tumours, the peritoneum is entered and the spleen and tail of pancreas mobilized and displaced forwards.

Large adrenocortical carcinomas should be excised together with the kidney: on the left side the spleen and tail of pancreas should be excised en bloc with the tumour.

Posterior Approach (*Fig.* 36.4)

The patient is placed prone on the operating table with support under the hips and shoulders so that the abdomen does not touch the operating table. Particular care is required for obese patients with Cushing's syndrome, whose skin and bones are easily damaged.

A posterior incision is made and the 11th or 12th rib excised. The adrenal gland is dissected free, and the adrenal vein ligated (*Fig.* 36.5). As for the lateral thoraco-abdominal approach, the right adrenal vein and adjacent vena cava are dissected with particular care to avoid injury.

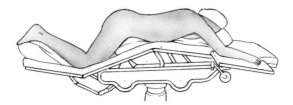

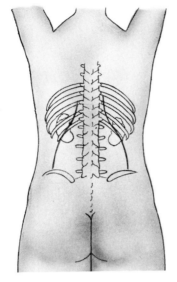

Fig. 36.4. The posterior approach. Careful positioning of the patient is important. On either side, extraperitoneal access is gained via the bed of the 11th or 12th rib.

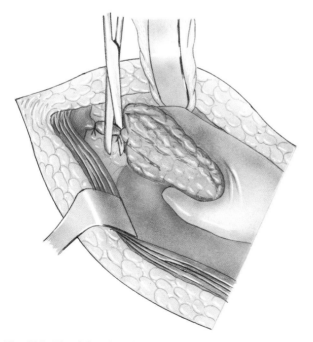

Fig. 36.5. The right adrenal gland is carefully dissected until the adrenal vein is identified and ligated.

Anterior Transperitoneal Approach

The anterior approach is used for phaeochromocytomas and for bilateral adrenalectomy for breast cancer. Either a subcostal transverse or a vertical incision may be used. The abdomen is opened and the viscera are carefully inspected and palpated.

The right adrenal is approached by mobilizing the hepatic flexure of the colon and displacing it downwards with upward retraction of the liver (*Fig.* 36.6).

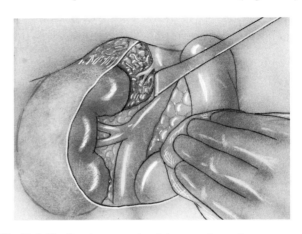

Fig. 36.6. The liver is retracted and the posterior peritoneum overlying the inferior vena cava incised. The short (0·5 cm) right adrenal vein enters the posterolateral surface of the vena cava and is dissected with great care.

The peritoneum over the gland is incised; excision proceeds as for the lateral thoraco-abdominal approach, with particular care during the ligation of the right adrenal vein (*Fig.* 36.7).

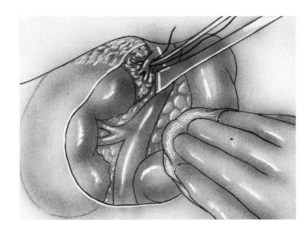

Fig. 36.7. Ligation of the right adrenal vein.

On the left side, the gastrocolic omentum is opened, and the gland exposed by incising the peritoneum overlying the lower border of the pancreas, and retracting the pancreas and splenic vein upwards (*Fig.* 36.8). The upper pole of the kidney and left adrenal are then in view, and the left adrenal vein is ligated (*Fig.* 36.9). Alternatively, the left adrenal

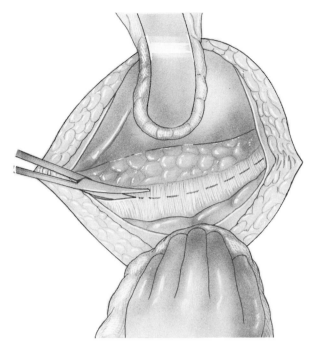

can be approached by mobilizing the spleen and tail of pancreas and displacing them downwards, or by incising the transverse mesocolon lateral to the inferior mesenteric vein to display the renal and hence the adrenal vein and gland.

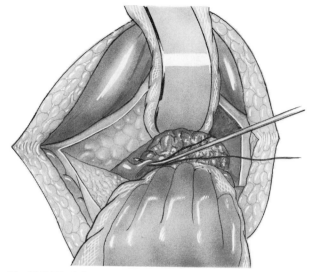

Fig. 36.8. Anterior aproach to the left adrenal gland by incising the gastrocolic omentum. The posterior peritoneum overlying the lower border of the pancreas is incised, and the pancreas and splenic vein are retracted upwards.

Fig. 36.9. The left adrenal is exposed and the adrenal vein is ligated at its confluence with the left renal vein.

FURTHER READING

Ahmed S. R., Shalet S. M., Beardwell C. G. et al. (1984) Treatment of Cushing's disease with low dose radiation therapy. *Br. Med. J.* **289**, 643–646.

Clarke D., Wilkinson R., Johnston I. D. A. et al. (1979) Severe hypertension in primary aldosteronism and good response to surgery. *Lancet* **1**, 482–485.

Edis A. J., Ayala L. A. and Egdahl R. H. (1975) *Manual of Endocrine Surgery*. Berlin, Springer-Verlag.

Ferris J. B., Brown J. J., Fraser R. et al. (1975) Results of adrenal surgery in patients with hypertension, aldosterone excess and low plasma renin concentration. *Br. Med. J.* **1**, 135–138.

Friesen S. R. (ed.) (1978) *Surgical Endocrinology, Clinical Syndromes*. Philadelphia, Lippincott.

Hunt T. K., Roisen M. F., Tyrell J. B. et al. (1984) Current achievements and challenges in adrenal surgery. *Br. J. Surg.* **71**, 983–985.

Leading Article (1977) Pituitary-dependent Cushing's disease. *Br. Med. J.* **1**, 1049.

Leading Article (1983) Primary aldosteronism: how hard should we look? *Br. Med. J.* **287**, 702–703.

Leading Article (1984) Iodobenzylguanidine for localisation and treatment of phaeochromocytoma. *Lancet*. 905–906.

Levine S. N. and McDonald J. C. (1984) The evaluation and management of phaeochromocytomas. *Adv. Surg.* **17**, 281–313.

Mathias C. J., Peart W. S., Carron D. B. et al. (1984) Therapeutic venous infarction of an aldosterone producing adenoma (Conn's tumour). *Br. Med. J.* **288**, 1416–1417.

Moldin I. M., Farndon J. R., Shepard A. et al. (1979) Phaeochromocytomas in 72 patients: clinical and diagnostic features, treatment and long term results. *Br. J. Surg.* **66**, 456–465.

Montgomery D. A. D. and Welbourn R. B. (1975) *Medical and Surgical Endocrinology*. London, Arnold.

Montgomery D. A. D. and Welbourn R. B. (1978) Cushing's syndrome: 20 years after adrenalectomy. *Br. J. Surg.* **65**, 221–223.

Scott H. W., Liddle G. W., Mullhevin J. L. et al. (1977) Surgical experience with Cushing's disease. *Ann. Surg.* **185**, 524–534.

Walker R. Milnes (1964) Phaeochromocytoma in relation to pregnancy. *Br. J. Surg.* **51**, 590–595.

Arterial, Cardiac and Venous Surgery

Chapter thirty-seven

The Abdominal Aorta and its Peripheral Branches

Sir Geoffrey Slaney and F. Ashton

CHRONIC OCCLUSIVE ARTERIAL DISEASE OF THE LOWER LIMBS

Clinical Assessment

Patients may present with claudication of varying degrees of severity in one or several of the major muscle groups in the legs. The calves are most commonly affected, especially in femoropopliteal occlusions, but symptoms may be confined to the anterior tibial muscles or those of the foot, particularly when the tibial vessels are affected. Numbness of the foot may occur after exercise. Proximal claudication in thighs and buttocks suggests aorto-iliac disease, but patients sometimes complain of fatigue or heaviness of the limb in exercise rather than claudication as such.

More extreme ischaemia is evidenced by pain at rest in the ankle or forefoot while further impairment of blood flow leads to gangrene, usually of the dry type in the toes, although local trauma to bony prominences, especially pressure, may cause ischaemic ulcers of the heel and the external malleolus.

Of the so-called 'signs of ischaemia' in the distal skin, hair loss is most unreliable, while punctate pigmentation and atrophy of the toe pulps, together with defective nail growth, usually reflect marked paucity of blood supply. Painful fissures may occur in the skin of the heel, and small cutaneous infarcts due to micro-emboli may rarely be seen.

These more extreme features of ischaemia are seldom seen with aorto-iliac disease alone and when present usually indicate coexistent distal disease in the femoropopliteal, tibial or distal vessels. In these cases a combination of aorto-iliac, femoral and tibial disease acts like resistances in series to reduce blood flow to extremely low levels. Moreover, very poor distal perfusion may occur even with minimal tibial artery disease, if there is simultaneous impairment of flow down both superficial femoral and profunda vessels; the resistance to flow in this situation being analogous to 'resistance in parallel'.

Pallor of the extremity on elevation with rubor on dependency are often seen with significant ischaemia; the elevation pallor being particularly marked after a period of exercise. With femoropopliteal or more distal disease pulses are usually absent, particularly in the more extreme degrees of ischaemia. However, well-collateralized proximal total occlusions and stenotic lesions associated with claudication alone may not be apparent because the distal pulses can often be felt, though these may disappear after brief exercise, revealing the true state of affairs. Clinical assessment of the femoral pulses is notoriously inaccurate and they may be judged normal in the presence of appreciable aorto-iliac disease, particularly when a reflected wave from a blocked femoral artery reinforces the amplitude. A bruit over the femoral or iliac arteries often clinches the diagnosis. If pulses do not weaken or disappear on exercise it is possible that the patient may have spinal stenosis—so-called 'cauda equina claudication'. However, the presence of backache, the occurrence of the pain on standing alone and the absence of neurological signs in the legs usually permit a distinction to be made. However, occasionally the differentiation can be difficult and warrant detailed neurological investigation. In the atypical case degenerative arthritis of the spine, hip or knee, disc syndromes and metastatic bone disease must be considered in the differential diagnosis of aorto-iliac occlusive disease.

Management

While clinical examination alone will often enable a sound assessment to be made in the majority of patients, supplemented by arteriography or other specialized techniques when surgery is contemplated, routine ancillary tests are essential in the management of these patients. While other manifestations of atherosclerosis, such as cerebral, cardiac, mesenteric and renal disease, may be evident from the history or clinical examination, other diseases are frequently present. Carcinoma of the gastrointestinal tract is common in this age group, as is carcinoma of the bronchus due to the almost invariable association of atherosclerosis with smoking. In our experience some 5 per cent of patients will have a coincident carcinoma and 18 per cent will have past or present evidence of peptic ulceration which may cause complications in the postoperative period.

Polycythaemia rubra vera is found in a small proportion of patients. Lesser degrees of polycythaemia are frequently due to smoking and chronic bronchitis and may have profound effects on viscosity in low-flow situations (Yates et al. 1979). Obviously primary polycythaemia and even its minor variants should be treated because of their deleterious effect on blood viscosity and thrombogenicity even if no arterial surgery is contemplated. Undetected or untreated following a reconstructive procedure, their effect may be disastrous. Primary thrombocythaemia may present with peripheral gangrene and lead to confusion with atherosclerotic gangrene but peripheral pulses tend to be present; however, the two conditions may coexist. Unsuspected raised platelet aggregation or adhesiveness can also jeopardize reconstruction and treatment with drugs may be considered; similarly a high level of fibrinogen with deficient fibrinolysis in the serum might militate against successful reconstruction.

The treatment of abnormal patterns of plasma lipids by diet or drugs seems rational whether or not surgery is undertaken, although the ultimate effect on the long-term success of arterial reconstruction remains uncertain. It is now widely accepted that smoking has a most potent aggravating effect on the progression of atherosclerosis and one recent study suggests that it is far more potent than hyperlipidaemia in this respect (Greenhalgh et al., 1980).

Concurrent diseases such as diabetes and hypertension must be borne in mind and while they do not contra-indicate surgery they increase the risks from sepsis, problems with hypoglycaemia and from untoward reaction to anaesthetic drugs. However, awareness and experience of these conditions by both surgeon and anaesthetist usually enable the patient to be safely treated.

It is generally considered important to treat previously undetected diabetes mellitus when dealing with patients with atherosclerosis. While it is undoubtedly correct to control the complications of the disease, it is not proven that treatment arrests the progression of the arterial disease. Diabetic patients have a significantly higher mortality rate than non-diabetics when followed for a decade or more postoperatively (DeWeese and Rob, 1977; Malone et al., 1977).

Renal Function

It is important to detect incipient or actual renal failure preoperatively. To the azotaemia of any major operation may be added the stress of aortic clamping which studies in the authors' Unit have shown always depresses renal function even if the renal vessels are normal; additionally, a preoperative aortogram may further depress renal function (Powis, 1975).

Myocardial Ischaemia

A previous history of angina, myocardial infarction or ECG evidence of ischaemia does not exclude vascular reconstruction, but in major aortic procedures it does, however, double the operative mortality rate. In distal reconstructions it affects the long-term prognosis, and of 329 autogenous vein bypass grafts which the authors performed, 125 had significant ECG evidence of ischaemia. Twenty-seven patients subsequently died from myocardial infarction during the

decade of follow-up. Of these 27 patients, 18 had ECG changes prior to surgery and 5 died with a patent graft (Grimley et al., 1979). The 10-year follow-up results reported by DeWeese and Rob (1977) demonstrated a mortality rate of over 40 per cent in patients with known myocardial ischaemia prior to surgery.

Pulmonary Disease

Severe chronic bronchitis seriously militates against abdominal aortic procedures, but an extracoelomic bypass may provide an excellent substitute with a low-operative risk because surgery can be accomplished under an epidural, local or light general anaesthetic. Preoperative blood gas estimations may be useful to establish a base line for a particular patient; for instance a high $P\text{co}_2$ may be 'normal' for a bronchitic patient and severe respiratory problems arise postoperatively if attempts are made to reduce such patients to accepted normal $P\text{co}_2$ levels.

Other Arterial Diseases

A previous history of stroke or the detection of an asymptomatic neck bruit do not in themselves contra-indicate surgery for leg ischaemia; indeed, mobility in a patient with a combined neurological deficit and ischaemic leg pain can be improved by a judicious arterial operation and would certainly be preferable to amputation.

The asymptomatic bruit may indicate carotid stenosis and a significant fall of blood pressure could possibly lead to occlusion of the vessel and stroke. It has been suggested that more information about the degree of stenosis should be sought by oculoplethysmography, ultrasound techniques, arterial scanning, or even carotid arteriography prior to leg surgery; carotid endarterectomy being indicated for carotid stenosis prior to any lower limb revascularization procedure. We have rarely adopted this line of management; indeed, Carney et al. (1977) have shown that the asymptomatic bruit relates poorly to the occurrence of postoperative stroke.

Evidence of widespread symptomatic arterial disease, a history of angina, previous strokes and the finding of bruits in the neck and abdomen may, on the other hand, contra-indicate major reconstructive surgery. The strength of such relative contra-indications must be weighed against the severity of the leg symptoms. While the risks of reconstructive surgery may be unacceptable for claudication alone they may be entirely justifiable when actual or threatened loss of the limb is present. However, in other instances an expeditious amputation may be the most satisfactory type of treatment.

Indications for Surgery

Consideration of the influence of coincident disease

on the general management of patients with arterial disease of the legs must be weighed against the indications for surgery which may be absolute or relative.

Absolute Indications

Ischaemic rest pain, ulceration and gangrene demand surgical relief, hopefully of a reconstructive nature. Sympathectomy may be helpful, and may avoid amputation for a time. Gross sepsis may rule out vascular replacement because of the risk of secondary haemorrhage in a patient who would otherwise merit reconstruction. If distal arterial surgery is impossible, either because there is no suitable 'run-off' or the limb is too septic or the patient too feeble, then amputation remains the only effective course.

Relative Indications

Patients with claudication alone should not be considered for surgery until at least 3 months after its onset and ideally even then only when smoking has been stopped for at least 1 month, since spontaneous improvement frequently occurs during this time. Severe claudication preventing the earning of a livelihood or, if the patient is retired, seriously interfering with daily tasks are strong indications since the patient's independence is jeopardized. Minor degrees of disability with claudication distances of 230 m or more causing but minor disturbances of the patient's life style or pastimes should be treated expectantly; many will improve by stopping smoking and reducing weight.

Patients who are considered to be serious candidates for reconstructive surgery can then be submitted to detailed investigation including arteriography, as a result of which the majority with an adequate 'run-off' will proceed to surgery. Other patients, who have no reconstructable vessels, with rest pain, gangrene or advanced ulceration usually require amputation but with rest pain alone sympathectomy may provide transitory relief in approximately 50 per cent. In our experience sympathectomy alone is not usually beneficial in cases with gangrene or ischaemic ulceration when there is major vessel occlusion, unless combined with a reconstructive procedure.

Severe claudicants without reconstructable vessels and without rest pain or gangrene may obtain some relief by Achilles tenotomy (Powis et al., 1971).

Sympathectomy does not usually help the pure claudicant although patients with severely ischaemic feet in addition may obtain such relief from symptoms in their feet as to be pleased with the result.

Arteriography

It has been well said that arteriography provides a 'road map' for the arterial surgeon; no proper assessment of the suitability of the patient for surgery is complete without it, though more recent techniques such as isotope angiology may, on occasion, render it unnecessary.

Since arteriography involves the cannulation of arteries it is not without risk and should not be employed until a decision regarding the necessity of the surgical management is made.

Digital subtraction angiography is less disturbing to the patient because there is less risk to the atherosclerotic artery and vasomotor instability after the angiogram is reduced.

While uniplanar arteriography can give useful information about total blocks and partial occlusions in one plane, biplanar arteriograms at right angles give more accurate information when assessing the degree of stenosis present. This facility is usually only available in specialized centres, but the incremental effect of a series of apparently minor stenotic lesions can frequently be demonstrated by pre- and post-exercise Doppler assessment or delayed flow times on isotope angiography (Hurlow et al., 1978).

In order to assess the relative importance of segmental aortic, iliac, femoral, popliteal and tibial disease it is important to visualize all these vessels on the arteriogram. The dye must therefore be injected into the aorta, either by the translumbar or retrograde Seldinger technique. The latter technique may fail because of tortuosity of the iliac vessels or may be impossible if the femoral pulses are not palpable (*Fig.* 37.1).

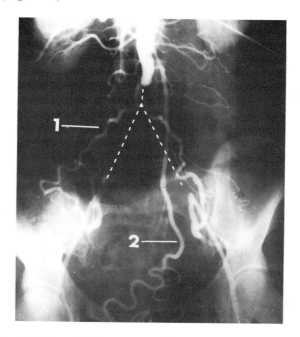

Fig. 37.1. A translumbar aortogram showing total aortic occlusion. The large iliolumbar (1) and inferior mesenteric (2) collaterals are well shown.

Progression of the dye down the arterial system is recorded by multiple exposures at known intervals from which flow rate can be judged but this information is better obtained by other methods such as isotope scanning. Indeed, there may be merit in timing the X-ray exposure by a bolus of injected radioisotope.

The arteriogram will reveal the position and extent of an occlusion and usually give some idea of the patency of the distal vessels, but it may not reveal the true state of these vessels because of inadequate filling. In such cases if the distal limb is very ischaemic surgical exploration may be the only way to determine distal patency.

Aortography will provide good information regarding its patency and the extent and type of occlusion can be seen. Potential operative difficulties can be evaluated and the probable best site for aortotomy assessed, subject to confirmation at operation when the arteriographic findings are integrated with palpation and actual observation of the aorta. Unsuspected aneurysmal disease may sometimes be revealed. Similarly, the successive iliac, common and superficial femoral, popliteal and tibial arteries are assessed.

An estimate, it is no more than that, of the degree of impedance to blood flow imposed in the superior vessels, aorta and iliacs, as opposed to the inferior vessels, the femoral and tibials, can be made. Other functional tests may decide this important point more scientifically.

This decision is important because in practical terms a choice has to be made whether to reconstruct the aorto-iliac segment, a major procedure, or whether merely to perform surgery distal to the common femoral artery. In practical terms additional distal occlusions are likely to be the most significant in terms of nutrition of the foot.

However, even when distal disease is significant haemodynamically, proximal disease may jeopardize the success of a distal reconstruction and must be dealt with first, followed by a distal reconstruction either at the same or a second operation. However, there is general agreement that amelioration of the proximal disease by aorto-bifemoral bypass graft frequently renders further surgery unnecessary, even when extensive femoropopliteal occlusion is present.

Dilatation of a proximal stenosis in the iliac vessels with a Grüntzig catheter may obviate the need for a proximal reconstruction and can be carried out prior to surgery at the time of arteriography. Alternatively, a stenotic iliac artery may be dilated by such a catheter after the common femoral artery is exposed during the femoropopliteal bypass operation. Fogarty (1981) has developed an ingenious dilatation balloon for this purpose which does not need prior passage of a guide wire which may be difficult.

The absence of significant proximal impedance to blood flow cannot be assumed because of a palpable femoral pulse. If there is an occlusion below this, pulse wave reflection from the obstruction may give rise to a deceptively strong impulse to the palpating fingers. Thus, when the common femoral artery is opened to anastomose the upper end of a femoropopliteal bypass, a disappointingly poor jet is all that can be obtained. If the bypass is continued without remedying this fault, it will fail.

Arteriographically determined knowledge of the state of the proximal vessels is therefore essential, supplemented when necessary by pressure studies.

Segmental Pressure Measurements in the Leg

1. Indirect Pressure Measurements

The ability of the Doppler ultrasound signal to detect movement of blood in the vessels is utilized in conjunction with a pressure cuff to measure pressure in the thigh and at the ankle. These pressures can be related to the blood pressure measured in the conventional way in the upper limb with a sphygmomanometer and expressed as a ratio, the brachial/ankle index (Yao et al., 1969).

Thus, the significance of arteriographically determined stenoses or occlusions at various levels in the leg arteries can be assessed, and the relative impedance to flow of a femoral artery stenosis can be compared to a stenosis or occlusion in the tibial arteries. The lesion having the greater pressure drop across it would by this test be imposing the greatest resistance to flow.

The test can be carried out at rest when low ankle pressures are usually associated with foot ischaemia; claudicants having higher ankle pressures at rest but testing after exercise might often reveal a marked drop in the latter group (*Fig. 37.2*).

Simple Doppler apparatus can be used to find the direction of flow in the inferior epigastric artery. Retrograde flow indicates a significant stenosis in the iliac segment.

2. Direct Pressure Measurements

The same principle may be used to decide which of the two sites is imposing the most significant resistance to flow. The pressure gradient from the aorta to the common femoral artery can be compared to the pressure gradient from common femoral to popliteal artery.

Pressure in the aorta may be measured directly by the Seldinger catheter or inferred from the pressure in the brachial artery measured by a cuff, provided there is no proximal aortic or subclavian artery disease. Pressure in the common femoral is determined by direct puncture.

In patients with claudication gradients measured at rest can be quite small, but these will increase when total leg flow is increased by exercise or more conveniently by intra-arterial injection of papaverine or phenoxybenzamine (Quinn, 1976).

Broadening of the spectrum of frequencies obtained from the common femoral arteries on ultrasound, with loss of the 'window' in the wave form,

Ward	ARTERIAL FLOW PROFILE		Q.E.H.

Patient identification label	Date of test	Diagnosis Operation Pre-op Post-op	

CLINICAL EVALUATION	Right	Left
Side affected		
Claudication distance (metres)		
Pre-gangrenous changes		
Gangrene		
PULSES: Femoral		
Popliteal		
Dorsalis pedis		
Posterior tibial		
BRUITS Carotid		
Femoral		
RESTING DOPPLER PRESSURES		
Brachial		
Thigh		
Calf		
Ankle		
RESTING PULSE VOLUME/MIN		
Brachial		
Upper thigh		
Lower thigh		
Calf		
Ankle		
Toes		

EXERCISE DOPPLER	B	A	B	A
Pre-exercise				
Post exercise 1 min				
2				
3				
4				
5				
6				
7				
8				
9				
10				

TREADMILL		
Claudication time		
Stopping time		

Fig. 37.2. A typical example of a proforma used in a vascular unit to record results of Doppler segmental pressure measurements together with clinical information.

indicates proximal stenosis. This indicates that significant stenosis exists which will interfere with flow and subsequent patency of a downstream graft.

'B' Scale Ultrasonic Scanning

'B' scale ultrasonic scanning to visualize intraluminal lesions has been developed (Mosersky et al., 1971) but is yet too expensive for general use.

Arterial Isotope Scanning

An injected intravenous bolus of pertechnetate can be followed with a gamma camera as it perfuses the ischaemic leg (Hurlow et al., 1977, 1978). Such records do not have the definition of contrast arteriography, but the ability to record the sequence of events on video-tape, and to play them back repeatedly, gives a deeper insight into the effect of the arteriographically displayed lesions on flow rate and distribution (*Fig.* 37.3).

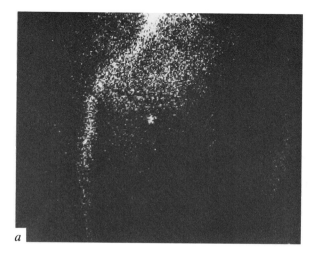

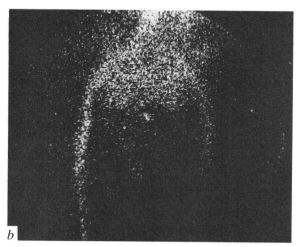

Fig. 37.3. *a*, Radio-isotope scan of patient with a left common iliac occlusion. *b*, After some delay the left femoral fills.

Occasionally in the feeble patient this investigation can replace arteriography with the advantage that the systemic effects, especially hypotension, that may follow arteriography are avoided. For example, sufficient visualization of a common femoral artery below a unilateral iliac occlusion can be obtained to determine that a femoro-femoral crossover or axillo-femoral bypass is feasible.

Anatomical Points in the Exposure of the Aorta and the Inferior Vessels

We prefer a long midline incision from xiphoid to pubis, the bladder having previously been emptied by a self-retaining catheter.

The peritoneal cavity is entered and the abdominal contents inspected for concomitant pathology, a most important step because of the high incidence of peptic ulcer and gastrointestinal cancer. The incision is spread to its fullest extent by a self-retaining retractor, and the transverse colon and mesocolon lifted up over the upper edge of the wound. The small intestine is displaced to the right over the right margin of the wound and there retained by an assistant. An incision is made in the posterior peritoneum between the duodenum and inferior mesenteric vessels which are often closely applied to the duodenum and if the incision is made to the left of them then the blood supply to the left colon will be damaged (*Fig.* 37.4).

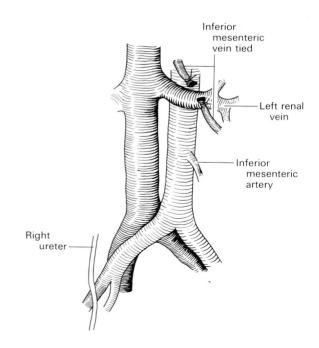

Fig. 37.5. *Above*, the inferior mesenteric vein has been tied and divided. *Below*, the right ureter has been exposed.

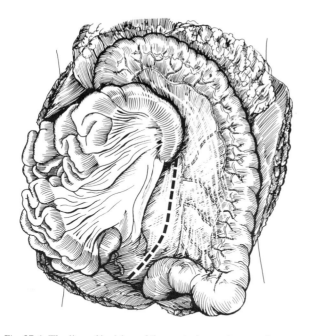

Fig. 37.4. The line of incision of the posterior peritoneum between the inferior mesenteric vessels and the duodenum.

The peritoneal incision is carried upwards to the left of the duodenum towards the inferior mesenteric vein which can be seen shining through the peritoneum in thin subjects. The vein can be tied and divided to improve access.

The incision is then carried downwards along the full length of the lower abdominal aorta on to and along the right common iliac artery after identifying

the right ureter where it crosses the bifurcation of the common iliac artery (*Fig.* 37.5). Lateral extension of this incision can be made to encircle the caecum, and if necessary upward along the right paracolic gutter so that the caecum and ascending colon together with the entire small intestine and duodenum can be mobilized and lifted upwards to expose the retroperitoneal great vessels, when looking, for example, for the source of retroperitoneal bleeding from whatever cause. However, such an exposure is not usually necessary for routine aorto-iliac surgery.

Left Renal Vein

Above and deep to the inferior mesenteric vein and closely applied to the anterior surface of the aorta is the left renal vein or its anterior moeity. Part or all of this vein may pass behind the aorta to drain into the inferior vena cava. It is embedded in the peri-aortic cellular tissue, sometimes adherent to the aorta and is very easily damaged. The left gonadal vein may be avulsed from it by careless retraction since its junction with the renal vein may be in front of the aorta. The left renal vein can be lifted on a tape to enable the origins of the renal arteries to be dissected out (*Fig.* 37.6a) or may be divided without permanently impairing renal function. Transection should be performed to the right of the gonadal vein between the termination of this vein and that of the left renal vein itself, so that venous return from the kidneys can pass into a more extensive collateral bed, including the gonadal and adrenal veins (*Fig.* 37.6b).

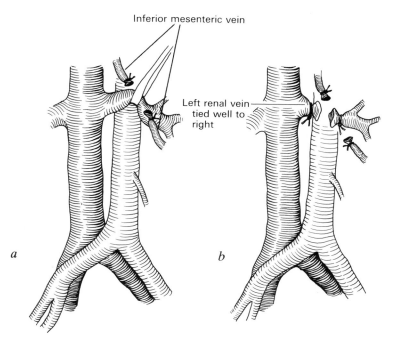

Inferior mesenteric vein

Left renal vein tied well to right

a   *b*

Fig. 37.6. The left renal vein may be lifted upwards on a tape (*a*) or divided (*b*).

Accessory Renal Arteries

Accessory renal arteries (lower polar vessels) may arise from the sides of the aorta and should normally be preserved.

Left Common Iliac Artery

The left common iliac artery is exposed by displacing and retracting the sigmoid colon and its mesentery downwards and to the left which gives good access to the proximal portion of the artery. The distal part of the left common iliac artery and the bifurcation may be better visualized, especially in the obese, by dividing the peritoneum lateral to the sigmoid and retracting the colon medially and upwards.

The loose but vascular peri-aortic tissue is then divided down to the true adventitial coat and further dissection carried out in this plane. This is usually easy but may be extremely difficult in some patients in whom there appears to be a sclerosis of this tissue, resembling retroperitoneal fibrosis.

Iliac Veins

The relationship of the iliac arteries to the veins is complex and intimate. The veins are thin walled, often closely adherent both to the diseased arteries and the parietes, and thus easily damaged. The right common iliac artery overlies the left common iliac vein, the confluence of the right and left iliac veins and in its lower part the right common iliac vein. The right external iliac artery lies at first anterior and then lateral to the vein. On the left the common and external iliac veins lie posteromedial to the artery, the external iliac vein lying medial to the artery in its lower part (*Fig.* 37.7).

These relationships should be borne in mind when passing tapes around the arteries and when applying clamps to them, since the veins may be torn easily. In some instances it may be safer and wiser to clamp the artery without formally dissecting it free from the vein. Because of the adherence of the thin vein walls to the pelvic wall, it may be difficult to pull the lips of a rent together with sutures. If the vein should be inadvertently damaged where it lies deep to the artery, the rent may be better visualized and haemorrhage more safely controlled by deliberately transecting the artery which can be replaced by the limb of the prosthesis.

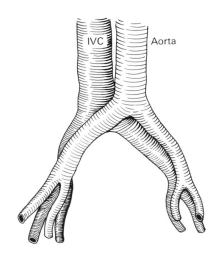

IVC   Aorta

Fig. 37.7. The relationship of iliac veins to arteries.

The origins of both internal and external iliac arteries are seen at the lower end of the peritoneal incisions, care always having been taken to mobilize the ureters out of harm's way.

Internal Iliac Artery

Extension of the incision in the peritoneum down the side walls of the pelvis enables the proximal parts of both internal iliac vessels to be seen. The internal iliac vein lies between the artery and the pelvic wall and can be readily damaged by careless passage of a forceps behind the artery.

External Iliac Artery

This vessel can be exposed by an incision in the peritoneum over it, and on the left the sigmoid colon should be retracted upwards and medially.

A possibly better alternative is to expose it extraperitoneally by stripping under the lower cut edge of the main peritoneal incision, which provides exposure as in the classic extraperitoneal approach. The vas can be pushed medially and inferiorly so as not to damage it. The external iliac artery is often extremely tortuous and may be displaced over the pelvic brim into the true pelvis and so may not immediately come to hand. However, its lower end as it is under the midpoint of the inguinal ligament is not so affected and it may be easily identified here. The close proximity of the vein, medially and posteriorly above, should not be forgotten. Division of the deep circumflex iliac vein which crosses the lower part of the artery may be necessary (*Fig.* 37.8).

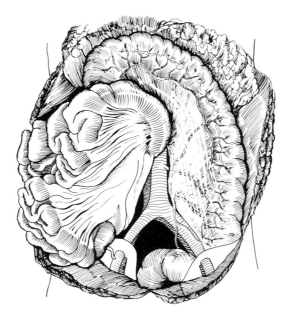

Fig. 37.8. Extraperitoneal exposure of the external iliac vessels with transperitoneal exposure of the aorta and common iliac arteries.

The ureter is swept upwards with the peritoneum. The gonadal vessels are displaced medially, as are the vas in the male and round ligament in the female.

Exposure of the Femoral Vessels in the Groin

We prefer a nearly vertical skin incision over the femoral artery. Its upper end should be above the inguinal ligament, over the vessels, and its lower end slightly more medially situated, particularly where the saphenous vein is to be exposed and removed for use as a bypass. It is a frequent beginner's mistake to make the incision too low since in the obese middle-aged person, the groin crease is considerably below the inguinal ligament. However, reference to the bony points of the anterior superior iliac space and the pubic tubercle will easily establish the level of the inguinal ligament running between them.

The skin divided, laterally placed tributaries of the saphenous vein often require to be tied and divided as they lie in the subcutaneous fat. Deeper dissection reveals the deep fascia, behind which the femoral vessels lie surrounded by a variable quantity of fat. To minimize division of lymphatics the dissection should be centred on the femoral artery and extended up and down rather than transversely.

Common Femoral Artery

Lateral to the common femoral artery lies the femoral nerve and care should be taken not to damage this when the vessel is isolated. Medially lies the femoral vein, but this should not normally need to be exposed unless the termination of the saphenous vein is sought prior to its ligation and removal.

The variable division of the common femoral into superficial and deep femoral arteries may be high, so that only a centimetre or so of common femoral can be displayed; or it may be low, well down in the femoral triangle. Do not hesitate to divide the inguinal ligament to provide better access.

Profunda Femoris Artery

The profunda femoris artery arises posterolaterally from the common femoral and can be displayed by careful dissection as it leaves the femoral triangle by passing between the pectineus and adductor longus muscles. Its finer branches are easily damaged. Large venous tributaries of the profunda vein pass across the artery from the lateral muscles and require division between ligatures as the profunda is followed into the medial part of the thigh. The adductor longus will also need to be divided. In this way several centimetres of the profunda artery can be displayed for endarterectomy and angioplasty.

Superficial Femoral Artery

The superficial femoral artery is seen as a direct continuation of the common femoral and can be displayed in its course across the femoral triangle to enter the subsartorial canal of Hunter, beneath the sartorius muscle.

Exposure of the superficial femoral artery in the subsartorial canal involves, after division of the skin, merely the splitting of the investing layer of deep fascia over the sartorius and the displacement of that muscle anterolaterally if the upper part of the artery is sought and posteriorly if the lower part of the artery is to be exposed. After displacement of the sartorius the strong fascial roofing of the canal is divided in the line of the artery.

Skin Sloughs in Thigh Incisions (*Fig. 37.9*)

If all that is required is to expose the artery then the skin incision should be over the vessel along the line following the anterior superior iliac spine to the adductor tubercle. It is better to use several small interrupted incisions than one long continuous one.

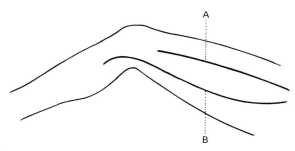

Fig. 37.9. A, The line of the incision to expose the artery. B, The line of incision to expose the vein.

However, if these skin incisions are made and the saphenous vein then sought through them, severe and often disastrous sloughs will occur in the skin edges posteriorly.

When it is proposed to use the saphenous vein in the arterial reconstruction, the skin incisions should be sited over the saphenous vein and having removed this then the deep fascia should be divided in the line of the skin incision and the artery found as above. Thus the vitality of the skin will not be impaired and subsequent healing facilitated.

Femoropopliteal Junction

At the lower end of the subsartorial canal the superficial femoral artery passes through the dense aponeurotic hiatus in the adductor magnus to become the popliteal artery. To expose the vessel here, having displaced the sartorius posteriorly, a variable number of aponeurotic and muscular fibres of the adductor magnus need to be divided. This arterial segment which is very prone to atherosclerotic disease can be reconstructed if required, but is usually better bypassed.

Upper Popliteal Artery (*Fig. 37.10*)

This vessel from the adductor hiatus to the level of the knee joint is revealed by displacing the sartorius muscle posteriorly and dissecting through the loose popliteal fat. The skin incision should be centred over the saphenous vein for the reasons previously stated.

Crossing the popliteal fossa is a branch of the popliteal artery to the sartorius and the saphenous nerve which should be preserved. The lower end of the vessel may be difficult to see and the exposure can be improved by dividing the medial head of the gastrocnemius; there is no need to reconstitute it subsequently.

Lower Popliteal Artery and its Bifurcation

The extreme lower end of this vessel can be displayed by an incision 1 cm behind the medial border of the upper tibia, skirting the saphenous vein and nerve and dividing the deep fascia in the line of the skin incision. With blunt dissection the space between the

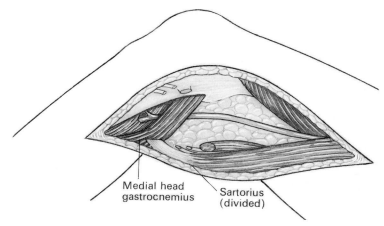

Medial head
gastrocnemius

Sartorius
(divided)

Fig. 37.10. Exposure of the upper popliteal artery does not necessitate division of the hamstrings as in the figure.

gastrocnemius and the soleus is entered and about 3–4 cm of the lower popliteal artery can be exposed just above its entry into the soleus tunnel. This exposure gives good and rapid access.

Full Exposure of the Popliteal Artery

This requires the joining up of the two previous incisions. The tendons of the sartorius, gracilis and semitendinosus are divided near to the tibia, followed by section of the much larger tendon of the semimembranosus and the medial head of the gastrocnemius (*Fig.* 37.11) thus opening the popliteal fossa in its full length (*Fig.* 37.12).

The saphenous nerve as it becomes superficial passing in close proximity to the lower end of the sartorius should not be damaged, as patients complain postoperatively of numbness and paraesthesia in the distribution of this nerve.

Anterior Tibial Artery

The anterior tibial artery is exposed by an incision midway between the tibia and fibula; it lies between tibialis anterior and extensor digitorum longus on the interosseous membrane. It is possible to perform bypass surgery to this vessel with this exposure taking the bypass through the interosseous membrane.

Posterior Tibial Artery

The posterior tibial artery is exposed by a skin incision behind and parallel to the medial border of the tibia. The investing fascia of the leg is divided in line with the skin incision. The soleus origin from the posterior aspect of the tibia is divided from the arch over the vessels above, downwards. Soleus and gastrocnemius are retracted posteriorly to reveal the posterior tibial vessels lying on the tibialis posterior and flexor digitorum longus. In its lower part the artery is only covered by skin and fascia.

Peroneal Artery

The peroneal artery can be exposed by resection of the shaft of the fibula over the desired length of vessel and incising the periosteum of its posteromedial aspect. An alternative is as for exposure of the posterior tibial artery, but the peroneal lies more laterally and in the substance of the flexor hallucis longus.

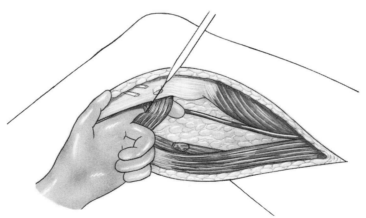

Fig. 37.11. The medial head of the gastrocnemius is hooked over the finger and divided.

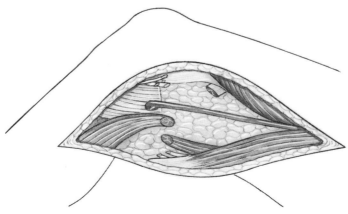

Fig. 37.12. The popliteal vessels leave the fossa under the arch of the soleus.

RECONSTRUCTION FOR AORTO-ILIAC DISEASE

Operations Available

The preferred operation is aorto-iliac or aorto-femoral bypass. Endarterectomy may be used with good long-term results for limited lesions, but recurrence is frequent, particularly in younger female patients. Bypass is quicker and is more likely to be adequate in the long term. With endarterectomy there is a tendency either not to endarterectomize a sufficient length of vessel or to have difficulty in deciding where to stop; in either event the operation requires extensive dissection of the aorto-iliac segments which may be too much for feeble elderly patients.

Lumbar sympathectomy may be added to the bypass or endarterectomy technique with the benefit of improving the skin circulation but not the claudication and possibly increasing flow across the operated segment. In the older enfeebled patient, variations of the bypass technique are used which avoid opening the abdomen, such as femoro-femoral bypass if the disease is limited to one iliac artery or unilateral or bilateral axillofemoral bypass (Blaisdell and Hall, 1963; Brief et al., 1975). All patients start an appropriate antibiotic on the evening prior to surgery.

Aorto-iliac or Aorto-femoral Bypass

This may be unilateral or bilateral if both iliacs are involved. The question of bypassing a mildly affected iliac artery while operating for the symptomatic other side is arguable but the general experience is that the less affected side will become symptomatic within 2–3 years. It is therefore usually wise to bypass both iliac vessels, although if the pressure gradient is small there is an increased risk that the prosthesis may clot. Prohibition of smoking postoperatively and the correction of lipid abnormalities by diet and drugs may prevent progression of the disease in the less affected side and recent studies have shown that of these cessation of smoking is the more important (Greenhalgh et al., 1980).

Aorto-femoral bypass is performed under general anaesthesia, with the patient supine and towels arranged for adequate access both to the abdominal midline and the femoral vessels. An incision from xiphoid to pubis is made and the aorta and iliac arteries exposed as described previously; we usually eviscerate the small intestine, but some prefer to pack it away behind retractors. Prior to clamping the vessels it is wise to systemically heparinize the patient using 1–2 mg heparin/kg body weight as this obviates secondary thrombosis in the distal tree. Though the majority of surgeons prefer a transabdominal operation, Helsby and Moosa (1975) strongly recommend the extraperitoneal approach and have reported encouraging results.

Proximal Anastomosis

The end-to-side or end-to-end technique may be used, the latter being particularly appropriate when the aorta is totally occluded, since it is much easier to carry out a thrombectomy with the aorta transected rather than via a longitudinal incision. Even when the aortic lumen is only partly occupied by thrombus and artheromatous debris, an end-to-end anastomosis may give superior long-term patency and is becoming the favoured technique in many clinics. Of course, with this technique the bypass principle is sacrificed together with the theoretical advantages of leaving the natural channel should it be necessary to remove the prostheses for some complication. Experience shows, however, that it is rare for the natural channel to provide an adequate alternative channel should it be necessary to remove the prosthesis.

Thrombus and atheromatous debris often extend up to the ostia of the renal vessels and careless clamping of the aorta just below these vessels may dislodge this material into the renal arteries, as may overzealous manipulation and dissection at this level.

If occlusion is complete no upper clamp is necessary until the aorta is transected: then with the suprarenal aorta controlled by pressure from one hand, thrombectomy can be accomplished with the other, either by squeezing the debris out or by using an instrument of the surgeon's choice; Desjardins' forceps are excellent for this purpose. When thrombectomy has been accomplished as shown by the free egress of blood on releasing the pressure of the left hand, a clamp can be applied infrarenally with the right. Some surgeons prefer, as an additional insurance against inadvertent dislodgement of debris into the renal arteries, to clamp them individually while these manoeuvres are being undertaken but this necessitates further dissection to expose their origin. Even though the lower cut end of the aorta is completely occluded it is wise to oversew it, since the rise in blood pressure in the vessels beyond the obstruction consequent on a successful operation may lead to bleeding around the thrombus or even its displacement.

If occlusion is incomplete the upper clamp should be applied at least 2 cm below the renal arteries and the lower aorta should be clamped between the inferior mesenteric origin and the aortic bifurcation to control back bleeding. The aorta is opened over 5 cm by a longitudinal curved incision which skirts the inferior mesenteric origin by 0·5–1·0 cm, so that the orifice of the vessel will not be included in the suture line. Temporary control by a sling or bulldog clamp on the mesenteric artery may be necessary, and back bleeding from the lumbar vessels can be prevented by bulldog clamps placed on them.

Atheromatous or thrombotic material is removed from the aortic lumen with forceps and it is wise to slacken the upper and lower clamps to allow the flushing out of loose material at the limits of the thrombectomy; it is most important that no loose flaps are left in the aortic lumen.

Preparation of the prosthesis

Most commercial bifurcation prostheses require drastic shortening of the main stem of the prosthesis otherwise the bifurcation will lie too low in the patient and produce an awkward splaying or even kinking of the limbs on their route to the iliac or femoral arteries.

After shortening the main stem, if the end-to-side operation is chosen, a taper must be cut so that the divided end is the same length as, or preferably slightly longer than, the aortotomy. It is most undesirable to have to stretch the cut end to fit the aortotomy as this imposes unnecessary tension on the sutures, fraying of the cut edge of the prosthesis and a 'dog-ear' suture line.

The prosthesis of the surgeon's choice is taken and if it requires preclotting the manufacturer's instructions should be faithfully observed prior to heparinization. Woven Dacron or Teflon require virtually no preclotting, other prostheses such as single or double velour need pre-immersion in clotting blood.

Silk should not be used as a suture material. Other non-absorbable materials such as monofilament polypropylene or braided polyester (Dacron) are satisfactory, but a gauge of 4/0 or 3/0 is the minimum. Suturing should commence at the most inaccessible spot, that is at the acute angle between the prosthesis and the aorta. It is convenient to use a double-armed suture with at least a 15-mm curved round-bodied or 'taper-cut' needle with the knot lying outside the lumen. Some prefer to make the first stitch a small mattress so placed as to appose the inner surfaces of prosthesis and aorta. In an end-to-end anastomosis the first suture is placed posteriorly and the anastomosis completed by a running 'one and over' stitch tied anteriorly.

In an end-to-side anastomosis the prosthesis should be 'matched up' to the aortotomy after the first stitch is tied and it is often convenient to use a temporary stay suture at the upper end of the aortotomy and the 'apex' of the prosthesis. Care should be taken not to obliterate the mouth of the inferior mesenteric artery while suturing and the final knot can be tied on the side opposite to this vessel. The suture line complete, upper and lower clamps are released and reapplied in turn to 'flush out' through the prosthesis any clot formed around the clamps or loose atheromatous material. It is wise to do this even if the patient has been systemically heparinized. The prosthesis is then irrigated in saline and sucked out via one of the limbs of the graft to remove all debris at the aortotomy site. The limbs of the prosthesis are then occluded and the clamps removed from the aorta.

The common femoral, proximal end of the superficial femoral, and profunda arteries are exposed as described previously. In order to pass the limbs of the prosthesis into the groin incision, it is necessary to make a tunnel retroperitoneally from the aorta to the groin beneath the inguinal ligament. The index fingers are the best instrument for this purpose, passed from above in front of the common iliac artery and behind the peritoneum and ureter to meet the index finger of the other hand passed upwards behind the inguinal ligament. There should be no hesitation in dividing the inguinal ligament if the tunnel is tight. The lower finger is best insinuated anterolateral to the common femoral artery, thus avoiding the inferior epigastric branch. The tunnel made, slightly curved, Roberts-type forceps are passed along it to seize the lower end of the prosthesis and to draw it down into the groin wound, taking great care not to twist the limb of the prosthesis in the process.

The Distal Implantation

The distal side of the implantation of the prosthesis may be just beyond the lower limit of arteriographically obvious disease, whether this be in the external iliac just above the inguinal ligament or below into the common femoral.

Because of the possibility of infection in a separate groin wound, it has been suggested that, if possible, the external iliac should be chosen. However, experience shows that superior haemodynamic results follow implantation into the common femoral because this vessel is wider than the external iliac, which is frequently rather inadequate in calibre to receive the blood from the prosthesis. Moreover, progressive occlusive disease is a frequent event in the external iliac artery. For all these reasons it is seldom satisfactory. Also, since in many cases the superficial femoral artery is blocked and the profunda femoris is the receiving channel, its orifice can be inspected and if necessary the common femoral incision can be carried down into the lateral aspect of the profunda to accomplish either an endarterectomy or widen the vessel by utilizing the tapered end of the prosthesis as a patch angioplasty. It is again important to check antegrade and retrograde flushing with subsequent irrigation to remove all fragments and clot prior to completion of the anastomosis.

Addition of Sympathectomy to Aorto-iliac Reconstruction

It is common practice to perform coincident bilateral or unilateral lumbar sympathectomy with such reconstructions with the benefit of an increased foot and skin circulation immediately postoperatively. This is particularly advantageous if toilet surgery is required for gangrenous toes.

The sympathetic chain can be easily felt against the vertebral column when the aorta is exposed, and is best identified by palpation initially which enables the overlying lymphatic chain to be pushed or swept aside. On the left side the lower end of the chain can be seized and a portion removed medial to the inferior mesenteric artery; that on the right is similarly dealt with by retracting the vena cava medially. Only 4–5 cm of chain need be removed and the upper end is conveniently marked by the application of a clip for future reference.

In our experience there is a significant incidence of post-sympathectomy neuralgia following the operation and although this fades after a variable period, it can be quite distressing in a few patients.

For this reason some believe that sympathectomy as an adjunct to aorto-iliac reconstruction is only indicated when there is associated femoropopliteal and tibial artery occlusive disease. In a number of such patients, the increased foot circulation may be so marked that the foot pulses may be palpable even though the superficial femoral artery is blocked.

Axillofemoral and Femoro-femoral Bypass

These operations are usually indicated to relieve occlusion in the aorto-iliac area in feeble patients or as an expedient following a catastrophe such as a septic aortic prosthesis. While the axillofemoral bypass can be performed either bilaterally or unilaterally with a side limb to the opposite common femoral artery for bilateral disease, obviously the femoro-femoral operation is only suitable for unilateral iliac disease (*Fig.* 37.13). Nonetheless, it is an effective operation despite the retrograde take-off of the prosthesis with regard to the direction of blood flow in the donor vessel (Crawford et al., 1975). Patency rates are better for femoro-femoral bypass than for unilateral axillofemoral bypass, and it is the preferred operation for unilateral disease in feeble patients (Eugene et al., 1977).

Patency rates for axillofemoral bypass are 50 per cent at 2 years and are improved if the graft is from one axillary artery to both femorals, presumably because of the increased graft flow (Logerfo et al., 1977). It is a *sine qua non* of axillofemoral grafting that there be no significant disease in the subclavian or axillary artery constituting the donor site. Symptoms attributable to 'stealing' of blood from the donor vessel are uncommon in both axillo-femoral and femoro-femoral bypass.

Percutaneous Transluminal Angioplasty

Percutaneous dilation of narrow or blocked arteries by the Dotter technique, and more recently by the Grüntzig balloon, has gained a degree of acceptance. The polyethylene balloon is passed along a previously introduced guide wire, to lie in the narrow region of the vessel. When inflated to very high pressures (1000 mmHg or more) dilatation occurs, which persists for a variable time thereafter. The procedure can be repeated if necessary.

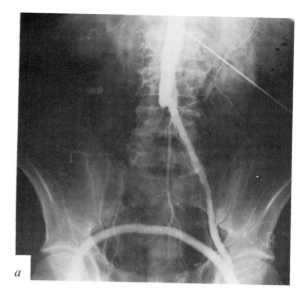

a

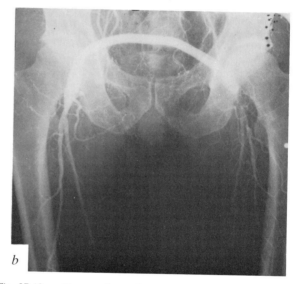

b

Fig. 37.13. *a*, Femoro-femoral crossover graft (10 mm Dacron). *b*, Same patient as above. There is disease in the lower left common femoral which necessitated a further distal grafting procedure.

Success rates reported are variable, being greater in the iliac segments than in the femoral. Thus Zeitler et al. (1983) found that with iliac dilatation an initial success rate of 85 per cent fell to 69 per cent on discharge from hospital while the femoral arteries showed a 74 per cent early patency falling to 31 per cent $2\frac{1}{2}$ years later. This was 26 per cent at 5 years.

Grüntzig and Kumpe (1979) had a success rate of 84 per cent for femoral dilatation and 92 per cent for iliac; by 2 years these figures were 72 and 87 per cent respectively. A 5 per cent distal embolization rate resulted. Only arterial stenoses, not occlusions, were treated and only femoropopliteal lesions of 10 cm or less were dilated. Various antiplatelet and anticoagulant drugs were used in the foregoing series.

Ring et al. (1982) reported a higher complication rate in a small series of 10 total occlusions. Successful dilatation occurred in four while two patients had embolization to the opposite leg.

COMPLICATIONS OF AORTO-FEMORAL BYPASS

Clotting of the Prosthesis

Patency of a graft immediately after implantation is maintained by an adequate blood flow through it and any factor that interferes with this may lead to clotting. Thus, hypotension due to oligaemia with peripheral vasoconstriction is a potent cause and similarly cardiogenic shock from myocardial infarction leads to failure. It is vital that blood loss is monitored during the operation and replaced; vasoconstrictor agents to raise blood pressure are harmful and have no place in the management of these patients. It is imperative that all clot and debris be removed from the prosthesis and contiguous vessels prior to the completion of the distal anastomoses. This was formerly a common cause of failure and has become much less frequent since the adoption of systemic heparinization.

A serious technical error causing kinking of a limb of the prosthesis is placing the bifurcation of the prosthesis too low because the stem of the graft was insufficiently shortened. Twisting the limb of the graft in passing it down the retroperitoneal tunnel is also easily done. Both these errors should be avoided, otherwise they may only be appreciated when prior to completion of the lower anastomosis the 'flush of blood' following temporary release of the clamp is clearly inadequate and may necessitate a complete revision of the graft.

Smallness in calibre of the distal vessels, particularly the profunda when the superficial femoral artery is blocked, can lead to early or late clotting in a graft limb. This can often be ameliorated by a 'profunda-plasty' including a tongue of the prosthesis to widen the profunda trunk. To these flow problems must be added any increased clotting tendency due to blood dyscrasias. These, notably polycythaemia rubra and thrombocythaemia, should be carefully excluded in the preoperative assessment of the patient.

Many surgeons now treat their patients postoperatively with low-dose aspirin and dipyridamole to reduce the risk of thrombosis (Goldman et al., 1983). A history of previous peptic ulceration would contraindicate the use of aspirin. Clinical trials are in progress.

There is a distinct relationship between early failure of the prosthesis and the presence of infection in it. The patient is often febrile, may have rigors and prior to occlusion of the prosthesis micro-emboli may be seen in the skin of the appropriate leg.

Thrombosis of a prosthesis associated with unexplained pyrexia in the early postoperative period is always highly suspicious of graft infection and should alert the clinician to the likelihood of this possibility. Although a systemic blood culture may be sterile, blood aspirated distal to the anastomosis may grow the causative organism.

Infection of the Prosthesis

Infection of the prosthesis is a grave complication often leading to loss of life or at least loss of the limb. Early infection shown by pyrexia which will not settle with perhaps a petechial rash on the skin of the legs probably arises as a result of infection introduced at operation. While the majority of vascular surgeons employ broad-spectrum antibiotics pre- and postoperatively to help to avoid this complication, others feel this confers no protection. Infection may also be blood borne from infected intravenous catheters, particularly when these have been in place for long periods and the strictest asepsis has not been used in their placement and management. It is wise to culture the catheter tips when these are removed. Knowledge of organisms and sensitivities thus revealed may be vital to the control of subsequent graft sepsis. Direct infection of a prosthesis may occur at any time from the bowel lumen. Bowel in close proximity to arterial anastomoses may become adherent; subsequent pressure necrosis of its wall leaves the prosthesis bathed in intestinal secretion and infection of the host artery and graft is certain. Such a condition has been called 'paraprosthetic fistula' by O'Mara and Imbembo (1977) (*Fig.* 37.14).

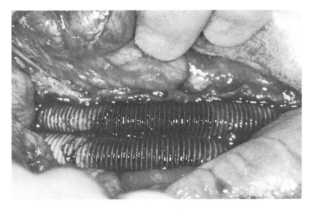

Fig. 37.14. Limbs of a bifurcation prosthesis stained with bile. There was no communication with the vascular lumen—so-called 'paraprosthetic fistula'.

Diagnosis of graft infection can be confirmed by culturing blood aspirated directly from the artery below the prosthesis and positive culture may be obtained in this way when routine venous samples are negative.

As mentioned above, infection may well lead to

clotting of the limb of the prosthesis. If it does not, once an anastomosis is infected either frank secondary haemorrhage occurs or a false aneurysm develops. Such a false aneurysm may become very large, often causing backache or abdominal discomfort. On the other hand, it may not obtain much size before it ruptures into the bowel lumen causing an aorto-enteric fistula.

Aortoduodenal and Aorto-enteric Fistula

The duodenum is most frequently involved in aortic suture line leaks of this type and there are many reports in the literature of aortoduodenal fistula following bypass and aneurysmectomy procedures.

The common history is that after an aortic reconstruction there is a complaint of melaena or haematemesis, often not of very severe degree, and this may be repeated several times over a period of weeks. The lapse of time between primary operation and the gastrointestinal bleeding can be anything from a week or two to several years. These relatively small gastrointestinal haemorrhages presage a subsequent fatal bleed and so any patient who has had an aortic reconstruction and then has melaena or haematemesis should be assumed to have a fistula until proved otherwise, though confirmation of the diagnosis may be difficult. Proof may come from barium studies or aortography which may show a false aneurysm, if not the fistula (*Fig.* 37.15). Gastroduodenal endoscopy may be helpful by excluding a peptic ulcer and confirming the presence of fresh blood in the second and third parts of the duodenum although actual identification of the fistula is rare.

Treatment is by urgent surgery. Since the prosthesis is infected most surgeons feel it should be removed and either the aortotomy closed, when it may be difficult to leave any sort of a lumen, or the aorta sewn off or ligatured. Blood supply to the legs is then restored by an axillo-bilateral femoral bypass, but the removal of the prosthesis and the later reconstruction should be separated by closure of the abdomen, sealing of the wound and a complete change of instruments, towels and gloves to lessen the risk of infection of the bypass.

Better than cure of this desperate condition is its prevention. As a general rule it is wise to cover exposed suture lines with peritoneum or omentum but it is probably better not to replace the duodenum back to its natural position over the aorta by siting a wedge of omentum between the two (*Fig.* 37.16).

Haemorrhage

Immediately postoperatively, haemorrhage is uncommon from the suture line and laparotomy for suspected intra-abdominal bleeding usually reveals the source to be an unligated vessel, usually a vein. Sometimes no source of bleeding can be found and in these circumstances the surgeon has to be content with merely removing the blood clot. Usually recovery is uneventful.

Late free haemorrhage into the peritoneal cavity is uncommon. After organization of the fibrous tissue around the prosthesis and host vessel any leak is generally contained by a slowly enlarging false aneurysm which, giving rise to pain, leads to timely investigation and treatment. Rupture of the prosthesis itself is rare and has occurred once in approximately 1000 aortic operations in our experience.

It is generally accepted that arterial sutures should be of non-absorbable synthetic material and Dacron or polypropylene are suitable. Silk undergoes degeneration and has been implicated in late suture line disruption and false aneurysm formation, though these complications have also been reported with synthetic sutures.

False aneurysm occurs occasionally in the groin due to leakage from the suture line between the prosthesis and host vessel. It is usually detected early because of the superficial position of the vessels by both patient and surgeon. Treatment is excision. The precaution of bacteriological swabbing of the tissues should be taken since low-grade infection may be present.

A suitable antibiotic should be used pre- and postoperatively.

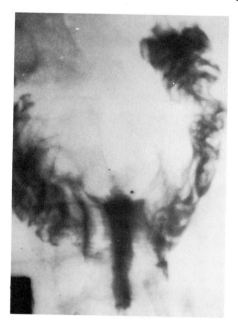

Fig. 37.15. Bifurcation prosthesis outlined by barium extravasated from duodenum in a patient with an aortoduodenal fistula.

RESULTS OF AORTO-ILIAC RECONSTRUCTIVE PROCEDURES

Although thrombo-endarterectomy is still performed for well-localized disease aorto-bifemoral bypass has become the standard procedure in many centres. The

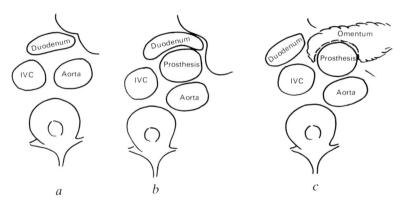

Fig. 37.16. *a*, Normal relationship of duodenum to aorta. *b*, To show the duodenum pressed against the graft after end-to-side anastomoses. *c*, Separation of duodenum from prosthesis by omentum to prevent pressure necrosis of duodenum.

results are inevitably influenced by case selection and the presence or absence of distal femoropopliteal disease but overall some 85 per cent or so of patients will have a satisfactory result 5 years later. The functional results are not so satisfactory in patients with associated distal disease as compared with those with aorto-iliac disease alone but, even in the former, revascularization of the profunda system usually suffices to produce marked symptomatic improvement and it is rarely necessary to perform a subsequent 'downstream' repair. These operations are, of course, major interventions but in most centres in the UK can be achieved with an appreciable, but acceptable, mortality rate of between 4 and 8 per cent (Dickinson et al., 1967; Irvine et al., 1972; Eastcott, 1973; Taylor, 1973; Helsby and Moosa, 1975; Baird et al., 1977).

RECONSTRUCTION OF THE ARTERIAL SYSTEM DISTAL TO THE GROIN

Owing to the small flows in these vessels compared with the aorta and iliacs the maintenance of patency after reconstruction is more complex and methods of reconstruction which are entirely satisfactory for the proximal vessels are not as successful and indeed may be frankly unsuitable when employed distally.

Reconstruction by endarterectomy of the blocked superficial femoral artery by either closed, such as ring stripper and gas endarterectomy, or open techniques does not give such good results as bypass with reversed autogenous saphenous vein (Sobel et al., 1966; Baddeley et al., 1968; DeWeese, 1971). The authors have performed 329 such operations with a 70 per cent 5-year patency rate (Grimley et al., 1979).

Late patency is influenced by the state of the 'run off' vessels and the site of implantation, being best when the vein is 5 mm or more in diameter, the implant site is above the knee and with patency of all three leg vessels—anterior and posterior tibial and peroneal arteries. The results become less satisfac-

tory with a graft less than 5 mm in diameter, the more distal implantation sites, such as the tibial vessels, giving patencies of 50 per cent at 2 years (Dardik et al., 1975; Davis et al., 1975).

Until recently synthetic grafts have had a bad reputation in the thigh and leg, results varying from 10 per cent patency at 1 year for woven Teflon (Ashton et al., 1962) to 15 per cent for Helanca Dacron at 5 and 6 years (Szilagyi, 1978). Better results have been reported for filamentous Dacron (Sauvage et al., 1978) and for velour Dacron (Cooley et al., 1978).

Expanded PTFE (polytetrafluoroethylene) gives higher patencies than previous synthetic grafts, depending on the state of the 'run-off' distally, and whether the graft terminates above or below the knee.

With above-knee implantations patencies can approach close to those of autogenous saphenous vein—the 'gold standard' of femoropopliteal grafting results. This is particularly so when results include patencies of successful thrombectomies of clotted PTFE tubes. Thrombectomy seems to be particularly easy and successful with PTFE grafts and reports of multiple thrombectomies in the same patient abound in the literature; the record seems to be 13 times.

Julian et al. (1982) report similar patency for saphenous vein and PTFE at 4 years of 41 and 30 per cent respectively (six thrombectomies were performed in the PTFE grafts) for patients with claudication, whereas in patients with a poor 'run off'—one tibial vessel or an isolated popliteal segment—51 per cent of autogenous veins and 12 per cent of PTFE grafts were patent.

Distal implantation to the tibial vessels gives patencies of 55 per cent for saphenous vein and 7 per cent for PTFE at 3 years according to Yeager et al. (1982), whereas this rises to 65 and 53 per cent respectively for femoropopliteal grafts at the same times since implantation.

Glutaraldehyde tanned human umbilical vein grafts have gained acceptance. Although expensive, delicate and needing special care in their use, their patency approaches that of saphenous vein grafts for claudication. Cranley and Hafner (1982) found 81 per cent patent at 5 years; this fell to 74 per cent for grafts for severe ischaemia. Grafts to the tibial segment had a patency of only 24 per cent. Thrombectomy was successful in 12 out of 16 attempts on clotted umbilical vein grafts in this series.

Comparable patency for PTFE in these groups was 65 per cent at $4\frac{1}{2}$ years for claudication, falling to 41 per cent for severe ischaemia particularly where below-knee implants were used.

Dardik et al. (1980) reporting on 361 reconstructions found a 76·4 per cent patency for femoropopliteal operations at 3 years falling to 39·8 per cent for femoropopliteal bypasses over the same period. However, Klimach and Charlesworth's (1983) experience was less fortunate showing a 9 per cent patency at 2 years for 112 patients who had femorotibial grafts. Occasional aneurysm formation is reported (Giordano and Keshinian, 1982).

In situ saphenous vein grafting with destruction of the valves has theoretical haemodynamic advantages—wide proximally tapering distally with possible reduction of turbulence—and was suggested by Rob and first reported by Hall (1962) using valve avulsion. Leather et al. (1981a, b) reported 85 per cent patency rates at 3 years using valve incision.

Increased vein utilization compared with the reversed techniques is among the advantages claimed for the procedure which also permits appropriate size matching to small tibial vessels. Natural vein tributaries allow convenient double distal implantation in patients with two patent distal vessels, theoretically increasing 'run-off' and therefore graft patency (Simms et al., 1982). Longer-term results show similar patencies for the two methods of vein bypass grafting—41 and 43 per cent at 10 years (Connolly and Kwaan, 1982).

In summary, modern techniques have provided a reasonable synthetic alternative for the saphenous vein in the 25 per cent or so of patients who do not have a satisfactory vein, at least for short blocks from the groin to the lower end of the adductor canal, particularly if the 'run off' is good.

For those patients with poor 'run off', one vessel or isolated popliteal segments, the saphenous vein reversed or *in situ* is still the best operation, although in some hands the human umbilical vein gives reasonable results.

Reconstruction of the proximal part of the profunda femoris artery by endarterectomy and vein patch with the object of increasing the flow around the occluded superficial femoral artery has been employed with some success (Martin et al., 1968; Martin and Bouhoutsos, 1977).

Biplanar angiography is necessary to show significant stenosis of the origin or first part of the profunda vessel, and best results seem to attend surgery for short occlusions. Longer endarterectomy down as far as the second or third branch has been employed

successfully, however, and may be worth while if no other reconstruction is feasible.

Success has also been claimed for this procedure even when no radiographic stenosis has been demonstrated, on the reasoning that since the arterial tree increases in cross-section with arborization, proximal surgical widening must reduce resistance to flow. We have not been convinced by this and, after trial, feel that only a radiographic stenosis of the profunda merits surgery. Even then unless the distal profunda branches can be seen to link up with the popliteal artery the results seem to us to be frequently disappointing.

Of course, if the popliteal artery is patent then a femoropopliteal bypass would be possible which will ameliorate symptoms much more effectively than increasing the collateral flow. However, it has been argued that in the young patient with rapidly advancing atherosclerosis a successful femoropopliteal bypass, although relieving symptoms dramatically, will accelerate the disease process distally and so lead to rapid failure with possible loss of the limb. Profundaplasty, while not relieving claudication entirely, does not raise the distal blood pressure to normal levels and so the advance of the atherosclerotic process is not so rapid and a longer life for the limb is obtained. There is considerable force in this argument for the young claudicant. However, if the underlying atherosclerotic process can be controlled by diet and cessation of smoking then the more direct revascularization is likely to bring greater satisfaction to patient and surgeon, though in general the disease is always more aggressive in the younger patient below the age of 50 (Bouhoutsos and Martin, 1973).

Concept of Limb Salvage

Since many distal bypasses are performed for the relief of rest pain, ulceration and gangrene, which are associated with extensive disease of the tibial vessels, patency rates are often low. However, it is common experience that if patency is maintained for a sufficient period for ulcers and toe and foot amputations for gangrene to heal, then in spite of occlusion of the graft the original symptoms may not recur. Thus, patency rates of the graft may be of the order of 50 per cent or less at 5 years but salvage rates (the percentage of limbs that would otherwise necessitate amputation) are commonly reported as 60–70 per cent.

Indications for Operation

Ischaemic rest pain, gangrene, threatened or actual, and ulceration are absolute indications, and figure more frequently as indications for surgery than with aorto-iliac disease. Claudication is a relative indication but, because of the less satisfactory long-term results of arterial reconstruction distal to the groin, should be crippling before surgery is considered.

Femoropopliteal Bypass with Autogenous Saphenous Vein

With the patient supine the affected limb is flexed at the knee and thigh and externally rotated (*Fig. 37.17*). Support is given by a pillow below the knee that the saphenous nerve is not damaged as it lies with the vein below the knee. The upper end of the vein is divided just distal to the saphenofemoral junction, but the lower end is not detached until the artery has been exposed, and the length of vein required for the bypass ascertained.

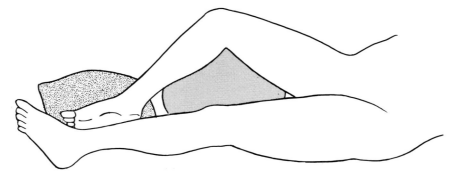

Fig. 37.17. The position of the patient on the operating table for femoropopliteal bypass.

and inadvertent extension prevented by a sandbag against the top of the foot. It is always wise to protect the heel with a plastic foam pad. As previously stated the thigh incision is placed directly over the saphenous vein, not the femoral artery, so that shallow undercutting of the skin is avoided as this leads to necrosis of the skin edges and it is better to use several short incisions rather than one long one. It is often not realized how posteriorly placed the saphenous vein is on the medial side of a fat thigh (*Fig.* 37.18).

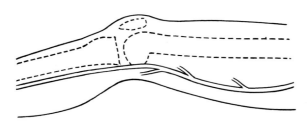

Fig. 37.18. The saphenous vein lies well posteriorly on the medial side of the thigh.

The upper end of the vein is exposed by a slightly oblique incision starting over the common femoral artery just below the inguinal ligament, and finishing over the upper end of the saphenous vein. In the obese elderly patient the inguinal ligament lies above the apparent groin crease and this should be allowed for. Thigh and groin incisions may suffice to obtain adequate vein length for short arterial obstructions, but if the reconstruction must extend to the knee joint or below, then the incision passes over the medial side of the knee joint to lie just behind the tibia.

The vein is dissected out using a combination of blunt and sharp dissection, taking care to ligate and divide all side branches. Care should also be taken

The common femoral artery is exposed through the upper incision and the proximal parts of the superficial and deep femorals exposed and taped ready for clamping.

The popliteal artery below the block is dissected out. If the upper part of the vessel was thought to be suitable on the arteriogram it is approached by displacing the sartorius muscle posteriorly and incising the underlying fascia. The popliteal space is entered and the vessel seen and secured after dissecting through the fat. It can then be palpated and its suitability for anastomosis determined. On the other hand, if it is decided that the lower popliteal artery is the best site for implantation the incision is extended, and the lower popliteal space entered by dividing the deep fascia. Blunt dissection between the tibia anteriorly and the gastrocnemius posteriorly reveals the neurovascular bundle from which the artery can be isolated. This limited exposure can be increased by dividing the hamstring tendons and the medial head of the gastrocnemius. Exposure of the posterior tibial artery is simply performed by division of the soleus arch and the origin of the soleus muscle from the posterior surface of the tibia.

After choosing the lower implantation site, the saphenous vein is detached at its lower end so that sufficient length is obtained to span the occlusion, remembering to straighten the knee temporarily before deciding on the length necessary, otherwise the graft will be unduly tight when the leg is extended postoperatively. This is not necessary when the implantation sites are above the knee. A 2-cm length of artery is isolated and clamped. The patient may be systemically heparinized with 1 mg/kg body weight or regional heparinization achieved by injecting 25 mg (2500 units) distally.

The lower implantation is done first, a longitudinal arteriotomy being adequate; it is not necessary to excise a portion of the artery wall. The vein graft, irrigated with heparinized saline and the absence of unligated side branches confirmed, is reversed and anastomosed to the arteriotomy, after an incision to 'spatulate' the end. A fine 5/0 or 6/0 non-absorbable double-armed suture is used, beginning at the acute or upper end. A simple over-and-over technique is followed and the anastomosis is left incomplete at its most accessible part.

The vein graft is passed subcutaneously upwards for anastomosis to the common femoral artery. If the lower anastomosis is below the knee it is probably desirable to pass the vein through the popliteal fossa and then subcutaneously or subfascially in the thigh, otherwise if the vein lies subcutaneously on the medial side of the knee, it produces an acute bend as it passes deeply to the popliteal artery. Twisting of the vein graft can be avoided by temporarily occluding it just above the lower anastomosis and distending it with saline prior to passing it upwards.

The upper anastomosis is accomplished in a precisely similar fashion to the lower but is completed after checking ante- and retrograde bleeding. It is then possible, prior to completing the lower anastomosis, to 'flush' the graft with blood, and to note from the vigour of the jet from the incomplete lower anastomosis whether or not there has been a technical error in the surgery. Any clot forming behind the clamps is removed in this way and after allowing a 'bleed back' by slackening the clamps on the popliteal vessel the anastomosis is rapidly completed and all clamps are removed. Temporary pressure soon leads to haemostasis from suture holes but occasionally an extra suture may be required. It is our practice to leave the wound open for 15–30 minutes in case early failure occurs.

Some surgeons take the precaution of on-table arteriography at this point to check that there is no deformity of the graft or the anastomoses and if such is shown the doubtful area is explored. Others are content with blood flow readings measured with an electromagnetic flowmeter. Figures for flow regarded as satisfactory are variable but of the order of 70–200 ml/min.

The wounds are closed with resuturing of divided muscles with non-absorbable sutures. Drainage is usually indicated and should be of the closed type.

Postoperative Care

Apart from the general care of a recovering anaesthetized patient, a close watch should be kept on the leg and foot. If the graft is continuing to function the foot which may be quite cool immediately after the operation will become gradually warmer. Pulses may not reappear until several hours after the operation, or may not reappear at all where there is severe tibial artery disease. Even so, gradually increasing warmth, filling veins and pinkness of the foot indicates a functioning graft.

Plethysmographic flow measurements indicate an increasing flow in the calf as the distal circulation opens up, becoming maximal at 24 hours (Wellington et al., 1966).

Complications

The two most important complications are graft occlusion and infection.

Graft Occlusion

EARLY OCCLUSION

This may be due to technical error in the surgery, in that one or other anastomosis may be severely narrowed often from a band of adventitia caught up in the suture, or an atheromatous plaque may be loosened and obstruct the lumen, particularly at the lower end. The authors' pause of 20 minutes after completion of the bypass reveals many of these errors by failure of the graft on the table. Others perform peroperative angiography on the functioning graft. Renwick et al. (1968) noted an 18 per cent early failure rate prevented by the use of this technique.

Flows may be measured electromagnetically and shown to fall off as the graft thromboses.

Whatever method of fault detection is used its correction there and then will avoid early return of the patient to the operating theatre. Poor 'run-off' or an inadequate vein (less than 4·0 mm diameter at the narrowest point) may also be responsible. If the vein is inadequate, its replacement with a synthetic of the modern type such as velour Dacron or expanded PTFE artery overcomes the immediate problem.

It is often worth while if all the above factors except poor 'run-off' can be excluded in a failure within hours of the bypass graft, to repeat the operation, clearing out recent clot. The observations of Wellington et al. (1966) lend support to the idea that several hours may need to elapse before a sufficiently adequate flow in the graft exists to obviate clotting. Repetition of the grafting procedure may achieve this degree of flow where it was not obtained after the first operation. It is therefore essential to maintain a stringent observation of the patient postoperatively to detect and correct failure as soon as it occurs.

LATE FAILURE

This may be due to advancing atherosclerosis in the arterial tree below the graft or sometimes to stenoses developing in the graft or at the lower end. This situation can only be detected prior to occlusion of the bypass by regular follow-up with arteriography—an expensive undertaking. As a compromise, regular clinical follow-up may reveal the return of claudication or weakening pulses in the elapsing years and these clinical suspicions, confirmed by Doppler ultrasound examination, then make further angiographic studies justified.

Since many patients, particularly smokers, have increased platelet adhesiveness, it follows that the risk of late thrombosis of the graft may be increased by smoking so that it should be discouraged. Platelet adhesiveness is reduced by aspirin and dipyridamole and so many patients are put on these drugs. Though clinical effectiveness is not proven, early platelet deposition is reduced (Goldman et al., 1983).

Infection

Frank wound sepsis should be rare with adequate technique. Sloughing of wound edges may occur if the skin is badly undercut, but graft infection even in these cases is uncommon.

Some infections may arise from transection of lymphatics draining a gangrenous or ulcerated area, and in such cases, at least, the appropriate prophylactic antibiotics started just prior to surgery may avert a disaster.

When it is suspected that the graft is infected some security against loss of life from secondary haemorrhage is given by a firm pad and bandage over the area, while the appropriate antibiotics are administered in large doses. Cross-matched blood should be ready for immediate use. Bleeding from an anastomosis in the presence of sepsis requires removal of the graft with oversewing or ligature of the host vessel. This may well result in loss of the limb, but anything less may jeopardize the patient's life.

Other causes of early postoperative bleeding are suture fracture, a blown-off ligature from a vein graft branch, or even rupture of a very thin-walled section of the graft. All may be managed by instant control of bleeding by pressure, blood transfusion and early return to the theatre. Here the fault can be corrected but it is also essential to make sure that clotting of variable degree, especially in the distal tree, has not occurred as a result of local pressure and hypotension. The passage of a Fogarty catheter may suffice but if doubt remains an on-table angiogram may be invaluable.

ACUTE ISCHAEMIA OF THE LEGS

Diagnosis

The diagnosis of acute arterial ischaemia of the legs may be easy or difficult. A story of sudden pain in the leg followed by paraesthesia and numbness, together with a 'useless' feeling in the limb, is classic and when physical examination reveals pallor and coolness of the extremity in which anaesthesia and paresis are present, it only remains to demonstrate that the pedal pulses are absent to clinch the diagnosis.

Acute venous thrombosis with swelling and lilac discoloration of the limb is not a likely cause of confusion even when pulses cannot be clearly felt owing to subcutaneous oedema.

However, the clinical picture is not always so definite. Many acute arterial occlusions do not have a clear history of sudden onset, particularly in the elderly and those with heart failure, and pain may be minimal or absent. Long-standing atherosclerotic arterial disease may lead to absent pulses contralaterally, in the so-called 'good' limb, and there is no physical sign which has so much observer error. Startling pallor of the limb may be replaced later by congestion with some proximal mottling, due to dependency of the limb with passive venous filling. Fortunately, skin anaesthesia or reduced sensation and muscle weakness remain a reliable indication of tissue ischaemia. It is important to remember that dead or dying toes can be moved by the long extensors and flexors lying in the better perfused, more proximal limb so that the fact that toes can be moved does not negate other evidence of severe limb ischaemia.

It follows that the most valuable signs of ischaemia in the limbs are reduced sensation and movement, in the absence, as is usually the case, of a major nerve lesion. Furthermore, the anaesthesia associated with a major nerve injury follows an anatomical pattern while that due to ischaemia is of the 'glove-and-stocking' variety.

Later Signs and Symptoms of Acute Ischaemia

The progression of ischaemic changes in the limb depends on how completely the blood supply is shut off. In acute thrombosis where the collaterals have already begun to develop due to prior atherosclerosis there is usually gradual improvement after the onset of occlusion. Following acute arterial embolism some limbs may demonstrate similar spontaneous improvement. Indeed, occasionally there may be a sudden dramatic spontaneous improvement with return of hitherto absent peripheral pulses, so-called 'pseudo-embolism'. This puzzling condition is usually due to the transient impaction of an embolus at a major bifurcation followed by its disintegration and the passage of the fragments into large intermuscular arteries as the profunda femoris and the peroneal, leaving the main axial vessels patent. In the majority of instances, however, progressive deterioration occurs. Extreme ischaemia may result if the iliac or femoral arteries are involved in an aortic dissection causing an abrupt cessation of distal blood flow.

When tissue blood flow falls below its critical level the early pallor is followed by purple blotching unaffected by pressure and indicating extravasation. The affected muscles, notably those in the calf, harden and become tender progressing to rigor mortis with fixed plantar flexion and forced dorsiflexion of the foot causes severe pain. These are the signs of irreversible tissue damage heralding the loss of the limb and treatment which aims to restore the circulation at this stage is unlikely to be successful. Moreover, it may possibly endanger the life of the patient by precipitating renal failure due to tubular necrosis. It is therefore a nicety of good clinical judgement to decide when the limb is irretrievably lost and proceed to primary amputation.

Determination of the Likely Cause of Arterial Obstruction

In the usual clinical situation occlusion may be due to embolism, acute thrombosis on an atheromatous lesion or dissection. The varieties of traumatic arterial lesion are discussed later.

The most common cause of acute arterial insufficiency is embolism; the least common, dissection. The mode of onset of the ischaemia with sudden pain in the limb favours a diagnosis of embolism rather than acute thrombosis. Certainly the development of collaterals associated with atherosclerotic narrowing tends to reduce the severity of the ischaemia and a history of claudication prior to the acute episode suggests that the occlusion is likely to be thrombotic rather than embolic. The distinction is important because the management of thrombosis is essentially conservative.

The limb affected by an aortic dissection extending to involve the iliofemoral segment is often profoundly ischaemic because the dissecting process blocks off the potential collaterals such as the lumbar and iliolumbar vessels. Permanent ischaemic changes soon develop and early revascularization must be attempted if the patient is not fatally ill. A history of severe chest and back pain, sometimes with evidence suggesting transient or permanent major vessel occlusion elsewhere such as hemiparesis, anuria or abdominal pain, makes dissection highly suspect as a cause of the ischaemic limb. Sometimes, however, the patient having had a total aortic dissection presents only with an ischaemic leg with chest or back pain being minimal.

The Place of Arteriography

Arteriography has no part to play in the routine management of embolism in the emergency situation. On the other hand, suspected acute thrombosis mandates arteriography: first, because attempts to relieve the situation with a Fogarty catheter may have disastrous consequences and, second, because correction of the occlusion will require a formal bypass or endarterectomy procedure. It is also desirable to ascertain the site and extent of 'run-off' vessels.

In the case of leg ischaemia complicating dissection, arch angiography is desirable to establish the origin of the dissection, but if it is not immediately available, or the general condition of the patient contra-indicates it, angiography may be deferred until after the threatened limb has been revascularized.

Management of Arterial Embolism of the Lower Limb

The advent of the Fogarty balloon catheter has revolutionized the management of arterial embolism since not only has it simplified the operative procedure but it may be attempted under local anaesthesia if indicated (Fogarty et al., 1971). Ninety per cent of arterial emboli originate within the heart—within the left ventricle, most commonly, as a sequel to myocardial infarction or from the left atrium, often fibrillating, secondary to atherosclerotic or rheumatic heart disease. But it must be remembered that some 10–15 per cent of all arterial emboli have a non-cardiac source, usually from aneurysms or atherosclerotic plaques arising in major vessels.

Although the mortality associated with arterial embolectomy has fallen in recent years it is still formidable and of the order of 20 per cent. This is usually related to the underlying cardiac conditions, being higher in patients with recent cardiac infarction, especially those over the age of 60.

Timing of Intervention

In gravely ill patients seen early, within 2 hours after embolism has occurred, a conservative approach may be practised. The patient should be heparinized to prevent clotting beyond the embolus and thus aid collateralization. Heparin 10 000 units i.v. administered by the practitioner who first sees the patient is always good treatment, whatever course is adopted, provided that the surgeon is informed. The patient must be reviewed at least hourly after this; improvement in colour, temperature, surface anaesthesia and muscle power permit continuation of the regimen. Failure to improve or deterioration of the condition of the limb indicates that this line of treatment should be abandoned forthwith and arterial flow restored by surgery. If significant symptoms associated with skin anaesthesia or hypo-aesthesia and muscle weakness persist after 6 hours of embolism, surgery is mandatory unless the patient is in danger of death and a deliberate decision is taken to sacrifice the limb. These considerations apart, in the majority of patients immediate surgery should be undertaken if the signs of ischaemia are present. A useful rule is that if the patient has been able to walk, however little, prior to the embolic episode, then surgery is indicated.

Embolectomy

Late embolectomy

By this is meant the removal of emboli days, weeks or even months after embolization. It follows that the limb must have survived the acute episode and is viable, although its function is limited. The results of late embolectomy are reported as encouraging but in our experience such patients are best treated by prior arteriography and standard reconstructive measures. This is not to say that small pieces of embolus in 'run-off' vessels cannot be successfully removed in conjunction with a bypass or endarterectomy.

Late embolectomy in the sense of embolectomy carried out late in the acute episode, when muscle stiffening and permanent skin staining have taken place, is attended by very poor results (*Fig.* 37.19).

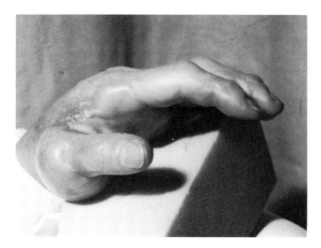

Fig. 37.19. The results of delayed restoration of arterial flow. Arterial repair 24 hours after traumatic thrombosis of the axillary artery. The skin survived with blistering and was anaesthetic but the muscles were dead. Late result was a classic Volkmann's ischaemic contracture.

In the presence of such physical signs the operation may be regarded not only as futile but possibly dangerous. Should flow be maintained in the ischaemic limb, which is not usually the case, renal failure from the absorption of tissue breakdown products may occur. This is analogous to the crush syndrome and may lead to a fatal outcome.

Technique

LEVEL OF ARTERIOTOMY

The artery usually opened for embolectomy is the common femoral. This is because the most frequent site of lodgement is at its bifurcation and furthermore this arteriotomy allows adequate removal of emboli from the bifurcation of the aorta downwards as far as the tibial vessels with use of the Fogarty balloon catheter. The artery is relatively easy to expose and its lumen of sufficient calibre not to be narrowed by suturing.

THE OPERATION

Having exposed the vessel under general or local anaesthesia together with its two terminal divisions, the deep and superficial femoral arteries, it may be evident that pulsation is absent, or if present is not expansile, but longitudinal. Always remember that soft clot transmits pulsation.

The main vessel and its branches are isolated with tapes; small side branches are controlled with heavy silk slings. Occlusion of the vessels can be accomplished with traction on the tape alone while an arteriotomy is made with a small-bladed knife. Clamps should not be used at this stage to avoid fragmentation of the embolus.

The arteriotomy should start on the anterior surface of the common femoral, a little above the origin of the profunda, and be carried downwards short of entering the superficial femoral origin. It should only be as long as is necessary to pass the embolus through it—no greater in length than the diameter of the common femoral artery. As the embolus comes into view slackening the upper tape will often result in its extrusion at the upper end. If not, gentle traction with Desjardins' forceps may produce it; alternatively, milking of the vessel from above may be successful. The gush of blood from above is controlled by traction on the upper tape and a clamp is then applied to the artery. Even if these manoeuvres are successful it is wise to pass a balloon catheter proximally in case some non-obstructive clot or thrombus is adhering to the upper vessel walls and which, if not removed, may lead later to occlusion. The deflated, previously tested catheter is passed proximally with one hand while the other controls bleeding by pinching the vessel with the tape, the assistant having removed the upper clamp. When the catheter is felt to have entered the aorta after the passage of about 30 cm the balloon is inflated and the catheter gently withdrawn. As the balloon engages in the mouth of the common iliac artery it is often necessary to deflate it slightly to avoid intimal damage as it passes distally to the arteriotomy site. For this reason the syringe maintaining the balloon pressure should always be controlled by the surgeon withdrawing the catheter who has a more finite sense of the precise pressure required than the assistant (*Fig.* 37.20).

Following removal of clot and embolus the upper clamp is reapplied. Attention is now turned to the superficial femoral artery and the embolus may now be lifted out from it, again aided by traction with forceps, 'milking' the artery or 'pumping' the thigh. A retrograde flow of blood may indicate distal patency, but in any case a Fogarty catheter with a 1·0-ml capacity balloon should always be tested and passed down the superficial femoral as far as it will go, and then withdrawn with the balloon inflated. It is often possible to pass the Fogarty catheter downwards as far as the ankle so that very small fragments of embolus and clot are removed. It is important not to damage the intima by excessive traction and inflation and to this end it is possible to inflate the balloon only partially while it is in the small-diameter distal tree, and as it is drawn proximally, to inflate it further gradually. This can be done with one hand, fragments of embolus and clot appearing at the arteriotomy

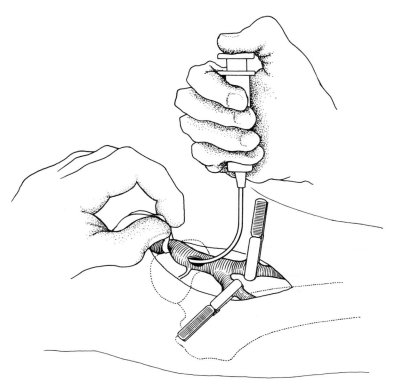

Fig. 37.20. Instrumentation of the iliac vessels, bleeding controlled by pinching tape.

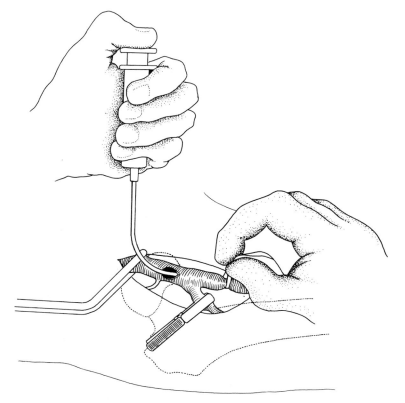

Fig. 37.21. Instrumentation of femoral artery. Friction of balloon completely under control of surgeon.

(*Fig.* 37.21). The distal vessel is then filled with a few ml of heparin saline and clamped and a similar manoeuvre is carried out on the profunda femoris artery this time using a 0·5-ml balloon catheter.

Repeated 'flue brushing' of the arteries should be avoided but each vessel may need two or three attempts before patency is restored.

Finally, the arteriotomy is closed with a fine 4/0 or 5/0 synthetic non-absorbable suture starting above and, prior to the completion of the suture line, allowing a small 'flush' of blood from each of the vessels in turn, by slackening the clamps to displace any clot which might have formed behind them.

'SADDLE' EMBOLUS

When the embolus is astride the aortic bifurcation, as the term implies, both legs are ischaemic and the femoral pulses are absent. More frequently the embolus fractures at the bifurcation and unequal pieces impact lower down in the arterial tree, often at the common femoral bifurcation or lower,

Both common femoral vessels should be exposed and that of the most ischaemic leg is opened first. Before passing the balloon catheter, however, the opposite common femoral should be clamped if it is still pulsatile, to obviate the risk of displacing some of the embolus into the distal tree of the less affected side. Having dealt with the worst affected leg, prior to closing the arteriotomy on this side, the embolectomy procedure is repeated on the less affected leg and then both arteriotomies are closed.

Occasionally it is impossible to remove the saddle embolus from below because of its firm consistency as when it is composed of myxomatous tissue. Removal by aortotomy is then necessary or if the patient is unfit for this, some form of extracoelomic bypass—axillofemoral—will be indicated. Failure to negotiate tortuous iliac arteries with the Fogarty catheter is more common but if it can be accomplished on one side at least and flow restored to one common femoral, then a 10-mm woven Dacron cross-over graft to the opposite common femoral resolves the difficulty in a simple way (*Fig.* 37.22).

Problems of Embolectomy

Although embolectomy can be a very simple procedure, the mortality remains high, particularly that of saddle embolus. This is due to the associated severe and often mortal cardiac disease. The heart may be unable to provide the additional output required consequent on the reopening of a large part of the vascular bed with its attendant reactive hyperaemia and also metabolites from the legs may tip the already electrically unstable heart into ventricular fibrillation. It is wise therefore to unclamp each femoral artery sequentially in case of saddle embolus, and to infuse bicarbonate peroperatively.

Similarly, there are good haemodynamic reasons why tight mitral stenosis with pulmonary oedema should be relieved by valvotomy prior to, or synchronously with, saddle embolectomy.

Failure to Restore Circulation after Embolectomy

Embolectomy should be undertaken early, before irreversible tissue changes have occurred, preferably within 6 hours of the event; the later it is performed the more likely is failure to occur. If operation is undertaken within 8 hours there is an 85 per cent probability of recovery of full function, but after 12 hours the percentage of successes falls sharply (Martin et al., 1969). Reocclusion of the main vessels after an apparently successful operation may be due to failure to perfuse the smaller arterial side-branches from which clot was never removed and indeed cannot be removed. Damage to the main vessel intima by too vigorous balloon catheterization or by prolonged contact with clot may also cause secondary thrombosis. Coexisting atherosclerotic lesions in the arteries predispose to failure of embolectomy and poor flow in the vessels postoperatively due to cardiac failure may lead to clotting of what otherwise could be a satisfactory revascularization.

Fasciotomy

It is always wise to perform this if the limb has been ischaemic for longer than 6–8 hours. The purpose of fasciotomy is to lower the pressure in the osseoaponeurotic compartments of the leg, dividing the deep fascia and allowing the swollen muscle to bulge into the subcutaneous compartment. Muscle swelling arises as a result of the imbibition of fluid into the anoxically damaged muscle when blood flow is restored. This swelling leads to a considerable rise in pressure in the compartment concerned with venous embarrassment producing further congestion and oedema. Complete sloughing of the muscle may result.

Fasciotomy can be carried out by the 'closed' method through short skin incisions, splitting the fascia with narrow scissors throughout the length of the compartment and all compartments in the leg should be thus treated. Open fasciotomy dividing the skin and fascia throughout the length of the compartments is likely to lead to infected large wounds and is best avoided.

Management of Acute Arterial Thrombosis

The severity of ischaemia in the legs in acute arterial thrombosis is likely to be less than that due to embolism or dissection because progressive collateralization, due to reduction in main vessel flow as the causative atherosclerotic lesions develop, exerts a protective effect. Indeed, the most frequent acute thromboses—those in the femoropopliteal segment—often are not reported to the doctor immedi-

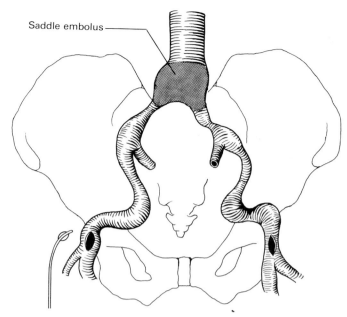

Saddle embolus

Fig. 37.22. Negotiation of tortuous vessels may be helped by putting a slight curve on the catheter and stillette.

ately, the patient subsequently seeking advice following a sudden decrease in claudication distance.

Occasionally, however, the clinical picture is much more urgent, with all the symptoms and signs of acute ischaemia necessitating emergency treatment. There is usually, but not invariably, a history of claudication prior to the acute episode of deterioration and the limb though clearly ischaemic is usually viable. Such cases usually respond well to initial full heparinization, possibly supplemented by the infusion of low molecular weight dextran, and once the immediate crisis recedes a routine arterial assessment can be undertaken.

Rarely the signs and symptoms may be so acute that the condition may be difficult to differentiate from embolism. Indeed, sometimes one suspects that a small embolus may have initiated the thrombosis, and either the aorta or the more distal vessels may be affected. The more distal acute thromboses such as those affecting the superficial femoral, if associated with profound ischaemia, will be found to extend distally to include the whole of a large part of the popliteal or even tibial vessels.

In practical terms this means that arteriography is necessary to define any distal vessel suitable for graft implantation, because any attempt at balloon catheterization in thrombosis secondary to atherosclerosis is doomed to failure. The operation indicated is one of the reconstructive variety used for chronic leg ischaemia, usually some form of bypass.

In acute aortic thrombosis, where conservative measures fail, arteriography is not so essential, although, if circumstances and time permit, it may be helpful. This is because the common femoral arteries are rarely involved in the thrombotic process. Satisfactory management includes the ascertainment of patency of the common femorals at a first stage of the operation, followed by bifurcation grafting as for chronic aorto-iliac disease. One of the alternatives for this operation, such as axillofemoral bypass already described, may have to be used in the poor risk patient.

Management of Acute Leg Ischaemia due to Aortic Dissection

Dissection involving the lower aorta, iliac or femoral vessels is usually an extension of a major dissection starting in ascending aorta arch or descending thoracic aorta (*Fig.* 37.23). A few start in the abdominal aorta. Acute leg ischaemia occurs in a proportion of patients. In our series of 41 cases, acute ischaemia of one or both legs occurred in 15; 2 of these were moribund on arrival, but 13 patients required operation to attempt to restore the circulation to the legs. Nine of these patients subsequently died as a result of complications of the dissection; usually cardiac tamponade, or after operation to cure the dissection such as ascending aortic transection, with graft interposition. However, there were 4 survivors in whom a satisfactory revascularization of the legs was obtained. Two additional patients recovered spontaneously from acute leg ischaemia.

The management of these patients is overshadowed by the Damoclean sword of high aortic dissection. Most give a history of severe retrosternal and back pain, some may be hypotensive and *in extremis*. Abdominal tenderness from gut ischaemia, anoxia,

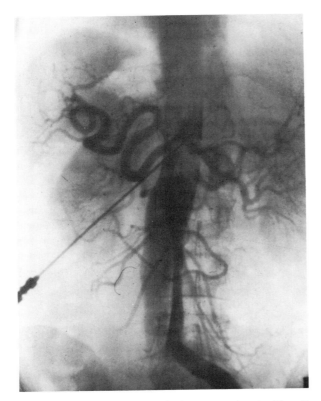

Fig. 37.23. Aortogram showing the lower aorta involved in a dissection originating in the ascending aorta. The left common iliac artery is completely obstructed. (Taken prone.)

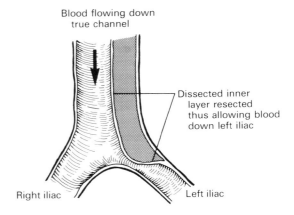

Fig. 37.24. Diagram to show the mode of obstruction of iliac artery by an aortic dissection and the method of relieving it.

or true paraplegia may also be present, but in the authors' experience is not common. The typical presentation is that of a patient with obvious acute ischaemia of one or both legs and with a clear story of chest and back pain. They may or may not be hypertensive. The degree of ischaemia is out of proportion to the elapsed time since the onset and muscle hardening may well be present with a length of history of only 3–4 hours.

As regards treatment it is not likely that a surgical attack on the origin of the dissection in the proximal aorta will result in viable legs and any undue delay may cause irreversible damage to the tissues, resulting in loss of one leg or both legs.

The line of management adopted is to control the blood pressure, if hypertensive, with a variant of the Wheat et al. (1965) regimen, and to expose and open the lower abdominal aorta. By resection of a portion of the dissected layer and a combination of distal balloon catheterization it is possible to restore flow to the legs. It is important to prevent a sudden rise in blood pressure when the aorta is clamped (*Figs.* 37.24, 37.25).

After this procedure the patient is returned to the intensive care ward and the origin of the dissection managed according to its exact site and complications. If aortography shows an ascending or arch dissection hypotensive therapy may be employed. The

development of tamponade or acute aortic incompetence demands proximal aortic surgery using cardiopulmonary bypass if the patient's life is to be saved. Post-subclavian dissection can usually be followed conservatively on hypotensive therapy with serial chest radiographs, to detect undue enlargement of the descending aorta.

Occasionally, the presentation may be of leg ischaemia with no history to suggest dissection. The dramatic onset mimics embolization. On common femoral arteriotomy no embolus is found, the vessel either being empty and collapsed or containing clotted blood. If the dissection actually involves the artery, particoloured streaking—normal colour alternating with the dark purple of the dissected wall—may be seen. Balloon catheterization should be tried proximally to establish re-entry and if a reasonable jet of blood can be obtained from above the arteriotomy can be closed; if not, the aorta must be exposed and dealt with as described above.

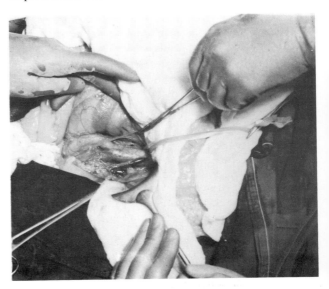

Fig. 37.25. Dissection of aorta exposed at bifurcation level. The upper iliac artery is normal, the lower one is the seat of dissection.

Acute Ischaemia due to Arterial Injury

Arterial injury should be suspected when, after trauma to the limb, there are signs of ischaemia or evidence of reduced perfusion as shown by weak or absent pulses. If there is doubt as to whether a pulse is present or not, for practical purposes it should be assumed to be absent.

Usually the trauma is severe and often there are fractures or dislocations present. Particular fractures associated with arterial injury are supracondylar of the femur and severe fracture-dislocations of the knee, but any fracture with severe displacement may be responsible. Laceration, complete transection or thrombosis of the artery may result. Kicks or crushing injury over the line of the vessels may lead to traumatic arterial thrombosis or partial rupture with the formation of false aneurysms.

Penetrating injuries by knives or bullets over the course of a known vessel should be suspected of having damaged that vessel, particularly if gross or continued bleeding is present. Bleeding may have stopped and a large haematoma be evident, which may be pulsatile. The degree of limb ischaemia is variable and sometimes there is a bruit which indicates an acute arteriovenous fistula.

Management of Acute Arterial Injury

Digital or other direct pressure over an actively bleeding site will arrest bleeding while the patient is resuscitated with intravenous plasma expanders and preferably blood. Exploration of such an actively bleeding wound is mandatory and urgent. If a major vessel has obviously been damaged then proximal control is gained by exposure of the vessel above the wound, distal pressure preventing bleeding meanwhile. In this way orderly haemostasis can be achieved prior to deliberate exploration of the wound and the avoidance of 'smash and grab' techniques.

When the wound is not actively bleeding following resuscitation, arteriography will show if there is a major vessel injury or not. The dye may be seen to enter the veins in arteriovenous fistula either directly or via a false aneurysm. If no fistula is present a false aneurysm may be shown (*Fig.* 37.26).

Once the general condition of the patient is satisfactory, and there is evidence that a major vessel has been damaged then urgent exploration is mandatory. This is especially true if a false aneurysm is present as these usually enlarge remorselessly, only the very small minority spontaneously clot. If they are left to enlarge they frequently become infected and repair is then fraught with the risks of secondary haemorrhage (*Fig.* 37.27).

Though the classic management of arteriovenous fistulas has been conservative, this was in the hope that an adequate collateral circulation would develop prior to ligation. With the techniques of modern arterial surgery available there is no advantage in

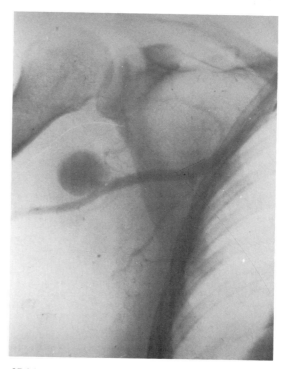

Fig. 37.26. False aneurysm of axillary artery shown on arteriography. Large haematoma in axilla but pulses still present distally.

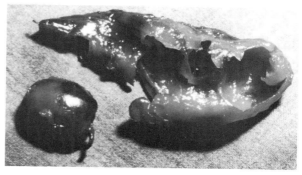

Fig. 37.27. False aneurysm of posterior tibial artery. Remorseless enlargement has resulted from rupture of the false capsule several times resulting in an irregular elongated cavity.

waiting and repair of both artery and vein, if necessary with vein grafting, is safe, swift and satisfactory.

Where there is no external wound and the story is one of a blow or kick over a major vessel followed by the development of a painful swelling, it is likely that the vessel has torn and blood extravasated; a false aneurysm may develop from this, so that the swelling becomes pulsatile and enlarges. The patient is frequently elderly with atherosclerotic vessels. Early repair should be performed (*Fig.* 37.28).

Traumatic Arterial Thrombosis and 'Arterial Spasm'

Direct violence to the artery of the closed type may not lead to complete disruption but to traumatic

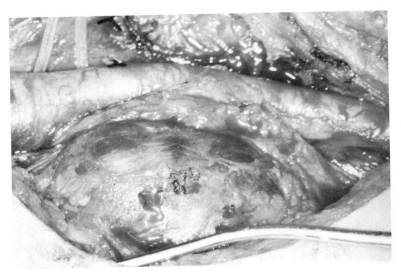

Fig. 37.28. False aneurysm of a branch of the profunda femoris artery, with the main femoral vessel bowed over it. Cure consisted of excision of the aneurysm with ligation of the feeding vessels.

arterial thrombosis. This condition also occurs after trauma to the artery by crushing or angulation at fracture sites or by piercing—sometimes by needles and catheters in the pursuance of X-ray and cardiac catheterization techniques. Iatrogenic injury is the most common form of arterial injury in most UK civilian experience.

The part of the arterial wall which is least resistant to trauma is the intimal layer, so that when an artery is crushed, angulated sharply or struck a severe blow, the intima may be disrupted while the adventitia remains intact, although bruised. With advancing age atherosclerosis results in an even greater disparity in resistance of the arterial coats to trauma. The intima may be calcified, covered with thrombus and infiltrated with lipid, extending a variable distance into the media. The adventitial layers and outer parts of the media are relatively unaffected. Not only is the aged intima thus more liable to damage, but temporary arrest of flow through the vessel may result in clotting owing to loss of its antithrombotic properties.

The zone of intimal disruption is the seat of primary thrombosis. Clotting occurs upwards to the major branch above and downwards to the most significant re-entrant collateral, where the inflow of blood is sufficient to prevent further clotting (*Fig.* 37.29).

Energy is lost from the blood perfusing the collateral bed and so the blood pressure in the vessel beyond the block is lower than that above, resulting in a tapering appearance from above down as the vessel is inspected. Early on, the recent clot above and below the zone of intimal disruption may transmit the pulse wave and so lead to the false impression that the vessel is patent, merely being in a state of contraction or 'spasm' below the contusion. The accumulation of blood and oedema beneath a tight

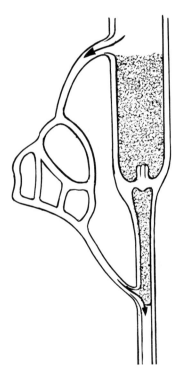

Fig. 37.29. Acute traumatic arterial thrombosis. The tapering 'spasm-like' appearance of the vessel is due to a disparity of intraluminal pressures above and below the thrombus.

investing fascia prior to exposure may accentuate this narrowing of the vessel and the vessel calibre may increase as a result of division of the fascia in the course of the operation (*Fig.* 37.30).

The authors have never in their experience of 160 civilian arterial injuries seen a case of undoubted arterial spasm. That is where arterial insufficiency has been caused by active contraction of the arterial

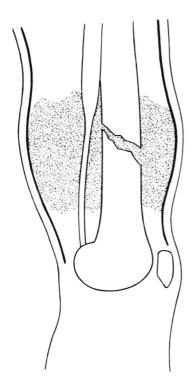

Fig. 37.30. Haematoma and oedema under the tight fascia also compress the vessel.

wall persisting unremittingly until relieved by the application of dilatory drugs to the wall of the vessel. In every case of 'spasm' which we have explored intimal rupture with superadded thrombosis has been found (*Fig.* 37.31).

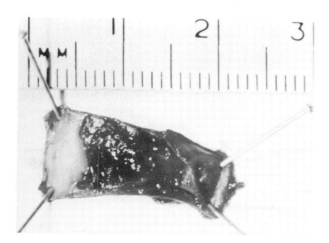

Fig. 37.31. Portion of artery removed for traumatic arterial thrombosis showing on the left relatively normal intima. There is disruption of the intimal layer elsewhere covered by clot.

Diagnosis

A high personal 'index of suspicion' that traumatic arterial thrombosis is likely or possible after reduction of a severely displaced fracture or fractures at particular sites should lead to examination of the circulation of the limb afterwards. Similarly, blows or crushing injury over the main vessels or instrumentation of them for diagnostic purposes should be followed by positive exclusion of arterial injury. It is a good clinical rule to assume the worst until proved otherwise (*Fig.* 37.32).

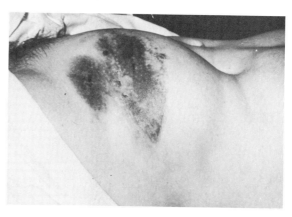

Fig. 37.32. Large haematoma in left groin caused by crushing with half-ton transformer. Both common femoral arteries were thrombosed and were replaced by vein grafts.

If circulatory impairment is evident as shown by the signs and symptoms of ischaemia previously discussed and especially if, in addition to absent pulses, pallor and coolness of the limb, there is impairment of sensation and movement then exploration of the vessel is mandatory.

Since an accompanying nerve injury is quite possible in a traumatized limb, less reliance can be placed on variation of sensation and movement than is the case in the non-traumatized patient. But it is worth repeating that ischaemic anaesthesia is of the 'glove-and-stocking' type. When seriously in doubt as to whether depressed sensation in the foot is due to nerve injury or insufficient perfusion, arteriography may be helpful (*Fig.* 37.33).

If the condition of the limb permits the use of inflatable cuffs, ankle pressure obtained by the Doppler velocity instrument can be useful in management. If the resting ankle pressure is above 60 mmHg, it is unlikely that the limb will come to harm, even if there is an arterial thrombosis. This technique is especially useful when pulselessness and coolness follow instrumentation of arteries for pressure and X-ray studies.

Management

As with spontaneous acute limb ischaemia an urgent decision has to be made as to the likely fate of the limb if nothing is done. Coincident, extensive, nerve and bone or joint injuries may sometimes be so severe that primary amputation is justified but this is rare in contemporary civilian practice. Procrastination is

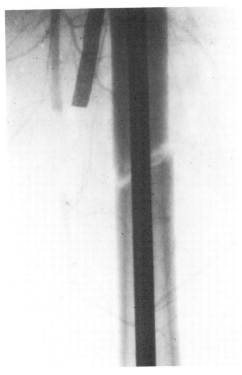

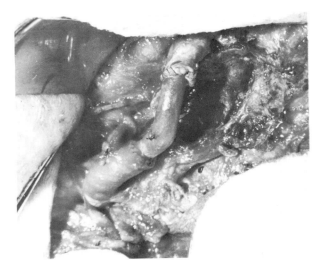

Fig. 37.34. Thrombosed portion of artery excised. Vein graft replacement.

Fig. 37.33. Arteriogram of a fixed fractured femur in an 18-year-old motorcyclist. The sciatic nerve was found to be damaged at the nailing operation. The region of thrombosis is shown and was resected and replaced by a saphenous vein graft.

indefensible for in our experience limbs are still lost by the erroneous concept of arterial spasm (Ashton and Slaney, 1970). Irretrievable damage may occur while this illusory state is treated by the futile administration of vasodilators, such as papaverine or flow promoters such as dextran. If ischaemia exists then it is due to organic arterial occlusion and early exploration is mandatory. Conservative optimistic expectancy is quite unwarranted. Of course, a collateral circulation *may* open up, but one cannot anticipate it, and when eventually the failure to improve becomes all too evident, permanent damage to the limb tissues may already have been done. When in doubt, urgent exploration of the vessel must be the clinical rule. It is wiser to 'look and see' than 'wait and see'; better by far a negative exploration than a dead leg.

Operative management is by resection of the damaged section of artery and usually its replacement by a reversed vein graft (*Fig.* 37.34). While there is no objection to simple 'end-to-end' arterial suture where no appreciable loss of vessel length occurs as in clean transection with a sharp knife, vein grafting is preferable to simple arterial suture because undue tension in the suture line is avoided and there is no temptation to restrict the excision of the damaged portion, so jeopardizing the result from later thrombosis. Ligation of arterial side-branches to allow

easier approximation of the proximal and distal vessels is also unnecessary and leaving these vessels in continuity safeguards the patency of the repair. Tangential loss of part of the arterial circumference, usually due to avulsion of a large side-branch, may be best repaired by utilizing a vein patch (*Fig.* 37.35).

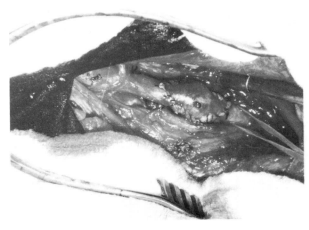

Fig. 37.35. Short segment of arterial thrombosis treated by thrombectomy and vein patch.

The saphenous vein is most convenient for a graft and may be taken from the same leg if there is no reason to suspect that this will cause venous insufficiency. Otherwise it should be taken from the opposite undamaged leg and this should certainly be done if there is concomitant damage to the major vein of the limb, particularly if there is extensive soft tissue disruption. This is especially true if the injury is at popliteal level as this is a particularly critical site both for arterial blood supply and venous drainage.

TECHNIQUE OF VEIN GRAFTING

After removing an adequate length of vein, it is distended with heparinized saline and reversed so that the valves will not impede arterial blood flow. It is important to keep the suture line stretched as the anastomosis proceeds by placing and tying a suture at each end of the suture line; if the vessels are small, three sutures may be thus used to avoid constriction of the anastomosis—the so-called 'triangulation procedure'. After completing one side the anastomosis can be rotated through 180° by passing the stay suture behind the vessel, so presenting the opposite side for suture (*Fig.* 37.36).

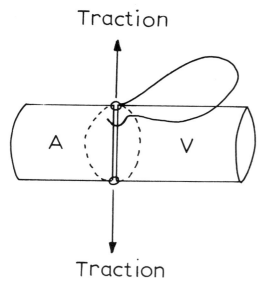

Fig. 37.36. A useful method of vein graft suture.

Prior to the completion of the anastomosis, it is wise to pass a balloon catheter proximally and distally to remove any clot which has formed during the period of cessation of the circulation (*Fig.* 37.37). This also has the effect of dilating the distal vessel and a little heparinized saline may be instilled after this manoeuvre prior to reapplication of the clamps while the anastomosis is completed. Fracture reduction and fixation should be undertaken prior to arterial repair because attempts at reduction afterwards may lead to tearing of the suture line. An approach to artery and bone can often be made through the same incision.

REPAIR OF DAMAGED VEINS

Repair of major vein injuries should always be performed rather than ligation, particularly where the popliteal vein is concerned or there is massive soft tissue trauma. Repair may be by lateral suture of laceration, or may require interposition vein grafts from the opposite limb (Rich et al., 1970).

Of 18 patients with combined popliteal artery and vein injuries in whom no venous repair was attempted, 12 patients developed complications including 4 with massive oedema of the leg. By contrast, of 26 other patients with vein injuries, 21 of whom had venous repair, none developed massive oedema (Sullivan et al., 1971).

ANEURYSMAL DISEASE OF THE LEGS

While it is customary to consider under this heading popliteal and femoral aneurysms as entities it should be appreciated that often the patient is suffering from a generalized dilatation of the arterial tree. These common regional aneurysms are therefore merely local exacerbations of this generalized condition. Thus popliteal aneurysms are frequently bilateral and often associated with aneurysms of the aorta and iliac arteries; femoral aneurysms are rarer but uniform femoral dilatation is more often present.

Aneurysms anywhere frequently contain stasis thrombus on their walls which is attached to a varying degree. Mobility of the part wherein the vessel lies is thus likely to detach this thrombus with resultant distal embolization.

Femoral Aneurysm

Common femoral aneurysms are less frequently met with than popliteal aneurysm, but may be seen in association with aortic and iliac aneurysm.

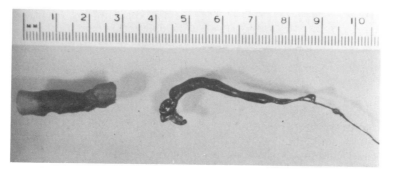

Fig. 37.37. An excised piece of damaged artery (*left*). Thrombus removed by suction prior to completion of the suture line (*right*).

They may give rise to pain in the groin when large and occasionally cause distal embolization in the legs, but the normal presentation is that of a pulsatile mass in the groin.

Management

When large (greater than 4 cm in diameter), they are best excised. A vertical incision is made along the line of the vessels, the upper end extending above the upper limit of the aneurysm. The inguinal ligament is divided and the spermatic cord and peritoneum pushed upwards to expose the external iliac artery. Proximal control of the aneurysm is thus gained.

Dissection should be kept close to the aneurysm to avoid the femoral nerve laterally and the femoral vein medially, which may be closely adherent. The profunda and superficial femoral arteries are exposed in the usual manner and after regional or systemic heparinization, the vessels are clamped above and below and the aneurysm opened. The sac can be excised, but in large aneurysms where the vein and nerve are densely adherent to the sac the technique of an inlay prosthesis can be safely used leaving the sac *in situ*.

Every effort should be made to connect the profunda femoris as well as the superficial femoral into the reconstruction. Fortunately, this is usually easy in that these two vessels commonly arise close together (*Fig.* 37.38).

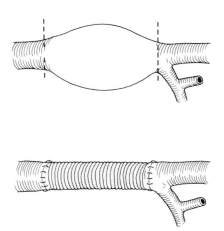

Fig. 37.38. Excision of common femoral aneurysm and replacement with Dacron prosthesis.

A Dacron graft woven, knitted or velour of about 10 mm diameter is a suitable replacement and it is sutured with non-absorbable sutures end to end to the external iliac artery above and end to end to the common stem of the profunda and superficial femoral vessels.

Alternatively, autogenous saphenous vein can be used, but the diameter is usually rather small

although the panel graft technique of Linton (1973) can then be used to increase the diameter.

Superficial Femoral Aneurysms

These are altogether less common in isolation but may be part of a femoropopliteal aneurysmal dilatation (*Fig.* 37.39). If in isolation they rarely give rise to embolization and make their presence known by enlarging steadily and giving rise to pain. They are treated by excision and replacement with prosthesis; an 8·0-mm Dacron tube is usually satisfactory in the thigh in these patients and remains patent whereas in obliterative disease it is not so satisfactory and is likely to occlude. Autogenous saphenous vein can also be used although we have seen a few subsequently become aneurysmal, particularly in diabetic patients.

Popliteal Aneurysm

Diagnosis

This is difficult in the early stages when the aneurysm is small and enclosed in the firm box of the popliteal fossa, but its presence should always be suspected if the popliteal pulse is unusually easy to feel. Indeed, they may not achieve a very large size when a pulsating lump at the back of the knee makes the diagnosis obvious (*Fig.* 37.40). However, even when quite small the aneurysm may give rise to devastating symptoms, notably those of acute ischaemia of the foot, due to thrombosis of the aneurysm. It is unusual for total thrombosis of the aneurysm to occur without prodromal symptoms, frequently as the appearance of small blue areas with hyperaemic margins in the skin of the foot, secondary to cutaneous infarcts due to micro-embolization (*Fig.* 37.41). Such areas may occur in the toes from embolization of the digital arteries and cause diagnostic difficulty (Downing et al., 1985).

These events may go on for a considerable time—months or years until the tibial vessels themselves become blocked and claudication then develops. Later still, the flow through the aneurysm itself may be so impeded by distal embolization of the 'run-off' vessels that clotting occurs and when this happens the collateral circulation is usually so poor that acute ischaemia of the foot results.

This was not the case when, as a deliberate manoeuvre, the aneurysm was made to clot by ligation, classically that of the Hunterian ligation. If this was performed early before distal circulatory silting-up had occurred then cure of the lesion by clotting was possible with preservation of a reasonable blood supply to the foot. Indeed, Hunterian ligation with sympathectomy has been employed in this century to treat popliteal aneurysm with good results (Richard and Learmonth, 1942).

Popliteal aneurysms steadily enlarge, pressing on

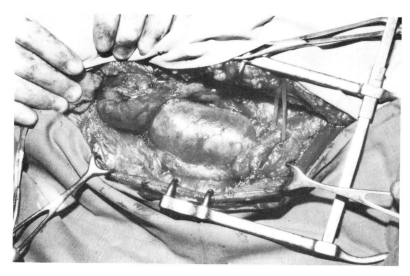

Fig. 37.39. Aneurysm of superficial femoral artery.

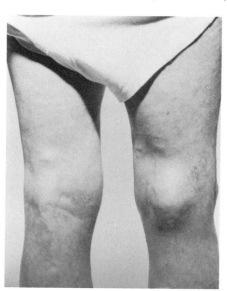

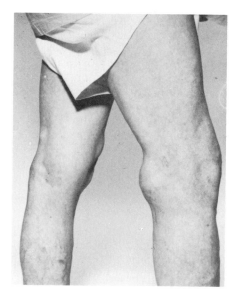

Fig. 37.40. Classic appearance of popliteal aneurysm.

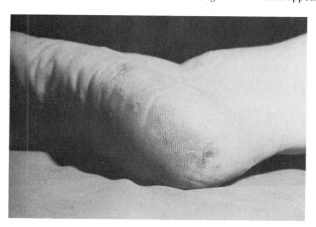

Fig. 37.41. Micro-embolization of the skin of the heel of a patient with a popliteal aneurysm.

surrounding structures so that impedance of venous return may give rise to oedema of the ankle and superficial venous prominence. Aching at the back of the knee may also occur. Bilocular aneurysms may occur with the upper portion enlarging and presenting as a swelling on the posteromedial part of the thigh (*Fig.* 37.42).

Leakage from the aneurysms occurs late and is often confined by the strong fascia, so that a steadily enlarging false aneurysm brings attention to the part which is the seat of considerable pain. This, combined with reddening of the overlying skin, may be mistaken for an infective process. Final rupture leads to intense local swelling with oedema and suffusion of the leg and foot.

Pedal pulses are present in uncomplicated popliteal aneurysm even when distal embolization has begun.

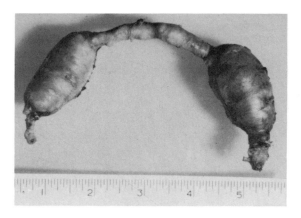

Fig. 37.42. Double popliteal aneurysms.

When the aneurysm has enlarged the foot pulses may become less easy to feel, no doubt due to the absorption of the pulse wave by the so-called 'windkessel' effect constituted by the elastic reservoir of the lesion. As distal embolization proceeds the distal pulses may eventually disappear.

Arteriography should be employed not only to show the aneurysm, but also to demonstrate the state of the distal vessels as these may then be occluded at various levels and the aneurysmal process may involve the bifurcation of the posterior tibial artery. The proximal extent of the process which may extend well up into the femoral artery can also be seen, enabling the proximal implantation side for a graft to be chosen. Ultrasound has been used to demonstrate the dilated vessel (Scott et al., 1977).

Treatment

Modern treatment includes a direct attack on the aneurysm with restoration of the circulation by reversed autogenous saphenous vein graft. It can be taken from the ipsilateral leg, since the condition is frequently bilateral and the contralateral vein may well be needed later for the opposite side. Synthetic grafts have no place for arterial replacement behind the knee because the failure rate is high.

The choice of incision is immaterial being either medial, using the incision used to harvest the vein as for femoropopliteal bypass, or midline posterior, which affords better access to a large aneurysm which may be densely adherent to vein and nerve. In this case a separate incision is necessary for the vein removal. Involvement of the femoropopliteal segment usually indicates a medial approach.

The aneurysm can be excised, which may be technically difficult due to the adherence previously mentioned, and the reversed vein is then sewn end to end to the vessel above and below. Due to the general enlargement of the vessels already alluded to and in order to effect a satisfactory anastomosis it is often necessary to spatulate the vein above, and sometimes below, in order to 'match up' the suture line. A fine 5/0 or 6/0 non-absorbable suture should be used.

Probably an easier and safer alternative to excision is bypass of the aneurysm with the reversed saphenous vein through a medial incision. End-to-side anastomosis above and below is performed and the operation concluded with ligature of the popliteal artery above and below the aneurysm, the ligatures being within the span of the bypass. This operation is now the authors' choice and infection of the aneurysm contents, which might be thought likely, does not seem to occur.

When the aneurysm is very large or has a false moiety, the leg being tense and bruised, proximal control via an incision over Hunter's canal with exposure and clamping of the femoral artery is wise. Similarly, the inferior vessels are sought and controlled.

The extravasated blood and clot can then be entered and the aneurysm opened. After evacuation of the thrombus any vessels leaving the sac which may be back-bleeding can be suture-ligated from within the sac and the reversed saphenous vein can then be anastomosed end to end to the main vessel where it enters and leaves the sac.

When the patient has an acutely ischaemic leg and foot, the presumption is, and it should be supported by arteriography, that the main outflow is occluded by thrombus. The procedure therefore includes an attempt to remove this distal thrombus by the use of the balloon catheter.

Having treated the clinically presenting aneurysm, no time should be wasted in dealing with any contralateral lesion which may be asymptomatic. Indeed, it is ironical that the best results attend the treatment of this side rather than the presenting leg in which the distal circulation may have been nearly destroyed before the patient was seen.

DIGITAL GANGRENE ASSOCIATED WITH PALPABLE PEDAL PULSES

Digital gangrene associated with easily palpable pedal pulses is a frequent cause of diagnostic dilemma, often resulting in unsatisfactory and ill-advised management. It is important to appreciate at the outset that if the pedal pulses are patent then gangrene of the toes must be due to occlusion of the small arteries in the foot or digits and that, as elsewhere, this is secondary to either embolism or thrombosis. With the possible exception of ergot poisoning or iatrogenic disasters with vasoconstrictor drugs such as ergotamine and adrenaline, digital gangrene due to vasospasm alone is not a tenable proposition. For practical purposes, therefore, frank digital gangrene excludes purely vasospastic states such as primary Raynaud's disease. It only then remains to decide whether the digital artery occlusion is embolic or thrombotic in origin, since this not only indicates the probable diagnosis but has an important bearing on case management (*Table* 37.1).

Table 37.1. Clinical features of small vessel occlusion

Embolic	Thrombotic
Unilateral	Frequently bilateral
Often repetitive	Often symmetrical
Progressive and serious	Remission and relapse
Surgery indicated	Management medical
Results good	Results poor

Digital gangrene due to distal embolization from a proximal source is usually unilateral and its appearance in an otherwise well-vascularized limb should always make one suspicious, especially if it is accompanied by evidence of small cutaneous infarcts or areas of discoloration of varying age. A likely proximal source should then be sought (*Fig.* 37.43). Another striking clinical feature of small vessel embolization is the repetitive nature of the attack resembling closely those of transient cerebral ischaemic attacks associated with carotid bifurcation lesions. Further showers of emboli are likely to produce serious sequelae by diffuse obliteration of the peripheral arterial tree which result in extensive gangrene necessitating a major amputation (Anderson and Richards, 1968; Slaney and Hamer, 1973). Although it has long been recognized that distal embolization may complicate atherosclerotic plaques or aneurysms arising in the aorta and major vessels, appreciation that identical situations occur in the peripheral arteries is comparatively recent. Confirmation of the clinical diagnosis by arteriography followed by expeditious and appropriate reconstructive surgery removes the source of emboli, often with gratifying results (*Fig.* 37.44).

Thrombotic digital gangrene is usually a manifestation of an underlying systemic disorder of which diabetes mellitus remains the commonest, but it may occasionally complicate acute hypovolaemic states especially if these are associated with septicaemic shock. In contrast to embolic phenomena thrombotic gangrene is quite frequently bilateral, often symmetrical, and the clinical course is one of remission and relapse (*Figs.* 37.45–37.47). A wide range of disorders may present in this fashion but clinically they may be divided into five groups with considerable areas of overlap (*Table* 37.2).

It is important to appreciate that the vascular

Table 37.2. Aetiology of thrombotic small vessel occlusion

Systemic disorders	Diabetes mellitus, scleroderma, rheumatoid arthritis, disseminated lupus erythematosus
Vasopathies	Raynaud's phenomena, Buerger's disease, polyarteritis nodosa, giant cell arteritis
Blood disorders	Polycythaemia, lymphomas, coagulopathies, macroglobulinaemia
Physical	Trauma, cold, heat, radiation, chemicals
Drugs	Ergot, adrenaline

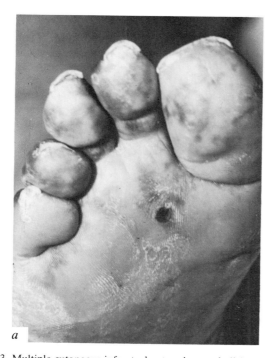 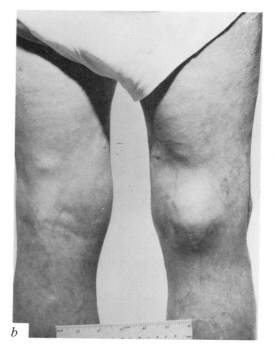

a   *b*

Fig. 37.43. Multiple cutaneous infarcts due to micro-emboli from an aneurysm of the right popliteal artery. Note also the asymptomatic left popliteal aneurysm subsequently treated to prevent a repetition of these events.

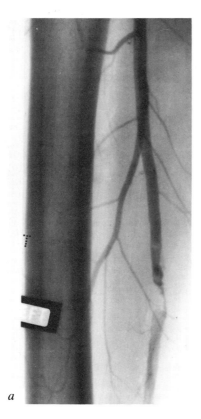
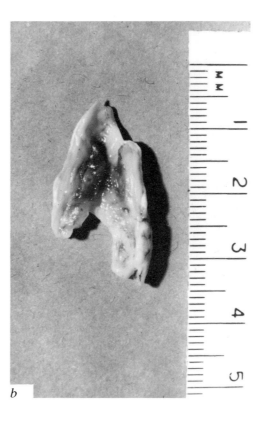

Fig. 37.44. *a*, Atherosclerotic plaque giving rise to micro-emboli, which caused ischaemic lesions in toes. *b*, Plaque and loosely adherent thrombus removed at operation. Complete resolution of pedal lesions following endoarterectomy and vein patch angioplasty combined with sympathectomy.

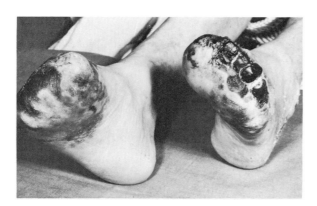

Fig. 37.45. Bilateral amputation of all toes for gangrene due to macroglobulinaemia. Initial remission followed by relapse and further bilateral symmetrical gangrene.

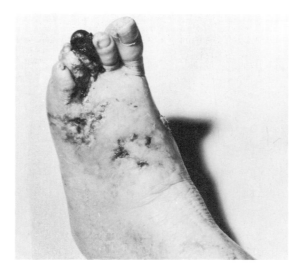

Fig. 37.46. Digital gangrene and cutaneous infarct in disseminated lupus erythematosus.

lesions may be the presenting features of these systemic disorders and precede their general manifestations by many months and sometimes years. During this latent period the majority, if not all, of the recognized serological screening tests may remain deceptively normal (Baddeley, 1965; Johnston et al., 1965). If pedal pulses are present the management of most of these lesions is conservative, though toilet surgery possibly combined with sympathectomy may be required. The institution of appropriate and intensive

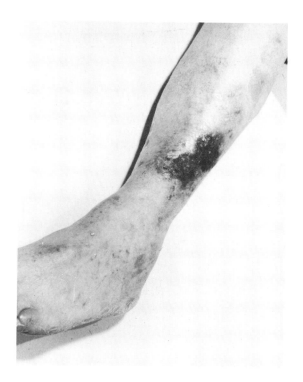

Fig. 37.47. Cutaneous infarcts in polycythaemia rubra vera.

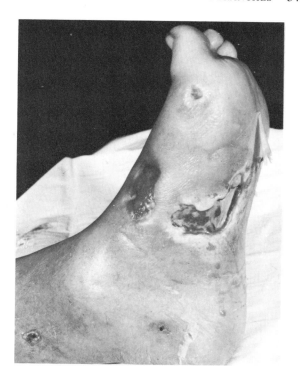

Fig. 37.48. Extensive ulceration in rheumatoid vasopathy. Complete resolution with intensive medical treatment.

medical treatment may occasionally result in dramatic improvement (*Fig.* 37.48). As in so many other situations the best results are achieved when physicians and surgeons sharing a common interest work in close collaboration in the management of these difficult and perplexing problems.

REFERENCES

Anderson W. R. and Richards A. M. (1968) Evaluation of lower extremity muscle biopsies in the diagnosis of atheroembolism. *Arch. Path.* **86,** 535–541.

Ashton F. and Slaney G. (1970) Arterial injuries in civilian surgical practice. *Injury* **1,** 303–313.

Ashton F., Slaney G. and Rains A. J. H. (1962) Femoropopliteal arterial obstructions: late results of Teflon prostheses and arterial homografts. *Br. Med. J.* **2,** 1149–1152.

Baddeley R. M. (1965) The place of upper dorsal sympathectomy in the treatment of primary Raynaud's disease. *Br. J. Surg.* **52,** 426–430.

Baddeley R. M., Ashton F. and Slaney G. (1968) A comparison of autogenous vein bypass grafts with vein patch angioplasty. *Surg. Gynecol. Obstet.* **127,** 503–508.

Baird R. J., Feldman P., Miles J. T. et al. (1977) Subsequent downstream repair after aorto-iliac and aorto-femoral bypass operations. *Surgery* **82,** 785–793.

Blaisdell F. W. and Hall A. D. (1963) Axillary femoral bypass for lower extremity ischaemia. *Surgery* **54,** 563–568.

Blumenberg M. D. and Gelfand M. L. (1977) Failure of knitted Dacron as an arterial prosthesis. *Surgery* **81,** 493–496.

Bouhoutsos J. and Martin P. (1973) The influence of age on prognosis after arterial surgery for atherosclerosis of the lower limb. *Surgery* **74,** 637–640.

Brief D. K., Brener F. J. and Alpert J. (1975) Crossover femoro-femoral grafts followed up for 5 years or more. *Arch. Surg.* **110,** 1294–1299.

Carney W. I., Stewart W. B., De Pinto D. J. et al. (1977) Carotid bruit as a risk factor in aorto-iliac reconstruction. *Surgery* **81,** 567–570.

Connolly P. T. and Kwaan J. H. (1982) In situ vein bypass. *Arch. Surg.* **117,** 1551–1557.

Cooley D. A., Wukasch D. C., Bennett J. G. et al. (1978) Double velour knitted Dacron grafts for aorto-iliac vascular replacements. In: Sawyer P. N. and Kaplitt M. J. (eds) *Vascular Grafts.* New York, Appleton-Century-Crofts.

Cranley J. J. and Hafner C. D. (1982) Revascularization of the femoro-popliteal arteries using saphenous vein, PTFE and umbilical vein grafts. *Arch. Surg.* **117,** 1543–1557.

Crawford F. A., Sethi G. K., Scott S. M. et al. (1975) Femoro-femoral grafts for unilateral occlusion of aortic bifurcation grafts. *Surgery* **77,** 150–153.

Dardik H., Dardik I. I., Sprayregen S. et al. (1975) Patient selection and improved technical factors in small vessel bypass procedures of the lower extremity. *Surgery* **77,** 249–254.

Dardik H., Ibraham I. M., Jarrall M. et al. (1980) Three year experience with a glutaraldehyde stabilised umbilical vein for limb salvage. *Br. J. Surg.* **67,** 229–232.

Davis R. C., Davies W. T. and Mannick J. A. (1975) Bypass vein grafts in patients with distal popliteal artery occlusion. *Am. J. Surg.* **129,** 421–425.

DeWeese J. A. (1971) Results of thromboendarterectomy vs. venous bypass grafts In: Dale W. A. (ed.) *Management of Arterial Occlusive Disease*, Ch. 8. Chicago, Yearbook Medical Publishers.

DeWeese J. A. and Rob C. G. (1977) Autologous vein grafts 10 years later. *Surgery* **82,** 775–786.

Dickinson P. H., McNeill I. F. and Morrison J. M. (1967) Aorto-iliac occlusion. A review of 100 cases treated by direct arterial surgery. *Br. J. Surg.* **54,** 764–770.

Downing R., Grimley R. P., Ashton F. et al. (1985) Problems in the diagnosis of popliteal aneurysms. *Proc. R. Soc. Med.* **78,** 440–444.

Eastcott H. H. G. (1973) *Arterial Surgery*. London, Pitman Medical, pp. 87–90.

Eugene J., Goldstone J. and Moore W. S. (1977) Fifteen year experience with subcutaneous bypass grafts for lower extremity ischaemia. *Ann. Surg.* **186,** 177–183.

Fogarty T. J., Chin A., Shoor P. M. et al. (1981) Adjunctive intra-operative arterial dilatation. *Arch. Surg.* **116,** 1391–1398.

Fogarty J. M. and Keshinian M. D. (1982) Aneurysm formation in human umbilical vein grafts. *Surgery* **91,** 343–345.

Fogarty T. J., Daily P. O., Shumway N. E. et al. (1971) Experience with balloon catheter technique for arterial embolectomy. *Am. J. Surg.* **122,** 231.

Giordano J. M. and Keshinian M. D. (1982) Aneurysm formation in human umbilical vein grafts. *Surgery* **91,** 343–345.

Goldman M. D., Simpson D., Hawker R. J. et al. (1983) Aspirin and dipyridamole reduce platelet deposition on prosthetic femoro-popliteal grafts in man. *Ann. Surg.* **198,** 713–716.

Greenhalgh R. M., Laing Susan P., Cole P. V. et al. (1980) Progressive atherosclerosis following revascularization. In: Bernhard V. M. and Towne J. B. (eds) *Complications in Vascular Surgery*. New York, Grune & Stratton, pp. 21–40.

Grimley R. P., Obeid M. L., Ashton F. et al. (1979) Long term results of autogenous vein bypass grafts in femoro-popliteal arterial occlusion. *Br. J. Surg.* **66,** 723.

Grüntzig A. and Kumpe D. A. (1979) Technique of percutaneous transluminal angioplasty with Grüntzig balloon catheter. *Am. J. Radiol.* **132,** 547–552.

Hall K. V. (1962) The great saphenous vein used in situ as an arterial shunt after extirpation of the vein valves. *Surgery* **86,** 453.

Helsby R. and Moosa A. R. (1975) Aorto-iliac reconstruction with special reference to the extraperitoneal approach. *Br. J. Surg.* **62,** 596–600.

Hurlow R. A., Chandler S. T. and Strachan C. J. L. (1977) Correlation between arteriography and isotope angiology in aorto-iliac disease. *Br. J. Surg.* **64,** 291–292.

Hurlow R. W., Strachan C. J. L. and Chandler S. T. (1978) The assessment of aorto-iliac disease by static isotope angiology. *Br. J. Surg.* **65,** 263–266.

Irvine W. T., Booth R. A. D. and Myers K. (1972) Arterial surgery for aorto-iliac occlusive vascular disease. Early and late results in 238 patients. *Lancet* **i,** 738–741.

Johnston E. N., Summerly R. and Birnstingl M. (1965) Prognosis in Raynaud's phenomenon after sympathectomy. *Br. Med. J.* **i,** 962–964.

Julian T. B., Louiseau J. M. and Stremple J. F. (1982) PTFE or SV as a femoro-popliteal bypass graft. *J. Surg. Res.* **32,** 1–6.

Klimach O. and Charlesworth D. (1983) Femorotibial bypass for limb salvage using human umbilical vein. *Br. J. Surg.* **70,** 1–3.

Leather R. P., Shah M. D., Buchbinder D. et al. (1981a) Further experience with the saphenous vein used in situ for arterial bypass. *Am. J. Surg.* **142,** 506–510.

Leather R. P., Shah D. M. and Karmody A. M. (1981b) Infrapopliteal arterial bypass for limb salvage; increased patency and utilisation of the saphenous vein used in situ. *Surgery* **90,** 1000–1007.

Linton R. R. (1973) *An Atlas of Vascular Surgery*. Philadelphia, London and Toronto, W. B. Saunders.

Logerfo F. W., Johnson W. C., Corson J. D. et al. (1977) A comparison of the late patency rate of axillo-bilateral femoral and axillo-unilateral femoral grafts. *Surgery* **81,** 33–40.

Malone J. M., Moore W. S. and Goldstone J. (1977) Life expectancy following aorto-femoral arterial grafting. *Surgery* **81,** 551–555.

Martin P. and Bouhoutsos J. (1977) The medium term results after profundaplasty. *Br. J. Surg.* **64,** 194–196.

Martin P., Renwick S. and Staphenson C. (1968) On the surgery of the profunda femoris artery. *Br. J. Surg.* **55,** 539–542.

Martin P., King R. B. and Stephenson C. B. S. (1969) On arterial embolism of the limbs. *Br. J. Surg.* **56,** 882–884.

Mosersky D. J., Hopkinson D. E., Baker D. W. et al. (1971) Ultrasonic arteriography. *Arch. Surg.* **103,** 663–667.

O'Mara C. and Imbembo A. L. (1977) Paraprosthetic-enteric fistula. *Surgery* **81,** 556–566.

Powis S. J. A. (1975) Renal function following aortic surgery. *J. Cardiovasc. Surg.* **16,** 565–571.

Powis S. J. A., Skilton J. S., Ashton F. et al. (1971) Place of Achilles tenotomy in the treatment of severe intermittent claudication. *Br. Med. J.* **3,** 522–523.

Quinn R. O. (1976) Assessment of peripheral vascular disease. M.D. Thesis, University of Glasgow, pp. 107–130.

Renwick S., Royle J. P. and Martin P. (1968) Operative angiography after femoro-popliteal arterial reconstruction. Its influence on early failure rate. *Br. J. Surg.* **55**, 134–136.

Rich N. M., Hughes C. W. and Baugh J. H. (1970) Management of venous injuries. *Ann. Surg.* **171**, 724.

Richard R. L. and Learmonth J. R. (1942) Lumbar sympathectomy in the treatment of popliteal aneurysm. *Lancet* **i**, 383–384.

Ring E. J., Freeman D. B., McLean G. K. et al. (1982) Percutaneous recanalisation of common iliac artery occlusion; an unacceptable complication rate? *Am. J. Radiol.* **139**, 587–589.

Sauvage L. R., Berger K., Wood S. J. et al. (1978) The U.S.S.C.I. Sauvage filamentous vascular prosthesis: rationale clinical results and healing in man. In: Sawyer P. N. and Kaplitt M. J. (eds) *Vascular Grafts*. New York, Appleton-Century-Crofts.

Scott W. W., Scott P. P. and Sander R. C. (1977) B scan ultrasound in the diagnosis of popliteal aneurysms. *Surgery* **81**, 436–441.

Simms M. H., Jones B. G., McCollum C. N. et al. (1982) Does anastomosis to two tibial arteries improve flow in femoro-crural bypass. *Br. J. Surg.* **69**, 676–689 (Abstract).

Slaney G. and Hamer J. D. (1973) Arterial embolism. In: Birnstingl M. (ed.) *Peripheral Vascular Surgery*. London, Heinemann.

Sobel S., Kaplitt M. J., Reingold M. et al. (1966) Gas endarterectomy. *Surgery* **59**, 517–521.

Sullivan W. G., Thornton F. H., Baker L. H. et al. (1971) Early influence of popliteal vein bypass in the treatment of popliteal vessel injuries. *Am. J. Surg.* **122**, 528–531.

Szilagyi D. E. (1978) Long term evaluation of an arterial substitute made of Helance Dacron. In: Sawyer P. N. and Kaplitt M. J. (eds) *Vascular Grafts*. New York, Appleton-Century-Crofts, p. 218.

Taylor G. W. (1973) Chronic arterial occlusion. In: Birnstingl M. (ed.) *Peripheral Vascular Surgery*. London, Heinemann.

Wellington J. C., Olslewski V. and Martin P. (1966) Hyperaemia of the calf after arterial reconstruction for atherosclerotic occlusion. *Br. J. Surg.* **53**, 180–184.

Wheat M. W., Palmer R. F., Bartley T. D. et al. (1965) Treatment of dissecting aneurysms of the aorta without surgery. *J. Thorac. Cardiovasc. Surg.* **50**, 364–371.

Yao S. T., Hobbs J. T. and Irvine W. T. (1969) Ankle systolic pressure measurements in arterial disease affecting the lower extremities. *Br. J. Surg.* **56**, 676–679.

Yates C. J. P., Berent A., Andrews V. et al. (1979) Increase in leg blood flow by normovolaemic haemodilution in intermittent claudication. *Lancet* **ii**, 116–118.

Yeager R. R. A., Hobson R. W., Jamil Z. et al. (1982) Differential patency and limb salvage for PTFE and ASV in severe lower extremity ischaemia. *Surgery* **91**, 99–103.

Zeitler E., Richter E. I., Roth F. J. et al. (1983) Results of percutaneous transluminal angioplasty. *Radiology* **146**, 57–60.

Chapter thirty-eight

Abdominal Aortic Aneurysms

R. N. Baird

INTRODUCTION

An aneurysm is a permanent localized dilation of an artery. Aneurysms have been feared since Galen's time because of the risk of rupture. The first successful replacement of an aortic aneurysm was achieved in Paris by Dubost et al. in 1951, by extraperitoneal excision and replacement with an aortic homograft. In the following 10 years, the procedure was simplified using a synthetic Dacron tube implanted within the opened aneurysm sac which was left in place. This standardized operation gave good long-term results and has become deservedly popular in the past 25 years. Today, specialist units report elective operative mortalities of 1–2 per cent, rising to 6–8 per cent in city-wide returns from routine vascular surgical audits. These results owe much to better identification of predictive factors associated with poor outcomes, and to finely tuned surgical, anaesthetic and intensive care. Despite these advances, the operative mortality of repair following rupture remains at 40–50 per cent, due mainly to pulmonary, cardiac and renal failure. These intractably bad results, and the unpredictability of rupture, have encouraged preventive operations so that most aneurysms are now dealt with electively.

SURGICAL ANATOMY

The aorta below the renal arteries is most commonly involved. Larger aneurysms may extend to the iliac arteries. Aortic tributaries at this level include paired lumbar arteries, median sacral and inferior mesenteric arteries. The infrarenal neck of the aneurysm is close to the inferior vena cava, left renal vein and lumbar veins, and is covered by the fourth part of the duodenum. A plexus of autonomic nerves covers the aortic bifurcation. The iliac arteries are crossed by the ureters and are closely adherent to, and sometimes inseparable from, the iliac veins.

PATHOLOGY

Abdominal aneurysms exist in up to 2 per cent of the elderly male population and are primarily aortic, fusiform and atherosclerotic, unlike those in centuries past that were mainly syphilitic. The pathogenesis is unknown, apart from one or two tantalizing clues. Collagen and elastin are the main strength-giving components of the arterial wall, and they can be degraded by collagenase and elastase, both of which are found in increased concentrations in aneurysm patients. Congenital aneurysms in patients with connective tissue abnormalities such as Marfan's and Ehlers–Danlos syndromes have weakened or absent collagen cross-links. In some animals in whom spontaneous aneurysms occur, namely *Blotchy* mice and pigs, there is a deficiency of an enzyme, lysyl oxidase, which is essential for elastin cross-linking. The enzyme contains copper and the animals have deficient copper metabolism. In humans, there is abnormal copper metabolism in the rare Menkes' syndrome, in which tortuous, dilated arteries and reduced arterial wall elastin have been found. Tilson (1982) has found decreased hepatic copper levels in 13 patients with abdominal aneurysms compared with a similar number of patients with atherosclerotic occlusive disease.

In about 10 per cent of abdominal aneurysms, there is a dense peri-aortic fibrotic reaction, indistinguishable from retroperitoneal fibrosis. The aorta, ureters and vena cava may be involved. They have been labelled 'inflammatory' because of the histology, high ESR and response to steroid therapy.

CLINICAL FEATURES

Most abdominal aneurysms do not give rise to symptoms, and are discovered by the patient as a central pulsating abdominal tumour. Others come to light on abdominal palpation during a routine medical check-up or during examination for a non-specific abdominal or back pain. The aneurysm may be seen on an abdominal radiograph as calcification in the wall of the sac. The pulsating mass may visibly displace the anterior abdominal wall in a thin patient.

On palpation, the aneurysm may be tender and the convex left border is easily felt; the right border and the upper edge and are often delineated with less certainty.

Confirmation comes from abdominal ultrasound which clearly shows the dilated aortic wall, lumen and mural thrombus (*Fig.* 38.1), and gives accurate anteroposterior diameters. The upper limit of the aneurysm often overhangs the renal arteries and this important relationship is not shown well by ultrasound. The origin of the superior mesenteric artery is a reliable landmark, and if the aortic diameter at this level is normal, the aneurysm can be assumed for practical purposes to be infrarenal. The lower extent of the aneurysm can usually be imaged, whether at the aortic bifurcation or extending into

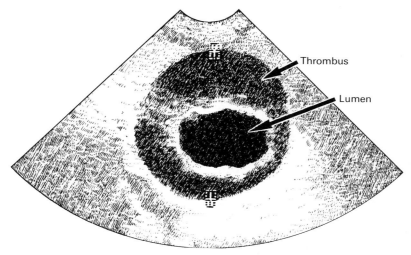

Fig. 38.1. Diagram of ultrasound scan of an abdominal aneurysm showing cursors measuring its anteroposterior diameter, as well as the lumen and mural thrombus.

the iliac arteries. The differential diagnoses are with a tortuous but normal-sized aorta and a retroperitoneal, pre-aortic mass, such as a lymphoma, and each can be identified by ultrasound.

Aneurysms Less than 4 cm in Diameter

The risk of rupture of small aneurysms, less than twice the size of a normal abdominal aorta (2 cm), is so low that operative replacement is seldom justified. Enlargement is monitored by repeating the scan in 1 year's time or if symptoms develop. Serial studies show that the average growth rate of a small aneurysm is 0·5 cm/year.

Aneurysms Greater than 6 cm in Diameter

Large aneurysms are potentially lethal and a Dacron replacement should be inserted unless there are good reasons for not doing so.

Aneurysms of Intermediate Size (4–6 cm)

An aneurysm of intermediate size should be dealt with in an otherwise fit, thin, motivated patient provided that a straightforward operative replacement is forecast and an experienced surgical team is available.

SELECTION FOR OPERATION

Broadly speaking, a patient with an aneurysm is likely to do well if he or she feels healthy, walks unaided and can respond sensibly to an explanation of the benefits and risks of operation.

Many patients have coexisting disease. This in itself does not disqualify them from having the aneurysm repaired. Hypertension, angina, diabetes and a previous myocardial infarct are often acceptable risks, provided that hypertension and diabetes are moderate, whether requiring drugs or not, angina is mild and stable, and any myocardial infarct has occurred more than 6 months earlier. Good surgical results can also be obtained in combined dilating and occlusive arterial disease. In these circumstances an arteriogram is recommended to outline distal vessels.

An aneurysm is suspected of extending above the renal arteries if the pulsatile mass extends high into the epigastrium on abdominal palpation, if abdominal ultrasound shows a dilated suprarenal aorta, and if a dilated thoracic aorta is shown on a chest radiograph. Arteriograms will show the upper limit of the aneurysm (Fig. 38.2) and CT scanning will clearly show its extent. Pre-aortic structures such as a horseshoe kidney and inflammatory aneurysms are well shown by CT scanning.

Adverse factors include preoperative breathlessness at rest, whether of pulmonary or left ventricular origin, right heart failure, a recent myocardial infarct (within 6 months) and a host of system failures, degenerative and neoplastic diseases. Operations for aortic aneurysm should only be undertaken in those with a worthwhile future ahead of them who have reserves of physical and mental strength to recover from a complex major procedure.

Efforts should be made to improve coexisting disease; the obese should lose weight; smokers should abstain; hypertension should be controlled.

PREOPERATIVE ASSESSMENT

A detailed history-taking and examination are undertaken several days preoperatively to assess fitness for operation. Routine investigations include urinalysis, haemoglobin, platelets, urea and electrolytes, chest radiograph and electrocardiogram.

Further investigations are done selectively: arterial gases and pulmonary function tests if there is a risk

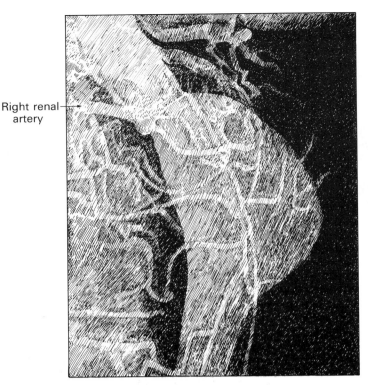

Right renal artery

Fig. 38.2. Diagram of lateral view of an arteriogram of an aortic aneurysm showing the right renal artery arising from aorta of normal diameter above the aneurysm.

of ventilatory failure; creatinine clearance, intravenous urography and angiography if poor renal function is suspected; and prothrombin time, platelet function and clotting screen where indicated.

The assessment is used to identify predictive factors of serious or fatal postoperative complications. Indices of cardiac risk such as those devised by Goldman et al. (1977) have been used to quantify the effects of predictive factors on outcomes following operations.

PREPARATION FOR OPERATION

Six units of *whole* blood are made available. There is no place for the use of packed cells to replace intraoperative blood loss in arterial surgery.

ECG electrodes are attached. Peripheral and central venous lines, an arterial line, a thoracic epidural and a urinary catheter are inserted. In high-risk cases a Swan–Ganz catheter is used. The patient is placed on a warming blanket.

Perioperative antibiotics are administered intravenously in three doses of a cephalosporin 8-hourly starting at the induction of anaesthesia.

RUPTURED ANEURYSMS

Without operation, virtually all patients with rup-

tured aneurysms die. Hypovolaemic shock causing damage to the heart, kidneys and lungs is the most common cause of death. Since surgery offers the only hope for survival, it should seldom be withheld.

Once the diagnosis has been made, a large-bore intravenous line is inserted, blood taken for a 10-unit cross-match, and the patient transferred directly to the operating theatre. The fall in blood pressure can *only* be corrected by controlling and clamping the aorta above the site of rupture. Because of this, the highest standard of professionalism is required by all concerned to get the patient onto the operating table as quickly as possible. The abdominal incision is made immediately and the aorta controlled while an endotracheal tube is inserted. Once the aortic clamp is safely applied, the patient is resuscitated and the operation proceeds expeditiously but with less urgency once the emergency has passed. In a desperate situation where bleeding is uncontrollable the measures indicated in *Fig.* 38.3 should be adopted.

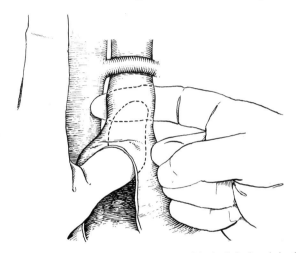

Fig. 38.3. Ruptured aortic aneurysm. With the left thumb in the aorta, mobilization is achieved by encircling the normal aorta with the right index finger, following which a clamp may be applied by the operator or the assistant.

OPERATIVE TECHNIQUES

Aortic Aneurysm

Incision

A transverse upper abdominal incision provides excellent access, can be readily extended towards the left chest for high aneurysms, heals well and has minimal risk of an incisional hernia. A long midline incision is a satisfactory alternative.

Findings

The gallbladder is checked for gallstones. The duodenum is inspected and the oesophageal hiatus and stomach are palpated. The colon is examined throughout its length. If carcinoma of the stomach or colon is discovered, the neoplasm should be resected and the aneurysm left unoperated. Duodenal scarring, hiatus hernia and diverticular disease are frequently encountered. They are carefully noted and do not preclude aneurysm repair. The small bowel is reflected to reveal the aneurysm. The size is measured with a ruler to compare with the preoperative investigations and any localized weakness is noted.

Procedure

The posterior parietal peritoneum is incised vertically to provide direct access to the aneurysm between the fourth part of the duodenum and the inferior mesenteric vein. The incision is continued upwards to reveal the left renal vein. The neck of the aneurysm is initially cleared on the left side and in front. Attention is then turned to the right side of the infrarenal aorta. A quadrilateral space is developed by gentle blunt dissection between the aorta and the cava with the renal vein above and the aneurysm below (*Fig.* 38.4). Finally, the posterior aspect of the aorta is cleared *in direct vision* to ensure that the lumbar vessels are avoided.

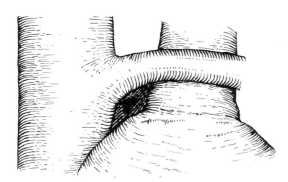

Fig. 38.4. Diagram showing dissection of the neck of the aneurysm. A space is developed between the right side of the aorta and the vena cava, with the left renal vein above and the aneurysm below.

The peritoneum is then incised downwards, skirting to the right of the inferior mesenteric artery to avoid its left colic branches, as far as the common iliac arteries. They are often normal or slightly dilated, and are exposed sufficiently to be controlled. The femoral pulses are palpated in the groins to ensure that intraluminal thrombus has not been dislodged distally by the dissection.

A tubular Dacron prosthesis is selected and preclotted. Its diameter is usually between 16 and 20 mm, though a full range of sizes from 12 to 25 mm should be available. A prosthesis of *knitted* manufacture is soft, easy to sew and becomes well incorporated after implantation. There is an initial blood loss from the porosity of the material until the interstices are sealed with fibrin and platelets. Grafts of *woven* manufacture are virtually impervious to blood loss and in consequence are preferred where there are anxieties about preclotting and blood loss.

Heparin, 5000 units, is administered by central venous line and the aorta and iliac arteries are clamped and the aneurysm opened. Intraluminal thrombus is removed (*Fig.* 38.5) and back-bleeding

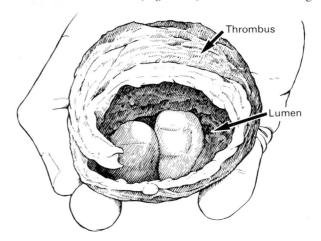

Fig. 38.5. Removal of intramural thrombus from within the aneurysmal sac.

from any of the lumbar, median sacral and inferior mesenteric arteries is controlled by suture ligation. Dilute heparin/saline solution (10–20 ml) is instilled into the clamped iliac arteries to minimize the risk of thrombosis in the absence of flow.

The graft is anastomosed to the intrarenal aorta using a 2/0 or 3/0 continuous Prolene suture. The aortic clamp is released to check that the suture line is intact (*Fig.* 38.6). The graft is reflected upwards

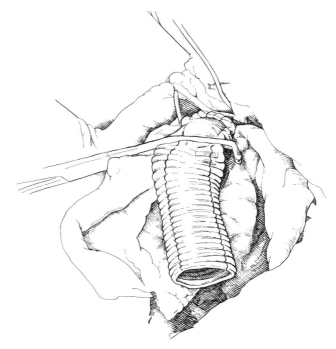

Fig. 38.6. Checking the front of the top anastomosis. Note the opened aneurysmal sac left in place.

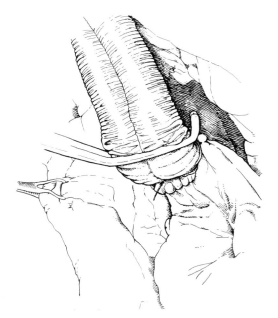

Fig. 38.7. The posterior part of the top anastomosis being checked so that any additional suture can be inserted under direct vision.

to check the posterior part of the anastomosis (*Fig.* 38.7) while it is readily accessible. The upper anastomosis may prove difficult. Rarely, it may be necessary to divide the left renal vein in order to expose the upper end of the resected aorta. Should this prove necessary, renal function will almost certainly be retained as the collateral venous drainage of the kidney is excellent.

The distal graft is trimmed to size and anastomosed to the aortic bifurcation with continuous 3/0 Prolene (*Fig.* 38.8). Prior to completion of the suture line

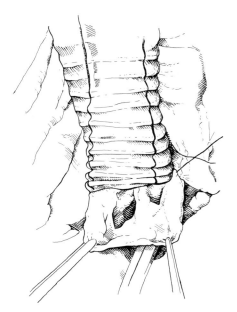

Fig. 38.8. The lower anastomosis partly completed at the aortic bifurcation.

the clamps are momentarily released to clear any thrombus or loose atheroma before flow is restored.

Declamping is done slowly, in patient cooperation with the anaesthetist, to minimize the hypotension that accompanies a reduction in afterload. When the clamps are finally released and normal arterial pressure restored, haemostasis is checked and the Dacron graft is covered by the aneurysm sac (*Fig.* 38.9) and

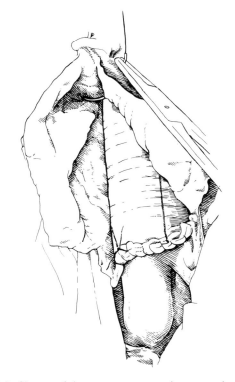

Fig. 38.9. Closure of the empty aneurysmal sac over the Dacron prosthesis on completion of the anastomoses.

the posterior peritoneum closed. The femoral pulses are palpated once more to ensure that the arterial supply of the legs has been restored to normal.

At this stage, further consideration is given to dealing with any other problems concurrently, e.g. gallstones, inguinal hernia, etc.

The position of the nasogastric tube is checked and the foot pulses checked by palpation, Doppler or pulse volume recordings and the abdomen closed with a continuous strong nylon suture.

Aorto-Iliac Aneurysm

Large aortic aneurysms frequently extend to the common iliac arteries. They are similarly amenable to operative repair, but require a bifurcation graft (*Fig.* 38.10) instead of a simple tube. In these circumstances, the limbs of the bifurcation graft are anastomosed to the common iliac, external iliac or common femoral artery depending on the extent of the aneurysm.

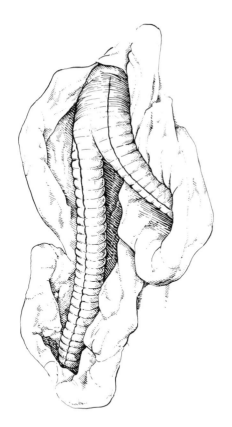

Fig. 38.10. A bifurcation prosthesis for an aneurysm involving the aorta and both iliac arteries.

Suprarenal Aorta

Control of the aorta at the level of the diaphragm is occasionally required for the repair of aortic rupture or injury and for high aneurysms. It is achieved by compression of the aorta on the lumbar spine, by clamping in the hiatus via the lesser sac, or by intraluminal occlusion using a Foley balloon catheter. The occlusion time should be as short as possible (<30 minutes) to minimize ischaemic damage to the kidneys.

These techniques afford limited access for repairs at renal artery level. Aneurysms of the upper segment of the abdominal aorta are best approached posterolaterally by Crawford's technique; after incising the peritoneum lateral to the left colon and developing a plane behind the colon, spleen, pancreas and left kidney. The aorta is opened longitudinally well behind the left renal artery orifice and a woven Dacron tube sewn into the aorta above the neck of the aneurysmal sac. Oval opening(s) are made in the graft to accommodate the origins of the coeliac axis, superior mesenteric and renal arteries and anastomoses are completed with circumferentially running sutures. Finally, the distal aortic anastomosis is performed.

Horseshoe Kidney

A horseshoe kidney is uncommonly encountered. In the straightforward case, the renal arteries are normal, the isthmus does not have an independent blood supply and there are no accessory renal arteries. Access to the neck of the aneurysm is obtained by reflecting the left kidney and isthmus upwards and to the right, and a Dacron replacement is undertaken. If there is a complicated anomaly, the feasibility of aneurysm replacement depends on the numbers and locations of accessory renal arteries, and in some cases with multiple vessels, reconstruction may not be possible.

Inflammatory Aneurysm

Another uncommon operative finding is an aneurysm encased in marble white retroperitoneal fibrous tissue, the so-called inflammatory aneurysm. This fibrous tissue has to be cut into to free the duodenum, and to find the limits of the sac. Thereafter grafting proceeds as described earlier. The retroperitoneal reaction resolves postoperatively and the ureter and the vena cava need not be freed. Occasionally, the reaction is so dense and extensive that it is safer to leave the aneurysm unresected.

Ruptured Aneurysm

Abdominal aneurysms rupture intraperitoneally, retroperitoneally and rarely into the vena cava or duodenum. The first operative priority is to apply an arterial clamp safely to normal aorta between the neck of the aneurysm and the renal arteries. Following this, the blood pressure picks up immediately and improves the perfusion of the heart, kidneys and brain. If direct clamping is impossible, control of the suprarenal aorta is obtained and the situation reassessed. Thereafter Dacron grafting proceeds as described earlier.

If an aortocaval fistula is present, venous bleeding occurs when the aneurysmal sac is opened. The fistula is usually small and is controlled by direct pressure while being sutured from within the wall of the aneurysm sac. Care is taken to avoid squeezing atheroma and thrombus through the fistula into the vena cava as a pulmonary embolism can result.

Rupture of an aneurysm into the duodenum presents as gastrointestinal bleeding. At operation the fistula is disconnected, the duodenum closed, the aneurysm replaced by a Dacron graft and omentum interposed to prevent recurrence.

POSTOPERATIVE CARE

In fit, elective cases, awakening from anaesthesia is straightforward and the patient is observed in the recovery area of the operating theatre for 3–4 hours before the arterial line is removed and the patient is returned to the ward. During this time, hypertension may need treatment with incremental doses of intravenous labetalol or hydralazine, or by a top-up of epidural analgesia.

Less fit elective cases are booked into the intensive care unit so that arterial line monitoring is continued overnight. During this time, the legs become rewarmed. Pulses, Doppler ankle pressures and pulse volume recordings are checked. As the patient rewarms and vasodilates, the need for a gentle top-up transfusion of 1–2 units of blood should be considered. Hypovolaemia is manifest as a fall-off in hourly urinary output, arterial and central venous pressures. If a sluggish urinary output persists after volume replacement and there is no intra-abdominal blood loss, an intravenous dose of Lasix (frusemide) usually brings an ample reward.

All ruptured cases should be treated in the intensive care unit postoperatively because of the morbidity and mortality of the operation in these circumstances. They are at risk of multisystem failure and the respiratory system is particularly vulnerable from pre-existing disease and the adverse effects of pulmonary oedema resulting from intraoperative transfusion of large fluid volumes. Frequent blood gas estimations are made and treatment includes oxygen therapy, nebulizers and physiotherapy. Endotracheal intubation and ventilation with positive end-expiratory pressure are used to relieve the severest hypoxaemia.

COMPLICATIONS

Early Complications

The main early complications are those of all arterial surgery, namely bleeding, thrombosis and embolism.

Reactive *haemorrhage* from a suture line is suspected if there is a continuing transfusion requirement within hours of operation, and leads to hypotensive collapse if untreated. At re-exploration, the anastomoses are inspected and additional sutures placed. Sometimes an active bleeding point is not identified.

Graft or *distal artery thrombosis* is suspected if the limb(s) fail to rewarm postoperatively. Loss of femoral artery pulsation in the groin will prompt a return to the operating theatre for clearance with a balloon catheter.

Embolism is an intraoperative complication in which atherothrombotic material (*see Fig.* 38.5) is propagated distally when the aneurysm is being dissected free of surrounding structures. The toes become acutely painful, discoloured and ischaemic despite good pedal pulses. The condition is known by the picturesque name of 'trash-foot'. The buttocks are also affected. The embolic material rests beyond the reach of a balloon catheter. Heparin and dextran may help, and the toes recover from all but the most extensive emboli.

Lymph fistula is a tiresome occasional sequel of any groin incision in which the femoral arteries are exposed. The groin incision becomes red, swollen and discharges copious volumes of clear lymph towards the end of the 1st postoperative week. Cultures may yield staphylococci and other organisms. Treatment usually consists of antibiotics, rest and elevation of the limb. The fistula may take up to 6 weeks to dry up completely. Throughout this period there is anxiety lest the Dacron prosthesis should become infected. A more aggressive approach is to cover the femoral artery and Dacron with the sartorius muscle by transposing it medially, freeing its proximal attachment from the anterior superior iliac spine and tacking it lightly to the inguinal ligament over the prosthesis. The fistula usually dries up when this is done.

Rare complications include graft infection and colon ischaemia following ligation of the inferior mesenteric artery. General postoperative complications affect the cardiac, respiratory and renal systems. As ever, prevention is infinitely better than cure. For example, the risk of respiratory complications is minimized by stopping smoking and preoperative physiotherapy, avoiding intraoperative pulmonary oedema caused by fluid overload and relieving postoperative pain by thoracic epidural to encourage deep breathing and coughing.

Aneurysm patients usually have diseased coronary arteries which can become thrombosed causing myocardial ischaemia or infarction. Excess intraoperative blood loss and inadequate replacement increase the chance of this happening.

Late Complications

The main late complications are myocardial infarction, false aneurysm and secondary aorto-enteric fistula.

Myocardial infarction is the commonest cause of death after aneurysm operations. Its prevalence dominates the survival curves to such an extent that some specialized centres, notably Hertzer's group at the Cleveland Clinic (Diehl et al., 1983), advocate preliminary coronary artery bypass in selected patients before the aneurysm is dealt with.

Anastomotic false aneurysms arise years later from suture line weakening of the wall of the host artery. Silk used in the anastomoses was at one time a contributory factor. False aneurysms are noted most commonly in the groins, but also occur at more deeply sited anastomoses. Good results are obtainable from local repair.

Aorto-enteric fistulas occur rarely after aneurysm repair. An intra-abdominal suture line forms the link between the arterial and gastrointestinal systems, resulting in haematemesis. Delays in recognizing the diagnosis are frequent. The most common fistula is between the upper aortic anastomosis and the fourth part of the duodenum. At operation, the aorta and graft are controlled, the fistula disconnected, the enteral aspect closed and separated by omentum from the aorta. Thereafter, opinions are divided on how the aortic deficit should be handled. Conservative surgeons simply close the defect in the Dacron–aorta anastomosis. A more radical approach is to remove the entire Dacron graft on the grounds that it must be infected, ligate the aorta and restore blood flow to the legs by an axillo-bifemoral bypass. However, the aortic stump may become disrupted later, creating a difficult situation.

REFERENCES

Diehl J. T., Cali R. F., Hertzer N. R. et al. (1983) Complications of abdominal aortic reconstruction. An analysis of perioperative risk factors in 557 patients. *Ann. Surg.* **197**, 49–56.
Dubost C., Allary M. and Oeconomos N. (1951) A propos du traitement des aneurysmes de l'aorte. *Mem. Acad. Chir.* (Paris) **77**, 381–384.
Goldman L., Caldera D. L., Nussbaum S. R. et al. (1977) Multifactorial index of cardiac risk in non-cardiac surgical patients. *N. Engl. J. Med.* **297**, 846–850.
Tilson M. D. (1982) Decreased hepatic copper levels. A possible chemical marker for the pathogenesis of aortic aneurysms in man. *Arch. Surg.* **105**, 338–344.

FURTHER READING

Brown S. L., Blackstrom B. and Busuttil R. W. (1985) A new serum proteolytic enzyme in aneurysm pathogenesis. *J. Vasc. Surg.* **2**, 393–399.
Crawford E. S. and Cohen E. S. (1982) Aortic aneurysm: a multifocal disease. *Arch. Surg.* **117**, 1393–1400.
Delin A., Ohlsén H. and Swedenborg J. (1985) Growth rate of abdominal aortic aneurysms as measured by computed tomography. *Br. J. Surg.* **72**, 530–532.
Fielding J. W. L., Black J., Ashton F. et al. (1981) Diagnosis and management of 528 abdominal aortic aneurysms. *Br. Med. J.* **283**, 355–359.
Malins A. F., Goodman N. W., Cooper G. W. et al. (1984) Ventilatory effects of pre- and postoperative diamorphine. A comparison of extradural with intramuscular administration. *Anaesthesia* **39**, 118–125.
Sethia B. and Darke S. G. (1983) Abdominal aortic aneurysm with retroperitoneal fibrosis and ureteric entrapment. *Br. J. Surg.* **70**, 434–436.

Chapter thirty-nine

Perfusion Techniques in Cardiac Surgery

J. S. Bailey

Special techniques are needed during surgery on the heart and great vessels to maintain tissue viability, to avoid massive blood loss and to prevent air embolism. These techniques involve the extracorporeal maintenance of a circulation, artificial oxygenation of blood and modification of tissue metabolism by chemical and physical means.

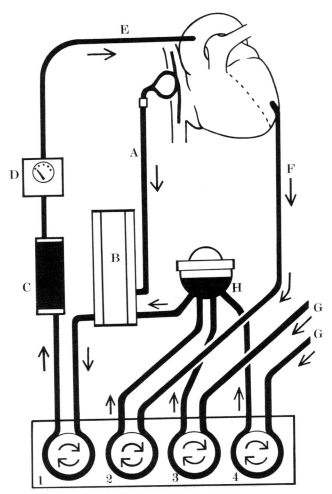

Fig. 39.1. Diagram of standard extracorporeal circulation for cardiac surgery. Blood draining from the venae cavae syphons (A) into an oxygenator (B) when it is taken by a roller pump through a heat exchanger (C) and a filter on the arterial line (D). It is then returned to the ascending aorta (E). Left ventricular vented blood (F) and cardiotomy sucker blood (G) are returned to the cardiotomy and debubbling reservoir (H) by roller pumps and then passed to the oxygenator for further recirculation. The heat exchanger is frequently incorporated with the disposable oxygenator.

EXTRACORPOREAL CIRCULATION (*Fig.* 39.1)

If, for anatomical reasons, the heart must be excluded from the circulation during surgery, tissue viability can be maintained by providing an artificial circulation. This circulation must provide blood of good quality and sufficient quantity to all organs for the duration of surgery. No absolute parameters of quality and quantity exist. Individual tissues vary in their needs and further modification of need can be obtained by interfering with metabolic activity chemically or by lowering the temperature.

Cardiopulmonary Bypass

Blood is removed from either the right atrium or the superior and inferior venae cavae, artifically oxygenated and returned at physiological pressure to the arterial tree. In addition, shed blood is harvested and returned to the extracorporeal circulation.

Cardiotomy Suckers

Once the patient has been anticoagulated any blood shed can be returned to the extracorporeal circuit. Roller pumps are used to provide suction and return the blood to a cardiotomy reservoir from which it flows through a filter into the oxygenator. Many alternative sucker ends have been designed to minimize the trauma to the blood caused by the sudden acceleration of a blood and air mixture into the suction end. Haemolysis is produced by this suction, however applied, and it should therefore be kept to a minimum.

Constituent Parts of the Extracorporeal Circuit

Pumps

Twin roller pumps are almost universally used to provide perfusion and suction for extracorporeal circulation. Haemolysis is minimized if the rollers are set to be just non-occlusive on the Silastic tubing on which they run.

Oxygenators

These work on many different principles of gas-to-blood interface, but three are commonly used: bubble oxygenators, rotating disc oxygenators and membrane oxygenators.

Heat Exchangers

Reusable heat exchangers of many designs exist. The important properties are low priming volume, low blood flow resistance and removal of any danger of contamination of the blood path by the water. Currently they may be included in the oxygenator or are available as disposable equipment. Tubing and flexible reservoirs are made of polyvinyl chloride. Rigid reservoirs and tube connections are made of polycarbonate. The gradual introduction of completely disposable equipment has been promoted because of the need for and difficulty of adequate removal of all protein from reusable equipment.

Priming Fluids

The extracorporeal circulation can be filled with as simple a solution as 5 per cent dextrose or as complicated a substance as whole blood. The lowered viscosity generated by blood dilution minimizes blood damage. This dilution can be safely performed to a lowest packed cell volume of 20 per cent calculated from the patient's circulating volume and the priming volume of the extracorporeal circulation used. While recognizing enormous individual preferences among users, it is usual to include a mixture of crystalloid and colloid. *Table* 39.1. is an example.

Table 39.1

25% of volume	Plasma or plasma substitute (Haemaccel)
75% of volume	Balanced electrolyte solution (Plasmalyte) Corrected to approximately pH 7·4 with 8·4% NaHCO$_3$

Preparation for Bypass

1. Monitoring

After induction of anaesthesia and endotracheal intubation, preparation is made for measurement of:
1. Arterial blood pressure.
2. Venous blood pressure.
3. Temperature.
4. Urine output.
5. ECG.

Since these monitoring sites will be maintained for 24 hours or longer, scrupulous sterility must be maintained in placing cannulas and catheters and fixation of dressings must be planned to maintain their sterility. It is a convenient practice to undertake full skin preparation of operating site and monitoring sites at the same time.

2. Position on Operating Table

Most open heart surgery is undertaken through a midline sternum-splitting incision. The patient lies supine on the operating table. If temperature regulation is to be undertaken, a water blanket is placed under the patient. It is of particular importance in open heart surgery to protect pressure points. The length of time taken and pathological circulation during bypass make skin necrosis more likely. In the supine position, the back of the head, scapulas, posterior ischial spines, sacrum and heels take most pressure. Morbidity from foot drop is also a recognized hazard from the weight of the feet producing plantar flexion.

3. Skin Preparation and Draping

Skin preparation begins 48 hours before surgery with chlorhexidine baths. Povidone-iodine is a good skin preparation. Towelling the operation site will vary with the needs of the theatre team. A proprietary sterile adhesive polythene sheet is often used to cover the residual skin after draping is completed.

Operation

The skin is incised from the suprasternal notch to 3 cm below the xiphoid process, in the midline. The incision is deepened with diathermy down to and through the periosteum of the sternum (*Figs.* 39.2, 39.3).

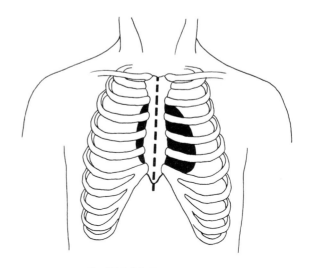

Fig. 39.2. Median sternotomy.

The two halves of the rectus abdominis muscles are separated by diathermy of the linea alba and a plane developed behind the xiphoid process which is divided in the midline by heavy scissors. This separates the xiphoid slips of the diaphragm so that a finger can be introduced behind the lower part of sternum into the mediastinum.

The skin is retracted at the top corner and the deep fascia incised to expose the clavicular heads of sternomastoid and the deep aspect of the sternum and sternothyroid muscles. These are separated in the midline after dividing the interclavicular ligament, and the finger can then be passed into the anterior

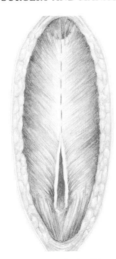

Fig. 39.3. Median sternotomy. The incision is marked out on the sternum and the linea alba is opened prior to sternotomy.

mediastinum behind the upper part of the manubrium.

The sternum is now divided using a pneumatic or electric-powered saw. Should neither of these be available, the Gigli saw is very useful (*Fig.* 39.4).

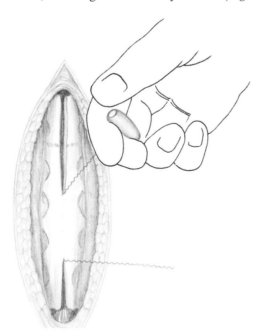

Fig. 39.4. Median sternotomy using the Gigli saw.

During division of the sternum, the anaesthetist holds the lungs still in expiration to avoid entering the pleura.

The sternal edges are held back by a self-retaining sternal spreader, revealing the deep thoracic fascia overlying the medial extensions of the pleura and the pericardium, and splitting to invest the thymus or its adult remnants in the upper part of the mediastinum.

The loose connective tissue forming this fascial layer is swept off the pericardium. Over the thymus it is more condensed and formal division of the superficial and deep layers is need to mobilize the thymus, especially in children. Care at this stage will prevent injury to the innominate vein which crosses the upper part of this dissection receiving short thymic veins. The level of the innominate vein varies, being lower in patients with short necks.

The pericardium is now opened by a vertical incision in the midline. At the lower end it fuses with the diaphragm and the peritoneum as a single sheet. With care the layers can be separated and the incision continued down through pericardium and diaphragm leaving the peritoneum intact. This manoeuvre provides considerably increased exposure of the diaphragmatic part of the heart from the inferior vena cava towards the left ventricular apex.

The edges of the pericardium are picked up in 'stay sutures' and fixed to the edges of the incision in the chest wall or to the sternal spreader, according to preference.

Cannulation (*Fig.* 39.5)

Blood is returned from the extracorporeal circulation either to the ascending aorta, femoral artery or external iliac artery. Of these, the ascending aorta is generally preferred.

Collection of venous blood is most simply undertaken from the right atrium direct. To be complete, retrieval must be through a large-bore cannula (12·5 mm ID) and from an undistorted atrium. In addition, the cardiac incisions made must be confined to the systemic side of the heart in the absence of abnormal communication between left- and right-sided chambers.

If cardiac surgery demands retraction of the heart to distort the right atrium, separate cannulas must be passed from the right atrium retrograde into superior and inferior venae cavae. If, in addition, the right atrium or ventricle is to be incised, or communication exists between right- and left-sided chambers, in addition to separate caval cannulation occlusive tapes must be placed around the cavae to stop blood loss or air entrainment after cardiotomy. This anatomical situation allows collection of all venous return except that from the coronary sinus, which must be collected by a separate atraumatic suction apparatus.

Before cannulation, the patient must be heparinized, using 3 mg heparin/kg body weight, initially and reinforced during surgery.

Air Removal

While the chest is opened, the perfusionist will be priming and de-airing the extracorporeal circulation. Bubbles tend to adhere to the plastic components of the apparatus and can be removed by percussion during a high-flow internal circulation.

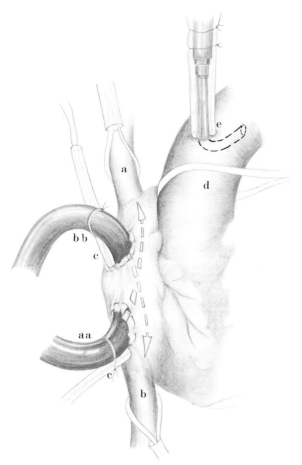

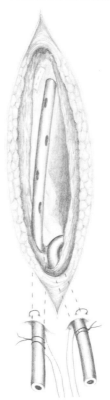

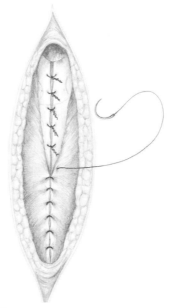

Fig. 39.5. Cannulation for cardiopulmonary bypass. The superior (a) and inferior venae cavae (b) are snared and cannulated individually (aa and bb). The cannulas are secured by the snares (c). The ascending aorta (d) is cannulated; the aortic cannula (e) must point away from the aortic valve and care is taken that it does not enter the innominate or internal carotid artery.

After introduction of the aortic cannula, the clamp which is in place is removed slowly and blood allowed to fill the cannula, and its connecting tube. Slow air displacement prevents frothing. Connection must then be made between the extracorporeal circulation and the cannula in such a manner that bubbles are not enclosed.

Finally the tubing is placed where it will not interfere with surgery and fixed to the drapes. At this stage, it is vital to check free communication between the lumen of the aorta and the extracorporeal tubing. This is indicated by a free swing of the pressure gauge in the arterial line of the pump circuit.

Closure (*Figs.* 39.6, 39.7)

At least two drains must be left in the mediastinum. These are introduced through separate stab incisions each side of the midline below the costal margin. One will lie within the pericardium to the left of the inferior vena cava between the curve in the dia-

Fig. 39.6. Median sternotomy, closure. Pericardial and anterior mediastinal drains are inserted.

Fig. 39.7. Median sternotomy, closure. The sternum is wired with interrupted sutures and the superficial tissues are carefully closed.

phragm and the ventricle to end in the posterior part of the pericardial space.

The second, which must have multiple side-holes, lies the full length of the anterior mediastinum from the suprasternal notch, deep to the sternum and superficial to the pericardium. The pericardium may be closed and the sternal edges brought together with interrupted wire sutures. The deep fascia is then securely closed. The linea alba is closed with non-absorbable sutures and care is necessary for incisional hernia is a well-known complication of this exposure.

Myocardial Preservation

Aortic valve replacement demands aortic cross-clamping and dissection close to the coronary ostia. Under these circumstances no coronary arterial flow can occur. Various methods of myocardial preservation have been adopted at different times by different surgeons.

1. Warm Ischaemia

Surgery is undertaken as swiftly as possible during the ischaemic cardiac arrest. Like all tissue, the myocardium will tolerate a period of ischaemia with progressive damage as time extends. At 37°C this is not recommended for longer than 10 minutes.

2. Cold Ischaemia

When the temperature of the myocardium is lowered, ischaemia can be tolerated for longer periods. Clearly experimental work in humans cannot be used to decide absolute levels. Increasing clinical experience suggests that 1 hour can be tolerated at 20°C and 2 hours at 15°C. Various methods of obtaining myocardial cooling are used by cold coronary perfusion, by epicardial cooling, by endocardial cooling or combinations of these three. Whatever method is used, it is vital that the method described by the original proponent is used in detail rather than a personal approximation. Whole body cooling will inevitably produce myocardial cooling, but direct measurement of the myocardial temperature must be included to ensure adequate cooling of heart muscle.

3. Chemical Cardioplegia

In asystole the myocardium is resistant to ischaemia for longer than when rhythmic contraction or ventricular fibrillation is occurring. This can be produced by anti-arrhythmic drugs such as lignocaine or procaine and by high concentrations of potassium ions. Many recipes have been successfully used, and argument continues about the added value of steroids and mannitol and other ions such as calcium. The combination of chemical cardioplegia with cold is commonly used in modern practice.

The solution, as given in *Table* 39.2, is infused into the coronary arteries at a perfusion pressure of approximately 100 mmHg measured at the aortic root.

When the aortic valve is competent the solution

Table 39.2

Cardioplegic solution		
1000 ml Plasmalyte 148 (Baxter)		
Sodium	140	mmol
Potassium	5	mmol
Magnesium	1·5	mmol
Chloride	98	mmol
Acetate	27	mmol
Gluconate	23	mmol
Plus additives:		
Potassium chloride	20	mmol in 10 ml
Sodium bicarbonate	17	mmol in 17 ml
Methyl prednisolone	500	mg in 8 ml
Dextrose 50%	50	ml
This solution is stored and used at 4°C.		

can be perfused through a wide-bore needle into the ascending aorta after the aorta has been clamped. When the aortic valve is incompetent the aorta must be opened after clamping and the solution instilled directly into the coronary ostia by hand-held coronary cannulas, 600 ml into the left and 400 ml into the right. If ischaemia of longer than 1 hour is needed, further infusions should be performed at the end of each hour. Properly applied, this technique produces rapid onset of electrical silence. At the end of the procedure, when air has been removed from the heart, the aorta is unclamped. Usually slow sinus rhythm returns within a minute. In a heart with severe preoperative myocardial decompensation, activity may return as ventricular fibrillation requiring electrical defibrillation.

4. Selective Coronary Perfusion (now rarely used)

This method of myocardial preservation during aortic valve replacement was popular for many years among surgeons, and proved very successful. However, it is now more or less universally accepted that the myocardial preservation provided by cold cardioplegia is superior to that offered by coronary artery perfusion. When surgery is undertaken with a closed aorta coronary perfusion continues, and the heart beats. If the whole venous return is captured by the venous drainage, no ejection occurs. However, cardiac movement may impede accurate surgery and myocardial tone will demand traumatic retraction for exposure. Similar conditions can be obtained with the aorta open and the coronary ostia individually cannulated. If myocardial contraction embarrasses surgery electrical fibrillation may be added.

Decompression of the Heart

Distension of the left ventricle may produce irreversible myocardial damage and must be prevented. Damage to the lungs is produced by persistent elevation of the left atrial pressure. For these two reasons, the left ventricle should usually be vented during cardiopulmonary bypass.

1. Apical Venting of the Left Ventricle (*Fig.* 39.8)

The most convenient method of introduction of a vent involves placing a square stitch in the left ventricle, making a stab incision at its centre, dilating this and introducing a suitable multiple side-holed vent.

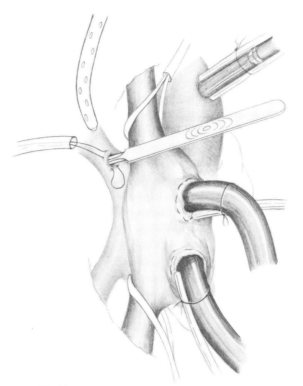

Fig. 39.9. Transatrial venting of the left ventricle.

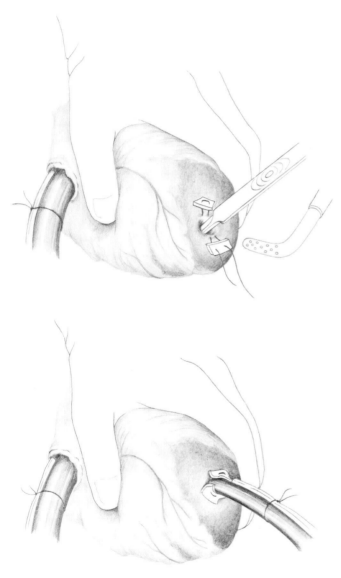

Fig. 39.8. Left ventricular venting.

2. Transatrial Venting of the Left Ventricle (*Fig.* 39.9)

If the apex is inaccessible, because of preoperative adhesions or in the presence of severe left ventricular hypertrophy, apical venting may be difficult or dangerous; the vent can be introduced through a purse-string placed in the anterior wall of the right superior pulmonary vein and advanced to enter the left ventricle across the mitral valve.

Blood from the vent is returned to the extracorporeal circulation after filtration, and the option of gravity drainage or active suction by a roller pump must be offered.

Surgery during Circulatory Standstill without Cardiopulmonary Bypass

If the superior and inferior venae cavae are occluded as they enter the right atrium there will be complete inflow occlusion of the heart, which will empty with cessation of cardiac output. The venous pressure will rise and arterial pressure fall, and the heart will continue to contract.

The brain will survive 3 minutes of inflow occlusion at 37 °C and during this time pulmonary commissurotomy and removal of large pulmonary emboli can be undertaken.

Longer periods of circulatory standstill can be tolerated at lower temperatures. Cooling to 30 °C can be safely done by surface cooling but this method is obsolete in cardiac surgery, as at this temperature only 10 minutes of cerebral ischaemia is tolerated. If longer periods of arrest are required, lower temperatures are demanded and must be produced by core cooling on bypass. This technique is of special value in small children.

Profound Hypothermia for Circulatory Standstill

Using conventional cardiopulmonary bypass with a heat exchanger in the circuit allows progressive cooling of the perfusate and consequent cooling of the patient. The brain temperature can be indirectly assessed by a temperature probe either in the nasopharynx adjacent to the basisphenoid or in the external auditory canal where it must be insulated by wax from the ambient air. When the predetermined 'brain' temperature is reached, the pumps are stopped, cardiac inflow prevented by occlusion of the venae cavae and clamping of the aorta and main pulmonary artery, and the heart is emptied through the atrial cannula which is then removed.

During 'suspended animation' thus produced, surgery can be undertaken in a totally relaxed, bloodless heart unencumbered by cannulas.

Total circulatory standstill can be survived for 45 minutes at 20°C and 90 minutes at 15°C measured in the nasopharynx or external ear.

At the end of surgery, air is evacuated from the heart which is filled with blood or crystalloid solution, the cannulas are replaced, the extracorporeal circulation restored and rewarming undertaken by gradual warming of the circulating blood. Once rewarming is complete and normal, cardiac activity is restored, the bypass is discontinued and the heart decannulated.

Profound Hypothermia with Autogenous Oxygenation (Drew Technique) (Fig. 39.10)

This method of inducing profound hypothermia using the patient's lungs for autogenous oxygenation was introduced in 1959. With this technique the patient may be cooled to 15°C at which temperature circulatory arrest is instituted by ceasing perfusion and occluding the superior and inferior venae cavae. At this temperature surgical procedures may be undertaken for maximum periods of 90 minutes. This technique has proved of immense value in cardiac surgical procedures on infants and children and did, in fact, anticipate the technique of profound hypothermia using an oxygenator. There is little doubt that the use of profound hypothermia with circulatory standstill is a most useful method in the cardiac surgery of infants and children but with the advent of high-quality membrane oxygenators profound hypothermia with autogenous oxygenation is used by few surgeons. For coronary artery surgery this technique can be used with continuing bypass without cooling.

INTRA-AORTIC BALLOON COUNTER-PULSATION

Low cardiac output may follow open heart surgery or myocardial infarction. Improvement in left ventricular function can be gained by diastolic pressure augmentation which alters the pressure/time relationship in the aortic route in such a way that there is an opportunity to maximize diastolic coronary flow.

Diastolic Pressure Augmentation

A balloon in the descending aorta immediately distal to the left subclavian artery is alternately inflated and deflated by a pump triggered by the ECG. The con-

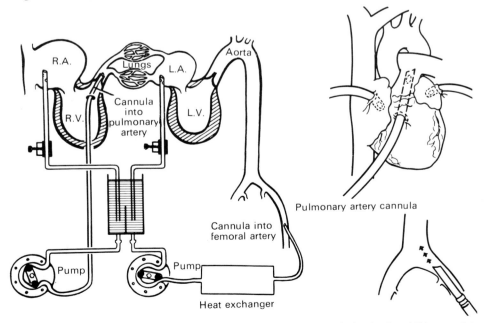

Fig. 39.10. Profound hypothermia with autogenous oxygenation (the Drew technique). In addition to right atrial drainage and systemic arterial return, it is necessary to cannulate separately the main pulmonary artery and the left atrial appendage in order to perfuse the lungs which will oxygenate blood during total bypass.

trols of the device allow the precise timing of this action so that the inflation and deflation times and intervals can be varied.

Diastolic augmentation is achieved by deflating the balloon in systole creating a volume equal to the balloon volume into which the LV can eject unhindered, followed by diastolic inflation which augments the diastolic filling of the aorta by the volume in the balloon with an inevitable increase in pressure.

Equipment

One of several available dedicated consoles is used to activate the pump to pump air in a primary circuit which compresses a balloon in a rigid cylinder. The balloon in the cylinder is connected by a catheter to the intra-aortic balloon and this secondary system is filled with CO_2 or helium. The low viscosity of the latter allows the use of finer catheters and will allow the pump to follow the ECG at faster heart rates. Balloons are made as single- or twin-chamber devices.

Methods of Balloon Introduction

Conventionally the balloon is introduced from the common femoral artery either at open operation or by a percutaneous Seldinger technique. When peripheral arterial or lower aortic disease impedes the balloon during advancement from the femoral artery a single-chamber balloon is introduced from the ascending aorta. This technique is obviously only of use when counter-pulsation is to be used following thoracotomy.

Femoral Artery Introduction

The common femoral artery is exposed through a vertical skin incision immediately inferior to the inguinal ligament, by incision of the roof of the sub-sartorial canal. The balloon and catheter are laid from the patient's left midclavicular point to the inguinal ligament and a ligature used to mark this length for introduction. The common femoral, superficial femoral and deep femoral arteries are isolated with slings and clamped.

An 8 mm vascular graft is threaded over the balloon and catheter. The common femoral artery is incised longitudinally and the balloon inserted up to the marking ligature and the common femoral sling tightened. Balloon pumping can now begin.

The vascular graft is sutured to the arteriotomy with two continuous 5/0 Prolene sutures. Corded tape tied tightly around the vascular graft prevents leakage and the vascular clamps and slings are removed. The graft is buried by closing the skin and the catheter allowed to emerge from the lower end of the incision.

Following completion of counter-pulsation the

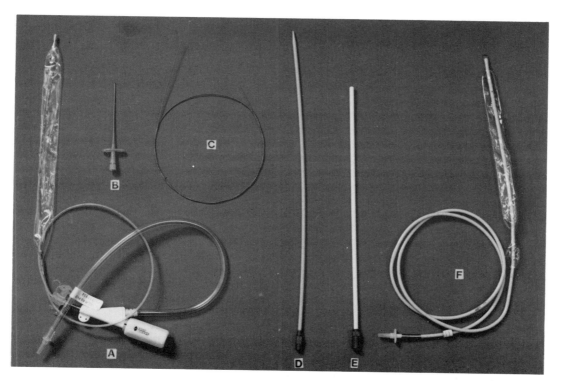

Fig. 39.11. Balloons and introducers for percutaneous introduction of intra-aortic balloon.

incision is reopened and the balloon removed. The femoral artery is cleared proximally and distally by femoral embolectomy procedures. The graft is trimmed to leave a flap which is closed to create a patch angioplasty.

Percutaneous Femoral Introduction (*Fig.* 39.11)

This is undertaken by first measuring the catheter and balloon length and marking as before. The balloon is introduced through an intra-arterial sheath which is itself introduced over a guide wire after dilatation of the arterial puncture site by a cannulated tapering dilator introduced over the guide wire.

When counter-pulsation is no longer required the balloon is removed and firm pressure over the arterial puncture for 10 minutes usually controls bleeding.

Ascending Aorta Introduction

This is used when the support is required following surgery and the balloon cannot be passed up the aorta because of aorto-iliac atheroma.

Two concentric purse-string sutures are applied to the ascending aorta. The ends are drawn through 5-mm polythene tubing to act as tourniquets. The single-chamber balloon is introduced through the centre of these and directed round the aortic arch. The purse-strings are tightened and secured with heavy ligature clips.

The skin only is closed leaving the balloon catheter emerging from the lower end of the incision. The incision is covered with a sterile adhesive 'drape'.

When counter-pulsation is no longer needed the chest is opened, the balloon removed, the aorta closed by tying the purse-string and the chest is closed formally.

FURTHER READING

Drew C. E. and Anderson I. M. (1959) Profound hypothermia in cardiac surgery. *Lancet* **i**, 748.

Drew C. E., Keen G. and Benazon D. B. (1959) Profound hypothermia. *Lancet* **i**, 745.

Gibbon J. H. (1954) Application of mechanical heart and lung apparatus to cardiac surgery. *Minn. Med.* **37**, 171.

Lillehei C. W., Cohen M., Warden H. E. et al. (1955) The direct vision intracardiac correction of congenital anomalies by controlled cross circulation. *Surgery* **38**, 11.

Chapter forty

Congenital Heart Disease

J. D. Wisheart

INTRODUCTION

History

The surgical treatment of congenital abnormalities of the heart and great vessels began in 1937, when Robert Gross, in Boston, successfully ligated a patent ductus arteriosus. Just after the Second World War, Alfred Blalock described the systemic-to-pulmonary artery shunt, known by his name, to relieve the effects of Fallot's tetralogy; this was the first palliative procedure for an intracardiac anomaly. Further such palliative procedures were developed, and in addition the relief of such simple abnormalities as valvular pulmonary stenosis using closed techniques was described by Holmes Sellors and Brock, in London. Definitive correction of intracardiac abnormalities awaited the development of cardiopulmonary bypass by Gibbon in 1954, and of moderate hypothermia which permitted short periods of circulatory arrest. For some abnormalities the philosophy of two-stage correction prevailed for many years, with palliation being advised in early life, to be followed by total correction later. During the past 15 years the refinement of techniques of bypass and hypothermia has enabled total correction of many intracardiac abnormalities to be carried out in infancy.

The foundations of paediatric cardiac surgery are:
1. Precise preoperative diagnosis.
2. Reliable and refined techniques of cardiopulmonary bypass.
3. Accurate methods of surgical repair.
4. Rational methods of intensive postoperative care.

Preparation for Surgery

Once the complete diagnosis has been established a decision to operate may be considered and taken. The next step is to advise the parents, setting out fully the potential benefits and risks of the operation in both the long and short term. Essential dental treatment should be completed well before admission, which should be at least 2 days before the operation to enable all the necessary investigations and preparations to be made. Prophylactic antibiotics are used for 48 hours or longer, beginning with the induction of anaesthesia.

Surgical Techniques

Approach to the Heart

In extracardiac operations right or left thoracotomy is commonly used and this approach is fully described elsewhere. For intracardiac repair access is virtually always by median sternotomy (*see* Chapter 39).

The midline incision extends from immediately below the suprasternal notch to the xiphisternum; it is deepened to expose the sternum and linea alba. The sternum is divided vertically using heavy scissors or a mechanical saw and the two halves separated using a spreader. After the thymus has been divided and cleared from the pericardium superiorly, and the anterior fibres of the diaphragm cleared inferiorly, the pericardium may be opened by a vertical midline incision. The cut edges of the pericardium are sutured to the skin.

Cannulation

The heart is inspected and a 3-mm tape is passed around the aorta using a plane within the aortic sheath. In preparation for cannulation a double purse-string of 4/0 or 5/0 Prolene is placed in the ascending aorta just proximal to the innominate artery. Further single purse-strings of 3/0 or 4/0 Prolene are placed in the right atrial appendage and on the lateral wall of the right atrium near the inferior vena cava, for venous cannulation. Before cannulation the presence of a left superior vena cava and a patent ductus arteriosus are excluded. Arterial and venous cannulas are selected, which are of a suitable size to accommodate the perfusion flows. After total body heparinization (3 mg/kg) the aortic cannula is inserted, and is connected to the bypass machine following careful displacement of all air bubbles. The venous cannulas are then inserted through the right atrium and passed into the cavae; when they are connected cardiopulmonary bypass may begin. Most forms of bypass in children utilize some degree of cooling, and while the temperature is being reduced 3-mm tapes are placed around the cavae and 'snugged' so that all venous return, other than coronary venous blood, is removed from the heart. A 'vent' sucker is placed in the left ventricle and all blood is returned from the heart or pericardium to the pump.

Management of the Operation

To carry out an accurate repair it is helpful to have a still heart and a bloodless field, which is usually achieved by cross-clamping the aorta; it is therefore also necessary to take steps to protect the myocardium from potential ischaemic damage. Thus, immediately after cross-clamping the aorta cardioplegic solution at 4 °C is injected into the aortic root. This solution contains potassium (K^+) at a concentration of 16 mmol/L which leads to the immediate cessation of both mechanical and electrical activity by the heart. Its low temperature, combined with topical cooling with cold isotonic crystalloid solution also at 4 °C, lowers the myocardial temperature which should be maintained below 20 °C while the aorta is cross-clamped. These measures minimize the damage which may be done to the myocardium during the period of ischaemia, by reducing oxygen requirement. A more sophisticated technique for myocardial protection uses blood as the vehicle to deliver the cardioplegia to the myocardium. Thus, ideal circumstances for precise and accurate operating may be combined with a high degree of myocardial protection.

Management in Infancy

The organization of the operation described above had been found unsuitable in infants, partly because the trauma of the surgical approach and cannulation often led to hypotension or cardiac arrest and, second, because long periods of bypass were poorly tolerated. These difficulties were largely overcome by a technique popularized by Sir Brian Barratt-Boyes in 1969; the effects of circulatory embarrassment before bypass are reduced by initial surface cooling, and the period of bypass is shortened by the use of profound hypothermia and circulatory arrest. Thus bypass is only used to complete the cooling, to achieve rewarming and for whatever time is required to achieve stability of cardiac performance. This technique is fully described in Chapter 39.

Withdrawal of Bypass and Closure

Once the repair is complete and the cardiotomies closed, full rewarming of the patient is achieved. Cardiac action will be restored but it is unlikely that blood will be ejected into the aorta as the cavae are still snared and the systemic ventricle vented. Care must be taken to ensure that all air has been removed from the heart and aortic root, and to do this two important rituals should be carried out. First, a small needle vent which sucks blood and bubbles back to the pump, or simply a freely bleeding hole, is placed at the highest point of the ascending aorta. Second, the anaesthetist should inflate the lungs while the surgeon elevates the apex of the heart, permitting blood and air to be expelled through the site of insertion of the ventricular vent. The caval snares are now released and the ritual repeated. Ejection may occur when the heart is replaced and will increase as the vent suction is reduced. The aortic needle vent should continue to suck, or the hole to bleed, for 5–10 minutes after ejection has started.

After removal of the aortic needle vent the bypass flow is gradually reduced and then stopped as the heart maintains the circulation. The volume of blood transfused from the pump will be determined by the left or right atrial pressure, which is commonly 12–15 mmHg at this stage, and by the systolic arterial pressure which should be maintained at not less than 70–80 mmHg immediately after bypass. Once the circulation is stable the perfusion cannulas should be removed; the effects of heparin may then be reversed by giving protamine.

Prior to closing the chest, surgical haemostasis must be achieved throughout the wound from the heart to the skin edge. When it is desired, a catheter is placed to monitor left atrial pressure, otherwise the right atrial pressure measurement is used. Drains are placed in the pericardium, the retrosternal space and in a pleural cavity if it has been opened. Temporary pacing wires are sutured to the surface of both the right atrium and the right ventricle. The pericardium is closed with interrupted sutures. The sternum is approximated with wire or heavy non-absorbable sutures, and the superficial layers are closed accurately.

Postoperative Care

The postoperative intensive care of infants and small children is a team discipline, involving anaesthetic, cardiology and nursing staff, in addition to the surgical team who have the central and coordinating responsibility. Inasmuch as it is not taken for granted that any physiological system will function properly after bypass, the structure of intensive care is designed to monitor and support, if necessary, each individual system, but chiefly the cardiovascular and respiratory systems. Great attention to detail is required in observing these small children whose condition may change very rapidly, and in the accurate ordering of all treatment and dosages.

Reception in Intensive Care

When the patient arrives from theatre the nursing staff are informed of the surgical procedure and the various drains, pacing wires and monitoring cannulas are identified. In the case of infants or small children the environmental temperature must be high to minimize heat loss and it may be convenient to use a cot with an overhead heater. The monitoring lines are immediately connected (*Fig.* 40.1) so that the lines are maintained patent by continuous flushing with heparinized Hartmann's solution, or half-normal saline in very small children. Artificial ventilation is advisable until stability is assured, or more commonly for longer. A nasotracheal tube is more suitable than an endotracheal tube for long-term ventilation in children. Care of the airway must be rigorously maintained by regular instillation of saline (0·2–1 ml) followed by suction, to avoid obstruction of the nasotracheal tube by inspissated secretions—a

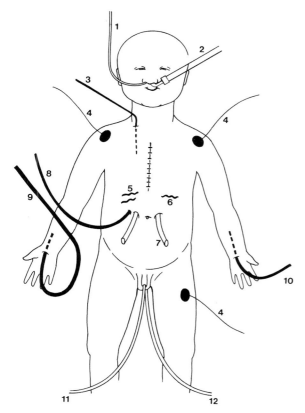

Fig. 40.1. Postoperative monitoring. 1, Nasogastric tube. 2, Naso-tracheal tube for ventilation. 3, Central venous cannula. 4, Electrodes for ECG. 5, Atrial pacing wires. 6, Ventricular pacing wire. 7, Pericardial and mediastinal drains. 8, Left atrial catheter. 9, Radial artery catheter. 10, Peripheral intravenous catheter in back of hand. 11, Urinary catheter. 12, Rectal temperature probe.

real danger in a small-calibre airway. A chest radiograph is immediately carried out and blood specimens sent for haemoglobin, packed cell volume, platelets, urea, electrolytes and sugar estimation, and for a coagulation screen.

Management in the First 24 Hours

It is wise to note initially the weight (kg), the body surface area (m^2) and the estimated circulating volume (70–80 ml/kg) for the child. All blood loss is usually replaced volume-for-volume (with plasma if the packed cell volume exceeds 40). If additional blood is required to maintain the cardiac output in the presence of a normal or a low left atrial pressure, it is convenient to order this in increments of approximately 2–5 per cent of the estimated circulating volume; 0·5–1 ml of 13·4 per cent calcium chloride should be given with each 100 ml of blood.

Total clear fluid intake is severely restricted and for the day of operation is 20 ml/m^2/hr; this should be increased by 25 per cent if the patient is nursed under an overhead heater.

Supplementary potassium is usually needed and may be calculated as 10 mmol/m^2/24 hr on the day of operation, if urine is being passed and potassium levels are within the normal range. Intravenous potassium may only be given diluted and infused over a half to one hour. Minimum urine output should be 0·5 ml/kg/hr. It is important to discuss the operation and progress of the child with the parents as early as possible.

Early Complications

1. BLEEDING

Excessive bleeding may require replacement to such an extent that the complications of massive transfusion may ensue. Re-exploration to secure surgical haemostasis should be carried out if the blood loss exceeds 10 per cent of the estimated blood volume in the first hour or 20 per cent in the first 4 hours, and so forth (*Fig.* 40.2). These rules should still apply if clotting is abnormal and the appropriate coagulation factors should be given during the surgical procedure.

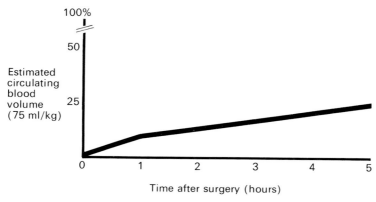

Fig. 40.2. Postoperative blood loss. The level of accumulated blood loss after the operation which indicates the need for reoperation. Blood loss is expressed as a percentage of the estimated circulating volume.

2. TAMPONADE

Tamponade is the collection of blood and clot around the heart, limiting diastolic ventricular filling and leading to a fall in cardiac output and usually a rise in atrial pressure. This condition may be rapidly fatal but is completely treatable if the diagnosis is made and immediate re-exploration carried out—in the bed if need be.

3. LOW CARDIAC OUTPUT

If the cardiac output is low and both hypovolaemia and tamponade are excluded, then an inotropic drug should be used by continuous intravenous infusion; dopamine is widely used and may be combined with a vasodilator such as sodium nitroprusside or glyceryl trinitrate. Alternatives include dobutamine and adrenalin.

4. DYSRHYTHMIAS

A variety of atrial and ventricular dysrhythmias and disorders of rate may occur. It is essential to exclude possible underlying causes such as hypokalaemia, hypoxia, metabolic or respiratory acidosis, digoxin toxicity or beta-adrenergic infusion, hypovolaemia or tamponade. If none of these factors is present then empirical therapeutic measures should be instituted.

Later Postoperative Management

As the patient progresses the framework of care described above may be progressively relaxed. Spontaneous breathing may be restored, using intermittent mandatory ventilation and continuous positive airway pressure for a time if needed; oral intake may be resumed, the monitoring arrangements withdrawn and the drains removed. A stable chronic therapeutic regimen designed to counter heart failure should be established if required.

PATENT DUCTUS ARTERIOSUS

Physiology and Natural History

Isolated patency of the ductus arteriosus is the second most common congenital cardiac anomaly accounting for 12 per cent of the total. The ductus connects the aorta—usually just distal to the origin of the left subclavian artery—to the pulmonary artery just to the left of its bifurcation (*Fig. 40.3a*). Blood passes from the aorta to the pulmonary artery. Spontaneous closure of the ductus is usual in the first few days of life, but if still patent it rarely closes later than the 3rd month. In infancy left ventricular failure may develop, but usually a patent ductus is discovered as an incidental finding in an otherwise asymptomatic child. In 5–7 per cent of cases pulmonary vascular resistance will eventually rise sufficiently to cause reversal of the shunt, while in those who survive to middle age aneurysmal dilatation or calcification of the duct may occur. Bacterial endarteritis may complicate 1 per cent of cases.

Anatomy

The ductus is thin walled and conical in shape with its wider part at the aortic end; a fold of pericardium

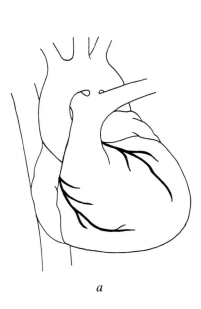

a

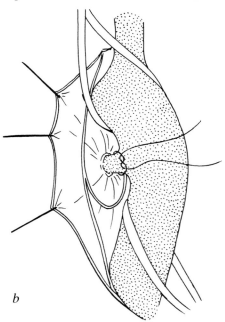

b

Fig. 40.3. Ligation of patent ductus arteriosus. *a*, The PDA in relation to both the aorta and the pulmonary artery. *b*, The ductus is ready for ligation, and its relation to the vagus nerve and to its recurrent laryngeal branch is shown.

overlies the pulmonary end. It is closely related to the vagus nerve and its recurrent laryngeal branch. Where there are anomalies of the aortic arch the ductal anatomy may vary considerably.

Diagnosis and Indications for Operation

Special investigations are not needed when a patent ductus arteriosus presents with a classic clinical picture in childhood. Cardiac catheterization may be required when: (1) any unusual clinical feature or possible associated abnormality is present; (2) the level of pulmonary vascular resistance needs to be measured; (3) the patent ductus arteriosus presents in infancy or in adult life.

Surgery should normally be carried out between the 2nd and 5th years, or at any time if complications are present. In the presence of severe pulmonary hypertension with shunt reversal, surgery is contra-indicated.

Operative Surgery

Operative Technique

The object of surgery is to divide or ligate the duct, which may be approached using a left lateral thoracotomy at the level of the fourth intercostal space. With the lung retracted forwards and downwards the aortic arch, left subclavian artery and descending aorta, together with the phrenic and vagus nerves, may be seen and a thrill may be felt over the ductus. A vertical incision is made into the aortic sheath extending from the left subclavian artery to well below the level of the ductus. The aortic sheath is reflected forwards, using both sharp and blunt dissection, and is maintained in position by stay sutures which also serve to keep the left lung out of the immediate operative field. The posterior part of the aortic sheath is dissected and tapes passed around the aorta. The anatomy of the arch and ductus may now be confirmed (*Fig. 40.3b*). Further dissection in the same plane will safely reflect forwards the vagus and recurrent laryngeal nerves, and will also permit all aspects of the ductus to be demonstrated. A right-angled dissecting instrument may now be passed behind the ductus; if this is difficult the aorta may be lifted forwards using the tapes, and the dissection behind the ductus completed under direct vision. The effect of 'test-clamping' the duct should be observed; the arterial pressure will normally rise a little and the heart rate remain stable. In the presence of known pulmonary vascular disease the pulmonary artery pressure should be measured before and after clamping; if it fails to fall the operation should be abandoned. Two ligatures of no. 1 linen or 2-mm braided silk are passed around the ductus and the aortic end ligated first (*Fig. 40.3b*). Secure ligation is made safe by temporary reduction of the aortic pressure which is easily achieved by cross-clamping the aorta proxi-

mal to the ductus for the 20 seconds needed to apply the first two throws to the knot. A second ligature is applied to the pulmonary end of the ductus.

Other Techniques

1. DIVISION OF THE DUCTUS

This is most easily carried out by applying a side-biting clamp to the aorta at the origin of the ductus and a straight clamp to its pulmonary end. The cut ends may be secured by running sutures of 4/0 or 5/0 Prolene (*Fig. 40.4a*).

2. CLOSURE OF A DUCTUS ASSOCIATED WITH INTRACARDIAC ANOMALIES

In these circumstances the ductus should be closed at the time of total correction. Control of the ductus should be obtained prior to instituting cardiopulmonary bypass in order to avoid loss of perfusion to the lungs. The anterior approach to the heart permits the pulmonary artery end of the ductus to be identified and ligated (*Fig. 40.4b*); alternatively the ductus may be closed from within the pulmonary artery after cardiopulmonary bypass has been established.

3. CLOSURE OF A CALCIFIED OR ANEURYSMAL DUCTUS

No direct approach is appropriate in these circumstances. The safest technique is to use cardiopulmonary bypass and to open the descending aorta between clamps, so that the orifice of the duct may be closed by a patch under direct vision.

Results

Operative mortality in children is less than 0·5 per cent but may be slightly higher in infants, adults or in the presence of pulmonary hypertension. The long-term results are usually excellent in terms of symptoms and cardiac performance. Recanalization is extremely rare.

COARCTATION OF THE AORTA

Physiology and Natural History

A coarctation is a localized severe narrowing, usually at the level of the aortic isthmus just distal to the origin of the left subclavian artery (*Fig. 40.5a*). It accounts for 6 per cent of congenital cardiac anomalies.

There may be a pressure gradient of 40–60 mmHg across the coarctation. The resulting proximal hypertension causes left ventricular hypertrophy with ischaemia and fibrosis of the myocardium which eventually leads to left ventricular failure. Aneurysms may develop on the intracranial and intercostal

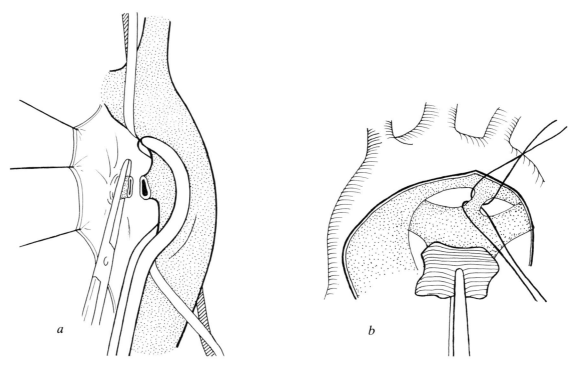

Fig. 40.4. *a*, Division of patent ductus arteriosus. The ductus is divided and the cut ends will now be sutured. *b*, Closure of ductus from anterior approach. After dissecting along the pulmonary artery, the ductus is demonstrated and ready for ligation, prior to going on to cardiopulmonary bypass.

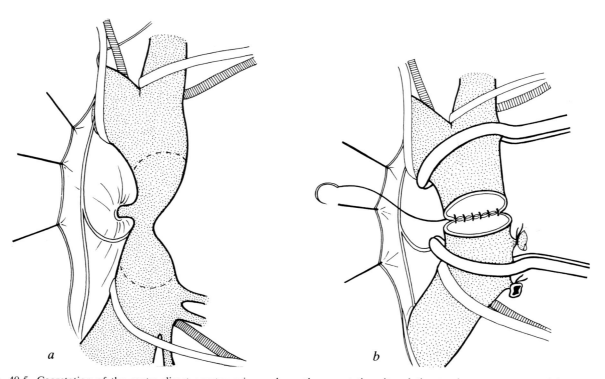

Fig. 40.5. Coarctation of the aorta: direct anastomosis. *a*, shows the coarctation, its relation to the vagus nerve and its recurrent laryngeal branch, the ligamentum arteriosum and the intercostal arteries. The proposed lines of resection are indicated. *b*, The aorta has been clamped, the intercostal arteries divided and the coarctation resected. Direct end-to-end anastomosis, using a simple continuous stitch, is being performed.

arteries or the aorta. Distally the circulation is maintained by many collaterals and the resulting flow has either dampened or absent pulsations which are thought to stimulate the renal mechanisms contributing to the hypertension.

Rarely an isolated coarctation leads to left ventricular failure or it threatens life in infancy. More commonly childhood is free of symptoms but life is threatened later by the mechanisms already described which lead to an average life expectation of about 40 years.

Anatomy and Classification

The luminal narrowing of a coarctation is caused by the narrowing of the aortic wall as seen on external inspection of the vessel, and an internal shelf or diaphragm, which together may limit the opening to 1 or 2 mm in diameter. Coarctations are usually divided into two groups: first, those which are approximately at the same level as the ligamentum arteriosum, called 'juxtaductal', and which are seen in children and adults; second, those which are proximal to the ductus, called 'preductal', which are seen in infants. In the latter group there is a longer segment of narrowing between the origin of the left subclavian artery and the patent ductus arteriosus which is continuous with the descending aorta and transmits blood from the pulmonary artery to the lower half of the body. Abnormalities of the aortic valve, the mitral valve or a patent ductus arteriosus may be associated with a coarctation.

Diagnosis and Indications for Operation

The diagnosis in children is a clinical one based on the classic findings of elevation of the blood pressure, absent or weak and delayed femoral pulses, with evidence of periscapular collaterals. If there is doubt about any of these findings, full investigation should be carried out. In infants and adults cardiac catheterization should be performed to measure the pressure gradient, to demonstrate by aortography the anatomy of both the coarctation and the collaterals, and to clarify any associated abnormalities.

Surgical treatment is required for virtually all patients with coarctation. In the symptomatic child elective operation may be planned in the year prior to going to school or if the diagnosis is made later the operation should not be delayed. In infancy persistent left ventricular failure due to the coarctation alone or in association with other anomalies requires urgent surgical treatment.

Operative Surgery

In 1945 both Gross and Crafoord, independently, treated patients with coarctation by resection and end-to-end anastomosis. This technique remains the most widely used in children and adults, although some surgeons prefer the plastic method first described by Vosschulte. The special problems presented by infants are probably best met by the subclavian 'flap' method, first described by Waldhausen, and which has been popularized in the U.K. by Hamilton.

Operative Techniques

The coarctation is approached through a long, left lateral thoracotomy, usually at the upper border of the 5th rib. Division of the muscles of the chest wall is time consuming and tedious as each enlarged collateral vessel must be individually ligated. Carefully controlled hypotension using trimetaphan or sodium nitroprusside is helpful. A long vertical incision is made in the aortic sheath extending from the left subclavian artery to below the coarctation. Carefully preserving the plane of the dissection, the anterior flap is reflected forwards together with the vagus and its recurrent laryngeal branch. The dissection of the aorta proximal to the coarctation may be completed and tapes passed around the left subclavian artery and the arch of the aorta distal to the left common carotid artery (*Fig. 40.5a*). Enlarged mediastinal branches of the aorta may cause troublesome bleeding if not carefully identified and secured. Distal to the coarctation, dilated, tortuous and thin-walled intercostal arteries pass from the aorta to the chest wall; occasionally one or two pairs of these will need to be controlled or divided.

Vascular clamps are placed on the aorta above and below the coarctation and before incising the narrowed segment it should be confirmed that it is not still being filled through an uncontrolled or unidentified branch. By digital examination or by formal manometry of the aorta distal to the clamp, it should be shown that there is satisfactory pressure in the descending aorta.

1. END-TO-END ANASTOMOSIS

The lines of resection were determined prior to application of the clamps and the coarctation should be excised (*Fig. 40.5a*). Usually the two ends may be brought together using 3/0, 4/0 or 5/0 Prolene and the posterior part of the anastomosis may be constructed with a simple running stitch (*Fig. 40.5b*). The anterior part may be completed by a further continuous suture or by interrupted sutures in smaller children. The anaesthetist should be warned prior to removing the clamps so that the hypotensive agent may be stopped and blood may be available in the event of severe haemorrhage from the suture line.

2. AORTOPLASTY

This method avoids a circumferential aortic suture line by reconstructing the aorta with a gusset inserted across the narrow segment. After clamping the arch

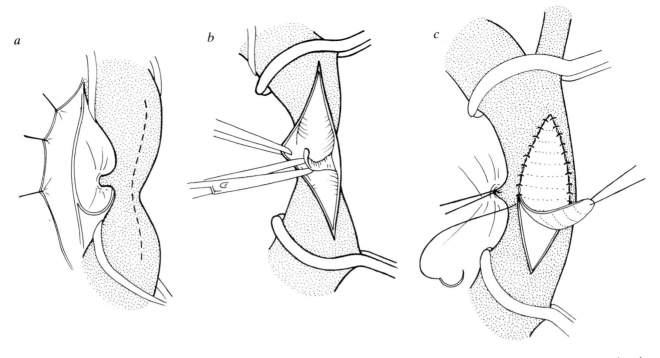

Fig. 40.6. Coarctation of the aorta: aortoplasty. a, Shows the proposed line of incision across the coarctation. *b.* After opening the aorta, the 'diaphragm' is excised. *c,* The aortotomy is closed using a gusset of woven Dacron.

of the aorta and the left subclavian artery, a vertical incision is made in the aorta beginning near the origin of the left subclavian artery and extending down across the coarctation and into the descending aorta (*Fig.* 40.6*a*). The diaphragm within the aorta at the level of the coarctation is excised (*Fig.* 40.6*b*). A large oval patch of woven crimped Dacron is cut from an arterial tube graft and sewn into the resulting defect using continuous runs of Prolene sutures (*Fig.* 40.6*c*).

3. TUBE GRAFT

If it is not possible to bring the ends together easily, then the gap should be bridged using a circumferential graft of woven crimped Dacron of the appropriate size (*Fig.* 40.7).

4. SUBCLAVIAN FLAP OPERATION

A circumferential suture line in infants commonly leads to recurrent obstruction at this site due to failure of growth of the anastomosis. This is avoided by a plastic operation using a gusset of living autologous tissue, namely the left subclavian artery which is divided proximal to its first branch. A vertical incision across the coarctation is extended into the left subclavian artery, which is thus changed from a tube to a flap (*Fig.* 40.8*a*). This flap is turned down and sewn into the defect across the coarctation using a fine Prolene continuous suture (*Fig.* 40.8*b*).

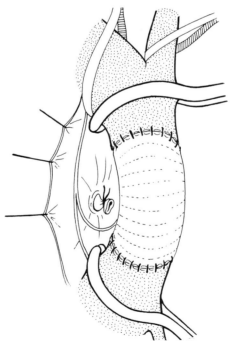

Fig. 40.7. Coarctation of the aorta: tube graft. The graft is shown after its insertion has been completed. It bridges the gap between the two ends of the aorta.

USE OF LEFT ATRIOFEMORAL BYPASS

When the collaterals are inadequate it may be necessary to preserve the distal circulation by left atrio-

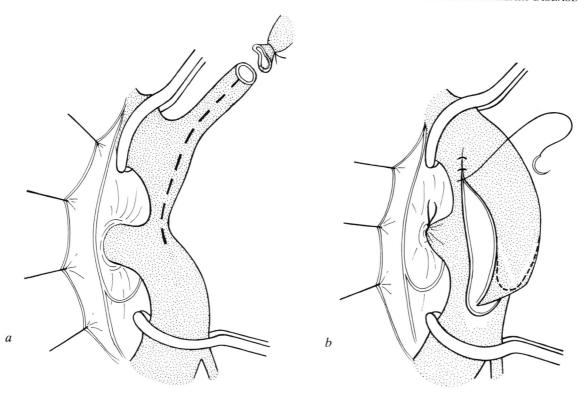

Fig. 40.8. Coarctation of the aorta: subclavian flap operation. An infantile or preductal coarctation is shown. *a*, The distal subclavian artery has been ligated and the aorta clamped: the proposed incision across the coarctation and into the left subclavian artery is shown. *b*, The 'flap' of subclavian artery is being sutured into the aortic defect.

femoral bypass or Gott shunt (*see* Chapter 43). Bypass should be used if after clamping the aorta the pressure of the descending aorta is less than 40–50 mmHg.

Results

The operative mortality for uncomplicated coarctation in childhood or the teenage years is less than 2 per cent, but in adults may be slightly higher due to technical problems arising from the degenerative changes in the aortic wall. The chief cause of operative death in these patients is severe haemorrhage. In infants where the coarctation is associated with other major anomalies, the mortality for the operation, which may include other palliative procedures, may be as high as 10–25 per cent. Important complications include haemorrhage from the aorta or chest wall, recurrent laryngeal nerve palsy, chylothorax, or rarely renal failure or paraplegia. Local infection, either blood-borne within the aorta or outside the aorta, may have serious consequences, particularly if prosthetic material has been used in the repair. A syndrome of crampy abdominal pain mimicking an acute abdomen is described and attributed to mesenteric arteritis due to the presence of

a pulsatile flow for the first time. This is usually associated with a high blood pressure immediately after operation. In the early postoperative period if systolic pressure is greater than 170 mmHg or diastolic greater than 110 mmHg the blood pressure should be reduced by pharmacological means. The blood pressure does not fall immediately after the operation and it may not reach its final level until 6–12 weeks later.

CONGENITAL AORTIC STENOSIS

Physiology and Natural History

Aortic stenosis accounts for about 6 per cent of all congenital heart disorders. The obstruction causes elevation of left ventricular pressure with resulting left ventricular hypertrophy, ischaemia and fibrosis. This may be sufficiently severe to threaten life in either infancy or childhood.

Anatomy and Classification

The obstruction may be valvar, subvalvar or supravalvar. In valvar aortic stenosis there may be two or three cusps, rarely one or four; the cusps themselves may be thin and pliable or thick and rigid. The commissures are usually fused and the annulus itself may be small. When the obstruction is subvalvar it is either a discrete diaphragm of fibrous tissue a few millimetres below the aortic valve or it may be caused by hypertrophic obstructive cardiomyopathy. Supravalvar obstruction is rare and is caused by a narrowing of the aorta at or just above the sinus ridge.

Diagnosis and Indications for Operation

If the patient is symptomatic or the electrocardiogram indicates severe left ventricular hypertrophy, catheterization should be carried out. Manometry and left ventricular angiography will permit both the severity and site of stenosis to be identified. Gradients of 60–80 mmHg in the presence of symptoms and ECG changes in children are indications for surgical relief of the obstruction. In infants smaller gradients may indicate important obstruction. The objects of surgery are to relieve the obstruction and thereby to protect the left ventricular myocardium from the damage that would follow persistent obstruction.

Operative Surgery

Operative Techniques

1. VALVAR

With cardiopulmonary bypass, moderate hypothermia and a short period of ischaemic arrest, the aortic valve may be exposed by an oblique incision in the aorta (*Fig.* 40.9*a*). The fused commissures should be carefully and accurately incised but no closer to the annulus than 2 mm, in case aortic incompetence

should occur (*Fig.* 40.9*b*). When this has been done the subvalar region should be inspected. The aortic incision may be repaired by continuous stitches of 3/0 or 4/0 Prolene.

2. SUBVALVAR

Access to the obstruction is through the aorta and aortic valve as described above. The subvalvar region is exposed by careful retraction of the valve leaflets and annulus, avoiding pressure on the upper part of the interventricular septum, lest the conducting tissue should be temporarily injured. If a discrete diaphragm is present it may be carefully excised by a mixture of some sharp, but predominantly blunt dissection, carefully avoiding any injury to the interventricular septum or mitral valve (*Fig.* 40.10).

The indications for surgical relief of hypertrophic obstructive cardiomyopathy are uncertain at present as beta-blockade is the mainstay of management.

3. SUPRAVALVAR

These rare anomalies require major reconstruction of the proximal aorta which may also involve the annulus or the ostia of the coronary arteries.

Results

Aortic valvotomy is best regarded as a palliative operation, carried out in order to preserve life and to protect the left ventricular myocardium. Although immediate relief of stenosis is usually good the obstruction may recur after an interval or the operation may be complicated by aortic incompetence. For either of these two reasons further surgery may be required in a high percentage of cases. When surgery is required early in infancy results are much less good and the operative mortality remains high.

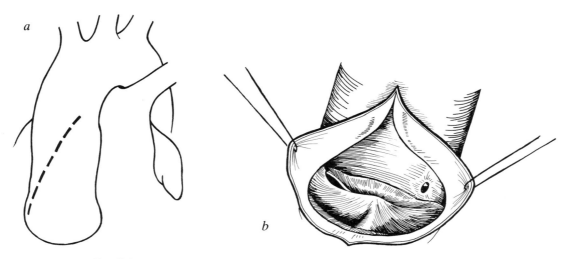

Fig. 40.9. Valvar aortic stenosis. A bicuspid, stenotic valve is shown.
a, Incision for an oblique aortotomy. *b*. The left coronary ostium is seen posteriorly.

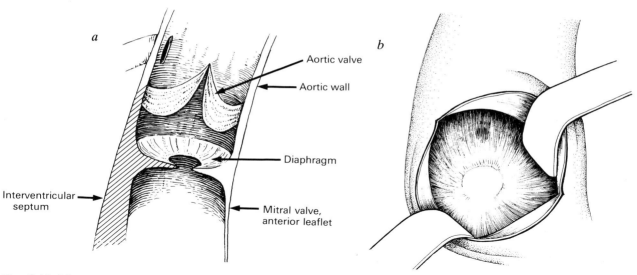

Fig. 40.10. Discrete Subvalvar aortic stenosis. *a*, A schematic cross-section showing the obstructive diaphragm a few millimetres below the aortic valve. *b*, The diaphragm as seen through the aortotomy with the valve cusps retracted.

PULMONARY STENOSIS

Physiology and Natural History

Pulmonary stenosis accounts for 9 per cent of all congenital cardiac abnormalities. There is a pressure gradient between the body of the right ventricle and the pulmonary artery resulting in hypertrophy of the right ventricle. Tiredness and shortness of breath are common and cyanosis may occur when a patent foramen ovale is also present. In severe cases, right ventricular failure, ventricular dysrhythmias, syncope or premature death may occur.

Anatomy and Classification

The obstruction may be valvar, infundibular or supravalvar. In valvar stenosis the commissures, which are partly adherent to the wall of the pulmonary artery, are fused. In infundibular stenosis hypertrophy and fusion of muscle bands impinge on the outflow tract of the right ventricle. This is a dynamic obstruction which is severe in systole.

Diagnosis and Indications for Operation

At cardiac catheterization the pressure gradient is measured and the level of the obstruction defined by angiography. Any associated abnormalities are demonstrated. The stenosis may be classified as mild if the gradient is less than 50, moderate if it is between 50 and 100, and severe if it is greater than 100 mmHg. Mild pulmonary stenosis rarely requires operation but severe obstruction should be surgically relieved. Moderate stenosis should be relieved if it is associated with symptoms and evidence of advanced hypertrophy of the right ventricle. Occasionally, a neonate presents with life-threatening pulmonary stenosis.

Operative Surgery

Relief of pulmonary valvar stenosis was devised by Holmes Sellors and Brock at about the same time, in 1947, using an instrument passed through the wall of the right ventricle to dilate the pulmonary valve. Semi-open methods using inflow occlusion and moderate hypothermia have also been used. Since cardiopulmonary bypass has become safe, open methods have been nearly always used. However, in recent years it has become possible to relieve some forms of pulmonary stenosis by balloon valvoplasty.

Operative Technique

1. VALVAR STENOSIS

First, the presence of a patent foramen ovale should be excluded by exploration through a small incision in the right atrium; if present it should be closed. The valve is approached by a longitudinal incision in the pulmonary artery (*Fig.* 40.11*a*). The commissures are freed from the wall of the pulmonary artery using fine scissors, enabling complete commissurotomies to be performed (*Fig.* 40.11*b*). The arteriotomy is repaired with a continuous suture of 4/0 or 5/0 Prolene.

If the valve cusps are thickened, partial or complete excision may be needed to relieve the obstruction. The resulting pulmonary incompetence is said to be well tolerated, whereas it is known that important residual obstruction is not.

In a moribund neonate there may be a place for performing a closed valvotomy using dilating instruments passed through the wall of the right ventricle.

2. INFUNDIBULAR STENOSIS

The infundibulum is exposed by a transverse ventri-

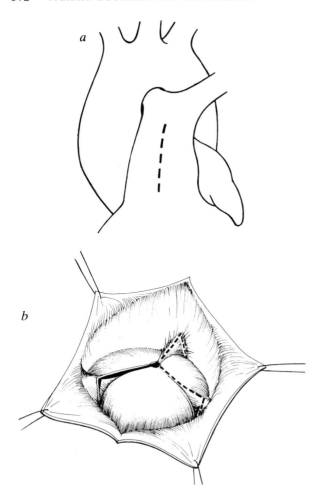

Fig. 40.11. Valvar pulmonary stenosis. A tricuspid pulmonary valve with fused commissures and a small central orifice. The broken lines indicate where the commissures are freed from the arterial wall and then divided. One commissure is already divided (*b*). *a*, Line of incision in pulmonary artery.

culotomy across the right ventricular outflow tract, carefully sited to avoid the coronary arteries. Obstructing bands of infundibular muscle, often covered with thickened endocardium, are incised or excised taking care to avoid perforating the interventricular septum or damaging the subvalvar structures of the tricuspid valve.

If the obstruction takes the form of a 'tunnel' below the pulmonary valve it may be necessary to enlarge the infundibulum using a gusset of autologous pericardium or woven Dacron.

3. SUPRAVALVAR STENOSIS

Supravalvar stenosis is not common in isolation but may occur with other abnormalities, such as Fallot's tetralogy. It is best dealt with by enlarging the narrowed area with a gusset, preferably of autologous pericardium, using a fine suture of 4/0 or 5/0 Prolene.

Results

The operative mortality in children should be not more than 2 per cent, although it may be higher in infants. An excellent result is nearly always achieved.

ATRIAL SEPTAL DEFECTS

Physiology and Natural History

Atrial septal defects account for 10 per cent of congenital cardiac anomalies. There is a communication between the two atria, resulting in a left-to-right shunt. Isolated atrial septal defects rarely threaten life in infancy or childhood, but symptoms may develop in adult life and average survival is to the fifth decade.

Anatomy and Classification

There are three types of atrial septal defect (ASD):
1. Secundum atrial septal defect.
2. Primum atrial septal defect (partial atrioventricular canal).
3. Sinus venosus defect.

The *secundum defect* is the most common and usually lies in the fossa ovalis, but may extend to the inferior vena caval orifice, the lateral atrial wall or the upper part of the atrial septum; it is commonly 2–3 cm in diameter. It never extends as far posteriorly or inferiorly as the coronary sinus or the tricuspid valve. A 'patent foramen ovale' is the name given to a probe-patent communication between the atria and it should be included in the group. However, it exists in 10–20 per cent of normal people and is only of significance when associated with other lesions, particularly pulmonary stenosis.

The *primum ASD* lies in the posteroinferior part of the septum and is immediately adjacent to the tricuspid and mitral valve orifices, and also, therefore, to the conducting tissue as it passes from the atrioventricular node to the interventricular septum. The size of the defect varies and when there is virtually no interatrial septum, the condition is known as 'common atrium'. In addition to the ASD there is a cleft in the anterior leaflet of the mitral valve causing mitral incompetence. The primum ASD is due to failure of development of the septum primum and is an incomplete form of a more complex anomaly which includes both atrial and ventricular septal defects, as well as defects of the endocardial cushions which cause abnormalities in both mitral and tricuspid valves.

The *sinus venosus defect* lies high in the atrial septum and the right upper pulmonary vein may empty into the right atrium or superior vena cava.

Diagnosis and Indications for Operation

Children with a secundum ASD or a sinus venosus defect are usually free of symptoms. The diagnosis may be made clinically but should be confirmed by catheterization. If the pulmonary to systemic flow ratio is greater than 2:1 the ASD should be closed, generally before school age. When adults present with an ASD it should be closed in order to reduce the effects of atrial fibrillation and to prevent further progression of pulmonary vascular disease.

Children with a primum ASD frequently have shortness of breath and increased tiredness. The diagnosis is suggested by the clinical findings of an ASD plus mitral incompetence together with the characteristic electrocardiogram. It should be confirmed by catheterization and left ventricular angiogram, which will demonstrate the classic 'goose neck deformity' of the left ventricle and the severity of the mitral incompetence. These defects should always be repaired.

Operative Surgery

Operative Techniques

1. SECUNDUM ASD

This is an operation of low risk (less than 1 per cent) in which there is a particular danger of air embolism. Any possibility of ejection by the left ventricle must be prevented while the heart is open; thus either the heart should be fibrillated or the aorta should be cross-clamped with either ischaemic or chemical cardiac arrest, while the defect is being closed.

Prior to bypass the heart is inspected and anomalies of the right pulmonary veins are sought. The atrium should be opened by an incision at the base of the appendage which extends towards the inferior vena cava (*Fig. 40.12a*). The ASD is identified and the adjacent parts of the septum and fossa ovalis are inspected for additional defects or fenestrations. The defect is closed, usually by a continuous suture (*Fig. 40.12b*). Care must be taken not to distort the orifice of the inferior vena cava. Occasionally very large defects require a patch of pericardium or Dacron for satisfactory closure.

So that all air may be removed, the heart should be fibrillated as the aortic clamp is removed. This permits full precautions to be taken before the heart may eject.

2. PRIMUM ASD

The object of this operation is to repair the mitral valve, close the ASD with a patch without causing heart block and to prevent the occurrence of air embolism.

Following the application of the aortic cross-clamp and administration of cardioplegia the right atrium is opened. The abnormal anatomy is inspected and the diagnosis confirmed (*Fig. 40.13a*); care is taken to exclude a ventricular septal defect lying below the atrioventricular valves. The mitral valve is repaired

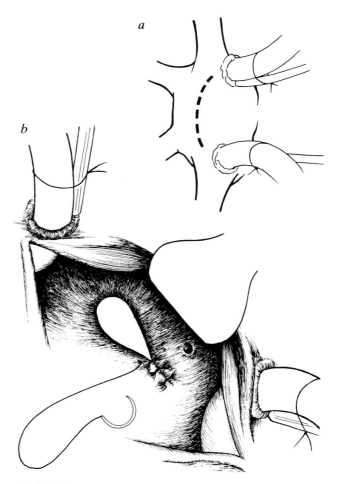

Fig. 40.12. Secundum atrial septal defect. *a*, Incision in right atrium to expose the defect. *b*, A secundum ASD being closed by a continuous suture.

first by approximating the edges of the cleft with interrupted sutures of 4/0 or 5/0 Prolene (*Fig. 40.13b*).

The ASD is always closed with a patch, using either autologous pericardium or thin Dacron. It is of prime importance to avoid damaging the conduction tissue while inserting the patch. The atrioventricular node lies between the coronary sinus and the tricuspid valve (*Fig. 40.13a*), while the bundle of His lies close to the tricuspid valve as it passes superiorly to enter the interventricular septum. A still heart and a bloodless field are the necessary conditions for precise suturing and avoidance of heart block, and these may be achieved by either of two techniques. The patch may be sutured to the attachment of the anterior leaflet of the mitral valve, the left side of atrial septum inferiorly and onto the edge of the defect to the right of the coronary sinus (*Fig. 40.13c*). Alternatively, the patch may be sutured to the attachment of the tricuspid valve until the suture line is inferior to the atrioventricular node and the coronary sinus; it is then carried around the floor of the right atrium so

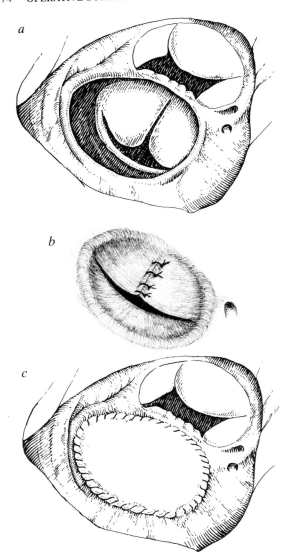

Fig. 40.13. Primum atrial septal defect. *a,* The right atrium is open and the tricuspid valve is seen anteriorly. The septal defect is immediately adjacent to the tricuspid valve and the mitral valve, which with its cleft anterior cusp may be seen through the defect. The position of the atrioventricular node is indicated, lying between the coronary sinus and the tricuspid valve. *b,* The cleft is closed with interrupted sutures. *c,* The septal defect is closed with a patch sutured to the attachment of the anterior leaflet of the mitral valve.

that the coronary sinus drains to the left atrium. Either way the patch may be securely inserted and the conducting pathways preserved.

3. SINUS VENOSUS DEFECT
The sinus venosus defect is closed with a patch ensuring that pulmonary venous blood drains to the left atrium.

Results
The mortality for repair of secundum ASD is less

than 1 per cent and there should be close to normal cardiac function ensuring both a satisfactory length and quality of life thereafter. The mortality for repair of primum ASD is slightly higher and is between 2 and 5 per cent. In these cases the future is determined chiefly by whether or not heart block has been avoided, and also by the severity of the mitral valve lesion. Thus a very small percentage may require permanent pacemaking, or replacement of the mitral valve later in life.

VENTRICULAR SEPTAL DEFECTS

Physiology and Natural History

Ventricular septal defects are the most common congenital cardiac anomaly, accounting for 25 per cent of the total. Blood passes from the left to the right ventricle in volumes determined by the size of the defect and the relative resistances in the pulmonary and systemic vascular beds; this results in a high pulmonary blood flow. The natural history of the condition is complex; spontaneous closure may occur in some, but in others life may be threatened early in infancy by left ventricular failure; after infancy the development of progressive obliterative, pulmonary vascular disease may lead to a rising pulmonary vascular resistance. This will initially cause a reduction and may eventually lead to a reversal of the shunt flow (Eisenmenger syndrome). These structural changes may become advanced before teenage years in 15–25 per cent of patients. Aortic incompetence, infundibular pulmonary stenosis and bacterial endocarditis may also occur, resulting in an expectation of life of 25–30 years if the ventricular septal defect is not closed.

Anatomy and Classification

The ventricular septum may be divided into three portions—inlet, outlet (or infundibular) and trabecular (or muscular) as shown in *Fig.* 40.14*a*. Each part is contiguous with part of the membranous septum. Defects may be classified as perimembranous, infundibular or muscular (*Fig.* 40.14*b*). The perimembranous defect is due to a deficiency of muscle around the membranous septum and the central fibrous body forms part of the rim of the defect. The defect may extend into the trabecular, the outflow or the inflow portions of the septum, and thus perimembranous defects may be subdivided on this basis. The perimembranous defects are always contiguous with the annulus of the tricuspid valve and the bundle of His always passes along the inferior margin of the defect before dividing into the right and left bundles to descend in the muscular septum. The infundibular defect lies above the crista supraventricularis and below the aortic and pulmonary valves. It is not related to the conducting tissue. Muscular defects

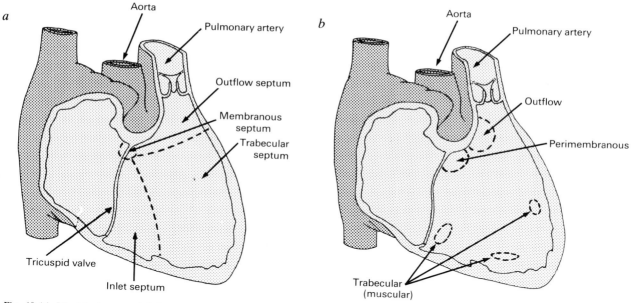

Fig. 40.14. Ventricular septal defects: classification. *a*, The three parts of the ventricular septum—the inlet, the trabecular and the outflow portions, each of which impinges on the membranous septum. *b*, The sites of different types of defect, perimembranous outflow and trabecular.
(*Fig.* 40.14 has been redrawn after Anderson R. H. and Becker A. E. (1983) In Stark J. and deLeval M. (eds) *Surgery for Congenital Heart Defects*. London, Grune and Stratton).

may be single or multiple and are situated in any part of the trabecular septum.

Diagnosis and Indications for Operation

The diagnosis may be demonstrated by cardiac catheterization and left ventricular angiography; this also enables the level of pulmonary blood flow and pulmonary arterial resistance to be calculated.

Surgical closure is not required if the pulmonary blood flow does not exceed twice the systemic flow and the pulmonary vascular resistance is low. If the pulmonary flow is higher than this, the defect should be closed, usually between the ages of 2 and 4 years. Earlier surgical treatment will be required if left ventricular failure in infancy does not respond to medical treatment, or if the baby fails to thrive. If very high pulmonary blood flow or elevated pulmonary artery pressure, or both, are noted early in life, they suggest the possibility of the early development of pulmonary vascular disease and the defect should be closed not later than at 18–24 months of age in these patients. If the patient is cyanosed due to shunt reversal, closure of the defect is contra-indicated.

Operative Surgery

In 1952 Muller and Dammann described how the effects of a ventricular septal defect (VSD) could be palliated by constriction of the pulmonary artery; thus by increasing the resistance to flow through the pulmonary artery the shunt flow is reduced, as is the volume load on the left ventricle. The development

of pulmonary vascular disease is at least partly prevented by the reduction in pulmonary blood flow. With cardiopulmonary bypass, techniques of closure of the defect became established and satisfactory in older children; pulmonary artery banding was reserved for infants. In the past decade cardiopulmonary bypass has become safe in infants and initial corrective surgery is now the treatment of choice in all age groups. Pulmonary artery banding is reserved for infants in whom the VSD is associated with other complex malformations.

Operative Technique for Closure of VSD

Perimembranous VSD may be approached through the right atrium and tricuspid valve or through the right ventricle.

1. TRANSATRIAL APPROACH

This approach has the advantage of avoiding an incision in the right ventricular muscle. The right atrium is opened by an incision passing from the base of the atrial appendage towards the inferior vena cava, thus exposing the tricuspid valve. The septal leaflet of the valve is retracted posteriorly and to the right, permitting the VSD to be visualized. A series of double-armed sutures of 4/0 Mersilene, buttressed with small pledgets of Teflon felt, are placed in the margin of the defect. Beginning inferiorly, where the bundle of His is close to the defect, the stitches are carefully placed through the attachment of the septal leaflet of the tricuspid valve. Proceeding clockwise, care must be taken to avoid the aortic valve which is close to the defect; proceeding anticlockwise from the tricuspid valve, once the papillary muscle of the conus has been passed, stitches may be placed deeply into the muscular margins of the defect. Each stitch is passed through a knitted Dacron patch which is slid into position and the sutures carefully tied. Alternatively a continuous suture may be used incorporating the same precautions.

2. TRANSVENTRICULAR APPROACH

If access through the right atrium is unsatisfactory the transventricular approach is used. The right ventricle is opened with a transverse incision at the level of the VSD, after carefully noting that no major branches of the coronary arteries will be injured (*Fig. 40.15a*). The edges of the ventriculotomy are gently retracted, the crista supraventricularis and tricuspid valve are immediately noted and the VSD may then be identified behind and below the crista and above the tricuspid valve (*Fig. 40.15b*). The papillary muscle of the conus lies posterior to the tricuspid valve. Looking through the defect, the cusps of the aortic valve may be seen. Sutures are placed as described previously and the defect closed with a patch. The ventriculotomy is closed with two layers of simple continuous sutures of 4/0 Prolene; each bite includes the whole thickness of the right ventricular wall.

3. CLOSURE OF OTHER TYPES OF VSD

Infundibular defects lying above the crista supraventricularis should be repaired through the ventricle with a patch. As the conducting tissue is not at risk a simple continuous suture may be used. In the past,

muscular defects were approached through the body of the right ventricle but the coarse trabecular pattern of the right side of the septum makes identification difficult and closure uncertain. It is now widely accepted that these should be approached using a 'fish-mouth' incision at the apex of the left ventricle. By this route both single and multiple defects may be identified and closed securely.

RESULTS

The operative mortality in children ranges from 2 to 5 per cent and is now only a little higher in infants. In nearly all, the symptomatic result is excellent but, where it was present preoperatively, pulmonary vascular disease is likely to persist. An excellent result may be defined as secure closure of the defect, a symptom-free life and a pulmonary artery pressure at or near normal levels; if this is to be obtained operation should be carried out at not later than 2–4 years of age and in some cases before 2 years. Late complications include a residual or recurrent VSD, complete heart block, persistence of important pulmonary vascular disease and bacterial endocarditis.

Operative Technique for Palliative Surgery: Pulmonary Artery Banding

This procedure is carried out through a left lateral thoracotomy at the upper border of the 4th rib. The pericardium is opened in front of the phrenic nerve and the great vessels are identified (*Fig. 40.16a*). A right-angled dissecting instrument may be placed in the transverse sinus behind the pulmonary artery and passed forwards in a plane already established deep to the aortic sheath: 2-mm braided silk (ductus silk) is used to constrict the artery. Particular care is

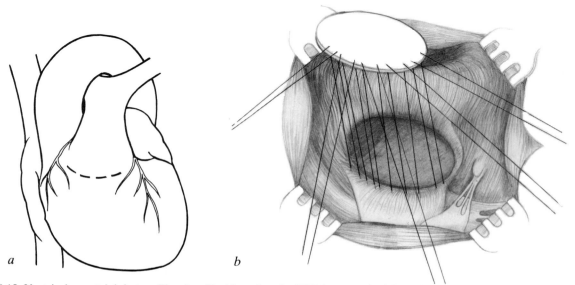

Fig. 40.15. Ventricular septal defect. *a*, The site of incision when the VSD is approached through a right ventriculotomy. *b*, Closure. A view of a membranous defect from the right ventricular aspect. Sutures have been passed through the attachment of the cusp of the tricuspid valve, and then through the patch.

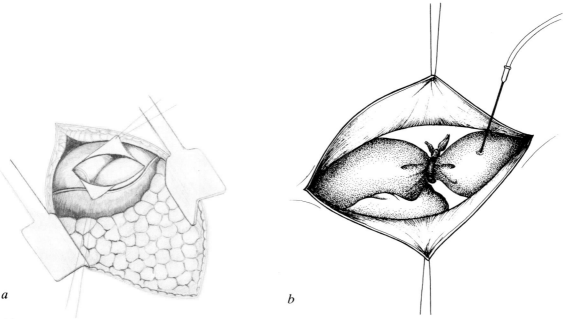

Fig. 40.16. Ventricular septal defect: palliation by banding the pulmonary artery. *a*, The pericardium has been opened in front of the left phrenic nerve, exposing the left atrial appendage and the pulmonary artery. *b*, The pulmonary artery is constricted and the pressure is being measured beyond the band.

required when there is also transposition of the great arteries as the coronary arteries arise higher than usual and are very close to the level of the band. Two methods may be used to secure the constricting band to the correct degree of tightness. Mustard and his colleagues have derived a formula relating the circumference of the band to the baby's weight; this rather arbitrary approach worked well in their hands but has not been widely applied. More commonly the band is progressively tightened until the pulmonary artery pressure beyond the constriction is reduced to 30 or 40 mmHg. If the arterial pressure, heart rate and systemic oxygenation remain stable and satisfactory then the band should be secured; if not, it must be loosened and secured at the tightest level consistent with stable haemodynamics (*Fig.* 40.16*b*).

The band itself must be secured to the pulmonary artery with at least three interrupted sutures to prevent its distal migration to the bifurcation, which would cause catastrophic obstruction to pulmonary blood flow. The pericardium is closed with interrupted sutures.

RESULTS

The mortality in children over 6 months with a simple VSD is substantially less than 5 per cent but in more complex conditions or infants under 6 months it rises to 10 per cent or more. Ideally the band will control the haemodynamic state until the child is ready for total correction, which will include reconstruction of the pulmonary artery. Occasionally the VSD will close spontaneously, when reconstruction of the pul-

monary artery alone will be required. Alternatively the constriction may be inadequate, in which case earlier intervention will be needed.

FALLOT'S TETRALOGY

Physiology and Natural History

Fallot's tetralogy is the most common cyanotic cardiac anomaly, accounting for 12 per cent of the total. Classically it is described as having four abnormal features: a ventricular septal defect, pulmonary stenosis, the aorta straddles the ventricular septum and right ventricular hypertrophy.

The abnormal circulation is determined by the VSD and pulmonary stenosis. In the face of severe stenosis the right ventricle ejects part of each stroke volume to the lungs and part through the VSD to the aorta. Thus the pulmonary blood flow is reduced and that small volume of oxygenated blood is mixed with the desaturated blood passing through the VSD resulting in arterial desaturation and cyanosis. When the myocardium contracts with greater velocity, the infundibular component of the pulmonary stenosis will be more severe, causing an acute episode of even more severe hypoxia.

Life may be threatened by hypoxia in infancy or early childhood in a substantial proportion of cases. The remainder divide into two groups: the majority, whose condition deteriorates steadily leading to death in the teenage years, and a small minority with milder forms of the anomaly, who survive into adult life. In addition to hypoxia these children suffer from polycythaemia, cerebral thromboses and abscesses.

Anatomy and Classification

The ventricular septal defect is perimembranous in position and large, approximating to the size of the aortic valve annulus. The pulmonary stenosis is complex and is the key to the surgery of this anomaly. Invariably there is severe infundibular obstruction due to hypertrophy, thickening and fusion of the muscle bands in this area. This aspect of the obstruction is progressive, although the infundibulum is also structurally hypoplastic from birth. At valvar level there is commonly, but not always, obstruction due to fusion or thickening of the cusps. The annulus of the valve is nearly always hypoplastic, often less than half the size of the aortic annulus, and contributes importantly to the obstruction. Finally, a discrete supravalvar obstruction may occur as a stenosis of the main, right or left pulmonary arteries. The main pulmonary artery is frequently small, its size being related to the size of the valve ring. Anomalies of coronary arteries are reported in as many as 9 per cent of cases and are of surgical importance if the anomalous vessel crosses the right ventricular outflow tract.

Diagnosis and Indications for Operation

The diagnosis is made at cardiac catheterization when the anatomy of the VSD and right ventricular outflow tract is demonstrated. Surgery is required when hypoxia is severe, whether episodic in early life or more progressive later.

Operative Surgery

The history of the surgery of this condition virtually encompasses the history of cardiac surgery. Prior to cardiopulmonary bypass Blalock and Taussig realized that the life-threatening hypoxia could be relieved by increasing pulmonary blood flow. In 1945 they introduced the systemic-to-pulmonary artery shunt using the subclavian artery—the first palliative operation. In 1962 Waterston described the ascending aorta to right pulmonary artery anastomosis as an alternative in infancy to the Blalock–Taussig shunt which was technically difficult and often thrombosed in that age group. This operation has been widely used with good early palliation, but recently it has been shown to cause severe deformation of the right pulmonary artery due to kinking at the anastomosis. This results in unilateral perfusion of the right lung through the shunt and severe technical problems at eventual total correction. Brock sought to palliate this condition by increasing pulmonary blood flow by relieving the pulmonary stenosis. His technique was a closed procedure using a dilator, bougies and a punch to resect infundibular muscle. In his hands

excellent results were achieved, but most surgeons found it a difficult and dangerous operation.

The two-stage philosophy of palliation and later correction for Fallot's tetralogy has been questioned by those who advance the policy of primary correction in those infants in whom surgical intervention is necessary. Some surgeons report brilliant results in infancy, but others have not found this to be a successful policy and persist with palliation in the first 2 years of life and total correction later.

Operative Technique for Total Correction

When cardiopulmonary bypass is begun, any systemic to pulmonary artery shunt is ligated or divided. A patent foramen ovale is closed or excluded through a small incision in the right atrium. The site for right ventriculotomy is selected and a vertical incision is made avoiding the coronary arteries, and their important branches (*Fig. 40.17a*). The intraventricular anatomy is carefully inspected and the abnormal muscle bands of the outflow tract are identified and divided or, where appropriate, muscle is excised (*Fig. 40.17b*). Care must be taken to avoid perforation of the free wall of the right ventricle or the interventricular septum, or damage to the papillary muscles of the tricuspid valve or to the aortic valve. Once adequate infundibular resection has been completed the VSD may be seen and repaired in the manner described elsewhere (*Fig. 40.18*). The pulmonary valve may be inspected from below, or if necessary from above, using a separate pulmonary arteriotomy. Commissurotomy or excision of thick cusps should be performed.

The next stage of the correction remains the most difficult. There may be important residual pulmonary stenosis due to hypoplasia of the infundibulum and the valve ring. In the past if the surgeon did not expect this to be a problem then the right ventricle was closed, bypass withdrawn and the pressures measured in the right and left ventricles. If the right ventricular pressure exceeded 0·65–0·70 of the left ventricular pressure in the absence of a high pulmonary vascular resistance, and the right exceeded the left atrial pressure, then important residual pulmonary stenosis was said to be demonstrated and reconstruction of the right ventricular outflow tract was needed. Today, a more precise indicator of the need for this additional procedure is the size of the pulmonary annulus, as measured with bougies before closing the right ventricle. Kirklin has published tables relating annulus size to age or surface area and which indicate the probability of needing further measures to relieve pulmonary stenosis. If these are not needed the ventriculotomy is closed incorporating a small Dacron gusset simply as a technique to avoid further restriction of the outflow tract. If the annulus size indicates that further measures are needed then reconstruction of the right ventricular outflow tract is carried out by extending the vertical incision across

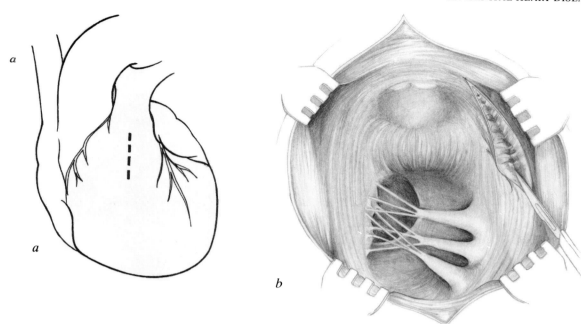

Fig. 40.17. Fallot's tetralogy. *a*, Site of vertical incision in right ventricle. *b*, Infundibular resection. Through an incision in the right ventricle, there may be seen the pulmonary valve, the hypertrophied infundibular muscle and crista supraventricularis and the VSD. Resection of infundibular muscle is being carried out.

the pulmonary valve ring into the main pulmonary artery as far as the bifurcation (*Fig.* 40.19). A large gusset of Dacron or pericardium is sutured into this defect to enlarge the outflow tract, the pulmonary annulus and the pulmonary artery. The pulmonary incompetence resulting from this is believed to be well tolerated in the long term.

RESULTS

The operative mortality for total correction in childhood remains around 10 per cent in most centres,

but in some reports is as low as 5 per cent. The most common mode of operative death is low cardiac output. Late mortality is low and a great majority of patients display excellent physical and educational development and capabilities.

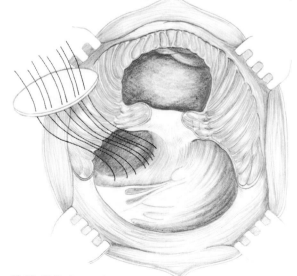

Fig. 40.18. Fallot's tetralogy: patch closure of ventricular septal defect. Extensive infundibular resection has been completed. The septal defect is being closed using a patch, as previously described.

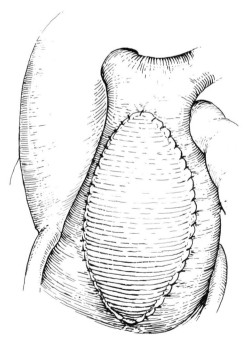

Fig. 40.19. Fallot's tetralogy: reconstruction of right ventricular outflow tract. The vertical incision in the right ventricle has been extended across the annulus of the pulmonary valve, and into the pulmonary artery. The outflow pathway from the right ventricle is enlarged by closing the defect with a patch or gusset.

Operative Techniques for Palliative Surgery

1. BLALOCK–TAUSSIG SHUNT

This, the first palliative operation, remains the most important and widely used. Patients under 2 years of age, with severe cyanosis or severe cyanotic attacks due to Fallot's tetralogy, should be considered for a Blalock–Taussig shunt if it is not the policy of the unit to carry out total correction at that stage. The subclavian artery is selected on the side of the innominate artery. (It is most important not to insert an arterial pressure monitoring cannula in the distribution of the artery to be divided.) The chest is opened at the upper border of the 4th or 5th rib and the lungs retracted gently downwards. The pulmonary artery is identified and freed as far proximally as possible, and distally beyond the origin of the first upper lobe branch. On the right it may be necessary to divide the azygos vein. The subclavian artery is dissected carefully from its origin to beyond its first branches where it will be divided. On the right it should be freed from, and withdrawn through, the loop formed by the vagus nerve and its recurrent laryngeal branch, permitting its origin to be fully mobilized (*Fig.* 40.20*a*). The mediastinal tissues may be carefully dissected and divided to form a bed for the artery as it passes to the pulmonary artery which is now clamped proximally and snared distally. A vertical arteriotomy may be made and the anastomosis constructed with either interrupted or continuous sutures of 6/0 Prolene (*Fig.* 40.20*b*). When the clamps are released a thrill will be a palpable over the anastomosis. If it is necessary to use the subclavian artery arising directly from the aorta, the danger of kinking at its origin may be avoided by using a plastic technique described by Castaneda.

The modified Blalock–Taussig operation is a subclavian artery-to-pulmonary artery shunt using a 5-mm diameter Goretex graft. The subclavian artery remains in continuity and the graft is anastomosed end to side to each artery. In addition to the obvious advantage of maintaining the integrity of the subclavian artery, there is a high incidence of graft patency even in neonates, and therefore many regard this method as the technique of choice. The approach to the right and left Blalock–Taussig shunts (whether classic or modified) at the time of total correction is shown in *Fig.* 40.21.

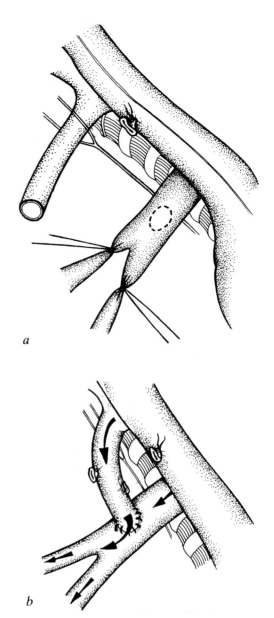

Fig. 40.20. Fallot's tetralogy: palliation with right Blalock–Taussig shunt. *a*, The right subclavian artery is divided and its relationship to the vagus nerve and its recurrent laryngeal branch is shown. The right pulmonary artery is controlled distally by snares and the site of arteriotomy for the anastomosis is shown. *b*, The subclavian artery is withdrawn through the loop formed by the vagus nerve and its branch, and is anastomosed to the pulmonary artery.

2. WATERSTON SHUNT

This operation is used rarely outside the neonatal period or early infancy. A right thoracotomy is performed and the pulmonary artery dissected as for a Blalock–Taussig shunt, taking care to preserve the phrenic nerve. The superior vena cava is mobilized, retracted forwards and the pericardium entered. The right convex border of the ascending aorta is seen and preparations are made to perform a side-to-side anastomosis between the posterior part of the ascending aorta and the anterior part of the right pulmonary artery, in such a way that the pulmonary artery is not deformed. A side-biting clamp is applied to isolate a segment of the aorta and cross-clamp the pulmonary artery in one bite. Corresponding incisions are made in the aorta and in the pulmonary artery so that the communication will not exceed 3 mm in a neonate, or 4 mm in an infant, and the anastomosis constructed with continuous runs of 6/0 Prolene (*Fig.* 40.22).

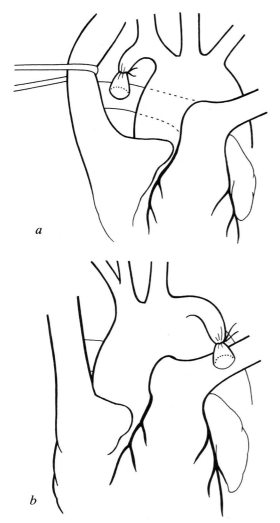

Fig. 40.21. Fallot's tetralogy: ligation of Blalock–Taussig shunt at operation for total correction. Right- (*a*) and left-sided (*b*) anastomosis.

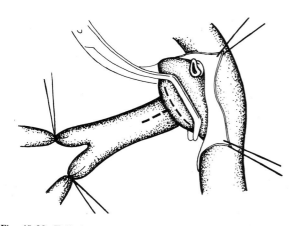

Fig. 40.22. Fallot's tetralogy: palliation with Waterston's shunt. The pericardium is opened, exposing the ascending aorta. Both the ascending aorta and right pulmonary artery are controlled by a side-biting clamp, while the distal pulmonary artery is controlled by snares. The sites of incision in the aorta and the right pulmonary artery are shown.

RESULTS

The mortality of palliative surgery beyond 6 months of age is not greater than 5 per cent. Below that age it may be 10–25 per cent. With the Blalock–Taussig operation an inadequate or thrombosed shunt may occur, while excessive flow causing left ventricular failure is rare. With the Waterston shunt excess flow is common.

TRANSPOSITION OF THE GREAT ARTERIES

Physiology and Natural History

Although only accounting for 5 per cent of all congenital cardiac anomalies, transposition of the great arteries is the most common cyanotic condition presenting at birth. In transposition, the aorta arises anteriorly from the right ventricle and the pulmonary artery posteriorly from the left ventricle. Thus there are two circulations in parallel—while the systemic circulation is desaturated the pulmonary is fully saturated and survival can only occur because limited mixing occurs across an ASD. Untreated, 80–90 per cent of babies born with this condition will not survive until their first birthday, death being chiefly due to hypoxia.

Anatomy and Classification

An ASD alone is present in 70 per cent of cases and in the remaining 30 per cent an ASD, or VSD and pulmonary stenosis are found. Rarely more complex associations of anomalies are present.

Diagnosis and Indications for Operation

Cardiac catheterization permits a firm diagnosis to be made and any associated abnormalities to be identified. If the ASD could be enlarged permitting increased mixing and improved systemic oxygenation, then the immediate threat to life would be averted. Attempts to achieve this by operative means carried a high mortality and have been superseded by the balloon atrial septostomy devised by Rashkind, which is carried out at the time of catheterization and is virtually free of serious hazard. This procedure permits survival to the 2nd year of life in the great majority of babies, so that definitive surgery may be performed between 9 and 15 months of age.

Operative Surgery

Blalock and Hanlon described the technique of closed operative atrial septostomy in 1960. Although it carried a high mortality it remained the only palliation for this condition, until Rashkind introduced his balloon septostomy in 1966. It is now only rarely used as many surgeons will proceed to an open corrective operation if the balloon atrial septostomy fails.

When surgeons first addressed the problem of 'correction' of simple transposition of the great arteries it was believed that 'anatomical correction' by switching the great arteries would be technically impossible due to the proximal origin of the coronary arteries. Therefore the alternative concept of redirecting flow at atrial level was formulated; pulmonary venous blood is directed to the tricuspid valve, the right ventricle and aorta, and systemic venous blood to the mitral valve, the left ventricle and the pulmonary artery. In the late 1950s and the 1960s various techniques to achieve this goal were described, the most notable being that of Senning which used the patient's own atrial tissue and that of Mustard using autologous pericardium or Dacron as the new interatrial septum or 'baffle'. Following Mustard's description of his operation in 1964 it gained popularity and was increasingly widely applied in the early 1970s when intracardiac surgery in infants became more safe. In 1977 Quaegebeur et al. described a modified Senning operation which is now widely practised. Thus, definitive surgery for transposition of the great arteries now takes the form of either the Mustard or the modified Senning operation, both of which achieve physiological but not anatomical correction.

In 1968 Rastelli devised an ingenious approach to anatomical correction for children with transposition of the great arteries, a ventricular septal defect and pulmonary stenosis. He suggested that the ventricular septal defect should be closed in such a way that the left ventricle drained through it to the aorta, the pulmonary valve being closed off. The right ventricle was then connected to the pulmonary artery by an external valved conduit and the atrial septal defect closed. In 1975 Jatene performed the first successful anatomical correction of transposition of the great arteries by arterial switch, with reimplantation of the coronary arteries into the new aorta (Jatene et al., 1976). *Figure* 40.23 shows one method of performing this operation, which may only be done when the left ventricular pressure is high, indicating that the left ventricle will be able to support the systemic circulation immediately after the operation. Thus the operation has an established role in the correction of transposition of the great arteries and a ventricular septal defect. The possibility of using the technique for simple transposition of the great arteries in the neonatal period while pulmonary vascular resistance and hence left ventricular pressure are still high, is presently being explored.

Operative Technique for Definitive Surgery

THE MUSTARD OPERATION

The new interatrial septum or baffle may be made from autologous pericardium or Dacron and is carefully prepared to the shape preferred by the surgeon—rectangular, dumbell shaped or trouser shaped. It is convenient to cannulate the superior vena cava directly and the inferior vena cava as close to the inferior caval atrial junction as possible. The right atrium is opened by an incision extending from the base of the appendage towards the inferior vena cava. The intra-atrial anatomy is carefully inspected and the remains of the intra-atrial septum excised (*Fig.* 40.24); its raw edges are oversewn with interrupted sutures of 5/0 Mersilene or Prolene. The coronary sinus may be cut back into the left atrium if necessary to enlarge the opening between the two atria; marker sutures are inserted above the opening of the right upper and below the opening of the right lower pulmonary vein. The baffle is inserted using a 5/0 Prolene continuous suture. One edge is sutured around the pulmonary veins with a U-shaped suture line which is open towards the right. The other edge is sutured to the remnant of the atrial septum and continued in either direction around the caval orifices as shown in *Fig.* 40.25a. Thus, systemic venous blood will flow deep to the baffle (as the surgeon sees it) to the mitral valve while pulmonary venous blood will flow forward over the baffle to the tricuspid valve. The pulmonary venous pathway may be narrow at the level of the old intra-atrial septum, and it may be enlarged by inserting a gusset of pericardium or Dacron into a further incision from the original atriotomy extending posteriorly between the right pulmonary veins (*Fig.* 40.25b).

THE SENNING OPERATION

This operation is most easily performed using a single venous cannula, profound hypothermia and circulatory arrest. The right atrium is opened with a vertical incision 4 mm anterior to the crista terminalis (*Fig.* 40.26a). The atrial septum is mobilized as a flap based on its right lateral attachment (*Fig.* 40.26b); this flap is then attached to the left lateral wall of the left atrium in front of the pulmonary veins and behind the mitral valve, completing the suture line in the roof and floor of the left atrium (*Fig.* 40.26c). The atrial septal defect is closed with a patch or by direct suture as appropriate. The exit for pulmonary venous blood is created by opening the left atrium at its junction with the right pulmonary veins (*Fig.* 40.26d); this opening may be enlarged by extending the incision onto a pulmonary vein. The systemic venous pathway is now constructed by using that part of the right atrial wall which lay posterior to the original incision and suturing it to the remnant of the atrial septum and around the caval orifices (*Fig.* 40.26d); thus caval blood passes to the mitral valve. The pulmonary venous pathway is constructed using that part of the right atrial wall which is anterior to the original incision, and its edge is sutured over the superior vena cava and inferior vena cava and around the edge of the incision in the right pulmonary veins, thus allowing pulmonary venous blood to pass forward to the tricuspid valve (*Fig.* 40.26e). When performing the final suture line it is important to avoid damage

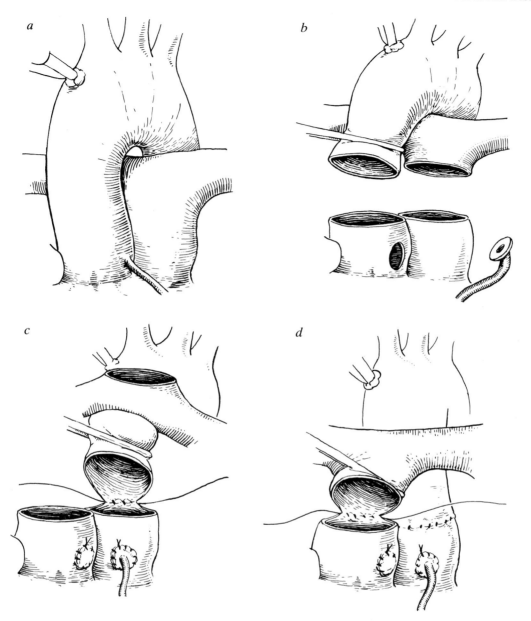

Fig. 40.23. The arterial switch operations or anatomical correction for transposition of the great arteries. *a,* The abnormal anatomy with anterior aorta. *b,* Both vessels transected and coronary ostia excised with a cuff of aorta. *c,* Aorta repositioned behind the bifurcation of the pulmonary artery. The coronary arteries are reimplanted into the new aorta, and the original defect closed with a patch. *d,* The nearly finished work.

to the sinuatrial node and to avoid constricting the suture line which passes over the cavae; the suture line around the pulmonary veins is completed using interrupted sutures.

RESULTS

The operative mortality for either of these operations is close to 5 per cent regardless of age. The great majority of children have an excellent result enjoying normal physical growth and ordinary education. Because it is a physiological and not an anatomical correction it may be regarded as a definitive, not a corrective procedure. It may be for this reason that three possible late complications may occur. First, there may be a high incidence of dysrhythmias, most commonly junctional rhythm, following the extensive atrial incisions and suturing; it is possible that this may lead to late sudden death in a very small number of patients. Second, narrowing of the newly constructed pathways may occur, leading to obstruction of the superior vena cava or pulmonary venous pathway; the latter is invariably fatal without further surgery to revise the pathway. Those who use the

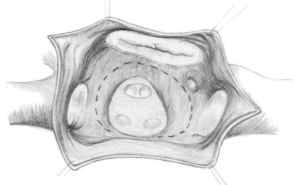

Fig. 40.24. Transposition of the great arteries: the Mustard operation. The left atrium and pulmonary veins may be seen through the ASD. The dotted line indicates the line of resection of the atrial septum.

Senning operation believe that pathway obstruction will be much less common than following the Mustard procedure; much longer follow-up is necessary, however, before this hope can be confirmed. Finally, the fundamental assumption that the right ventricle and tricuspid valve can support systemic pressures indefinitely remains unproved. However, 10-year follow-up after the Mustard operation indicates that 85–90 per cent of children are alive and well, and it is hoped that currently performed Mustard and Senning operations will yield even better results.

Operative Techniques for Palliative Surgery

The Blalock–Hanlon closed operative septectomy is carried out through a right anterolateral thoracotomy and the pericardium entered immediately in front of the phrenic nerve. Snares should be placed on the right pulmonary artery and veins. A side-biting clamp is placed on the septum including some wall of the right and left atria and the orifices of both right pulmonary veins. Two incisions are made parallel to the septum, one anterior and the other posterior. The septum is grasped and drawn to the right as the side-clamp is partly released. A section of septum is now excised, leaving an interatrial septal defect of substantial size.

RESULTS

This operation is rarely performed now, but the operative mortality was as high as 45 per cent in the late 1960s.

LESS COMMON ANOMALIES

Total Anomalous Pulmonary Venous Drainage

In this condition the pulmonary veins are usually confluent and drain to the right atrium via the left innominate vein, the coronary sinus or the inferior vena cava, and not to the left atrium. Blood reaches the left side of the heart through an ASD. There may also be obstruction at some point on the pulmonary venous pathway. This condition nearly always threatens life in early infancy and corrective surgery is designed to anastomose the common pulmonary venous chamber to the left atrium. The operative mortality is between 30 and 50 per cent. The late results are encouraging.

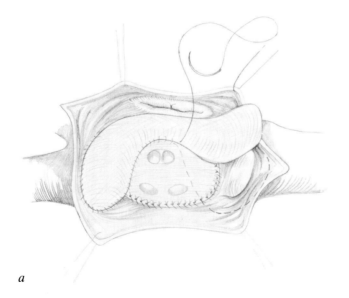

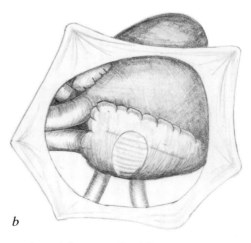

a

b

Fig. 40.25. Transposition of the great arteries: the Mustard operation. *a*, The cut edges of the resected atrial septum are oversewn with interrupted sutures. The new baffle is partly inserted; the SVC pathway is complete and the IVC pathway is being constructed. *b*, The pulmonary venous pathway has been enlarged by making a transverse incision from the atriotomy, backwards between the right pulmonary veins. The defect is closed with a patch or gusset of Dacron or pericardium.

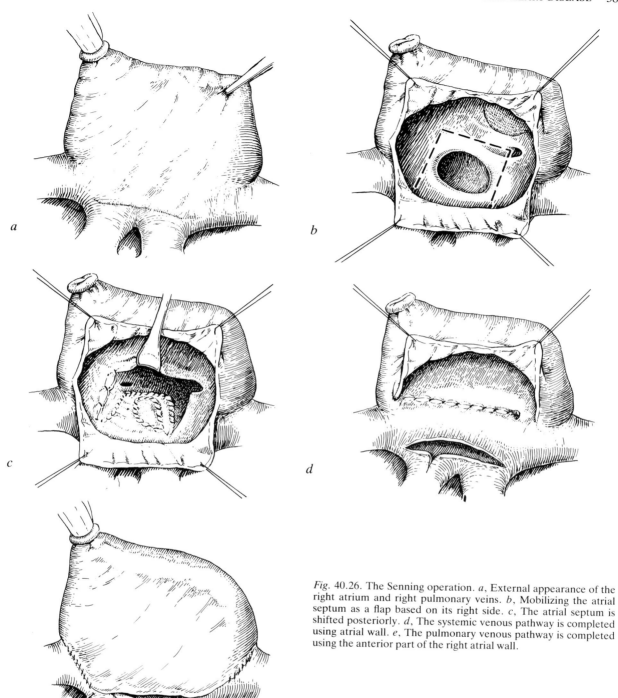

Fig. 40.26. The Senning operation. *a*, External appearance of the right atrium and right pulmonary veins. *b*, Mobilizing the atrial septum as a flap based on its right side. *c*, The atrial septum is shifted posteriorly. *d*, The systemic venous pathway is completed using atrial wall. *e*, The pulmonary venous pathway is completed using the anterior part of the right atrial wall.

Persisting Truncus Arteriosus

In persisting truncus arteriosus one great vessel only leaves the heart and a VSD is always present. The pulmonary arteries arise directly from this vessel and, therefore, blood flow to the lungs is high and is at a high pressure. Life is threatened by left ventricular failure and pulmonary vascular disease in infancy. Palliative measures have been disappointing and anatomical correction with a valved conduit from the right ventricle to the pulmonary artery, together with closure of the VSD, is currently the treatment of choice.

Tricupsid Atresia

In tricuspid atresia there is no communication from the right atrium to the right ventricle and blood passes to the left atrium through an ASD. If the great vessels are normally related there is usually severe pulmonary oligaemia, as the only sources of pulmonary blood flow are a patent ductus arteriosus and bronchial collaterals. If there is also transposition of the great arteries a large VSD is usual, with high pulmonary flows and pressures, which may lead to heart failure and pulmonary vascular disease. Palliative measures are often required in infancy and are designed to either increase or reduce the pulmonary blood flow, as indicated. The best approach to physiological correction is to perform the Fontan operation later in childhood; in this procedure the right atrium is anastomosed to the pulmonary artery or vestigial right ventricular outflow tract, either directly or using a tube conduit.

Ebstein's Anomaly

In Ebstein's anomaly there is an abnormal tricuspid valve which is displaced into the right ventricle; the part of the right ventricle which lies between the actual and usual sites of the tricuspid valve is thin walled and aneurysmal; there is usually an ASD. Hypoxia, dysrhythmias and right-sided heart failure may develop during childhood or early adult life. Correction involves repair or replacement of the tricuspid valve, exclusion of the abnormal part of the right ventricle and closure of ASD. The conducting system is at risk. The operative risk is between 10 and 25 per cent.

Complete Atrioventricular Canal

In complete atrioventricular canal there is a composite defect involving both the atrial and ventricular septa and the mitral and tricuspid valves. Correction involves reconstruction of the atrioventricular valves and both the atrial and ventricular septa. The procedure is complex and the most important complications are residual mitral incompetence and heart block.

Aortic Arch Abnormalities

In double aortic arch the trachea and oesophagus lie between the right and left arches and are compressed, causing stridor which usually presents in infancy. The diagnosis is based on a barium swallow which shows an indentation due to the abnormal aortic anatomy. Aortography may confirm the precise aortic anatomy and the condition is treated by division of the lesser of the two arches through a left thoracotomy.

In interruption of the aortic arch there is always a VSD and a patent ductus arteriosus which fills the descending aorta. Left ventricular failure presents in infancy and is usually life threatening. At operation continuity of the aorta may be restored with either biological or prosthetic materials, and is occasionally successful, but a high operative risk is involved. The VSD is closed and the ductus divided.

FURTHER READING

Barratt-Boyes B. G., Simpson M. and Neutze J. M. (1971) Intracardiac surgery in neonates and infants using deep hypothermia with surface cooling and limited cardiopulmonary bypass. *Circulation* **43–44**, Suppl. 1–25.

Blackstone E. H., Kirklin J. W., Bradrey E. L. et al. (1976) Optimal age and results in repair of large ventricular septal defects. *J. Thorac. Cardiovasc. Surg.* **72**, 661–679.

Chiariello L., Agosti J., Ulad P. et al. (1976) Congenital aortic stenosis. *J. Thorac. Cardiovasc. Surg.* **72**, 182–193.

Danielson G. K., Exarhos N. D., Weidman W. H. et al. (1971) Pulmonic stenosis with intact ventricular septum. *J. Thorac. Cardiovasc. Surg.* **61**, 228–234.

Hamilton D. I., DiEusanio G., Sandrasagra F. A. et al. (1978) Early and late results of aortoplasty with a left subclavian flap for coarctation of the aorta in infancy. *J. Thorac. Cardiovasc. Surg.* **75**, 699–704.

Jatene A. D., Fontes V. F., Pallista P. P. et al. (1976) Anatomic correction of transposition of the great vessels. *J. Thorac. Cardiovasc. Surg.* **72**, 364–370.

Kirklin J. W. and Karp R. B. (1970) *The Tetralogy of Fallot*. Philadelphia, Saunders.

Lincoln J. C. R., Deverall P. B., Stark J. et al. (1969) Vascular anomalies compressing the oesophagus and trachea. *Thorax* **24**, 295–306.

McMullan M. H., McGoon D. C., Wallace R. B. et al. (1973) Surgical treatment of partial atrioventricular canal. *Arch. Surg.* **107**, 705–710.

Panagopoulos P. G., Tatooles C. J., Aberdeen E. et al. (1971) Patent ductus arteriosus in infants and children. *Thorax* **26**, 137–144.

Quaegebeur J. M., Rohmer J., Brom A. G. et al. (1977) Revival of the Senning operation in the treatment of transposition of the great arteries. *Thorax* **32**, 517–524.

Stark J. and deLeval M. (1983) *Surgery for Congenital Heart Defects*. London, Grune and Stratton.

Stark J., deLeval M. R., Waterston D. J. et al. (1974) Corrective surgery of transposition of the great arteries in the first year of life. *J. Thorac. Cardiovasc. Surg.* **67**, 673–681.

Tawes R. L., Aberdeen E., Waterston D. J. et al. (1969) Coarctation of the aorta in infants and children. *Circulation* **39–40**, Suppl. 1, 1–173 to 1–184.

Chapter forty-one

Acquired Heart Disease

G. Keen

SURGERY OF THE PERICARDIUM

Pericardial Aspiration

Aspiration of the pericardium is required for either diagnostic purposes, when a small amount of fluid is removed for examination, or for the relief of large pericardial effusions which may be causing circulatory embarrassment or pericardial tamponade. These effusions may be pus or blood, or may be inflammatory or transudatory effusions.

Pericardial aspiration should not be undertaken lightly, for patients requiring this are usually very ill, and cardiac arrest may be precipitated even by experienced operators. This procedure should be carried out under sterile conditions and adjacent to facilities for immediate resuscitation and exploratory thoracotomy. This last remark applies particularly to patients undergoing pericardial aspiration for the relief of pericardial tamponade caused by stabbing, for these dangerously ill patients readily undergo cardiac arrest during this procedure.

The patient is sat up at an angle of 45°. The site of insertion of the needle is between the left border of the xiphisternum and the right border of the 6th left costal cartilage (*Fig.* 41.1). A local anaesthetic

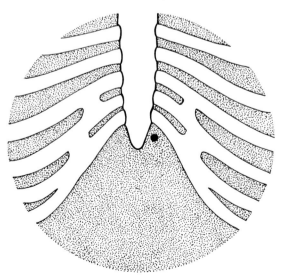

Fig. 41.1. Site for pericardial aspiration.

is introduced into the subcutaneous tissues and skin and injected down to the pericardium. The patient is monitored with electrocardiography during this procedure and this is watched very carefully for evidence of arrhythmias. Some advocate that the aspiration needle be used as an exploring electrode, contact with the heart producing an altered electrical complex, although the value of this refinement is doubtful. The aspiration needle should be strong, and at least 12 cm in length, attached to a three-way tap and a 20-ml syringe. A plastic cannula is an alternative. From the site of insertion into the skin it is passed upwards and backwards at an angle of 45° to a point midway between the patient's shoulder blades (*Fig.* 41.2). While being inserted, continuous

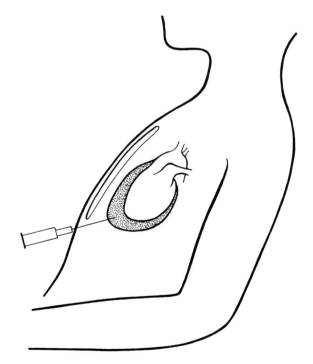

Fig. 41.2. Ideal position of patient for pericardial aspiration.

negative suction is applied at the syringe, and when pericardial fluid is withdrawn further insertion is terminated. The scratchy sensation of the heart moving against the end of the needle is unforgettable and when this is felt the needle must be withdrawn a little.

Treatment of Chronic Pericardial Effusions

Such effusions may be inflammatory or malignant or may occur as an event during renal failure. Although repeated pericardiocentesis may provide temporary relief from the effusion, it is justified in some circumstances to advise surgical decompression. This may be achieved by removal of a large pericardial window. The pericardium is approached by anterior left thoracotomy through the 5th intercostal space. As large a portion as possible of pericardium anterior to the phrenic nerve is then excised, taking care to ensure haemostasis at the cut edges, which may, in inflammatory situations, be exceedingly vascular. It is, however, preferable to resect the pericardium as completely as is possible in these patients, for this is a more definitive procedure than the creation of a simple window and it is more likely to have long-term benefits for the patient.

CHRONIC CONSTRICTIVE PERICARDITIS

Constrictive pericarditis is the terminal stage of a chronic inflammatory process which produces a fibrous, thickened and often calcified restrictive coat around the heart. This constricting layer prevents diastolic relaxation of the heart which in turn gives rise to the physical signs and symptoms of constrictive pericarditis. The cause of this condition was at one time considered to be tuberculous but more frequently it is the end result of a pyogenic or viral infection, of previous trauma, or it may be a rare late complication of haemorrhagic pericarditis. The diagnosis is made clinically, radiologically and at cardiac catheterization.

Surgical Treatment

The aim of surgery is to remove as completely as possible the fibrous layer and both serous layers of the pericardium. Although the thickened and calcified layer may envelop the entire heart, the deleterious effect of constrictive pericarditis is largely on ventricular relaxation. The object of surgery is to release both ventricles and as a secondary procedure to turn attention to removal of the pericardium covering the atria. The pericardium over the atria, although part of the process, rarely obstructs emptying of the atria, although some cases have been reported in which constricting bands are said to have caused narrowing at the atrioventricular ring. Again, some patients have been shown to have constricting rings of pericardium around the superior and inferior vena caval entrances into the heart, which may require attention.

Surgical Approach

The approach for the removal of the constricted and adherent pericardium may be either median sternotomy, left thoracotomy or bilateral anterior thoracotomy. Median sternotomy has the advantage that the right atrium and ventricle and the venae cavae may be safely cleared of pericardium together with the lateral aspect of the left ventricle and the inferior surface of the heart. Nevertheless, using this exposure it is frequently extremely difficult and sometimes dangerous to gain good access to the posterior aspect of the left ventricle and of the left atrioventricular groove. Since it is most important to completely decompress the left ventricle, it is considered by many that extended left thoracotomy is the exposure of choice in this condition. The incision is made through the bed of the 5th left rib. This exposure gives an excellent view of the whole of the lateral and inferior border of the heart and enables safe clearing of the left ventricle, left atrium, inferior surface of the heart and of the right ventricle to be achieved. However, the unilateral left anterior thoracic approach, although adequate for limited decortications, is considered by some to be inadequate for the more radical pericardiectomy preferred by most surgeons. Furthermore, inadequate exposure does not allow complete removal of the pericardium and does not permit the operator to handle effectively any emergency such as major haemorrhage from the right atrium or right ventricle. The extent of pericardial resection can be determined only at operation and poor results can invariably be attributed to insufficient removal of pericardium. Should left thoracotomy be chosen as the approach, and if it is then discovered that further access is required, the incision may be extended across and transecting the sternum, entering the right 4th intercostal space.

The author favours median sternotomy, with the patient in the supine position on the operating table and with the arms by the side. Should left thoracotomy be chosen, the patient should be placed in the supine position but with the arms at right angles to the side and supported by appropriate operating table fittings. The incision will then extend from the left midaxillar line to the left border of the sternum and enter the 4th intercostal space following subperiosteal stripping of the upper border of the 5th rib. Should further access be necessary, the sternum is transected with a Gigli saw, the internal mammary vessels on either side of the sternum are doubly ligated and divided and the incision then extended into the right 4th intercostal space. Median sternotomy gives the patient a far more comfortable postoperative course than does bilateral thoracotomy. It is clear that there is no ideal operative approach for this condition.

When the surgical field is exposed, it is important to select a portion of the pericardium, to begin the dissection, which is less tightly attached to the underlying heart. The important hazards of this operation are damage to the coronary arteries and the opening of a cardiac chamber. Although the heart can be repaired, perhaps with difficulty, damage to a major coronary artery is extremely serious. With the development of a plane of cleavage, scissors, knife and blunt dissection will gradually extend the dissection away from the incision. Dissection proceeds initially over the left ventricle, and after the development

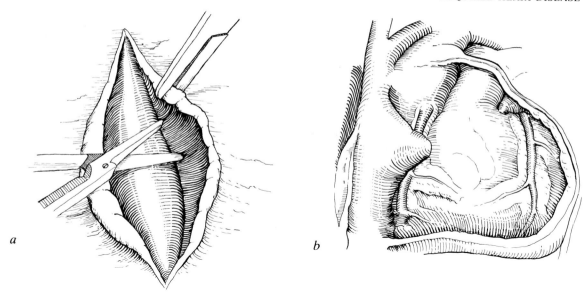

Fig. 41.3. Constrictive pericarditis. Blunt dissection of the pericardium from the right and left ventricles.

of a long incision in the enveloping pericardium which is then undermined (*Fig.* 41.3*a*), the ventricle bulges out in an unrestrained fashion, allowing immediate improvement in the patient's cardiac output. The thickened pericardium may contain layers of organizing and crumbling purulent contents, and in many instances the pericardium is heavily calcified and up to 1 cm thick. The use of bone shears is frequently necessary to complete the procedure. As much pericardium as possible is cleared from the left ventricle, followed by the right ventricle, the left atrioventricular groove and the right atrium. Should an opening into or even through the myocardium occur, it is controlled by sutures supported by Teflon felt pledgets. Should the atria be opened prior to release of the ventricles, the persistent high intra-atrial pressures will precipitate serious bleeding, difficult to control other than by a swab applied and held in place until ventricular release of the pericardial constriction allows some fall in venous pressure. Care is taken to avoid damage to the phrenic nerves, which may be difficult to identify in the inflammatory process.

The base of the heart is cleared backwards across the diaphragm for as far as it is accessible. Following removal of the thickened pericardial layer, the surface of the myocardium should be carefully examined, for there may be a considerable amount of thickened, semi-opaque serous membrane which remains to constrict the action of the heart, and this membrane must then be attended to. The myocardium is more readily seen through this membrane and a point is chosen, where no coronary vessels are seen, to begin the dissection. With patient gauze and knife dissection this layer may eventually be removed piecemeal, completing relief of the condition. Following pericardiectomy, there will be considerable oozing from the denuded myocardial surface but this

readily ceases with prolonged gauze pressure (*Fig.* 41.3*b*).

The use of cardiopulmonary bypass during pericardiectomy has some advocates. This undoubtedly complicates an otherwise usually straightforward procedure, and the heparinization required will increase the operative and postoperative haemorrhage. At the present time the majority of surgeons prefer to undertake this operation without the assistance of cardiopulmonary bypass.

ACQUIRED DISEASE OF THE MITRAL VALVE

Mitral Stenosis

Assessment
It is remarkable that the symptoms frequently bear little relation to the degree of mitral stenosis. Some patients with extremely severe stenosis may continue to work almost entirely without symptoms whereas others with moderate stenosis may be extremely dyspnoeic on effort. Although in many patients the physical signs and symptoms may correlate with the degree of severity, other more objective methods of assessing mitral stenosis are required.

The most important of these are the mitral valve gradient and the pulmonary wedge or left atrial pressure measured at cardiac catheterization, both at rest and on exercise. At this investigation measurement of the pulmonary vascular resistance and an assessment of the tricuspid valve and of the aortic valve are also important. Echocardiography is routinely conducted to ensure that the patient's symptoms are not due to an atrial myxoma, and will offer reliable evidence of the degree of stenosis, the rigidity and thickness of the valve cusps and of the presence of calcification. Unfortunately, intra-atrial thrombi are not readily detectable using echocardiography, although myxomas are readily diagnosed by this means. Left ventricular ciné-angiocardiography ensures the detection of mitral regurgitation. In those with few or no symptoms, but in whom very high left atrial pressures are recorded, operation should be advised despite apparent wellbeing, for they may develop serious or fatal pulmonary oedema in response to stress, exercise, pregnancy or on alteration from sinus rhythm to atrial fibrillation.

Treatment

Following the earliest successful closed mitral valvotomy undertaken by Souttar in 1925, the operation was largely abandoned until 1949, when Bailey, Harken and Brock demonstrated independently the value of closed digital commissurotomy (Harken et al., 1948; Bailey, 1949; Baker et al., 1950). This operation has since been undertaken successfully in hundreds of thousands of patients with rheumatic mitral stenosis. Modifications of the technique of valvotomy, such as the use of small intracardiac knives and later the introduction of mechanical dilators, produced a more successful mitral commissurotomy, developing the standard operation for the next 25 years. With the development of open heart surgery and the current extremely low risk associated with its use, it seems clear that open commissurotomy using cardiopulmonary bypass has in most cardiac surgical centres emerged as the operation of choice and has superseded closed valvotomy almost entirely. This seems surprising when one considers the long-term relief from symptoms obtained by countless patients who have undergone closed mitral valvotomy in the past. Many long series of patients treated by closed valvotomy have been studied and these demonstrate that a large proportion are free of, or are greatly relieved of, symptoms for as long as 15 years, and that when further operation is required the subsequent open valvotomy or open mitral valve replacement is done with comparative ease and safety.

There is no doubt that in the past many patients were submitted to closed mitral commissurotomy when the valve was clearly unsuitable for this operation due to calcification, mitral regurgitation or extreme rigidity. In the presence of a rigid valve, even a full-length commissurotomy will not result in reduction of left atrial pressure, for a high left atrial pressure is required to open the rigid cusps. Nevertheless, with careful clinical examination, cardiac catheterization and angiocardiography, together with echocardiography, it should be possible to separate those whose purely stenotic, mobile and fibrous valves will be suitable for closed valvotomy from those whose rigid or calcified valves will require re-

placement using cardiopulmonary bypass. There is, however, the important risk of intraoperative embolism to be considered, for in many patients with chronic rheumatic heart disease and atrial fibrillation, intra-atrial thrombosis and the organization of these clots within the atrial appendage commonly occur. There is no doubt that the risk of intraoperative dislodgement of such thrombi is greater during closed surgery than it is during open heart surgery. It is unfortunately the case that there are younger patients, in sinus rhythm, who may harbour thrombi within the atrial appendage which may be dislodged during closed valvotomy.

Nevertheless, having excluded those with a rigid or calcified valve, those with associated important aortic or tricuspid valve disease, and others in whom intra-atrial thrombosis is likely, there remain a considerable number of patients with pure stenosis of a fibrous, mobile valve who are suitable for closed valvotomy. It is this group of patients in whom there is a predictably extremely low operative mortality and low morbidity and in whom relief of symptoms will be extremely prolonged, in many cases for 10–15 years. One danger of open commissurotomy is that inspection of the valve may persuade the surgeon that the valve is unworthy of salvage and it may consequently be removed and replaced by a prosthetic valve, perhaps unnecessarily. There seems little doubt that very many valves which have been successfully opened by closed procedures would, if viewed at open heart surgery, have been removed and replaced by a prosthetic valve, due to their unpromising appearance.

Nevertheless, the assessment of patients for closed mitral valvotomy and the undertaking of this operation are becoming less frequent each year and it is likely that future generations of cardiac surgeons will be unfamiliar with this procedure and resort universally to open operations on the mitral valve under all circumstances and will consider closed mitral valvotomy to be obsolete. Open valvotomy offers certain advantages over closed valvotomy. There is little doubt that closed valvotomy will not relieve the obstruction caused by fusion of the subvalvar mechanism and it is in this group of patients, perhaps 20 per cent of those with mitral stenosis, that open valvotomy is so successful. Under vision, separation of the chordae tendineae which are fused to the underlying papillary muscles, débridement of calcium and selected annuloplasty are now possible. At the present time, therefore, it is fair to say that the previously widely undertaken operation of closed mitral valvotomy is rapidly giving way to open valvotomy. It is necessary to appreciate that the majority of patients with rheumatic mitral stenosis live in developing countries, and there is little doubt that closed valvotomy will be the operation of choice in those regions for very many years to come. It is inevitable that open heart surgery will not be universally available in poor countries for at least another generation.

Mitral Valvotomy in Pregnancy

From time to time, a previously asymptomatic patient develops pulmonary oedema in the last trimester of pregnancy, and mitral stenosis is shown to be responsible. There is little dispute that for reasons of safety, for both the mother and the unborn child, closed mitral valvotomy is the operation of choice.

Closed Mitral Valvotomy

With improved selection of patients, the great majority of closed mitral valvotomies are carried out without complication. Nevertheless, there is the occasional patient prepared for closed valvotomy who is found at operation to be unsuitable, due to excessive valve calcification, intra-atrial thrombosis or the presence of previously undetected mitral regurgitation, or unsuspected atrial myxoma. Rarely, there may be an accident at the time of closed surgery, producing a serious tear of the left atrial wall or overwhelming mitral regurgitation. For these reasons, it is an advantage to have immediate pump stand-by so that the operation can be converted from a closed procedure to cardiopulmonary bypass without delay.

PREOPERATIVE PREPARATION

It is safe to discontinue digoxin 24 hours prior to surgery, for many patients on this drug tend otherwise to experience significant postoperative bradycardia with consequent problems of management. Should the patient be in severe heart failure, it may be necessary to continue diuretic therapy up to the time of operation.

It is generally agreed that all patients with atrial fibrillation who are to be submitted to mitral valvotomy should be adequately treated by an anticoagulant such as warfarin for some months prior to surgery. This will frequently prevent further deposition of left atrial thrombus and enable soft thrombus, which is already within the atrial appendage and the atrium, to organize and adhere to the left atrial wall. Unfortunately, despite therapeutically maintained levels of anticoagulant therapy, there have been frequent instances of cerebral or peripheral embolism occurring during mitral valvotomy, and it is the unpredictability of this complication that prompts surgeons away from closed valvotomy and to consider open mitral valvotomy using cardiopulmonary bypass to be the lesser risk. It is wise to maintain therapeutic levels of warfarin through the operation and to continue indefinitely postoperatively, for if anticoagulant therapy is discontinued several days prior to surgery in order to diminish operative bleeding, further thrombi might form within the left atrial appendage with possible disastrous results.

THE OPERATION

The patient is placed on the operating table lying on the right side, rotated backwards at about 30°. The incision is a left anterolateral thoracotomy extending from 5 cm from the midline, passing underneath the left breast and extending just distal to and below the angle of the left scapula. The chest is opened through the 5th left intercostal space. The pericardium is opened vertically posterior to the phrenic nerve and this incision extends from the diaphragm up to the pulmonary artery. Stay sutures are inserted into the edges of the pericardium to expose the left side of the heart and the pulmonary veins.

It is useful to measure the left atrial pressure and the pulmonary artery pressure at operation and to record these before and following valvotomy.

It is necessary that the left atrial appendage is handled as little as possible during the preliminary manoeuvres, for it is within this part of the left atrial chamber that soft, mobile thrombus may be loosely adherent. It is usual to place a purse-string of heavy Mersilene at the base of the appendage to aid control of the operation and finally to obliterate the appendage when it is tied. When this purse-string suture is inserted, care should be taken that only the epicardium is picked up with the needle, for penetration of the atrium at this stage may cause severe bleeding should the left atrial pressure be very high, which is usually the case. A plastic tube is slid on to the purse-string to act as a snare. The tip of the appendage is gently grasped with forceps and is opened with scissors. The appendage is then lightly grasped with the finger and thumb and forceps are placed on the edge of this incision, allowing the escape of 100 ml or so of blood, enabling loose thrombus to be washed out. The right lubricated index finger is then introduced into the left atrial appendage and the left atrium. It may be necessary to tighten the purse-string but usually the finger will fit snugly through the incision and obstruct the left atrial appendage adequately, ensuring that bleeding does not occur.

The finger is then passed to the mitral valve, where the pathology and function are assessed. Should the preoperative assessment prove to be correct, the valve will feel mobile and there will be a tightly stenotic orifice which will not admit the tip of the finger, the edges of the stenosis being fibrous and rolled. The valve should be palpated for calcium, its extent determined, and the atrium just proximal to the valve carefully assessed for mitral regurgitation, which is often difficult. Even in the presence of marked mitral regurgitation a jet may not be palpable, whereas mild regurgitation through a fine jet may readily be noted. If during the introduction of the finger large amounts of thrombus are palpated, it is wise to withdraw, ligate the purse-string and to abandon the closed procedure at this stage. The risk of producing massive systemic or cerebral embolism is so real that the operation should be conducted either at the time or later using cardiopulmonary bypass under safe conditions.

Similarly, should more than a trivial amount of mitral regurgitation be encountered, the closed operation should be abandoned, for mitral valve replacement will be the operation of choice.

Should unsuspected calcification be detected in the valve, a decision needs to be made at the time whether or not mitral valvotomy should be undertaken by the closed procedure. This operation carries the risk that fragments of calcium may be carried into the systemic circulation with possible serious consequences. Furthermore, calcification of the valve implies that the valve is probably more rigid than expected and that closed valvotomy will produce an indifferent and only short-term result. Nevertheless, numerous patients with calcific mitral stenosis have undergone successful mitral valvotomy with excellent long-term results. Despite this experience it is probably wiser to convert the operation from a closed procedure to an open operation, should valve calcification be more than trivial.

Hopefully, the selection of the patient has avoided either a calcified valve, a regurgitant valve, or the presence of much interatrial thrombus, and the operation can now be completed.

The original operation of mitral commissurotomy was that of opening of the adherent commissures using the finger, and was undertaken in many patients seemingly successfully for some years. Nevertheless, it is now clear that very few patients are suitable for finger commissurotomy, for the valve is usually too thickened and fused for this to be successful. In earlier days the use of small knives, which were attached to the index finger and introduced into the heart to cut the commissures, was fashionable, and certainly many patients benefited from such an operation. Nevertheless, many more patients were given important mitral regurgitation due to either an inadvertent cut into a cusp or division of the chordae tendineae

below the valve. Finger commissurotomy and the use of intracardiac knives are now considered to be both dangerous and ineffective in the majority of patients. It is now the invariable practice of all surgeons to use a dilator within the mitral valve, the usual instrument being the Tubbs dilator.

A tiny stab is made at the apex of the left ventricle in the small muscular area placed between the fat surrounding the anterior descending branch of the left coronary artery and the marginal artery, using a fine artery forceps. This is enlarged with heavier artery forceps or a sound, following which the closed dilator is passed into the left ventricle. It is passed up to the mitral stenotic orifice from below, passing through into the left atrium to meet the tip of the right index finger (*Fig.* 41.4). It is important that the instrument be passed completely into the heart, for opening of the Tubbs dilator with part of its opening mechanism within the left ventricular wall may cause tearing of this wall and serious haemorrhage. At this stage it is wise to take an extra precaution to ensure that, should a piece of calcium or clot be dislodged, these will not enter the cerebral circulation. The anaesthetist is therefore asked to compress both common carotid arteries for a 30-sec period while the valvotomy is being undertaken. This compression ensures stasis of the arterial circulation to the head for this period, and it is hoped that pieces of calcium or thrombus will be swept around the aortic arch into the descending aorta. The dilator is then opened, and whether this is undertaken gradually, as several movements, or as one swifter movement is a matter for debate. It is the author's practice to use one swift movement with the dilator set at 4 cm, and it is remarkable that mitral valvotomy almost invariably occurs in the line of the fused commissures. The dilator is then withdrawn from the valve but remains in the ventricle while the valve and subvalvar appara-

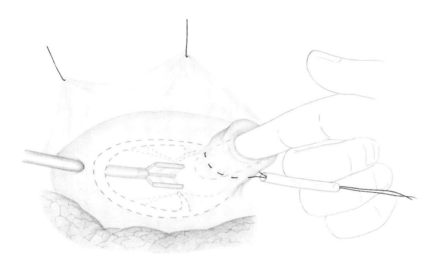

Fig. 41.4. Closed mitral valvotomy. The Tubbs dilator is passed through the apex of the left ventricle towards the tip of the finger introduced through the left atrial appendage.

tus are palpated to estimate the degree of residual stenosis and to determine whether or not regurgitation of the valve has been produced. It is sometimes necessary to reintroduce the dilator into the valve for further commissurotomy.

Closed valvotomy is an operation which should not be overdone, for if the valve is split completely to the ring and both commissures are totally separated, interference with the support of the leaflets to the valve ring and cardiac skeleton may follow with consequent severe mitral regurgitation. Following satisfactory valvotomy, the closed dilator is withdrawn from the left ventricle and the resultant wound is covered with a small swab for several minutes. This usually seals spontaneously but it is wise to reinforce its closure with two sutures of 3/0 Mersilene. The finger is withdrawn from the left atrial appendage and as this is done the purse-string is tied, which obliterates the left atrial appendage.

During the early years of this operation there was great controversy over the management of the atrial appendage. Many believed that the appendage should be carefully sutured and left for use at second and subsequent valvotomies, but there is no doubt that this diverticulum is an ideal site for further thrombus formation and possible embolic complications from this. It is now the practice of all surgeons to either amputate and suture the appendage or to ligate it, which obliterates this potentially dangerous backwater.

Following valvotomy the left atrial and pulmonary artery pressures are again measured and in the majority of patients a dramatic fall in left atrial pressure will have been obtained. The pericardium is irrigated and loosely closed with interrupted sutures. It is important that the pericardium be closed to avoid herniation of the heart postoperatively. The chest is closed with an intrapleural drain.

OPERATIVE COMPLICATIONS

Apart from the complications which may beset any surgical or cardiac surgical operation the particular complications of closed mitral valvotomy are traumatic mitral incompetence and systemic embolism.

1. *Traumatic mitral incompetence*: In a patient with pure mitral stenosis, the left ventricle is a small atrophic chamber. Should even moderate mitral incompetence be produced during valvotomy the sudden increase in work required by this ventricle may overwhelm it, resulting in acute left ventricular failure with pulmonary oedema and congestive cardiac failure. This complication is seen from time to time and if mild to moderate is readily controlled by medical treatment using digoxin, diuretics and bed rest. Given time the left ventricle will hypertrophy and cope adequately with this amount of mitral regurgitation.

Severe degrees of traumatic mitral incompetence

may produce almost instant pulmonary oedema and require emergency mitral valve replacement with the use of cardiopulmonary bypass if the patient is to survive. This serious situation is very uncommon and has not been encountered in a personal experience of over 1000 closed mitral valvotomies.

Between these two extremes is the occasional patient in whom more than moderately severe mitral regurgitation is produced and who remains in severe congestive failure with pulmonary oedema postoperatively and who will require mitral valve replacement using cardiopulmonary bypass within a few days of the first operation. The author has had this experience in one patient only.

2. *Systemic embolism*: This may take the form of cerebral embolism of thrombus or of calcium, or of peripheral arterial embolism into a limb or mesenteric vessels. Invariably the thrombus which lodges peripherally originates from within the left atrium or the left atrial appendage. Occasionally small fragments of calcium produce showers of fine emboli within the brain with neurological effects which may be transient or permanent.

Following completion of closed mitral valvotomy, and after the patient is turned onto his or her back, all peripheral pulses are palpated and a comparison made with the records of pulses which were present or absent preoperatively. The limbs are watched carefully over the subsequent few hours to note coldness, pallor, loss of sensation or loss of movement. The most common embolic complication is that of saddle embolism of the aortic bifurcation which is readily diagnosed by the complete absence of femoral pulses and of distal pulses in the lower limbs, pallor and perhaps mottling of the legs, together with coldness, loss of sensation and paralysis. The treatment of this condition is removal of the offending obstructing emboli by the use of Fogarty balloon catheters passed retrograde up both femoral arteries.

Mesenteric vascular occlusion is a consequence of left atrial thrombi travelling to the mesenteric vessels. The diagnosis and treatment of this condition are considered elsewhere (*see* Chapter 17).

POSTOPERATIVE MANAGEMENT

Those patients with poorly compliant lungs associated with either pulmonary oedema or marked pulmonary hypertension are best managed for 24 hours postoperatively using intermittent positive-pressure ventilation via an endotracheal tube. This is certainly safer than immediate extubation, allowing patients to breathe as best they can, for many will become tired and have difficulty in ventilating their stiff lungs with consequent anoxia and hypercapnia. In the early days of mitral valve surgery many of the so-called 'unexplained' immediate postoperative deaths were doubtless due to hypoventilation, anoxia and retention of carbon dioxide.

Digoxin is restarted on the 1st postoperative day and diuretics with potassium supplement are given as necessary.

SECOND AND SUBSEQUENT VALVOTOMIES

There is no indication for a second or subsequent mitral valvotomy being undertaken as a closed procedure. Although in the past many surgeons undertook subsequent closed valvotomies, there are many good reasons for avoiding this. It is probable that many years have elapsed since the first valvotomy, during which the process of thickening, shortening and perhaps calcification of the valve has continued, making it less likely that further closed valvotomy will be as successful as the first operation. Furthermore, there is little doubt that re-exploration of the mitral valve by the closed method, bearing in mind the adhesions and absence of left atrial appendage, is a more dangerous operation than that undertaken originally, and many cardiac surgeons who have attempted a number of second closed valvotomies have faced massive and at times uncontrollable haemorrhage during this operation.

MANAGEMENT OF SEVERE HAEMORRHAGE DURING MITRAL VALVOTOMY

Should a large tear in the appendage of the left atrium occur during valvotomy, the situation may arise where the friable and tense left atrium is difficult or impossible to suture. In these circumstances, fatal haemorrhage may be prevented only by the surgeon keeping a finger or fingers within or controlling the atrium by pressure. If valvotomy can be completed, the reduced left atrial pressure may enable repair to be completed. Otherwise, this potentially extremely serious situation must be controlled by conversion of the operation to an open procedure using cardiopulmonary bypass. A useful method of controlling haemorrhage temporarily is the introduction of a large balloon catheter of the Foley type through the tear and inflating it fully within the atrium. Traction on this catheter from without will effectively seal the atrium for as long as it remains in place, enabling the patient to be prepared for cardiopulmonary bypass, should control and suture still elude the surgeon.

TRANSVENOUS BALLOON VALVOTOMY

A recent innovation has been that of closed mitral valvotomy using a dilating balloon. A catheter is introduced percutaneously into the femoral vein and passed into the right atrium puncturing the septum whence it is introduced into the mitral orifice. The attached balloon can then be forcibly dilated with fluid producing an apparently successful mitral valvotomy.

This is a very early report and it is not possible at the present time to speculate whether or not this will become routine clinical practice.

Open Mitral Valvotomy

This operation is undertaken using full cardiopulmonary bypass. Access to the mitral valve may be gained through a left thoracotomy, right thoracotomy or median sternotomy. Access via left thoracotomy is ideal when, during an attempt at closed valvotomy, it is necessary to institute cardiopulmonary bypass. Venous return may be obtained by inserting a cannula into the right ventricle or into the right atrial appendage, with arterial return into the descending aorta or left femoral artery. This approach is also useful should a left atrial myxoma be discovered during an exploration for apparent mitral stenosis.

Approach to the mitral valve via a right thoracotomy was popular at one time in patients who had previously had surgery undertaken through the left chest and in whom pleural adhesions were to be anticipated, but this approach is now obsolete.

The mitral valve is now almost invariably approached by a median sternotomy. This exposure allows surgery to be undertaken on the mitral valve, the aortic valve and the tricuspid valve and furthermore allows adequate manipulation of the left ventricle for the purpose of expelling air, a procedure which remains incomplete when surgery is undertaken through a right thoracotomy. To explore the mitral valve after median sternotomy a long incision is made in the left atrium extending from the right upper lobe pulmonary vein well down and parallel to the interatrial groove and towards the inferior vena cava (*Fig.* 41.5). This gives excellent access to the mitral valve when using appropriate retractors. On rare occasions when the left atrium is tiny, adequate exposure may be undertaken by incising the right atrium in the horizontal plane and extending this incision back across the septum towards the tricuspid valve, also in the horizontal plane—the exposure of Dubost. Although this approach allows good visualization of the mitral valve under some circumstances, it has the disadvantage that the septal incision or its repair may interfere with atrioventricular conduction and cause permanent heart block, and furthermore the very thin portion of the septum surrounded by the annulus ovale may be difficult to resuture. The atrial cavity is carefully examined for thrombi. From time to time an extremely large thrombus occupying much of the chamber and extending into the pulmonary veins is present, and it is important that this thrombus is removed as completely as possible. Usually there is a plane of cleavage between the organized thrombus and the atrial wall, and when this is entered, and with care, the thrombus may be removed, very often in one piece.

When the thrombus is completely removed, the atrium and ventricle are irrigated with saline solution to ensure that fragments do not remain. At this stage

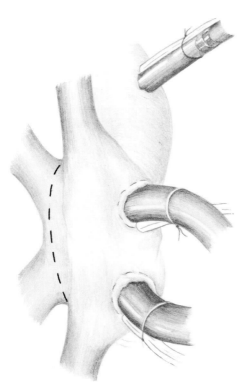

Fig. 41.5. Open mitral valvotomy. The line of incision into the left atrium is parallel and posterior to the right atrium, care being taken to avoid incision too far laterally into the pulmonary veins.

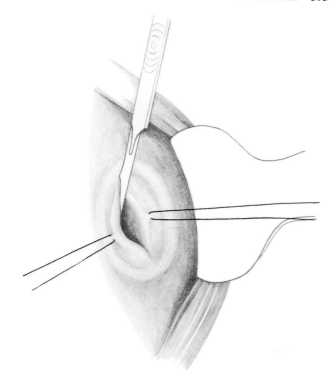

Fig. 41.6. Open mitral valvotomy. The cusps of the mitral valve are retracted with stay sutures and this facilitates exposure for accurate commissurotomy.

it is wise to obliterate the orifice of the left atrial appendage using a fine continuous suture to ensure that postoperative thrombosis does not originate within the appendage, with the danger of subsequent embolization. Great care must be taken when placing this suture, for too deep an insertion may damage the circumflex coronary artery or vein in the atrioventricular groove. The insertion of a suture into the anterior and posterior leaflets of the valve is a valuable aid to the demonstration of the stenosis of the valve and of its subvalvar pathology (*Fig.* 41.6). Horizontal traction is applied to these sutures, following which careful incision of the fused commissure can be undertaken safely. The fused commissure usually presents as a wrinkled furrow considerably thicker than the adjacent valve cusps.

The introduction of a right-angled clamp beneath the fused commissures and between the chordae aids in separation and accurate division of the commissure. The commissure is cut a few mm at a time and after each cut the valve cusps and the chordae are carefully separated to avoid damage with consequent regurgitation. In many instances the valve can be widely opened by cutting both commissures and it may be noted that there is little if any chordal fusion, enabling a competent, mobile, almost full-sized valve to be obtained. Unfortunately, in some instances the valve will be thickened with early calcification and with considerable subchordal fusion. Whereas it was until recently the common practice to replace such

a valve, there is now a distinct leaning towards conservation of the mitral valve if at all possible, for it is clear that the patient's own mitral valve, perhaps imperfect, is far more serviceable than any prosthesis so far designed. In these patients, careful commissurotomy and removal of calcium with forceps will demonstrate the subchordal problem, and splitting of the chordae with a sharp knife or scissors may enable the valve to be separated into a good anterior and posterior leaflet, each with good chordal support mechanism (*Fig.* 41.7). It may be that during this procedure one or two chordae are divided but in these the valve may still be satisfactorily repaired by the placement of a few sutures in the edge of the unsupported part of the valve. At the end of this procedure it is most important to evacuate thrombus, calcium and air from the heart before ejection into the aorta begins and the bypass is discontinued.

PREVENTION OF AIR EMBOLISM DURING MITRAL VALVE SURGERY

In any operation which widely opens the left heart, such as aortic or mitral valve replacement, considerable amounts of air may be trapped in the pulmonary veins and the chambers of the left side of the heart, and unless great care is taken this air will be ejected through the aortic valve when the heart takes over following the termination of cardiopulmonary bypass. It is important to anticipate this problem by

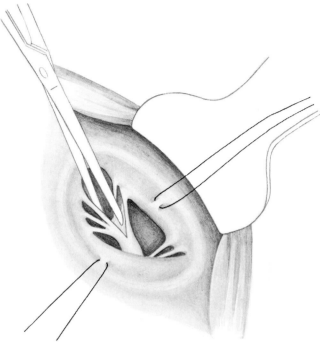

Fig. 41.7. Open mitral valvotomy. Following commissurotomy the fused chordae and papillary muscles may be carefully split.

the use of good left ventricular venting tubes and with a supra-aortic needle vent, both of which are aspirated prior to terminating the bypass and prior to release of aortic cross-clamps. Cerebral air embolism, which was at one time a serious complication of cardiac surgery, has now been almost completely eliminated by careful attention to these details.

Acquired Mitral Regurgitation

Principal Causes
1. Rheumatic fever.
2. Subacute bacterial endocarditis.
3. Prolapse of the cusps, especially the posterior, with herniation into the left atrium, the so-called 'floppy valve syndrome'.
4. Ruptured chordae associated with myxomatous degeneration of the mitral valve.
5. Mitral regurgitation following myocardial infarction due to either rupture of a papillary muscle, or due to so-called 'papillary muscle dysfunction'.
6. Following mitral valvotomy, either closed or open.
7. Mitral regurgitation associated with closed chest injuries.
8. Congenital clefts. Although these are not acquired, they may present in adult life and appear to cause acquired mitral regurgitation and will be considered in this chapter (McGoon operation).

Until recently the operation of choice for mitral regurgitation was replacement of the valve with a prosthesis. However, the long-term complications of mitral valve replacement have made surgeons increasingly willing to conserve the patient's own mitral valve and there is no doubt that with careful attention to the valve, and an appropriate annuloplasty or ring insertion, many seriously regurgitant valves may be rendered quite competent.

Operation is undertaken via median sternotomy using full cardiopulmonary bypass. The left atrium is opened posteriorly to the right atrium by a vertical incision and, following exposure of the valve and its examination, a decision is made concerning its reconstruction or removal. Reconstruction of the valve is made possible by several manoeuvres. Clefts may be sutured and pieces of calcium removed. Following this the valve cusps may be thinned out by planing off layers of thickened material, and the cusps may then appear much more pliable. Nevertheless, the valve often remains incompetent due to the inability of the shrunken cusps to meet during systole. This problem may be corrected by some form of annuloplasty. The annuloplasty may be undertaken by the insertion of a circumferential purse-string suture after the De Vega method for tricuspid valve annuloplasty. When this is tightened the valve edges may approximate more readily to produce a competent valve.

A more satisfactory way of narrowing the mitral ring is the insertion of a Carpentier ring. The size of ring to be chosen is determined by the use of sizing obdurators and it is recommended that the sizing obdurator which covers the anterior cusp should conform to the size of ring to be selected. The mitral ring will then be reduced in size to that of the anterior cusp of the mitral valve which will then readily obstruct the mitral orifice during systole, preventing mitral regurgitation (*Fig. 41.8*).

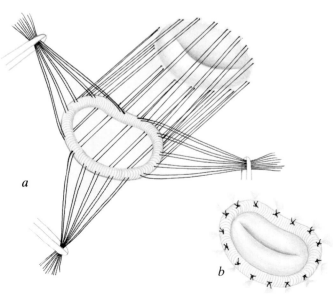

Fig. 41.8. Carpentier ring used for narrowing the mitral annulus when the valve leaflets and the subvalvar mechanism are otherwise intact.

Mitral Valve Replacement

Should it prove impossible to preserve the valve the cusps should be excised together with their associated chordae tendineae and tips of the papillary muscles. Care should be taken to leave a 2-mm ring of mitral valve at the ring, for complete removal of the mitral valve, especially anteriorly where the ring is not very well in evidence, may result in sutures cutting out of the thin muscle (*Fig.* 41.9). Although the tips of

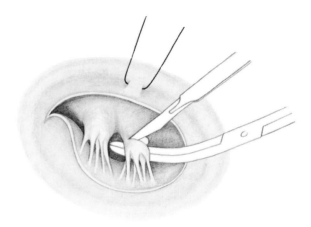

Fig. 41.11. Mitral valve replacement. The papillary muscle is divided just proximal to the insertion of the chordae.

those situations where the valve ring seems inadequate it is probably safer to use interrupted sutures, supported where necessary with Teflon felt buttresses (*Fig.* 41.12).

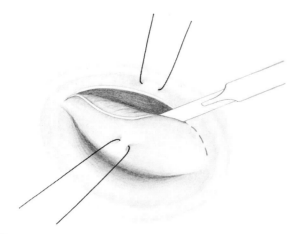

Fig. 41.9. Mitral valve replacement. Traction on stay sutures facilitates accurate resection of the anterior cusp of the mitral valve.

the papillary muscles must be removed, care should be taken when the valve is elevated to expose the papillary muscles that the left ventricular wall is not tented inwards, with consequent damage to or rupture of the ventricular wall during excision of the papillary muscle (*Figs.* 41.10, 41.11). It is now the practice of most surgeons to fix the valve using a continuous suture of 2/0 polypropylene, although in

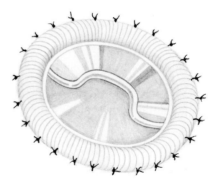

Fig. 41.12. Mitral valve replacement. The mitral valve prosthesis (Bjork–Shiley) is sutured into the mitral ring using interrupted non-absorbable sutures.

Following suture of a prosthetic valve into position it is important that it is made incompetent, otherwise the beating left ventricle may eject air into the aorta before an opportunity has occurred to evacuate this air. This is achieved by passing a fine Foley balloon catheter across the valve from the atrium into the ventricle and inflating the balloon. This will prevent the ball or disc closing and will enable free ventricular air to be ejected back into the atrium. This catheter is removed only after the atrium has been closed around it and air has been completely evacuated from all cardiac chambers (*Fig.* 41.13).

Acute Infections of the Mitral Valve

This serious illness presents as acute or subacute bacterial endocarditis of the mitral valve. The responsible organism is frequently *Streptococcus viridans* which usually originates in dental sepsis. This organ-

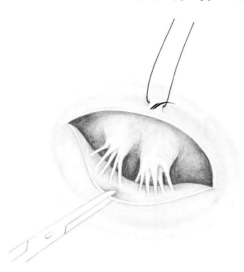

Fig. 41.10. Mitral valve replacement. Following detachment of the anterior cusp of the mitral valve from the ring, the papillary muscles are seen.

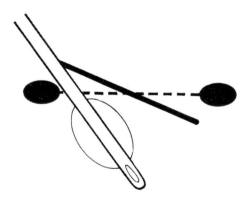

Fig. 41.13. Mitral valve replacement. The use of a Foley balloon catheter (as shown) is advised during mitral valve replacement. By rendering the valve incompetent, air contained in the ventricle is displaced back into the atrium, whence it may be removed during atrial suture.

ism may produce subacute infection of the valve but acute bacterial endocarditis is more likely to be caused by an organism such as *Staphylococcus aureus*. While the patient may slowly develop congestive cardiac failure, allowing an intensive 4–6-week course of the appropriate intravenous antibiotics prior to valve replacement, there are occasions when mitral regurgitation is so severe that the patient will clearly not survive to enable this long antibiotic therapy to be undertaken. In these, emergency mitral valve replacement is necessary to save life, in the face of the real risk of implanting a prosthetic valve into an infected mitral valve ring.

Assessment of Tricuspid Valve

At the beginning of any open operation on the mitral valve, prior to starting bypass, digital examination of the tricuspid valve is essential. This will demonstrate the presence of previously unsuspected tricuspid valve stenosis or regurgitation, the latter being either functional or organic. Should this valve be haemodynamically seriously abnormal, attention to it is mandatory, for otherwise, following an otherwise successful mitral valve operation, the patient may develop a serious or fatal low output state.

Management of Open Mitral Valve Operations in the Presence of Significant Aortic Regurgitation

Aortic regurgitation of either mild or moderate degree is present in many patients with mitral valve disease. In itself the aortic regurgitation may not be haemodynamically significant but during cardiopulmonary bypass the leak back through the valve into the non-beating left ventricle may cause problems.

The torrent of blood regurgitating into the left ventricle will create difficulties of visualization during the mitral valve operation, and this was a serious problem when it was customary to operate on the beating heart at normal temperatures. However, now

that open mitral valve surgery is undertaken with aortic cross-clamping and the use of cold cardioplegia (*see* Chapter 39), the leaking aortic valve no longer presents a problem during perfusion. However, for the efficient production of a cold paralysed heart it is necessary for the aortic valve cusps to be fairly competent in order that the coronary arteries may be perfused with the injected cold solution. Should the valve be incompetent the solution will run back into the left ventricle and not perfuse the coronary arteries. This state of affairs is obvious as the aortic root will not become tense during the injection and furthermore the heart will not cool. In these circumstances it is therefore necessary to open the root of the aorta and to inspect the aortic valve. If the valve is found to be only mildly diseased, cold cardioplegia may be proceeded with by injection of the cold solution individually down both coronary arteries. If, however, the aortic valve is clearly far more diseased than was previously considered, it will be necessary to excise the aortic valve and replace it in addition to any contemplated mitral valve surgery.

ACQUIRED DISEASE OF THE TRICUSPID VALVE

The tricuspid valve may be affected by stenosis or incompetence, usually part of the rheumatic process which affects the mitral valve and perhaps the aortic valve. A significant degree of tricuspid stenosis may affect perhaps 5 per cent of patients with mitral valve disease, but tricuspid regurgitation is more commonly seen. Tricuspid regurgitation may be organic with fibrous retraction, shortening and thickening of the leaflets by the rheumatic process or it may be functional and follow dilatation of the tricuspid valve ring associated with right ventricular dilatation consequent on pulmonary hypertension. It is unfortunately the case that serious tricuspid stenosis or regurgitation may pass unnoticed during cardiac catheterization and even clinical examination, and for this reason it is always necessary to palpate the tricuspid valve prior to cardiopulmonary bypass during open mitral valve surgery. Tricuspid stenosis is rarely amenable to separation of the commissures, for in these patients the cusps are thickened and shortened, and any such operation to relieve stenosis usually results in regurgitation. It is necessary under these circumstances to perform, in addition, some form of annuloplasty.

Tricuspid Regurgitation

Tricuspid regurgitation is rarely amenable to any form of surgery to the cusps alone. Fortunately, the tricuspid ring is suitable for annuloplasty either by De Vega annuloplasty or by the ring annuloplasty of Carpentier. The annuloplasty introduced by De Vega is an excellent method of narrowing the tricuspid valve orifice in patients with tricuspid regurgitation, whether this be functional or pathological. The annuloplasty occupies about three-quarters of the circumference of the tricuspid ring, avoiding the area adjacent to the coronary sinus where lies the atrioventricular conducting bundle. A suture is introduced into the tricuspid valve ring and passed as a purse-string three-quarters of the way around the ring where it emerges (*Fig. 41.14a*). It is then inserted into a Teflon felt buttress and retraces its steps back to the original point of insertion of the suture where it is again buttressed. This suture which is of heavy Prolene or heavy Ethiflex is gradually tightened over a 20-mm diameter sound and, when it sits snugly over this, it is tied. The valve will then be seen to be competent (*Fig. 41.14b*).

Aortic Stenosis

Although aortic stenosis should be detected in childhood, it is more commonly detected in adult life with the development of calcific aortic stenosis. It is likely that the majority of patients with calcific aortic stenosis have calcified a congenitally stenotic or abnormal valve. The valve is frequently bicuspid or, if tricuspid, one cusp is larger than the others or there may be rudimentary commissures. Such an abnormal valve produces turbulence of flow through and around it and over the years the deposition of platelets and fibrin add to the rigidity of the valve which becomes thickened, fibrosed and later calcified. Rheumatic fever is a common cause of aortic stenosis with thickening and fibrous fusion of the commissures and is fre-

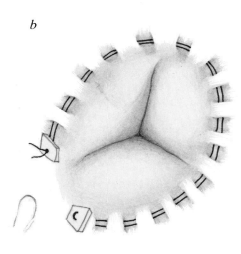

Fig. 41.14. De Vega annuloplasty suture to narrow the tricuspid orifice.

The Carpentier ring annuloplasty is undertaken in much the same way as with the mitral valve. However, bearing in mind the dangerous area adjacent to the atrioventricular conducting bundle, this ring is incomplete and takes up the slack in three-quarters of the ring only. This is a most successful method of annuloplasty.

Tricuspid Valve Replacement

It is unfortunately the case that although many patients have undergone successful tricuspid valve replacement, it is in this situation that valve dysfunction and early thrombosis of the prosthetic valve, despite adequate anticoagulation, are common.

ACQUIRED AORTIC VALVE DISEASE

Aortic valve disease is common and there seems to be no shortage of patients who require surgery for aortic stenosis or regurgitation.

quently associated with rheumatic disease of the mitral valve.

Aortic Regurgitation

The causes of aortic regurgitation are:
1. Calcific aortic stenosis and incompetence.
2. Rheumatic aortic incompetence.
3. Subacute bacterial endocarditis.
4. Syphilis of the root of the aorta and aortic valve.
5. Dissection of the root of the aorta.
6. Marfan's syndrome.
7. A complication of rheumatoid arthritis and ankylosing spondylitis.
8. Traumatic aortic incompetence.

In some of these conditions, such as syphilis, dissection and Marfan's syndrome, the aortic valve is not primarily at fault. It is the associated pathology of the root of the aorta which causes dilatation and disruption at the aortic ring which produces regurgitation.

Aortic regurgitation may be associated with an ascending aortic aneurysm which often involves the aortic ring and the origin of the coronary arteries, together with the ascending aorta as far as, if not distal to, the innominate artery. Such aneurysms are frequently seen in association with Marfan's syndrome and syphilitic aortitis, and of course dissection has its own peculiar pathology.

Assessment

Many patients with aortic stenotic and regurgitant murmurs may have no symptoms and it is necessary to assess these patients clinically and haemodynamically before suitable advice may be given.

Radiological examination will disclose the size of the heart, and of the aorta, valve calcification and the vascularity of the lung fields, together with an assessment of degrees of pulmonary venous congestion denoting heart failure.

Electrocardiography is an important investigation in aortic valve disease. Left ventricular hypertrophy is commonly seen and the various criteria for determining hypertrophy are well documented. Associated evidence of ischaemic heart disease will indicate the need for coronary arteriography.

Cardiac catheterization will establish the level of the gradient across the aortic valve, the left atrial pressure, pressures in the left ventricle and the pulmonary vascular resistance, and when these are considered a fair understanding of the patient's haemodynamic state will be possible. Angiocardiography will assess incompetence at the aortic and mitral valves and left ventricular function. Echocardiography will help in the assessment of left ventricular function and also estimate the orifice size and function of the aortic valve. In most adults who are to be considered as candidates for aortic valve surgery, coronary arteriography is considered necessary. Certainly in those patients with associated angina pectoris, such an investigation is mandatory. It is sad to replace an aortic valve in a patient who dies and is discovered at autopsy to have previously unsuspected and important coronary artery disease.

The decision to operate is more readily made in those with symptoms, for it is known that patients with aortic valve disease who are experiencing anginal pain, syncopal attacks, or have evidence of left ventricular failure, have an exceedingly poor life expectation, variously estimated at between 1 and 3 years.

Subacute bacterial endocarditis may be a slow process and may respond to a prolonged course of intravenous antibiotics prior to valve replacement. However, as with endocarditis of the mitral valve cardiac failure may be so severe that emergency aortic valve replacement in the presence of a possibly inadequately sterilized aortic valve is sometimes necessary, and it is inevitable that the risk of reinfection of the prosthetic aortic valve must be taken.

Surgical Treatment of Acquired Aortic Valve Disease

Closed valvotomy by means of dilators introduced through the left ventricle is obsolete.

Aortic valve surgery is now invariably an open procedure conducted using cardiopulmonary bypass, and presents the need for some form of myocardial protection, because exposure of the aortic valve requires cross-clamping of the aorta with consequent deprivation of natural coronary artery perfusion.

Methods of Left Ventricular Protection and Support during Aortic Valve Surgery
See Chapter 39.

Surgical Approach to the Aortic Valve
The aortic valve is invariably approached via median sternotomy and using full cardiopulmonary bypass and cold cardioplegia (*see* Chapter 39). The ascending aorta is mobilized and cross-clamped. The aortic incision is either a vertical hockey stick-shaped incision or a transverse incision in the aorta 1 cm above the right coronary orifice. The valve, if fibrous, is readily excised but in the presence of calcific aortic stenosis care is required when removing the cusps and calcium from the aortic root. Particular attention should be paid anteriorly at the commissure between the non-coronary and right coronary cusps, for it is at this site that the atrioventricular conducting bundle enters the ventricular septum and it is here that it may be damaged with the production of complete heart block. When the aortic ring is ready to receive the valve the appropriate valve size is estimated by the introduction of graded obturators which are supplied with the particular valve to be used. Interrupted sutures of Ethibond are used and where the valve ring is weak or not very much in evidence support using Teflon felt buttresses is advised (*Fig.* 41.15).

In the presence of an ascending aortic aneurysm a preclotted woven Dacron aortic graft is required in addition to aortic valve replacement. This graft may be placed distal to the coronary arteries, but should their orifices be involved in the aneurysm complete replacement of the ascending aorta, with reimplantation of the coronary arteries into the graft, is required (*Figs.* 41.16–41.18).

Dissection of the aorta with aortic regurgitation is primarily a disease of the aorta and frequently the valve is entirely normal, the regurgitation being produced by loss of support of the valve from its ring. It is usually necessary to replace the ascending aorta with a woven Dacron graft and it is sometimes possible to resuspend the patient's own aortic valve to the ring and to the graft. However, although this is desirable it is often safer to replace the aortic valve together with the ascending aorta in this situation, with or without transfer of coronary ostia to the graft.

Similarly, syphilitic aortic incompetence and the aortic incompetence associated with Marfan's syn-

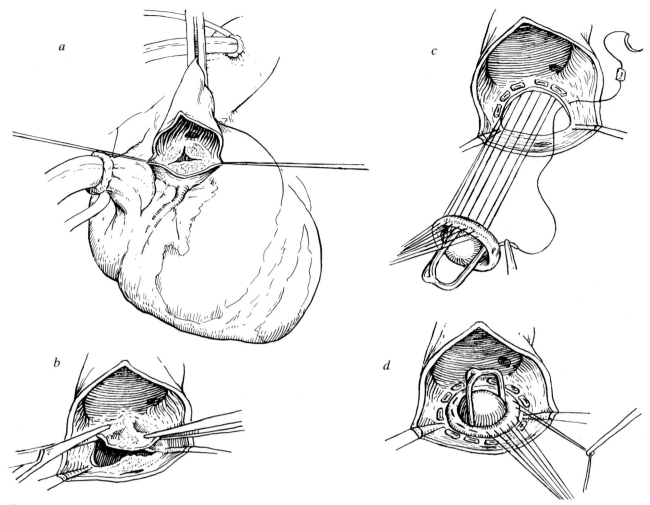

a

b

c

d

Fig. 41.15. Aortic valve replacement using Starr–Edwards ball valve. After removing the leaflets and decalcifying the ring the valve in this case is inserted using mattress sutures buttressed with Teflon felt supports.

drome will usually require resection and graft replacement of the ascending aorta together with aortic valve replacement.

Replacement of the Ascending Aorta using an Intraluminal Shunt

The recent introduction of an intraluminal device which may be tied into the ascending aorta has obviated the need in many cases to undertake formal removal and replacement of the ascending aorta with a Dacron tube. The intraluminal device is inserted into the ascending aorta and its upper and lower ends are tied in place with a circumferential ligature. The use of the intraluminal shunt is precluded in those patients in whom concomitant aortic valve replacement and reimplantation of the coronary arteries are necessary.

Combined Aortic and Mitral Valve Replacement

This operation is frequently undertaken. It is impor-

tant to replace the mitral valve first, for if the aortic valve is dealt with initially the consequent rigidity and fixation of the aortic root create difficulties in mobilizing the mitral valve and its replacement.

Hypertrophic Obstructive Cardiomyopathy

This condition has gained increasing attention in recent years. It is a muscular obstruction of the left ventricular outflow tract, characterized by marked hypertrophy in the left ventricle, particularly in the interventricular septum. During systole the hypertrophic outflow tract muscle almost completely obstructs left ventricular ejection. Fortunately, the majority of these patients respond to medical treatment, usually with beta-blocking drugs. In some patients, however, despite medical treatment, symptoms remain severe and haemodynamic and angiographic evidence of severe outflow obstruction remains. In these, resecting some of the obstructing left ventricular muscle via a supravalvar aortotomy (*Fig.* 41.19) or a combined supravalvar and transventricular

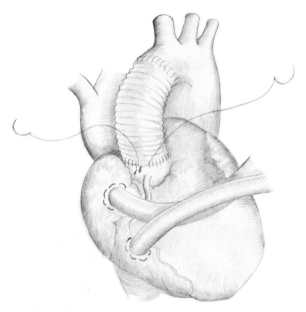

Fig. 41.16. Ascending aortic aneurysm complicating aortic regurgitation. The aortic valve prosthesis has been implanted in the usual way. A woven Dacron graft is used to replace the ascending aortic aneurysm but as is usual with simple aneurysms in this situation it has been possible to spare the proximal portion of the ascending aorta bearing the coronary arteries.

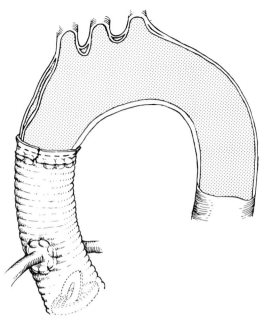

Fig. 41.18. Dissecting aneurysm of the ascending aorta. A composite graft of woven Dacron with which is incorporated an aortic prosthesis is sutured directly to the aortic root below the coronary ostia. The coronary ostia are then sutured directly to small holes cut into the woven Dacron graft.

approach has achieved relief of symptoms and has been associated with a diminution or almost complete obliteration of the measured haemodynamic gradient. Although surgical management of this condition may relieve the obstruction, it in no way influences the underlying pathology, and operative treatment is best reserved for patients with severe symptoms who have not responded to medical treatment.

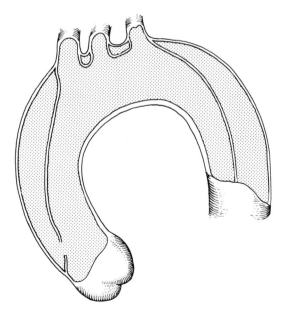

Fig. 41.17. Dissecting aneurysm of the ascending aorta. The aneurysm has been opened and its anterior aspect removed demonstrating separation of the layers both proximally and distally, and in this situation the orifices of the coronary arteries are frequently involved. It is necessary to oversew the divided proximal and distal aorta with continuous sutures supported by Teflon felt prior to insertion of a composite graft.

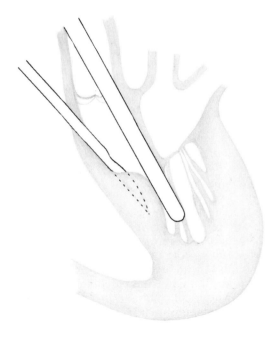

Fig. 41.19. Hypertrophic obstructive cardiomyopathy. Resection of subvalvar muscle mass is safer when the spatula introduced via the ascending aorta protects other structures.

ARTIFICIAL HEART VALVES

The ideal replacement heart valve has the following characteristics:
1. Central laminar flow.
2. Absence of turbulence.
3. Resistance to thrombus formation or the attraction of platelet and fibrin aggregates.
4. Resistance to wear or deterioration in function.

Artificial valves are of two basic types, the prosthetic valve and the biological valve.

Prosthetic Valves

These are of two main varieties—the caged ball valve and the horizontal tilting disc valve.

These valves are manufactured from a non-ferrous metallic frame which is covered by artificial fabrics incorporating a sewing ring and containing a ball or disc which may be of silicone rubber, metal or pyrolitic carbon. These valves have a primary orifice, a secondary orifice and a tertiary orifice, an understanding of which is important when one considers the choice of a valve.

1. The primary orifice is the diameter of the annulus which is retained following excision of the diseased valve.

2. The secondary orifice is the diameter of the blood passage through the valve itself and this will depend largely on the thickness of the sewing ring.

3. The tertiary orifice is the effective orifice through which blood may flow following ejection through the valve and this will depend on the size of the ball in the cage or on the angle of tilt of the pivoting disc.

Furthermore, the size of the aorta or ventricle distal to the valve will determine whether or not the disc or the caged ball obstructs blood flow during systolic ejection. The valves in common use are the Starr–Edwards caged ball valve, the variations of which have stood the test of time, and several types of tilting disc valve, notably the Bjork–Shiley tilting disc valve and the Lillehei–Kaster valve (*Fig.* 41.20).

Whether or not a caged ball valve is used in preference to a tilting disc valve is often a matter of personal preference. It should be said, however, that the presence of a large caged ball valve within the left ventricle in mitral valve replacement may well interfere with left ventricular function, and erosion of the left ventricular muscle by the struts of such a valve has been recorded. For these reasons many surgeons who use prosthetic valves in this situation prefer the use of a tilting disc valve, which has very little protrusion into the left ventricle. On the other hand, the presence of a caged ball valve in the ascending aorta does not interfere with the function of the valve although it may rarely obstruct a very narrow aorta. When the valves are compared there is little doubt that the secondary orifice of the pivoting disc valves, such as the Bjork–Shiley and Lillehei–Kaster valves, is considerably larger than the secondary orifice in the Starr–Edwards valve of similar primary orifice diameter. This is an important factor when one considers mitral valve replacement, for it is essential that this valve opens at a very low pressure and that blood passes through as wide an orifice as possible, and with little turbulence.

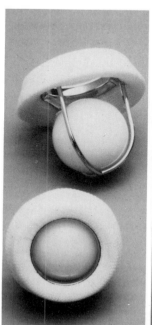
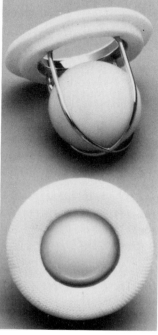

a

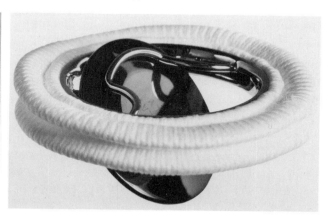

b

Fig. 41.20. *a*, Starr–Edwards valves. Left, Aortic. Right, Mitral.

b, Bjork–Shiley mitral valve.

Biological Valves

The valves now in use are homograft human aortic valves, valves prepared from calf pericardium, valves prepared from dura mater, valves prepared from fascia lata, and mounted porcine xenograft valves. With the exception of the cadaver human aortic valve, the porcine xenograft valve and the pericardial valve, those others mentioned are used very rarely and, following the disappointing experience with human fascia lata valves in the mitral and aortic positions, there is uncertainty concerning the prolonged life expectancy of dura mater valves. The great attraction of the human aortic valve or of the pig valve is its conformity with the principles of the ideal valve. It opens centrally with laminar flow and does not attract thrombus, platelets or fibrinogen and therefore requires, apart from the first few weeks postoperatively, no long-term control with anticoagulants.

Unmounted homograft aortic valves have been used with very great success by a handful of experienced surgeons in selected centres, but few are trained in this particular technique. The mounted porcine xenograft of either the Hancock or Carpentier type (*Fig.* 41.21) is very much easier to insert than are unmounted human aortic homografts. These valves are factory prepared, already sutured to flexible metal and fabric stents stored in buffered glutaraldehyde, and are inserted in much the same way as are prosthetic valves.

Biological vs Prosthetic Valve Replacement

The introduction of the biological valve (aortic homograft, bovine pericardial, mounted porcine xenograft) was particularly welcome to cardiac surgeons for, being far less prone to thrombo-embolic problems, they do not require the patient to be anticoagulated, with the attendant risks of this treatment. It was therefore not surprising that following the introduction of factory-mounted biological valves these were inserted into numerous patients. Unfortunately, after the passage of a few years it became clear that biological valves had their own disadvantages, particularly that of variable durability. It became clear that the insertion of biological valves into children (in whom chronic anticoagulation therapy is very difficult for both doctor and child) was frequently accompanied by early degeneration and calcification of the valve which was usually severe enough to require replacement with a prosthetic valve. Adults are not immune from the complication of calcification and furthermore with the passage of time more reports are emerging of these valves thickening, becoming stenotic or the cusps rupturing and producing regurgitation. It is claimed that the degeneration of biological valves is usually a very slow process, associated with gradual deterioration of the patient, enabling doctors to diagnose and treat valve failure in good time and before the patient becomes very ill. This, unfortunately, is not always the case for some patients who appear to be well, then deteriorate and die very quickly and are subsequently shown to have extensively calcified and stenotic biological valves. Furthermore, rupture of a cusp of a biological valve may occur suddenly with early deterioration and death of the patient.

There is no doubt that the factory-made prosthetic valve is extremely durable and the modern valve rarely, if ever, suffers from ball variance or from valve failure, although a small batch of prosthetic valves recently exhibited strut failure and fracture with release of the disc into the circulation with fatal consequences for a few patients. Despite this, however, it is safe to say that the factory-produced prosthetic valve is far more durable than the biological valve and the insertion without complication of such a valve into a patient is likely to provide the patient with a well-functioning valve for very many years and possibly the remainder of his or her lifetime. It must be emphasized, however, that the long-term anticoagulation required for the safe maintenance of the prosthetic valve is accompanied by significant mortality and morbidity caused by anticoagulant related haemorrhage (*see below*).

The biological valve is particularly suited for the elderly in whom the criterion of long-term durability

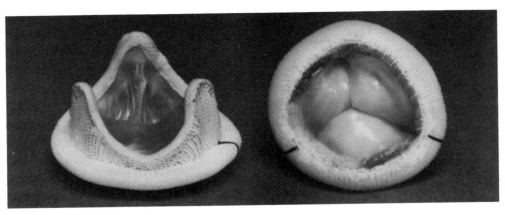

Fig. 41.21. Mounted porcine xenograft for mitral position (Carpentier–Edwards).

is not a primary consideration for it is particularly in these patients that it is desirable, if at all possible, to avoid anticoagulation. It is the view of some cardiologists that the biological valve should be favoured when operating on women of childbearing age in order to avoid anticoagulants, some of which may be teratogenic.

There is no ideal valve for all patients and it is largely consideration of the individual patient and the experience of the individual surgeon which will determine the choice of valve. Bearing in mind the problems which may arise with either biological or prosthetic valves it is certain that cardiac valve replacement should not be undertaken lightly and if it is at all possible to preserve the mitral valve this should be attempted.

Complications of Artificial Valve Replacement
Both prosthetic and biological valves are subject to similar postoperative complications.

1. *Thrombo-embolic Events*
There is no doubt that all prosthetic heart valves are liable to attract thrombi, platelets and fibrin with consequent risk of obstruction of the valve by clot and the embolization of this clot to peripheral vessels or to the central nervous system. For this reason, and with few exceptions, patients bearing a prosthetic valve must inevitably be treated with anticoagulants for life. Other drugs, such as aspirin and dipyridamole (Persantin), are used in an attempt to avoid the use of anticoagulants but at the time of writing their use is not well established. Biological valves are far less likely to produce thrombo-embolic complications and consequently anticoagulants are used for the 1st month postoperatively to allow endothelization of the fabric and of the sutures and are then discontinued.

2. *Anticoagulant-related Morbidity and Mortality*
It is inescapable that of any group of patients who are on lifelong anticoagulant therapy, a small but significant number will suffer haemorrhage which may be cerebral, retroperitoneal or gastrointestinal. Although some of these, particularly those with gastrointestinal or retroperitoneal haemorrhage, will cause no permanent problems, those patients suffering cerebral haemorrhage will usually die. It is also the case that it is not necessarily those patients whose anticoagulant control has gone wildly wrong who will experience such a disaster, for many patients with cerebral bleeding are shown to have their anticoagulant control at therapeutic levels. This problem has, of course, prompted many surgeons away from the use of prosthetic valves and towards the universal use of tissue valves, which in many cases do not require anticoagulant therapy.

3. *Infection*
All artificial valves, whether prosthetic or biological, are liable to septic complications. This disaster usually becomes apparent some weeks after the patient leaves hospital and is associated with a regular fever and evidence of septicaemia. Although in many instances the infection may be cured by the vigorous use of intravenous antibiotics over a prolonged period, it may be necessary to replace such a valve on account of septicaemia, valve failure, or for both these reasons.

4. *Paravalvar Leak*
This complication follows detachment of the sewing ring from the patient's own valve ring, and usually occurs very shortly after operation. It may be associated with infection or be due to the cutting out of a suture from a weak area or a region from which calcium has been inadequately removed. This complication may produce cardiac failure and resuture or replacement of the valve will be necessary. More frequently heart failure is not severe but the regurgitant jet may result in haemolytic anaemia and mild jaundice. If this is not severe the patient may be maintained by the use of iron, but frequently valve resuture or valve replacement is required.

5. *Fatigue and Wear of the Valve*
The earlier models of prosthetic valves were liable to many complications such as ball variance which resulted in splitting and sometimes escape of the silicone ball from the cage, rupture of struts, wearing and fragmentation of the cloth covering the struts, and fracture or escape of the disc from low profile valves. Although these complications are still from time to time reported they are now fortunately rare. Such wear may be suspected in a patient who has remained well for some years postoperatively and who develops signs of cardiac failure. In these circumstances, early cardiac catheterization or echocardiography should be undertaken to establish the function of the prosthetic valve and, if shown to be faulty, replacement may be a matter of urgency.

6. *Degeneration of Biological Valves*
Biological valves such as homografts, xenografts, or those valves designed from fascia lata, dura mater or pericardium, have an excellent appearance and function well when inserted. Unfortunately, some have not stood the test of time and particularly unfortunate was experience with fascia lata valves when used in the mitral position. In a large number of patients the cusps of this valve underwent thickening and retraction with consequent severe regurgitation. Other biological valves have undergone late calcification or rupture of the cusps. In some instances, late degeneration has been attributed to the method of

sterilization of the valve, whether by freeze drying, irradiation or the preservation in unsuitable buffer media or unsuitable antibiotics. It is now the practice to use almost fresh human homograft aortic valves, and in those centres where this has been practised the incidence of breakdown of homograft aortic valves is now very low. The mounted porcine xenograft valve is preserved in buffered glutaraldehyde and seems to stand up extremely well, although after several years of use occasional case reports are now emerging of calcification, stenosis, or rupture of the cusps. Degeneration in biological valves will result in either stenosis or more usually regurgitation at the valve which is readily diagnosed both clinically and by cardiac catheterization. When such degeneration has been demonstrated there is no alternative but to replace the valve.

CARDIAC TUMOURS

Metastatic tumours of the heart may be detected either clinically or at autopsy, but with few exceptions surgery plays no part in their management. Likewise primary malignant tumours of the heart are rarely amenable to surgical excision.

The common tumour of the heart is the benign atrial myxoma that arises from the annulus ovale and protrudes into the left atrium, where it may fill the cavity and then project through the mitral valve. This tumour may arise from a similar site in the right atrium but those on the left side are ten times more frequently seen.

These tumours may cause obstructive, embolic or systemic disturbances and their diagnosis is sometimes long delayed, being frequently mistaken for mitral stenosis or heart failure. When suspected, the diagnosis is confirmed by echocardiography and angiocardiography.

Treatment

The treatment of this condition is urgent surgical removal, for increasing delay increases the likelihood of tragic embolism.

Operation

These tumours are invariably removed using cardiopulmonary bypass. The left atrium is approached as for mitral valve surgery, i.e. via median sternotomy. However, on those rare occasions when a left atrial myxoma is diagnosed during left thoracotomy, under the mistaken diagnosis of mitral stenosis, the operation may be converted into an open heart procedure through the left chest, as described on p. 594, and removal of the myxoma undertaken at that time.

The serious hazard of this operation is the danger of fragmentation of the myxoma with consequent peripheral and cerebral emboli. It is therefore advised that, while the tumour is being handled, the heart is arrested by cold cardioplegia and cross-clamping the aorta during this procedure, lest an uncontrolled heartbeat eject fragments of tumour into the aorta. When the left or right atrium is involved, the tumour is noted to be friable and gelatinous, with a mixture of solid and cystic elements. It should be removed whole if possible and the use of a large spoon is helpful in this situation. The tumour will be seen to originate from a pedicle on the annulus ovale. It is advised that a disc of the atrial septum bearing this pedicle be removed and that the resultant atrial septal defect be sutured. Failure to remove completely the pedicle of the tumour has been regarded as contributory to recurrence of this tumour. The atrium and ventricle are carefully washed out to remove remaining loose fragments. The atrium is repaired, air evacuated from the heart and aorta, and bypass terminated, allowing the heart to take over the circulation.

SURGICAL TREATMENT OF ISCHAEMIC HEART DISEASE

After many false starts spanning the past 45 years, the surgical treatment of ischaemic heart disease at last seems rational and is based more on objective assessment rather than on the previous purely subjective complaints of the patient. Advances in treatment have been stimulated by the development of selective coronary arteriography, good ciné-angiocardiography, and well-developed techniques of echocardiography, which enable an accurate diagnosis to be made of both structure and function. Furthermore, postoperative objective studies have been undertaken in many who have undergone surgical treatment for either angina pectoris or the complications of myocardial infarction, making available an enormous amount of data assessing the value of this treatment. Although there is little doubt that operations for the relief of ischaemic heart disease have been undertaken in many doubtful situations and on many occasions, the passage of time will enable a more rational assessment and it is hoped that in due course a better understanding of the indications and anticipated results of such treatment will be available. Ischaemic heart disease presents to the surgeon in the following ways:
1. Angina pectoris.
2. The complications of myocardial infarction, which are left ventricular aneurysm, ventricular septal defect or mitral regurgitation.

Treatment of Angina Pectoris

Although the diagnosis of angina pectoris may readily be made by good history taking, it is well established that many patients with the typical clinical features of angina pectoris prove on investigation to have a perfectly normal coronary arterial tree. It may be that in some of these patients the condition of coronary arterial spasm does exist, but it is also likely that in some their symptoms are due to other conditions such as hiatus hernia, pancreatitis or gallbladder disease. There remains a group of patients in whom full investigation will detect no such abnormality.

It is clear that the aorto-coronary bypass procedure can restore generous blood flow to ischaemic myocardium but it cannot revitalize dead muscle or make scar tissue contract. The operation was originally offered to patients with severe but stable angina, refractory to medical treatment, and in most patients the results are truly dramatic—85 per cent relieved of angina with an operative mortality of less than 2 per cent. Exercise tolerance is usually improved but there is no good evidence that, in the majority, survival is prolonged beyond that associated with good medical management. However, there are reliable data suggesting that patients with triple vessel disease who receive complete revascularization and those with left main coronary disease who have successful operations, will gain an increased life expectation.

Indications for Operation

The patient with disabling angina pectoris unresponsive to a good clinical trial with nitrites and beta-blocking drugs should be considered for surgery, prior to which selective coronary arteriography is, of course, mandatory. It is important to consider the degree to which the angina affects the patient's lifestyle. Clearly, the pain experienced by an elderly patient and regarded as tolerable will, in a younger person, possibly interfere with his or her work and lifestyle to such a degree that surgical relief is indicated.

Coronary arteriography will demonstrate the number and location of blocks and it seems that obstructions of less than 50 per cent of the diameter of the coronary artery are haemodynamically insignificant. In most patients with angina pectoris the operation is not urgent other than the conditions of pre-infarction or unstable angina and critical stenosis of the left main coronary artery. In the latter condition angina is often severe and the patient is liable to massive and fatal infarction at any time.

Surgical Treatment

Operations of historical interest, such as cardio-omentopexy, scarification of the pericardium, the Beck operations of arterialization of the coronary sinus, and the Vineberg operation of implantation of the freely bleeding internal mammary artery into the myocardium are no longer practised and are not described. The overall poor results of these operations, coupled with the unwarranted enthu-

siasm of many surgeons, prejudiced many cardiologists against operative intervention for coronary artery disease and delayed the emergence—in some centres for many years—of the modern and effective operation of coronary artery bypass grafting, using reversed lengths of autogenous saphenous vein.

Coronary Artery Bypass Grafting

This operation was introduced by Favaloro in 1969. Lengths of the patient's own long saphenous vein are reversed and implanted proximally into the ascending aorta and distally beyond the blocked segment of the coronary artery. The operation is undertaken using cardiopulmonary bypass and, almost invariably, cold cardioplegia.

OBTAINING THE SAPHENOUS VEIN FOR GRAFTING

The vein may be taken from either the thigh or the leg. Whether the vein from the thigh or leg is to be preferred is a matter of controversy but since many patients require multiple grafts it is often necessary to use the full length of the saphenous vein. The vein may be obtained either through one long incision or through multiple short incisions (*Fig. 41.22a*). The vein is then tested for leaks by distending it with the patient's own heparinized blood or Ringer's solution. Distension of the vein in addition to identifying further leaks will reveal any twists or narrow segments when one of the side-branches has been ligated too close to the main vessels (*Fig. 41.22b*). The vein is carefully cleaned of adventitia and segments with aneurysmal dilatations are discarded.

ISOLATING THE CORONARY ARTERY (*Fig. 41.23*)

The site of block of the artery has been previously determined at coronary arteriography, and may be frequently palpated as a hard mass along the line of the coronary vessel. Having identified the coronary artery, a linear incision is made into the vessel using a fine pointed scalpel, extended to about 0·75 cm in length with fine pointed Potts scissors (*Fig. 41.23a*).

The vein to be grafted is bevelled to 45° using scissors, and care is taken to ensure that the vein is inserted in a reverse direction so that the venous valves open during flow from the aorta into the coronary artery. The vein is sutured to the open coronary artery using continuous 6/0 Prolene (*Figs. 41.23b, c*). Fine Prolene is particularly suited for this operation for loops of sutures need not be drawn tight until the whole suture line is placed, and with a little traction the suture line is watertight without kinking or damage by the suture. Care must be taken to avoid purse-stringing the anastomosis. Before completing the anastomosis, fine plastic or silver probes are passed to confirm patency.

Access to the right coronary artery is best obtained by retraction of the right atrium and its cannulas to

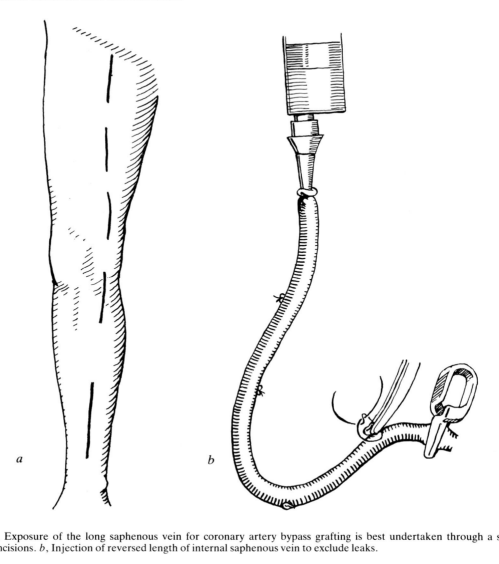

Fig. 41.22. *a*, Exposure of the long saphenous vein for coronary artery bypass grafting is best undertaken through a series of short longitudinal incisions. *b*, Injection of reversed length of internal saphenous vein to exclude leaks.

the right, and at the same time retraction of the right ventricle to the left and cephalad. Access to the marginal branches of the circumflex artery is readily obtained by elevation of the apex of the heart to the right and towards the patient's right shoulder.

The site for anastomosis is best decided prior to operation by carefully studying the coronary arteriogram. It is usually sufficient to place one graft on the anterior descending artery, although further grafts to one or more of its diagonal branches may also be required. It is usually not possible to implant a graft into the circumflex artery for this lies deep in the atrioventricular groove, usually deep to the corresponding vein. It is usual to place one or more grafts to the lateral or obtuse marginal branches of this vessel. The right coronary artery may require disobliteration of a long atheromatous core, following which grafting may be undertaken to the main right artery or the posterior descending branch.

Following the distal anastomoses the veins are anastomosed to the ascending aorta. The ascending aorta is grasped with a vascular side-clamp and either a 5-mm hole is punched or a 5-mm slit is made with a sharp scalpel, both of which leave a clean-cut orifice on which to sew the vein. It is possible to insert two veins into the same segment of aorta which is isolated by the side-clamp. Care is taken to perform the upper anastomosis at a site where kinking is avoided. Right coronary grafts usually lie best when joined to the right side of the ascending aorta whereas anterior descending and circumflex grafts lie best on the left side of the ascending aorta. Left-sided grafts to the anterior descending, diagonal or marginal arteries may sometimes lie more comfortably when taken in the transverse sinus behind the ascending aorta and pulmonary artery and anastomosed to the right side of the ascending aorta. A continuous suture technique is very appropriate for the proximal end of the graft using 5/0 Prolene. While the upper anastomoses are undertaken the aortic cross-clamp is

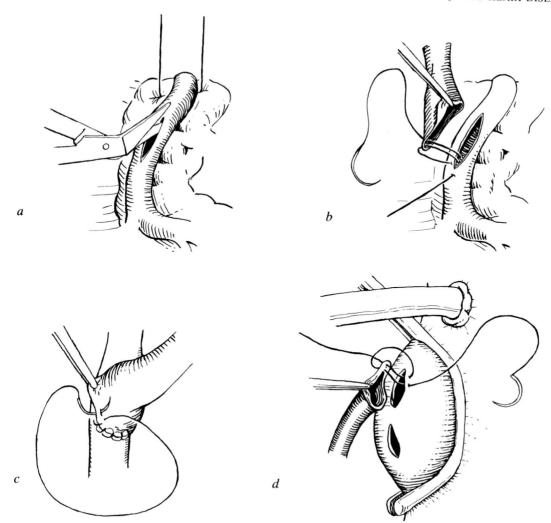

Fig. 41.23. Technique of anastomosis of saphenous vein to coronary artery and of saphenous vein to ascending aorta. *a*, Following isolation of the chosen coronary artery an initial small incision is made with a pointed scalpel, following which a 6-mm incision is made with fine vascular scissors. *b*, *c*, Anastomosis is undertaken using continuous 6/0 or 7/0 Prolene as an everting suture. *d*, Anastomosis of saphenous vein to ascending aorta using a side occlusion clamp. The anastomosis is undertaken with continuous 5/0 or 6/0 Prolene as an everting suture.

released, following which the heart will rewarm and either commence spontaneous beating or require electrical defibrillation. It is the practice of some surgeons to undertake the aortic anastomoses prior to cardiopulmonary bypass and to undertake the distal anastomoses following the commencement of bypass (*Fig.* 41.23*d*).

Having completed the grafts, it is desirable to measure the flow using electromanometric devices. It is generally considered that a flow of at least 50 ml/min will ensure a patent graft, although far higher flows are frequently recorded (*Fig.* 41.26).

Although it has in the past been popular to provide as many as four or five separate vein bypass grafts implanted in the aorta and the recipient coronary arteries, the more recent tendency is to use perhaps only two anastomoses at the aortic end and to tailor the distal vein into sequential anastomoses, with perhaps a side-to-side anastomosis between the obtuse marginal artery and the vein continuing around the base of the heart to terminate in an end-to-side anastomosis in the posterior descending branch of the right coronary artery. By various ingenious permutations as many as six sapheno-coronary anastomoses may be undertaken with perhaps two or three segments of vein.

RESULTS

In good hands at least 80 per cent of such bypass grafts remain patent 3 years following operation, but success relates directly to the experience of the operating surgeon.

Coronary Artery Bypass Grafting using the Internal Mammary Artery (*Fig.* 41.24)

With the considerable experience available following the widespread use of the internal mammary artery during the Vineberg operation of intramyocardial insertion of a freely bleeding internal mammary

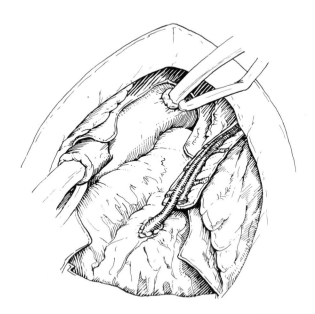

Fig. 41.24. Coronary artery bypass grafting using the internal mammary artery. Mobilized pedicle of the internal mammary artery, internal mammary vein and associated chest wall tissues are brought down, following which the end of the internal mammary artery is carefully bevelled and anastomosed to the opened left anterior descending coronary artery using continuous 7/0 Prolene sutures.

artery, many surgeons were familiar with the technique of isolating the internal mammary artery from the chest wall. It was but a small step for surgeons to anastomose the distal end of the internal mammary artery to the coronary arteries using very fine suture material.

The internal mammary artery is isolated from the chest wall in a pedicle consisting of extrapleural tissues containing the internal mammary artery and vein, ligating or clipping the intercostal branches and tributaries. Although it is usually possible to bypass a block in the anterior descending coronary artery or the diagonal vessels only, more experienced surgeons are able, using both internal mammary arteries, to bypass two or more blocked coronary vessels and have in addition used this vessel for sequential grafting of up to four coronary arteries.

The advantage of the internal mammary is not only that of availability but it has been shown that over periods as long as 10 years the internal mammary–coronary artery anastomosis remains patent more frequently than do similar anastomoses undertaken using reversed lengths of internal saphenous vein.

The native internal mammary artery grows and is able to deliver a far greater flow as time goes on and it is likely that more surgeons will in future utilize the internal mammary artery for at least some of the grafting undertaken at surgery (Green, 1984).

Endarterectomy (*Fig.* 41.25)

It is frequently the case that a coronary artery, usually the right, is almost completely blocked by a large length of atheroma. It is usually possible to remove

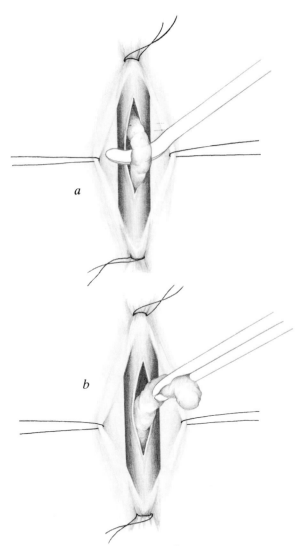

Fig. 41.25. Coronary endarterectomy.

a long sausage-like piece of this atheromatous deposit following incision into the artery, following which saphenous vein grafting may be undertaken. The atheroma may be removed either with fine dissecting instruments or by the use of carbon dioxide gas injectors.

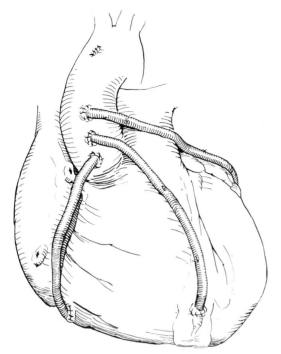

Fig. 41.26. Coronary artery saphenous vein bypass grafts. Three separate grafts have been inserted into the left anterior descending coronary artery, the obtuse marginal branch of the left circumflex artery, and the right coronary artery as it turns round the base of the heart towards the posterior descending coronary artery.

Percutaneous Transluminal Coronary Angioplasty

This recently introduced technique (Grüntzig et al., 1979) is a technique whereby coronary artery atheromatous obstructions may be dilated via a balloon introduced into the coronary artery at cardiac catheterization and is undertaken by either the physicians or radiologists skilled in this technique.

A fine guide wire is introduced via the femoral artery and is passed up the aorta and introduced into the orifices of the left or right coronary artery. A fine catheter is threaded over this guide wire and is passed through the coronary artery block using the image intensifier. With the injection of dye into the coronary artery the block can be readily identified and the balloon placed in an ideal situation, following which it is forcibly dilated by the injection of a small amount of saline.

In many instances the dilatation of the atheromatous plaque is dramatic, converting a serious or almost complete obstruction of a coronary artery into a less obstructed vessel. It is rarely, if ever, possible to completely restore the lumen to normal but initial reports, extending over a period of several years, indicate that the relief of angina may be maintained for a prolonged period and at the same time further coronary arteriography may demonstrate the relief of obstruction to be well maintained over a period of several years. Several vessels may be dilated at the same sitting. Although ideally suited for the dilatation of coronary blocks, this technique may usefully be applied to those patients who have had previous surgery and in whom the current angina is caused by stenosis at the anastomoses between the saphenous vein and major coronary artery.

It is not yet possible to assess the influence of percutaneous transluminal coronary angioplasty on the volume of surgical operations undertaken for coronary artery disease. At the present time dilatation is reserved for one or two vessels only although in very skilled hands three or four vessels are being dilated at one sitting. So far, very few centres have staff trained in this technique and the influence on the volume of surgery is minimal. However, as it emerges that this is a fairly safe and successful technique, it is clear that this treatment will in due course be available in all major cardiac centres. It is likely that this technique will be reserved for patients with one- or two-vessel disease and that fewer operations for one- or two-vessel disease will be undertaken by surgeons, the operation of aorto-coronary bypass being reserved for patients requiring four or more grafts.

Whether patients in the future are treated by surgeons, or by physicians, will in no way make either of them less busy for the foreseeable future, for there are clearly far more patients requiring relief of coronary artery obstruction than there are facilities, surgeons or physicians available to treat them.

COMPLICATIONS

The important complication is dissection of an important coronary artery with the production of early myocardial infarction. Should dissection of the vessel occur during percutaneous transluminal coronary angioplasty it is imperative that the patient is transferred to the operating theatre immediately for formal aorto-coronary venous bypass operation. For this reason the medical operation of percutaneous transluminal coronary angioplasty is undertaken only in hospitals where cardiac surgeons are immediately available with a vacant operating theatre to deal with this complication.

Recurrence of Angina following Coronary Artery Bypass Grafting

Although this may be due to progression of disease, the most likely cause is obstruction of the vein grafts, which may in turn be due either to complete thrombosis of the vein or more likely to obstruction at the anastomosis. This latter complication when occurring early is probably associated with a technical fault, for despite the many variables involved, it seems that a good initial anastomosis in the presence of good 'run-off' offers the patient the best chance of late patency of the graft. Recurrence of angina requires further coronary arteriography and, if indicated, further bypass grafting.

Surgical Treatment of Complications of Myocardial Infarction

Infarction followed by necrosis and fibrosis may damage the ventricular septum, its free wall or the papillary muscles. Damage and perforation of the septum will result in a post-infarction ventricular septal defect which is an acute condition resulting in very severe congestive heart failure. Necrosis of the free wall of the left ventricle may result in fatal perforation into the pericardium but may frequently produce a left ventricular aneurysm. Although the aneurysm may appear much larger than the ventricle itself, it must be remembered that the original lesion which produced the aneurysm consisted of no more than perhaps 20 per cent of the ventricular wall. Damage to the papillary muscle by either rupture or dysfunction will result in mitral valve regurgitation.

Post-infarction Ventricular Septal Defect

This is a serious condition. Although the patient may be in very severe heart failure, it is frequently surgically unwise to attempt closure of the defect earlier than 2 weeks following the myocardial infarction. The edges of the defect are otherwise oedematous and necrotic and it is unlikely that they will hold sutures. If the patient's condition allows a waiting period of 2 weeks following the myocardial infarction, the edges of the acquired ventricular septal defect will usually become thickened and fibrous. The defect may occur anywhere in the septum and when the anterior descending coronary artery has been obstructed the defect is often anterior and low in the septum and may be difficult to find from the right ventricular aspect where it may be overlain by large trabeculae and papillary muscles. The defect may be sutured but it is probably wiser to close the defect using a Dacron patch held in place by interrupted non-absorbent sutures, or with a sandwich of two patches of Teflon outside the heart.

Left Ventricular Aneurysm

Although aneurysms may appear on the left border of the heart, they are best approached via median sternotomy using cardiopulmonary bypass. The patients are often in a poor condition and, following the rapid establishment of cardiopulmonary bypass, dissection of the pericardium from the aneurysm may then proceed. It is unwise to attempt dissection earlier for this may produce troublesome arrhythmias and furthermore there is the real danger of perforating the very thin aneurysm before cardiopulmonary bypass is established, or of dislodging thrombi into the circulation.

When on full bypass a left ventricular vent is inserted through the aneurysm. Aspiration of this vent collapses the aneurysm which appears as a saucer in the left ventricle and the extent of the aneurysm is then clearly defined.

During excision of the aneurysm it is important to leave in place a rim of fibrous tissue to enable sutures to hold well. The interior of the heart is carefully examined and frequently large amounts of adherent thrombus will be found which require removal. At the same time the septum is examined for a previously undetected ventricular septal defect. While the aneurysm is being excised it is usual to cross-clamp the aorta to ensure that any detached thrombi in the left ventricle are not carried into the general circulation and to protect the heart by the use of cold cardioplegia. Following removal of the wall of the aneurysm and removal of clots from the ventricle, the aortic clamp may then be opened, allowing continuous coronary perfusion and normal heart action (*Figs.* 41.27, 41.28).

Closure of the Ventricle

This is achieved using continuous and interrupted sutures of heavy Prolene, taken in two layers. Support of these sutures with Teflon felt buttresses is usually necessary (*Fig.* 41.29).

Mitral Regurgitation

Mitral regurgitation following myocardial infarction may be due to so-called 'papillary muscle dysfunction' or to rupture of a necrotic papillary muscle. In any event, these patients are extremely seriously ill and although their only hope is mitral valve replacement, using cardiopulmonary bypass, the results of this treatment are poor, reflecting the gravity of the condition which is treated.

PULMONARY EMBOLISM

Treatment of Massive Pulmonary Embolism

Whereas the treatment of massive pulmonary embolism was until recently a choice between operation or treatment with anticoagulants, the subject has been further complicated by the introduction of powerful thrombolytic enzymes used intravenously, of which streptokinase is the most favoured. The protagonists of anticoagulant and thrombolytic therapy appear convinced that few patients now need surgical removal of pulmonary emboli and that the great majority of these patients will survive with this conservative management.

On the other hand, the view of many physicians and surgeons is that the simplicity of removal of these large obstructing emboli and the urgency of this operation must inevitably be the preferred treatment in the collapsed and possibly dying patient. These apparently opposing views are not irreconcilable.

Although the direct removal of massive pulmonary emboli from the pulmonary artery was first attempted by Trendelenburg in 1908, few successes were reported until the advent of cardiopulmonary bypass.

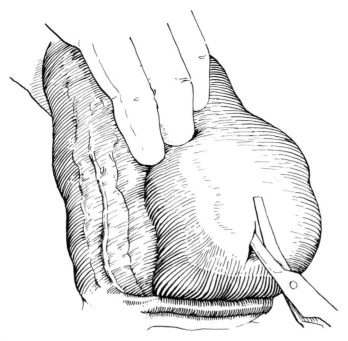

Fig. 41.27. Opening into left ventricular aneurysm. This aneurysm is on the base of the heart in the territory supplied by the right coronary artery and the heart has been elevated and turned backwards to expose the aneurysm.

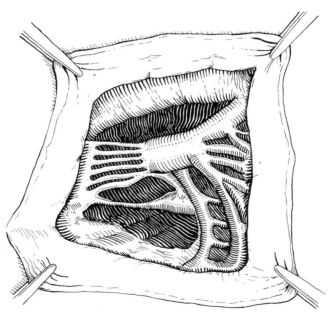

Fig. 41.28. The left ventricular aneurysm has been opened and much of it excised apart from a 1-cm rim of fibrous tissue around its edge for secure suturing. The interior of the heart and the papillary muscles of the left ventricle are shown.

Pulmonary Embolectomy

Indications

The criteria for surgical intervention will vary and in some centres little time is lost in operating on patients who in other centres would be treated conservatively for a further period. It is, of course, important that the diagnosis be established, for all of the following conditions have been mistakenly treated as massive pulmonary embolism and submitted to surgery:

1. Myocardial infarction, or myocarditis.
2. Postoperative septic shock.
3. Postoperative low output state.

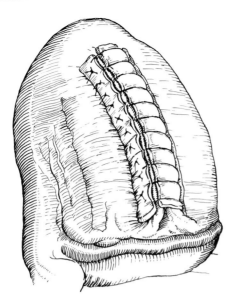

Fig. 41.29. Closure of left ventricular aneurysm using heavy Prolene sutures buttressed with Teflon felt supports; these sutures may be interrupted or continuous.

4. Mesenteric vascular occlusion.
5. Acute pericarditis.
6. Acute pancreatitis.

The diagnosis is best established by pulmonary arteriography, together with lung scanning, but these facilities may not always be available. It is not always the case that these patients present with so-called 'typical' physical findings and patients may suffer with major pulmonary embolism, having a normal jugular venous pressure. Electrocardiography is frequently of very great assistance, a recent change of axis from left to right being significant. No reliance whatsoever should be placed on the appearances at chest radiography, for many patients dying with massive pulmonary embolism have an apparently normal plain chest radiograph. The timing of operation is important, for published figures indicate that the chance of survival is poor for patients who have their operation following resuscitation from an episode of cardiac arrest.

Arbitrary definitions and levels of 'shock', hypotension, oliguria or even anuria are referred to in the literature when the indications for surgical intervention are discussed. If the patient is allowed to deteriorate before surgery is recommended this reflects the conservative approach of many clinicians. On the other hand, operative intervention on a diagnosis alone in a reasonably fit patient will clearly produce excellent operative results, albeit at the expense of some unnecessary surgery. These disparate views are reflected in the excellent results of this operation in some hands and the poor experience of others. It is clear that to await a prolonged period of severe hypotension, oliguria or anuria is to court disaster. Once considered, operation should be undertaken as soon as possible, and in an institution where those familiar with cardiothoracic surgery are present or available the timing of such an operation should be fairly well defined and the operative results acceptable.

Methods

Pulmonary embolectomy may be undertaken in one of two ways:
1. Using cardiopulmonary bypass.
2. Using inflow occlusion without cardiopulmonary bypass.

1. USING CARDIOPULMONARY BYPASS

General anaesthesia should be induced very carefully, for the patient's circulation may be maintained only by intense peripheral vasoconstriction. If this compensatory effect is abolished by the hasty administration of intravenous anaesthetics and relaxants, further hypotension and cardiac arrest may occur.

Full cardiopulmonary bypass is instituted following median sternotomy (*Fig.* 41.30). The main pulmonary artery is opened vertically above the valve and the clot is removed with forceps and suction. Desjardins' common bile duct forceps are very useful for their angles make it possible to explore the distal

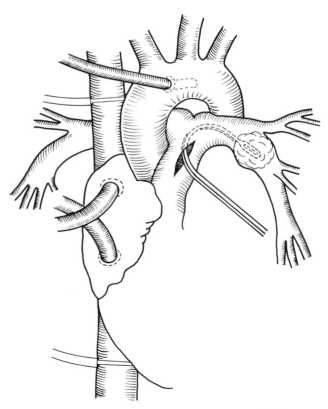

Fig. 41.30. Pulmonary embolectomy using cardiopulmonary bypass. Desjardins' fully curved bile duct forceps are very useful for grasping distal thrombi.

branches of both the right and left pulmonary arteries in order to secure clots. The right and left pleural cavities may be opened to enable the lungs to be gently massaged in order to extrude further thrombi in a retrograde direction, and at this stage forced ventilation of the lungs by the anaesthetist is useful to this end. When all clots have been removed the interior of the right ventricle and right atrium should be inspected and if necessary explored, for large coiled-up thrombi are often impacted in these chambers. The pulmonary artery is closed with a fine continuous suture and the patient gradually weaned from bypass.

Following this procedure it is considered by some surgeons that attention should now be turned to the inferior vena cava to undertake a procedure that will hopefully prevent further peripheral and pelvic thrombi from reaching the heart (*see* p. 657).

2. USING INFLOW OCCLUSION

Whereas pulmonary embolectomy using cardiopulmonary bypass is ideal, many patients present with major pulmonary embolism in hospitals where cardiac surgeons and cardiac surgery are not available. Although cardiac surgeons have from time to time travelled together with their equipment to undertake embolectomy in such hospitals, it is clear that this is unlikely to become a routine procedure. It is also clear that it is usually not possible to transfer such patients to cardiac surgical centres. It is, however, possible for cardiac surgeons or general surgeons to undertake pulmonary embolectomy in hospitals lacking the equipment for cardiopulmonary bypass and using the simplest of equipment.

Median sternotomy is undertaken using a Gigli saw, which is usually available in most general hospitals. The pericardium is opened vertically, and following a period of oxygenation of the patient with 100 per cent oxygen for several minutes, the superior and inferior venae cavae are occluded using shod intestinal clamps (*Fig.* 41.31). The heart is allowed to beat for a further 10–15 seconds to empty it of blood and the pulmonary artery, which is usually bulging and tense with clot, is incised vertically for 3 cm just above the pulmonary valve. This incision will be rewarded by the expulsion of a certain amount of blood together with masses of old and organizing thrombus. As much as possible is removed from the distal pulmonary arteries using Desjardins' clamps and the heart is massaged in order to milk further thrombus from the right ventricle. At the moment of caval occlusion the clock is watched carefully, and after a period of 2 minutes the superior vena caval clamp is removed, allowing the heart to fill with blood and to eject from the incision in the pulmonary artery. At that moment the pulmonary artery incision is occluded with a Satinsky or similar clamp, and the inferior vena caval clamp is then removed. To facilitate the reapplication of the Satinsky clamp, stay

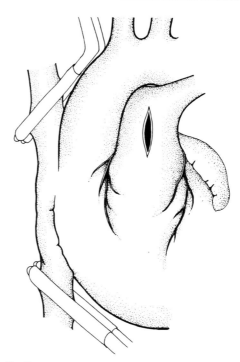

Fig. 41.31. Pulmonary embolectomy without cardiopulmonary bypass. Inflow occlusion by caval clamping is well tolerated for several short periods.

sutures of 4/0 Mersilene are placed in the pulmonary artery prior to its incision. The circulation is thus restarted and it is likely that the administration of inotropic drugs such as adrenaline, isoprenaline or dopamine will be required. Following a further period of 5 minutes of resumed circulation with both cavae unclamped, the Satinsky clamp is again removed, allowing a further 2-minute period of exploration of the pulmonary artery.

In most patients one or two periods of pulmonary artery exploration will enable the majority of thrombus to be removed and following the final application of the Satinsky clamp the pulmonary artery is repaired using the previously placed stay sutures as a continuous running stitch.

Although undertaking pulmonary embolectomy by caval occlusion is less satisfactory than it is with the use of cardiopulmonary bypass, it remains the only hope for the majority of patients requiring pulmonary embolectomy, for it is unrealistic to advocate cardiopulmonary bypass when in the majority of instances it is not available.

Acknowledgement

The editor wishes to thank W. B. Saunders Company of Philadelphia and Dr Denton Cooley of the Texas Heart Institute for permission to copy and modify the following illustrations in this chapter: *Figs.* 41.3, 41.15, 41.22, 41.23, 41.25, 41.27–41.29.

REFERENCES

Amoury R. A., Bowman F. O., Jr et al. (1966) Endocarditis associated with intracardiac prostheses. *J. Thorac. Cardiovasc. Surg.* **51**, 36.

Bailey C. P. (1949) The surgical treatment of mitral stenosis (mitral commissurotomy). *Dis. Chest* **15**, 377.

Bailey C. P., May A. et al. (1957) Survival after coronary endarterectomy in man. *JAMA* **164**, 641.

Baker C., Brock R. C. et al. (1950) Valvulotomy for mitral stenosis. *Br. Med. J.* **1**, 1283.

Barratt-Boyes B. G., Roche A. H. G. et al. (1969) Aortic valve replacement—a long-term follow-up of an initial series of 101 patients. *Circulation* **40**, 763.

Beck C. S. (1948) Revascularization of the heart. *Ann. Surg.* **128**, 854.

Berger S. and Salzman E. W. (1974) Thromboembolic complications of prosthetic devices In: Spaet T. (ed.) *Progress in Haemostasis and Thrombosis, Vol. II.* New York, Grune & Stratton, p. 273.

Bradley M. N., Bennett A. L., III, et al. (1964) Successful unilateral pulmonary embolectomy without cardiopulmonary bypass. *N. Engl. J. Med.* **271**, 713.

Braun L. O., Kincaid O. W. and McGoon D. C. (1973) Prognosis of aortic valve replacement in relation to preoperative heart size. *J. Thorac. Cardiovasc. Surg.* **65**, 381.

Braunwald E., Lambrew C. T. et al. (1964) Idiopathic hypertrophic sub-aortic stenosis. *Circulation* **30**, Suppl. 4, 1.

Cooley D. A., Leachman R. D. et al. (1973) Diffuse muscular sub-aortic stenosis: surgical treatment. *Am. J. Cardiol.* **31**, 1.

Cutler E. C. and Levine S. A. (1923) Cardiotomy and valvulotomy for mitral stenosis. *Boston Med. Surg. J.* **188**, 1023.

Favaloro R. G. (1969) Saphenous vein graft in the surgical treatment of coronary artery disease: operative technique. *J. Thorac. Cardiovasc. Surg.* **58**, 178.

Green G. E. (1984) Internal mammary–coronary anastomosis for myocardial ischaemia. In: Sabiston D. C. and Spencer F. C. (eds), *Gibbon's Surgery of the Chest*, 4th ed. Philadelphia, Saunders, pp. 1451–1458.

Grüntzig A. R., Senning A. and Siegenthaler W. E. (1979) Non-operative dilatation of coronary artery stenosis. *N. Engl. J. Med.* **301**, 61–68.

Hammermeister K. E. (1983) *Coronary Bypass Surgery.* New York, Praeger.

Harken D. E., Ellis L. B. et al. (1948) The surgical treatment of mitral stenosis. *N. Engl. J. Med.* **239**, 804.

Holman E. and Willett F. (1955) Results of radical pericardiectomy for constrictive pericarditis. *JAMA* **157**, 789.

McGoon D. C. (1960) Repair of a mitral insufficiency due to ruptured chordae tendineae. *J. Thorac. Surg.* **39**, 357.

Miller G. A. H., Sutton G. C. et al. (1971) Comparison of streptokinase and heparin in treatment of isolated acute massive pulmonary embolism. *Br. Med. J.* **2**, 681–684.

Moor G. F. and Sabiston D. C., Jr (1970) Embolectomy for chronic pulmonary embolism and hypertension. Case report and review of the problem. *Circulation* **41**, 701.

Muller W. H., Jr., Dammann J. F., Jr et al. (1960) Surgical correction of cardiovascular deformities in Marfan's syndrome. *Ann. Surg.* **152**, 506.

Mullin M. J., Engelman R. M. et al. (1974) Experience with open mitral commissurotomy in 100 consecutive patients. *Surgery* **76**, 974.

Pluth J. R. and McGoon D. C. (1974) Current status of heart valve replacement. *Mod. Concepts Cardiovasc. Dis.* **43**, 65.

Robinson M. J. and Ruedy J. (1962) Sequela of bacterial endocarditis. *Am. J. Med.* **32**, 922.

Roe B. B., Edmunds H., Jr et al. (1971) Open mitral commissurotomy. *Ann. Thorac. Surg.* **12**, 483.

Sabiston D. C., Jr and Wolfe W. G. (1968) Experimental and clinical observations on the natural history of pulmonary embolism. *Ann. Surg.* **168**, 1.

Sauvage L. R., Wood S. J., Eyer K. M. et al. (1963) Experimental coronary artery surgery: preliminary observations of bypass venous grafts, longitudinal arteriotomies and end-to-end anastomoses. *J. Thorac. Cardiovasc. Surg.* **46**, 825.

Selzer A. and Cohen K. E. (1972) Natural history of mitral stenosis: a review. *Circulation* **45**, 878.

Sharp E. H. (1962) Pulmonary embolectomy: successful removal of a massive pulmonary embolus with the support of cardiopulmonary bypass. A case report. *Ann. Surg.* **156**, 1.

Sones F. and Shirey E. K. (1962) Cine coronary angiography. *Mod. Conc. Cardiovasc. Dis.* **31**, 735.

Souttar H. S. (1955) Correspondence to Blades B. Intrathoracic surgery (lungs, heart and great vessels: surgical management of diseases of the oesophagus), 1905–55. *Int. Abstr. Surg.* **100**, 413.

Speller D. C. E. and Mitchell R. G. (1973) Coagulase-negative staphylococci causing endocarditis after cardiac surgery. *J. Clin. Pathol.* **26**, 517.

Starr A. and Edwards M. L. (1961) Mitral replacement: clinical experience with a ball valve prosthesis. *Ann. Surg.* **154**, 726.

Starr A., Grunkemeier G. L. and Lambert L. E. (1977) Aortic valve replacement. A ten-year follow up of non cloth covered vs cloth covered caged ball prostheses. *Circulation* **56** (suppl. 2), 133.

Stinson E. B., Griepp R. B. et al. (1974) Clinical experience with a porcine aortic valve xenograft for mitral valve replacement. *Ann. Thorac. Surg.* **18**, 391.

Stinson E. B., Griepp R. B. and Oyer P. E. (1977) Long term experience with porcine valve xenografts. *J. Thorac. Cardiovasc. Surg.* **73**, 54.

Trendelenburg F. (1908) Ueber die operative Behandlung der Embolie der Lungenarterie. *Arch. Klin. Chir.* **86**, 686.

Vineberg A. M. (1946) Development of an anastomosis between the coronary vessels and a transplanted internal mammary artery. *Can. Med. Assoc. J.* **55**, 117.

Wallace R. B., Londe S. P. et al. (1974) Aortic valve replacement with preserved aortic valve homografts. *J. Thorac. Cardiovasc. Surg.* **67**, 44.

Zacharias A., Grones L. K. et al. (1975) Rupture of the posterior wall of the left ventricle following mitral valve replacement. *J. Thorac. Cardiovasc. Surg.* **69**, 259.

Chapter forty-two

The Aortic Arch

D. A. Cooley, D. A. Ott and G. J. Reul Jr.

The operative management of pathological conditions of the aortic arch and its major branches has remained a particular challenge to the surgeon. Several major problems may be encountered while attempting operative repair. Because the great vessels arising from the aortic arch provide the cerebral blood flow, manipulation of these vessels during operation may result in severe neurological complications. Clamping the arteries during reimplantation or shunting procedures without the proper support may result in permanent neurological damage from cerebral ischaemia. Manipulation of the arteries may release atherosclerotic debris, or air may be introduced causing cerebral embolization. Proximal and distal clamping of the transverse aorta without support results not only in cerebral ischaemia but also in ischaemia to most vital structures, that is, the spinal cord, abdominal viscera, the kidneys and, proximally, ischaemia to the heart. Without careful placement of clamps or sutures, damage to other anatomical structures such as the recurrent laryngeal nerve, the venous drainage or the oesophagus may occur.

Most pathological conditions of the transverse arch and its branches have generalized involvement of the proximal and distal arteries and aorta, so that haemostasis and adequate restoration of flow are difficult. This, along with supportive measures during repair, may result in excessive bleeding. Furthermore, there are other operative risk factors in most patients such as old age, generalized arteriosclerosis, coronary arteriosclerosis, hypertension with early renal failure and/or chronic obstructive pulmonary disease.

In discussing the operative management of aortic arch lesions, solution to these problems is stressed.

SURGICAL ANATOMY

The thoracic aorta is divided into the ascending, transverse arch and descending aorta. The transverse aortic arch is that portion of the thoracic aorta which extends from the origin of the innominate artery or whichever is the first major great vessel to the last great vessel. In most cases, the last great vessel is the left subclavian artery. The distal portion of the aortic arch is also demarcated inferiorly by the ductus arteriosus or its remnant the ligamentum arteriosum. At the most distal portion of the transverse arch, the recurrent laryngeal nerve crosses over the ligamentum arteriosum. The reflexion of the pericardium extends to the level of the origin of the innominate

artery. The innominate vein overlies the uppermost portion of the aortic arch and the origin of the innominate artery. The trachea and oesophagus are immediately posterior to the ascending aorta and arch (*Fig.* 42.1).

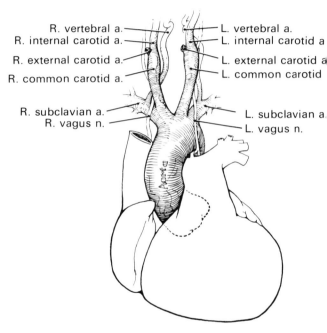

Fig. 42.1. The anatomy of the aortic arch and great vessels is shown. The transverse aortic arch is that part of the aorta which lies in between the first and last great vessel.

PATHOLOGY

The major pathological lesions discussed here are aneurysms and occlusive lesions of the arch and/or its branches. Traumatic lesions may occur either by deceleration injuries with blunt trauma or by penetrating and perforating injuries caused by various missiles or sharp instruments. The approach to traumatic lesions of this area is similar to the approach for the other pathological lesions. Several reviews have been written on this subject (Reul et al., 1973; 1974; Reul, 1976; Schaff and Brawley, 1977).

The pathology of aneurysms and occlusive lesions of the arch and great vessels is of particular significance and in some instances quite different from aneurysms and occlusive lesions in other areas of the vasculature.

ANEURYSMAL AND OCCLUSIVE LESIONS

Aneurysms

A clinically applicable classification of arch aneurysms on an anatomical basis is difficult since there has been confusion with regard to terminology (see Table 42.1). Fusiform aneurysms involve the entire

Table 42.1. Types of arch aneurysm

Anatomical classification
  Saccular
  Fusiform
  Dissecting
  Pseudo-aneurysm
Aetiological classification
  Congenital
    Marfan's syndrome
    Ehlers–Danlos syndrome
    Poststenotic from congenital lesions
Degenerative
  Arteriosclerosis
  Cystic medial necrosis
  Fibromuscular intimal hyperplasia
Inflammatory
  Syphilis
  Mycotic
  Postoperative infection
Mechanical
  Dissecting
  Iatrogenic—catheterization,
    cannulation, etc.

circumference of the aorta and usually have a more ovoid configuration. In a sacciform aneurysm, the defect in the aortic wall is confined to a portion of the circumference, whereas the remainder of the aortic wall is uninvolved.

Other considerations in management of the aneurysm are whether it is of a dissecting type in which a double lumen is present or whether the aneurysm is not a true aneurysm but a false aneurysm which is not composed of all layers of the aorta. Most dissecting aneurysms are fusiform; however, some may be saccular. False aneurysms, on the other hand, are frequently saccular and rather extensive. Arteriosclerotic aneurysms are usually fusiform, while most syphilitic aneurysms are saccular.

Another useful classification is based on the aetiology: congenital, degenerative, inflammatory or mechanical. The congenital type of aneurysms most commonly found in the thoracic aorta are those associated with Marfan's syndrome and rarely aneurysms from the Ehlers–Danlos syndrome. In addition, some aneurysms of the aortic arch may occur as a result of poststenotic dilatation because of obstructing congenital lesions or due to pseudo-coarctation of the aorta. These may occur in severe cases of supravalvular aortic stenosis, congenital aortic stenosis or cases of coarctation of the thoracic aorta. These are rare,

since the aorta most commonly becomes dilated or tortuous in these conditions.

In developed countries degenerative aneurysms of the thoracic aorta are most commonly seen in older patients, while in underdeveloped countries inflammatory aneurysms are more common and seen in younger patients. In the United States, the most common cause of degenerative aneurysm is arteriosclerosis. In most instances, other portions of the thoracic or abdominal aorta are involved, the most common site being the infrarenal abdominal aorta. When the arch is involved, arteriosclerosis is most frequently associated with uncontrolled hypertension and other risk factors associated with generalized arteriosclerosis. There may also be occlusive lesions of the great vessels and their branches. Fortunately, in most instances when the aortic arch is involved with arteriosclerosis there is merely a dilatation, and other aneurysms of the aorta take precedence. There usually is a large amount of arteriosclerotic debris and clot inside the aneurysms. This may result in cerebral embolization.

Another type of degenerative process resulting in aneurysm formation is cystic medial necrosis. The media and, in most cases, the elastic lamina of the aorta degenerate and are replaced by necrotic cystic material. Medial necrosis may also occur and is more common without cyst formation. This type of degenerative process may be associated with dissection and formation of a saccular or fusiform dissecting aneurysm. Pathological findings are similar to those of Marfan's syndrome.

In the great vessels fibromuscular intimal hyperplasia may also result in aneurysm formation. This is probably due to poststenotic dilatation resulting from the stenotic lesions.

Of the inflammatory lesions causing aneurysm formation, the most commonly associated condition has been syphilis. Although syphilitic lesions of the aortic arch have become rare in this country, they are common in other countries. The syphilitic aorta is somewhat different grossly from the arteriosclerotic aorta because the aorta is thickened from chronic inflammation and there may be several layers of calcium and gummatous deposits. There usually is a large amount of debris present in these aneurysms again acting as a potential source for embolization. The entire aorta is usually involved making proximal and distal anastomosis somewhat difficult. The origin of the great vessels may also be involved with occlusive lesions.

Another type of inflammatory aneurysm is the mycotic aneurysm. True mycotic aneurysms of the aortic arch are quite rare. Marasmic implantations are spared in this area probably because of the high blood flow. Rarely, following arch replacement or great vessel surgery, a postoperative infection may occur resulting in an infected graft or pseudo-aneurysm formation. Usually the surrounding structures are also involved, i.e. lungs, heart, oesophagus.

These are extremely difficult problems to treat because of the vital structures involved.

Dissecting aneurysms may be classified as mechanical with respect to aetiology. These are perhaps the most difficult problems to manage surgically. The lesions may be quite complex, involving the entire aorta and extending into the great vessels. If the aneurysm is acute, the consistency of the aorta is altered by oedema and inflammation. The presence of a double lumen also weakens the aortic wall making suturing difficult. Dissection may extend into the aortic root causing dehiscence of the aortic valve, necessitating aortic valve replacement and/or coronary artery reimplantation.

The most common causes of dissecting aneurysm of the aortic arch are medial degeneration and necrosis of the thoracic aorta, resulting in a mechanical tearing of the intima and a large false lumen or haematoma confined by a partial layer of media and adventitia. There may or may not be a re-entry site. Degeneration from arteriosclerosis has been the commonest cause of dissection in our series. The arteriosclerosis is associated with hypertension. Syphilitic lesions rarely cause dissection. Post-traumatic deceleration injuries of the thoracic aorta may cause retrograde or antegrade dissection into the aortic arch.

Iatrogenic manipulations such as cardiac catheterization or cannulation for cardiopulmonary bypass may also cause aortic arch dissection. Because they are acute, they may be difficult problems to manage.

Dissecting aneurysms of the aortic arch may originate with an intimal tear of the ascending aorta. The aneurysm may dissect into the entire distal aorta involving the arch, the descending thoracic aorta and abdominal aorta (type 1). In most instances these aneurysms can be managed by replacing the ascending thoracic aorta and obliterating the distal lumen just proximal to the arch.

The most difficult dissections to handle are the acute dissections which occur when a type 3 descending thoracic aortic aneurysm ruptures retrograde into the arch, ascending aorta and coronary arteries (Reul et al., 1975).

Type 1 dissecting aneurysms involving the aortic arch require arch resection only when they cannot be controlled by proximal or distal aortic surgery—that is, false lumen obliteration by resecting the ascending aneurysm portion. If the major great vessels are involved as indicated by loss of pulse or neurological deficit, then limited surgical intervention by bypass to the involved vessel may be done along with repair of the distal or proximal thoracic aorta. If the arch portion is dilated and is aneurysmal with a large haematoma or a thin outer layer, that is, if potential rupture is apparent, then arch replacement should be done.

In chronic dissecting aneurysms of the aortic arch, occasionally a large dilatation, causing respiratory obstruction or a potential danger of rupture, may be an indication for surgical intervention (Grande et al., 1984).

Occlusive Lesions

Occlusive lesions of the great vessels of the aortic arch are most commonly caused by arteriosclerosis. The arteriosclerotic plaques are localized usually to the sites of origin of the great vessels. Frequently other branches of the great vessels are involved such as the subclavian artery, vertebral artery and internal or external carotid arteries.

Syphilis rarely may cause areas of obstruction of the great vessels and is usually associated with generalized aortic disease (Duncan and Cooley, 1983c).

A unique type of obliterative process of the great vessels has been described by Takayasu (1908). Hypoplasia of the great vessels with obliteration of the lumen may occur in far advanced disease (Fig. 42.2). It is most commonly described in young females of Oriental descent (Shimizu and Sano, 1951). The pathological conditions causing occlusive lesions of the aortic arch have been described as the 'aortic arch syndrome' (Duncan and Cooley, 1983a, b, c).

Clinical Picture

Aneurysms of the aortic arch like aneurysms of other areas are frequently asymptomatic. For symptoms to occur, the aneurysm must be large. Actual erosion into the sternum may occur with long-standing aneurysms, in particular the syphilitic type. Pain from pressure of the aneurysm on the sternum or surrounding structures is probably the most common presenting symptom (Kampmeier, 1938). Symptoms of hoarseness or chronic 'brassy' cough may occur by stretching or damage to the left recurrent laryngeal nerve which passes over the ligamentum arteriosum. Respiratory symptoms associated with chronic respiratory distress and in some cases acute respiratory distress have been described (Lefrak et al., 1972). Compression of the trachea may occur because of expansion of the aneurysm in a posterior direction.

If haemoptysis occurs, it usually is a distressing sign, since this may indicate erosion of the aneurysm into the pulmonary parenchyma or bronchi. In most instances when frank haemoptysis appears in association with an arch aneurysm, rupture is imminent.

Some patients have the sensation of a large mass in their neck, and this may be associated with dysphagia when the aneurysm compresses the oesophagus during swallowing.

Dissecting aneurysms of the aortic arch that are associated with aneurysms of the ascending or descending aorta may be diagnosed because of the presenting symptoms common to dissecting aneurysms of these areas, that is, pain, cough, dyspnoea, loss of pulse or neurological signs.

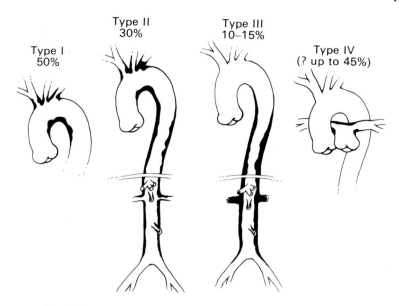

Fig. 42.2. A simplified classification of Takayasu's syndrome is illustrated. The incidence of the various types is shown.

With occlusive lesions of the great vessels, cerebrovascular symptoms are the most common. Stroke, transient ischaemic attacks or localized neurological signs or any combination may occur depending on the blocked vessel. In some instances, the occurrence of a transient ischaemic attack is not from the vascular obstructive lesion, but from embolization of debris from an ulcerative plaque. Most arteriosclerotic plaques of the great vessels, however, are not ulcerated as opposed to the common occurrence of ulcerative plaques of the internal carotid artery at the common carotid artery bifurcation.

Occlusion of the origin of the subclavian artery may result in the 'subclavian steal syndrome' because the ipsilateral vertebral artery supplies blood to the upper extremity in a retrograde manner by way of intracranial collateral arteries, in particular the basilar system and posterior circulation. This is most frequently an angiographic finding rather than a true clinical syndrome, because in most cases cerebrovascular symptoms associated with exercise of the ipsilateral extremity occur infrequently. On the other hand, in some instances vertebrobasilar insufficiency may be associated with these lesions, and corrective surgery may abolish the symptoms. True claudication of the hand may also occur depending on the collateral circulation and the level of obstruction. Gangrene of the upper extremity is extremely rare with occlusive lesions of the aortic arch, and may be related to distal embolization of necrotic debris from an aortic arch aneurysm or ulcerative plaques of the great vessels.

Diagnosis

Although both aneurysmal and occlusive lesions may be diagnosed with a strong index of suspicion and careful observation of the patient's signs and symptoms, the hallmark of diagnosis is angiography. Plain chest radiographs may show a large superior mediastinal mass in patients with transverse arch aneurysm and, in most cases, there is deviation of the trachea to the right, although deviation of the trachea to the left may also occur. Pulsation of the sternal notch or sternum may be present with large aneurysms.

Angiography not only determines the definitive diagnosis of aneurysms of the transverse arch, but also aids to determine the type of approach, the extent of repair and the type of support for surgery. Good arteriograms will determine the presence and the extent of the dissection. The origin of the arch vessels can also be evaluated for obstruction. Further study may be essential to demonstrate the coronary arteries to rule out occlusive disease or to demonstrate the aortic root and aortic valve function.

There is some danger in aortography. In dissecting aneurysms, the dissection may be extended or perforated by the catheter. A small test dose injection should be done to determine whether the catheter is in the true lumen or in the false lumen so that rupture or further dissection may not occur. Immediate surgery may be indicated if sudden rupture or cardiac tamponade occurs during the time of angiography.

In occlusive lesions, a plain chest radiograph may demonstrate calcium in the aortic arch or its branches. On auscultation, bruits may be present in the neck at the area of the level of stenosis or obstruction. Distal pulses may be decreased, and an occluded artery may take on a cord-like pulseless character.

Occlusive lesions may be demonstrated by angiography with a variety of techniques which visualize the aortic arch and the take-off of the major branches. In addition, since more distal lesions or intracranial lesions may cause the same symptoms, views of the bifurcation of the common carotid artery and intracerebral circulation in both anterior–posterior and lateral positions should be taken. In many cases, occlusive lesions of the great vessels are only demonstrated when complete cerebral vascular studies are done to rule out other causes of extracranial cerebral vascular disease of a more distal nature, such as occlusive lesions of the internal carotid or vertebral arteries. If proper arch studies have not been done prior to surgery for distal lesions, occlusive lesions of the arch vessels may be suspected when poor antegrade blood flow is obtained on release of the clamp on the common carotid artery.

Operative Management

Surgical Approach

There are several surgical approaches to the aortic arch and its branches (*Fig. 42.3*). We prefer to utilize the simplest possible approach causing the least dis-

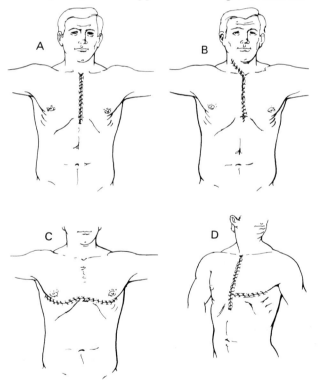

Fig. 42.3. The standard approaches for surgical treatments of aneurysms of the aortic arch are shown. A, Small- or moderate-sized aneurysms which do not extend far distally into the thoracic aorta can be treated by median sternotomy. B, If a bypass must be done to the great vessels, a neck extension to the right or left can be done. C, For large aneurysms of the ascending aorta, arch and descending thoracic aorta, a bilateral anterior thoracotomy provides sufficient exposure. D, In some instances when a median sternotomy has already been accomplished, a sideward extension through the 3rd or 4th interspace must be done to obtain control of the descending thoracic aorta if involved with aneurysm.

ability. In aneurysms of the aortic arch which do not extend far distally into the descending thoracic aorta and are not massive, median sternotomy with occasional extension into the neck (to the right or left) is the incision of choice. With a large aortic arch aneurysm, a bilateral transverse thoracotomy through the 3rd interspace is done to expose the entire ascending aortic arch and descending thoracic aorta and origin of the great vessels. This allows for treatment of large dissecting aneurysms in which the distal thoracic aorta must be repaired to obliterate the distal lumen or to control the saccular dilatation distally. Occasionally extension of the median sternotomy to the left 3rd or 4th intercostal space is necessary to further control the distal thoracic aorta, especially in emergency situations.

With occlusive lesions of the aortic arch and its great vessels, a median sternotomy is usually adequate to bypass innominate or left carotid arteries with a bypass originating in the aortic arch. In most instances, occluded vessels may by bypassed from extracranial vessels when they are not involved in the disease process. A large variety of different bypass combinations have been utilized in the treatment of single or multiple occlusions of the neck vessels. The surgical approach for each of these procedures is through the standard incision utilized for exposure of the arteries.

Type of Support

Perhaps the most important determinant to a good result in surgery of the aortic arch is the type of circulatory support during the operative procedure. Multiple techniques have been described for supporting cardiopulmonary, cerebral and renal function during operative repair of aortic arch aneurysms. Circulatory support may be divided into three basic types: (1) conventional cardiopulmonary bypass (Gwathmy et al., 1958; Muller et al., 1960; Hu et al., 1964; Larmi and Pentti, 1974; Panday et al., 1974), (2) cardiopulmonary bypass with cerebral extracorporeal perfusion (Cooley et al., 1957; DeBakey et al., 1957; Pearce et al., 1969; Philips and Miyamoto, 1974) and (3) hypothermia with circulatory arrest (Barnard and Schrire, 1963; Nicks, 1972; Griepp et al., 1975; Ott et al., 1978; Livesay et al., 1982, 1983; Speir et al., 1982). The first two techniques have been used in the past, but the third technique is now preferred.

CONVENTIONAL CARDIOPULMONARY BYPASS

The conventional cardiopulmonary circuit is established. The cavae are cannulated through the atria for venous return and the femoral artery for arterial return. The aneurysm is bypassed by a Dacron graft placed from the ascending aorta to the descending aorta in an end-to-side fashion. Partial occlusion clamps are used so that aortic interruption is not necessary. While circulation is maintained through the original thoracic aortic aneurysm, the arch vessels are bypassed individually in an end-(graft)-to-side-(artery) fashion during a short period of occlusion of the grafted artery. The distal circulation of the arch vessels can be supported at this time by an internal shunt. The proximal ends of the Dacron grafts placed to the great vessels are then placed to the previously placed graft between the proximal and distal aorta. After all the bypasses are accomplished, the aneurysm is resected between the Dacron graft, the proximal and distal aortic stumps are oversewn and continuity of the aortic arch is established by releasing the clamps. Any combination of anastomoses may be done in this fashion.

There are several disadvantages to this technique. Proper cerebral protection is not achieved during the occlusion period for the bypass grafts, and it is usually difficult to place good intraluminal shunts. The procedure is also complicated by the large number of anastomoses, in some instances into the very poor tissue of the great vessels or aorta. The proximal and distal stumps of the aorta are difficult to close with good haemostasis.

CARDIOPULMONARY BYPASS WITH CEREBRAL EXTRACORPOREAL PERFUSION

This second technique is similar to the first; however, cerebral protection is attempted by cerebral perfusion through either a single roller pump for all the great vessels or through individual roller pumps with flow-regulated lines to each individual great vessel (*Fig.* 42.4). An end-to-end thoracic graft can be placed rather than a side-to-side graft as with the first technique. The femoral artery is cannulated for conventional cardiopulmonary bypass. The right axillary artery is cannulated. This provides retrograde perfusion to the right subclavian artery and the right carotid artery through the innominate artery. A third cannula is placed directly in the left carotid artery to perfuse the left carotid circulation. Perfusion through the separate cannulas then supports cerebral circulation while the aortic arch is resected and continuity re-established and the aortic arch reconstructed with Dacron grafts or reimplantation. Cerebral arterial perfusion pressures may be monitored by bilateral temporal artery catheters or other indirect techniques.

The major disadvantage of this technique is that the cerebral circulation cannot be accurately regulated since the cerebral circulation is not self-regulatory. Flows at different levels from 50 to 300 ml/kg/min have been recommended in each individual artery. Frequent neurological complications have occurred in the practice of this technique because of too much or too little perfusion, and possibly because of micro-emboli generated by the perfusion process. The multiple cannulas are cumbersome. Also, there is a high margin of error for introduction of air along with debris or other complications attendant on multiple artery cannulation.

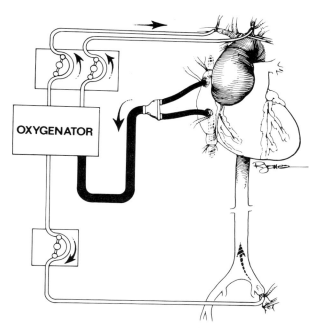

Fig. 42.4. A second method of cerebral protection is illustrated. Conventional cardiopulmonary bypass is established and extra pumps or the same roller pumps are utilized for perfusion of the great vessels. In this case, the one separate roller pump and cannula serve the right axillary artery which perfuses the right carotid artery in a retrograde manner. A second roller pump and cannula is placed in the left carotid artery. The pumps are individually regulated with low flow. Since the cerebral blood flow is not self-regulatory, this technique can be hazardous and also it is quite complex.

HYPOTHERMIA WITH CIRCULATORY ARREST

The third technique of support is that of moderate total body hypothermia by core cooling followed by total circulatory arrest (*Fig.* 42.5). In this technique, the femoral artery and in some instances the ascending aorta are cannulated, and core cooling is accomplished to a temperature of approximately 20°C. For anticipated short periods of circulatory arrest (less than 30 minutes), core temperature of 20°C is sufficient. In anticipated longer periods, the core temperature may be reduced to 16°C. Usually, the temperature falls below the level at which cold perfusion is discontinued, and may be 2–4°C lower after the circulation is arrested. In some instances, application of ice bags to the scalp will ensure a lowered cortical temperture and may be indicated for longer periods of circulatory arrest. When the temperature has been reduced to the desired level, arterial perfusion is discontinued at the same time that the venous outlet line is occluded. When possible, the aortic arch vessels are cross-clamped to prevent air entrapment in those vessels, but this manoeuvre is not essential. The aneurysm is opened, and internal inspection of the aortic arch ensues. A plan of reconstruction is decided, and rapid restoration of the internal vessels by endoaneurysmorrhaphy is done (Cooley, 1984).

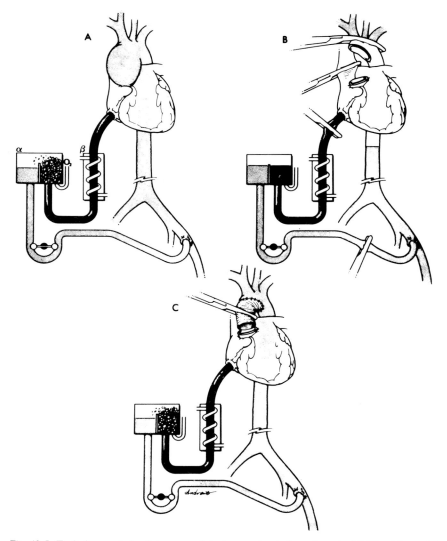

Fig. 42.5. Techniques of circulatory arrest during moderate hypothermia (20 °C) with partial exsanguination.

Recently we have continued a very low flow perfusion, approximately 10 cm³/kg body weight, during this period to ensure some circulation to the lower half of the body and prevent air entrapment. Once restoration of circulation has been accomplished by the distal anastomosis, perfusion becomes possible into the arch vessels by clamping the aortic graft. Air is evacuated from the arterial system, and retrograde perfusion of the femoral artery to the cerebral circulation is restored. The proximal anastomosis to the ascending aorta or the aortic annulus is then completed during the period of rewarming. Cardiac preservation may be enhanced during this period by further hypothermia or introduction of cardioplegic solution if aortic valve replacement is necessary.

We have used all three techniques described above and have found that moderate body hypothermia with total circulatory arrest is a superior supportive technique during arch replacement. It has become a simple method of cerebral protection and is associated with the lowest rate of complications.

We have not routinely utilized internal shunts for treatment of aneurysms or occlusive lesions of the great vessels. The extrathoracic approach to most of these lesions offers a superior form of protection and an uncomplicated course. On occasion, in conjunction with other cardiac surgical procedures, innominate artery or carotid artery reconstruction has been undertaken, and in these instances the bypass grafts may be placed easily from the ascending aorta to the distal artery. On rare occasions, in these procedures, total circulatory arrest with deep hypothermia has been utilized; however, if the systemic metabolic conditions are maintained during a short episode of occlusion of a great vessel, cerebral complications can be avoided without the use of shunts. If a shunt is utilized, care must be taken that distal dissection and introduction of air or debris do not occur.

Operative Technique for Arch Aneurysms

The operative technique depends on the type of circulatory support utilized during occlusion of the great vessels in repair of aortic arch aneurysms. Our preferred method has already been stated, as have other methods of reconstruction of the aortic arch. Whenever possible the simplest approach should be utilized, and this is to allow the arch vessels to be retained on the distal aortic segment so that one anastomosis accomplishes repair of the entire aneurysm (*Fig.* 42.6). This approach can be utilized in instances when the great vessels are not occluded by plaques.

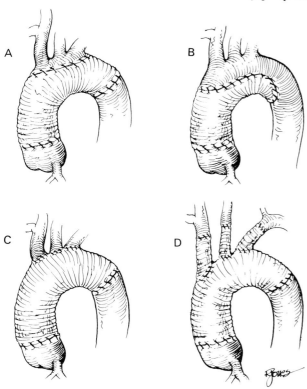

Fig. 42.6. Different types of arch repair are shown. A, the arch has been replaced with a Dacron graft and the great vessels placed to the Dacron graft as one unit. B, The inferior portion of the arch aneurysm has been resected, and a single anastomosis is used for the entire distal aorta with its great vessels. C, Separate reimplantation of each artery is done to the graft which has been used to replace the transverse arch. D, Bypass or interposition grafts are done from the transverse arch graft to the great vessels individually. Grafts have been fabricated which avoid the proximal anastomosis of graft to graft. This technique is reserved for cases where the arch vessels are severely involved with aneurysmal or occlusive disease in conjunction with an aortic arch aneurysm.

In some instances, if the vessels are occluded by plaques, endarterectomy may be done to one or two or all of the great vessels. The proximal anastomosis can be achieved by anastomosis to an area usually above the annulus, and in most instances of pure arch aneurysm the aortic valve is not involved. When, however, the aortic valve is involved, replacement rather than resuspension is done as based on our pre-

vious experience. Reimplantation of the coronary arteries can be done by a variety of techniques (Kidd et al., 1976). Saphenous vein grafts may be done to either the right or left coronary system, or reimplantation of the right coronary artery and left coronary artery may be accomplished.

We prefer to use a tightly woven Dacron graft (Meadox*) of large enough size to fit snugly into the inner lumen of the aorta. Size must be equilibrated to both the proximal and distal aorta and when a single distal anastomosis is utilized with all the arch vessels, a 26- or 30-mm graft is most frequently used. A multifilament-coated Dacron suture is used for the anastomosis. Because of the great problems with haemostasis in these patients, careful anastomotic techniques must be utilized. We prefer a single running suture for the entire anastomosis.

Dissecting aneurysms originating in the ascending aorta (type A) should all be managed by the open technique, utilizing induced hypothermia and circulatory arrest (Cooley and Livesay, 1981; Speir et al., 1982; Livesay et al., 1983). In the acute dissection, cross-clamping of the aorta is contra-indicated, since it lacerates the internal lumen, and this prevents an adequate repair. Open distal anastomosis is essential for an adequate repair of an acute dissection and also facilitates repair in a chronic lesion. Usually the distal anastomosis may be done proximal to the origin of the arch vessels. The graft may be telescoped into the true lumen of the aorta to ensure that the direction of the major blood flow is centrally placed. Extension of the dissection into the descending aorta is common, but if the site of origin of the dissecting process is repaired, the distal dissection usually becomes quiescent. Surgical removal of residual dissection is technically almost impossible and may lead to complications due to compromise of blood supply to the spinal cord or kidneys. Thus, the concept of treatment for dissections is to repair the site of origin and to prevent acute rupture into the pericardial sac with tamponade. Also, restoration of aortic competence is necessary. When commissures are detached from the aortic wall by the dissecting process, then reattachment and reconstruction of the valve are essential. In severe valve disruptions, the valve may require replacement with a prosthesis.

Operative Technique for Occlusive Lesions

The operative technique for occlusive lesions differs from that of arch replacement because flow does not have to be interrupted through the entire transverse arch. The basic techniques of reimplantation, endarterectomy and bypass have been utilized in the past. Reimplantation of a great vessel, after resection of the diseased portion, may be done; however, it is technically difficult because in most instances the aor-

* Meadox Medicals Inc., P.O. Box 530, Oakland, New Jersey 07436, USA.

tic arch is arteriosclerotic so that anastomosis may be difficult. In addition, not enough length of the distal vessel can be obtained following resection of the diseased segment.

Another technique is that of endarterectomy of the diseased artery. The artery is opened over the area of blockage and the intimal plaque carefully removed. This can be done only in selected cases where the arterial occlusive lesion is a short isolated segment and there is no severe distal or proximal disease. Therefore, it is preferred in younger patients who do not have diffuse arteriosclerosis. We have utilized it in several instances of isolated innominate artery stenosis.

Perhaps the most useful and simple technique is that of bypass of the diseased vessel utilizing either an extrathoracic or intrathoracic approach (*Fig.* 42.7). The approach chosen depends on the accompanying lesions and the general condition of the patient, along with the distal and proximal anatomical disease. Any combination of techniques is possible and is left to the imagination of the vascular surgeon. In general, we prefer to use a double velour Dacron graft (Meadox) for these bypasses. The graft is usually 7 or 8 mm in diameter. A multifilament-coated Dacron suture is utilized for both anastomoses. Bifurcation grafts or specially designed grafts may be used for multiple distal anastomoses from one proximal anastomosis on the aorta. An inverted 12×7-mm double velour bifurcation graft may be utilized to bypass two vessels from the ascending thoracic aorta. In the case where endarterectomy may be done in conjunction with the bypass procedure, such as a carotid endarterectomy with carotid subclavian bypass, the distal portion of the bypass graft may function as a large patch graft over the endarterectomized segment and the proximal portion led to the subclavian artery.

In the 'aortic arch syndrome', most often bypasses must be done from the ascending aorta because of the multiple vessel involvement and the length of the stenotic lesions. In some instances distal vessels are completely occluded and bypass may be done to one or two non-major distal arteries, such as the vertebral artery or external carotid artery, to increase the collateral circulation (*Fig.* 42.8). Frequently the ascending

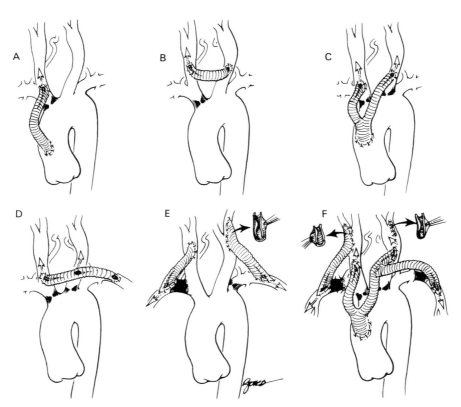

Fig. 42.7. The various types of extrathoracic and intrathoracic bypass graft techniques for the treatment of occlusive lesions of the great vessels are shown. A, Ascending aorta to innominate artery bypass is done through a transthoracic approach. B, The same lesion can be treated by left carotid to right carotid bypass. This avoids the intrathoracic approach. C, An inverted Y bifurcation graft is shown from the ascending aorta to the innominate artery and left carotid. D, With the similar obstruction as C, an extrathoracic approach can be used by placing a Dacron graft from the left subclavian artery to both carotid arteries. E, Carotid subclavian bypass is shown for treatment of either carotid or subclavian occlusive disease. On the left carotid, carotid endarterectomy is done and the Dacron graft acts as a long patch graft over the endarterectomized segment and is placed to the subclavian artery. F, Bilateral carotid endarterectomies have been done as staged lesions and the bypass grafts placed as shown. The extrathoracic or intrathoracic approach to these lesions should be individualized for each individual case.

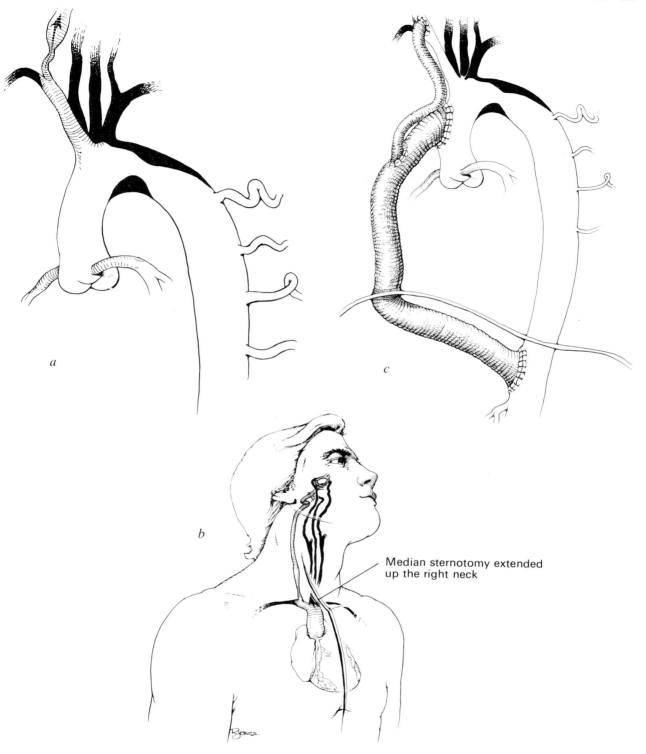

Median sternotomy extended
up the right neck

Fig. 42.8. A complicated case of Takayasu's disease is shown diagrammatically. *a*, Complete occlusion of the great vessels is shown. The only artery supplying the cerebral circulation is a tortuous and dilated right vertebral artery arising from a right innominate artery. In addition, there is a coarctation of the aorta. *b*, The surgical approach to this lesion is shown. A median sternotomy with extension to the right neck was done. The large tortuous vertebral artery can be seen to be the only artery supplying the brain. *c*, Treatment of the coarctation was done by anterior approach through a median sternotomy as previously seen. A Dacron graft was placed from the ascending aorta to the abdominal aorta just below the diaphragm. The bypass graft was then placed from the aortic graft to the vertebral graft. The remaining arteries were characteristically small and hypoplastic and could not be bypassed. This offers an alternative technique to a difficult problem of Takayasu's syndrome.

aorta is likewise involved, and the proximal anastomoses may be quite difficult.

Results

During the past 30 years 1775 patients have undergone surgical repair of aneurysms involving the thoracic aorta at the Texas Heart Institute. In 843 patients the aneurysm was limited to the ascending aorta (AATA) with or without involvement of the aortic valve. This group (AATA) included patients with acute and chronic dissections, non-dissecting aneurysms and those patients with Marfan's syndrome. Operative mortality was 16·5 per cent (139 patients).

Aneurysms of the descending thoracic aorta (ADTA) occur with a similar frequency, there being 734 cases in the Texas Heart Institute series. Prior to 1974 the operative mortality for ADTA, including acute and chronic dissection and non-dissecting aneurysms, was 20·6 per cent (75/363). Recent advances in technique have accounted for an improvement to the present mortality of 8–11 per cent (Livesay et al., 1985).

Aneurysms involving the aortic arch are less common than those limited either to the ascending or to the descending thoracic aorta. One hundred and ninety-eight patients with such aneurysms have been operated on at the Texas Heart Institute. Because of problems related to air embolization, bleeding and the need of continued cerebral perfusion, aneurysms of the aortic arch were felt to be beyond the realm of surgical therapy as recently as 25 years ago. Overall surgical mortality for these otherwise fatal aneurysms has been as high as 37 per cent, but the recent institution of techniques using moderate hypothermia and circulatory arrest has decreased the operative mortality for resection of arch aneurysms to 10 per cent (Livesay et al., 1983). The haemorrhagic, neurological, renal and pulmonary complications have likewise been reduced dramatically by adoption of the technique of moderate body hypothermia followed by total circulatory arrest.

Results in surgical repair of occlusive lesions of the great vessels of the aortic arch have been good. The ultimate result is determined by the many previously stated factors; however, with the techniques of endarterectomy, bypass or reimplantation, the mortality rate is less than 1 per cent and related to the extent of the disease process and general condition of the patient. It is obvious that for a simple carotid–subclavian bypass, the mortality rate is virtually negligible. In more complex cases, such as the aortic arch syndrome where multiple bypasses are done, from diseased proximal segments to diseased distal segments, the mortality is somewhat higher. The incidence of transient neurological problems is less than 5 per cent and permanent neurological problems less than 2 per cent with the operative techniques described above. Long-term patency rates approach 90 per cent, and 85 per cent of the patients experience relief of symptoms without recurrence. Since the lesions are so varied, an individual approach to each patient with regard to prognosis and choice of operation must be exercised.

REFERENCES

Barnard C. N. and Schrire V. (1963) The surgical treatment of acquired aneurysm of the thoracic aorta. *Thorax* **18**, 101–115.
Cooley D. A. (1984) Endoaneurysmorrhaphy revisited. *Texas Heart Inst. J.* **11**, 8–9.
Cooley D. A. and Livesay J. J. (1981) Technique of 'open' distal anastomosis for ascending and transverse arch resection. *Cardiovasc. Dis., Bull. Texas Heart Inst.* **8**, 421–426.
Cooley D. A., DeBakey M. E. and Morris G. C. (1957) Controlled circulation in surgical treatment of aortic aneurysm. *Ann. Surg.* **146**, 473–486.
DeBakey M. E., Crawford E. S., Cooley D. A. et al. (1957) Successful resection of fusiform aneurysm of aortic arch with replacement by homograft. *Surg. Gynecol. Obstet.* **105**, 657–664.
Duncan J. M. and Cooley D. A. (1983a) Surgical considerations in aortitis with special emphasis on Takayasu's arteritis. *Texas Heart Inst. J.* **10**, 233–247.
Duncan J. M. and Cooley D. A. (1983b) Surgical considerations in aortitis. II. Mycotic aneurysms. *Texas Heart Inst. J.* **10**, 329–335.
Duncan J. M. and Cooley D. A. (1983c) Surgical considerations in aortitis. III. Syphilitic and other forms of aortitis. *Texas Heart Inst. J.* **10**, 337–341.
Grande A. M., Eren E. E., Hallman G. L. et al. (1984) Rupture of the thoracic aorta: emergency treatment and management of chronic aneurysms. *Texas Heart Inst. J.* **11**, 244–249.
Griepp R. B., Stinson E. B., Hollingsworth J. F. et al. (1975) Prosthetic replacement of the aortic arch. *J. Thorac. Cardiovasc. Surg.* **70**, 1051–1063.
Gwathmey O., Pierpont H. C. and Blades B. (1958) Clinical experiences with the surgical treatment of acquired aortic vascular disease. *Surg. Gynecol. Obstet.* **107**, 205–213.
Hu Y. U., Shank T. Y. and Wy Y. K. (1964) Surgical treatment of aneurysm of the thoracic aorta. *Chin. Med. J.* **83**, 740.
Kampmeier R. H. (1938) Saccular aneurysm of the thoracic aorta: a clinical study of 633 cases. *Ann. Intern. Med.* **12**, 624–651.

Kidd J. N., Reul G. J. Jr, Cooley D. A. et al. (1976) Surgical treatment of aneurysms of the ascending aorta. *Circulation* **54**(6), Suppl. III, 118–122.

Larmi T. K. I. and Pentti K. (1974) Resection of the transverse aortic arch. *J. Thorac. Cardiovasc. Surg.* **68**, 70–75.

Lefrak E. A., Stevens P. M. and Howell J. F. (1972) Respiratory insufficiency due to tracheal compression by an aneurysm of the ascending, transverse, and descending thoracic aorta: successful surgical management in a 76-year-old man. *J. Thorac. Cardiovasc. Surg.* **63**(6), 956–961.

Livesay J. J., Cooley D. A., Duncan J. M. et al. (1982) Open aortic anastomosis: improved results in the treatment of aneurysms of the aortic arch. *Circulation* **66** (Suppl. 1), 122–127.

Livesay J. J., Cooley D. A., Reul G. J. Jr., et al. (1983) Resection of aortic arch aneurysms: a comparison of hypothermic techniques in 60 patients. *Ann. Thorac. Surg.* **36**, 19–28.

Livesay J. J., Cooley D. A., Ventemiglia R. A. et al. (1985) Surgical experience in descending thoracic aneurysmectomy with and without adjuncts to avoid ischemia. *Ann. Thorac. Surg.* **39**, 37–46.

Muller W. H., Warren W. D. and Blanton F. S. (1960) A method for resection of aortic arch aneurysms. *Ann. Surg.* **151**, 225–230.

Nicks R. (1972) Aortic arch aneurysm: resection and replacement: protection of the nervous system. *Thorax* **27**, 239–245.

Ott D. A., Frazier O. H. and Cooley D. A. (1978) Resection of the aortic arch using deep hypothermia and temporary circulatory arrest. *Circulation* **58** (3), Suppl. 1, 1227–1231.

Panday S. R., Parulkar G. B., Chauker A. P. et al. (1974) Simplified technique for aortic arch replacement: first stage right subclavian to left carotid bypass. *Ann. Thorac. Surg.* **18**, 186–190.

Pearce C. W., Weichert R. F. and del Real R. E. (1969) Aneurysms of aortic arch: simplified technique for excision and prosthetic replacement. *J. Thorac. Cardiovasc. Surg.* **58**, 886–890.

Philips P. A. and Miyamoto A. M. (1974) Use of hypothermia and cardiopulmonary bypass in resection of aortic arch aneurysms. *Ann. Thorac. Surg.* **17**, 398–404.

Reul G. J., Jr. (1976) Vascular injury and arteriovenous fistula. In: Sabiston D. C. (ed.) *Practice of Surgery: Cardiovascular Surgery*, Ch. 5. Maryland, Harper & Row, pp. 15–16.

Reul G. J., Jr, Beall A. C., Jr, Jordan G. L., Jr et al. (1973) The early operative management of injuries to the great vessels. *Surgery* **74**, 862–873.

Reul G. J., Jr, Cooley D. A., Hallman G. L. et al. (1975) Dissecting aneurysm of the descending aorta: improved surgical results in 91 patients. *Arch. Surg.* **110**, 632–640.

Reul G. J., Jr, Rubio P. A. and Beall A. C., Jr (1974) The surgical management of acute injury to the thoracic aorta. *J. Thorac. Cardiovasc. Surg.* **67**, 272–281.

Schaff H. V. and Brawley R. K. (1977) Operative management of penetrating vascular injuries of the thoracic outlet. *Surgery* **82**(2), 182–191.

Shimizu K. and Sano J. (1951) Pulseless disease. *J. Neuropathol. Clin. Neurol.* **1**, 37.

Speir A. M., Grey D. P. and Cooley D. A. (1982) Resection of the aortic arch with moderate hypothermia and temporary circulatory arrest. *Texas Heart Inst. J.* **9**, 311–320.

Takayasu M. (1908) Case of queer changes in central blood vessels of retina. *Acta Soc. Ophthalmol. Jap.* **12**, 554.

Chapter forty-three

The Descending Thoracic Aorta

G. Keen

Operations on the descending thoracic aorta are indicated for acute traumatic rupture, acute dissections and for chronic aneurysms, but a common indication is for the resection and anastomosis of coarctation of the aorta. The surgical management of coarctation of the aorta is dealt with in Chapter 40 but much of this present chapter is appropriate to the management of coarctation in certain circumstances.

Operations on the descending thoracic aorta are complicated by the need to cross-clamp the aorta high up and at the same time prevent left ventricular strain and to protect the kidneys, spinal cord and abdominal viscera from the effects of ischaemia. In experimental animals aortic cross-clamping at this level without bypass results in a marked rise in left ventricular, left atrial and pulmonary artery pressure, and if aortic occlusion is maintained for longer than about 20 minutes at normal temperatures the risk of paraplegia becomes very great (Kahn, 1970; Taber, 1970; Keen, 1972).

In the first reported successful repair of traumatic rupture of the aorta (Passaro and Pace, 1959) the surgeon cross-clamped the aorta of a 30-year-old man without bypass for a 17-minute period, during which he sutured a 3 mm tear at the isthmus. He noted that the heart became grossly distended and the electrocardiograph pattern bizarre, with conduction defects and T-wave inversion, and that the proximal blood pressure rose to 200 mmHg. Although the patient survived, this experience was sufficiently worrying to persuade the surgeon to recommend hypothermia on future occasions. Others have stated that patients in whom restorative surgery is undertaken rapidly have no need of bypass support, but the development of paraplegia in some cases following this technique hardly commends this advice (Crawford et al., 1970). Moreover, it takes no account of possible renal damage, especially in the elderly.

PARAPLEGIA AND AORTIC SURGERY

In 1972, Brewer et al. studied a collected series of 12 532 cases of repair of coarctation of the aorta which were complicated by 51 instances of severe neurological damage, usually paraplegia, an incidence of 0·41 per cent or about 1 in 240 cases. In addition, they discovered a total of eight patients with this condition who developed paraplegia without surgical operations. They carefully reviewed this complication from the standpoint of the blood supply of the spinal cord and it is this blood supply and its variations which may determine whether or not a patient having descending aortic surgery is likely to be at risk of neurological damage.

ANATOMY (*Figs.* 43.1, 43.2)

The traditional concept of the blood supply to the spinal cord is that the anterior spinal artery forms a single continuous channel which flows uninterrupted from the cervical to the lumbar region. There are, however, many variations. The first accurate description of the circulation of the spinal cord was reported by Adamkiewicz (1882) and Kadyi (1886, 1889). They showed that the anterior spinal artery is not a continuous vessel and that not every intercostal vessel in the thoracic region will have a radicular branch to supply the anterior spinal artery.

The anterior spinal artery is divided into end arteries at several levels making possible a functional division of the blood supply to the cord. The upper division, which is the upper cervical and thoracic regions, is supplied by branches of the vertebral arteries which form the anterior spinal artery and by a number of spinal arteries which vary in location, the most constant branch accompanying a radicular branch of C4 and which receives its blood supply from the superior intercostal vessels. The middle division from the middle of the lower thoracic region of the cord has the poorest segmental blood supply and is usually dependent on one radicular artery which commonly arises from T7, T8 or T9.

The lower or lumbar division is supplied almost exclusively by the unpaired great radicular artery of Adamkiewicz and this artery shows considerable variation. When it arises from a lower thoracic intercostal vessel the branch to the middle division may be absent and when the great radicular artery arises in the lumbar region the blood supply to the lower thoracic cord is poor in the absence of T7–T9 radicular branches. Under normal circumstances, there is little exchange between the territories of the various radicular arteries, and variations in number and origin of important radicular arteries may result in an inability of the anterior spinal artery to function as a collateral. In effect, occlusion of intercostal vessels may be harmless in one patient and dangerous in another.

Although these anatomical variations are of particular importance in the management of coarctation of the aorta, they are of course most relevant when undertaking surgery for traumatic and degenerative

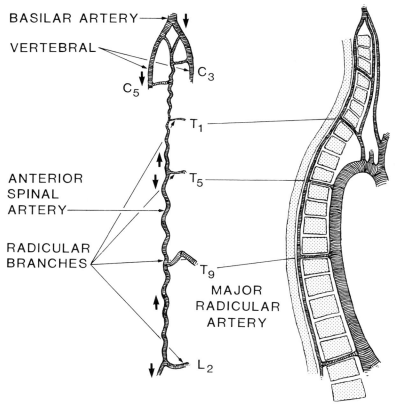

Fig. 43.1. Segmental blood supply of the anterior spinal arteries via the radicular branches of the intercostal and other aortic vessels together with a supply from the vertebral arteries. The anterior spinal artery is shown as a continuous vessel but common variations make the continuity of the anterior spinal artery precarious and undependable.

conditions of the aorta. It is important that the surgeon determines whether the collateral circulation is adequate in the distal aorta after cross-clamping, and it is clear that the only safe measure is that of recording intra-aortic pressures in the descending aorta during surgery. Although the majority of patients with coarctation of the aorta will maintain a high distal pressure after cross-clamping (i.e. above 50 mmHg mean), all, or nearly all patients with surgery for acquired conditions, and who have no collateral circulation, will produce no distal aortic pressure following cross-clamping. It is clear that those patients with coarctation of the aorta, who after cross-clamping produced little or no distal pressure, and all patients having surgery for acquired diseases will need some form of bypass.

Laschinger et al. in 1983 undertook an investigation of the experimental and clinical assessment of the adequacy of partial bypass in the maintenance of spinal cord blood flow during operations on the thoracic aorta using spinal cord impulse conduction (somatosensory-evoked potentials). This group found no significant changes in spinal cord blood flow or somatosensory-evoked potentials in any animal with a distal aortic pressure greater than or equal to 70 mmHg. With a pressure of 40 mmHg, normal flow and somatosensory-evoked potentials were maintained in five of the six experimental animals. Loss of somatosensory-evoked potentials, with simultaneous loss of spinal cord blood flow at the level of T6, occurred in one dog. Restoration of distal aortic pressure to 70 mmHg in all animals resulted in immediate return of somatosensory-evoked potentials and loss of somatosensory-evoked potentials routinely occurred in animals with a distal aortic pressure less than 40 mmHg. They concluded that maintenance of a distal aortic pressure greater than 60–70 mmHg will uniformly preserve spinal cord blood flow in the absence of critical intercostal exclusion. Should distal aortic pressure be inadequate, early reversible changes in the somatosensory-evoked potentials will alert the surgeon and failure to institute measures to reverse these changes may result in paraplegia.

In those centres where extensive experience of descending aortic surgery has been obtained, some surgeons advocate descending aortic surgery without the use of left heart bypass or some form of shunting. It must be borne in mind that this small and select group of surgeons operates with extreme rapidity thus avoiding prolonged periods of spinal cord ischaemia. For the majority of surgeons, however, who

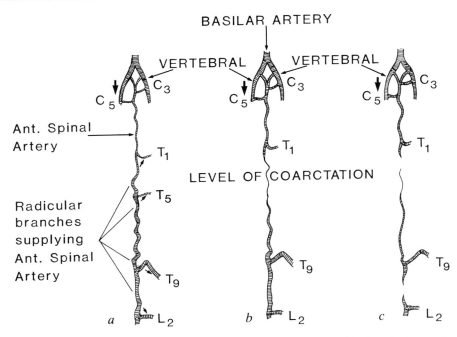

Fig. 43.2. Variations in the supply to the anterior spinal artery. In (*a*) the spinal artery is supplied by many good radicular vessels but in (*b*) there is clearly limitation of anterior spinal artery flow between T1 and T9. In (*c*), owing to the poor radicular supply from the intercostal vessels, there is discontinuity in the anterior spinal artery between T1 and T9 and again between T9 and L2, and it is in such cases that the spinal cord is endangered during operations on the descending thoracic aorta. The large radicular artery at the level of about T9 (the artery of Adamkiewicz) is a very constant and reliably large branch to the lumbar cord.

have less experience but who from time to time necessarily undertake these operations, such surgery without bypass is reckless.

LEFT ATRIOFEMORAL BYPASS

Left atriofemoral bypass (Cooley et al., 1957; Gerbode et al., 1957) is employed in many cases in which surgery of the descending thoracic aorta is undertaken. This technique allows satisfactory operating conditions, preventing proximal hypertension and left ventricular strain during aortic cross-clamping and also ensuring adequate renal and spinal cord perfusion. Heparinization and its reversal by protamine pose no undue problems, but should intra-abdominal or intracerebral bleeding be taking place heparinization might aggravate this. The patient is positioned on the operating table in the right lateral position—that is, with the left chest uppermost—with the pelvis rotated 45° backwards and the left hip joint fully extended, the chest being thus exposed for full thoracotomy and access provided to the femoral vessels. The left femoral artery is first prepared for cannulation and the chest is opened widely through the 4th intercostal space. Before mobilization of the aorta the pericardium is opened posteriorly to the phrenic nerve and the left atrial appendage snared by a purse-string. These precautions allow for immediate left

atriofemoral bypass should haemorrhage occur during dissection of the acute aortic rupture. A large-bore cannula is introduced into the left atrium, whence blood is drained by gravity into an open reservoir and thence returned via a roller pump to the femoral artery. Heparinization is required in a dosage of 1 mg/kg body weight and is subsequently reversed with protamine in similar dosage. A distal flow rate of 40 ml/kg body weight per minute ensures adequate decompression of the proximal aorta with adequate perfusion of the kidneys and spinal cord. During perfusion the radial arterial pressure should be maintained at 80 mmHg and urine should be passed. A modification of left atriofemoral bypass has been described in which a pulsatile pump containing porcine valves and tubing coated with a non-thrombogenic compound are used, thus avoiding the use of heparin (Connolly et al., 1971).

MODERATE HYPOTHERMIA

Moderate hypothermia at 30 °C, which has now been superseded by bypass procedures, was used when surface cooling had an important place in cardiac and vascular surgery. Although several successful cases of suture of ruptured aortas and resection of thoracic aneurysms have been reported, the period of safe aortic occlusion in these conditions is so unreliable and variable and the risk of ventricular fibrillation during the surface cooling of badly injured people is so high that the use of this technique is no longer advised (Neville et al., 1968).

FEMORAL VENOUS-TO-ARTERIAL OXYGENATION

Femoral venous-to-arterial oxygenation was described in 1968 in the treatment of 19 patients who underwent resection of aneurysms of the descending aorta or the repair of ruptured aortas (Neville et al., 1968). A large-bore catheter is inserted into the inferior vena cava via the femoral vein, whence blood is drained into a disposable bubble oxygenator and returned to the femoral artery. This allows a measured perfusion of the lower part of the body during aortic cross-clamping and decompresses the upper aortic segment. It has the additional advantage of removing cannulas and tubing from the operative field and avoids cannulation of the left atrium. Although the use of this method does not seem to be widespread, it offers an attractive alternative to left atriofemoral bypass.

ARTERIAL SHUNTS

In 1970 Molloy reported the successful repair of ruptured thoracic aorta in three patients with the use of a left ventriculo-aortic shunt (*Fig.* 43.3). A plastic cannula was used, one end of which was inserted into the left ventricle at its apex and the other into the descending thoracic aorta below the site of trauma. The only complication reported was clotting of blood in the cannula on one occasion. The advantages of this method are the avoidance of heparinization on the one hand and the avoidance of elaborate bypass procedures on the other. It is extremely simple and it may well be that it will ultimately be favoured as the procedure of choice in the repair of traumatic rupture of the descending aorta. However, great care must be taken to ensure that the cannula does not pass back into the left atrium, or flow will cease.

Another author (Kahn, 1970) described the use of a similar type of temporary plastic shunt inserted at one end into the ascending aorta and at the other into the descending aorta in operations to repair traumatic rupture of the aorta (*Fig.* 43.4), but reported the occurrence of paraplegia in one patient which may have been due to too small a diameter of shunt. A further report (Gott, 1971) described the use of a shunt from the left subclavian artery to the left femoral artery using a plastic tube lined with a nonthrombogenic substance.

At the present time most surgeons are veering away from complicated extracorporeal systems, utilizing left ventriculo-aortic bypass, or subclavian-aortic bypass, with the Gott plastic shunt which is internally heparin-bonded and non-thrombogenic (Keen, 1972).

ACUTE DISSECTION OF THE AORTA

Acute dissection of the aorta is a specific clinical and pathological entity. The underlying aetiology is degeneration of the elements of the media which may be localized or diffuse, so-called 'cystic medial necrosis'. The cause of the initial tear in the intima and the media is not understood although severe hypertension is often associated with this disease. The tear usually occurs in the ascending aorta 2 to 3 cm above the aortic valve or in the region of the ligamentum arteriosum or in the abdominal aorta. More rarely, the tear originates in the transverse arch of the aorta. The layers of the aorta are then dissected by the forceful torrent of blood, usually at the junction of the

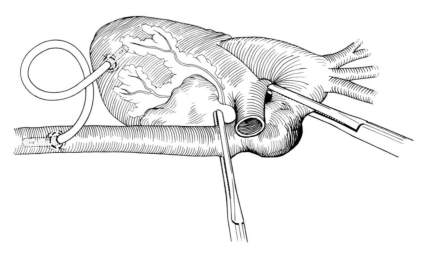

Fig. 43.3. Left ventriculo-aortic shunt using heparinized bonded shunt. This is a most useful procedure when dealing with traumatic rupture of the descending aorta (Molloy).

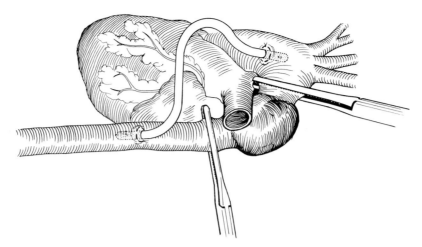

Fig. 43.4. Aorto-aortic shunt using heparinized bonded shunt. The shunt is inserted into the ascending aorta and into the femoral artery or the descending aorta, and is a most useful method of dealing with large aneurysms of the descending thoracic aorta.

middle and outer thirds of the media, which may progress to involve part or all of the circumference of the aorta and may extend for a short or a long distance along the aorta. Dissection of the entire aorta may occur quickly or in stages and the intramural channel may rupture back into the lumen at another level or may rupture externally causing fatal haemorrhage into the pleural or abdominal cavity or into the pericardium causing fatal tamponade. In chronic cases the dissection channel may heal and may become endothelialized and many instances are recorded where such healed dissections are found at routine autopsy in elderly patients who have died of unrelated disease. Dissection may extend along the larger branches of the aorta, interfering with the blood supply to the kidneys, limbs or brain. The intercostal and lumbar arteries are frequently torn or separated by splitting of the aortic wall and paraplegia is a common consequence of such injury. A localized and rapidly increasing dilatation may occur, particularly in the descending aorta.

Classification

DeBakey and his colleagues in 1965 introduced a classification of dissections of the aorta.

Type I DeBakey (Stanford type A) (Fig. 43.5)

The dissection which has arisen in the ascending aorta has extended distally and throughout the remaining aorta including the arch, descending aorta and major terminal branches, and is often associated with aortic regurgitation.

Type II DeBakey (Stanford type A)

The disease is limited to the ascending aorta and ori-

ginates from a transverse tear in the intima which usually begins just above the aortic valve and is also associated in many cases with acute aortic regurgitation.

Type III DeBakey (Stanford type B)

The dissection arises in the descending thoracic aorta usually at or just distal to the origin of the left subclavian artery extending distally for a varying distance.

Since this description there has been a variety of other classifications, including the Stanford classification, but from the point of view of the surgeon the type II affects the ascending aorta and type III affects the descending aorta. These are entirely separate conditions and require an entirely different surgical approach.

Acute Dissection of the Ascending Aorta (type II DeBakey)

This subject, together with its effect on competence of the aortic valve, is dealt with in Chapters 41 and 42.

Acute Dissection of the Descending Aorta (type III DeBakey)

The clinical picture is usually characteristic and the diagnosis is readily made by aortography. Recently, the use of the CT scan has shown that dissections can be accurately diagnosed and furthermore accurately localized, avoiding in many instances the need for aortography.

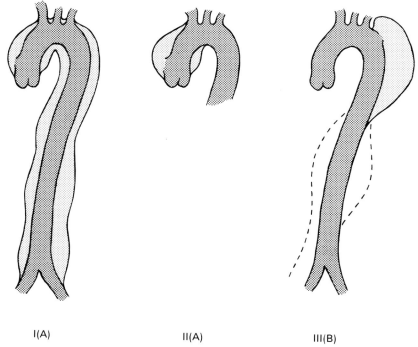

I(A) II(A) III(B)

Fig. 43.5. Classification of aortic dissections: types I, II, III DeBakey; types A and B Stanford.

Treatment

The surgical management of acute dissection of the aorta was rationalized by DeBakey et al. in 1955 and although the surgical mortality at that time was high it has progressively declined and in those units where this disease is managed surgically and frequently the results are now very good indeed, achieving an acceptably low mortality for what is an otherwise highly lethal disease. In 1965 Wheat intoduced the concept of the medical management of acute dissections of the distal aorta (Wheat et al., 1965). He maintained that progression of a dissection was the consequence of the extremely high blood pressure and was associated with a very high pulse pressure. He also maintained that if the mean blood pressure could be reduced and if the bounding pulse pressure could also be reduced, the progress of dissection would be arrested and healing would be expected in many patients who would, therefore, survive without what was at that time a very risky operation.

The selection of cases for such conservative management should be very carefully supervised by a team consisting of both surgeons and physicians, for the complications of dissection such as aortic rupture with haemopericardium, haemothorax, together with the dangers of obstruction, occlusion or separation of one or more aortic branches, causing myocardial infarction, stroke, paraplegia, intestinal, renal or distal limb ischaemia, are very real and their development or impending development might indicate the need for emergency operation. The advocates of a universal surgical attack on this disease

criticize the conservative approach, for it is their view that should one of these complications develop rapidly it is by that time probably too late to save the patient, and since these complications are so common the risk should be avoided. On the other hand, Wheat and his associates point out that a large number of patients who are treated conservatively do survive without operation, and since the patient group under discussion is often elderly and otherwise unfit, conservative management should be considered in all patients with acute dissections of the descending thoracic aorta.

It is, however, necessary to say that acute dissections arising in and involving the descending thoracic aorta, which are associated with progressive extension, occlusion of vital arteries, significant aortic dilatation or leak, should be treated by immediate surgery, and that patients with any form of aortic dissection, either acute or chronic, complicating Marfan's syndrome are candidates for surgical treatment because of the high incidence of recurrent dissection and rupture. However, in elderly patients in whom there is clinical and radiological evidence of a localized dissection of the descending thoracic aorta without any of these complications, it is reasonable to conduct a trial of hypotensive therapy. It is essential that when such conservative management is undertaken, the patient is treated in the intensive care unit. An indwelling radial artery cannula is inserted in order to monitor the arterial pressure and the patient is treated actively with beta-blockers, and afterload reducers such as sodium nitroprusside. The intention is to maintain the mean pressure at a low enough level hopefully to prevent further extension of the tear but at the same time to maintain an adequate pressure for the patient to perfuse his or her own vital organs.

It is now clear that although a great number of these patients will be managed safely only by operative intervention, at the same time a large number of patients will respond satisfactorily and do leave hospital with a healed or healing dissection following the careful use of conservative treatment.

Operative Management (*Fig.* 43.6)

Dissections of the descending aorta are approached through an extended left posterolateral thoracotomy. It is necessary to resect the descending aorta containing the intimal tear if possible, and an appropriate size Dacron graft is inserted to restore aortic continuity. Certainly at the distal end of aortic resection and to some extent at the proximal end, the aorta will be separated into layers which will require initial circumferential resuturing prior to the insertion of a Dacron graft (*Fig.* 43.6*b*). The native aorta, especially distally, is extremely friable and often requires Teflon felt support to prevent sutures cutting through. Although many experienced surgeons advocate the undertaking of this operation using aortic cross-clamping without using any adjuncts to avoid distal ischaemia or to provide proximal decompression, it is the view of others that some form of support such as left atriofemoral bypass, femoral vein to femoral artery bypass, or the use of heparin-bonded shunts, should be used to avoid the complications of distal ischaemia or proximal cardiac overload. In view of the friability of tissues and severe haemorrhage associated with heparinization, many experienced surgeons undertake this operation using aortic cross-clamping without any form of bypass and very good results are recorded in their reports. It must, however, be pointed out that these selected groups of experienced surgeons are technically able to insert the aortic Dacron graft very rapidly, thus avoiding neurological and other complications. Unhappily the great majority of acute dissections of the descending aorta are treated in units lacking the experience of these large series of patients and in these cases the period of aortic cross-clamping will usually be prolonged. It is then recommended that some form of circulatory support such as left atriofemoral bypass or the use of heparin-bonded shunts should be used to avoid complications of distal ischaemia or proximal cardiac overload.

INTRALUMINAL PROSTHESIS (*Figs.* 43.7, 43.8) (Sariel et al., 1978)

A modification of aortic replacement is the recent introduction of the intraluminal prosthesis. This consists of a low-porosity woven Dacron tube with expanded polypropylene ends which are grooved to accept a peri-aortic tape and these ends are covered with Dacron velour. These prostheses are manufactured in varying lengths and diameters (*Fig.* 43.7). The prosthesis may be introduced into the ascending

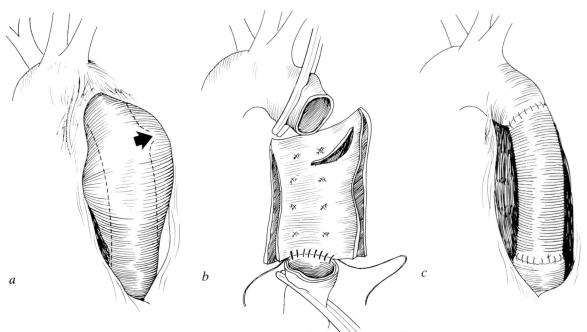

Fig. 43.6. Operative management of acute dissection of the descending thoracic aorta. The segment bearing the tear (*a*) is isolated (*b*) and replaced with a Dacron graft (*c*). Intercostal vessels are sutured and the separated distal and proximal aortic layers are sutured into one layer prior to graft replacement.

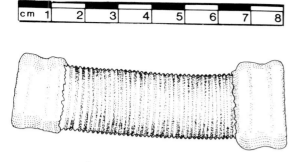

Fig. 43.7. Intraluminal prosthesis.

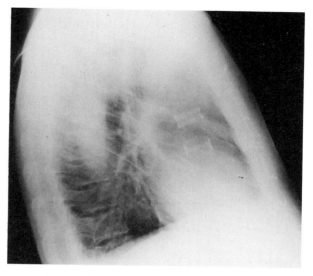

Fig. 43.8. Lateral chest X-ray of intraluminal prosthesis which has been inserted in the ascending aorta to repair acute dissection of the aorta.

or descending aorta in patients with localized dissections or traumatic tears. When used in the ascending aorta, full cardiopulmonary bypass with aortic cross-clamping and cold cardioplegia are required. When used in the descending thoracic aorta, aortic cross-clamping and some form of left heart bypass are considered mandatory by most surgeons. When controlled, the aorta is opened longitudinally and the intraluminal prosthesis placed within the true lumen across the pathological or traumatic tear following which the peri-aortic tapes are tied above and below thus securing the prosthesis. The aortic wall is then sutured over the prosthesis anteriorly (*Fig.* 43.8).

Although this prosthesis has been recently introduced, there are now several encouraging reports and if in the long term this prosthesis appears to have no disadvantages, it will offer a real advantage in the reduction of aortic cross-clamp time and in the amount of blood loss, as long and often leaky anastomotic suture lines are avoided.

The concept of the intraluminal prosthesis is not new, being introduced by Carrel in 1912 and Blakemore et al. in 1942. In 1951 Hufnagel introduced such a prosthesis carrying a ball valve into the descending thoracic aorta and this was used extensively in patients during the early 1950s. Although this valve was frequently obstructed by clots, there were few difficulties associated with the tube itself.

Acknowledgement

Figs. 43.1. and 43.2 have been copied with kind permission of C. V. Mosby from the article by Brewer et al. (1972).

REFERENCES

Adamkiewicz A. (1882) Die Blutgefasse des Menschlichen Ruckenmarkes. I. Teil. Die Gefasse der Ruckenmarksubstanz. II. Teil. Die Gefasse der Ruckenmarkoberflache. *Sitz. Akad. Wiss. Wein. Math. Natur. Klass.* **84**, 469; **85**, 101.

Blakemore A. H., Lord J. W., Jr and Stefko P. L. (1942) The severed primary artery in the war wounded. *Surgery* **12**, 488–508.

Brewer L. A., Fosburg R. G., Mulder G. A. et al. (1972) Spinal cord complications following surgery for coarctation of the aorta. A study of 66 cases. *J. Thorac. Cardiovasc. Surg.* **64**(3), 368–381.

Carrel A. (1912) Results of the permanent ventilation of the thoracic aorta. *Surg. Gynecol. Obstet.* **15**, 245–248.

Connolly J. E., Wakabayashi A., German J. C. et al. (1971) Clinical experience with pulsatile left heart bypass without anticoagulation for thoracic aneurysms . *J. Thorac. Cardiovasc. Surg.* **62**, 568–576.

Cooley D. A., DeBakey M. E. and Morris G. C. (1957) Controlled extra-corporeal circulation in surgical treatment of aortic aneurysm. *Ann. Surg.* **146**, 473–486.

Crawford E. S., Fenstermacher J. M., Richardson W. et al. (1970) Reappraisal of adjuncts to avoid ischaemia in the treatment of thoracic aortic aneurysms. *Surgery* **67**, 182–196.

DeBakey M. E., Cooley D. A. and Creech O., Jr (1955) Surgical considerations of dissecting aneurysms of the aorta. *Ann. Surg.* **142**, 586.

DeBakey M. E., Henly Walter S., Cooley D. A. et al. (1965) Surgical management of dissecting aneurysms of the aorta. *J. Thorac. Cardiovasc. Surg.* **49**, 130–147.

Gerbode F., Braimbridge M., Osborn J. J. et al. (1957) Traumatic thoracic aneurysms: treatment by resection and grafting with the use of an extra-corporeal bypass. *Surgery* **42**, 975–985.

Gott V. L. (1971) Discussion of paper by Connolly et al.

Hufnagel C. A. (1951) Aortic plastic valvular prosthesis. *Bull. Georgetown Univ. Med. Centre* **4**, 128–129.

Kadyi H. (1886) Uber die Blutgefasse des Menschlichen Ruckenmarkes. *Anat. Ann.* **1**, 304 (1889, Lemberg: Gubrynowicz and Schmidt).

Kahn D. R. (1970) Discussion of paper by Crawford et al.

Keen G. (1972) Closed injuries of the thoracic aorta. *Ann. R. Coll. Surg. Engl.* **51**, 137–156.

Laschinger J. C., Cunningham J. N., Jr, Nathan I. M. et al. (1983) Experimental and clinical assessment of the adequacy of partial bypass in maintenance of spinal cord blood flow during operations on the thoracic aorta. *Ann. Thorac. Surg.* **36**, 417–426.

Molloy P. J. (1970) Repair of the ruptured thoracic aorta using left ventriculo-aortic support. *Thorax* **25**, 213–222.

Neville W. E., Cox W. D., Leininger B. et al. (1968) Resection of the descending thoracic aorta with femoral vein to femoral artery oxygenation perfusion. *J. Thorac. Cardiovasc. Surg.* **56**, 39–42.

Passaro E. and Pace W. G. (1959) Traumatic rupture of the aorta. *Surgery* **46**, 787–791.

Sariel G. G., Ablaza M. D., Suresh C. et al. (1978) Use of a ringed intra-luminal graft in the surgical treatment of dissecting aneurysms of the thoracic aorta. *J. Thorac. Cardiovasc. Surg.* **76**, 390–396.

Taber R. E. (1970) Discussion of paper by Crawford et al.

Wheat M. W., Palmer R. F., Bartley T. B. et al. (1965) Treatment of dissecting aneurysms of the aorta without surgery. *J. Thorac. Cardiovasc. Surg.* **50**, 364–371.

Chapter forty-four

The Peripheral Veins

D. Negus

Disorders of the peripheral veins provide a large proportion of a general surgeon's work. Disorders of the veins of the upper limbs are rare, and this account will be largely confined to the veins of the lower limbs. Varicose vein operations, being common and not usually presenting much technical difficulty, are usually left to the end of operating lists, and to the least experienced surgeons. A high recurrence rate is not surprising. Venous ulcers, similarly, may be relegated to a dressing clinic run largely by nurses, with equally poor results. Both conditions respond well to a logical approach, and it is hoped to present such an approach in this chapter. Modern views on the prevention and management of deep vein thrombosis—still only too common a complication of surgical operation—are presented.

SURGICAL ANATOMY OF THE VEINS OF THE LOWER LIMB

A detailed account is given in Dodd and Cockett's *The Pathology and Surgery of the Veins of the Lower Limb* (1976), and the descriptions which introduce each section of this chapter seek only to emphasize points of special surgical significance.

The venous drainage of the superficial tissues of the leg is by three main routes—the long and short saphenous veins and the perforating veins. Valves direct blood flow both proximally and into the deep veins. The paired venae comitantes of the three main lower leg arteries converge to form the popliteal vein, which also receives soleal and gastrocnemius tributaries, and then ascends the thigh as the superficial femoral vein. Venous blood is directed proximally by the numerous valves, and propelled by the powerful contractions of the calf muscles.

The long and short saphenous veins have relatively thick muscle coats, but the walls of their tributaries are thin and dilate to form varices following incompetence of the valves, and consequent high pressure, in the main trunks. Knowledge of the anatomy of these veins is essential for effective surgery.

VARICOSE VEINS

Varicose veins are divided into two main groups: primary familial varicose veins and the less common varices which are secondary to post-thrombotic deep and perforating vein incompetence. Most primary varicose veins are associated with valve incompetence of the long or short saphenous veins. Much less common are vulval and pudendal varices, varices secondary to arteriovenous fistula formation, and those associated with the Klippel–Trenaunay syndrome.

Dilated venules (venous flares or stars, telangiectasia) are common. These dilated cutaneous venules are *not* varicose veins, and are only of cosmetic importance.

Rare among rural Africans and Indians, varicose veins are seen only too often in industrialized Western society. Inherited collagen and smooth muscle deficiencies seem to be the principal aetiological factors. A collagen defect has been demonstrated in the walls of varicose veins (Svejcar et al., 1963) and the same defect is present in undilated leg veins and in the arm veins of the same subject. Smooth muscle deficiency has also been demonstrated (Rose, 1986).

Catabolism of connective tissue in patients with primary varicose veins is greater than in normal controls (Buddecke, 1975) and this seems to be related to increased local lysosomal enzyme activity (Niebes and Laszt, 1971) and to increased serum levels of these enzymes (Niebes and Berson, 1973). Venous dilatation secondary to wall weakness prevents the valve cusps meeting and reflux then increases the dilatation. The valves themselves are not damaged, in contrast to post-thrombotic recanalization.

The familial nature of primary varicose veins is undisputed. In the author's clinic, questioning reveals a close blood relative with varices in nearly every case. This familial tendency to varices may be increased by occupations involving prolonged standing.

Primary varices often appear initially during the first pregnancy. They often disappear after childbirth, only to reappear and persist during and after the second pregnancy. Obvious predisposing causes are generalized smooth muscle relaxation resulting from high oestrogen levels, increase in circulating blood volume, and perhaps also the bulk of the gravid uterus.

Symptoms and Complications

The commonest symptom is aching, particularly after prolonged standing. Night cramps may also be a complaint.

Varicose eczema is common. Treatment is by olive oil massage and support stockings or tights until operation.

Very superficial varices may bleed, and this may

be catastrophic unless the patient or a companion elevates the limb and compresses the bleeding point. Early operation is indicated.

Superficial thrombophlebitis is quite common and may propagate to involve the deep veins. Ascending thrombophlebitis of the long or short saphenous vein is an indication for emergency surgery.

Venous ulceration is not a common complication of primary varicose veins (Homans, 1916), and responds well to pressure bandaging and ligation of the incompetent veins. The management of venous ulcers is described below, with the post-thrombotic syndrome.

Symptomless varicose veins, of cosmetic importance only, do not often require active treatment.

The differential diagnosis of lower limb pain is important. A patient may present with obvious varices, but with symptoms resulting from arterial insufficiency, osteoarthritis of the knee or hip, sciatica or other neurological disorder. Such possibilities must always be kept in mind and excluded by examination.

Management

Management of primary varicose veins may be:
1. Conservative—by elastic stockings or tights.
2. Surgical.
3. By injection sclerotherapy.

1. *Conservative*

Elastic stocking support is indicated in the following circumstances:
  a. Pregnancy.
  b. Old age.
  c. Cardiac or respiratory disease, or other condition contra-indicating active treatment.
  d. Obesity, while losing weight sufficiently for active treatment.
  e. Long hospital waiting lists for surgery.

Elastic stockings are contra-indicated in the presence of peripheral arterial insufficiency. Suitable elastic stockings or tights are made by Elbeo and Haynes. Severe cases may require stronger stockings (Sigvaris, Scholl Duoten or Jobst).

2. *Surgery*

Surgery is indicated in roughly two-thirds of patients presenting to a varicose vein clinic. The indications are:
  a. Long or short saphenous vein incompetence.
  b. Above-knee varices.
  c. Varices associated with post-thrombotic deep and perforating vein incompetence.
  d. Recurrent varices (usually).

In addition, a number of patients whose varices are otherwise suitable for injection sclerotherapy request surgical treatment. Some of the reasons given are: previous unsuccessful injections; relative or friends with poor results; dislike of prolonged bandaging.

CONTRA-INDICATIONS

These are, of course, the same as the indications for conservative management, e.g. pregnancy, old age, cardiac or respiratory disease or other debility, and obesity.

The contraceptive pill should be stopped at least 6 weeks before surgery.

3. *Injection Sclerotherapy*

Indications and contra-indications are described in that section (*see* p. 648).

Principles of Treatment

The successful treatment of varicose veins is based on two principles:

1. *Control 'Leak Points'*

These are the long and short saphenous terminations and the perforating veins. Some surgeons advocate simple saphenous ligation without stripping; but a dilated long or short saphenous vein may subsequently fill from other tributaries. These veins should therefore be stripped when incompetent, though the long saphenous need not be stripped below knee level.

2. *Remove or Sclerose Varices*

Once superficial veins have become thin walled and dilated, they will remain so even after adequate 'leak point' control. Varices may either be avulsed or injected.

Recurrent varicose veins result from failure to fulfil these criteria.

Surgery of the Long Saphenous Vein

Surgical anatomy

The long saphenous vein and its tributaries can be thought of as two tridents (*Fig.* 44.1).

In the groin the important tributaries are the antero-lateral and posteromedial veins of the thigh. Smaller tributaries are the superficial and deep external pudendal veins, and the superficial epigastric and circumflex iliac veins. Just below the knee the medial and lateral prongs are the anterolateral vein and the posterior arch vein (of Leonardo da Vinci). The important medial calf direct perforating veins communicate with the posterior arch vein and *not* with the main long saphenous vein. These tributaries commonly become varicose; the main long saphenous

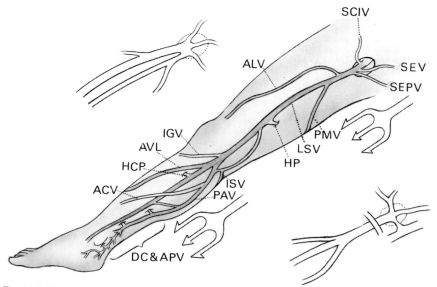

Fig. 44.1. The long saphenous vein and its tributaries. *Insets:* duplication of the long saphenous vein (*upper*), aberrant superficial external pudendal artery (*lower*), SCIV, Superficial circumflex iliac vein; SEV, Superficial epigastric vein; SEPV, Superficial external pudendal vein; ALV, Anterolateral vein of thigh; PMV, Posteromedial vein of thigh; LSV, Long saphenous vein; HP, Hunterian perforator; IGV, Infragenicular vein; ISV, Intersaphenous vein; HCP, High calf (Boyd's) perforator; AVL, Anterior vein of leg; PAV, Posterior arch vein (of Leonardo da Vinci); ACV, Anterior crural vein; DC & APV, Direct calf and ankle perforating veins.

stem is only occasionally dilated and varicose in the lower leg. There is usually also a small medial tributary which communicates with the short saphenous vein, and this can lead to confusion in diagnosis.

The long saphenous vein is accompanied by the saphenous nerve, which is closely applied to the vein in the lower one-third of the leg, where it may be damaged by the passage of a stripper.

At the ankle the long saphenous vein lies *in front of* the medial malleolus. The posterior tibial artery passes behind this bony landmark. Failure to remember this very elementary anatomical point has resulted in the femoral artery being stripped out on more than one occasion.

Important Anatomical Variations

The tributaries of the long saphenous vein terminate with extraordinary variation, and successful surgery depends on their thorough demonstration. The long saphenous vein itself may be duplicated, and may sometimes join the common femoral vein deep to the crossing external pudendal artery (*Fig.* 44.1). Occasionally a high bifurcation of the common femoral artery results in the profunda femoris artery being medial to the femoral vein. This can lead to confusion, particularly in exposure of the femoral vein in the treatment of deep vein thrombosis.

Examination of the Patient

All patients with varicose veins must undergo a general physical examination and, as in other surgical clinics, the urine must be tested on the first visit. In a single year, the author diagnosed osteoarthritis, peripheral arterial insufficiency, lumbar disc lesion, Parkinson's disease, hypertension and diabetes in patients referred specifically to a vein clinic.

Abdominal examination to exclude pelvic tumour or other abnormality must never be omitted. The legs, including the peripheral pulses, are quickly examined with the patient lying on the examination couch, but the veins can only be examined properly with the patient standing. This is carried out with a rubber-covered, 30 cm high 'mounting block'. The surgeons sits opposite on a low chair. A good light is essential (*Fig.* 44.2). Allow at least 30 seconds for the veins to fill. Look for groin varices, which may be collaterals in iliac vein stenosis, and make sure that no varices are pulsating (arteriovenous fistula). Note the distribution of varices, and look for dilatation of the long or short saphenous trunks. Varices on the 'gaiter area', a 'venous flare' over the medial malleolus, pigmentation, induration or ulceration, all indicate direct perforator incompetence.

Special Tests

The 'cough impulse' is useful in assessing competence of the proximal long saphenous vein.

Percussion with a finger feeling for the impulse is carried out both from distal to proximal, and in the reverse direction.

The Trendelenburg test, feeding vein control by

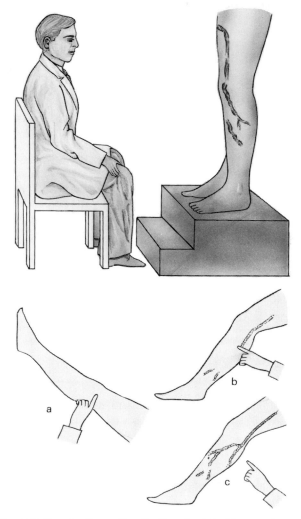

Fig. 44.2. Examination and localization of points of incompetence.

one or several rubber tourniquets, can be useful for distinguishing varices secondary to long saphenous incompetence from those resulting from perforating vein incompetence; but the authors finds it quicker and more accurate to control sites of incompetence, 'leak points', with one or two fingers. As in the Trendelenburg test, the patient lies with the leg elevated while finger control is applied, and then stands upright. Varices are observed to fill either before or after the controlling finger is removed (*Fig.* 44.2). The accuracy of this test can be increased by using Doppler ultrasound to detect reflux flow.

This outpatient examination is repeated in the ward shortly before surgery. Veins and 'leak points' are then accurately marked with an indelible felt tip pen.

Phlebography is only likely to be necessary in the investigation of recurrent varicose veins. It is more frequently necessary in the mangement of the post-thrombotic syndrome, and is considered in that section (p. 650).

Operation

General anaesthesia is usual in the UK, though local anaesthesia is perfectly possible and is more widely used elsewhere.

The patient is positioned with the legs widely abducted on a padded board, and the operating table is tilted 10° head downwards.

Povidone-iodine skin preparation has the advantage of not washing away the skin marks—an occurrence guaranteed to cause extreme irritation to the surgeon, and an inadequate operation.

1. *The groin incision* (*Fig.* 44.3). A skin crease incision is made 3 cm below the inguinal ligament, extending laterally for about 5 cm from the adductor longus origin. This landmark is easy to feel, even in the obese, and must always be identified. An incision shorter than 5 cm may be possible in the very

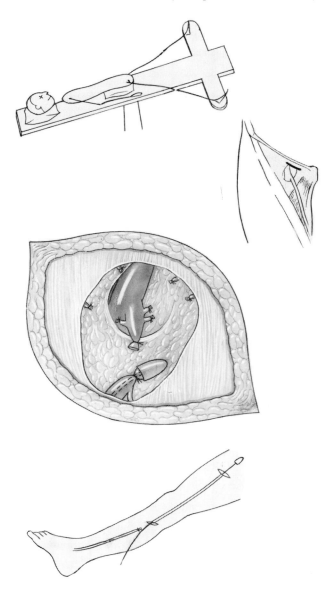

Fig. 44.3. High saphenous ligation and strip.

thin; a longer one is necessary in fat patients. As in other branches of surgery, strict rules cannot be laid down; sufficient to remember the phrase: *accurate, adequate access*. The incision should err on the high rather than the low side. In operating on recurrent varicose veins, a longer 'hockey stick' type of incision may be necessary (*see Fig.* 44.11).

2. The deep layer of superficial fascia and a number of small blood vessels and lymphatics are divided, and the long saphenous vein is identified. This must be followed to its termination at the foramen ovale, usually just proximal to the crossing superficial external pudendal artery. Every tributary is carefully dissected out and divided between ligatures (*Fig.* 44.3). Good retraction and light are particularly important at this stage. Failure to control these tributaries is the most common cause of recurrent varicose veins in the thigh.

3. The long saphenous vein and its divided tributaries are then followed through the cribriform fascia which is best divided by careful sharp dissection rather than being pushed off. Blunt dissection is likely to cause bleeding from torn small tributaries. The common femoral vein is exposed and carefully inspected. A deep external pudendal vein is found entering its medial border in about 10 per cent. This is most easily controlled by ligation in continuity, using an unabsorbable ligature on an aneurysm needle (*Fig.* 44.3).

4. Finally, or earlier if it helps in the dissection of tributaries, the long saphenous vein is divided between artery forceps 1 cm proximal to the saphenofemoral junction. Identification must be absolutely certain; in very thin patients the superficial femoral artery can be mistaken for the vein, and this mistake has resulted in amputation. A single, carefully tied 1/0 black silk ligature at the saphenofemoral junction is perfectly safe in most cases, but a wide junction should be doubly ligated or a transfixion stitch used (*Fig.* 44.3).

The Stripping Operation

A Myers metal stripper or one of its modifications may be used, or a plastic disposable stripper may be preferred.

How far should the long saphenous vein be stripped, and in which direction? In most patients, the varicose calf tributaries of the long saphenous vein join the main trunk just below the knee. The long saphenous vein itself is usually normal below this level, lower medial varices most often being related to perforating vein incompetence. Except in occasional cases, therefore, it is quite sufficient to strip down to the upper one-third of the lower leg (*Fig.* 44.3). Much discussion has taken place on the pros and cons of stripping upwards or downwards, and this argument chiefly relates to the risk of saphenous nerve damage. The nerve is closely applied to the vein in the lower one-third of the leg, and if this

section of vein is varicose and requires stripping, there is less risk of nerve damage if it is carried out in a proximal direction. In the vast majority of patients it is quite unnecessary to strip this lower one-third, and by avoiding it there is little risk of nerve damage whichever route is used.

The stripper is best passed down the vein from the groin incision, and identified under the skin in the upper one-third of the leg. If a Cockett incision is necessary for perforator ligation, the stripper can be brought out through this. Otherwise a small incision is made over the stripper end. The veins is identified, divided and ligated, and the stripper brought out. The vein is secured at each end with linen thread ties. The stripper is then left *in situ* until other procedures (avulsion of varices, ligation of perforators) have been completed, and the actual stripping is performed later, just before the leg is finally bandaged.

Avulsion of Varices

Varices are wormed out through small incisions placed over the most dilated points of the tributaries (*Fig.* 44.4). These incisions are usually placed

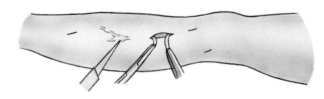

Fig. 44.4. Avulsion of varices.

5–7·5 cm apart. By using a pointed (no. 11) scalpel blade and pointed scissors to dilate the wound, very small (2 mm) incision are sufficient. The vein is found and brought to the surface with mosquito forceps, and then held and pulled out by the more sturdy Dunhill forceps. Intermittent steady pulls are used. A sharp tug will tear the vein. Between 5 and 7·5 cm of vein are easily avulsed through each incision. Firm pressure is applied for a few minutes. Ligation is not usually necessary.

Perforating Vein Surgery

Calf, and occasionally thigh, perforating vein incompetence frequently accompanies long or short saphenous incompetence in the aetiology of primary varices. This subject is considered later (pp. 657, 661).

Wound Closure and Bandaging

Subcuticular 3/0 Prolene is used for closing the groin incision, except in the obese, in whom interrupted 2/0 nylon sutures should be used. Very small avulsion incisions, if dry, can be closed with Steristrips. Residual oozing will, however, dislodge these, and a single 3/0 Prolene stitch should be used for each incision. Lower leg perforator incisions are more liable to break down than the others, and interrupted 3/0 Prolene sutures are used.

Small incisions are covered by Elastoplast squares; Mepore dressings are more comfortable for the larger incisions.

The leg is bandaged with 10- or 15-cm crêpe bandages (for details, *see under* Complications) and the groin wound covered with gauze dressings and Elastoplast.

The patient returns to the recovery room, and then the ward, with the foot of the bed elevated.

One or Both Legs?

We have found that most patients prefer to have both legs operated on at the same session—preferring some additional temporary discomfort to more prolonged treatment. Many surgeons prefer to operate on one leg at a time, but I have not found this necessary, except in the elderly or when extensive surgery (particularly perforating vein exploration in the postthrombotic syndrome) is performed.

Postoperative Care

Active movement in bed is encouraged. The patient walks around the bed within 24 hours of the operation, and thereafter for 5 minutes every hour on the hour. Each day the time is increased until full mobilization is achieved in 2 or 3 days. Sitting in a chair beside the bed is strongly discouraged. Pain is controlled with analgesics as necessary.

The bandages are removed after 24 hours and are replaced by medium-weight elastic stockings.

Most patients are fit to go home in 3–4 days, wearing their stockings. Day surgery is practised in some centres, but this precludes operating on both legs at the same session. We have found that most patients prefer to get the whole thing over at one session, and to spend a few days in hospital.

Groin sutures are removed as an outpatient, 7–8 days, and lower leg sutures 9–12 days postoperatively.

Stockings are worn continuously for 2 weeks, and then for increasingly shorter periods, being discarded altogether after about 3 weeks. Most patients return to work 2–3 weeks after operation.

Complications of High Saphenous Ligation and Stripping

1. Groin haemorrhage occasionally results from a slipped saphenofemoral ligature. It should never happen if the precautions mentioned above are followed.

2. Damage to the common femoral vein can usually be repaired without serious after-effects, using a partial occluding clamp and fine silk sutures. A good sucker is essential here.

Division of the femoral artery, or an abnormal pro-

funda femoris artery, can happen, particularly when the operator is inexperienced. The torn vessel must be controlled with finger pressure, and a vascular surgeon obtained. With the patient anticoagulated, the artery is properly exposed and controlled between clamps, and repair effected with arterial sutures, usually 4 or 5/0 Prolene.

3. Wound sepsis is rare, provided haematoma formation is avoided (*see below*). Superficial groin wound infection responds rapidly to antibiotics.

4. Saphenous neuritis is not a significant complication if stripping is limited to the upper third of the lower leg.

5. Other nerves, e.g. the lateral popliteal, may occasionally be damaged during the avulsion of varices. Awareness of this possibility, and reasonable care, should prevent this complication.

6. Deep vein thrombosis and embolism are very uncommon, except following perforator exploration, when prophylactic low-dose subcutaneous heparin should always be given (*see below*).

7. Haematoma and bruising in the track of the stripped long saphenous vein are common when above-knee bandaging is employed. Lymphatoma or lymph fistula in the groin wound may occur occasionally. Both these complications can be avoided by the following technique.

Redivac drainage of the long saphenous track

Above-knee bandages are notoriously difficult to keep in place, particularly when postoperative mobilization is started. Knee bending soon works these bandages loose. Haematoma formation and ecchymoses on the medial surface of the thigh are common. This complication can be avoided by attaching a narrow suction (Redivac) drain with 30 cm of perforations to a drilled-out stripper acorn by a 3/0 silk stitch.

The drain is drawn into the long saphenous track until its lower perforations are at, or just above, knee level. Holding the proximal end firmly, the stripper is detached with a sharp pull. The leg is then elevated and bandaged with a 10- or 15-cm crêpe bandage from the base of the toes to the knee (*Fig.* 44.5). A second bandage may be necessary above the knee, particularly if multiple varices have been avulsed; this is removed 24 hours postoperatively. The lower leg bandage is then covered with Tubigrip stockinet to keep it in place, and active walking is encouraged.

The Redivac drain remains in place until there is no more drainage—usually about 48 hours.

8. The last 'complication' to be remembered is that of recurrent varicose veins—the result of inadequate surgery.

Surgery of the Short Saphenous Vein

Surgical Anatomy

The short saphenous vein extends from the posterior

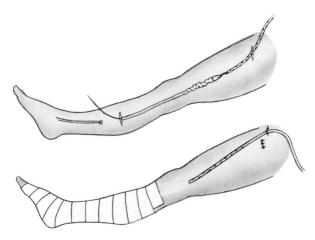

Fig. 44.5. Long Redivac drainage of the long saphenous track.

border of the lateral malleolus to the popliteal fossa, where it (usually) joins the popliteal vein. It perforates the deep fascia in the lower third of the calf, and then lies deep until its termination. It is often joined by a perforating vein which penetrates deeply between the twin bellies of gastrocnemius.

A number of tributaries join it in the popliteal fossa. Important ones are the persisting postaxial vein, which runs up the middle of the posterior surface of the thigh, and a tributary joining the long saphenous vein (*Fig.* 44.6).

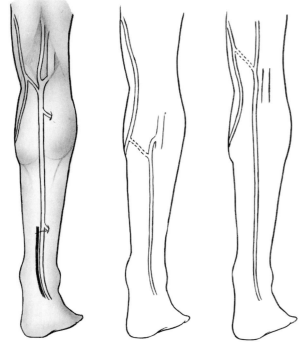

Fig. 44.6. The short saphenous vein. Low and high terminations.

In its lower third, the short saphenous vein is accompanied closely by the sural nerve, which must be identified and preserved.

Anatomical Variations

The short saphenous vein is very variable in its termination. The most common variation is the high termination (33 per cent) (Kosinski, 1926). The vessel ends in the centre of the thigh (persistent postaxial vein) either in muscle veins or by joining the long saphenous vein. The low termination occurs in about 9 per cent. The vein either terminates in the long saphenous vein, or joins gastrocnemius veins below knee level (*Fig.* 44.6). Its termination may then be missed when the conventional popliteal skin crease approach is used. Preoperative 'varicography' (phlebography by injecting a varix) can prevent such mistakes (Hobbs, 1980).

Short Saphenous Ligation and Stripping

Incompetence of the short saphenous vein may occur alone, but more often accompanies long saphenous incompetence. The two procedures are then carried out under the same anaesthetic.

Examination and preoperative vein marking are carried out as described for the long saphenous vein.

1. The patient lies face downwards with the chest and abdomen resting on pillows. The legs are widely abducted on a padded board. Remember to warn the anaesthetist in good time, so that the patient is intubated and ventilated (*Fig.* 44.7).

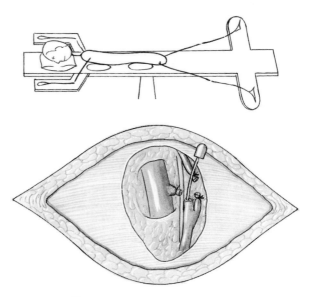

Fig. 44.7. Short saphenous ligation.

2. The popliteal fossa is explored through a 7–10-cm long skin crease incision. As for long saphenous exposure, be careful not to place this too low. Superficial vessels are controlled and the deep fascia is opened in the line of the incision. The sural nerve is identified and preserved and the vein is easily found lying in loose popliteal fat between the two heads of gastrocnemius.

3. The vein is divided between ligatures, and then the *knee is flexed* by an assistant. This important step enables thorough exploration of the popliteal fossa by relaxing the gastrocnemius and other muscles. The vein is carefully traced to its termination (feel for the pulsation of the popliteal artery), all tributaries being ligated and divided. Look carefully for a high or low termination. The short saphenous vein is then ligated as closely as possible to the popliteal vein, using 2/0 black silk (*Fig.* 44.7).

4. The stripper is passed distally down to the lower calf or ankle and tied to the vein with linen thread. The sural nerve is carefully dissected free. Stripping is postponed until other procedures—avulsion of varices, etc.—have been completed. These have already been described.

Stripping is followed by bandaging and postoperative care is as for the long saphenous vein.

Complications

These are infrequent. Haemotoma formation is prevented by bandaging, and with reasonable care neither wound infection nor nerve damage should occur.

Inadequate surgery will result in the 'complication' of recurrent varices.

Surgery of the Perforating Veins

Surgical Anatomy

The perforating veins are those veins, other than the long and short saphenous, which penetrate the deep fascia, passing from the subcutaneous venules into the deep veins. A number of unimportant 'indirect' perforating veins enter the muscles in the upper half of the lower leg before joining the deep veins. Clinically much more important are the 'direct' perforating veins of the lower half of the leg and ankle, usually three on the medial side, which communicate with the posterior arch vein, *not* the long saphenous vein, and one or two laterally (*Fig.* 44.8). Each contains a valve, which directs blood from the superficial to the deep veins (Thomson, 1979).

Incompetence of the higher direct perforators (Hunterian perforator, Boyd's perforator and the gastrocnemius perforator) will cause varices, but not ulceration.

Incompetence of the direct perforating vein valves may be associated with primary varices. This is often accompanied by long or short saphenous incompetence. The perforators may not be detected at the first operation, and later become apparent when recurrent varices develop. 'Secondary' perforating vein incompetence may follow local trauma, thrombophlebitis and recanalization. Post-thrombotic deep vein incompetence is nearly always associated with perforating vein incompetence, and results eventually in liposclerosis and ulceration.

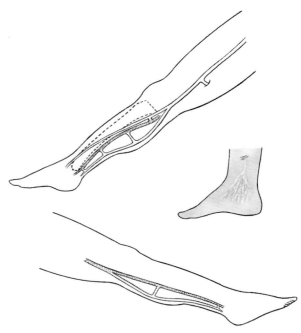

Fig. 44.8. The principal perforating veins and the 'ankle venous flare'. Deep veins are stippled.

The upper and middle medial direct calf perforators are most often incompetent; the lateral, peroneal perforator less commonly; and the lowest medial perforator, which lies behind the medial malleolus, very rarely.

Indications and Contra-indications

The indications and contra-indications for the treatment of varicose veins secondary to perforator incompetence are identical to those which follow long or short saphenous incompetence.

Injection sclerotherapy is indicated if there is little or no long or short saphenous incompetence.

Post-thrombotic perforating vein incompetence is considered with the management of the post-thrombotic syndrome (p. 657).

Examination and Investigation

Again this is as described for long saphenous incompetence. 'Leak points' can be controlled by finger pressure. Phlebography may be indicated in the post-thrombotic syndrome, and before operating on recurrent varices where perforator incompetence is suspected. It is not otherwise usually necessary. Doppler ultrasound is a simple and accurate method of locating incompetent perforating veins; pressure on the calf muscles with the patient standing produces a characteristic noise at points of incompetence (Miller, 1974).

An important physical sign, which must always be looked for, is the 'ankle venous flare' (*Fig.* 44.8; *see also Fig.* 44.20). These radiating venules, over the medial, or more rarely the lateral, malleolus are the single most important indication of incompetence of the direct lower calf and ankle perforators.

Operation

Patient preparation and anaesthesia have been described. A head-down tilt (about 10°) is important to reduce bleeding.

1. Incompetent Medial Calf Perforating Veins

These veins, the most common of the direct perforating veins, can be approached by the medial approach developed by Cockett (1955) from Linton's (1938) operation; or by the posterior 'modified seam' incision. The latter is indicated where there is much medial induration or healed ulceration, and is described with the post-thrombotic syndrome.

THE MEDIAL APPROACH

a. The incision is placed one finger's breadth behind the posterior border of the tibia, and extends from 2·5 cm above and behind the medial malleolus to nearly halfway up the leg (*Fig.* 44.9). The perforating veins may be approached extrafascially, but the

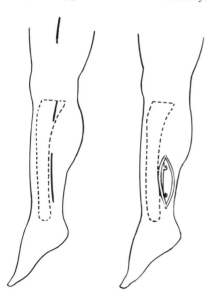

Fig. 44.9. Cockett's approach to the calf and ankle perforating veins and the incisions for Boyd's perforator and the Hunterian perforator.

author prefers the subfascial (Linton, 1953) approach which avoids undercutting skin.

b. The anterior flap of deep fascia is elevated and the perforating veins identified as they pass forwards close to the posterior border of the tibia. With a little dissection they can be traced down to their junction with the posterior tibial veins. This manoeuvre prevents branches being missed. The veins are either

divided between catgut ligatures or, if very short and inaccessible, underrun with a 0 linen thread suture on an aneurysm needle. By gently stripping the muscles from the deep fascia, other perforators, e.g. the gastrocnemius perforator, can be found and ligated.

c. The deep fascia does not need to be closed. The skin is closed with interrupted 2/0 Prolene sutures. An incompetent long saphenous vein can easily be found under the upper end of this incision and stripped down to it; and this is therefore the ideal approach for medial perforating vein incompetence associated with long saphenous incompetence.

2. Lateral Calf Perforator Incompetence

The approach is similar to the medial operation. Alternatively, this vein can be controlled through the posterior modified seam incision (*see below*).

3. High Medial Calf Perforator (Boyd's Perforator) Incompetence

This is approached through a similar longitudinal incision (*Fig.* 44.9)

4. Other Gastrocnemius Perforators

Lateral or posterior gastrocnemius perforators are similarly approached. The posterior calf perforator is usually associated with short saphenous incompetence, and is ligated at the same time as this vein is stripped.

5. The Hunterian Perforator

Recurrent varicose veins not infrequently arise from a lower thigh (Hunterian) perforator which was missed at the original operation. The vein is approached by a longitudinal medial thigh incision about 7·5 cm long (*Fig.* 44.9). Varicose branches are traced to the main feeding vein, which must be followed down, deep to sartorius, to the main vein in Hunter's canal. A number of small muscle veins may have to be divided in this approach. The Hunterian perforator is ligated close to the neurovascular bundle.

6. The Tensor Fascia Lata Perforator

This rare perforator communicates with the muscular veins of the thigh to cause varices on its lateral aspect, which are prominent in the Klippel–Trenaunay syndrome. Treatment is by exploration and ligation.

Postoperative Care and Complications

These are similar to those for other varicose vein operations with two important exceptions.

The medial incision is usually slow to heal. Interrupted sutures must be used and not removed before 12 days or so. If the incision is made through indurated subcutaneous tissue, scar ulceration is likely. Bandages or elastic stockings may be necessary for several weeks, or even a month or two; but provided the deep vein valves are competent, permanent elastic support is not usually necessary (cf. post-thrombotic syndrome).

Subfascial exploration is followed by a high incidence of deep vein thrombosis, particularly where the operation is being performed for post-thrombotic venous incompetence. Anticoagulant prophylaxis is therefore indicated, a convenient method being calcium heparin 5000 units 12-hourly by subcutaneous injection.

Injection Sclerotherapy

Injection sclerotherapy acts by sclerosing short segments of superficial varices. It has been suggested that these should be related to incompetent perforating veins (Fegan, 1967) but this is not essential. By injecting into a collapsed vein and applying immediate and prolonged pressure, venous sclerosis is produced—the final result being a thin, scarred vein. Failure to apply adequate and prolonged pressure leads to thrombosis, which is lumpy, painful and may become recanalized.

Indications

1. Injection sclerotherapy is indicated in the treatment of below-knee varices *without* long or short saphenous incompetence. Patients with such incompetence may sometimes request injection sclerotherapy rather than operation, because they wish to avoid being admitted to hospital. This treatment will usually produce good initial results, but such patients should be warned that recurrent varices are likely in 3–5 years' time (Hobbs, 1968) and these will then require further treatment.

2. Incompetent perforating veins respond well to injection sclerotherapy (Hobbs, 1974), providing that they can be identified accurately. This is often not possible in the presence of post-thrombotic induration.

Contra-indications

1. Long or short saphenous incompetence.
2. Above-knee varices (compression difficult to apply and maintain).
3. Veins very close to arteries (e.g. posterior tibial).
4. A history of allergy.
5. Induration or ulceration.
6. Pregnancy.
7. Contraceptive pill.
8. Any contra-indication to prolonged bandaging, e.g. arterial insufficiency.

9. General debility and inability to walk for any reason.
10. Obesity should be corrected before injections.
11. Avoid injecting in very hot weather, when prolonged bandaging (and lack of baths if both legs are treated at once) can be intolerable.

About one-quarter to one-third of patients with primary varicose veins are suitable for injection sclerotherapy.

Technique

The collapsed vein technique introduced by Fegan (1967) is important. The sclerosant—sodium tetradecyl sulphate (STD) 3 per cent—is almost universally used, and has generally superseded ethanolamine oleate.

1. The patient stands on a 'mounting block' and veins are carefully marked with a felt tip pen (*Fig.* 44.10). Particular attention is paid to the sites of varicose dilatation and perforating vein incompetence.

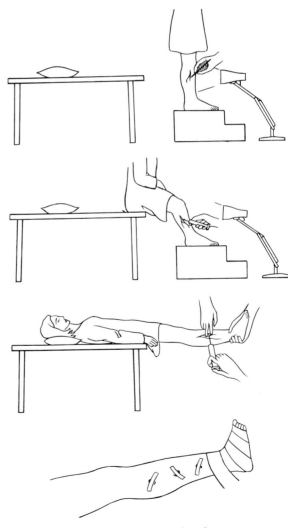

Fig. 44.10. Injection sclerotherapy.

2. The patient sits at the end of the examination couch, with the legs hanging over the end. The surgeon sits opposite on a low stool. One or two pillows are placed halfway along the examination couch. A good light is essential.

3. The needle (no. 16) is inserted in the vein. Care is taken that the blood drawn back into the syringe is venous, e.g. dark in colour and *non-pulsatile*.

4. The patient leans backwards on the pillows, elevating the leg with help from the assistant. The surgeon controls the vein above and below the injection site, and injects between 0·25 and 0·5 ml of sclerosant.

5. A small cottonwool pad mounted on an Elastoplast strip is immediately applied by the assistant.

6. The patient sits, lowering the legs, and the procedure is repeated on the next marked site. Large or dilated varices can often be injected without the leg being lowered.

Two ml of STD per leg per session are a safe upper limit.

7. Immediately the last injection has been given, the leg is elevated and bandaged with 10- or 15-cm Elastocrêpe which is covered with Tubigrip stockinet.

8. The patient is instructed to walk for about 1·5 km (1 mile) immediately, and thereafter for about 5 km (3 miles) a day. The patient is also advised to avoid prolonged standing, and to report to the clinic at once if the bandages become too loose, too tight or at all uncomfortable.

9. The patient is seen again after 1 week. The bandages are removed, scurfy skin washed away (we have found a plastic washing-up bowl essential to this part of the treatment!) and the legs inspected. Remaining varices are injected, and cotton wool pad pressure is reapplied. Any lumpy thrombi are evacuated through small incisions under local anaesthesia. The legs are rebandaged, and the patient seen once more in 2 weeks or 1 month, depending on the size and extent of the varices. Total bandaging time should be 5 or 6 weeks for extensive varices, but can be shortened to 3 weeks where only a few small varices are injected.

Complications

1. A painful thrombus results from the vein being distended during the injection, or inadequately compressed afterwards. If not evacuated by a stab incision through a bleb of local anaesthetic, a brown stain will result. These usually fade, but may take up to 3 years to do so.

2. Extravenous injection can be avoided by *always* drawing back blood into the syringe before injecting. Never inject if in doubt. Extravasation of sclerosant may cause skin ulceration.

3. Sensitivity reactions may occur, usually at the second course of injections. Anaphylactic shock and death, though very rare, have been reported. Adrena-

line, hydrocortisone and antihistamines must be available.

4. Deep vein thrombosis and pulmonary embolism are avoided by never injecting more than a small volume of sclerosant at any one session (2 ml per leg per session), and by brisk walking immediately after the injections.

5. Accidental *arterial* injection has occurred, and has caused peripheral gangrene. Attempts to inject the lower calf perforators, which lie close to the posterior tibial artery, are particularly dangerous. *Always* draw blood back into the syringe, make certain it is dark in colour and non-pulsatile, and *never* inject if at all in doubt.

Venous Flares

These are of cosmetic importance only, and the best treatment is often simple advice on cosmetic masking creams. Injection sclerotherapy can be performed using a long-barrelled 1-ml syringe and a 27 or 30 SWG needle and a suitable sclerosant. STD 3 per cent is too strong and is liable to produce inflammation and brown stains. It can be used diluted to 1 per cent, but a better sclerosant is Sclerovein (hydroxypolyaethoxydodecan and trichlorisobutyl alcohol in aqueous solution, 0·5–2 per cent). At present this is not formally approved for use in the UK, though it is widely used in Switzerland, Germany and Holland (Scleremo is used in France). A good light is essential, and some form of magnification desirable. Patience is the greatest necessity. Compression bandaging is required for 1 week only. Residual brown staining may take weeks, or even months, to resolve.

Those not prepared to undertake a time-consuming cosmetic procedure, with a proportion of poor results, should not embark on this treatment.

RECURRENT VARICOSE VEINS

Recurrent varicose veins may occasionally be true recurrences after accurate surgery, but by far the majority are the results of inadequate surgery, or of injection sclerotherapy performed in spite of the contra-indications which have been described.

Careful examination may be sufficient, but very often ascending phlebography is required to delineate 'leak points'. On occasion this may be supplemented by 'unconventional' phlebography, in which the contrast is injected directly into the varix, and its passage to the deep vein followed with the image intensifier ('varicography').

Groin and Thigh Recurrence

This most often results from inadequate surgery, one or more tributaries of the saphenous vein having been missed.

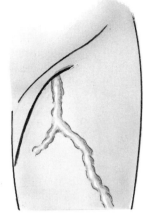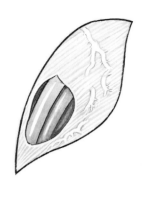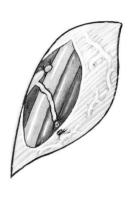

Fig. 44.11. Operation for recurrent varices of the long saphenous system.

The region of the saphenofemoral junction is approached through a long, if necessary 'hockey stick' incision (*Fig.* 44.11). Rather than a difficult and dangerous dissection through dense scar tissue, it is best to approach the medial border of the superficial femoral vein well below the foramen ovale. The saphenofemoral junction is thus approached from below, and can be identified and ligated without much difficulty (*Fig.* 44.11). Varicose tributaries are avulsed through small incisions. Occasionally the whole long saphenous vein has been inadvertently left *in situ*, and this must be stripped out.

Recurrent Popliteal Varices

These results from inadequate short saphenous surgery. The mass of varices must be divided and the stump of the short saphenous vein identified and ligated flush with the popliteal vein.

Recurrent Lower Leg Varices

If small, or resulting from previous injection sclerotherapy, these can be avulsed or injected. Be careful to exclude previously missed long or short saphenous incompetence, and deal with these veins as necessary. Most often, recurrent lower leg varices are the result of perforating vein incompetence which was either overlooked at the original operation or has developed since that time. Varicography (phlebography by direct injection into a varix) is usually necessary for a proper demonstration of these 'leak points', which may include the Hunterian perforator. They can then be approached and ligated as has been described.

VULVAL VARICES

Vulval and pudendal varices are uncommon complications of pregnancy. They are varicose tributaries of the pudendal and obturator veins. Although they can be so large as to obstruct vaginal delivery and make Caesarean section necessary, they almost always disappear after parturition. Treatment is therefore usually conservative, by an appropriate pad and elastic pants. Occasionally they persist, causing premenstrual pain. Both injection sclerotherapy and surgery have been recommended. The latter—multiple avulsions through small incisions lateral to the vulva—gives good results.

'Pseudo'-pudendal varices are dilated branches of the long saphenous vein, and are readily treated by high saphenous ligation.

Groin varices may be collaterals for iliac vein obstruction. These must not be interfered with.

DEEP VEIN THROMBOSIS AND THE POST-THROMBOTIC SYNDROME

Surgical Anatomy

The deep veins of the lower leg are the paired venae comitantes of the anterior and posterior tibial and the peroneal arteries, the gastrocnemius veins and the soleus venous arcades. They all join to form the popliteal vein (*Fig.* 44.12) which also receives the short saphenous vein. The main veins are profusely valved, but the soleus arcades dilate at intervals into sinusoids. These important vessels, with a total capacity of about 140 ml, act as reservoirs or 'ventricles' for the calf muscle pump. They are also a common site of thrombus initiation.

The calf and ankle direct perforating veins penetrate the deep fascia to join the posterior tibial vein medially and the peroneal vein on the lateral side.

The deep veins of the calf are profusely valved. Contractions of the calf muscles, enclosed in their tight fascial sheath, force venous blood proximally, and their relaxation draws blood from superficial to deep along the direct perforating veins (*Fig.* 44.13) (Negus, 1970). Post-thrombotic recanalization results in valve incompetence and 'pump failure'. The high ambulatory venous pressures are transmitted to the vulnerable ankle skin and subcutaneous tissues along the incompetent dilated direct perforating

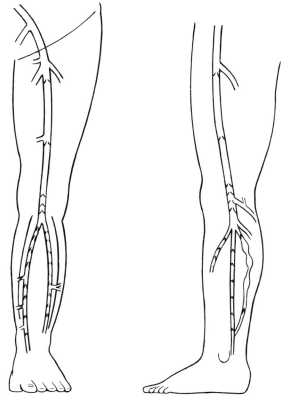

Fig. 44.12. Diagrammatic representation of the deep veins of the leg.

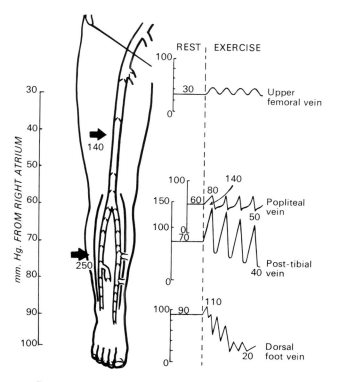

Fig. 44.13. Pressure profiles in the veins of the normal leg.

veins with a net outflow from the deep compartment of 60 ml/min (Bjordal, 1981), and this leads to the sequence of venular dilatation and fibrin deposition which ends in venous ulceration (*see* Venous Ulcers).

The superficial femoral vein has few tributaries apart from the Hunterian perforator, some muscle veins and the profunda femoris, which joins it to form the common femoral vein. The profunda is an important collateral in superficial femoral thrombosis and occlusion.

The common femoral vein receives the termination of the long saphenous vein and also, in many cases, a deep pudendal branch. The common femoral and iliac veins are usually valveless.

Surgical interest in the iliac veins and inferior vena cava is chiefly related to the predominantly left-sided incidence of iliac vein thrombosis and of post-thrombotic stenosis or occlusion (Cockett and Thomas, 1965), and also in the difficulty often encountered in left common iliac thrombectomy. These phenomena have a common cause, the anatomical anomaly of compression and 'band' or 'spur' formation at the mouth of the left common iliac vein (*Fig.* 44.14). This is found in about 20 per cent of the otherwise normal adult population, and is the result of the lumbar lordosis forcing the left common iliac vein forwards against the overlying right common iliac artery (Negus et al., 1968a). Following thrombosis at this point, band formation and compression of the left common iliac vein prevent adequate recanalization, and the resulting stenosis obstructs venous return from the leg.

Important collaterals are the internal iliac veins and their tributaries, the iliolumbar trunk, which anastomoses with the vertebral venous plexus and the uterine and ovarian veins. These collateral veins dilate, but may be inadequate to conduct the high venous outflow of an exercising leg, particularly after hysterectomy.

Little need be said of the inferior vena cava, except that its main tributaries below the renal veins, the paired lumbar veins, constitute a hazard for the unwary in lumbar sympathectomy and aorto-iliac surgery. Congenital abnormalities include paired cavae, a left-sided cava and occasionally complete absence of the inferior vena cava.

Deep Vein Thrombosis

Thrombosis and thrombophlebitis can affect both superficial and deep veins. The commonest cause of superficial thrombophlebitis is intravenous cannulation. 'Clotted drips' can be prevented to a considerable extent by the addition of heparin (1000 units/L) to the infusion (Tanner et al., 1978). Thrombophlebitis migrans may be the first sign of Buerger's disease. Spontaneous thrombophlebitis is a common complication of varicose veins, and emergency high saphenous ligation is sometimes necessary.

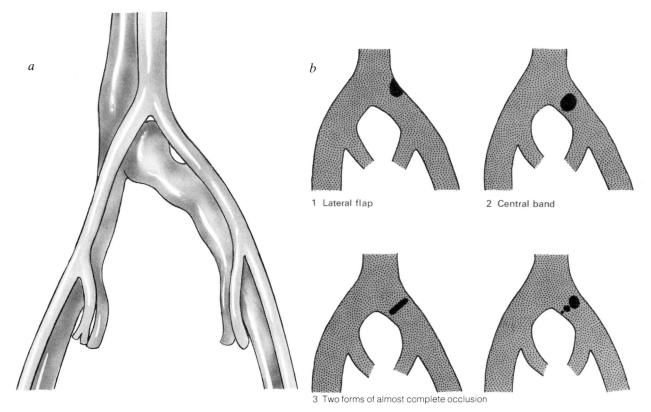

a

b

1 Lateral flap   2 Central band

3 Two forms of almost complete occlusion

Fig. 44.14. *a*, Compression of the termination of the left common iliac vein. *b*, The variety of 'bands' which are found in otherwise normal veins.

Venous thrombosis is rare in the upper limb. Axillary vein thrombosis may result from prolonged extension of the arm over the head.

Lower limb deep vein thrombosis may occur spontaneously. It sometimes indicates occult cancer and, rarely in younger patients, results from a congenital deficiency of fibrinolytic or antithrombin III activity. More commonly, it may follow superficial thrombophlebitis in varicose veins.

Most often, deep vein thrombosis occurs as a complication of bed rest and major illness (particularly myocardial infarction) or trauma, whether surgical or accidental. Careful questioning will often reveal an episode of half-forgotten trauma preceding an episode of 'spontaneous' deep vein thrombosis. Pregnancy and the puerperium are still predisposing causes, but to a much smaller extent since the introduction of early activity. The sensitive ^{125}I-fibrinogen uptake technique has shown an incidence of 25–30 per cent of small, clinically insignificant thrombi after major thoracic or abdominal surgery (Flanc et al., 1968; Negus et al., 1968b). Head and neck, upper limb and breast surgery, and hernia repair, have a very small incidence indeed. Hip operations and lower limb fractures carry a high (50–70 per cent) risk of isotope-detected thrombi. Of the 25–30 per cent fibrinogen-detected 'mini-thrombi' which follow major abdominal or thoracic surgery, about 2.7 per cent produce physical signs.

Clinically evident pulmonary embolism occurs in about 1.3 per cent of general surgical patients, and is fatal in about 0.4 per cent. Hip surgery has a much higher incidence, 2 or even 3 per cent in some series. These figures (Salzman, 1978) are all very approximate. Of deep vein thromboses, 85 per cent are confined to the calf and only a minority propagate to, or arise in, the femoral or iliac veins, apart from those which are associated with hip surgery. Iliofemoral venous thrombosis most commonly affects the left leg (Negus, 1970).

Venous thrombo-embolism is much less common in underdeveloped countries than in the industrialized Western world.

Prevention of Postoperative Deep Vein Thrombosis

The risk of developing postoperative deep vein thrombosis increases with the following factors:
1. A past history of deep vein thrombosis.
2. Malignancy.
3. The contraceptive pill.
4. Major abdominal or thoracic surgery (rare in upper limb, thyroid, breast surgery, etc.).
5. Hip and lower limb fracture or surgery, particularly hip replacement.
6. Obesity.
7. Polycythaemia, thrombocythaemia, hyperfibrinogenaemia and raised blood viscosity.

Methods of Prevention

1. Obesity should be reduced by dieting.
2. Constipation, with subsequent 'straining at stool', should be corrected by diet and aperients.
3. *Early ambulation* must *never* be forgotten with the introduction of more 'sophisticated' measures. Active exercise in bed and deep breathing are encouraged at all times, with early ambulation on a regular basis (5 minutes' walking around the bed every hour, on the hour, with steadily increasing times and distances). Sitting for long periods is discouraged.

MECHANICAL METHODS

a. Passive: TED 'anti-embolism' stockings reduce the incidence of postoperative deep vein thrombosis by 50 per cent (Holford and Bliss, 1976) and significantly reduce the incidence of fatal pulmonary embolism (Wilkins et al., 1952). Knee-length stockings seem to be as effective as thigh-length ones (Negus and Nicholson, 1986). Elevation of the foot of the bed may also be helpful.

b. Active: Intermittent calf compression by inflatable plastic leggings (Sabri et al., 1971; Hills et al., 1972) and electrical calf muscle stimulation (Browse and Negus, 1970) reduce the incidence of ^{125}I-fibrinogen detected thrombi. Neither method has yet been submitted to large-scale clinical trial to determine its effectiveness in preventing fatal pulmonary embolism.

PHARMACOLOGICAL METHODS

a. Full anticoagulation with warfarin or dindevan effectively prevents postoperative deep vein thrombosis, but it is usually contra-indicated after major surgery.

b. Subcutaneous heparin, given at 10 000 units 8–10 hours preoperatively, followed by 2500 units 8-hourly postoperatively until mobilization or discharge, effectively prevents postoperative venous thrombo-embolism. (Sharnoff et al., 1962; Sharnoff and DeBlasio, 1970.) Regular dose monitoring by means of a modified Dale and Laidlaw coagulometer prevents bleeding or haematoma formation.

This regimen has been simplified to a dose of 5000 units of subcutaneous heparin preoperatively, followed by 5000 units 8- or 12-hourly for 7 days without monitoring coagulation times (Kakkar et al., 1972). Deep vein thrombosis and fatal pulmonary embolism are effectively reduced (An International Multicentre Trial, 1975) but haematoma formation at the injection site is quite common and severe postoperative bleeding occasionally occurs (Britton et al., 1977). This method should not be used where a significant raw area is left, e.g. prostatectomy, abdominoperineal resection of rectum, etc.

c. Low molecular weight dextran, 500 ml during and after operation and 500 ml the following day, is probably less effective in preventing isotope-detected thrombi, but reduces the incidence of fatal pulmonary embolism as effectively as low dose subcutaneous heparin (Kline et al., 1975). The intravenous route is an advantage in patients undergoing thoracic or abdominal surgery, who require intravenous fluids for several days postoperatively. Circulatory overloading can occur, but is usually corrected without difficulty, by stopping the infusion and administering diuretics. Dextran should be avoided in patients with any impairment of renal function. Acute anaphylaxis has been described, but is extremely rare.

Intravenous heparin in the very low dose of 1 unit/kg/hr (micro-dose intravenous heparin) reduced the incidence of isotope-detected deep vein thrombosis from 22 to 4 per cent in two randomized controlled trials (Negus et al., 1980; Negus and Friedgood, 1986). The heparin must be dissolved in normal saline, which is then 'piggy-backed' into the dextrose infusion line, as it is rapidly denatured in dextrose solution. This method is simple, safe and inexpensive.

Diagnosis of Deep Vein Thrombosis

The development of more 'sophisticated' methods has not reduced the need for regular and thorough examination of patients' legs. It is not only after operation that patients are at risk. Those admitted for investigation not uncommonly develop deep vein thrombosis and even fatal embolism.

Important physical signs are calf tenderness and ankle oedema. Extensive deep vein thrombosis may exist with moderate pitting oedema of the ankle as the only physical sign. An increase in calf temperature may be present, but usually only serves to confirm the physical signs; and Homans' sign is generally held to be of little value (Negus, 1978).

An unexplained low-grade pyrexia may indicate occult deep vein thrombosis, but many patients with deep vein thrombosis have some other, infective cause for the pyrexia. Conversely, major pulmonary embolism can occur without pyrexia or other physical signs (Negus and Rickford, 1975).

Most deep vein thromboses are confined to the calf veins and extensive femoral and iliofemoral thromboses, which are responsible both for major pulmonary embolism and for the most severe cases of post-thrombotic syndrome, are relatively less common.

There is no difficulty in diagnosing massive occlusive iliofemoral deep vein thrombosis. Both thigh and calf are tensely swollen and the skin is pale ('phlegmasia alba dolens'). Rarely venous hypertension may lead to peripheral cyanosis and even to distal gangrene ('phlegmasia caerulea dolens'). Massive thrombotic occlusion of the inferior vena cava is fortunately rare, and then often associated with terminal carcinomatosis.

Diagnostic Methods

1. ASCENDING PHLEBOGRAPHY

This is the single, most accurate method. Injection of contrast medium is made into a dorsal foot vein, monitored by image intensifier and recorded on serial films by means of a rapid cassette changer (*Fig.* 44.15). Recent developments in non-irritant contrast media (metrizamide, etc.) have improved the comfort and safety of phlebography. Petrochanteric phlebography may occasionally be necessary to delineate the iliac veins.

2. DOPPLER ULTRASOUND

Ultrasound can detect major venous obstruction (e.g. popliteal to iliac veins) (Evans and Cockett, 1969). It is rapid and simple, but not entirely reliable.

3. ^{125}I-FIBRINOGEN UPTAKE

This depends on the incorporation of isotope-labelled human serum fibrinogen (obtained from hepatitis-free donors) into developing thrombus. Any increase in radioactivity is detected with a scintillation counter. It is very accurate in the calf and lower thigh (Flanc et al., 1968; Negus et al., 1968b). Many of the thrombi so detected are small and of doubtful clinical significance.

4. ISOTOPE-LABELLED ALBUMIN

The albumin concentrates in sites of thrombus formation, and this can be delineated with a gamma camera. Neither this method, nor any of the following, is used to any significant extent in the UK at present.

5. INFRA-RED THERMOGRAPHY

Developing thrombus shows up as a 'hot spot'. The instrument is unfortunately very expensive.

6. PLETHYSMOGRAPHY

A vein obstructed by thrombus collapses more slowly than a normal vein when an occluding pressure cuff is released and this results in a slower than normal fall in calf muscle volume. This can be measured directly by a strain gauge or by air-filled cuffs, or indirectly by changes in electrical conductivity (impedance plethysmography).

Other methods have been described, but only the first three described above are used to any extent at the present time: phlebography—for definitive diagnosis; Doppler ultrasound—for rapid screening; ^{125}I-fibrinogen—for research.

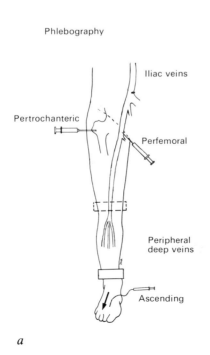

Phlebography

Iliac veins

Pertrochanteric

Perfemoral

Peripheral
deep veins

Ascending

a

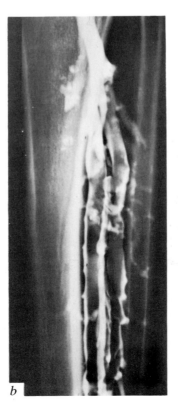

b

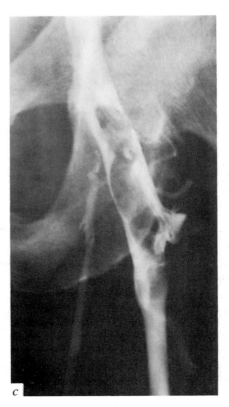

c

Fig. 44.15. *a*, Ascending phlebography. *b*, Thrombus in the calf and *c*, femoral veins.

Conservative Management of Established Deep Vein Thrombosis

Anticoagulation remains the most important measure in the treatment of thrombo-embolic disease. Pulmonary embolism must *always* be treated by full anticoagulation, whether the source of the emboli is detected by phlebography or other methods or not.

Anticoagulants

Intravenous heparin is given as a continuous infusion using an appropriate pump (40 000 units in 24 hours), and a loading dose of warfarin (usually 10–15 mg) is given at the same time. The heparin is continued until warfarin anticoagulation is achieved—usually after 3 days. Pulmonary embolism should be treated for 5–6 days with heparin. Daily clotting time (or accelerated clotting time) estimation is important because 'heparin resistance' sometimes develops by the formation of antibodies, and a daily dose of up to 80 000 units may then be necessary to maintain full anticoagulation. This is arbitrarily defined as a level of anticoagulation between two and three times a normal control. Warfarin dosage is similarly maintained by serial prothrombin times, and warfarin anticoagulation is continued for a minimum of 3 months. Recurrent pulmonary embolism may sometimes require permanent anticoagulation.

Fibrinolytic Agents

Urokinase and streptokinase have an important role in the treatment of massive pulmonary embolism when given through a catheter in the pulmonary artery (Miller and Sutton, 1970). Their place in the treatment of peripheral venous thrombosis is less well established. Fresh occluding thrombus can be lysed sufficiently to improve venous blood flow and good result have been obtained in cases of severe iliofemoral thrombosis (Browse et al., 1968) and in massive inferior vena caval thrombosis. Local infusion by an indwelling catheter gives the best results. Both urokinase and streptokinase are expensive. The latter, though the less expensive, is antigenic. Steroid cover is therefore required, and a second course cannot be given. Fibrinolysis is, of course, contraindicated by recent surgical operation or trauma, and this excludes most patients with postoperative deep vein thrombosis. A course of fibrinolytic therapy is always followed by full and prolonged anticoagulation.

Surgical Treatment of Deep Vein Thrombosis

Surgical procedures are divided into 'pulling out' procedures—thrombectomy—and 'locking in' procedures to prevent further embolism—venous ligation, plication or occlusion by clips or umbrellas.

Successful treatment depends on accurate knowledge of both the site and the degree of fixity of the thrombus. Adherent thrombus usually presents with limb swelling. Pulmonary embolism indicates nonadherent thrombus, with a risk of further embolism. Doppler ultrasound is useful for rapid assessment, but precise diagnosis depends on phlebography, and this investigation is mandatory in the management of pulmonary embolism.

Anticoagulation, which must be properly controlled, remains the most important method of treatment. Surgical thrombectomy is only indicated for the removal of phlebographically non-adherent thrombus in the iliac or upper femoral vein, or in an attempt to relieve the gross venous obstruction of phlegmasia cerulea dolens. Plication of the superficial femoral vein is indicated to prevent possible embolism from extensive, non-adherent femoral vein thrombus, following incomplete or doubtfully complete femoral thrombectomy; in the prevention of further emboli in an adequately anticoagulated patient with recurrent pulmonary emboli from calf or popliteal thrombosis; and in the treatment of patients with lower leg thrombosis in whom anticoagulants are contra-indicated.

Interruption of the inferior vena cava is not often indicated. Partially adherent common iliac thrombus and recurrent pulmonary embolism from internal iliac thrombosis are the most common indications.

Fibrinolytic therapy by urokinase or streptokinase is an alternative to femoral or iliac thrombectomy, in patients who have no recent history of trauma, whether accidental or surgical.

Venous Thrombectomy

INDICATIONS

1. Non-adherent iliofemoral thrombus shown by phlebography (usually in patients presenting with pulmonary embolism).

2. Phlegmasia cerulea dolens, where peripheral ischaemia is threatening the viability of the limb.

CONTRA-INDICATIONS

Partially adherent thrombus is unlikely to be completely removed and rapid or eventual rethrombosis is very common, and the operation is then a waste of time. Thrombectomy is less likely to be successful in the left iliac veins (cf. Surgical anatomy).

The operation is, of course, contra-indicated in those patients unfit for surgery. Fibrinolytic therapy should be considered as an alternative, provided there has been no surgery or trauma within 7 days.

THE OPERATION

Preoperative phlebography is mandatory. Local anaesthesia can be used, but general anaesthesia is preferable.

The patient is placed as for long saphenous high ligation and strip (legs apart with a head-down tilt).

Blood for transfusion should be cross-matched and available. Heparin should be stopped 1½–2 hours before the operation.

1. The incision: a longitudinal groin incision is made over the femoral vessels.

2. The superficial femoral artery is identified by its pulsation and is exposed by dividing the superficial fascia and femoral sheath (*Fig.* 44.16).

3. The superficial femoral vein is found on the medial side of the artery, and dissected proximally to the level of the inguinal ligament. The profunda femoris and other smaller tributaries are controlled by fine plastic slings (*Fig.* 44.16*a*).

4. Intravenous heparin (5000–8000 units) is given and the veins are occluded by soft 'bulldogs' or small DeBakey clamps.

5. A transverse incision is made in the superficial femoral vein 0·5 cm below the junction of the profunda femoris (*Fig.* 44.16*a*). A no. 8 or 10 Fogarty balloon catheter is passed proximally into the inferior vena cava. The balloon is inflated and the catheter withdrawn, bringing thrombus with it (*Fig.* 44.16*c*). The procedure is repeated until no more thrombus is extracted. The vein is flushed out with heparin/saline solution (1000 units heparin to 250 ml saline). The procedure is repeated in the distal superficial femoral vein (*Fig.* 44.16*d*). Valve resistance can be overcome by inflating the vein with normal saline flushed through a catheter passed alongside the Fogarty balloon catheter. Thrombus extraction can be helped by winding an Esmarch bandage tightly round the leg from ankle to thigh. Heparin/saline solution is similarly flushed into the distal vein.

6. The venotomy is closed with a continuous 4/0 Prolene or silk suture.

7. If distal thrombectomy has been incomplete, as is usually the case, superficial femoral vein interruption ('locking in') is performed to prevent further pulmonary embolism.

8. The incision is closed in layers with suction drainage. Anticoagulation is continued for at least 3 months.

COMPLICATIONS

The obvious complication is haemorrhage, but with careful suturing this is rare. Control is by pressure and reversal of anticoagulation.

Superficial wound infection responds to antibiotics and dressings.

The most common complication is rethrombosis, which is not uncommon in spite of prolonged and adequate anticoagulation. The reason is that even 'loose' thrombus is usually partially adherent, and this irremovable thrombus forms the nucleus for further thrombosis. For this reason the operation is only comparatively rarely indicated.

Venous interruption—superficial femoral plication

INDICATIONS

1. Recurrent pulmonary embolism arising from the lower leg in spite of adequate anticoagulation.

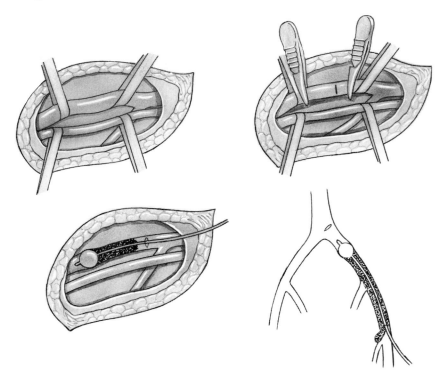

Fig. 44.16. Fogarty embolectomy of the superficial femoral and external iliac veins.

2. Following superficial femoral venous thrombectomy (which is usually incomplete).

3. Lower leg thrombosis when anticoagulants are contra-indicated, e.g. active peptic ulceration.

THE OPERATION

The patient's position, preparation, incision and exposure are the same as for venous thrombectomy.

1. The superficial femoral vein is controlled by small soft clamps or bulldogs immediately below the junction of the profunda femoris.

2. Two or three 3/0 silk sutures are placed between the anterior and posterior walls of the vein (*Fig.* 44.17).

3. The incision is closed with Redivac drainage.

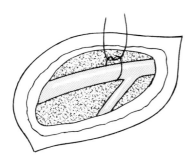 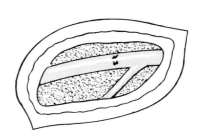

Fig. 44.17. Ligation and plication of the superficial femoral vein.

COMPLICATIONS

Apart from the usual complications, rethrombosis is always a risk. Prolonged anticoagulation is therefore mandatory.

Inferior vena caval interruption

INDICATIONS

1. Non-adherent internal or common iliac thrombosis, particularly with recent pulmonary embolism.

2. Incomplete removal of partially adherent iliac thrombosis.

3. Recurrent pulmonary embolism; source not demonstrable by phlebography.

METHODS

A number of plastic clips have been described. There is a small risk of their opening later, and also of aortic pressure necrosis. Inferior vena caval plication is preferable, but this operation has now been largely superseded by inferior vena caval filters (Mobin–Uddin umbrella and Kimray–Greenfield filter) which are passed to the infrarenal inferior vena cava through a small incision in the jugular vein under X-ray control. Withdrawal of the introducer opens the umbrella, which has tiny claws to hold it in position (*Fig.* 44.18*c,d*). The Kimray–Greenfield filter

design is claimed to provide more secure fixation in the caval wall and less risk of thrombus occlusion.

Inferior vena caval plication

1. The inferior vena cava is approached through a retroperitoneal muscle-splitting incision, as for right lumbar sympathectomy (*Fig.* 44.18).

2. The infrarenal cava is mobilized, care being taken not to tear any lumbar veins.

3. A short segment (2–3 cm) of the vein is controlled between soft occluding clamps.

4. Three or four interrupted 2/0 silk sutures are placed between the anterior and posterior walls of the vein.

5. The clamps are removed and the abdominal wall is closed in layers using chromic catgut. A Redivac drain is left *in situ*.

Full anticoagulation is continued for at least 3 months.

COMPLICATIONS

Haemorrhage or sepsis should not occur if the operation is properly prepared and wound closure is meticulous.

Inferior vena caval and iliac thrombosis may result from inadequate postoperative anticoagulation. This can lead to hypovolaemic collapse due to venous blood entrapment in the lower limbs. Urokinase infused into the thrombus through an indwelling catheter has been used successfully to lyse the thrombus and restore venous return.

Venous Ulcers, Perforating Vein Incompetence and the Post-Thrombotic Syndrome

Venous ulceration is the direct result of an increase in ambulatory venous pressure, most often in the supramalleolar network of veins which communicate with the direct calf and ankle perforating veins. Primary varicosity of the long or short saphenous systems rarely causes ulceration, even when long-standing.

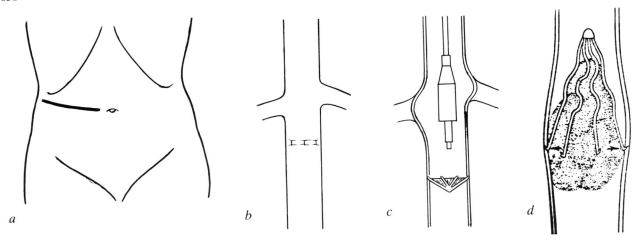

Fig. 44.18. Inferior vena caval plication. *a*, Incision. *b*, Final appearance. *c*, The Mobin–Uddin umbrella. *d*, The Kimray–Greenfield filter.

True varicose ulcers are variable in situation and are small, shallow and easily healed (Homans, 1916).

By contrast, ulcers which result from incompetence of the direct perforating veins of the lower leg are more constant in position—most commonly just above the medial malleolus—more extensive in area, deeper and surrounded by induration and pigmentation.

Lateral ulcers also occur in relation to the incompetence of the peroneal perforating veins, and circumferential ulcers are not uncommon.

Direct perforating vein incompetence may arise from one of the following causes, or a combination of these:

1. Following local thrombophlebitis, which in turn usually follows an injury (*Fig.* 44.19).

2. Associated with primary long or short saphenous incompetence.

3. Following deep vein thrombosis and recanalization of the deep and perforating veins of the lower leg. This is the post-thrombotic syndrome. Popliteal and femoral vein recanalization and incompetence lead to hydrostatic distension of the deep calf veins; and ulceration resulting from such extensive thrombosis is likely to be more severe and resistant to treatment than that following localized calf vein incompetence.

The first physical sign indicating incompetence of one or more direct perforating veins is the 'ankle venous flare', a network of small dilated veins which form a triangle over the medial (or less commonly lateral) malleolus. The responsible incompetent perforating vein is found about 3 cm above the apex of this triangle. These dilated venules are the result of high ambulatory venous pressure, which is transmitted through the incompetent direct perforating veins by contractions of the calf muscles (Cockett and Jones, 1953) (*Fig.* 44.20). This, in turn, leads to high pressure at the venular end of the cutaneous capillaries. The capillaries themselves proliferate and dilate,

so that gaps appear between their endothelial cells, and through these erythrocytes and fibrinogen 'leak out' into the surrounding tissue spaces. Haemosiderin deposition leads to this typical pigmentation, and the fibrinogen precipitates to form a 'fibrin cuff' around the capillaries, which interferes with the transfer of oxygen and metabolites to the surrounding tissues (Jarrett et al., 1976). This results in woody induration or 'liposclerosis', and subsequent skin necrosis and ulceration. A relatively poor arteriolar supply in the gaiter area of the lower leg is an additional factor.

It cannot be emphasized too strongly that incompetence of the *direct* perforating veins in the lower third of the leg is responsible for venous ulceration. Indirect perforating veins may also become incompetent, but these are situated in the upper two-thirds of the lower leg, where the ambulatory venous pressures are not so high. Their incompetence may result in local varices, but they are rarely, if ever, responsible for ulceration.

Patients with venous ulcers resulting from direct perforating vein incompetence can be conveniently divided into four groups (*Fig.* 44.21):

1a. Those whose ulcers are secondary to incompetent direct calf perforating veins with little or no deep vein incompetence. These respond well to perforating vein ligation and do not usually require prolonged elastic stocking support.

1b. Those whose perforating vein incompetence is accompanied by post-thrombotic popliteal and femoral, as well as calf, deep vein incompetence. These patients need permanent elastic stocking support as well as ligation of perforating veins. Operations to transpose or replace damaged deep valves are being developed and may become an alternative to stockings in suitable patients.

2. Those with iliac vein stenosis following iliofemoral venous thrombosis. This is usually left-sided (*see* Surgical Anatomy) and has been called the 'iliac

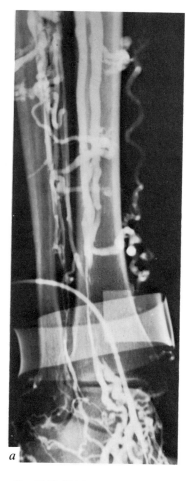

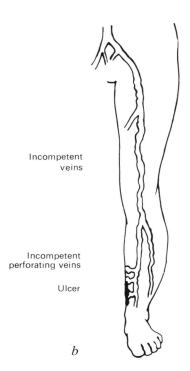

Incompetent
veins

Incompetent
perforating veins

Ulcer

a   *b*

Fig. 44.19. Phlebogram showing deep calf and perforating vein incompetence.

compression syndrome' (Cockett and Thomas, 1965). These patients are a very small proportion of those with the post-thrombotic syndrome. They all eventually develop peripheral deep vein incompetence (group 3) and leg ulcers (Negus, 1970). But most present before ulceration has developed, complaining of 'bursting pain' on walking. This 'venous claudication' (Negus, 1968) results from the high ambulatory venous pressure produced by proximal venous obstruction, which must be relieved if this distressing symptom is to be alleviated.

3. Patients with both iliac vein stenosis and peripheral deep and perforating vein incompetence constitute the most intractable subgroup of the post-thrombotic syndrome.

Management of Venous Ulcers

Management is considered under four headings:

1. Heal the ulcer; and at the same time exclude ulcers arising from other causes. These include traumatic ulcers, rheumatoid ulcers, diabetic ulcers, tropical sores, Martorell's (hypertension) ulcers,

syphilis, tuberculosis, steroid treatment and ischaemic ulcers from arterial insufficiency.

2. Diagnose the underlying venous abnormality. Doppler ultrasound is very useful, and phlebography is only necessary in complicated cases.

3. Control the 'leak points'. All incompetent perforating veins and saphenous veins must be occluded, usually by surgery. Occasionally injection sclerotherapy is sufficient. Surgical relief of venous stenosis (group 3) is also necessary in this least common type of post-thrombotic syndrome.

4. Continued elastic stocking support in patients with deep vein incompetence. The patient's continued cooperation is a most important factor in obtaining a good long-term result.

1. *Ulcer Healing*

This is based on four principles:

    a. Control infection.

    b. Avoid irritation.

    c. Remove debris.

    d. Counteract venous hypertension.

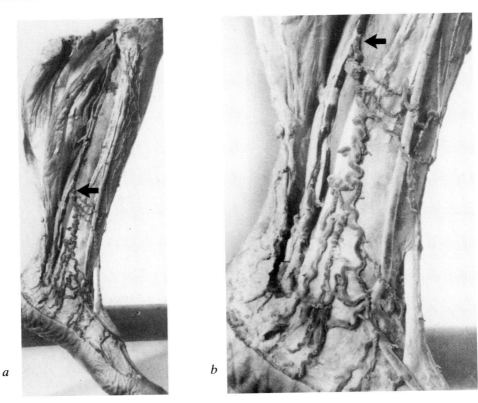

Fig. 44.20. a, Medial calf dissection showing dilated veins of 'ankle venous flare' communicating with posterior tibial vein through incompetent perforating vein. b, Enlargement; note the venules crossing the long saphenous vein without communicating with it. (Anatomy Museum, Royal College of Surgeons of England).

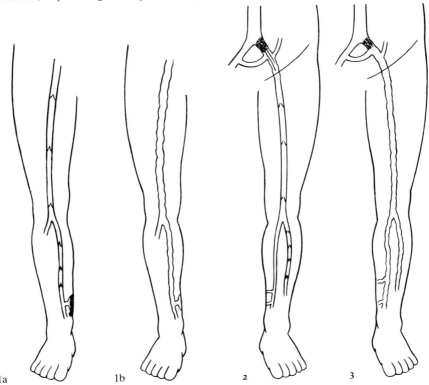

Fig. 44.21. The four main groups of perforating and deep vein incompetence and obstruction.

a. A bacteriological swab is cultured and antibiotic sensitivities determined, following which a 2-week course of the appropriate antibiotic is given systemically.

b. Steroids and other local applications are avoided. These frequently cause sensitivity reactions and delay healing.

c. The skin around the ulcer is cleaned daily with olive oil to remove loose flakes, and this is followed by half-strength hypochlorite solution if infected, otherwise by distilled or boiled water. The ulcer is then dressed with a single layer of non-adhesive dry dressing (NADD), followed by several layers of dressing gauze. Melolin and medicated dressings must be avoided. Slough in large chronic ulcers responds well to Debrisan (dextranomer) powder.

d. Venous hypertension is counteracted by:

i. Firm pressure bandaging. Elastocrêpe bandage with Tubigrip stockinet drawn over it is usually satisfactory. Large ulcers or large legs may require the stronger Elastoweb or Dickson–Wright bandages. The bandages are removed at night and a light dressing only is used.

ii. Elevation of the foot of the bed by 15–20 cm. Legs must be elevated when reading or watching television.

iii. Prolonged standing is avoided. Walking, with good elastic compression, is encouraged.

With these measures, most ulcers will heal within 2 or 3 months and only the most intractable—usually in the elderly—need to be treated by bed rest and elevation. Skin-grafting (pinch-grafts) is necessary in about 20 per cent.

2. *Diagnosis of the Underlying Venous Abnormality*

EXAMINATION AND INVESTIGATION

Clinical examination is as described in the surgery of varicose veins. Doppler ultrasound has already been described in the diagnosis of perforating vein incompetence. This simple method is also of great value in detecting reflux down the femoral and popliteal veins (Sumner, 1977) and phlebography is reserved for cases of suspected deep vein stenosis (*see Fig.* 44.19). Iliac vein stenosis may require phlebography by the perfemoral or pertrochanteric route.

Deep vein incompetence results in a high ambulatory foot venous pressure, but foot venous pressures, which involve cannulation, have now been largely superseded by photoplethysmography, which provides the same information in a non-invasive manner (Miles and Nicolaides, 1981).

Femoral venous pressure studies must always be performed in the investigation of suspected iliac vein stenosis. Significant stenosis with inadequate collaterals is indicated by a resting venous pressure above the normal 8–10 mmHg and an exercising pressure-rise of more than 2 mmHg in the horizontal position (Negus and Cockett, 1967).

3. *Operative Surgery*

A. PERIPHERAL DEEP AND PERFORATING VEIN INCOMPETENCE—PERFORATING VEIN LIGATION

Indications and contra-indications: The operation is indicated in most patients with post-thrombotic ulceration. The ulcer must be healed first by the measures which have been outlined, and obesity may require a period of dieting. Old age or infirmity may contra-indicate surgery. These patients form the 'hard core' of those attending ulcer clinics. Perforating vein injection has been recommended (Fegan, 1967; Hobbs, 1968) but the author's experience is that subcutaneous induration usually makes this difficult and unreliable.

The posteromedial subfascial approach: Perforating vein ligation may be performed through the medial approach which has been described. However, post-thrombotic subcutaneous induration and a relatively poor arteriolar distribution in this area make the medial incision slow to heal and liable to break down. The posterior subfascial approach (Dodd, 1964) avoids both medial and lateral indurated areas. Good access is afforded to the medial and lateral perforators, and the incision heals well.

The patient is intubated and placed face downwards as for short saphenous surgery. The incision is placed 2·5 cm medial to the midline, and the lower end is swung still more medially in order to avoid the Achilles tendon (*Fig.* 44.22*a*). (Painful skin adherence to the Achilles tendon caused the earlier 'seam' incision to be abandoned.)

Avoiding the sural nerve, the deep fascia is incised along the length of the incision. By retracting gastrocnemius laterally and then medially, the subfascial compartment is opened sufficiently to identify the medial and lateral direct perforating veins (*Fig.* 44.22*b*). These are either divided and ligated, or ligated in continuity using 2/0 linen thread on an aneurysm needle. The skin is closed with interrupted nylon sutures.

Long and short saphenous high ligation and stripping are performed at the same operation if these veins are incompetent.

Aftercare is as described for varicose veins, but mobilization is likely to be slower and convalescence more prolonged. The sutures should not be removed for 10 or 12 days. Bandaging is continued until healing is complete; and the bandages are then replaced by properly measured and fitted elastic stockings.

Complications: Wound infection is not common and responds well to antibiotics and dressings. Deep vein thrombosis is a considerable risk in these patients who have usually already suffered from at least one episode. Prophylactic subcutaneous calcium heparin, 5000 units 8-hourly, is therefore given for 7 days.

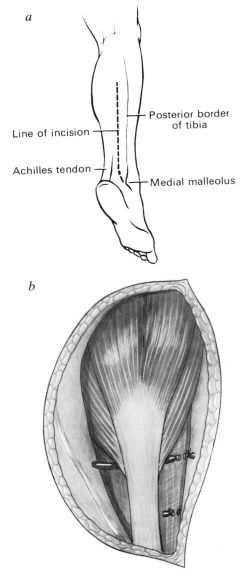

Fig. 44.22. Dodd's posteromedial subfascial approach for direct perforating vein incompetence.

B. ILIAC VEIN STENOSIS

Post-thrombotic venous stenosis most often occurs at the mouth of the left common iliac vein (*see* Surgical Anatomy). In spite of the development of collateral veins, functional obstruction to venous return often persists, producing venous hypertension and 'venous claudication'.

Examination and investigation: The affected leg may show no varices or ulceration, but is usually generally enlarged. Calf and thigh circumference is an inch or so greater than the normal leg. Careful inspection of the groin will often show dilated superficial collateral veins. A history of 'venous claudication' and inability to mark time at one step a second for more

than 3 minutes, also indicate significant iliac stenosis (Negus, 1968).

The site and extent of the stenosis are demonstrated by iliac phlebography, femoral venous pressure studies being performed at the same time. These have already been described.

Indications and contra-indications: These operations are relatively new and untried, and a significant failure rate is expected. Only patients with severe symptoms of 'venous claudication' and 'bursting pain' should be considered. Elderly, unfit or obese patients, or those whose lives are completely sedentary, are not suitable candidates for these procedures. Stenosis must be demonstrated by phlebography and venous pressure measurements.

The Operations:

i. *The Palma or Dale Operation:* Long saphenous cross-over graft using the contralateral saphenous vein, was first described by Palma and Esperon (1960), and subsequently by Dale and Harris (1968). The saphenous vein is tunnelled through the suprapubic fat (*Fig.* 44.23*a*). Improved results have been

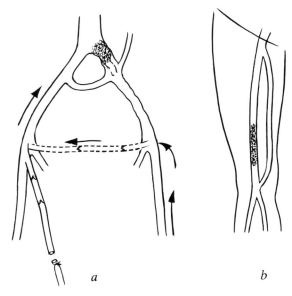

Fig. 44.23. Post-thrombotic occlusion of the left common iliac vein. *a*, The Palma–Dale operation for iliac vein obstruction. *b*, The Husni operation for superficial femoral obstruction.

claimed following the addition of a temporary arteriovenous fistula (Vollmar, 1977) which both improves flow in the maturing vein graft and helps dilate it. The fistula is closed after 4–6 months. Eight mm PTFE (Gortex) can be used in the absence of a suitable vein.

ii. Other procedures which have been devised to relieve iliac vein obstruction include perivenous scar tissue stripping (Wanke et al., 1956) and vein angioplasty at the caval bifurcation, but these have now generally given way to saphenous cross-over.

C. SUPERFICIAL FEMORAL VEIN STENOSIS

Post-thrombotic superficial femoral vein stenosis with inadequate collateral formation is a rare cause of lower leg swelling and intractable ulceration. The stricture can sometimes by bypassed by anastomosing the long saphenous to the popliteal vein (Husni, 1971) (*Fig.* 44.24).

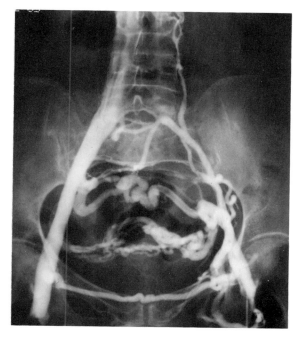

Fig. 44.24. Perfemoral iliac venogram showing post-thrombotic left common iliac occlusion with extensive cross-pelvic collateral veins (sacral, uterine and pudendal).

Complications: The most common complication is graft occlusion and failure to relieve the obstruction.

4. *Continued Support and Supervision: the Results of Treatment*

Continued firm elastic stocking support and regular supervision are essential to achieve good long-term results in most of these patients. Those with only localized perforating vein incompetence do not require permanent elastic stockings, but those with venographic or Doppler ultrasound evidence of deep vein incompetence must wear permanent knee-length compression stockings. Correction of deep vein incompetence by valve transposition (Queral et al., 1980) is not widely practised in the UK at present.

This regimen has been shown to give a good long-term result in 85 per cent of patients (Negus and Nicholson, 1986) and this confirms Arnoldi and Haeger's (1967) figures. Exclusion of patients with rheumatoid arthritis (and vasculitis) improves the success rate to over 90 per cent. This figure falls to 65 per cent if patients neglect to wear firm elastic stockings continuously, or fail to attend follow-up clinics (Cranley, 1975). If no postoperative support is provided at all, recurrent ulceration is inevitable in patients with extensive deep vein incompetence (Burnand et al., 1976).

Suitable elastic stockings are the Scholl 'Duoten' stocking for the less severe; and the Sigvaris stocking for those with extensive deep vein incompetence. These must be measured and fitted accurately. Below-knee stockings are usually sufficient.

It may be necessary for patients to change their employment from a standing to a sedentary occupation; but walking, tennis, golf and other pursuits are usually possible and should be encouraged.

The measures outlined above are intended for the relatively young and fit. Very old or frail patients are not suitable for surgery, and continued support and ulcer dressing are the only sensible approach.

RARE VENOUS ABNORMALITIES

1. Arteriovenous fistulas may produce large pulsatile varices. Generalized enlargement of the limb is often present.

Treatment is by surgical excision in localized cases; or by embolization during selective angiography.

2. The Klippel–Trenaunay syndrome consists of port-wine staining (capillary haemangioma) of the lateral aspect of the thigh, associated with enlargement of the underlying superficial veins. Arteriovenous fistula formation and limb enlargement may also be present.

3. Cutaneous capillary haemangiomas. Flat port-wine stains are treated by cosmetic creams or, rarely, by plastic surgery. 'Strawberry marks' (raised capillary haemangiomas) usually regress spontaneously.

4. Localized cavernous haemangiomas can be excised, but diffuse cavernous haemangiomas are too extensive. Investigation by phlebography must precede any decision on the advisability of surgery.

REFERENCES

Arnoldi I. C. and Haeger K. (1967) Ulcus cruris venosum—crux medicorum? *Lakartidningen* **64**, 2149.
Bjordal R. I. (1981) Circulation patterns in incompetent perforating veins of the calf in venous dysfunction. In: May R., Partsch H. and Staubesand J. (eds) *Perforating Veins*. Munich: Urban & Schwarzenberg.
Britton B. J., Finch D. R. A. et al. (1977) Low dose heparin. *Lancet* **ii**, 604.
Browse N. K. and Negus D. (1970) Prevention of postoperative leg vein thrombosis by electrical muscle stimulation. An evaluation with ^{125}I-labelled fibrinogen. *Br. Med. J.* **3**, 615–618.
Browse N. L., Thomas M. L. et al. (1968) Streptokinase and deep vein thrombosis. *Br. Med. J.* **3**, 717–720.

Buddecke E. (1975) Altersveränderungen der Proteoglykane. *Verh. Dtsch. Ges. Pathol.* **59**, 43.

Burnand K. G., O'Donnell T. et al. (1976) Relation between postphlebitic changes in the deep veins and results of surgical treatment of venous ulcers. *Lancet* **i**, 936–938.

Cockett F. B. (1955) The pathology and treatment of venous ulcers of the leg. *Br. J. Surg.* **43**, 260–278.

Cockett F. B. and Elgan Jones D. (1953) The ankle blow-out syndrome. A new approach to the varicose uicer problem. *Lancet* **1**, 17–23.

Cockett F. B. and Thomas M. L. (1965) The iliac compression syndrome. *Br. J. Surg.* **52**, 816–821.

Cranley J. J. (1975) *Vascular Surgery. Vol. II. Peripheral Venous Disease.* Hagerstown, Md: Harper & Row.

Dale W. A. and Harris J. (1968) Cross-over vein grafts for iliac and femoral venous occlusions. *Ann. Surg.* **168**, 319.

Dodd H. (1964) The diagnosis and ligation of incompetent ankle perforating veins. *Ann. R. Coll. Surg. Engl.* **34**, 186–196.

Dodd H. and Cockett F. B. (1976) *The Pathology and Surgery of the Veins of the Lower Limb.* Edinburgh, Churchill Livingstone.

Evans D. S. and Cockett F. B. (1969) Diagnosis of deep-vein thrombosis with an ultrasonic Doppler technique. *Br. Med. J.* **2**, 802–804.

Fegan W. G. (1967) *Varicose Veins: Compression Sclerotherapy.* London, Heinemann.

Flanc C., Kakkar V. V. et al. (1968) The detection of venous thrombosis of the legs using ^{125}I-labelled fibrinogen. *Br. J. Surg..* **55**, 742–747.

Hills N. H., Pflug J. J. et al. (1972) Prevention of deep vein thrombosis by intermittent pneumatic compression of calf. *Br. Med. J.* **1**, 131–135.

Hobbs J. T. (1968) The treatment of varicose veins. A random trial of injection-compression therapy versus surgery. *Br. J. Surg.* **55**, 777–780.

Hobbs J. T. (1974) Surgery and sclerotherapy in the treatment of varicose veins. *Arch. Surg.* **109**, 793–796.

Hobbs J. T. (1980) Peroperative venography to ensure accurate sapheno-popliteal vein ligation. *Br. Med. J.* **280**, 1578.

Holford C. P. and Bliss B. P. (1976) The effect of graduated static compression on isotopically diagnosed deep vein thrombosis of the leg. *Br. J. Surg.* **63**, 157.

Homans J. (1916) The operative treatment of varicose veins and ulcers, based upon a classification of these lesions. *Surg. Gynecol. Obstet.* **22**, 143–158.

Husni E. A. (1971) Venous reconstruction in postphlebitic disease. *Circulation* **44**, Suppl. 1, 147.

An International Multicentre Trial. (1975) Prevention of fatal postoperative pulmonary embolism by low doses of heparin. *Lancet* **ii**, 45–51.

Jarrett P. E. M., Burnand K. G. et al. (1976) Fibrinolysis and fat necrosis in the lower leg. *Br. J. Surg.* **63**, 157.

Kakkar V. V., Corrigan T. et al. (1972) Efficacy of low doses of heparin in prevention of deep-vein thrombosis after major surgery. *Lancet* **2**, 101–106.

Kline A., Hughes L. E. et al. (1975) Dextran 70 in prophylaxis of thromboembolic disease after surgery: a clinically orientated randomized double-blind trial. *Br. Med. J.* **2**, 109–112.

Kosinski C. (1926) Observations on the superficial venous system of the lower extremity. *J. Anat.* **60**, 131–142.

Linton R. R. (1938) The post-thrombotic ulceration of the lower extremity: its etiology and surgical management. *Ann. Surg.* **107**, 582–593.

Linton R. R. (1953) The post-thrombotic ulceration of the lower extremity: its etiology and surgical treatment. *Ann. Surg.* **138**, 415–430.

Miles C. and Nicolaides A. N. (1981) Photoplethysmography; principles and development. In: Nicolaides A. N. and Yao J. S. T. (eds) *Investigation of Vascular Disorders.* New York, Churchill Livingstone.

Miller G. A. H. and Sutton G. C. (1970) Acute massive pulmonary embolism. Clinical and haemodynamic findings in 23 patients studied by cardiac catheterization and pulmonary arteriography. *Br. Heart J.* **32**, 518–523.

Miller S. S. (1974) Investigation and management of varicose veins. *Ann. R. Coll. Surg. Engl.* **55**, 245–252.

Negus D. (1968) Calf pain in the post-thrombotic syndrome. *Br. Med. J.* **2**, 156–158.

Negus D. (1970) The post-thrombotic syndrome. *Ann. R. Coll. Surg. Engl.* **47**, 92–105.

Negus D. (1978) Diagnosis of deep vein thrombosis: results of a survey. *J. R. Soc. Med.* **71**, 796–799.

Negus D. and Cockett F. B. (1967) Femoral vein pressures in post-phlebitic iliac vein obstruction. *Br. J. Surg.* **54**, 522–525.

Negus D., Fletcher E. W. L. et al. (1968a) Compression and band formation at the mouth of the left common iliac vein. *Br. J. Surg.* **55**, 369–374.

Negus D. and Friedgood A. (1986) Further studies on micro-dose intravenous heparin in the prevention of post-operative deep vein thrombosis. Unpublished observations.

Negus D. and Nicholson E. A. (1986) Are knee length elastic compression stockings as effective as thigh length in preventing post-operative deep vein thrombosis? Unpublished observations.

Negus D., Pinto D. J. et al. (1968b) The reliability of the ^{125}I-labelled fibrinogen uptake method in the diagnosis of occult deep-vein thrombosis. *Br. J. Surg.* **55**, 858.

Negus D. and Rickford C. R. K. (1975) In: Ruckley C. V. and MacIntyre I. M. C. (eds) *Venous Thromboembolic Disease.* Edinburgh, Churchill Livingstone.

Negus D., Friedgood A. et al. (1980) Ultra-low dose intravenous heparin in the prevention of post-operative deep vein thrombosis. *Lancet* **i**, 891–894.

Niebes P. and Laszt L. (1971) Influence in vitro d'une série de flavonoïdes sur des enzymes du métabolisme des mucopolysaccharides de veines saphènes humaines et bovines. *Angiologia* **8**, 297–302.

Niebes P. and Berson I. (1973) Determination of enzymes and degradation products of mucopolysaccharide metabolism in the serum of healthy and varicose subjects. *Bibl. Anat.* **11**, 499.

Palma E. C. and Esperon R. (1960) Vein transplants and grafts in surgical treatment of the post-phlebitic syndrome. *J. Cardiovasc. Surg.* **1**, 94.

Queral N., Whitehouse W. M., Jr, Flim W. R. et al. (1980) Surgical correction of chronic deep venous insufficiency by valvular transposition. *Surgery* **87**, 688.

Rose S. S. (1986) Some thoughts on the aetiology of varicose veins. *J. Cardiovasc. Surg.* **27**, 534–43.

Sabri S., Roberts V. C. et al. (1971) Prevention of early postoperative deep vein thrombosis by intermittent compression of the leg during surgery. *Br. Med. J.* **4**, 394–396.

Salzman E. W. (1978) Paper read to the Royal Society of Medicine, London, March 1978.

Sharnoff J. G. and DeBlasio G. (1970) Prevention of fatal postoperative thrombo-embolism by heparin prophylaxis. *Lancet* **ii**, 1006–1007.

Sharnoff J. G., Kass H. H. and Mistica B. A. (1962) A plan of heparinization of the surgical patient to prevent postoperative thromboembolism. *Surg. Gynecol. Obstet.* **115**, 75–79.

Sumner D. S. (1984) In: Rutherford R. B. (ed.) *Vascular Surgery* 2nd ed. Philadelphia, Saunders.

Svejcar J., Prerovsky I., Linhart J. et al. (1963) Content of collagen, elastin and hexosamine in primary varicose veins. *Clin. Sci.* **24**, 325–330.

Tanner W. A., Delaney P. V. et al. (1978) A reduction in intravenous cannula sepsis. *Br. J. Surg.* **65**, 355.

Thomson H. (1979) The surgical anatomy of the superficial and perforating veins of the lower limb. *Ann. R. Coll. Surg. Engl.* **61**, 198–205.

Vollmar J. (1977) In: Hobbs J. T. (ed.) *The Treatment of Venous Disorders*. Lancaster, MTP.

Wanke E. R. et al. (1956) *Chirurgie der grossen Körpervenen*. Stuttgart, Thieme.

Wilkins E. R., Mixter G., Stanton J. R. et al. (1952) Elastic stockings in the prevention of pulmonary embolism: a preliminary report. *N. Engl. J. Med.* **246**, 360–364.

Chapter forty-five

Portal Hypertension

K. E. F. Hobbs

INTRODUCTION

Most patients with portal hypertension present to the surgeon because of acute or recent major gastrointestinal haemorrhage from ruptured oesophageal or, rarely, rectal varices. Occasionally surgeons are consulted by colleagues for advice on management of a patient with proved varices secondary to portal hypertension, which have not bled, or for surgical help in the management of ascites and portosystemic encephalopathy.

AETIOLOGY

Various authorities classify portal hypertension in different ways (Hobbs, 1985; Crossley et al., 1985). It follows increased resistance to the flow of portal blood at any level. Common causes are extrahepatic portal vein thrombosis, presinusoidal occlusion in the region of the portal triad, cirrhosis in which portal hypertension is associated with hepatocellular disease and increased resistance to the venous drainage of the liver (Budd–Chiari syndrome). World wide, the commonest cause is presinusoidal intrahepatic narrowing due to schistosomiasis. However, in the West the commonest cause is secondary to the various types of cirrhosis. In these patients the immediate problems associated with the portal hypertension may be complicated by poor liver cell function resulting in impaired synthesis of albumin and clotting factors. Additionally the spleen may enlarge and produce hypersplenism and thus thrombocytopenia.

As portal hypertension develops, anastomotic channels between the portal and systemic circulations dilate. Portal blood is then shunted through these channels into the systemic circulation, bypassing the liver. Toxic nitrogenous products absorbed from the gut then enter the systemic circulation without detoxification in the liver. This leads to portosystemic encephalopathy (PSE), especially if there is hepatocellular damage. When the shunts between the two venous systems lie in the submucosa of the oesophagus or the rectum, they then sometimes rupture and produce massive haemorrhage. The factors contributing to this rupture are unknown.

INDICATIONS FOR SURGICAL INTERVENTION IN THE MANAGEMENT OF PROBLEMS ASSOCIATED WITH PORTAL HYPERTENSION

There is no evidence to support surgical intervention in patients with oesophageal varices which have not bled. However, surgery can contribute to the management of patients with:
1. Haemorrhage from oesophageal varices and occasionally rectal varices.
2. Ascites.
3. Portosystemic encephalopathy (PSE).

1. Emergency Control of Haemorrhage

When patients present with a major acute upper gastrointestinal haemorrhage, resuscitation and diagnosis must be carried out at the same time. Ideally these patients should be treated in a specialist gastroenterology unit with medical and surgical staff in attendance. If such a department does not exist then early medical, surgical and radiological consultation is mandatory.

Diagnosis

If haemorrhage is continuing at the time of admission adequate monitoring and resuscitation are necessary. Continuous measurements of arterial and central venous pressures and urine flow are essential. Initially sodium-free colloid, blood, fresh frozen plasma and platelets are required to maintain the circulation and encourage clotting.

Concurrently the cause of the haemorrhage needs to be found. History and clinical examination may suggest portal hypertension with or without liver disease, but it must be remembered that even when portal hypertension secondary to cirrhosis exists many patients have a very high incidence of bleeding from lesions other than oesophageal varices. This is especially so in countries in which alcoholic liver disease is a common cause for the portal hypertension. However, in the United Kingdom, once a patient has proved oesophageal varices, a major upper gastrointestinal haemorrhage is usually from this source. Perhaps the best investigation is upper gastrointestinal endoscopy, but if facilities for this do not exist upper gastrointestinal radiology remains a valuable investigation.

The next step in management requires accurate diagnosis of the cause of the portal hypertension and should follow soon after the initial bleeding has been controlled. Haematological and liver function tests and portal venous angiography, either directly by splenic puncture or indirectly observing the venous phase of coeliac and superior mesenteric angiograms, are essential. In this way both the severity of hepatocellular disease and portal venous patency will be detected and often the presence of any liver malignancy will be revealed. If time and clinical condition permit then a percutaneous needle liver biopsy should be carried out. Additional tests are needed to find out if the patient is Australia antigen positive.

Conservative measures

Once severe bleeding from ruptured oesophageal varices has been confirmed, the initial management should be conservative. Emergency surgery carried out by an inexperienced team in the middle of the night is very hazardous and carries a high mortality. Conservative measures include treatment with vaso-active drugs such as parenteral Pitressin (vasopressin), given either as a bolus or slowly intravenously, tamponade of the varices using the Sengstaken balloon tube or variceal injection with sclerosant solution either using an oesophagoscope or through a transhepatic portal catheter.

Usually simple resuscitation and Pitressin infusion will stop the bleeding initially. Any recurrence or continuation should be treated with the Sengstaken tube. This should control the bleeding long enough to allow the correct decision to be taken regarding future treatment. Since these patients are very sick this next step can be difficult and ideally should be carried out in a major specialist centre.

The use of the Sengstaken tube has its advocates in the emergency situation although serious complications such as damage to the oeosphagus and aspiration pneumonitis are well recognized. Most users would argue that this should only be used as a prelude to more definitive action. A valuable modification of the Sengstaken tube is a four-lumen tube. Through one lumen gastric aspiration is carried out and through a second the upper oesophagus is aspirated in an attempt to reduce salivary spill into the lungs. The other two connect with balloons which are positioned one in the stomach and the other in the lower oesophagus. The tube should be stored in a refrigerator and passed cold. This makes its passage much easier since it is more rigid. When the lower part is in the stomach the gastric balloon is inflated. The tube is then gently withdrawn until resistance of the balloon can be felt against the cardia and with a little tension the tube is fixed to the skin of the cheek by adhesive tape or gentle traction of about 1 kg is made by means of an apparatus attached to the patient's head. The oesophageal balloon may then be inflated. While the tube is in place, stomach contents and the upper oesophagus must be aspirated at frequent intervals.

Variceal sclerosis

If despite these measures bleeding continues then some argue that despite lack of conclusive evidence the next step is to attempt to sclerose the varices.

There are two techniques for this. Under fluoroscopic control using percutaneous transhepatic catheterization of the portal vein it is possible to guide a catheter into both the coronary and short gastric veins. Clotting agents such as absolute alcohol or thrombin plugs can then be injected. In a few expert hands it has proved to be an excellent technique for acute control of haemorrhage.

Another and now very popular method to produce sclerosis of the varices is to inject them directly with ethanolamine oleate with a needle introduced through a rigid Negus oesophagoscope or a flexible endoscope. Several attempts are often necessary to stop bleeding and the hospital admission mortality in published series is between 20 and 30 per cent (Terblanche et al., 1983). Death is usually due to multiple organ failure in these very sick patients but is sometimes the result of uncontrolled haemorrhage.

Further measures

If all these methods fail or it becomes necessary for long-term management to attempt a more radical surgical procedure, there are three possibilities:

   a. Direct oesophageal surgery at thoracotomy with ligation of the varices within the oesophagus.
   b. Ligation of the veins feeding the varices at the oesophago-gastric junction by gastric, oesophago-gastric or oesophageal transection with reanastomosis.
   c. Portal venous decompression.

Indications for the various surgical procedures, the surgical techniques and the results of surgery are discussed later.

2. Ascites

With the advent of modern diuretics and intravenous albumin preparations very few patients with ascites are resistant to medical treatment. For those who are, a catheter shunt has been described by LeVeen and his colleagues (1974). It consists of a catheter containing a valve, one end of which is placed in the peritoneal cavity and the other end passed subcutaneously to the neck where it is inserted into the subclavian vein. The ascitic fluid can then flow into the subclavian vein. The results are often dramatic with rapid weight loss and diuresis but the shunts tend to occlude quickly and may produce disseminated intravascular coagulation. Although occluded shunts can be recanalized, this is often unnecessary for periods as long as 1 year since the ascites does not reaccumulate quickly.

3. Portosystemic Encephalopathy (PSE)

Surgery is rarely indicated now in the treatment of PSE. However, total colectomy has been carried out in the past in some patients with PSE resistant to all conservative measures. Modern treatment includes control of protein intake, sterilization of the gut and oral laxatives such as lactulose.

SURGICAL TECHNIQUES USED IN THE MANAGEMENT OF OESOPHAGEAL VARICES

Thoracic Oesophageal Surgery

Emergency surgery on the thoracic oesophagus in acute variceal haemorrhage carries a 40 per cent mortality rate and so it is not a generally accepted technique for the control of acute bleeding. It may be of value very rarely in the management of young children with portal hypertension secondary to portal vein thrombosis when bleeding cannot be controlled although portosystemic shunting or sclerotherapy may be preferable. It may be the only feasible operation for patients who have had multiple abdominal procedures with resultant obliteration of all major portal vessels suitable for decompression surgery. Results of this operation carried out in the elective rather than the emergency situation seem to be better.

Technique

Under general anaesthetic the patient is positioned on the operating table in the lateral position lying on the right side to allow a left 8th rib thoracotomy. The chest is opened and the ribs spread with a self-retaining retractor. The lower lobe of the left lung is mobilized and gently retracted cephalad to expose the mediastinum below the hilum.

The mediastinal pleura is incised from lung hilum to diaphragm and the pulmonary ligament divided until the inferior pulmonary vein is seen. The oesophagus is identified and mobilized gently. Tapes are placed around the oesophagus at its upper and lower extremities. If any varices are actively bleeding non-crushing vascular clamps can be placed across the oesophagus at these sites too. A longitudinal incision

is made through the muscle coats exposing the mucous membrane and columns of vessels. One of two procedures can now be carried out. Either the oesophageal mucosa can be transected and then resutured or the lumen can be entered and the columns of varices oversewn. In the first procedure the tube of mucous membrane and varices is mobilized from the muscle layers, transected and resutured with catgut. A sample of the oesophageal lumen contents should be taken for microbiological culture. In the second procedure, after exposure of the mucous membrane, it is incised longitudinally (*Fig.* 45.1). The edges of the incision should be held with Babcock tissue forceps. A technique of cross-gartering is employed to oversew the columns of varices (*Fig.* 45.2). One advantage of this technique is that the columns can be followed downwards into the fundus of the stomach allowing ligation of some of the fundal varices too. Usually three columns of varices require ligating. The mucous membrane is sutured longitudinally after taking a microbiological swab from the lumen for culture.

At this stage in both procedures the muscle layer is closed gently with interrupted non-absorbable sutures. The pleura is not closed, in order to avoid the collection of a haematoma which could become infected. The chest is closed in a routine manner with a chest drain connected to an underwater seal. This should be removed as soon as drainage stops and the lung is fully expanded. A case can be made for a short course of antibiotics, such as cefotaxime and metronidazole, started at the time of surgery. However, the sensitivities of the organisms grown from the swabs taken during surgery may indicate a change in regimen in due course.

Ligation of Portal Vessels Feeding Oesophageal Varices

Several operations designed to ligate all the patent varices have been described. The operation of oesophago-gastric transection and reanastomosis described by Tanner (1954) and Milnes Walker (1964)

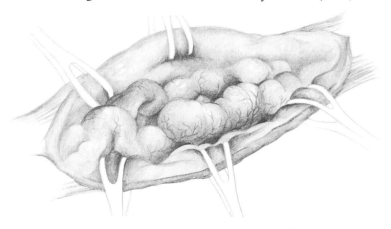

Fig. 45.1. Exposure of oesophageal varices at oesophagotomy.

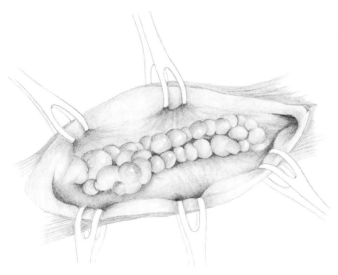

Fig. 45.2. Cross-gartering of oesophageal varices.

has proved popular, especially in the Middle East where schistosomal liver disease is the commonest cause of portal hypertension. The oesophagus is transected just above the cardia and bleeding is avoided by lightly clamping both ends of the divided oesophagus. The mucous membrane and muscular coats are resutured with continuous catgut sutures, ensuring that the large venous channels are included in the suture. Before completing the suture the lower clamp is released in order to make sure that all bleeding is controlled. It may be necessary to under-run one or two large veins. The muscle layers are then sutured separately.

Other techniques involve ligation of all the vessels along the greater and lesser curvatures of the stomach and splenectomy (Hassab, 1967) and even total oesophago-gastrectomy with colon replacement. These have produced excellent results in the hands of the surgeons describing them. However, all operations are difficult and haemorrhagic and when they involve oesophageal opening or transection carry the added serious risk of early suture line breakdown and fistula formation, usually a fatal complication in these very ill patients.

To overcome these problems and simplify the procedure a technique of oesophago-gastric transection and reanastomosis using a mechanical stable instrument or 'gun' (*Fig.* 45.3) has been practised (Johnson, 1978).

Through a left subcostal incision 5 cm of abdominal oesophagus are mobilized as for truncal vagotomy but the vagi do not need necessarily to be freed from the oesophageal wall (*Fig.* 45.4). The mechanical staple 'gun' with the largest size cartridge that will enter the oesophageal lumen is selected and introduced into the lower oesophagus (*Fig.* 45.5) via a gastrotomy. The entire oesophageal wall is encircled

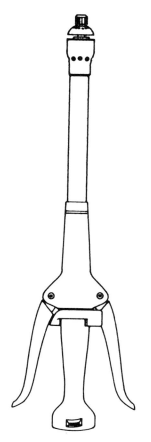

Fig. 45.3. Mechanical circular stapling instrument.

with a thick thread ligature and this is tied tightly between the separated staple cartridge and the anvil (*Fig.* 45.6). These are then approximated by turning a screw in the handle (*Fig.* 45.7) and the gun 'fired'

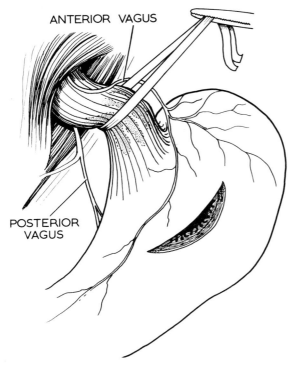

Fig. 45.4. Oesophago-gastric disconnection. Mobilization of abdominal oesophagus and gastrotomy prior to transection.

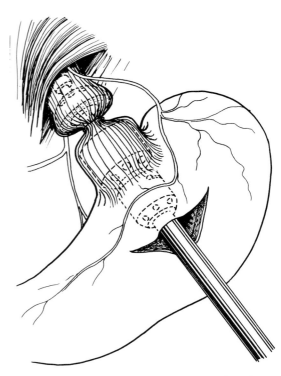

Fig. 45.6. Oesophago-gastric disconnection. Ligation of oesophagus between staple cartridge and anvil.

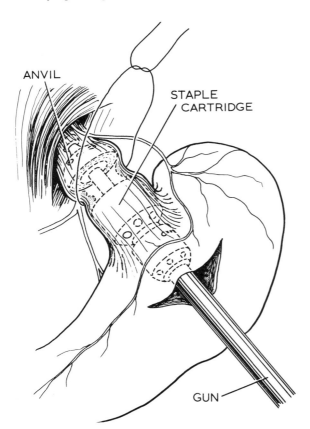

Fig. 45.5. Oesophago-gastric disconnection. Introduction of staple gun into the lower oesophagus.

(*Fig.* 45.8). This removes a complete circle of oesophageal wall and at the same time haemostatically staple-sutures together the two cut ends of the oesophagus.

Results of this technique are excellent. Operative blood transfusion is minimal and bleeding is always controlled. Mortality of the operation is 20–30 per cent which is comparable to that for other treatment methods. However, no study reports any death from continued variceal haemorrhage. In studies comparing this technique with endoscopic sclerotherapy it seems this may be the emergency surgical treatment of choice for these very sick patients, especially since this operation can be undertaken by an experienced surgeon whereas endoscopic sclerotherapy requires special equipment and expertise.

Portal Decompression

Principles

In order to reduce the blood flow through the dilated oesophageal varices, it would seem logical to suggest that a large portosytemic shunt should be constructed (Malt, 1976). The first operation of this type to be described was the end-to-side portacaval shunt (*Figs.* 45.9–45.11). Although this is successful in decompressing the portal system and stopping haemorrhage, nevertheless it is complicated by the development of severe PSE in about 30 per cent of patients.

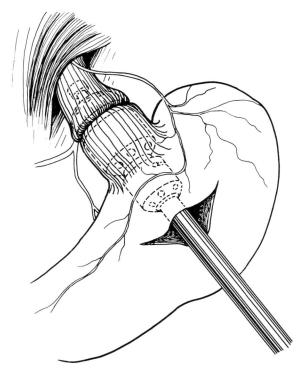

Fig. 45.7. Oesophago-gastric disconnection. Approximation of staple cartridge and anvil.

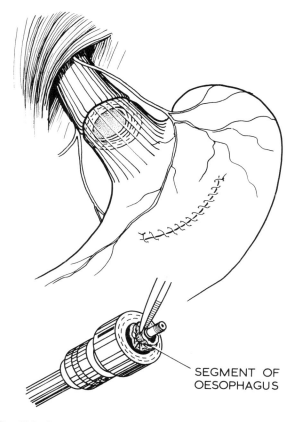

SEGMENT OF
OESOPHAGUS

Fig. 45.8. Oesophago-gastric disconnection. After firing the gun the stapled anastomosis and the removed segment of the oesophagus are shown.

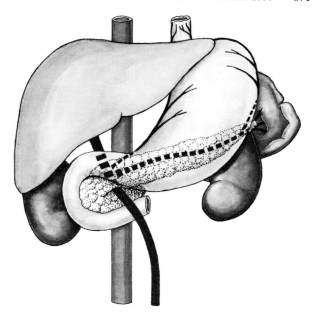

Fig. 45.9. Normal portal venous system.

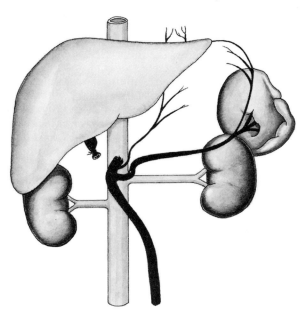

Fig. 45.10. End-to-side portacaval shunt.

In an attempt to overcome this, other shunts have been described which allow partial decompression of the portal system. These include the Linton splenorenal (Linton et al., 1947) (*see Fig.* 45.12) and Drapanas 'H' mesocaval shunts (*see Fig.* 45.16) (Drapanas, 1972). Unfortunately the theoretical advantages of such shunts have not been confirmed in clinical practice. On review of all published results it seems that providing that a good shunt is made which remains patent the likelihood of oesophageal rebleeding is reduced, but at the cost of a high incidence of PSE. Conversely, if the shunt does not allow

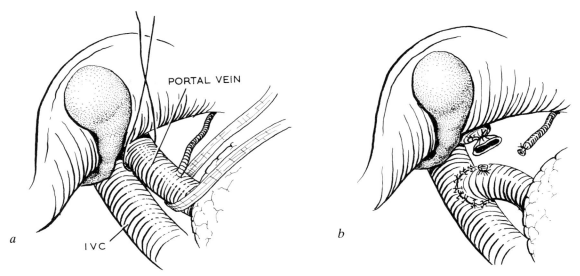

PORTAL VEIN

a

IVC

b

Fig. 45.11. Portacaval shunt. *a*, Retraction of the hilum of the liver exposes the inferior vena cava and the portal vein. *b*, The completed anastomosis.

adequate blood flow or if early thrombosis occurs then variceal rebleeding is common while encephalopathy is less.

A shunt which allows the theoretical ideal situation to be achieved, i.e. selected decompression of the oesophageal variceal bed while maintaining normal hepatic portal flow, is the Warren distal splenorenal shunt (*see Fig.* 45.20) (Warren et al., 1967). Some clinicians find this is associated with a lower incidence of PSE at least for 2 or 3 years after the operation. However, when patients with portal hypertension due to a common aetiology are studied the 5-year survival following any method of treatment, including conservative management, is about the same. It would seem, therefore, that portal decompression only serves to protect against further rebleeding and not to prolong life.

Emergency portal decompression

Portacaval decompression in the emergency situation to control acute haemorrhage has been proposed by some as the treatment of choice. Although there remain a few centres where this technique is practised (Orloff et al., 1980), most surgeons prefer to employ the techniques described above. Enthusiasts for this procedure argue that although the initial operative mortality is fairly high at 45–50 per cent the patient has had a definitive treatment for his or her problem and will have a low incidence of further bleeding episodes. However, this operation carried out on unselected patients is accompanied by a high incidence of PSE which most would regard as unacceptable.

Preoperative measures

In addition to standard preoperative measures it is

essential to carry out radiographic angiography in order to have a 'road map' and demonstrate the anatomy of the portal system before attempting shunt surgery. Some surgeons measure portal pressures and attempt to measure hepatic arterial portal venous inflow rate but these measurements are not essential. Good renal function is necessary for uncomplicated postoperative recovery and creatinine clearance studies are advised. Any clotting abnormalities should be corrected by giving vitamin K and if necessary fresh frozen plasma and sometimes platelets since these patients frequently have haemorrhagic tendencies. At least 6 units of blood should be crossmatched and arrangements made for the supply of platelets and fresh frozen plasma to deal with clotting problems encountered at the time of surgery. The patient should be as nutritionally fit as possible.

Peroperative measures

Standard monitoring techniques which are used for all major surgery are essential: these include careful measurement of blood loss, systemic pressure, central venous pressure and urine flow. In this way any deterioration can be recognized quickly and the appropriate therapy given to anticipate the problems of postoperative organ failure. Portal venous manometry is helpful since a satisfactory fall indicates if adequate decompression has been achieved.

Portacaval shunt (*Fig.* 45.10)

Under general anaesthetic the patient is positioned on the table supine with small pillows under the right shoulder and pelvis giving a slight rotation to the left.

A suitable incision is a right-sided extended

Kocher's subcostal incision. A self-retaining retractor is used to hold the wound edges widely apart and a good exposure of the hepatic hilum is usually possible. If the liver is grossly enlarged and cirrhotic then exposure of the hilum is more difficult.

Kocherization of the duodenum by dividing the peritoneum which binds it to the posterior abdominal wall is the first step. Retraction of the duodenum to the left exposes the inferior vena cava behind the second part. The anterior wall of the cava is exposed by dividing all the perivascular tissues and the dissection continued upwards until the lowest hepatic vein is encountered.

The peritoneum covering structures in the free edge of the lesser omentum is divided and the common bile duct identified anteriorly with the portal vein behind.

The portal vein is mobilized and stripped of periportal tissues between the bifurcation and the point it appears from the pancreas. Usually a side-branch, the coronary vein, requires ligating and dividing in order to gain a long length of portal vein. A tape is passed round it to make dissection easier. Attention is then redirected to the inferior vena cava and this too is cleared of any remaining adhesions especially in the region of the proposed anastomosis (*Fig. 45.11a*).

Two straight atraumatic vascular clamps are placed across the portal vein, one close to the liver and the second close to the pancreas. The vessel is divided close to the first liver end clamp and the cut edge tied or sutured with 3/0 Ethiflex. The clamp can then be removed.

The lumen in the free end of the portal vein is washed with heparinized saline to remove any clots. It is drawn towards the inferior vena cava and the end is trimmed to allow a smooth, non-kinked anastomosis. A Satinsky clamp is applied to the anterior wall of the inferior vena cava at the point of desired anastomosis. A piece of the anterior wall is removed, leaving a stoma the size of the portal vein. The end of the portal vein is then sutured to the incision in the inferior vena cava with 3/0 Ethiflex in one layer using conventional vascular suturing techniques (*Fig. 45.11b*). Prior to insertion of the final stitch the portal vein clamp is released momentarily allowing any clots to be flushed out and heparinized saline is flushed into the end before completing the anastomosis. The clamps are removed, haemostasis ensured and the muscle layers are closed en masse without a drain.

Proximal splenorenal shunt (*Fig. 45.12*)

A preoperative intravenous pyelogram is necessary before performing this procedure to ensure both right and left kidneys are present and functioning normally. If coeliac and superior mesenteric arterial angiography is employed for investigation of the portal anatomy then renal arteriography for the same purpose can be carried out then.

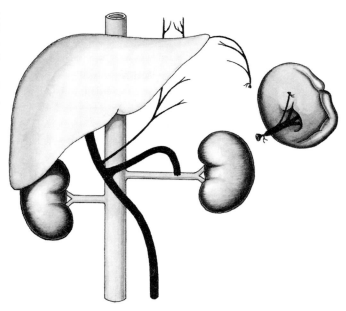

Fig. 45.12. Proximal splenorenal shunt and splenectomy.

Although the operation is possible through a left subcostal abdominal incision a left 8th rib thoracoabdominal incision with the patient lying in the right lateral oblique position is preferable. The value of this incision is to allow division of the costal margin which gives greater exposure of the spleen and splenic hilum which are often surrounded by very vascular adhesions, each of which needs dissection and ligation. The anterior end of the incision should cross the midline just above the umbilicus.

With wide wound retraction the spleen is steadily and gently mobilized and all vascular connections involving short gastric vessels ligated and divided. The splenic hilum is dissected in a similar way until artery and vein are clearly defined. The splenic artery is ligated and divided. Gentle squeezing of the spleen will allow a degree of auto-transfusion at this stage. The splenic end of the splenic vein is then clamped with a vascular clamp and divided distal to the clamp. The spleen is discarded.

Using a vascular clamp as a gentle retractor the splenic vein is dissected from the pancreas by ligation and section of the small pancreatic veins which connect them (*Fig. 45.13, 45.14*). These usually enter the splenic vein in pairs and haemorrhage from any one can cause problems since the ends are difficult to find once they have retracted into the pancreatic tissue. About 5 cm of vein must be mobilized.

The left renal vein is next identified immediately inferior and deep to the tail of the pancreas. Dissection of this vessel and the mobilized splenic vein is extended until a smooth anastomosis between the two is possible without any kinking. The renal artery should also be exposed. When haemostasis has been achieved the renal artery is controlled with a vascular clamp.

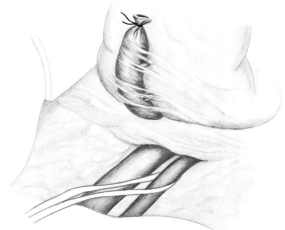

Fig. 45.13. Splenorenal shunt. The pancreas is shown with the divided splenic vein tightly bound to its posterior surface by small veins. The renal artery is taped prior to clamping.

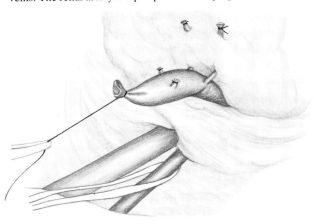

Fig. 45.14. Splenorenal shunt. The splenic vein is carefully mobilized by ligating its pancreatic tributaries.

The most proximal end of the mobilized segment of splenic vein is clamped and the distal clamp removed. The proximal clamp is released momentarily to flush out any clot and the lumen of the distal segment is then flushed with heparinized saline. A Satinsky clamp is placed on the side of the renal vein. A segment of wall of renal vein is removed. End-to-side splenorenal anastomosis is carried out using standard vascular techniques (*Fig.* 45.15). All vascular clamps are removed and the incision closed in layers without drainage.

Drapanas 'H' mesocaval shunt (*Fig.* 45.16)

With the patient supine with small pillows under the right shoulder and pelvis giving slight rotation to the left, a supra-umbilical transverse incision is made extending from the right anterior axillary line ending just to the left of the midline. After careful exploration of all abdominal viscera the edges of the incision are retracted, the omentum and colon packed cephalad and the coils of small bowel packed into the lower

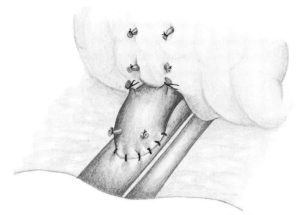

Fig. 45.15. Splenorenal anastomosis completed.

abdomen. The superior mesenteric artery is palpated through the exposed root of the transverse mesocolon and a horizontal incision made through the peritoneum from this point towards the right. With careful gentle dissection the superior mesenteric vein can be identified lying to the right of the superior mesenteric artery. During this dissection careful haemostasis is necessary and often many dilated lymphatic channels are cut. The superior mesenteric vein is then cleared as far proximally as possible and distally until its major branches are encountered. Usually about 5 cm of vein can be mobilized in this way.

The inferior vena cava is then identified by dissecting posteriorly through the transverse mesocolon lateral to the superior mesenteric vein. During this dissection the junction of the second and third parts of the duodenum is seen and retracted cephalad. When the inferior vena cava is identified a 5-cm length of its anterior wall is cleaned. This is then clamped with a Satinsky clamp and a piece removed

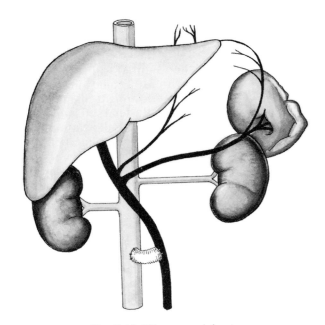

Fig. 45.16. 'H' mesocaval shunt.

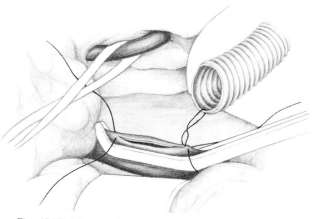

Fig. 45.17. Mesocaval shunt. The Dacron prosthesis is anastomosed to the inferior vena cava and the superior mesenteric vein is taped.

to allow an 18-mm Dacron graft to be sutured to it (*Fig.* 45.17, 45.18).

The graft is cut so that it will lie neatly below the loop of the duodenum and anastomose to the side of the superior mesenteric vein with slight tension.

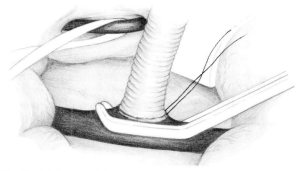

Fig. 45.18. Mesocaval shunt. Completed Dacron–caval anastomosis.

A second Satinsky clamp is applied to the right lateral wall of the superior mesenteric vein and again a piece removed. The Dacron graft is sutured to this (*Fig.* 45.19). Before the final sutures are inserted the graft

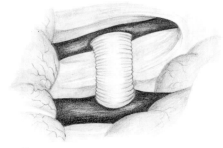

Fig. 45.19. Completed mesocaval shunt.

and venous lumina are washed with heparinized saline. The clamps are removed, haemostasis obtained and the wound closed without drainage.

Postoperative care

Postoperative careful systemic monitoring and maintenance of renal and liver function are necessary. When feeding is possible the initial protein intake should not exceed 10 g daily. When this is tolerated without any evidence of encephalopathy clinically or on electro-encephalography then this can be increased in 10-g amounts to a maximum of 40–50 g daily. If there is liver cell damage then severe sodium retention occurs and this should be appreciated when calculating sodium intake. Frequently very little, if any, is required and if given it will result in gross fluid retention. Although there is no definite evidence of its value, histamine H_2-receptor blocking drugs are given by some clinicians throughout the postoperative course in the belief that they will reduce any likelihood of postoperative upper gastrointestinal bleeding by reducing gastric acid production.

Despite all the precautions to prevent or reduce PSE, which include protein restriction and the administration of lactulose or neomycin, some patients do develop PSE following these shunt procedures. In an attempt to reduce this incidence a distal splenorenal shunt has been described.

Warren distal splenorenal shunt (*Fig.* 45.20)

Using a transverse upper abdominal incision the transverse colon is mobilized downwards away from the greater curvature of the stomach and the lower edge of the pancreas identified. This is rotated upwards and the segment of splenic vein between the superior mesenteric vein and inferior mesenteric vein branches identified. Other techniques for exposing this vessel have been described including one in which the splenic flexure of the colon is mobilized

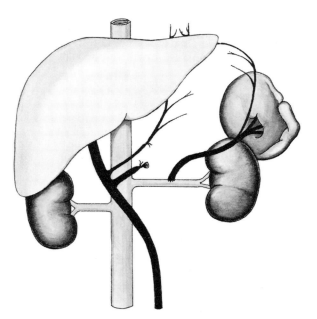

Fig. 45.20. Warren distal splenorenal shunt.

and together with the transverse and descending colon and base of mesentery gently swept towards the right.

The proximal superior mesenteric vein end of the splenic vein is identified, dissected off the pancreas, ligated and divided. The cut distal end of the splenic vein is anastomosed to the side of the left renal vein immediately below and deep to it. Any major tributaries of the portal vein which communicate with the oesophageal plexus, i.e. the coronary vein, are identified and ligated, although some authorities deny the need for this. This procedure allows decompression of the spleen and the venous plexus at the lower end of the oesophagus, while at the same time allowing the superior mesenteric vein blood to enter the liver still under high pressure.

Selection of Patients for Shunt Surgery

In view of the results of portal decompression the current opinion is to avoid shunt surgery for as long as possible. The decisions on the optimum time to create a portosystemic shunt and its nature are difficult. Many factors govern such a decision and they include:

1. Age of the patient.
2. Abode of the patient.
3. Occupation of the patient.
4. Cause of portal hypertension.
5. Liver cell function.

Young patients can undergo a major operative precedure with minimal complications. However, long-term follow-up studies of patients having decompression shunts in their youth for portal vein thrombosis with excellent liver cell function suggests that they do eventually develop a degree of portosystemic encephalopathy.

Patients who do not depend on their intellectual abilities for their livelihood and who live in an area removed from medical expertise and the ready availability of blood transfusion will require shunting as a life-saving procedure earlier than patients with a lifestyle and occupation that demand high intellectual capacity. Extrahepatic portal obstruction as the cause of portal hypertension with good liver cell function is associated with fairly uncomplicated tolerance of shunts, especially in the early days, whereas this is not so in the presence of severe liver disease. As the degree of hepatocellular disease advances so the prognosis of shunt surgery becomes worse. Patients with the worst prognosis of all are those with chronic active hepatitis. PSE precipitated by a bleeding episode or any drug therapy should caution against any shunt procedures.

In an attempt to measure the severity of hepatocellular damage a point scoring system has been devised as a modification of Child's grading of liver cell dysfunction (Pugh et al., 1973). Points are given for high bilirubin levels, low albumin levels, impaired clotting and the presence of ascites and encephalopathy. A high total score indicates severe liver cell damage and would tend to contra-indicate decompression surgery.

The choice of shunt is by no means simple although there is little evidence at the moment to suggest that there is any one technique that is better than any of the others. Unfortunately none of the conventional haemodynamic measurements gives any help in deciding on any specific shunt procedure. The distal splenorenal shunt does seem to have a significantly lower incidence of PSE than the other shunts, at least for 2 or 3 years following the procedure. However, complications such as portal thrombosis and massive ascites do develop and the long-term results of all shunt operations are similar.

Thus the surgeon should consider the patient's anatomy, his or her own expertise and training and technical simplicity. A familiar and technically straightforward operation performed at leisure is likely to have a less complicated postoperative course than an emergency, more complicated, unfamiliar procedure.

REFERENCES

Crossley I. R., Westaby D. and Williams R. (1985) Portal hypertension. In: Wright R. et al. (ed.) *Liver and Biliary Disease*, 2nd ed. London, Saunders, pp. 1283–1316.

Drapanas T. (1972) Interposition mesocaval shunt for treatment of portal hypertension. *Ann. Surg.* **176**, 435.

Hassab M. A. (1967) Gastro-esophageal decongestion and splenectomy in the treatment of oesophageal varices in bilharzial cirrhosis: further studies with a report of 355 operations. *Surgery* **61**, 169.

Hobbs K. E. F. (1985) The surgery of portal hypertension In: Wright R. et al. (ed.) *Liver and Biliary Disease*, 2nd ed. London, Saunders, pp. 1317–1328.

Johnson G. W. (1978) Simplified oesophageal transection for bleeding varices. *Br. Med. J.* **1**, 1388–1391.

LeVeen H. H., Christoudias G., Ip M. et al. (1974) Peritoneo-venous shunting for ascites. *Ann. Surg.* **180**, 580–591.

Linton R. R., Jones C. M. and Volwiler W. (1947) Portal hypertension. The treatment by splenectomy and splenorenal anastomosis with preservation of the kidney. *Surg. Clin. North Am.* **27**, 1162–1170.

Malt R. A. (1976) Portasystemic venous shunts. *N. Engl. J. Med.* **295**, 24.

Orloff M. J., Bell R. H., Hyde P. V. et al. (1980) Long term results of emergency portacaval shunt for bleeding oesophageal varices in unselected patients with alcoholic cirrhosis. *Ann. Surg.* **192**, 325–337.

Pugh R. N. H., Murray-Lyon I. M., Dawson J. L. et al. (1973) Transection of the oesophagus for bleeding oesophageal varices. *Br. J. Surg.* **60**, 646–649.

Tanner N. C. (1954) In: Discussion on portal hypertension. *Proc. R. Soc. Med.* **47**, 475.

Terblanche J., Bornman P. C., Kahn D. et al. (1983) Failure of repeated injection sclerotherapy to improve long term survival after oesophageal variceal bleeding. *Lancet* **ii,** 1328–1332.

Walker R. Milnes (1964) Oeosphageal transection for bleeding varices. *Surg. Gynecol. Obstet.* **126,** 585.

Warren W. D., Zeppa R. and Forman J. (1967) Selective trans-splenic decompression of gastro-esophageal varices by distal splenorenal shunt. *Ann. Surg.* **166,** 437–455.

Orthopaedic Surgery

Chapter forty-six

Basic Techniques in Orthopaedic Surgery

P. G. Stableforth

OPERATING ROOM TECHNIQUE AND EQUIPMENT FOR ORTHOPAEDIC PROCEDURES

Limb Preparation and Draping

While the usual methods of preoperative preparation and care prior to bone or joint procedures are no different from those employed by surgeons in other specialties, the long-lasting and serious consequences of sepsis following surgery on these structures make attention to detail vital during preparation and draping of the operative field.

When surgery is undertaken after injury, wounds are covered with sterile gauze swabs, and the scrubbed and gloved surgeon or assistant should wash the entire surgical area with a suitable detergent solution (such as Cetavlon 0·5 per cent in chlorhexidine 0·02 per cent) to remove all dirt, grease and loose scale from the part. The operative field is close clipped in preference to shaving, nails cut and nail folds cleaned if necessary. The wound is now irrigated with warm normal saline to remove all loose debris and the operative field is covered with a clean towel. The tourniquet is now applied if appropriate. The surgeon then rescrubs and gowns before undertaking the formal surgical skin preparation.

When surgery is to be undertaken on a limb that has been encased in a plaster-of-Paris cast, extra care is taken with skin preparation as there is likely to be maceration and there will certainly be keratin scale on the skin surface. The cast should be carefully bivalved and removed and the supported limb washed with a detergent solution, so as to remove all debris and loose scale. If the skin condition is poor a day or two spent on preparation with regular washing and the application of a non-greasy skin softener will often decrease later skin problems.

For many surgical procedures on the limb, access and handling are simplified if the part is draped so that the limb is freely mobile on the trunk, and thus can be repositioned at will during surgery. The application of the drapes, so as to avoid contamination of the surgical field, is something of an art that can only be perfected by practice.

Use of the Tourniquet

Surgery on the distal two-thirds of the limb can be made much simpler, safer and often speedier by undertaking surgery in a bloodless field, exsanguinated and controlled by a tourniquet. A pneumatic tourniquet applied over a smooth roll of wood wool around the upper arm or proximal thigh will most safely apply even pressure when inflated and minimize the risk of skin or nerve damage. When the cuff has been applied and fastened in position, the limb is exsanguinated with an Esmarch bandage rolled firmly from the end of the extremity up to the cuff. The cuff is then inflated to 50 mmHg above the measured arterial pressure and the encircling Esmarch bandage removed.

The limb should not be exsanguinated by a pressure bandage if surgery is undertaken for the biopsy or removal of malignant lesions or for acute sepsis, as malignant cells or bacteria may be squeezed into the general circulation. Similarly, the Esmarch bandage should be avoided when the limb has been immobilized in a plaster-of-Paris cast for 48 hours or more prior to surgery, as venous thrombi may be detached to form emboli. In these circumstances the limb should be elevated well above the heart level for a full 2 minutes before the proximally applied cuff is inflated.

The tourniquet should never be left inflated round the limb for more than 90 minutes before release. If it becomes clear that the surgical procedure will need a bloodless field for over 60 minutes, it is wisest to pack the wound, control bleeding by direct pressure, elevate the limb and release the tourniquet for 10 minutes. After this time, while the limb is still elevated, the tourniquet may be reinflated for a further period. Tourniquet 'paralysis', a patchy sensory and motor disturbance persisting hours or days after tourniquet release, may follow careless application or overinflation of the cuff, while gross limb swelling and a diffuse neurological disorder may follow an excessive period of tourniquet ischaemia.

The resulting neurological deficits should be carefully charted so that subsequent progress may be followed.

The limb care after tourniquet palsy is the same as that for any neurological disorder in that joints are protected from excessive stresses and are put through a range of movement exercises daily, while anaesthetic skin is protected from damage until sensory recovery recurs.

TENDON TRANSFER

Muscle weakness or paralysis from disease or injury may give rise to increasing deformity from muscle imbalance or from the action of body weight on unprotected joints. In some circumstances abnormal joint movement and instability may be controlled and the joint protected from progressive damage by the use of orthoses (splints).

If the joint is not degenerate, remains mobile and has healthy surrounding tissues, tendon transfers may restore muscle balance and preserve joint movement; if a joint is stiff, shows degenerative changes or if no suitable tendons are available for transfer, arthrodesis may be necessary.

Indications

Tendon transfer can only be undertaken where the disorder has left suitably strong muscles available for transfer such that surgery can be undertaken without creating new imbalances and where it is considered that there will be no later progression of the disease to disturb muscle balance. They are thus most commonly used:

1. Where a static state of muscle imbalance follows poliomyelitis, leprosy or similar motor nerve disorder.
2. When inoperable or irreparable nerve injury has produced paralysis and muscle imbalance.

Points of technique

Fixed joint deformities are usually a bar to tendon transfer and all joints across which the transfers are to act must be made supple prior to surgery. The tendon chosen must be of similar amplitude of excursion to the one that it is going to replace, should lie in healthy unscarred subcutaneous tissue and its line of pull should be as direct as possible from origin to new insertion.

The correct tension of the transfer may be difficult to judge, particularly where the tendon crosses more than one joint, but too little tension is the commoner fault.

Attachment of a Transferred Tendon to Bone

The selected site of tendon insertion into bone is exposed by subcutaneous dissection. The surface of the bone may be roughened with a gouge to encourage tendon adherence and the tendon simply sutured to periosteum. A much more secure fixation is achieved if a bone window is raised or a hole drilled through the bone to receive the tendon.

A double-ended stainless steel wire or strong nylon suture is interwoven through the tendon end. The two ends of the suture are passed through the bone on a strong needle or awl and pulled firmly so as to draw the end into the cavity within the bone. The sutures are tied off on the bone or over a gauze roll on the skin.

The tissues are carefully closed and the site of attachment protected by external splintage until sound healing is assured. This is usually 4–6 weeks

in the upper limb and twice that time in the lower limb. Where transfer has been undertaken for paralytic disorder, bracing may be necessary for 4–6 months to protect the new transfer and re-education of function may need a prolonged course of supervised physiotherapy.

BONE GRAFTING

The placing of strips or blocks of bone around fractures or across freshened joint surfaces in stabilization procedures remains an important technique in orthopaedic surgery. Bone stabilization can now usually be achieved by the use of metallic internal fixation devices so that cortical bone grafts are rarely used for this purpose and reliance is placed on onlaid grafts of cancellous bone to promote fracture healing and joint arthrodesis. It is useful to use corticocancellous grafts if thin strips of bone are needed as the rind of cortical bone provides structural stability to the cancellous and makes it easier to handle.

Indications

1. To stimulate healing in slow or un-uniting fractures, particularly those of the shafts of the long bones.
2. To achieve arthrodesis where an unstable or arthritic joint is to be stiffened.
3. For special stabilization procedures (e.g. in scoliosis).
4. To bridge the gap between bone ends in primary fracture management when injury has resulted in extensive bone loss.

Contra-indications

1. Avascular bone or gross soft tissue scarring. The bed in which the graft is to lie must have a rich blood supply to act as a base from which vessels may grow into and through the graft. Ideally all dead bone or heavily scarred soft tissue is excised to provide such a base prior to free bone grafting. If the overlying skin and subcutaneous tissue are heavily scarred, it may be helpful to transpose a cutaneous, myocutaneous or muscle flap over the bone surface following wide scar excision, though carefully compacted cancellous bone will revascularize and incorporate well in a healthy soft tissue or bone bed between rigidly immobilized bone ends even when left exposed in the wound.

Defects in soft tissue and bone may also be bridged by composite flaps or by free vascularized grafts in which vessels of the inlaid graft are anastomosed to local feeder vessels by microsurgical techniques.

2. Free movement of the bone ends. Bone healing depends on the establishment of a capillary granulation network across the fracture site or joint surface. Internal fixation or external splintage must be used if the fracture or the joint remains mobile.

3. Infection is only a relative contra-indication to cancellous bone grafting, as the graft may survive and lead to bone healing; however, the infecting organism must be known, the infection quiescent, and accessible sequestra removed and abscess cavities drained prior to grafting.

Sources of Bone

For most of the cancellous bone grafting procedures in adults the patient's own skeleton is the source of donor bone. The iliac crest is the most favoured site as it can provide a large volume of cancellous and corticocancellous bone, but smaller quantities of cancellous bone can be obtained from the interior of the volar aspect of the distal radius (if the graft is required for wrist surgery, scaphoid fracture grafting, etc.), from the interior of the greater trochanter or through the anterior cortex of the proximal end of the tibia (useful for grafting some tibial plateau fractures and other lower limb fractures).

The graft probably acts principally as a scaffolding through which granulation tissue can grow and if enough cortical bone cannot be obtained from the patient bone from another individual can be used. In some centres a bone bank is maintained and bone obtained from other donors is refrigerated in sterile conditions.

Commercially prepared bovine bone graft has been used with variable success, though the recent use of this material as a carrier for the patient's own bone marrow aspirate seems to hold promise as an alternative.

Approach to the Iliac Crest

Most cancellous bone is in the thick anterior one-third of the crest as far back as the gluteal ridge. In adults bone is abundant at this site but in the elderly patient osteoporosis may leave little suitable bone. Bone graft can also be taken from this site in a child if the crest epiphysis is first turned aside and finally reattached when enough bone has been obtained. The posterior one-third of the iliac wing is also a reliable source of bone and particularly useful for spinal fusion operations.

Anterior Approach (Fig. 46.1)

The patient is placed supine with a sandbag under the hip on the selected side to throw the anterior part of the iliac crest into prominence, or laid on his side.

A curved incision is made just below the prominence of the iliac crest to avoid later problems from pressure on a sensitive scar by a skirt waistband or trouser belt. The incision is deepened through the subcutaneous fat and the small vessels ligated.

If the abdominal muscles overhang, they are pulled upwards to expose that portion of the iliac crest

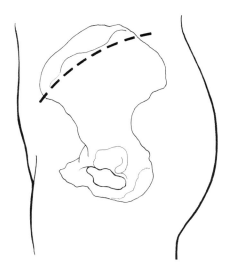

Fig. 46.1. Corticocancellous bone graft. (N.B. Incision is below the prominence of iliac crest.)

between the oblique muscle insertions above and the origin of the glutei below. A cut is made into the top of the iliac crest between these muscles.

The oblique muscles are stripped subperiosteally and reflected medially with a Bristow or similar broad elevator, and the iliacus stripped off the deep surface of the blade of the ilium. Bleeding from the raw bone surface is controlled by diathermy or bone wax; a large damp swab is spread out flat over the muscles and a broad retractor or copper strip used to hold them away from bone (*Fig.* 46.2).

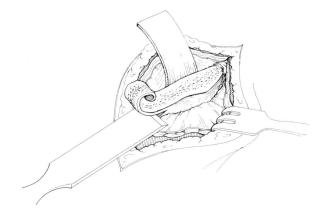

Fig. 46.2. Corticocancellous bone graft. The abdominal muscles are stripped down but the glutei as little as possible.

When a thick block of cancellous or corticocancellous bone is required, it is cut out as a window from the deep surface of the iliac blade; the area required is outlined with a 1-cm osteotome, the cuts deepened carefully and the block levered out and removed in one piece leaving the outer cortex of the bone intact.

If corticocancellous strips are needed, the skin and deeper tissues are retracted away to expose the iliac crest in profile, the anterior superior iliac spine is cleared of muscle and other soft tissue attachments and the muscles on the outer side of the iliac blade stripped down, and the cortical top of the crest removed.

A chisel, slightly wider than the iliac crest, will cut the graft mostly readily, although an osteotome is also satisfactory. Long, thin corticocancellous strips are raised as far back along the bone as is required, and are removed gently with Kocher forceps and laid between saline-soaked swabs in a kidney dish until needed. Strips of ideal thickness will curl a little on themselves as they are cut.

If additional cancellous bone is required it is removed with a narrow gouge or small curette. When enough bone has been obtained, bone wax is smeared along the bare surface until all bleeding is stopped. A suction drain is laid on the deep aspect of the iliac wing and the iliacus, gluteus and tensor muscles reapproximated to abolish any dead space. The fat layer and skin are carefully closed.

Application of Graft Bone (*Fig.* 46.3)

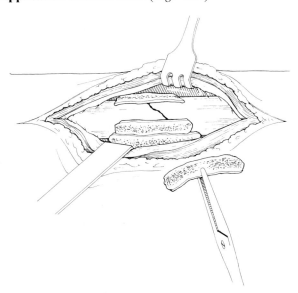

Fig. 46.3. Corticocancellous bone graft. The long strips of cancellous bone are laid subperiosteally over the undisturbed fibrous union.

The bone obtained is usually used as onlay graft, applied to the freshened bone surface. When grafting is undertaken for the treatment of a non-union of a fracture of the shaft of a long bone the Phemister–Charnley technique is employed.

The fracture site is approached through a suitable incision and the periosteum raised to expose the bone on either side of the non-union. This may be achieved by stripping with a suitable periosteal elevator, or the periosteum may be raised with a sharp osteotome so that small fragments of the superficial bone surface

remain attached to the periosteal flap. This 'petalling' may be followed by more rapid incorporation of the graft than if a simple subperiosteal strip has been undertaken. The fibrous union between the bone ends is not disturbed but the enlarged bone ends of the hypertrophic mobile non-union may be flattened with the osteotome to improve the bone contour and make it easier to apply a fracture stabilization plate or onlay graft; the bone graft strips are laid across the fracture site under the raised periosteum. The soft tissues are closed over the bone graft, the wound closed in layers and the limb again immbolized until fracture healing is clinically and radiologically confirmed.

Where the graft is used in a stabilization procedure as in arthrodesis of a joint, the articular surface is removed to expose fresh cancellous bone and the graft material packed in between and around the rawed bone ends, being firmly pushed or punched into place as compactly as possible. Some form of internal fixation or external splintage is used until bone healing is confirmed.

Postoperative

Strong analgesics will usually be required for 24 or 36 hours. The suction drain is then removed and the patient remobilizes as rapidly as his or her symptoms and condition permit. As only a limited dissection of the hip abductor muscles has been undertaken, severe pain on walking is not usually a problem but a stick may be helpful for the first few days.

Complications

Division of one or more posterior cutaneous branches of the lumbar nerves may produce hyperaesthesia or cutaneous insensitivity over the posterior half of the upper buttock. This usually lasts 9–12 months and slowly fades.

A haematoma may collect deep to the iliac blade. This will produce early postoperative pain with swelling, inflammation and tenderness, and fluctuation may be present. Such a haematoma should be drained to relieve symptoms and decrease the risk of subsequent infection. Primary reclosure of the wound after evacuation of the haematoma is usually possible.

Occasionally the sutures holding the abductor muscles in position may give way a few days after surgery causing local pain and swelling and a marked limp. Resuture of the muscles is not usually satisfactory and protection from the stresses of weight bearing by the use of crutches or a stick may be necessary until symptoms subside.

FRACTURE FIXATION

Many fractures, when they are insignificantly displaced, require neither open reduction nor internal fixation of the fragments and can be manipulated into an acceptable position and prevented from further displacement by external splintage. The acceptable limits of displacement are a matter for mature surgical judgement but by and large it is rarely necessary to undertake operative procedures on young children, whose bones remodel considerably with continuing growth, but more commonly so in adults in whom remodelling is very limited.

Comminuted fractures of the shafts of long bones may often be managed very satisfactorily by closed techniques, and considerable distortion of the healing bone may be compatible with excellent appearance and function provided that general alignment is restored. By contrast, primary open reduction and stable fixation are usually necessary in fractures which involve joints so that anatomical restoration of the articular surface may be followed by early remobilization which will give the best chance of recovery.

While wider use is now made of open reduction and internal fixation for suitable long bone fractures, experience has shown that primary fixation of open fractures is attended by an unacceptably high sepsis rate and thus, where possible, sound wound healing should precede internal fixation. There are, of course, injuries of the limb of such extent and severity that the bone may have to be stabilized to allow repair of the soft tissues if the limb is to be saved, but even here the use of external skeletal fixation has proved a valuable and safe alternative. The use of open reduction and internal fixation allows an accurate and stable fracture position to be achieved and this, in turn, allows early remobilization of the injured part, earlier restoration of function and earlier economic independence. Surgery, however, exposes the patient to the dangers of wound and bone sepsis while the tissues may be stripped of their blood supply and devitalized, thus increasing fibrosis and stiffness. Carefully planned incisions, gentle tissue handling and retraction, and meticulous attention to surgical technique are all vital. Careful haemostasis, the insertion of suction drains where dead space is unavoidable and the skilful application of postoperative dressings will all serve to minimize the complications.

Although the rigid 'no touch' technique of the older generation of orthopaedic surgeons is not widely employed, unnecessary handling of swabs, sutures, implants and the working ends of instruments is to be avoided. Experience has shown that the surgeon's gloves are frequently perforated if fracture fragments or Kirschner wires are handled during surgery, and in this type of procedure surgeons should wear two pairs of gloves as it is uncommon for both to be damaged.

Techniques of Internal Fixation (*Fig.* 46.4)

Fractures may be internally fixed following open reduction by a variety of devices.

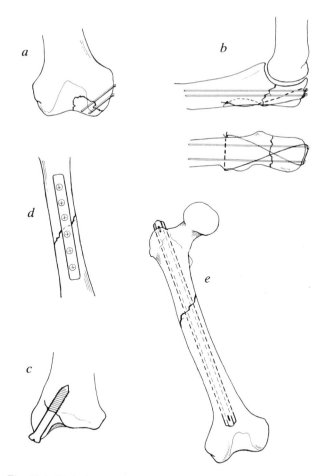

Fig. 46.4. Techniques of internal fixation. *a*, Transfixation with Kirschner wires. *b*, Wires and tension-absorbing band. *c*, Axial screw fixation. *d*, Rigid fixation with plate. *e*, Intramedullary nailing.

1. Fractures of small bones and comminuted fractures may be transfixed and held by Kirschner wires drilled through the fragments (finger bone fractures, fractures of the ends of the long bones, with articular surface involvement).

2. The fracture may be aligned by parallel Kirschner wires and muscle pull neutralized by a tension-absorbing band (fractures of the patella and olecranon).

3. Screws may be used to secure fracture fragments. These are inserted down pre-drilled holes and a thread path tapped through the bone prior to screw insertion. (This allows load spreading by use of square-shouldered long-thread non-self-tapping screws).

4. A plate may be applied over the periosteum across the fracture site and fixed with screws. Where possible at least three screws should lie along each side of the fracture (fractures of the shafts of the long tubular bones).

Cancellous and malleolar screws have large threads over their distal portions only. They hold well within cancellous bone and exert a lag compression effect (malleolar fractures, fractures of the tibial plateau, fractures of the greater tuberosity).

Cortical screws are threaded less coarsely, but along their whole length, exert no lag effect and should always hold on both cortices of the bone into which they are fixed, as they hold weakly in the cancellous interior.

5. Intramedullary fixation, a semi-rigid nail (Küntscher) or a pin (Rush) is inserted along the medullary cavity of a long bone; the cavity is usually enlarged by reaming before a Küntscher nail is inserted but no particular preparation is made if Rush pins are to be used.

The Küntscher nails can be up to 14 mm in diameter and are the only devices which can be used to fix the shafts of the long bones of the lower limb so as to allow unprotected weight bearing before fracture healing.

A detailed description of the many techniques of internal fixation would be inappropriate in this text and readers are referred to the manuals mentioned under Further Reading.

Postoperative Complications

The three major complications of surgery of fractures are skin necrosis, haematoma formation and sepsis.

Skin Necrosis

This may follow surgery through badly placed incisions especially where skin has been damaged at the time of injury, or may occur as a result of injudicious attempts to close wounds under tension following skin loss or where a bulky plate has been applied to the subcutaneous surface of a superficial bone. It may also follow post-traumatic swelling. Such necrosis may expose the plate and predispose to further problems.

Haematoma Formation

This should not be a problem provided care is taken to seal all damaged vessels prior to wound closure. If a tourniquet has been used during surgery it should be released prior to closure. A suction drain should lead from the deepest part of the wound, particularly if dead space remains after surgery, and should be removed 24–72 hours postoperatively. If a haematoma develops the patient should be taken back to the operating room and the wound completely reopened; the haematoma is evacuated and the wound resutured.

Infection

This may be a sequel to skin necrosis or to haematoma formation and usually occurs as a result of bacterial contamination of the surgical field. It may vary in severity from minor superficial wound redness to a fulminating infection with deep abscess formation. Elevation, immobilization of the part and the administration of appropriate antibiotics may suffice prior to suppuration, but wide exploration of the wound, irrigation and early or delayed resuture should be undertaken if pus has formed. The internal fixation device must be left if it is still secure and should not be removed until sound bone healing has occurred.

THE SHOULDER

Surface Anatomy

The rounded contour of the shoulder is produced by the bulge of the greater tuberosity under the deltoid muscle. The tip of the acromion can be felt above this and the acromioclavicular joint palpated two finger-breadths medially. The coracoid process can be felt on finger palpation about 1 cm below the junction of the middle and outer thirds of the clavicle, deep to the deltoid. If the shoulder is viewed from above the supraspinatus and subscapularis tendons lie under the deltoid muscle lateral to and in front of the tip of the acromion, as they pass from under that bone to their insertions on the tuberosities (*Fig. 46.5*).

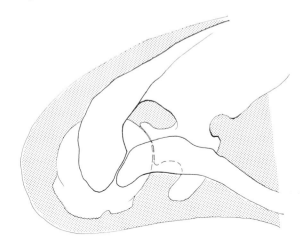

Fig. 46.5. Shoulder from above. From this view the tuberosities lie well lateral and anterior to the acromion.

Surgical Anatomy

The deltoid muscle clothes the whole of the shoulder joint, and whatever the approach the muscle needs to be split, reflected or detached to provide access.

The anterior approach allows wide exposure of the head and upper shaft of the humerus, the lesser tuberosity, the tendon of subscapularis and the glenohumeral joint. It provides access for elective surgical repair for recurrent dislocation, and is the favoured approach for open reduction of those few anterior or posterior shoulder dislocations and those fractures of the proximal humerus for which surgery is needed.

The upper end of the biceps muscle and the coracoid process are also accessible. In a thinner or poorly muscled patient shoulder flexion allows exposure of the joint without detachment of the clavicular fibres of the deltoid, and in the larger, more muscular patient the deltoid can be partially detached from its humeral insertion to improve access while preserving clavicular attachment.

Limited access for the repair of rotator cuff tears may be obtained by a split along the line of the deltoid fibres, provided that it extends for less than 2 cm into the muscle. A long deltoid splitting incision would jeopardize the axillary nerve as it runs the last part of its course transversely in that muscle.

Wider access for the treatment of rotator cuff tendon tears and for fractures of the greater tuberosity is obtained through a superior-posterior approach as the tendons of the cuff lie under the deltoid alone for the last 1–2 cm of their course to the tuberosity.

Indications for Surgery

Surgical exploration of the shoulder joint is indicated for:

1. Diagnostic biopsy of the synovium.
2. Treatment of recurrent dislocation of the shoulder.
3. In the management of some displaced fractures of the neck of the humerus.
4. Exploration of the rotator cuff tendons for the repair of extensive cuff tears.
5. Rarely for suppurative arthritis of the glenohumeral joint.

Prior to surgery, an anteroposterior X-ray of the shoulder joint, a lateral X-ray with the arm fully abducted or an axial X-ray of the scapula is essential.

Examination of the shoulder joint by contrast arthrography is valuable in assessment of the site and extent of rotator cuff tears.

Anterior Approach

Putti–Platt or Bankhart Repair for Recurrent Anterior Dislocation of the Shoulder

The skin incision is along the medial border of the deltoid from the lower palpable edge of pectoralis major to the coracoid process, and then turns sharply laterally along the anterior border of the clavicle and skirts the acromion as far round the shoulder as is required (*Fig.* 46.6). The incision is deepened below to allow exposure of the deltopectoral groove. The cephalic vein is either ligated distally, divided and removed, or is traced upwards and retracted medially to allow development of the deltopectoral cleft. Its proximal end should be handled gently as it may retract deep to the costocoracoid membrane and prove difficult to find and ligate. In the upper medial corner the deltoid and acromial branches of acromiothoracic arteries should be defined, controlled and divided.

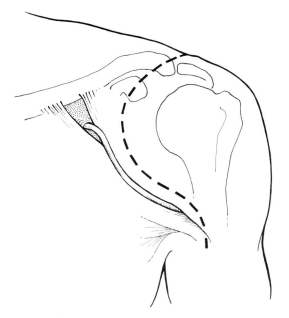

Fig. 46.6. Anterior approach to the shoulder joint. Relationship of structures to incision.

The deltoid is freed from the underlying loose connective tissue by finger dissection and its clavicular attachment defined. The muscle is divided sharply 1 cm from its insertion and bleeding controlled. The skin, subcutaneous tissue and deltoid are then turned laterally to expose the deeper structures. The coracoid process, the coracobrachialis and short head of biceps are identified. An incision down the lateral side of the muscles exposes the subscapularis above and teres major below as they pass transversely to the bicipital groove.

Access may be improved by division of the coracoid process or its attached muscles, which can then be retracted medially. The arm is externally rotated and the subscapularis muscle and tendon defined (above it blends unmarked, edge to edge, with supraspinatus, while below a leash or vessels lies transversely between it and teres major). Two or three stay sutures are placed in the musculotendinous junction so that the retracted muscle end can be found later, and the tendon divided 1 cm from its insertion into the lesser tuberosity. This tendon is thick and broad, and is blended on its deep surface with the joint capsule, from which it should be gently freed. The capsule is incised vertically to expose the head of the humerus, the glenoid fossa and labrum (*Fig.* 46.7).

The arm is manipulated to allow inspection of the humeral head and glenoid cavity. The anterior glenoid rim and labrum are more easily seen if a skid is passed carefully through the joint so that its tip engages behind the posterior glenoid lip and is angled to lever the humeral head laterally. If the capsule and cartilaginous labrum have been torn off the front of the neck of the scapula (the Bankhart lesion) this

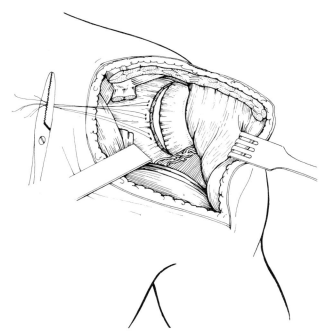

Fig. 46.7. Putti–Platt operation. Biceps and coracobrachialis have been divided and retracted. Stay sutures are in subscapularis which has been cut to expose the capsule.

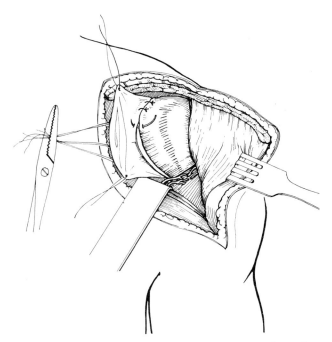

Fig. 46.8. Putti–Platt operation. The arm is in neutral rotation and by the side. The lateral cuff of subscapularis is sutured to the capsule at the glenoid rim.

can be revealed by gentle traction on the capsule. Surgical reattachment of the labrum can be difficult and should not be performed by a surgeon unfamiliar with the technique, and the Putti–Platt procedure, in which the slack anterior capsule is overlapped and reinforced with the subscapularis muscle, is preferred.

When the glenohumeral joint has been inspected the skid is removed. An assistant supports the arm in 10–15° of flexion, neutral duction and neutral rotation. Alliss tissue forceps are applied to the lateral flap of the capsule which is pulled medially to overlie the medial flap. The doubled capsule is secured with non-absorbable sutures. It should now not be possible to rotate the arm externally (*Fig.* 46.8).

The subscapularis muscle is retrieved by traction on its stay sutures and is pulled across to its tendon stump and sutured with interrupted non-absorbable stitches so as to provide a thick layer of muscle in front of the capsule. The coracoid process is reattached with a screw, or its muscle reattached with non-absorbable sutures.

A suction drain is left deep to the deltoid muscle and the muscle carefully reattached to its origin on the clavicle. A further drain is placed subcutaneously if the patient is fat, and the layers closed carefully.

Postoperative Care

The arm is held across the body in internal rotation and a greater arm sling is applied to support the

elbow. The arm is kept in this position for 6 weeks but the hand is put through the clothes and used from the start.

After 6 weeks the arm is remobilized, flexion initially, abduction and external rotation later. Full shoulder remobilization usually takes 4 months but it may be 6 months before range, strength and confidence are restored.

Exploration for Posterior Dislocation

Posterior dislocation of the shoulder may be associated with a fracture of the head of the humerus. Such a fracture, which can clearly be seen on an axial radiograph of the scapula or axillary view of the joint, may make closed manipulative reduction impossible. An open reduction through the anterior approach is then necessary. The deltopectoral approach described above is followed until the subscapularis tendon is identified. Part of the lesser tuberosity with the attached subscapularis tendon may be found to have been avulsed, allowing easy access to the front of the joint. The capsule is incised longitudinally, the haemarthrosis aspirated, and the joint irrigated free of blood clot. The head of the humerus is levered forwards from where it lies trapped behind the posterior lip of the glenoid so that it slips back into joint. If a large impaction fracture has occurred in the front of the humeral head, the lesser tuberosity bone fragment is trimmed and screwed into the humeral head defect. The wound is closed in the manner described above.

Postoperative Care

The arm is immobilized, supported with an arm sling. Use of the hand is permitted from the start and gentle shoulder remobilization is begun once wound healing has occurred.

Coraco-acromioplasty

This procedure may be undertaken:

1. For the relief of impingement pain in disorders of the rotator cuff or for subacromial bursitis.
2. To improve access for surgery on the rotator cuff or upper aspect of the shoulder joint.

The scapula is suspended from the clavicle by the coracoclavicular ligaments so acromionectomy does not affect the stability of the shoulder. Acromionectomy does, however, lead to some alteration in the appearance of the joint.

Surgical treatment should be reserved for those patients with complete acute tears of the rotator cuff and for those patients with other lesions who have failed to respond to a full trial of non-operative therapy.

Preoperative radiographs of the shoulder joint are necessary and where the diagnosis is in doubt contrast arthrography may be valuable.

The angled shoulder strap incision starts lateral to the biceps groove and tendon some 5 cm below the acromion and passes up medially to the acromioclavicular joint. A 1-cm cuff of periosteum is 'petalled' and detached from the anterior edge of the acromion and the deltoid split not more than 2 cm distally to expose the acromiclavicular joint and coracoacromio ligament. The rotator cuff tendons are guarded, the anterior portion of the acromion removed with a sharp osteotome and the coracoacromial ligament divided (*Fig.* 46.9); this ligament occasionally has two limbs at its clavicular end, and care must be taken that a complete ligament division

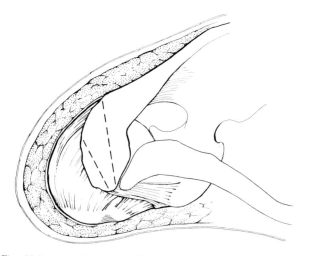

Fig. 46.9. Acromionectomy. Removal of the larger amount of bone prevents painful crowding of the rotator cuff, while the smaller resection gives access for repair.

has been undertaken. The rotator cuff and subacromial bursa can now be examined as the arm is placed in different positions. If impingement of the degenerate or torn portion of the supraspinatus tendon is found, a segment of the coraco-acromial ligament, any osteophytes on the underside of the acromioclavicular joint and not more than the anterior one-half of the acromion, are excised. It is occasionally necessary to excise the distal 1 cm of the clavicle to complete the decompression.

Small longitudinal splits in the tendon may be excised and oversewn, and larger tears repaired and reattached to a trough in the upper part of the humeral head if necessary. The deltoid is reapproximated to the periosteal cuff with non-absorbable sutures and sometimes holes need to be drilled through the bone to receive the sutures and make the reattachment more secure.

Postoperatively the limb is supported in a triangular sling and gravity-eliminated exercises can begin as the pain of surgery subsides. More vigorous range of movement exercises begin at 3 weeks.

EXPOSURE OF THE HUMERAL SHAFT

Surgical Anatomy

The head and neck of humerus are clothed by deltoid, which has to be peeled aside as previously mentioned if access is needed. The greater part of the shaft of the humerus is accessible anterolaterally just in front of the lateral intramuscular septum through the brachialis muscle, whose double innervation makes access through the muscle possible without denervation. The radial nerve which curves through the lateral intramuscular septum at the midshaft is protected by the posterolateral fibres of the brachialis that it innervates. No other important structures lie on this side of the humerus until the epicondyle is reached. The lateral epicondyle is easily palpable in all subjects, and the grooves that mark the position of the lateral intramuscular septum can usually be identified.

Indications for Exposure

1. Exposure and biopsy or curettage of lesions of the shaft of the humerus.
2. Open reduction and internal fixation of humeral shaft fractures, chiefly those associated with progressive radial nerve damage or fractures in bedridden patients whose supine position makes external splintage inadequate.
3. Exploration of the radial nerve for post-traumatic palsy.

Anterolateral Approach (Thompson)

Parts of this approach can be used as access to any part of the bone from the neck of humerus down to the lateral epicondyle. The skin incision starts over the distal one-half of the deltopectoral groove and continues down the lateral side of the biceps as far as its musculotendinous junction. The deep fascia is opened and the cephalic vein ligated proximally and distally. Proximally the humeral shaft is exposed between the deltoid and biceps, while below the deltoid insertion the brachialis is split longitudinally into medial and lateral halves and retracted to expose the bone (*Fig.* 46.10).

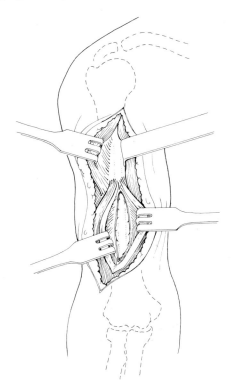

Fig. 46.10. Anterolateral approach to humeral shaft. The brachialis has been split at the lower end of the incision and the radial nerve lies hidden behind its lateral fibres.

More distal access to the anterior aspect of the shaft is obtained through the interval between brachialis and brachioradialis. The radial nerve is protected as it is reflected laterally with brachioradialis.

The radial nerve can be exposed in the distal half of the arm by this approach, and can be found as it leaves the musculospiral groove to lie first between triceps and brachialis and then between brachialis and brachioradialis until it enters the forearm (*Fig.* 46.11).

THE ELBOW

Surface Anatomy

In all but the fattest patient the two humeral epicondyles and the tip of the olecranon process of the ulna

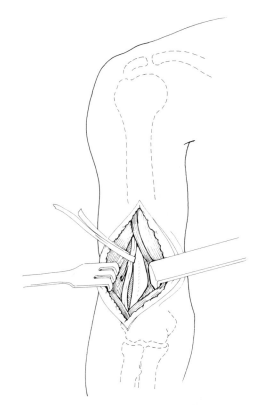

Fig. 46.11. Anterolateral approach to humeral shaft. The radial nerve has been exposed between brachialis and brachioradialis,

are easily palpable bony landmarks. This allows incisions to be placed safely for exploration of the joint without endangering the major nerves or vessels of the limb. The two epicondyles may, however, be displaced by injury or become totally obscured by swelling or haematoma and thus great caution must be then exercised.

Surgical Anatomy

The ulnar nerve can be palpated as it leaves the arm behind the medial epicondyle and passes distally to reach the interval between the two heads of flexor carpi ulnaris.

The radial nerve passes behind the midshaft of the humerus in the spiral groove, traverses the intramuscular septum and lies between brachioradialis and brachialis, where it may be located surgically, then passes within the supinator over the head and neck of the radius, into the forearm. The nerve is vulnerable to injury if an incision placed anterior to the line of the lateral intramuscular septum and epicondyle is extended distally for more than two fingerbreadths below the crease of the elbow joint.

The median nerve and brachial vessels lie deep in the cubital fossa under cover of the bicipital aponeurosis and are endangered with direct anterior approaches to the joint.

Indications for Surgery

Exploration of the elbow joint may be required for:

1. Diagnostic synovial biopsy or less commonly for synovectomy.
2. Excision or replacement arthroplasty in patients with rheumatoid arthritis.
3. Open reduction and internal fixation of displaced fractures of the humeral epicondyles or of the olecranon process.
4. Excision of the severely damaged radial head.
5. Surgical release of the trapped or stretched ulnar nerve producing numbness, paraesthesia or intrinsic muscle dysfunction in the hand.

Open Reduction and Internal Fixation of Fractures around the Elbow Joint .

Good quality anteroposterior and lateral radiographs of the elbow joint are essential in the management of elbow joint injuries. This is particularly true where internal fixation is being considered, as comminution of fracture fragments may pose problems if internal fixation is proposed, and damage to the articular surface may affect the decision to undertake surgery.

Exploration and Fixation of Olecranon Fractures

These fractures may be avulsions of the triceps insertion alone, or may involve the articular surface of the coronoid fossa, and may be associated with dislocation of the radial head. Study of these features on the preoperative radiographs is essential if good surgical results are to be achieved.

The patient is placed supine, the limb exsanguinated and a tourniquet applied high on the upper arm. If the triceps muscle is pulled down as the cuff is applied, the triceps tendon will be slack and fracture reduction aided.

The back of the elbow joint is exposed by a longitudinal incision passing to the lateral side of the olecranon process from 4 cm proximal to its tip and extending down the posterior subcutaneous border of the ulna 3 or 4 cm beyond the fracture site.

If the fracture does not involve the coronoid fossa and is only a triceps insertion avulsion, the bone fragment is excised and the insertion reattached to the proximal end of the ulna by sutures passing through drill holes in the bone.

In other circumstances the fracture haematoma is released, the fracture exposed and the bone ends cleared of blood clot with a bone curette. The elbow is extended to relax the triceps and the fragments are realigned to restore a smooth articular surface. The fracture is held reduced by a Tulloch Brown clamp or towel clip, and two 5-mm Kirschner wires drilled through the end of the olecranon to run longitudinally down the ulna across the fracture site parallel to each other and close to the coronoid articular surface. The ends of the wires are bent back, so that they may be buried in the soft tissues before wound closure (see Fig. 46.4).

An 18-gauge SWG wire is inserted as a figure-of-eight tension-absorbing band from the triceps insertion into the ulna distal to the fracture site. With the elbow extended, the wire is threaded deep to the triceps tendon of the olecranon, the ends crossed over each other on the posterior surface of the ulna, one is passed through a drill hole in the posterior cortex of the ulna, the loop is completed, and the wire tensioned and knotted. The elbow is then moved cautiously through its full range of movements to ensure that there is no mechanical block. The wound is closed in layers and a dry dressing, cotton wool and crêpe bandage applied.

Postoperatively the elbow is held flexed just above 90° and the arm supported in a sling. The dressings are reduced to a minimum at 48 hours and range of movement exercises commenced to restore both elbow and forearm function.

Complications

If the articular surface of the coronoid fossa cannot be accurately restored there will be permanent loss of elbow movement. Degenerative arthritis will occur as a result of progressive damage to the trochlea. The wires may back out of the bone unless they are carefully secured in the soft tissues. They will back into the olecranon bursa, and if they are causing a bursitis they should be removed once fracture healing is sound.

Lateral Approach to the Elbow (Kocher)

The upper part of this exposure gives access to the lateral epicondyle and the lower half to the head and neck of the radius.

Open Reduction of a Fracture of the Lateral Epicondyle

Displaced or malrotated fractures of the lateral epicondyle of the humerus in growing children should be accurately reduced so that the growth of the lateral bony structures continues and late valgus deformity avoided. The radiograph only shows calcified or ossified tissues, and the displaced fragment is always larger than the radiographic appearance would suggest.

The longitudinal incision is in the lateral plane, starting 5 cm above the epicondyle and passing down its bony prominence, then downwards and backwards towards the subcutaneous border of the ulna 5 cm below the elbow joint.

In the upper part of the incision the tip of the epicondyle is located and dissection continued between brachioradialis and the radiocarpal extensors anteriorly, and triceps posteriorly until the epicondylar fragment is identified; the fracture fragment is turned downwards and forwards with its attached muscles and the fracture surface cleaned and cleared of blood clot. It is rotated, replaced and fixed with a periosteal suture or fine Kirschner wire. The wound is closed in layers and a cottonwool and crêpe bandage applied.

The elbow is protected in a plaster-of-Paris back-slab. Range of movement exercises are begun at 3 weeks and full range usually restored by 3 months.

Excision of the Head of the Radius

The incision starts at the lateral epicondyle and passes downwards and backwards to meet the posterior border of the ulna 5 cm below the elbow joint (*Fig.* 46.12).

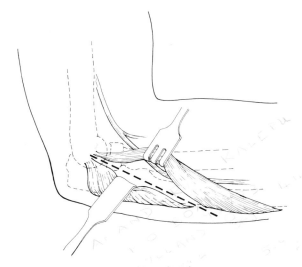

Fig. 46.12. Exploration of head of radius. The incision should be kept posterior to the radius to avoid the posterior interosseous nerve.

Dissection is deepened between anconeus posteriorly and extensor carpi ulnaris anteriorly until the radial neck is found. In surgery for fracture the haemarthrosis usually causes the synovium to bulge and guides the surgeon to the joint. The capsule and synovium are opened in the same line and the hae-marthrosis aspirated.

The radial neck is divided with a saw or bone cutters at the level of the annular ligament and the raw surface trimmed as the forearm is fully pronated and supinated. The wound is closed in layers.

Postoperatively the arm is supported in a sling and remobilization begun 48 hours after surgery. Full pronation/supination is usually restored but full elbow extension may not return.

Ulnar Nerve Release or Transposition

Symptoms of ulnar nerve dysfunction may occur as a result of pressure on the nerve as it passes between the two heads of flexor carpi ulnaris, as a result of bony pressure on the nerve as it lies behind the medial epicondyle, or as a result of cubitus valgus following

a lateral epicondyle fracture in childhood, with consequent irritation of the nerve.

Surgery may relieve sensory disturbance particularly paraesthesia, but motor weakness and wasting usually persist although they may be prevented from progression by surgery.

Prior to surgery anteroposterior and lateral radiographs of the elbow and a tunnel view of the medial epicondyle should be examined. If these show cubitus valgus or roughening of the posterior surface of the medial epicondyle, anterior transposition of the nerve should be undertaken. If the films show no such lesions simple nerve release should suffice.

Ulnar Nerve Release

The limb is exsanguinated and the tourniquet applied as high on the upper arm as possible. The patient is placed supine with the affected arm flexed and adducted across the chest or, alternatively, the arm may be placed on an arm table to allow exploration of the medial side of the joint.

The incision is centred on the medial epicondyle and extends proximally and distally 4–5 cm along the medial axis of the limb (*Fig.* 46.13). It is deepened

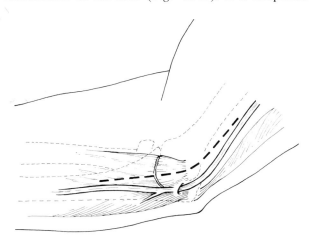

Fig. 46.13. Ulnar nerve transposition. The nerve to flexor carpi ulnaris must be freed with care. The common flexor tendons are shown cut near their origin.

above and behind the medial epicondyle until the ulnar nerve, recognizable by its longitudinal fasciculi and fine longitudinal blood vessels, is identified and isolated. The nerve is followed distally round the epicondyle to the interval between the bellies of flexor carpi ulnaris. The dissection must be carried out on the superficial aspect of the nerve and care must be taken to preserve the muscular branch to flexor carpi ulnaris, as it leaves the main trunk just above the elbow joint; the small leash of vessels at this level and the small articular branch from the nerve to the elbow joint may be sacrificed if necessary. The upper tendinous fibrous arcade through which the nerve enters flexor carpi ulnaris is divided to release the nerve of any tension there, and any other soft tissue bands are divided so that the nerve lies free from above the elbow joint to its tunnel (*see Fig.* 46.13).

Anterior Transposition of the Ulnar Nerve

The dissection described above is undertaken until the nerve has been freed. The nerve should then be transferred to lie in front of the medial epicondyle and lie either in the fatty subcutaneous tissues overlying the flexor muscle mass origin or deep to that mass in the plane of the brachial vessels and median nerve; subcutaneous transposition is technically the smaller operation, avoids the danger of nerve entrapment in a new bed, but leaves the nerve more exposed to the knocks of everyday activity than does the deeper intermuscular transposition.

For subcutaneous transposition a flap of the deep fascia in front of the epicondyle is developed as the nerve is approached to provide a broad sling to hold the nerve in its anterior position, while for intermuscular anterior transposition the common tendon of origin of the flexor muscles of the medial condyle is defined and divided so as to leave a tendinous cuff attached to the bone. The muscle block is very thick and may easily be incompletely freed and dissection should continue until the median nerve and brachial vessels are exposed at the front of the cubital fossa (*Fig.* 46.14).

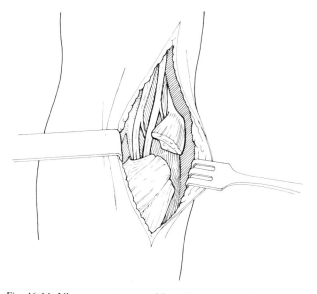

Fig. 46.14. Ulnar nerve transposition. The nerve and its branches to flexor carpi ulnaris have been brought in front of the common flexor origin which will be sutured over the transposed nerve.

The ulnar nerve, including its vulnerable motor branch to flexor carpi ulnaris, is now gently mobilized from its bed and is placed subcutaneously, or deep to the flexor muscles (*Fig.* 46.14). The elbow is now fully extended and the medial intramuscular septum and the ulnar origin of flexor carpi ulnaris divided

as necessary to allow the nerve to lie without tension in its new bed. The elbow is flexed and the flexor muscle mass reattached to its tendinous cuff of origin by mattress sutures of stout nylon or silk, so that the transposed nerve lies slackly in a new intermuscular plane.

The tourniquet is released and bleeding vessels controlled by pressure, diathermy or ligature as appropriate. A suction drain is placed in the deep layers and the wound closed in layers. A dry dressing, cottonwool and crêpe compressive bandage are applied to support the elbow at the right angle. The arm is supported in a sling. A plaster-of-Paris backslab is used to immobilize the elbow for the first 2 weeks after nerve transposition, but gentle remobilization may start immediately after simple nerve release. Active use of the hand and fingers is encouraged from the start.

Complications

If much handling of the nerve occurred at operation, symptoms of ulnar nerve dysfunction, particularly paraesthesia, may be increased for a time following surgery.

Elbow mobility and forearm strength are sometimes slow to recover after transposition of the nerve.

ANTERIOR EXPOSURE OF THE RADIAL SHAFT

This exposure is useful for biopsy of lesions of bone and for internal fixation or grafting of radial shaft fractures. Exposure of the head of the radius is best through the posterolateral approach described previously, but the exposure outlined here allows access to any part of the bone from the upper shaft to the radial styloid.

Anterior Approach (Henry)

The forearm is supinated and a longitudinal incision made where necessary on a line starting just lateral to the biceps tendon and extending down the medial border of brachioradialis as far as the radial styloid, and the deep fascia is opened.

Proximally the radial vessels are identified and the radial recurrent branches ligated and divided as they pass in a leash to the lateral muscles (*Fig.* 46.15).

The elbow is now flexed and the brachioradialis, radiocarpal extensors and radial nerve are defined and retracted laterally so as to expose the supinator. This muscle is freed from its attachment at the medial side of the radius and reflected laterally protecting the deep branch of the radial nerve.

More distally the brachioradialis and flexor carpi radialis are separated to expose the superficial branch of the radial nerve and the radial vessels which are retracted medially. Flexor pollicis longus and prona-

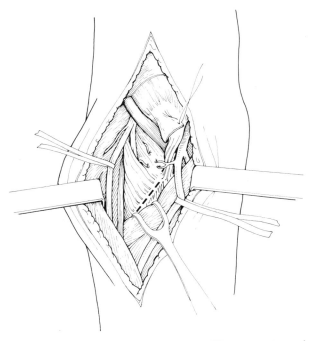

Fig. 46.15. Anterior approach to the radius. The recurrent vessels are divided. Brachioradialis and pronator teres separated to expose the radial shaft between supinator and flexor digitorum sublimis.

tor quadratus are stripped subperiosteally off their attachments on the anterolateral surface of the radius, and the bone is exposed. Following surgery the flexor pollicis and pronator muscles are re-attached to the soft tissues of the lateral border of the radius. The other muscles usually fall into place.

The deep fascia is closed as far as possible and the skin sutured.

THE HIP JOINT (*see* Chapter 47)
APPROACH TO THE SHAFT OF THE FEMUR

The whole of the shaft and supracondylar region of the femur can be conveniently exposed for biopsy of bone lesions or for the internal fixation of fractures by the posterolateral approach in which access to the femur is gained by detachment of the quadriceps from the anterior surface of the lateral intramuscular septum. This approach avoids division of any of the major muscles of the thigh, or damage to its nerve or blood supply. Access may be difficult in muscular patients with a bulky vastus lateralis.

Posterolateral Approach

The patient lies suitably supported on the sound side. The limb is prepared surgically and draped so as to allow free movement of the hip and knee joints.

A skin incision of suitable site and length is made along the palpable depression at the posterior border of the vastus lateralis. The fascia lata is incised in the line of skin incision, the vastus peeled forwards off the lateral intramuscular septum and retracted until the shaft of the femur is located at the attachment of the septum to the linea aspera (*Fig.* 46.16).

Two or three of the perforating branches of the profunda vessels will be found and should be ligated before division so as to avoid their retraction behind the linea aspera.

In the upper two-thirds of the incision the vastus

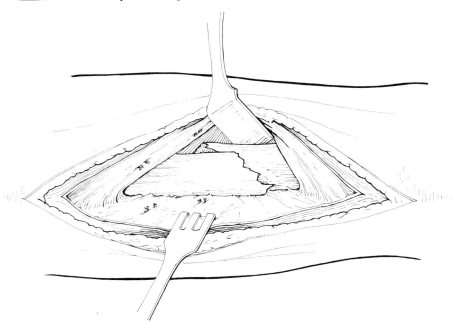

Fig. 46.16. The posterolateral approach to the shaft of the femur. The vastus lateralis has been stripped off the septum and two sets of perforating vessels ligated. The periosteum has been stripped from the femur by the fracture.

intermedius is peeled off the bone, and care must be taken to reflect both heads of the biceps posteriorly as dissection between the heads jeopardizes the sciatic nerve. Closure following surgery is by repair of the fascia lata, deep fascia and skin, and suction drains should be left in deep layers of the wound for 48 hours after surgery.

THE KNEE

This major joint is affected by a wide variety of inflammatory and infective disorders. Injury, particularly in the young male athlete, is common.

Surface Anatomy

In all except the fattest individual the general contours and bony landmarks of the joint are relatively easy to palpate. Anteriorly the quadriceps with the sweeping fibres of vastus medialis inserts into the upper border and corners of the patella and via the patellar tendon into the tibial tubercle. There is a fullness on either side of the tendon caused by the bulge of the patellar fat pad. The hollows on either side of the patella are lost if there is an effusion or thickening of the synovium.

The upper surface of the tibial flares is covered by capsule to whose deep surface are attached the menisci. The head of the fibula lies laterally and below the joint line. The lateral ligament and biceps tendon, both palpable in the thin subject, are attached to its upper margin. The lateral popliteal nerve can sometimes be felt under the skin as it passes forwards around the neck of the fibula. The medial ligament cannot be defined through the skin, but the three tendons of the pes anserinus can be felt as they cross the posteromedial corner of the knee to insert into the upper anterior tibial surface. The posterior structures of the knee are difficult to define when the joint is extended but are more easy to feel if the joint is flexed 30–40° to relax the muscles. If the patient is prone and the front of the tibia cradled by the examiner's elbow, an enlarged or thickened popliteal bursa can be felt overlying and between the heads of origin of the gastrocnemius.

Investigations

Clinical examination of the knee is supplemented by X-ray examination. Anteroposterior and lateral views should always be taken; the intercondylar anteroposterior view and the tangential 'skyline' view of the patellofemoral joint may provide additional information. Contrast arthrography of the knee may be of great value but is unlikely to prove useful unless the clinician has experience in the techniques and film appearances.

Arthroscopy allows wide examination of the interior of the knee joint, inspection of most of the articular surface, the menisci and the cruciate ligaments, and inspection and biopsy of the synovium. Operative arthroscopy, which includes the division of plicae, lateral patellar retinacular release, removal of loose bodies, trimming of irregular areas of articular surface and partial or total meniscectomy, is, in skilled and experienced hands, increasingly supplanting open surgery of the knee and reducing the length of hospital stay and postoperative disability.

Skill in the use of the arthroscope, and particularly operative arthroscopy, can only come from careful instruction and frequent use of the instruments.

Indications for Surgery

Exploration of the knee joint may be required for:
1. Removal of torn or degenerate menisci.
2. Inspection of the femoral condylar articular surface, the reattachment or removal of oestochondral fragments, and the drilling or trimming of an irregular articular surface.
3. Repair of cruciate or collateral ligament rupture.
4. Surgical synovectomy of the knee joint.
5. Surgical repair of the extensor mechanism, patellar fixation or patellectomy after injury.
6. Arthrodesis of the knee joint.
7. Joint replacement for degenerative or inflammatory arthritis.

Approaches to the Knee Joint

All approaches should respect the medial and lateral collateral ligaments and the lateral popliteal nerve. Damage to the quadriceps muscle or its expansions should be avoided.

Limited or wide exposure of most of the joint can be achieved anteriorly but adequate exposure of the tibial insertion of the posterior cruciate ligament, the posterior aspects of the femoral condyles or tibial plateau can only be obtained by exploration through the popliteal fossa.

Limited anteromedial or anterolateral low parapatellar incisions allow access for inspection of the menisci for their removal, or for trimming of the articular surface of the femur. Supplementary incisions to aid meniscectomy are described below. A more generous anterior parapatellar approach in which the incision skirts the patella and extends into the suprapatellar pouch is necessary for wide exposure of the femoral condyles, for surgery on the patella, the anterior cruciate ligament, or for surgical synovectomy of the knee.

Anteromedial or Anterolateral Parapatellar Approaches (Fig. 46.17)

These are used for surgery on the menisci and the medial approach is useful for the exploration and reattachment of osteochondral fractures, or for the drilling of the medial femoral condyle.

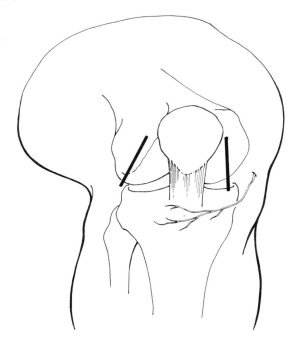

Fig. 46.17. Parapatellar approaches. The infrapatellar branch of the saphenous nerve is endangered if the medial approach is brought too low.

Medial Approach

The incision, nearly vertical, extends from the prominence of the medial femoral condyle downwards to not more than one finger-breadth below the upper edge of the tibial plateau. This lower limit will avoid damage to the infrapatellar branch of the saphenous nerve, which would be jeopardized by a longer incision. The incision is deepened through all layers to the synovial membrane. The membrane is picked off the femoral condyle before incision to allow it to balloon as air enters the joint and thus avoid knife damage to the condylar articular surface. The whole of the medial compartment can now be examined if retractors are placed medially behind the patellar tendon and fat pad and laterally between synovium and femoral condyle. A blunt hook is put round the inner edge of the meniscus to draw it forwards and allow wider inspection. As the knee is flexed and extended much of the medial femoral condyle, anterior cruciate ligament and posterior patellar surface can be seen. If the incision is extended upwards into the medial edge of the quadriceps tendon the patella can be retracted laterally and if it is held across as the knee is flexed it will lie without tension on the lateral side of the femoral condyle to allow access for the drilling and reattachment of osteochondral fragments, repair of the anterior cruciate ligament or reattachment of the fractured anterior tibial spine.

OPEN MEDIAL MENISCECTOMY

The anterior horn is pulled forwards with a blunt

hook and is freed from the tibia by a horizontal incision and from the capsule by vertical division of the meniscus at its attachment to the coronary ligament.

The meniscus flap is now gripped in toothed forceps and pulled medially so that the peripheral attachment can be identified (*Fig.* 46.18). Further

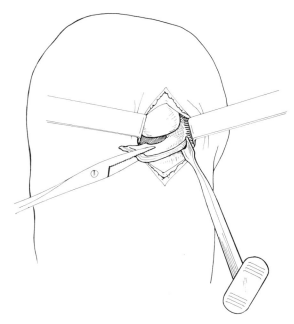

Fig. 46.18. Medial meniscectomy. The knife is cutting through the extreme outer edge of the meniscus and not in the coronary ligament.

mobilization is by vertical sweeps of the knife or by backward cuts with a Smillie knife while gentle tension is maintained on the meniscus.

When possible the meniscus is dislocated into the intercondylar space and the posterior attachment of the meniscus divided under vision. The view is often improved by full flexion of the knee or external rotation of the tibia. If the posterior horn of the meniscus still cannot be adequately seen a second, more posterior vertical incision is made just behind the medial collateral ligament. It is deepened down to the joint and care is taken to avoid the saphenous vein; the joint is opened and the attachments of the posterior half of the meniscus are defined and divided so that the meniscus can be freed from the posterior cruciate ligament and capsule.

The wound is closed in layers. A drain is rarely necessary after medial meniscectomy.

A cottonwool and crêpe compressive bandage is placed around the joint, and a plaster-of-Paris backslab applied to keep the knee in extension.

Lateral Approach

The low parapatellar approach slopes obliquely backwards and downwards to end 1–2 cm below the tibial plateau. The capsule is incised along the anterior edge of the iliotibial tract where it overlies the lateral femoral condyle. The thick fat pad is incised and the joint entered. The lateral meniscus, lateral femoral condyle, anterior cruciate ligament and patella surface can all be seen through this incision.

A wider exposure can be achieved by extending the incision into the suprapatellar pouch through the fibres of vastus lateralis.

OPEN LATERAL MENISCECTOMY

The broad anterior one-third of the meniscus is freed by incisions to mobilize it from the tibial plateau, and the anterior pole is detached from the intercondylar notch. The freed anterior portion is gripped in toothed forceps and the peripheral attachment of the meniscus identified and freed backwards to the non-attached portion at the lateral ligament and popliteus tendon by a combination of traction on the forceps and divisions of the attachments with a Smillie knife. The meniscus is dislocated into the intercondylar fossa and the posterior horn detached under vision.

If difficulty is experienced in removing the posterior horn a second vertical incision is made through all layers at the posterolateral angle of the joint, and deepened with care. The course of the lateral popliteal nerve is defined prior to incision so that it is not endangered.

Drainage may be necessary particularly if the meniscectomy has been difficult. The wound is closed in layers.

A cottonwool and crêpe compressive bandage is applied, and a plaster-of-Paris backslab from groin to ankle is used to encase the limb.

Post-meniscectomy Care

Intensive quadriceps drill begins 48 hours after surgery, and the patient is allowed up, partially weight bearing with crutches once control of the knee has been regained. Knee remobilization free of plaster is allowed from the 10th postoperative day, and function is usually restored 6–8 weeks from surgery.

Complications

1. HAEMARTHROSIS

This may develop following meniscectomy as a result of capsular bleeding or rarely as a result of damage to the genicular vessels, particularly the lateral inferior artery which passes around the knee at the level of the lateral meniscus.

Bleeding is less common if dissection is undertaken just within the attached margin of the meniscus rather than in the vascular coronary ligament.

Severe rest pain after meniscectomy is unusual and should it occur the dressings should be completely removed and the joint inspected. The haemarthrosis should be aspirated or the joint reopened surgically in the operating room under general anaesthesia. A suction drain is inserted and the wound closed. The limb is immobilized, the drain removed at 48 hours, and the usual postoperative regimen resumed.

Repeated development of a haemarthrosis may indicate development of a false aneurysm and the telltale pulsatile swelling should be sought.

2. INFECTION

This may range from an acute suppurative arthritis with an acutely swollen tender knee in a sick patient to a low-grade infection manifest by a slow postoperative recovery with persistent synovial thickening and delayed remobilization.

Aspiration of the joint, or repeated blood culture, may reveal the pathogen and aggressive treatment is necessary if joint mobility is to be restored.

Repeated aspiration of the joint or wide surgical re-exploration may be indicated.

3. PERSISTENT EFFUSION

This may follow too early or too vigorous remobilization of the knee. Quadriceps recovery is slow if incautious weight bearing has been permitted from the start.

A decrease in activity with avoidance of standing or weight bearing and intensive static quadriceps drill is all that is usually necessary to get the effusion to resolve.

Exposure of the Patella

This may be required for the internal fixation of transverse fractures, or for the patellectomy after trauma or in treatment of severe patellofemoral osteoarthritis.

While a transverse midpatellar incision gives satisfactory access, troublesome adhesions between skin and scar may hamper healing and remobilization and a curved longitudinal incision some 10 cm long, skirting the medial side of the bone is favoured. The incision is deepened through skin, superficial fascia, deep fascia, and composite flap retracted laterally to allow inspection of the knee joint and patella.

Wiring of Transverse Fractures of the Patella

The fragments are manipulated so that the patellar articular surface is perfectly restored and are held in position by a sharp-toothed clamp or towel clip. Two 4-mm Kirschner wires are drilled longitudinally down through the patella to stabilize the fracture, cut short, and the upper ends turned back to form a hook. The fracture fragments are then compressed by an 18-gauge SWG wire that is passed behind the quadriceps tendon, then down in front of the patella, across behind the patellar tendon and back anteriorly to complete a figure-of-eight. It is tightened and tied off. The placing of the wire in front of the patella provides the most effective transfer of pull of the quadriceps muscle to the tibia as the knee is actively extended.

Patellectomy

If the lateral expansions of the quadriceps mechanism are intact, then the patella should be enucleated through a vertically placed incision in its tendon fibres, and the defect repaired with strong absorbable sutures.

Where the lateral expansions have been torn and separated patellectomy should be undertaken through a transverse incision, and care taken to form a strong repair of the patellar mechanism, without reefing or overlapping of the lateral expansions as this would restrict postoperative knee flexion.

When wiring of the patella, or vertical incision enucleation has been undertaken remobilization of the knee may start once the wound is comfortable. If the lateral expansions have needed repair then immobilization in a backslab plaster-of-Paris cast for a period of at least 4 weeks is advisable to allow sound repair of the extensor mechanism.

Synovectomy of the Knee

This major surgical undertaking should only be performed where there are staff and facilities to carry out the taxing postoperative regimen. The procedure is most commonly required for rheumatoid synovitis which has not responded to a non-operative regimen of rest and drugs, where the bulky synovial membrane is causing pain and loss of movement in a stable and erosion-free knee; it may occasionally be performed for pigmented villonodular synovitis or for synovial chondromatosis.

Strictly speaking operation is an anterior synovectomy as the posterior recesses cannot be excised through the approach to be described.

The operation can be performed through a single long anteromedial approach, but access to the lateral side of the joint is poor, and separate shorter anterolateral and anteromedial parapatellar incisions allow better access to all recesses of the joint and lessen the need for vigorous retraction.

The incisions are deepened through the quadriceps expansion and dissection is started by development of the plane between the suprapatellar synovial pouch and surrounding tissues. The articularis genu muscle is divided and the pouch mobilized by scissors dissection downwards until the edge of the synovium can be dissected sharply from the femoral condyles. The knee is flexed and synovial clearance continues down both sides of the condyles where particular care is taken to excise the synovium that lies deep to the collateral ligaments, and in the recesses between the

capsule and tibial flares. The synovium lies under the menisci so that meniscectomy will be necessary to complete the synovectomy.

Finally, the synovium around the cruciate ligaments is excised and with the knee fully flexed all accessible synovium removed from the posterior part of the notch.

Where synovium has advanced onto an articular surface, as much of it as possible is removed by sharp dissection and the remnants grasped with bone nibblers and twisted off away from the intact cartilage while care is taken to avoid damaging healthy tissues. Throughout the operation the cartilaginous articular surface must be kept moist and not handled, abraded or scored.

All obvious bleeding points are diathermied, a suction drain is placed in the intercondylar notch and the joint carefully closed in layers. A bulky bandage and temporary plaster-of-Paris backslab are applied and the leg elevated on pillows. Static quadriceps drill and flexion within the dressing are started at 48 hours and free remobilization of the knee begins when the surgical reaction is lessening. If flexion range is not improving rapidly by the 4th week a gentle manipulation of the knee under anaesthesia is performed and the joint immobilized in a plaster-of-Paris cast in 90° of flexion. The patient works for extension from this rest splint which is finally discarded when full extension and 90° of flexion can be achieved during the physiotherapy session.

Complications

Healing of the tissues of patients with rheumatoid arthritis is always slow and sutures should be left for at least 3 weeks.

1. Wound disruption may occur if remobilization is begun too early or manipulation is undertaken too vigorously. The wound should be resutured at once and the joint immobilized until sound healing has occurred. Some loss of joint motion is then inevitable.

2. Postoperative haemarthrosis or joint infection may occur. The features and management are outlined in the section on meniscectomy (p. 697).

Arthrodesis of the Knee

This procedure is employed less frequently than in the past, as many joints previously arthrodesed are now suitable for total joint replacement.

Arthrodesis may still be required, however, where joint infection has progressed to painful fibrous ankylosis, and in some post-traumatic arthritis in younger patients where the demands on the joint are great and where stability and security are more important than mobility.

The most favoured method is that of Charnley, where planed tibial and femoral cancellous bone surfaces are held snugly in apposition by compression clamps.

Charnley Compression Arthrodesis of the Knee

If the arthrodesis is being undertaken for tuberculosis a midline anterior approach through the quadriceps tendon and patella is recommended. Through this wide exposure the patellar tendon can be freed, the capsule cleared and the tibial collateral ligaments divided. A complete synovectomy with excision of menisci, cruciate ligaments and infrapatellar fat paid is performed.

For other disorders requiring arthrodesis a transverse approach to the knee joint is favoured.

The patella is excised and the patellar expansions divided to expose the anterior aspect of the knee joint.

The collateral ligaments are divided to allow flexion of the knee and inspection of its interior. The menisci and the intercondylar tissues are excised. Access to posterior structures is aided if a bone lever is introduced behind the upper tibia to draw it forwards. The posterior third of the menisci and capsule of the joint are then exposed for excision.

A 1-cm thick wafer of bone and articular cartilage is removed from the upper surface of the tibia with an osteotome or oscillating saw to expose the cancellous bone of the upper shaft (*Fig.* 46.19). A similar 1-cm segment of bone and cartilage is removed from the distal end of the femur but the saw cut is aligned so that the joint will be arthrodesed in full extension.

The soft tissues are temporarily approximated while a Steinmann pin is inserted transversely across the upper end of the tibia parallel to the cut tibial surface, and in the plane of neutral rotation. It is introduced from the lateral side of the tibia to avoid damage to the lateral popliteal nerve.

The compression clamp is applied to this pin, and used as a guide to site the upper pin, which is drilled through the lower femur to lie parallel to the first. The second clamp is now applied, both are tightened and the wing nuts threaded down so as to provide compression.

The wound is closed in layers and a dry dressing bandage applied.

Postoperatively the limb is rested on a Thomas' splint, to allow reactionary swelling to settle, and the clamp kept snug. Once the wound has healed a long-leg plaster-of-Paris cylinder case is applied.

Four weeks from surgery plaster and clamps are removed and the pins withdrawn; a new cast is applied and the patient allowed full weight bearing. The leg is left free 8 weeks from surgery.

Medial Approach to the Knee Joint

This multi-purpose approach provides excellent exposure of all the structures on the medial and posteromedial aspects of the knee joint, and is used for exploration of the medial structures after injury, and allows inspection and repair of the medial collateral and capsular ligaments or medial meniscectomy after injury.

The patient lies supine with a large support under the pelvis of the uninjured side. The skin incision is gently curved or S-shaped, centred on the joint line on the medial side of the knee. It passes upwards and backwards, downwards and forwards for some 12 cm from this point. The incision is deepened and the long saphenous nerve and vein reflected with the posterior flap. The pes anserinus tendons and medial quadriceps expansion are exposed anteriorly, the fibres of the medial ligament centrally and the semitendinosus and gastrocnemius posteriorly. The knee joint can be entered by a vertical incision placed either in front of or behind the fan-shaped fibres of the medial ligament, and the whole of the medial ligament and posteromedial capsule can be visualized and repaired as necessary.

Posterior Approach to the Knee Joint

This approach is valuable for the repair of an isolated injury to the cruciate ligament, or for the removal of a popliteal bursa. The patient is turned prone and the limb draped to allow free movement of the knee.

The S-shaped incision is centred on the popliteal fossa, the transverse limb being at the level of the joint line with an extension downwards from its

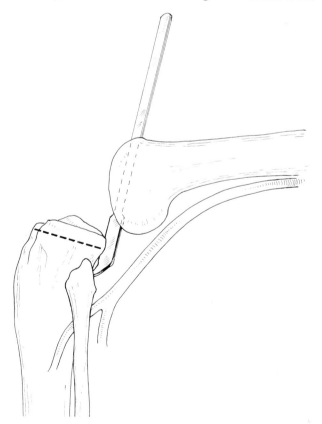

Fig. 46.19. Compression arthrodesis of the knee. The cruciate ligaments and the posterior capsule have been divided. The bone lever is placed behind the upper tibia to protect the vessels when the articular surface is removed.

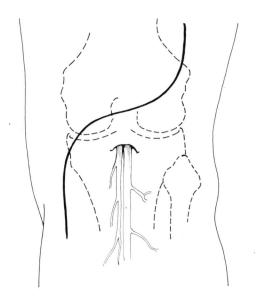

Fig. 46.20. Posterior approach to the knee joint. The posterior cutaneous nerve pierces the deep fascia with the short saphenous just below the joint and is followed in to reveal the posterior tibial nerve.

medial end and upwards from its lateral end (*Fig.* 46.20). The deep fascia is divided at the line of the skin incision, the posterior cutaneous nerve of the leg is identified and followed into the fossa. The medial head of gastrocnemius is defined up to its tendinous insertion into the femoral condyle and the tendon divided to leave a small cuff attached to the bone (*Fig.* 46.21). The medial edge of the muscle

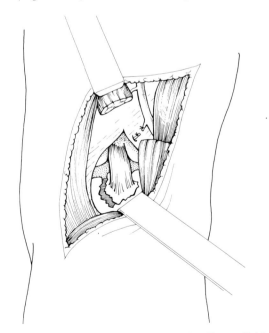

Fig. 46.21. Posterior cruciate ligament repair. The medial head of gastrocnemius has been divided—and pulled laterally—the middle genicular artery ligated, and the posterior capsule opened. The ligament has been pulled off the tibia by the injury.

belly is freed, and this and its nerve and blood supply reflected laterally to expose the back of the upper end of the tibia and the knee joint. The middle genicular vessels are identified, ligated and divided with care, and the superior medial genicular vessels sometimes also need to be divided to provide access. The back of the knee joint is opened by a vertical incision through the capsule and posterior oblique ligament, allowing a good view of the posterior part of the knee joint, and the insertion of the posterior cruciate ligament.

Closure of the incision is by repair of the posterior capsule and reattachment of the medial head of gastrocnemius to its tendinous cuff. Following closure a compressive bandage is applied.

Further aftercare will depend on the indication for surgery, and will include the application of a plaster-of-Paris cast if the posterior cruciate ligament has been repaired.

Arthroplasty of the knee

Over the past decade interposition arthroplasty of the joint has become an established procedure for the management of both unicompartmental and general osteoarthritis of the knee joint. The techniques are still evolving and readers are referred to the many recent articles on the topic as a description of techniques is inappropriate in a chapter on basic orthopaedic skills.

High Tibial Osteotomy

Indications

High tibial osteotomy is valuable in the management of early osteoarthritis of the knee when mobility is retained but pain, particularly night pain, is the problem. The operation should not now be performed for advanced osteoarthritis nor for rheumatoid arthritis when replacement arthroplasty is the treatment of choice.

A fixed flexion deformity of greater than 15°, total flexion less than 90°, gross liagmentous laxity, and obliterative arterial vascular disease in the leg are all contra-indications; the results of osteotomy are less predictable if the lateral compartment is the more severely affected.

Preoperative Evaluation

Clinical examination is supplemented by anteroposterior and lateral radiographs of the knee. An anteroposterior radiograph of the knee with the patient standing allows assessment of deformity on weight bearing.

Lateral Approach to the Upper Tibia

This is the approach of choice if arthritis is more

severe in the medial half of the knee joint, or affects both compartments equally.

The limb is prepared surgically in the usual fashion, is exsanguinated and a high thigh tourniquet applied. The skin incision extends from just in front of the neck of the fibula 15 cm upwards along the lateral side of the knee and lower femur. The knee is flexed so that the neurovascular structures fall posteriorly, and the incision deepened through the fascia lata. The peroneal nerve is identified and retracted gently, and the biceps tendon and the fibular collateral ligament dissected off the head of the fibula. The fibular head and neck are cleared of soft tissue and excised. The tibial flare is identified and the knee joint located (if necessary a short incision is made to expose the joint). The soft tissues are stripped anteriorly as far as the patellar tendon and subperiosteally behind the posterior tibial cortex. Bone levers are placed posterior and anterior to the bone to isolate it from the other structures.

A guide wire is passed transversely through the upper tibia to lie parallel to and 1 cm below the articular margin (*Fig.* 46.22). If it is necessary to remove

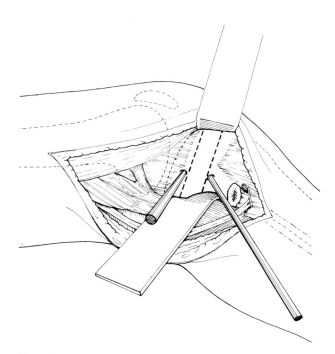

Fig. 46.22. High tibial osteotomy. The nerves and vessels are relaxed by knee flexion and protected by the broad retractor behind the tibial flare.

a wedge of bone to correct a varus deformity a second guide wire is inserted 1·5–2 cm below the first and angled up to meet its tip under the medial ligament, and an anteroposterior radiograph taken to check the position of wires and size of the wedge.

With the knee flexed to 90° a transverse tibial osteotomy is undertaken, or wedge of bone removed,

if indicated, by the use of a broad osteotome, power saw, and bone nibblers as seems appropriate. The osteotomy must be taken right across the tibia to the posteromedial cortex as failure to do this may result in fracture of the medial tibial plateau. A rim of medial cortex is left and is fractured manually, and a valgus stress applied to the tibia to close the wedge. A stepped or oblique staple is inserted across the osteotomy site to stabilize it.

A suction drain is placed behind the upper tibia, the biceps and fibular collateral ligament reattached to the neck of fibula or adjacent soft tissues, and the rest of the wound closed in layers.

Postoperative Care

A cottonwool and crêpe compressive bandage and padded plaster-of-Paris backslab are applied. The suction drain is removed 48 hours from surgery and a snug plaster-of-Paris cylinder cast applied when operative swelling has settled. Anteroposterior and lateral radiographs are now taken to assess the limb alignment. Weight bearing is allowed. The cast is removed at 5 weeks from surgery and remobilization then starts.

Complications

1. Bleeding around the surgical site may be considerable and if the suction drain is not working satisfactorily a deep or superficial haematoma may develop. It should be evacuated surgically.

2. The peroneal nerve should be handled with care. Vigorous traction may be followed by quite severe postoperative pain in the outer side of calf and ankle, and although this pain will subside spontaneously it may disturb convalescence. If handling has been particularly rough there may be transient paresis of the dorsi flexor and evertor muscles of the ankle. No particular measures are required for this as recovery is usually spontaneous.

3. Non-union of the tibia is uncommon, but it should be considered in any patient in whom severe pain persists at the osteotomy site following cast removal. A further period of immobilization in plaster usually allows union to occur, but a bone graft procedure may be necessary if signs of non-union develop.

EXPOSURE OF THE TIBIAL SHAFT

The direct approach to the subcutaneous border of the tibia allows access for exploration, biopsy of shaft lesions or for the internal fixation or grafting of diaphyseal fractures. There are occasions when severe skin damage or scarring makes the posterolateral approach desirable.

Posterolateral Approach

A high thigh tourniquet is applied and the patient is turned prone or semi-prone with the affected limb uppermost. A straight longitudinal incision is made along the skin depression that overlies the back of the fibula and deepened between the peroneal muscles and gastrocnemius and soleus to expose the posterior border bone. Flexor hallucis longus is stripped subperiosteally off the interosseous surface of the fibula to expose interosseous membrane (*Fig. 46.23*). The tibialis posterior is stripped from the interosseous membrane to expose the tibia.

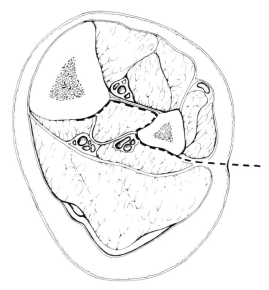

Fig. 46.23. Posterolateral approach to tibial shaft. This transverse section through the leg shows the access to the lateral and posterior surface of the tibia.

In this approach care must be taken to keep close to the fibula and avoid damage to the peroneal vessels, but provided that dissection remains between tibialis posterior and interosseous membrane the posterior tibial neurovascular bundle is not endangered. Once the tibia has been identified the distal three-quarters of its posterior surface are readily exposed by subperiosteal dissection.

At the end of surgery a suction drain is placed in the deepest part of the wound, the muscles are allowed to fall back into place and the fascia and skin are sutured.

A padded plaster-of-Paris backslab is applied over dressings, to keep the foot up to the right angle. The leg is elevated for 48–72 hours.

Complications

Swelling may be considerable after this procedure but is usually adequately controlled by high elevation of the foot.

THE ANKLE

Surface Anatomy

Unless obscured by oedema the bony contours of the ankle and hindfoot are usually easy to identify.

The tip of the medial malleolus is the lowest bony prominence on the inner side of the ankle and its anterior margin can be followed upwards to where it forms the slightly rounded upper bony margin of the ankle joint in front.

The lateral malleolus lies lower and more posteriorly than does the medial, a point to be remembered when drilling a screw from the lower fibula into the tibia just above the ankle mortice. The Achilles tendon passes in the midline posteriorly from the calf muscles to its insertion into the calcaneum. Between it and the lateral malleolus lies a small flat fat pad, but in the interval between the tendon and the medial malleolus lie the tendon of the flexor hallucis longus, the posterior tibial neurovascular bundle and the tendons of extensor digitorum longus and tibialis posterior.

This last grooves the back surface of the medial malleolus and may be damaged by an incision carried deeply behind or below the bone.

Indications for Surgery

Exploration of the joint may be required for:
1. Open reduction and internal fixation of displaced malleolar fractures, for ligament repair, or for the repair of the ruptured Achilles tendon after injury.
2. The removal of a loose body in the joint after talar dome fracture.
3. Synovial biopsy.
4. Arthrodesis of a painful arthritic joint or unstable joint from paralytic disorders.

Preoperative anteroposterior and lateral radiographs of good quality are essential before surgery is undertaken on the joint.

Approaches

After trauma a direct approach to a malleolar fracture usually gives adequate access but occasionally an extended posteromedial approach is required to inspect the back of the lower tibia.

Limited access to the ankle joint can be obtained anteromedially, but for wide exposure and inspection of the joint an anterolateral or a lateral approach after transverse division of the lower fibula is best.

Internal Fixation of a Fracture of the Malleolus

Most isolated fractures of the lateral malleolus can be managed adequately by closed methods as can many such fractures with associated ligament rupture; if talar shift persists after closed manipulation, fixation of the fibula and/or medial ligament repair may be needed.

Internal fixation of the displaced fracture of the medial malleolus is usually advised in adults and allows early remobilization. Bimalleolar fractures of the ankle may be difficult to reduce or control by plaster cast, and may require open reduction and internal fixation for satisfactory results.

The more complex injuries in which the inferior tibiofibular joint is disrupted and those in which the distal end of the tibia is fractured into the ankle joint, may also require open reduction and internal fixation, but surgery can be taxing and prolonged and should only be undertaken by the expert.

Medial Approach

Good access for treatment of a fracture of the medial malleolus is obtained from a gently curved longitudinal incision convex forwards centred on the base of the medial malleolus. The incision is deepened down to the periosteum and the skin and soft tissue swept back as a single flap to expose the fat at the anteromedial corner of the ankle joint, the medial surface and tip of the malleolus. The long saphenous vein and nerve course at the upper end of the incision and the tendon of tibialis posterior at its lower.

The fracture site is identified, the malleolar fragment gently disimpacted downwards so that inturned periosteum can be cleared, the fracture surfaces are cleaned and the underlying surface of the talus inspected for damage.

The fracture is reduced and held in apposition by a Tulloch Brown clamp or by a bone awl or Kirschner wire drilled across the fracture site. The fracture is stabilized with one or two screws inserted along prepared tracks, drilled from the tip of the medial malleolus upwards parallel and close to the articular surface (*Fig.* 46.24).

If the fracture of the medial malleolus is so comminuted that only a poor hold can be obtained on the bone by a screw, two longitidinal Kirschner wires, supplemented by a tension-absorbing band, may be used.

A check radiograph confirms that the metal has not penetrated the articular surface of the ankle joint.

The wound is closed in layers and a dry dressing and cottonwool and crêpe bandage applied. A plaster-of-Paris backslab to hold the foot at the right angle is then applied over the bandage.

Postoperative Care

The limb is elevated on a pillow and the foot of the bed is raised for the first 24–36 hours.

The dressings are then reduced and the cast removed daily to allow active remobilization. When a functional range of movement has been restored the patient is discharged with partial weight bearing on crutches.

Full weight bearing is allowed when bone union is confirmed on X-ray examination.

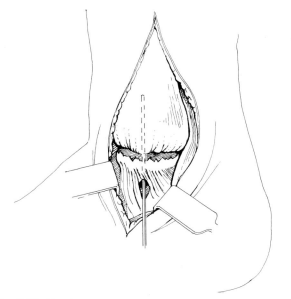

Fig. 46.24. Fixation of fracture of medial malleolus. The periosteum should be cleared and fracture reduced before the drill is inserted.

Posteromedial Approach

This exposure allows inspection of the posterior aspect of the lower tibia and back of the ankle joint.

The incision is placed vertically midway between the Achilles tendon and posterior border of the tibia and curves forwards below the medial malleolus.

It is deepened carefully to develop the interval between the flexor hallucis longus and the neurovascular bundle which is gently retracted medially to expose the back of the joint and lower quarter of the tibial shaft (*Fig.* 46.25).

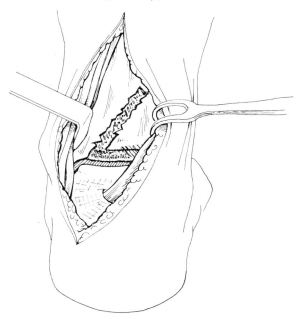

Fig. 46.25. Posteromedial approach to the lower tibia and ankle joint. The neurovascular bundle has been retracted medially.

Lateral Approach

The lateral malleolus and lower fibular shaft are exposed by a mid-lateral vertical incision deepened down to the periosteum. Avoid damage to the peroneal tendons which lie behind the malleolus. Fracture reduction is often easier if the foot is firmly everted and externally rotated during the manipulation. The fracture is stabilized by an axial screw or Rush pin or by two oblique cortical screws. A laterally placed buttress plate with at least two screws above and below the fracture site gives the best stabilization.

Repair of the Ruptured Achilles Tendon

Fresh ruptures may be repaired through a short posterolateral approach, while access for treatment of a long-standing injury may need a longer incision proximally into the calf.

The limb is exsanguinated and a tourniquet applied around the thigh. The patient is placed prone with pillows supporting the pelvis and shoulders.

The limb is prepared and draped from just above the knee so as to provide access to the whole back of the leg and the foot covered with a large surgical glove.

The longitudinal incision lateral to the Achilles tendon extends from the musculotendinous junction to the calcaneum, and is deepened into the fibro-fatty tissue on the deep aspect of the tendon. The rupture haematoma is entered and the shredded tendon ends defined and approximated by plantarflexion of the foot (*Figs.* 46.26, 46.27). The tendon is repaired with

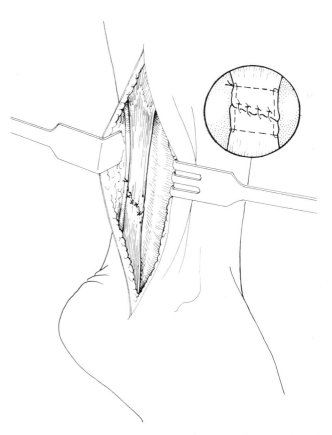

Fig. 46.27. Repair of Achilles tendon. The ankle is plantarflexed and the tendon repaired.

absorbable sutures. Catgut is best avoided as it may produce troublesome local reaction.

A suction drain is left in the dead space and the wound is closed in layers and a dry dressing applied; a padded incomplete plaster-of-Paris cast moulded to the leg from just below the knee to the metatarsal necks is applied and positioned to hold the foot in equinus.

Postoperative Care

The cast is completed when reactionary swelling has subsided and the patient allowed up with crutches non-weight bearing after 72 hours. At 3 weeks the foot is brought up to the right angle, a new cast applied and weight bearing is permitted. At 6 weeks the cast and sutures are removed and active foot and ankle remobilization begin. The heel of the walking shoe is raised 1.5–2 cm and weight bearing on a bare foot is forbidden. Normal shoe wear and bare foot walking are allowed 10–12 weeks from surgery.

Anterior Approach to the Ankle Joint

This approach gives good access for synovial biopsy and for arthrodesis of the ankle joint.

An anterior vertical skin incision is made from 8 cm

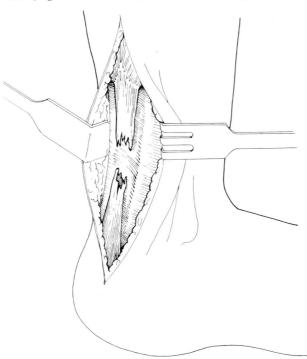

Fig. 46.26. Repair of Achilles tendon. If the ankle is in neutral there is a big gap between the tendon ends.

above to 4 cm below the ankle joint. The deep fascia is divided in the same line as the skin incision.

The interval between extensor hallucis longus and digitorum longus is identifed and developed to expose the front of the lower tibia and ankle joint and neck and body of the talus. The small anterior branches of the malleoli and tarsal arteries are ligated and a self-retaining retractor is inserted to pull extensor hallucis and the neurovascular bundle medially and the other tendons laterally.

Arthrodesis of the Ankle Joint (Charnley)

Although Charnley described a transverse approach for this operation it is suggested that the joint is exposed through the anterior approach described above. The cartilage of the lower tibia and dome of talus is excised with a broad flat osteotome or power saw, to leave two plane surfaces of cancellous bone such that the foot will lie in neutral or no more than 5° of equinus.

Two Steinmann pins are inserted transversely, one 2 cm above the distal end of the tibia and the other across the body of the talus, to allow application of clamps and compression of the cancellous surfaces. The wound is closed in layers and a cottonwool and crêpe bandage applied. The ankle and foot are supported by a carefully moulded backslab that does not foul the clamps.

If clamps are not available a much less stable alternative is to support the arthrodesis by a screw drilled from medial malleolus into the body of the talus.

Postoperatively the leg is elevated for 48 hours until reactionary swelling is subsiding. If clamps have been applied the wing nuts are snugged as necessary (initially every day) to keep the pins slightly bowed.

A new below-knee walking plaster-of-Paris cast is applied at 4 weeks and the clamps and pins withdrawn, and this cast is retained until there is clinical and X-ray evidence of sound bone union.

THE FOOT

Surgery for Disorders of the First Metatarsophalangeal Joint

Surgical procedures are undertaken on this joint for symptoms arising as a result of hallux valgus, hallux rigidus or as a part of a surgical programme for the forefoot problems of rheumatoid arthritis. Patients with hallux rigidus complain of pain localized to the first metatarsophalangeal joint, while those with hallux valgus also complain of bunion pressure symptoms, metatarsalgia and foot appearance.

Surgeons differ in the procedures that they favour on this joint, but the following should be considered.

1. Bunion removal alone will provide relief of symptoms for a short time only, and should be reserved for the more elderly patient with local pressure symptoms.

2. Keller's excision arthroplasty will provide good relief of bunion or joint symptoms, but will increase metatarsalgia, and the toe after this procedure tends to be shortened and floppy.

3. Osteotomy of the first metatarsal allows correction of toe deformity, but a period of immobilization in plaster-of-Paris is necessary after surgery.

4. Arthrodesis can be undertaken however severe the deformity, and is a good salvage procedure following other unsuccessful surgery. The angle at which the joint is stiffened must be carefully chosen, as the choice of shoe heel height will be restricted after surgery.

Surgery for disorders of this joint is undertaken through a dorsomedial incision, 6 cm in length parallel to and about 1 cm medial to the extensor hallucis longus tendon. The incision is deepened through all layers to the base of the proximal phalanx and the head and neck of the first metatarsal. Care is taken to avoid the dorsal branch of the digital nerve.

The full thickness of tissues including the adventitious bursa of the bunion is dissected off the exostosis to expose the head of the first metatarsal; the bursa is not excised as this may damage the blood supply to the medial skin.

Keller's Arthroplasty

The proximal one-third of the proximal phalanx is cleared of soft tissues and the flexor hallucis longus tendon is retracted away from the base of bone.

The exostosis on the first metatarsal head, the margin of which is visible on the articular face of the bone, is excised and osteophytes trimmed from the metatarsal head. The proximal one-third of the proximal phalanx is removed to leave a smooth plane joint surface.

The tendon of extensor hallucis longus is Z-lengthened if it seems tight. Gentle traction is applied along the toe and the capsule; adjacent soft tissues and skin are sutured.

The toe is dressed and a cottonwool and crêpe bandage applied to hold the toe in the corrected position.

This bulky bandage and the sutures are removed 3 weeks from surgery and intrinsic muscle re-education begun. The toe will take about 8 weeks to stabilize and may need to be strapped in varus during this period. An open shoe should be worn.

Mitchell Osteotomy

This operation will achieve lasting correction of hallux valgus, and is to be preferred particularly in the younger patient, in those with varus of the first metatarsal and those in whom the first metatarsophalangeal joint is supple.

The operation allows correction of valgus and leaves the toe of normal length and stability.

The dorsal medial approach is as described above, but the joint capsule opened by a distally based dorsal

Y-shaped incision. The medial side of the metatarsal head is cleared of capsule and periosteum and the exostosis excised from the side of the metatarsal head (*Fig.* 46.28). Two holes are drilled vertically 1 cm

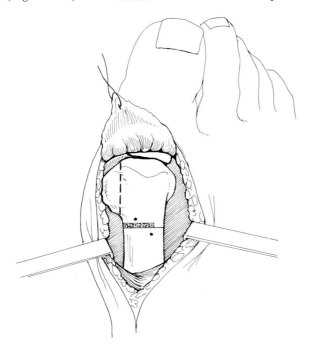

Fig. 46.28. First metatarsal osteotomy. The drill holes and the bone to be removed are shown.

apart through the neck of the metatarsal, the proximal to the lateral and the distal to the medial side of the bone. About 4 mm of the metatarsal neck are removed by a transverse osteotomy between the holes, leaving a lateral spike on the distal fragment. The head is displaced laterally so that the spike locks against the proximal fragment and a suture passed through the two holes secures the osteotomy, but care is taken neither to angle nor to displace the metatarsal head dorsally (*Fig.* 46.29).

The soft tissues are carefully sutured, the toe dressed and splinted in a few degrees of varus and plantarflexion. A protective plaster-of-Paris cast is applied when the swelling has subsided and walking is permitted. The cast is removed at 6 weeks when the osteotomy is clinically and radiologically united and intrinsic muscle re-education begins.

Arthrodesis

This is a valuable operation for the treatment of hallux rigidus and hallux valgus and as a salvage operation after other unsuccessful great toe surgery.

The dorsomedial approach is used. The first metatarsophalangeal joint exostosis is exposed and removed and the joint is dislocated.

The base of the proximal phalanx is removed with a saw to leave a plane vertical cancellous bone sur-

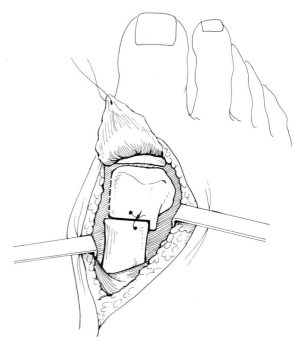

Fig. 46.29. First metatarsal osteotomy. The head and neck have been displaced laterally and the suture inserted and tightened.

face. The subchondral bone is often dense so that at least 0·5–1 cm of bone needs to be removed. The articular surface of the metatarsal head is now removed to leave a plane surface to match that of the proximal phalanx. The angle of this second cut is planned so that the toe lies in 5–20° of dorsiflexion at the joint, and in very slight valgus and medial rotation. The arthrodesis is best stabilized with a malleolar lag screw passed from the metatarsal head obliquely into the proximal phalanx so as to engage on its far cortex. If this is not available, two parallel Kirschner wires are passed obliquely across the arthrodesis.

The wound is closed in layers and a bulky dressing is applied. A below-knee walking plaster-of-Paris cast is applied when the reactionary swelling has subsided and weight bearing is commenced.

The cast is removed at 6 weeks when union has occurred and free walking is permitted.

Clawing of the Toes

Surgical correction of claw toes may be needed in the surgical management of patients with muscle imblance following poliomyelitis or as a result of spina bifida or one of the muscular dystrophies; in these disorders all five toes are usually affected. A number of patients of varied age present without evidence of any recognizable muscular disorder but with clawing of the lateral four toes, and minor if any involvement of the great toe.

Clawing of the toes is usually a painful deformity as the metatarsal heads are subject to great presure, with resultant metatarsalgia, while the skin over the flexed proximal interphalangeal joints and at the tips of the toes develops painful corns as they rub in shoes. While chiropody and attention to shoe comfort may be helpful, surgical correction to the toe deformity is often necessary. Where the toe deformities are manually correctable, tendon transfer is the appropriate treatment. The Girdlestone–Taylor operation is favoured for the lateral toes and the modified Jones' procedure for the great toe.

Where the deformity is limited to the lateral toes and is fixed, as is often the case with idiopathic deformity of adults, corrective interphalangeal arthrodesis is appropriate.

If a single, lateral toe is affected removal of the distal half or the whole of the proximal phalanx is easy and effective.

Arthrodesis of the Interphalangeal Joints of the Toes

It is usually necessary to fuse both interphalangeal joints of the second, third and fourth toes and the proximal interphalangeal joint of the fifth toe. A dorsal ellipse of skin and subcutaneous tissue is excised over the interphalangeal joint. The incision is deepened on each side of the toe to the mid-lateral plane (further plantar extension would jeopardize the neurovascular bundle). The extensor tendon is divided transversely and the collateral ligament of the joint divided at its insertion into the neck of the phalanx.

The joint is flexed to reveal its articular surfaces which are removed with bone cutters and nibblers and the medullary cavity of the phalanx base is entered with an awl, but when the head of the phalanx is excised a central part of the dorsal cortex is left to form a peg; the peg and the hole are then fashioned so that they lock snugly together when the toe is realigned.

The dorsal tissues are sutured with two or three stitches that pick up the extensor tendon as well as the skin, to give additional stability to the arthrodesis. If the straightened toe does not appear stable a Kirschner wire is drilled longitudinally down from toe tip to base of proximal phalanx.

If the toes do not lie dorsiflexed at the metatarsophalangeal joint subcutaneous extensor tenotomy and dorsal capsulotomy are undertaken to correct this deformity and the Kirschner wire is drilled into the metatarsal neck.

Postoperatively the toes and forefoot are bandaged firmly in the corrected position. The legs are elevated for 48–72 hours and plaster-of-Paris cast is then applied.

The plaster-of-Paris and wires are removed after 5 weeks and unprotected weight bearing is begun.

Tendon Transfer (Girdlestone–Taylor)

The tendon of extensor digitorum longus is exposed through a dorsolateral incision extending 3 cm distally from the neck of the metatarsal, and a blunt hook passed down the side of metatarsophalangeal joint to locate the flexor tendons. Hold the tendons with tissue forceps so that they cannot retract and divide them at their insertions, and suture them end-to-side to the extensor tendon (*Fig. 46.30*). The skin is sutured and dressings applied. A piece of orthopaedic felt is placed on top of the forefoot and toes and a well-padded plaster boot extending to the toe tips is applied. Weight bearing is permitted.

The cast is removed at 6 weeks.

Jones' Procedure for Clawing of the Great Toe

Expose the interphalangeal joint of the great toe, and extensor hallucis longus through a short incision centred over the joint. Divide the tendon just proxi-

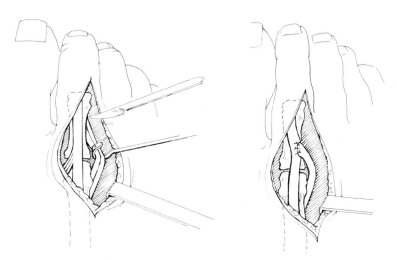

Fig. 46.30. Tendon transfer for claw toes.

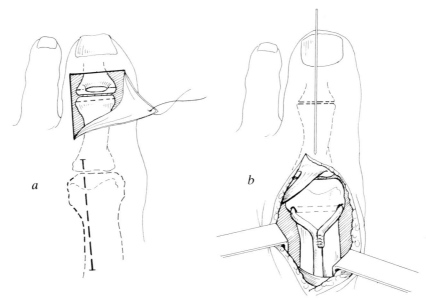

Fig. 46.31. Jones' transfer for clawing of great toe.

mal to the joint and excise the joint articular surfaces. Stabilize the bones with a Kirschner wire passed across the joint (*Fig.* 46.31*a*). Expose the neck at the first metatarsal through a 2-cm dorsomedial incision. Identify and retract the tendon of extensor hallucis brevis and excise carefully as much of the sheath of extensor hallucis longus as is possible through the incision. Use a 0·5-cm drill bit to make a hole from the inferomedial to dorsolateral surface of the metatarsal neck. Withdraw the extensor hallucis longus tendon with a hook into the proximal wound and pass a suture through its end. Pull the suture and tendon through the hole at the metatarsal neck and suture the tendon to itself on the dorsum of the bone (*Fig.* 46.31*b*). Close the skin incision.

Apply a padded below-knee plaster-of-Paris cast. Elevate the foot for 48–72 hours and then permit weight bearing. The plaster-of-Paris and wire are removed at 6 weeks and remobilization begins.

Proximal Phalangectomy .

Expose the proximal phalanx by a dorsal longitudinal incision which is deepened through the extensor tendon. Strip the shaft of the bone subperiosteally and grip the head in a towel clip. Clean the capsule of the proximal interphalangeal joint off the bone and apply traction along the bone to expose the soft tissues of the base of the phalanx. Remove these by sharp dissection and discard the phalanx. Suture the skin.

For 6 weeks postoperatively the toe should be strapped in line between the first and third toes so that it will tend to stiffen in this position.

FURTHER READING

Armstrong J. R. (1949) Excision of the acromion in the treatment of the supraspinator syndrome. *J. Bone Joint Surg.* **31B**, 436.

Bankart A. S. B. (1938) The pathology and treatment of recurrent dislocation of the shoulder joint. *Br. J. Surg.* **26**, 23.

Charnley J. (1951) Compression arthrodesis of the ankle and shoulder. *J. Bone Joint Surg.* **33B**, 180.

Charnley J. (1953) *Compression Arthrodesis.* London, Livingstone.

Charnley J. (1968) *The Closed Treatment of Common Fractures*, 3rd ed. Edinburgh, Churchill Livingstone, p. 247.

Charnley J. and Lowe H. G. (1958) A study of the end results of compression arthrodesis of the knee. *J. Bone Joint Surg.* **40B**, 633.

Crenshaw A. (ed.) (1971) *Campbell's Operative Orthopaedics*, 5th ed. Tourniquet Application, Surgical Technique, Chapters 2, 19. St Louis, Mosby.

Dickson F. D. and Diveley R. L. (1926) Operation for the correction of mild claw foot; the result of infantile paralysis. *JAMA* **87**, 1275.

Geens S., Clayton M. L., Leidholt J. D. et al. (1969) Synovectomy and debridement of the knee in rheumatoid arthritis. *J. Bone Joint Surg.* **51A**, 617.

Harmon P. H. (1945) A simplified surgical approach to the posterior tibia for bone grafting and fibula transference. *J. Bone Joint Surg.* **27**, 496.

Ingliss A. E., Scott W. N., Sculco T. P. et al. (1976) Ruptures of the tendo Achillis. *J. Bone Joint Surg.* **58A**, 990.

Jones R. (1916) The soldier's foot and the treatment of common deformities of the foot. Part II, Claw foot. *Br. Med. J.* **1**, 749.

Keller W. L. (1904) Surgical treatment of bunions and hallux valgus. *N. Y. Med. J.* **80**, 741.

Kocher T. (1911) *Text Book of Operative Surgery*. London, Black.

McLaughlan H. L. (1952) Posterior dislocation of the shoulder. *J. Bone Joint Surg.* **34A**, 584.

Mitchell C. L., Flemington J. L., Allen R. et al. (1958) Osteotomy-bunionectomy for hallux valgus. *J. Bone Joint Surg.* **40A**, 41.

Money B. F. and James J. M. (1976) Recurrent anterior dislocation of the shoulder *J. Bone Joint Surg.* **58A**, 253.

Müller M. E., Allgöwer M. and Willenegger H. (1970) *Manual of Internal Fixation*. Berlin, Springer.

O'Donoghue D. H. (1950) Surgical treatment of fresh injuries to the major ligaments of the knee. *J. Bone Joint Surg.* **32A**, 721.

Osborne G. (1967) In: Lloyd Roberts G. C. (ed.) *Clinical Surgery. Vol. 13, Orthopaedics*. London, Butterworths, p. 440.

Osmond-Clarke H. (1948) Habitual dislocation of the shoulder: the Putti–Platt operation. *J. Bone Joint Surg.* **30B**, 19.

Peebles R. E. and Margo M. K. (1978) Function after patellectomy. *Clin. Orthop.* **132**, 180.

Phemister D. B. (1947) Treatment of un-united fractures by onlay grafts without screws on the fixation and without breaking down of the fibrous nerves *J. Bone Joint Dis.* **29**, 946.

Ratliff A. H. C. (1959) Compression arthrodesis of the ankle. *J. Bone Joint Surg.* **41B**, 524.

Saunders R. (1973) The tourniquet: instrument or weapon. *The Hand* **5**, 119.

Smillie I. S. (1970) *Injuries of the Knee Joint*, 4th ed. Edinburgh, Livingstone.

Taylor R. G. (1951) The treatment of claw toes by multiple transfers of flexor into extensor tendons. *J. Bone Joint Surg.* **33B**, 539.

Thompson J. E. (1918) Anatomical methods of approach in operations on the long bones of the extremity. *Ann. Surg.* **68**, 309.

Trickey E. L. (1968) Rupture of the posterior cruciate ligament of the knee *J. Bone Joint Surg.* **50B**, 334.

Wilson J. N. (1966) The management of infection after Küntscher nailing of the femur. *J. Bone Joint Surg.* **48B**, 112.

Wilson J. N. (ed.) (1976) *Watson-Jones Fractures and Joint Injuries*, 5th ed. Edinburgh, Churchill Livingstone.

Chapter forty-seven

The Hip Joint

H. E. D. Griffiths

The majority of hip surgery can be carried out using three fundamental incisions; these are the antero-lateral or Smith–Petersen incision, the lateral approach to the upper femur and the posterior or southern approach.

Anterolateral or Smith–Petersen Incision

The patient is placed on the table in the supine position with a sandbag under the buttock.

Skin Incision (Fig. 47.1)
The skin incision is made along the line of the iliac crest about 1 cm distal to the inferior lip, starting posteriorly about the middle of the crest and passing anteriorly to just short of the anterior superior iliac spine. It is then carried distally along the line of the anterior border of the tensor fascia lata muscle for a distance of about 12 cm.

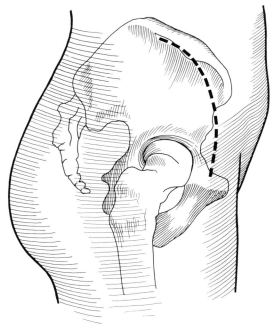

Fig. 47.1. Anterolateral approach to the hip joint. Skin incision.

FIRST LAYER
The fascia is incised over the tensor fascia lata muscle down to the bone in the region of the iliac crest in the line of the skin incision. This deepening is continued anteriorly, then distally, separating the tensor

fascia lata muscle from the sartorius muscle and preserving the lateral femoral cutaneous nerve, which lies on the medial side of this approach (*Fig. 47.2*).

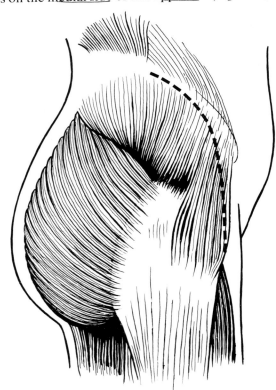

Fig. 47.2. Anterolateral approach to the hip joint. Muscle detachment.

SECOND LAYER
The incision is continued deeper between the ilio-psoas and the gluteus minimus muscles, taking the latter off the dorsum ilii, thereby exposing the rectus femoris muscle attachments to the anterior inferior iliac spine and its reflected head over the superior aspect of the hip joint capsule. These origins are detached, completing the exposure of the outer lip of the acetabulum, and the hip joint capsule (*Fig. 47.3*).

Lateral Approach to the Upper Femur
The patient is in the supine position. Radiographic control may be needed for any procedure carried out through this approach, in which case the patient should be on an orthopaedic table.

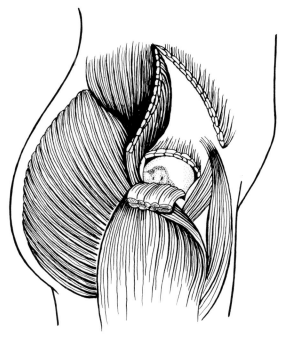

Fig. 47.3. Anterolateral approach to the hip joint. Exposure of hip joint.

Skin Incision

A mid-lateral incision is made in the skin along the line of the femur extending from the tip of the greater trochanter distally for 14–18 cm (*Fig.* 47.4).

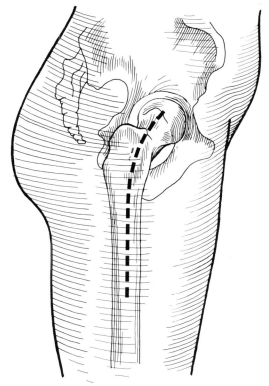

Fig. 47.4. Lateral approach to the upper femur. Skin incision.

FIRST LAYER

The fascia lata is incised in the same line as the skin, exposing the vastus lateralis muscle, applied to the lateral aspect of the femur (*Fig.* 47.5).

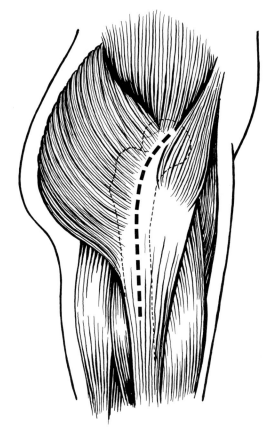

Fig. 47.5. Lateral approach to the upper femur. Muscle incision.

SECOND LAYER

An incision is now made in the vastus lateralis near its attachment to the trochanteric ridge and the intertrochanteric line. It is carried from anterior to posterior, about 1 cm distal to these landmarks until the muscle is interrupted at its femoral attachment by the passage of gluteus maximus fascia from above downwards into the femur. The incision is then carried down the line of the femur, through the fascial layer of the vastus. The muscle belly is then detached from the femur with a periosteal elevator and any bleeding from branches of the perforating vessels is easily controlled with diathermy. The curtain of the vastus so elevated is raised and can be retracted with bone spikes to expose the lateral aspect of the femur (*Fig.* 47.6).

This approach can be extended proximally by extending the skin incision in a slightly curved fashion proximally and anteriorly, deepening between tensor fascia lata and gluteus medius muscles, and then extending the second layer incision anteriorly along the intertrochanteric line. The approach to the an-

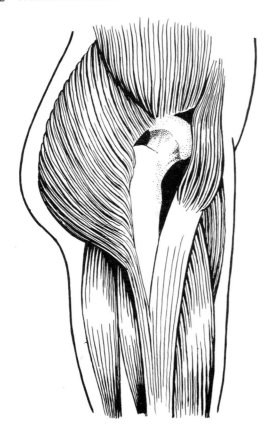

Fig. 47.6. Lateral approach to the upper femur. Femur exposed.

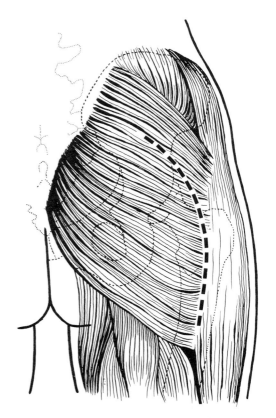

Fig. 47.7. Posterior approach to the hip joint. Skin and muscle incision.

terior aspect of the femoral neck and lesser trochanter is more complete.

Posterior or Southern Approach

The patient is placed in the mid-lateral position with two table supports, one in the middle of the lumbar spine posteriorly and the second against the symphysis pubis anteriorly. The placing of this anterior prop can be crucial, for if it is too low it interferes with proper flexion of the hip and this limits the ability both to dislocate the hip and to reduce a prosthesis. If it is too high it tends to press on the abdominal contents and embarrass the anaesthetic.

Skin Incision

The skin incision is made along the upper 5 cm of the femoral shaft in the mid-lateral line until the tip of the greater trochanter is reached. The incision then sweeps posteriorly over the buttock towards the posterior superior iliac spine for about 9 cm (Fig. 47.7).

FIRST LAYER

The fascia lata is divided over the upper end of the femur until the gluteal bursa is opened. The fibrous layer overlying gluteus maximus is then incised by continuing this incision posteriorly in the line of the skin incision. The horizontal fibres of gluteus maximus are separated by a sweep of the closed scissors, exposing the pad of fat overlying the short rotators and the sciatic nerve. A vessel is usually encountered just deep to the muscle at this point, which requires control with diathermy.

SECOND LAYER

The floor of the gluteal bursa is incised with scissors immediately posterior to the greater trochanter. The soft tissues here, including the fat pad, are then removed by a sweep of a dry swab from lateral to medial and in this manoeuvre the branches of the cruciate and trochanteric anastomotic vessels are laid bare, presenting themselves for diathermy. More medially the sciatic nerve is found embedded in the fat and this is preserved from damage (Fig. 47.8). The fat pad may be excised with scissors at the margin of the sciatic nerve, but this can cause troublesome bleeding and if it is not too voluminous it may be retained and retracted over the nerve as a protection.

THIRD LAYER

The short rotator muscles, so cleaned, are now divided with diathermy in the line of the acetabular

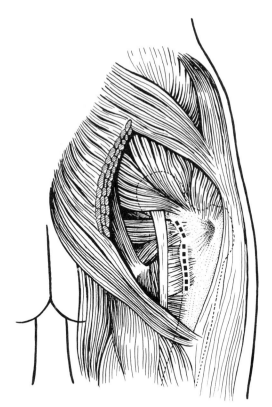

Fig. 47.8. Posterior approach to the hip joint showing exposure of sciatic nerve.

margin and about 1 cm distal from it. This division may include piriformis tendon superiorly and the upper 1 cm of the quadratus femoris muscle inferiorly. The latter cut often causes some troublesome bleeding from the cruciate anastomotic vessels. The hip joint capsule is exposed deep to these muscles.

OPERATIVE MANAGEMENT OF CONGENITAL DISLOCATION OF THE HIP

Open Reduction of the Hip Joint

Via the Smith–Petersen incision the capsule of the hip joint is exposed. Medial retraction of the neurovascular bundle reveals the psoas muscle and its tendon. This can be lengthened in a Z fashion, if required. The capsule is opened via a T-shaped incision, with the cross-piece made parallel to the acetabular margin and the vertical component along the anterosuperior border of the femoral neck. The femoral head is dislocated anteriorly through the defect, and the ligamentum teres is excised. The shape and size of the head and the acetabulum are noted. The presence or absence of an inturned limbus in the acetabular roof is also noted. The incision of the capsule from the acetabular margin is continued inferiorly until the inferior ligament of the acetabulum is divided. A small capsular vessel may require

diathermy at this point. This move allows the head to get into the most inferior part of the acetabulum. Any fat pad in the unoccupied depths of the acetabulum is removed with scissors.

The head is now reduced into this deepest part of the acetabulum by passing it under the limbus. The degree of internal rotation of the leg required to make the articular surface disappear into the acetabulum is noted and this is approximately the degree of anteversion of the femoral neck. It may be possible to evert the limbus, if it is inturned, by incising it anteriorly and posteriorly, and then gently levering it out as a lip to the acetabulum, by blunt dissection. The capsule is closed after excising redundant corners of the flaps. After wound closure the leg is immobilized by application of a double hip spica with the affected leg held in the desired position of internal rotation and the plaster will be completed with the knee bent to 90°. Extension to the knee only is required on the normal side.

Rotation Osteotomy (*Fig. 47.9*)

An osteotomy is performed in the intertrochanteric region to correct the degree of anteversion mentioned above, and to ensure that the head remains facing into the acetabulum when the child walks with the toe pointing to the front. The lateral approach to the femur is made with the child lying supine and the thigh supported on a small sandbag. The incision

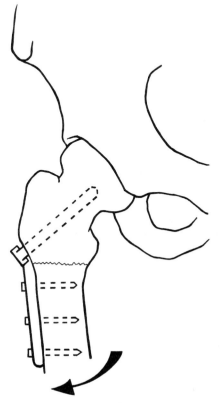

Fig. 47.9. Rotation osteotomy.

in the vastus lateralis is usually made in the line of the femur, rather than lifting the muscle as a curtain, which is described above. The periosteum is incised in the same line, and bone spikes are placed subperiosteally round the femur. A Coventry screw of appropriate length, 2–4 cm, is placed up the femoral neck over a guide wire inserted under the guidance of palpation of the femoral neck. A two- or three-hole plate is then bent to the line of the femur, avoiding varus or valgus, and is loosely bolted to the screw. The planned rotation is marked on the femur with an osteotome. The osteotomy is carried out with multiple drilling and completed with an osteotome. The lower fragment is rotated laterally through the same degree as the estimated anteversion and the plate is then screwed to the femoral shaft in this new position. After layer closure of the wound, the femur is immobilized in a single hip spica for a period of 4 weeks.

Pemberton's Acetabuloplasty

This is one of the commonly used methods of acetabular reconstruction, and is applicable to hips in which there has been a failure of proper development of the acetabular roof between the ages of 18 months and 12 years. The child is placed supine with a sandbag under the appropriate buttock, the upper part of the Smith–Petersen approach is used exposing the outer table of the iliac blade as far as the hip joint capsule, and the anterior inferior iliac spine. The iliac crest epiphysis is then dissected off the anterior half or two-thirds of the iliac crest, taking with it the abdominal and the iliacus muscles.

Trethowan bone spikes are inserted into the greater sciatic notch outside and inside the pelvis. The osteotomy is marked out with a small straight osteotome and extends from just above the anterior inferior iliac spine through the outer and inner tables of the pelvis, extending backwards, dipping inferiorly before it reaches the greater sciatic notch to meet the cartilage of the triradiate epiphysis of the pelvis (*Fig.* 47.10). The osteotomy is performed with a 1·5-cm curved osteotome, cutting first the outer then the inner tables and joining these cuts through the body of the pelvic bone. At the point when the osteotomy cuts disappear beneath the psoas muscle on the inner side, and the gluteal muscle on the outer side, the cut curves downwards so as to avoid breaking into the pelvic rim. The point at which the osteotomy reaches the triradiate cartilage is a matter of conjecture, but once the leaf of pelvic roof becomes pliable on trial bending down, a broad curved osteotome is advanced into the cut with gentle blows until the leaf descends, relatively easily, with the spreading forceps. This displacement is maintained by wedging a segment of bone, taken from the iliac crest in the region of the anterior superior iliac spine, into the gap. It is held by gouging shallow gutters in the cut surfaces of the osteotomy (*Fig.* 47.11).

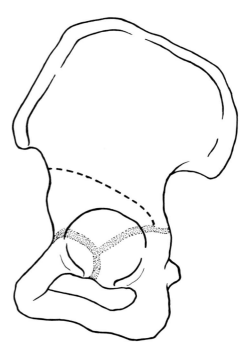

Fig. 47.10. Pemberton acetabuloplasty. Line of osteotomy.

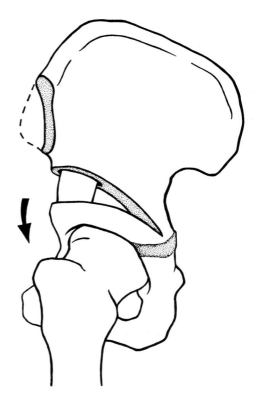

Fig. 47.11. Pemberton acetobuloplasty. Final position.

In opening the osteotomy it is essential that the leaf, consisting of the acetabular roof, should bend downwards and forwards, rather than the main body of the pelvic blade being forced upwards. To allow this to happen requires the femoral head to be removed from under the acetabular roof. It will require, in some cases, the opening of the hip joint capsule to allow the head to be subluxed inferiorly, thereby giving room for the acetabular roof to descend. The turning forwards and downwards ensures cover of the femoral head in the anteverted position, and there is no clear indication for rotation osteotomy following this operation. Closure of the wound is performed by sewing the epiphysis back to the iliac blade with a trocar pointed needle, the suture also picking up the abductor muscles and overlying fascia in one big bite. The remainder of the wound is closed in the usual manner. A plaster-of-Paris spica is applied for 2 months and then free mobilization is allowed with walking.

Salter's Pelvic Osteotomy

This is another operation for the acetabular side of a dysplastic hip, overcoming the objection that the Pemberton procedure deforms the acetabular roof. In this procedure the whole of the acetabulum is moved anteriorly and laterally over the dome of the femoral head to cover the defect in the acetabular development. The surgical approach is exactly as in the Pemberton's operation. Once the bone spikes are in the greater sciatic notch, they are manipulated to produce enough room to allow the passage of a Gigli saw, without damage to the superior gluteal vessels and nerve. The osteotomy extends from the greater sciatic notch forwards to a point just superior to the anterior inferior iliac spine.

Once again, to ensure that the acetabular roof moves forwards and downwards it is sometimes helpful to open the capsule to remove the femoral head pressure from the roof. In addition, the movement is best performed by grasping the iliac fragment with tongue forceps and pulling it forwards and downwards, rotating it about the symphysis pubis and steadying the remnant of the pelvis with the other hand. The new position is held by a wedge of bone cut from the crest in the region of the anterior superior iliac spine. In contrast to the Pemberton operation, the two-dimensional displacement causes the wedge to be unstable. It is secured by transfixing the osteotomy and the wedge with two or three Kirschner wires, passing them upwards through the acetabular lip, the wedge and the main body of the ilium. These are bent over as they protrude from the hip joint capsule and cut off. This prevents the wires migrating upwards into the iliac blade. Wound closure is carried out as in the Pemberton procedure. A plaster-of-Paris spica is applied and retained for 8 weeks.

Bosworth Shelf Operation

In the adolescent and young adult, this operation has proved successful in averting progressive subluxation in a hip in which acetabular dysplasia is established.

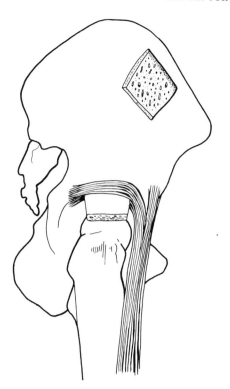

Fig. 47.12. Bosworth shelf operation.

The approach is via the Smith–Petersen incision, with the patient lying supine and the hip joint supported with a small sandbag. The iliac blade is stripped to expose the hip joint capsule, including the straight and reflected heads of the rectus femoris muscle. The aim is to insert a shelf of bone, corticocancellous in type, into the side of the pelvis, just above the articular surface of the hip joint, directing the free margin downwards and forwards. First, a trapezium of bone, slightly wider at one end than the other, and corticocancellous in thickness, is cut from the outer table of the iliac blade. It should measure a minimum of 5 cm long and 4 cm wide. Second, the superior articular margin of the acetabulum is located by opening the hip joint. About 0·5 cm above this an osteotome is driven medially and slightly posteriorly into the pelvis. A slight wedge of bone is then cut out to allow room for the insertion of the graft. The depth of insertion is about 1–2 cm. Third, the reflected head of rectus femoris is dissected free from the hip joint capsule and from the acetabular margin, but the proximal attachment is retained. To get the tendon free enough to allow the graft to pass underneath it, it may be necessary to separate it some way distally from the straight head of the muscle. The narrow width of the graft is then passed underneath the reflected head, cortical side downwards for ease of passage over the capsular tissue, and inserted into the defect made in the side of the pelvis (Fig. 47.12). Firm fixation may be assisted by packing fragments of cancellous bone into the defect, as well as the shelf.

The reflected head ensures the close application of the graft to the superior hip joint capsule. Wound closure is then carried out.

Weight bearing is best deferred for 6 weeks to avoid excessive strain on the graft in the early phase of incorporation. It is not essential for the hip to be immobilized, unless the stability of the graft is in doubt.

Pinning of Slipped Upper Femoral Epiphysis

In this condition the femoral epiphysis slips posteriorly and inferiorly, resulting in the neck of the femur moving superiorly and anteriorly while the capital epiphysis remains in the acetabulum (*Fig. 47.13*). The displacement is a slow one and is not

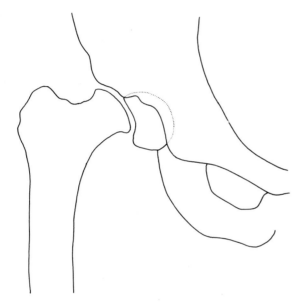

Fig. 47.13. Slipped femoral epiphysis.

usually amenable to any manipulative correction, either gradual or acute. The policy is to pin the epiphysis in the best position and await fusion of the epiphysis. The exposure is via the lateral upper femoral approach, and through this the outer aspect of the upper femoral cortex is exposed. Three pins, either guide wires, Moore's or Newman's pins, are inserted up the neck of the femur and into the epiphysis across the growth plate (*Fig. 47.14*). X-ray control is essential and an image intensifier is best, as one is able to advance the pins to a perfect position just short of the articular cartilage, to get the best grip on the epiphysis, without having to take two films every time a pin is moved. If the slip is marked, the most posterior of the pins may well have to pass outside the posterior part of the femoral neck, before entering the capital epiphysis. The passage of the pins can be difficult, as the bone is rather hard and it may be easier to insert them with a power drill. As the

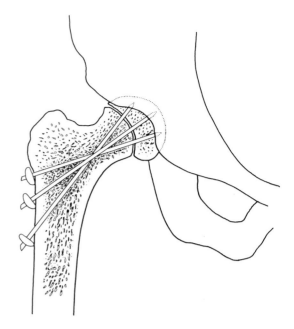

Fig. 47.14. Pinning of slipped femoral epiphysis.

condition may possibly be under a systemic endocrine influence, the effect of non-weight bearing may put the good hip under stress and cause it, in its turn, to slip. Hence it is acceptable to pin the contralateral femoral epiphysis prophylactically, and then in the convalescent phase the patient can be allowed to mobilize bearing full weight on this good hip. The pins are retained until there is radiological evidence of fusion across the upper femoral growth plate.

FRACTURES OF THE UPPER END OF THE FEMUR

Intertrochanteric Fractures

These are fixed with an implant angled at 135° with a screw nail up the neck of the femur attached to which, in the manner of a sleeve, is a plate of varying length. Most of these fractures can be reduced to a normal shaft neck angle of 135°. A more varus position may be unavoidable and thus a 125° appliance may be appropriate. The dynamic hip screw is an effective appliance, having slightly more scope than the Jewett fixed angle nail and plate, particularly when dealing with a very comminuted intertrochanteric fracture (*Fig. 47.15*).

The method of insertion is very similar to that for the nail and plate, with the patient placed on an orthopaedic table and using image intensification X-ray control. Reduction of the fracture is achieved by traction on the leg with some internal rotation, and the legs are then held in the foot rest. The leg is prepared and draped, following which the upper surface of the lateral aspect of the femur is exposed as described previously. The guide wire is inserted

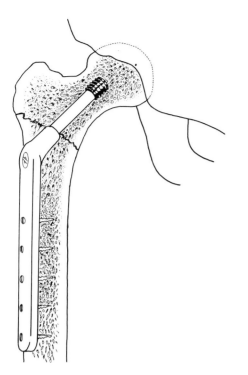

Fig. 47.15. Inter trochanteric fracture. Fixation using dynamic screw and plate.

up the neck of the femur in a central position via a template guide, which ensures an entry angle of 135°. It can be done either by hand or preferably on a power tool. It is advanced to within 1 mm of the subarticular bone margin under X-ray control and its interosseous length is measured. A dynamic hip screw 5 mm shorter than that is selected. The wire is now used as a guide for the special drill which is inserted up to the depth calculated for the nail length, making not only a channel for the screw itself, but a wider proximal channel to accommodate the sleeve of the plate. The screw is now inserted over the guide wire and checked in position with a radiograph. The wire is withdrawn and a four- or six-hole plate is slid over the base of the screw. The plate is attached to the shaft of the femur with screws and compression can be applied to the appliance by using a special small screw in the base of the main screw nail. The wound is closed by tacking down the vastus lateralis flap, inserting a drain in the sump deep to the fascia lata and finally that layer being closed with interrupted sutures. The patient is allowed to mobilize as soon as the general state permits and if any impaction occurs at the fracture site, the sliding nature of the screw allows it to take place in the correct line.

Subcapital Fracture of the Femur

This fracture is intracapsular and the head of the femur may well have an imperilled blood supply. An adequate fixation of the fracture ensures the best chance for the restitution of that blood supply and union of the fracture. In the case of the impacted undisplaced fracture it is sufficient to pin the head with a Smith–Petersen pin, or some simple screw fixation.

The patient is placed on an orthopaedic table with the affected leg slightly internally rotated. Under X-ray control a guide wire is inserted through the skin and deep tissues, and by palpation at the point of the wire, the lateral aspect of the femur is penetrated about 2 cm below the trochanteric ridge and at the midpoint between the anterior and posterior aspects of the shaft. The guide wire is then passed up the femoral neck and, under X-ray control, the point is brought to within 2–3 mm of the articular surface of the femoral head. The amount of wire in the bone is then measured by use of another guide wire placed against the extruded part. A Smith–Petersen pin is chosen, measuring the equivalent of the intraosseous wire, plus 1 cm to allow for some nail to remain outside the femoral shaft.

A small skin incision is then made where the guide wire penetrates the skin, and a Smith–Petersen pin of appropriate length is hammered home under X-ray control, to verify that it comes to rest in the same position as the guide wire.

Displaced fractures of the femoral neck require reduction before fixation is attempted. This is achieved by placing the patient on the orthopaedic table and manipulating the affected leg before it is tied into place. This manipulation consists of a gentle traction and internal rotation of the leg. Heavy traction is contra-indicated as it tends to over-reduce the fracture. Perfect reduction is difficult to achieve and the closed method can only achieve as good a result as the posterior neck cortex comminution allows. An open reduction may be attempted via a proximal extension of the lateral approach between the tensor fascia lata and gluteus medius muscles, the hip joint capsule being opened in the same line.

Pinning of this fracture is performed via an open approach to the lateral aspect of the femur. Guide wires are then inserted in a cross-wise fashion and over them Garden or Howse screws are inserted to give a firm fixation of the fracture (*Fig.* 47.16). After layer closure of the wound with suction drain, mobilization is immediately recommended. Check radiographs at 2 weeks will indicate the success of the fixation as, if there is any serious defect, it will be revealed by this time, with a redisplacement of the fracture. Undisplaced impacted fractures are satisfactorily treated also by this method of fixation.

There are indications for treatment of displaced subcapital fractures by femoral head replacement. Patients over the age of 70 are suitable candidates and in younger patients medical reasons may support replacement as being a better solution than the more problematic method of pinning the femoral head. Replacement is also indicated if pinning should fail for any reason.

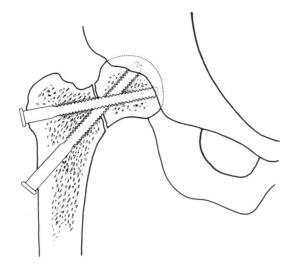

Fig. 47.16. Fixation of subcapital fracture of femur using screws.

The posterior approach is used with the patient lying in the mid-lateral position. After opening the capsule in a T fashion, the femoral neck is dislocated by internal rotation of the leg. The femoral head is removed from the acetabulum by impaling it with a 'corkscrew' and levering it out of the acetabulum with the help of a hip skid inserted inferiorly within the capsule. The femoral head is then measured and an appropriate prosthesis is selected. Two types are in common use, the Austin Moore and the Thompson prosthesis.

The Austin Moore prosthesis requires an intact calcar, sawn off about 1–2 cm proximal to the lesser trochanter. The cut is made at an angle, dictated by a template, with a mechanical reciprocating saw or a small hand pad saw. The face of the cut should look slightly anteriorly, about 15°. The shaft is then reamed carefully to make an accurate confined channel in the cancellous bone of the neck and shaft. The lateral part of this channel is deepened to the lateral cortex of the femur and greater trochanter in its upper part (and there may even be the need to broach this by use of an osteotome). This allows comfortable seating of the upper part of the prosthesis and spares excessive pressure on the calcar which may crack under the strain as the prosthesis is hammered home.

Finally the acetabulum is cleared of remnants of the ligamentum teres and synovium. The fit of the head in the acetabulum is checked and if correct the prosthesis is inserted down the shaft of the femur and hammered home until it sits on the calcar. Reduction is achieved by flexing the hip in the internally rotated position and then the prosthetic head is pushed into the acetabulum with the hand, or impactor, assisted by gentle external rotation of the leg.

The Thompson prosthesis requires the neck to be sawn off just proximal to the lesser trochanter at the angle dictated by the template or the prosthesis itself. The reaming is a more widespread hollowing of the femoral shaft to accept both the prosthetic stem and the cement. After checking the fit of the prosthesis in both the acetabulum and the femur, and that reduction is possible, the acetabulum is cleared of redundant soft tissue and debris. An obturator may now be placed down the femoral shaft to restrict the distal drift of the cement.

While the bone cement is being mixed by the assistant, a fine polythene catheter is inserted down the reamed femoral shaft. The cement, when ready, is pressed into the shaft with the fingers and thumbs, and blood will be seen to be displaced up the catheter as the pressure in the shaft increases. When the shaft is full of cement, the catheter is removed, the prosthesis inserted and then hammered home, ensuring that about 10° of anteversion is present. Surplus cement is removed, and a curved curette is a valuable instrument to clear the anterior aspect of the femoral neck which is now obscured by the large size of the femoral head. After a pause of about 9 minutes, during which the cement is curing, a reduction is carried out as described for the Austin Moore prosthesis. The capsular remnant is closed, if possible, on the acetabular side. The femoral end of the short rotators has usually failed to survive the dissection to clear the femoral neck and attempt at repair has no great value. The superficial layer of the fascia lata and the fascia over gluteus maximus muscle are then closed. A suction drain is inserted around the prosthesis and is brought out on the outer side of the thigh through the gluteus muscles. Mobilization may be started the following day with standing and walking. Sitting is usually deferred until the sutures are removed.

OSTEOARTHRITIS OF THE HIP

The surgical management of osteoarthritis of the hip falls into two groups, the conservative and the radical. The conservative procedure is McMurray's intertrochanteric osteotomy with internal fixation (*Fig. 47.17*). This operation is reserved for those hips affected with osteoarthritis which retain some joint space, a reasonably spherical head of femur and a range of flexion approaching, or more than, 90°. The operation is performed with the patient supine, supported under the appropriate buttock by a sandbag, but ensuring that anteroposterior X-ray facilities are available. The lateral approach is made to the upper end of the femur, extending proximally for a short way between the gluteus medius and the tensor fascia lata muscles. The area of the anterior intertrochanteric line is cleared of the vastus attachment, in addition to raising the curtain, as described in the lateral approach (p. 710). The lesser trochanter is located by the finger curling over the medial side of the femur and is usually much more posterior than anticipated. A bone spike is pushed through the hip joint capsule at a point above the trochanter and this constitutes

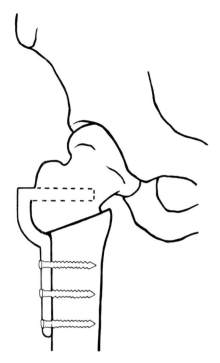

Fig. 47.17. McMurray's intertrochanteric osteotomy with internal fixation.

an aiming point for the osteotomy as well as retracting all the anterior soft tissues.

A broad bone lever is then placed under the femur at intertrochanteric level, acting as a retractor as well as the protector of posterior soft tissues when the osteotomy is carried out. Guide wires are inserted through the greater trochanter and through the lateral aspect of the femur, just below the trochanteric ridge. The former is horizontal and reaches the calcar, marking out the line of the blade of the Müller plate. The latter is oblique and marks the line of the osteotomy. The anteroposterior centring of the wire in the neck is controlled by placing a finger behind the neck to judge the correct line. The position of the wires is checked with anteroposterior radiographs. A Müller plate of appropriate length is selected and inserted along the line of the upper wire and immediately inferior to it. It is not yet hammered fully home.

Next the osteotomy is marked out in the line of the inferior wire, with an osteotome, and this wire is removed. The osteotomy is performed by making multiple drill holes in the area through both cortices, paying particular attention to the calcar region. It is completed with osteotomes; a narrow one is used in the calcar, attacking it from directly anteriorly. A broad osteotome is then driven across the shaft, lateral to medial, completing the cut. The fragments are freed by rotation. The upper fragment may cock up slightly, adopting the position of the flexion contracture. The shaft is displaced medially by the simple expedient of driving home the blade plate up to its

limit. Correction of external rotation deformity may then be made, and the shaft clamped to the plate of the apparatus.

Compression of the osteotomy is now carried out using the Müller apparatus, and some impaction of the shaft in the broad raw area of the upper fragment may take place. This avoids the necessity of cutting sections off either fragment to accommodate the flexion deformity correction. After completing the compression, the plate is screwed to the side of the femur, and the clamp is removed. Suction drainage is instituted before layer closure is carried out. Mobilization may begin immediately, and walking (non-weight bearing) is allowed as soon as discomfort permits. The plate is often quite prominent on the lateral aspect of the hip, and for comfort of the patient removal is recommended once the osteotomy is radiologically soundly united.

The radical approach to the problem of osteoarthritis is that of total hip replacement. There are many prostheses using high-density polyethylene cups and metal femoral heads on stems and two common ones among these are the Charnley (*Fig.* 47.18)

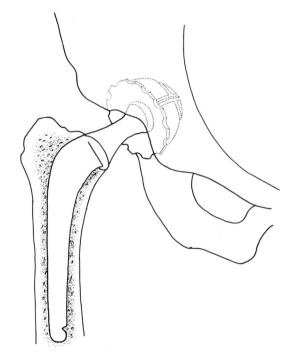

Fig. 47.18. Total hip replacement using Charnley prosthesis.

and the 'D' Series (Zimmer). The posterior approach is the simplest one for this operation, and is carried out with the patient firmly placed in the mid-lateral position on the table. The hip is exposed as previously described and before section of the short rotator a stay suture is placed in the obturator internus tendon to the lateral side of the sciatic nerve. The short rotators being divided, the suture folds the medial bulk of the rotators backwards over the sciatic nerve, thereby adding to its protection. Before the capsule is divided markings are made on the acetabular lip between the inferior gemellus and the quadratus femoris muscle with a diathermy burn. In line with this a companion burn is made in the posterior part of the greater trochanter and these are painted with gentian violet dye which persists throughout the operation. The hip is now dislocated, after division of the capsule, by full flexion in the first instance, gentle internal rotation and backward pressure on the femur via the flexed knee. A line of section in the femoral neck is marked out, being guided by either a trial prosthesis or a special template. This should give a small degree of anteversion in the cut face. The neck is severed using a reciprocating saw in the line of the mark and the head is removed. Redundant soft tissue is cleared from the acetabulum and an adequate view is obtained by retracting the femoral neck using a large bone hook.

Preparation of the acetabulum consists of removing the remains of the articular cartilage and all the soft tissues adherent to it thus producing an irregular articular surface which is stable and which will accept cement to produce satisfactory fixation of the cup. This is achieved by the use of the Charnley sharp spoon, the 'nutmeg grater' reamers and the small acetabular preparing drill. The prepared acetabulum is now measured, using the trial cup, and a choice is made between a small or a large cup with a long posterior wall. The appropriate cup is then placed on an introducer. The final preparation of the acetabulum is carried out using saline to irrigate, thereby cleaning away all the loose bone fragments and finally soaking the acetabulum in Betadine (povidone–iodine) or some other antiseptic solution. The acetabulum is then thoroughly dried and freshly mixed cement is pressed into the acetabulum making sure all the irregularities are evenly coated. The applicator is used to press the cup into position, giving about 10° of anteversion with 40–45° of lateral facing. Excess cement will be seen to ooze round the margin of the cup and this is removed with a spoon. The applicator is now removed from the cup and further cleaning of redundant cement is carried out. The position of the cup can be amended by using the fingers, and when a satisfactory position is achieved, a ball-ended punch is inserted into the cavity of the cup and a few gentle blows of the hammer ensures its proper impaction in the cement. The cup is now left untouched while the cement is setting, care being taken that the femur does not fall back against it, distorting the previously selected position.

When the cement is finally set, attention is then paid to the femoral shaft which is reamed out to accept the stem prosthesis. The 'D' Series has a

shoulder which sits on the appropriately cut calcar, whereas the Charnley, having no rim, may very likely sit within the cement cuff inside the neck. The preparation of the shaft is completed using the Charnley spoon, paying particular attention to hollowing out the bone in the region of the greater trochanter so that sufficient cement may be present round the upper end of the femoral shaft where the bone support is less obvious. The femoral shaft itself is also cleared of effete cancellous spicules which will give insufficient support to the cemented prosthesis. The cavity of the shaft is irrigated with saline to remove blood clot and other debris and the size of the cavity verified so that it will take the femoral component of the prosthesis. Various sizes of the prosthesis are available and a satisfactory one is selected that allows easy insertion into the shaft cavity, which will leave room for an adequate amount of cement and will come to rest easily in a few degrees of anteversion. In order to prevent cement drifting down the femoral shaft and not remaining in the upper part where it can support the prosthesis properly, a plastic stopper is inserted down the shaft to a depth of 14 or 15 cm.

After the final irrigation of the shaft, a fine catheter is placed into it and attached to the sucker. A dry swab is then pressed into the cavity of the shaft to maintain it in a dry, blood-free state until the cement is inserted. The cement is then mixed and when ready is pressed into the cavity, being assisted in its descent down the shaft by the suction exerted through the catheter. When the femoral shaft is full of cement the catheter is removed, and the prosthesis then pressed into the femoral cavity. Pressure is applied in order to achieve the most valgus position possible and about 10–15° of anteversion. Cement is cleared from round the neck of the prosthesis and the acetabulum and when the prosthesis is in the final stable position, the cement is allowed to set without interference by pressure from soft tissue or from introducing appliances. The acetabulum is then finally cleared of all debris and reduction achieved with appropriate manoeuvres of the leg, thumb pressure on the prosthetic head and by the assistance of a swab placed round the neck of the prosthesis. This latter is extremely valuable, particularly if reduction is difficult to achieve or if an imperfect reduction has taken place. After removal of the swab, the prosthesis is checked for a stable range of movement and the range is recorded. The wound is closed in layers with reconnection of obturator internus if possible. A suction drain is placed in the region of the prosthesis itself, and a second one outside the muscle layer in the fat. Weight bearing may commence the following day but sitting is discouraged until the wound is healed.

FURTHER READING

Adam A. and Spence A. J. (1958) Intertrochanteric osteotomy for osteoarthritis of the hip. *J. Bone Joint Surg.* **40B,** 219–226.

Bosworth D. M. (1960) Hip shelves in children. *J. Bone Joint Surg.* **42A,** 1223–1238.

Dunn D. M. (1964) Treatment of adolescent slipping of the upper femoral epiphysis. *J. Bone Joint Surg.* **46B,** 621–629.

Garden R. S. (1964) Stability and union in subcapital fractures of the femur. *J. Bone Joint Surg.* **46B,** 630–647.

Newman P. H. (1960) Surgical treatment of slipping of upper femoral epiphysis. *J. Bone Joint Surg.* **42B,** 280–288.

Nicola T. (1966) *Atlas of Orthopaedic Exposure.* Baltimore, Md, Williams & Wilkins.

Pemberton P. (1965) Pericapsular osteotomy of the ilium for treatment of congenital subluxation and dislocation of the hip. *J. Bone Joint Surg.* **47A,** 65–86.

Salter R. B. (1961) Innominate osteotomy in the treatment of congenital dislocation and subluxation of the hip. *J. Bone Joint Surg.* **43B,** 518–539.

Chapter forty-eight

The Hand

A. H. C. Ratliff

SURGERY OF INFECTIONS OF THE HAND

Surgical Anatomy

The Nail Fold Subungual Space

The subcuticular plane beneath the nail fold is potentially continuous at the sides of the nail with the subungual space deep to the nail. Infection may therefore easily spread under the nail and the resulting abscess cannot be drained effectively unless part of the nail is removed.

The Pulp Space

The proximal end of this space is closed by attachment of the deep fascia to the periosteum on the palmar aspect of the terminal phalanx. The interval between the skin and the anterior aspect of the distal phalanx is traversed by tough fibrous partitions which subdivide the space into separate compartments bounded anteriorly by skin, posteriorly by bone and on each side by fibrous septa. As a result, a localized pulp space infection can easily occur with a rise of tissue pressure and unwise lateral incision at the sides of the pulp space may be placed away from the core of the abscess.

The Thenar Space

This lies deeply under the radial half of the hollow of the palm in the interval between posteriorly the adductor pollicis muscle and anteriorly the flexor tendon of the index finger and lumbrical muscles. It is separated from the mid-palmar space by a fibrous septum that passes on to the metacarpal bone of the middle finger.

The Mid-palmar Space

This lies under the ulnar half of the hollow of the palm and it is bounded on the ulnar side by the fifth metacarpal bone and on the radial side by a septum attached to the front of the third metacarpal bone. It is important to appreciate that these infections are deep, very rare and often produce considerable oedema on the dorsum of the hand.

The Flexor Tendon Sheaths

The synovial flexor tendon sheaths are illustrated (*Fig.* 48.1). They extend proximally into the palm in the case of the thumb and little finger. In acute

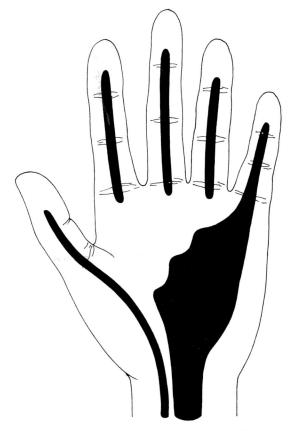

Fig. 48.1. The anatomy of the flexor tendon sheaths.

infective tenosynovitis pus is formed within the synovial sheath and it is confined by the limits of the sheath.

Treatment

Treatment consists of rest and antibiotics in the diffuse stage, and careful incision over the area of maximum tenderness when localization is obvious.

The bacteriology of hand infections is as follows (Sneddon, 1984):

80 per cent due to the staphylococcus alone.
10 per cent due to the haemolytic streptococcus.
 5 per cent due to both staphylococcus and streptococcus.
 5 per cent due to coliforms.

A very high percentage of the Gram-positive bacilli are sensitive to flucloxacillin (and the haemolytic streptococcus to penicillin); all the coliforms are sensitive to Septrin (sulphamethoxazole/trimethoprim).

The Localized Lesion

The area of maximum tenderness should be defined by palpation with a blunt probe immediately before surgery. A bloodless field is achieved by raising the arm for 2 minutes and then tying a thin piece of rubber tubing 5 mm wide round the base of the finger. For lesions proximal to a finger, general anaesthesia and a pneumatic tourniquet are recommended. Anaesthesia may be local ring block with 1 per cent Xylocaine (lignocaine) without adrenaline; alternatively, a general anaesthetic may be necessary particularly when there is a severe infection of the hand.

Pulp Space Infection

A localized abscess should be drained directly rather than by lateral incisions which traverse uninfected pulp tissue and are quickly narrowed by oedema. Often subcuticular pus is visible at the site of injury and demonstrates a collar stud abscess which leads to the compartment involved. Where there is evidence of subcuticular pus the overlying skin is removed with scissors and the cavity opened and thoroughly drained with sinus forceps. Drains are unnecessary; a dry dressing and sling are applied (*Fig. 48.2*).

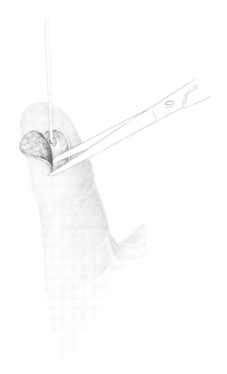

Fig. 48.2. Relief of pulp space infection.

Subcutaneous Infections of the Finger

When tenderness is superficial and localized, simple deroofing of the subcuticular lesions is required,

avoiding midline incisions. The tendon sheath must not be penetrated.

Acute Paronychia

Unilateral subcuticular lesions require deroofing with scissors, exploration with a blunt probe and drainage. If there is no pus under the nail bed, the nail is left intact, but if pus is seen beneath the nail, or if the nail base is loose, it should be lifted in its entire width and the base of the nail removed by cutting across with scissors (*Fig. 48.3*).

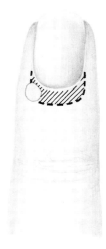

Fig. 48.3. Excision of paronychia.

Web Space Infection

This is usually due to an infected blister at the base of the fingers and more than one web may be involved. Cellulitis and oedema of the hand appear early, especially on the dorsum where the swelling can be seen separating adjoining fingers. The infected blister is entirely deroofed and the underlying cavity explored with sinus forceps. Where drainage is inadequate, a transverse incision is made opposite the affected web in the palm, a little proximal to the edge of the web. This does not endanger the tendon sheath but guarantees adequate drainage of the web space.

Tendon Sheath Infection

This is rare but inadequate or late treatment may lead to permanent stiffening of the entire finger. It should be suspected with the early onset of severe symptoms after a midline injury, the organism usually being the Streptococcus. The finger is uniformly red, hot and swollen, and held in moderate flexion, and attempts at extension of finger passively are resisted by severe pain. Tenderness is located to the line of the tendon sheath over the palmar aspect of the finger.

TREATMENT

With very early diagnosis, i.e. within 24 hours, treatment should be conservative. The patient must be admitted, the hand elevated and large doses of antibiotics are advised. In the author's experience these patients usually attend late, when the tendon sheath should be opened as an urgency. A transverse incision should be made through the site of the original trauma. In advanced cases the sheath should be opened proximally at the distal part of the palm and irrigated by catheters (*Fig.* 48.4). With adequate and early surgery the prognosis is now remarkably good.

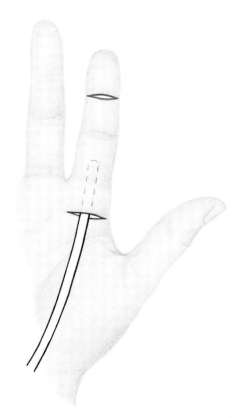

Fig. 48.4. Irrigation of infected flexor tendon sheath.

Bone Infection Associated with Neglected Terminal Pulp Infection

This is rare. Loose bone should be removed with forceps through the overlying sinus which is always present and the correct systemic antibiotics given for a minimum of 2 weeks.

MICROSURGERY

Microsurgery is now an established technique in surgery of the hand. High-quality operating loupes with a wide field of vision are now available. These are extremely helpful in surgery of Dupuytren's contracture and in the repair of flexor tendons. Many surgeons now use loupes for every operation of the hand. They give significant magnification for the epineural repair of digital nerves although higher magnification is desirable.

An operation microscope is an essential piece of equipment in any unit dealing with hand and peripheral nerve surgery. For ease of operating it is required that the microscope shall have a magnification of at least 25×. The microscope should have facilities for the assistant to sit directly opposite the surgeon; the focus and the magnification should be controlled by a foot. This enables the surgeon to maintain concentration on the operating field while adjustments are made. Microsurgical instruments must be kept separate from all other instruments and should only be used with magnification. Microscopes should be used for all nerve repairs as they allow an accurate alignment of the fasciculi within the nerve and accurate placement of the fine 10/0 sutures within the epi- or perineurium. The replantation of digits and limbs is now a well-accepted surgical procedure and at forearm, wrist and digital level the microscope is a necessity for vascular and neural repairs. (*See* Chapter 31.)

CARPAL TUNNEL SYNDROME

Aetiology

Compression of the median nerve within the carpal tunnel can be caused by any condition which diminishes the capacity of the tunnel. The common causes are primary or idiopathic and those in association with rheumatoid disease. Both the primary and rheumatoid forms are caused by increased bulk of the flexor synovium. The primary form has a peak incidence in middle life between the ages of 20 and 40 and women are affected more frequently than men. Symptoms may occur during pregnancy and resolve after confinement. Rare causes such as carpal dislocation, fracture, acromegaly or myxoedema should be remembered.

Symptoms

The patient is typically a woman who complains of a feeling of 'pins and needles' in the digits supplied by the median nerve, particularly the middle and ring fingers. The symptoms are characteristically worse at night. Rarely the condition may be progressive and the hand severely damaged with loss of sensitivity and appreciable motor weakness. Examination in the early stages may demonstrate no physical signs. The diagnosis is based on the history and exclusion of other neurological disorders.

Treatment

In some patients with a short history, particularly during pregnancy, it may be wise to observe progress before advising surgery. A night splint may be used as a diagnositc test. Injection of steroids into the tunnel may give relief but the effect is not reliable; there may be temporary improvement but this method of treatment is not recommended.

Operative Treatment

This consists of a complete division of all the retinaculum and should be carried out in all cases where the symptoms persist. Immediate and lasting relief almost always occurs. The operation is now usually performed from a day-stay ward and general anaesthesia with a pneumatic touniquet is advisable. The incision is demonstrated (*Fig.* 48.5). It is important

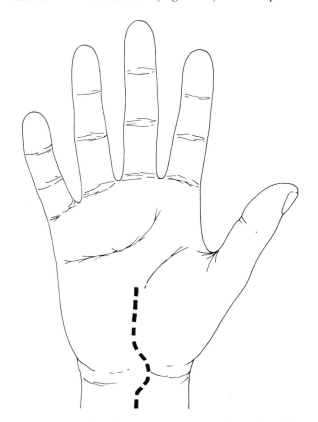

Fig. 48.5. Incision for decompression of carpal tunnel.

to avoid damage to the palmar cutaneous branch of the median nerve. A tiny incision is made longitudinally in the deep fascia at the proximal part of the incision, a director is then inserted underneath the flexor retinaculum and this is then divided with the nerve protected. The distal part of the division of the retinaculum should incline towards the ulnar side of the median nerve to avoid damage to the motor branch.

PRIMARY TREATMENT OF OPEN INJURIES OF THE HAND (INCLUDING AMPUTATIONS)

Principles

1. The efficiency of the primary treatment determines the fate of the injured hand. The care of the wound is all important and skin which has been avulsed or is dead must be replaced by grafting if fibrosis and contracture are to be prevented. Tendons and nerves can sometimes be left for secondary repair.

2. Injuries of the hand may be divided into two groups:

a. Crush injuries, where there is skin and soft tissue damage with difficulty in controlling oedema.

b. Incised wounds, where there may be damage to deep structures, e.g. tendon or nerve. The aim of primary treatment is to achieve healing of skin.

3. Meticulous attention to detail in postoperative management is essential to restore the maximum functional recovery. Joint stiffness must be prevented if at all possible.

Preoperative Preparation

General anaesthesia is acceptable but axillary block or local block may be used. Adrenaline must never be included with any anaesthesia injected into the hand.

Shaving, irrigation and gross débridement precede more careful cleaning with a mild detergent. Where grafts are necessary these should be taken from the flexor aspect of the forearm and the donor area sealed with an occlusion dressing. Antibiotics are not a substitute for correct surgical toilet.

Fingertip Injuries

1. *Subungual Haematoma*

Crush injuries of the distal phalanx frequently produce a haematoma underneath the nail which is extremely painful. Immediate relief can be obtained by trephining the nail with the heated end of a paper clip or the point of a fine-bladed scalpel. The haematoma is decompressed (*Fig.* 48.6).

2. *Nail Bed Injuries*

Slicing wounds which remove part of the nail bed but leave the nail root intact are best treated by split-skin graft immediately sewn into place.

3. *Partial Amputation of a Terminal Segment of the Finger*

If one of the vascular bundles has been left intact the distal portion of the finger should be sutured,

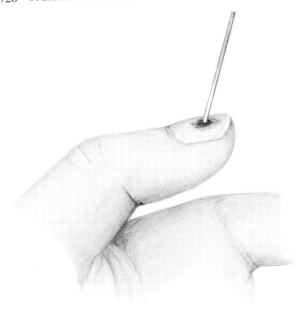

Fig. 48.6. Release of subungual haematoma.

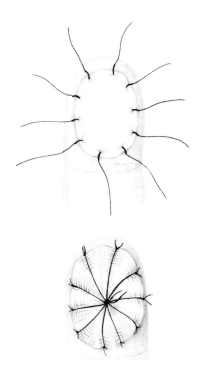

Fig. 48.7. Skin graft used to replace pulp skin.

even if the injury has damaged bone. If pulp, including some soft tissue, has been lost, especially with a slicing anterior injury, then a difficult decision has to be made. The alternative is to terminalize by cutting back enough bone to give adequate mobile skin cover or to retain by replacing the skin with a split-skin graft. The operation of thenar flap is now no longer recommended. Where there is loss of deep tissues then a full-thickness graft is necessary. The donor site is from either the volar surface of the forearm or the skin of the medial side of the arm above the medial epicondyle. The fat is dissected off with scissors and the graft sutured into position (*Fig.* 48.7).

Amputations

Indications

1. Injury.
2. Infection, for example disorganized and stiff fingers following sepsis.
3. Degeneration, for example a severe Dupuytren's contracture with a gross flexion deformity of the proximal interphalangeal joint.
4. Rarely for specialized problems, for example congenital abnormalities, vascular disease and neoplasm.

Painful Stumps

Amputation of a digit is often poorly performed in an accident department and the most common cause of pain after this operation is a sensitive stump with an adherent scar.

Levels of Amputation

Length should be preserved as far as possible, especially in the mutilated hand. The best levels are:

1. The terminal segment of the digit distal to the attachment of the sublimis tendon at the base of the middle phalanx.
2. In the index and little fingers, through the neck of the metacarpal. The cosmetic appearance of an amputation of the metacarpophalangeal joint of these digits is poor and particularly in women should not be performed.
3. In the middle and ring fingers through the base of the proximal phalanx.

Skin Flaps

Scars of a finger amputation should be transverse and dorsal, but provided there is a mobile stump with underlying subcutaneous tissue even a palmar suture line may be non-sensitive and satisfactory.

Nerves

Neuromas are inevitable. The individual digital nerves should therefore be carefully studied and shortened to ensure that they do not become adherent to skin. The nerves should be cut cleanly with a sharp knife or razor blade (*Fig.* 48.8).

Tendons

Tendons must not be sutured to each other across

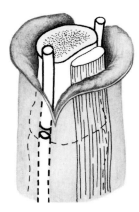

Fig. 48.8. When amputating the terminal part of a finger, the digital nerves must be cut back well proximally to avoid painful terminal neuroma adherent to the scar.

a stump otherwise a flexion deformity will occur in the adjacent joints.

Bones

Bone stumps should be cut short so that they do not cause tension in the overlying skin.

Vessels

The tourniquet should be removed before completion to ensure haemostasis. Minimal ligation is advised.

Amputations of the Thumb

These may be conveniently classified into two groups.

1. Where the amputation is distal to the metacarpophalangeal joint with adequate length. The principles of treatment are as described for amputation of the fingers.

2. Where the amputation is through the metacarpophalangeal joint or more proximal. Length is then inadequate and permanent and major disability may result. In these circumstances in an accident service primary closure of skin and soft tissue should be carried out by suture or free skin graft and later reconstruction may be necessary in the form of pollicization.

Multiple Amputations

As much of the hand as possible should be saved to provide some grip with a normal opposing thumb. Viable skin of a severely damaged and otherwise unpreservable digit can often be used to fill defects which would otherwise have to be treated by less satisfactory methods, such as grafting or the amputation of a flap from a distance. The intact little finger may be of considerable use in these severe injuries. The undamaged thumb is most valuable for power grip. Loss of both the index and middle fingers leads

to a severe disability since pinch grip is no longer possible.

Phalangeal Fractures (*Fig.* 48.9)

Displaced fractures of the phalanges, particularly the proximal phalanx, with open wounds are probably best treated by internal fixation by pinning if the

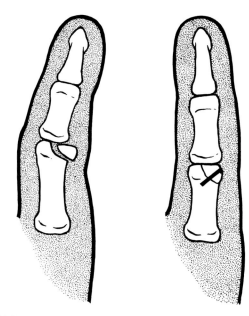

Fig. 48.9. Oblique fractures into the interphalangeal joint are best managed by open reduction of internal fixation.

finger is likely to survive. This allows early movement of adjacent joints. Wire is usually best introduced at the dorsal aspect of the head of the phalanx to one side of the midline and passed down to the base of the phalanx. Similarly, metacarpal shaft fractures often need to be internally fixed, preferably by a Kirschner wire if the wound is open. This allows early healing of skin tissue and reduces the need for external splintage.

Degloving Injuries

Avulsion of a skin cylinder of a digit occurs after a ring has been caught on a protruding hook. Complicated skin grafting is tempting to carry out, but usually the best treatment is primary amputation of the digit.

The palm may be caught on protruding objects leading to varying degrees of avulsion of skin. The plane of cleavage is usually between the subcutaneous tissues and palmar fascia. Flaps are raised which at first appear to have adequate arterial supply but frequently necrosis occurs with an underlying haematoma. The best primary treatment is to suture these flaps back into place. If there is the slightest sign of necrosis of tissue and it is well defined, it should be excised and later a thick split-skin graft performed.

Postoperative Management

A compression bandage in the correct position with elevation of the hand to prevent oedema is a basic need for all injured hands.

TENDON INJURIES IN THE HAND

Principles

1. Tendons heal rapidly when held in apposition, union being strong at about 4 weeks.

2. Tendons easily become adherent to surrounding tissues, thus limiting their gliding movement. A gentle and precise technique is therefore essential including a tourniquet, the use of fine instruments and suture material producing a minimum of tissue reaction.

3. Extensor tendons are enclosed in loose elastic tissue—the paratenon. The results of immediate repair are usually good.

4. Flexor tendons are provided with a sheath. Considerable retraction of the cut ends occurs when a tendon is divided within the sheath. Even in expert hands the suture of a tendon is likely to fail owing to adhesions, if performed inside the flexor sheath. In these circumstances a tendon graft is necessary.

5. Where there is no sheath, and retraction less likely, e.g. in the palm, immediate suture usually yields satisfactory results.

Extensor Tendons

Immediate repair is indicated for tendons divided in the proximal part of the hand and over the wrist. The method of suture for a cut extensor tendon in the finger is shown in *Fig.* 48.10.

Flexor Tendons

There are two flexor tendons in each finger, a superficial flexor which attaches to the base of the middle phalanx and the deep flexor which attaches to the base of the terminal phalanx. In the thumb there is one tendon, flexor pollicis longus. These tendons may be damaged in different sites in the hand and their management varies according to these sites. In view of the difficulties of tendon grafting, the inconsistency of results and the prolonged period off work often necessary, in recent years there has been a considerable swing towards the performing of primary tendon repair within the digital theca.

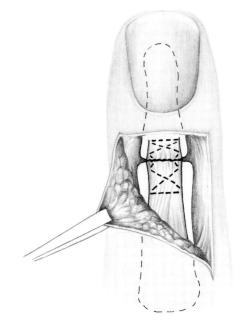

Fig. 48.10. Method of suture of divided extensor tendon in the finger.

Primary Flexor Tendon Suture in the Finger or Thumb (*Fig.* 48.11)

In view of the improved surgical technique possible with fine, delicate instruments, non-reactive suture material on atraumatic needles, aided by operating magnifying loupes, there have been several series in recent years which have reported good results from

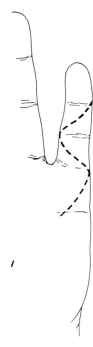

Fig. 48.11. Incision suitable for exposure of flexor tendon in the finger.

primary repair of flexor tendons. Strict criteria must be adhered to if good results are to be obtained.

Main Requirements

1. Only those wounds caused in a clean, incised manner—such as one sustained by a knife—are suitable.

2. There should be no preoperative interference with the wound by blind exploration in conditions of doubtful sterility.

3. Careful wound excision is required, with a minimum of handling of the tendons, and care should be taken that the vinculum is not damaged.

4. Operation should usually only be considered when it can be performed within a few hours after injury—in a well-equipped accident centre. Alternatively it may be done as a secondary procedure, preferably on the next operating list, if the original primary wound has been cleaned and closed and the wrist immobilized, fully flexed with a posterior plaster shell.

Operative Approach

The transverse or oblique laceration may need to be extended. The technique of suture is illustrated in *Fig.* 48.12.

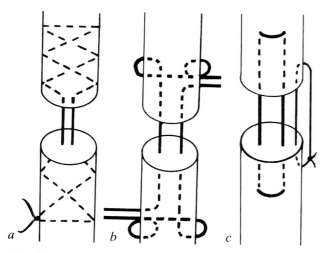

Fig. 48.12. Flexor tendon suture. *a*, Bunnell criss-cross stitch. *b*, Kessler grasping stitch. *c*, Simple apposition.

Kleinert Technique for Repair of Flexor Tendons in the Finger

Kleinert (1973) recommends the use of the Kessler stitch and suturing the tendon mainly on the volar or superficial aspect, so that the main blood vessels running on the dorsal aspect of the tendon and entering on the deep aspect are not disturbed. A continuous 6/0 Prolene suture is then used to hold the tendon ends accurately together. The repair of both tendons is recommended where these are divided and

the fibrous flexor sheath should be sutured if possible. Immobilization is required for a period of 3 weeks but in order to prevent rigid adherence at the site of injury a technique whereby elastic traction is applied to the nail of the affected digit has been introduced. On completion of surgery the wrist is immobilized with a dorsal plaster slab in the position of flexion sufficient to prevent any tension in the tendon with the wrist and metacarpophalangeal joints about 30° flexed. The traction is then applied through a rubber band attached to the front of the wrist with enough tension to put the digit through a range of flexion but not so strong as to prevent the digit extending to the limit allowed by the plaster (*Fig.* 48.13).

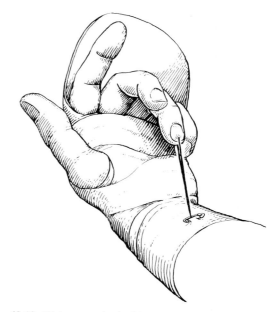

Fig. 48.13. Kleinert method of immobilization of sutured flexor tendon using elastic traction.

Flexor Digitorum Profundus in the Finger

If this tendon is divided alone in the distal part of the finger (*Fig.* 48.14, area 1) good results may be achieved by primary suture. Early delayed suture may be possible if the vincula are intact and retraction has been prevented. Tendon grafting using plantaris and retaining sublimis runs the risk of reducing flexion in the proximal interphalangeal joint and aims essentially for perfection. It is only indicated if an excellent result is desired and special experience is available.

Flexor Digitorum Profundus and Sublimis in the Finger

If both these tendons are divided (*Fig.* 48.14, area 2) then the finger flexes at the metacarpophalangeal joint and projects as a loose and useless digit. Surgical treatment is always necessary. The alternatives are

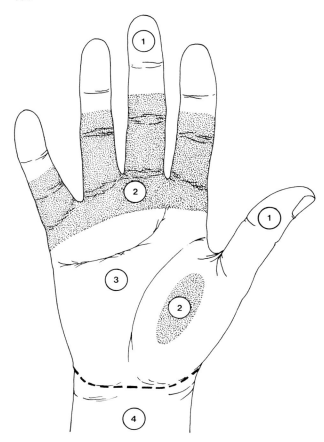

Fig. 48.14. At the unshaded areas primary suture of divided tendons is satisfactory but at the shaded sites primary suture is not usually recommended (but see text for recent advances).

primary suture wherever possible, as indicated above, or closure of the wound and tendon grafting a few weeks later.

Flexor Pollicis Longus

Distal division of flexor pollicis longus should be treated by immediate suture (*Fig.* 48.14, area 1). If the division is more proximal or the conditions for primary suture are not present then function can be restored by tendon grafting. The results of tendon grafting for the thumb are usually good.

The Palm

Suture of both the profundus and sublimis tendons at the same level may be followed by cross-union which limits action of the sublimis, i.e. flexion at the proximal interphalangeal joint. If the tendon ends are ragged then it is advisable to cut back sublimis and restrict the repair to the profundus.

Wrist

Immediate suture should always be performed providing the wounds permit. End-to-end sutures should be carried out using the Bunnell criss-cross stitch. All tendons with the exception of palmaris longus should be sutured.

Summary of Method of Repair of Flexor Tendon Division (in areas marked by numbers on *Fig.* 48.14.)

1. Primary suture should be performed if wound conditions are satisfactory. Otherwise the skin is sutured. Secondary suture, tendon graft or arthrodesis of the interphalangeal joint is performed later.

2. Primary suture providing the conditions permit (*see above*); alternatively a secondary graft.

3. Primary suture should always be performed providing that wound conditions are satisfactory.

4. Primary suture is highly desirable since delay may necessitate bridge grafting.

The Tendon Graft Operation

Graft Source

Two tendons are commonly used for a graft in flexor tendon surgery, namely palmaris longus and the plantaris. Each has advantages. Palmaris longus, when present, is adjacent in the same limb and is therefore convenient. Plantaris is sufficiently long to use as two grafts and has the advantage of being smaller and therefore runs more smoothly

Incisions in the digit and palm (Fig. 48.15)

Incisions in the fingers are classically made in the line joining the posterior end of the flexor crease, i.e. strictly mid-lateral. It must always be remembered that this is also the surface marking for the digital nerves and vessels and therefore great care should be taken to protect them.

Excision of the Digital Theca and Insertion of the Graft

The digital theca containing the tendons is fully exposed and then cut away leaving three bands to serve as pulleys. The profundus tendon and the proximal part of the sublimis tendon are completely removed. The graft is then inserted and attached to the distal phalanx (*Fig.* 48.16).

Tension of the Graft

The proximal suture of graft to motor tendon in the palm is finally performed (*Figs.* 48.17, 48.18). The tension must be carefully adjusted so that the finger lies at a slightly more flexed position than would appear correct in relation to the other fingers. Plaster is applied with the fingers flexed and the hand elevated.

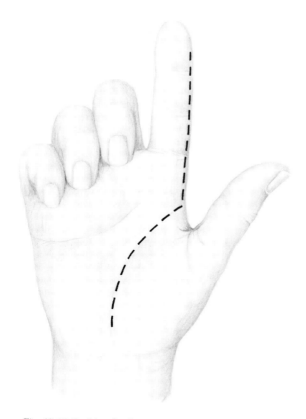

Fig. 48.15. Incision for flexor tendon graft to index finger.

Postoperative care

Immobilization in the plaster to relax the suture line is necessary for 3 weeks. Protective light splintage should be given for a further week to reduce the risk of the tendon junction giving way. Convalescence is prolonged and intensive physiotherapy is essential.

DUPUYTREN'S CONTRACTURE

Indications for Surgery

1. *Early:* Where there is a progressive contracture in the palm and a mild flexion deformity of the metacarpophalangeal joint. The prognosis is excellent with surgery at this stage.

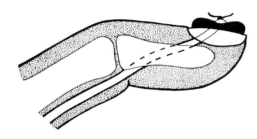

Fig. 48.16. Technique of insertion of flexor tendon graft through terminal phalanx.

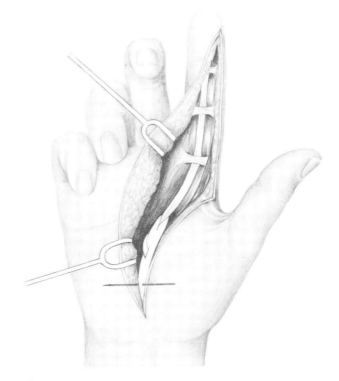

Fig. 48.17. Flexor tendon graft to index finger. Proximal suture.

2. With more *advanced* disease the decision for operation depends on the presence or absence of the inherited diathesis. The elderly patient with no diathesis will require very limited surgery, if any. However, a young patient with a strong Dupuytren's diathesis may require extensive reconstructive surgery; this case is likely to deteriorate rapidly and develop recurrences either at the site of operation or elsewhere in the hand.

It is important to explain to patients before operation the probable chances of cure.

1. A palmar nodule alone does not warrant surgery.

2. Metacarpophalangeal flexion deformity is almost always fully correctable by surgery.

3. Interphalangeal flexion deformity, particularly

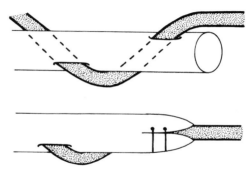

Fig. 48.18. Flexor tendon graft showing interlacing and suture of tendon graft.

if it is more than 60°, is often not fully correctable by surgery.

Types of Operation

Fasciotomy

This is reserved for the very elderly patient, otherwise unfit for major surgery, who has a localized flexion deformity.

Regional Fasciectomy

This is the most commonly indicated operation and is confined to removal from fingers and palm of all tissue macroscopically involved in the contracting process.

Extensive Fasciectomy

This includes excision of palmar aponeurosis from the whole width of the palm with all detectable digital disease. There is a greater risk of complications. There may be a 'dead space' in the palm after surgery with problems of haematoma, possible skin necrosis and delay in convalescence. Extensive fasciectomy is a major and difficult operation.

Skin Graft Replacement

This is the only method which has been proved to be capable of preventing local recurrence of Dupuytren's contracture. Its use is restricted to those digits where local recurrence has already occurred or where, in the presence of diathesis, local recurrence can be anticipated.

Amputation

It is surprising how often patients will not attend for consultation until they have a severe contracture of both metacarpophalangeal and, particularly, the proximal interphalangeal joint of the little finger. It has to be accepted that in some of these cases improvement is not possible, and that a well-judged amputation through the metacarpophalangeal joint will often lead to a shorter convalescence and be the wiser treatment.

Operative Principles

There are two essential principles in surgery for this condition: (1) maximum correction of deformity with excision of diseased tissue; (2) minimum delay in healing and recovery of movements.

Incisions are planned to produce: (a) maximum exposure of fascia to be dissected, (b) minimum risk of skin flap ischaemia and necrosis, (c) normal scar contractures without impeding joint excursion. There has been a recent trend away from multiple trans-verse incisions in the palm and fingers since these make dissection of underlying structures difficult. They are replaced with either S-shaped types of incision in the palm or longitudinal incisions with conversion of some of this scar to transverse by means of multiple Z-plasties. Fasciectomy involves a dissection of the digital nerves and care must always be taken especially where they pass in the distal part of the palm to the adjacent sides of the digits. An ischaemic field is obligatory in order to allow precise dissection.

Incision

Each case must be considered on its own merits depending on the exact position of the contracted bands in the palm and digits. Possible incisions employed are demonstrated in *Fig.* 48.19. It will be noted that part of the palmar incision is in the skin crease, thus assisting wound healing.

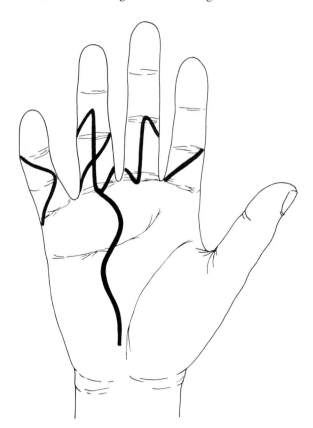

Fig. 48.19. Dupuytren's contracture. Choice of palmar and digital incisions.

Exposure and Removal of Thickened Aponeurosis

The skin edges are reflected by gentle dissection in the plane between dermis and palmar aponeurosis, care being taken to avoid 'button holing' the adherent skin. The contracted aponeurosis in the palm is displayed. As far as possible, all grossly thickened tissue should be removed but the dissection need not be carried too far proximal since this is unnecessary and is more likely to result in haematoma formation. If the skin flaps are reflected too widely then viability is endangered with a risk of skin necrosis.

Resection begins with a fasciotomy at the proximal end of the thickened exposed band. At this stage and before division digital nerves should be demonstrated, which run towards the interdigital clefts in close relationship with the aponeurosis. The lateral neurovascular bundle may be found with confidence as it lies along the anterior border of the lumbrical muscle in the middle and distal palm. Proximal fasciotomy allows immediate correction of the metacarpophalangeal deformity.

The flexor tendons are then exposed in the palm and dissection of the main band progresses distally. During removal deep extensions are found to pass down between the flexor tendons towards the front of each metacarpal; they should be excised by sharp dissection with careful retraction of the neurovascular bundles. Diseased tissue often distorts anatomy and damage to digital nerves may occur easily, especially as they run into the bases of the digits. The digital artery is almost as important as the digital nerves and must be preserved on at least one side of the digit during this tedious and often difficult dissection. The flexor sheath is often demonstrated but should not be excised. At the conclusion of the dissection the deeper structures of the palm, namely vessels, nerves and tendons, should be clearly displayed in the limited area of the wound and there should be no remnant of thickened aponeurosis.

At this stage complete correction of flexion deformity at the proximal interphalangeal joint may not have been achieved. This may be due to unprotected bands which must be sought out and reflected, but sometimes it is due to capsular joint contraction and cannot be corrected. In these difficult cases, where there is severe deformity of the proximal interphalangeal joint, the patients should be warned before the operation that they will be left with deformity at this joint or that possibly amputation may be necessary.

Closure

It is important that the tourniquet be removed and haemostasis secured. Drainage is not required.

Postoperative Management

Copious dressings of gauze are applied over the palm and round the affected finger which is held semiflexed. The palmar skin is thus prevented from any tendency to lift away from its bed. The hand is maintained elevated for the first few days after surgery. On the 4th day the bandage should be removed to ensure that the suture line is healthy with no haematoma. Sutures should not be removed earlier than 14 days after operation.

NERVE INJURIES

Peripheral Nerve Injuries at the Wrist and in the Hand

General Principles

Peripheral nerve injuries may be classified as 'open' or 'closed', or according to the histological nature of the nerve injury.

1. Lesions in continuity without distal axonal degeneration—neuropraxia—recovery rapid.
2. Lesions in continuity with distal axonal degeneration—axonotmesis—recovery follows the rate of nerve regeneration.
3. Nerve division—neurotmesis; degeneration distal to the division—no recovery. The pathology may be mixed.

Closed Nerve Injuries

Approximately 90 per cent of nerve injuries are lesions in continuity, neuropraxia or axonotmesis. These are usually the result of fractures and dislocations and attention is directed towards the care of the skeletal injury. A conservative policy is followed for the nerve injury in the expectation of recovery at a rate which is dependent on the pathology. These injuries are rare in the hand, for example a median nerve lesion after a dislocation of the lunate. Usually early exploration in peripheral nerve injury associated with closed fractures or dislocations is not indicated. Early exploration is indicated where pain or severe paraesthesia in the nerve distribution suggests persistent compression. Severe hand injuries with oedema and symptoms of median nerve compression should always be treated by carpal tunnel decompression, and freeing of the nerve.

Open Nerve Injuries

In the hand these are more common. In humans functional regeneration will not occur if there is a gap in excess of 1–2 mm. Following nerve division the nerve ends invariably retract and they must be approximated if there is to be any possibility of recovery. It is important to distinguish between two different processes:

1. Repair—a connective tissue phenomenon.
2. Nerve regeneration—a complicated process which can only occur if proximal axons are in close proximity to the distal nerve sheaths.

The decision to perform primary or secondary nerve suture is still debatable but is based on important prognostic factors. The prognosis of recovery after nerve division is influenced by:

1. The age of the patient—results of primary nerve suture in children are often good.
2. The level of nerve division. The more distal the lesion the better the prognosis.
3. The nature of the divided nerve. A pure sensory nerve or a pure motor nerve has a better prognosis than a mixed nerve.

4. The severity of the injury, both with regard to the extent of nerve damage and disturbance of blood supply.

Many advances have recently been made challenging the accepted teaching of early secondary repair. Microsurgery allows accurate insertion of fine sutures in primary repair and the careful removal of scar tissue with secondary nerve suture. Improved techniques have led to considerable debate concerning the relative merits of primary epineurial as against fascicular suture. The conclusion at present is that primary fascicular repair has not been proved to give statistically better results than simple epineurial repair and the latter is recommended. There has been a national improvement in the results of nerve repair as a result of these advances.

Primary repair should now be favoured, but only if the state of the wound and nerve allows and if the necessary surgical skill and technical surroundings are available. In the common transverse laceration due to injuries with a knife or glass just above the wrist (often with associated division of tendons), primary repair of both nerve and tendons is usually advisable. In small, incised wounds of the finger a digital nerve may be divided. Primary treatment should be nerve suture wherever conditions permit and particularly in the thumb, the lateral side of the index finger and the medial side of the little finger. Loss of sensation is especially important in the area supplied by these nerves. Late repair of divided digital nerves in the author's experience presents very difficult problems and the results are usually poor.

Secondary nerve repair is usually indicated when the circumstances are adverse:
1. When delay has occurred before wound treatment begins.
2. In complicated injuries or when there is considerable soft tissue damage.
3. In contaminated wounds.
4. In proximal nerve injuries.

In these circumstances scarring should be eliminated by isolating the site of nerve damage at the primary operation with a Silastic sheath, as advocated by McQuillan (1970).

Primary Repair (*Fig.* 48.20)

A tourniquet is essential and it must be released and bleeding stopped before the wound is closed. Suture is performed of the divided nerve by opposing the delicate epineurium with very fine wire or nylon (8/0–10/0), care being taken to ensure that the rotation is correct. After operation the nerve sutures should be protected for a period of 3 weeks by immobilizing with a dorsal plaster slab with the wrist flexed.

Delayed Nerve Repair

This is a completely different operation because of the distortion of normal anatomy and scarring which

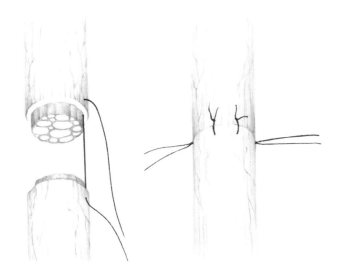

Fig. 48.20. Peripheral nerve suture.

results from a complex wound. The operation must be carried out under ideal theatre conditions and is usually time consuming. A long incision is essential and the nerve widely exposed above and below the lesion and mobilized. The inevitable neuroma must be resected with a razor blade until normal axons pout from the stump. Removal of the end bulbs leaves a gap. Suture must be performed without tension and gaps bridged by mobilization of the nerve, if necessary, high in the forearm. In nerve repair there is a critical resection length above which it is useless to bridge a gap. Nerve grafting is then necessary.

POSTOPERATIVE

The limb is splinted for 3–6 weeks to relieve suture line from tension.

MISCELLANEOUS HAND CONDITIONS

Bone Grafting of the Scaphoid for Un-united Fracture

This operation is indicated in un-united scaphoid fractures in young people, after an adequate period of immobilization in plaster, and where there is no evidence of degenerative changes in the wrist or avascular necrosis of the proximal pole.

The scaphoid is approached through an anterior incision lateral to the tendon of flexor carpi radialis (Russe operation). (*Fig.* 48.21). The fracture is exposed in the middle third of the bone, both fragments excavated with a small gouge (*Fig.* 48.22) and a block of cancellous bone from the iliac crest is punched into place across the fracture site. Bony union occurs in 80–90 per cent.

Herbert and Fisher (1984) have produced strong evidence to suggest that non-union of the scaphoid is related to uncontrolled instability at the site of fracture. They have described a new operative technique, using a double-threaded compression screw, especially designed to provide rigid fixation of all types of scaphoid fractures. The screw is simple to insert, providing special instrumentation and a jig are employed. This recent advance is likely to offer significant advantages over conventional techniques, particularly where there is early, delayed or non-union.

Arthrodesis of the Wrist

This operation is indicated for severe painful rheumatoid or osteoarthritis of the wrist. The joint should be fused in the position of function, i.e. 20° of dorsiflexion.

The approach is by a serpentine dorsal incision. The extensor tendons are retracted and a thorough excision of articular cartilage performed from the radiocarpal and intercarpal joints. A graft of corticocancellous bone is taken from the wing of the ilium, the donor site being chosen so that the graft is curved and fits into the dorsal hollow of the wrist when it is extended (*Fig.* 48.23).

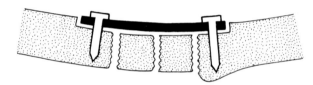

Fig. 48.23. Arthrodesis of wrist joint.

The ulnar and carpal joint is not touched and therefore rotation of the forearm is preserved. The wrist is immobilized in a plaster cast until fusion is sound, usually 12 weeks after operation.

Surgery of the Rheumatoid Hand

The rheumatoid hand can present in several stages:

1. The early phase with swollen painful tendon sheaths or joints.

2. The phase of unbalanced postures and movements, e.g. early ulnar deviation or hyperextension of the proximal interphalanageal joints.

3. The phase of developing fixed deformity by bony fusion or fibrosis ankylosis.

4. The phase of severe destruction with dislocation and gross loss of function.

The indications for surgery fall naturally into three stages:

1. *Early:* where there is minimal damage to joints or tendons. Operative treatment is confined to synovectomy with the aims of relief of pain, the arrest of further joint or tendon damage and the removal of impediments to movement.

2. *Intermediate:* Where damage is fairly advanced. These include repair of ruptured tendons, release of

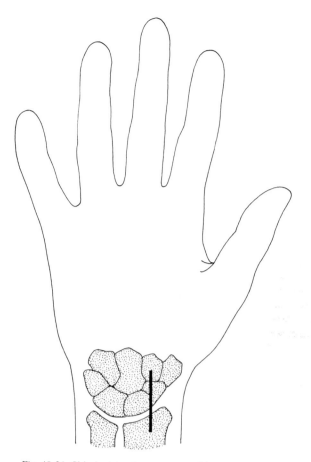

Fig. 48.21. Skin incision for exposure of fracture scaphoid.

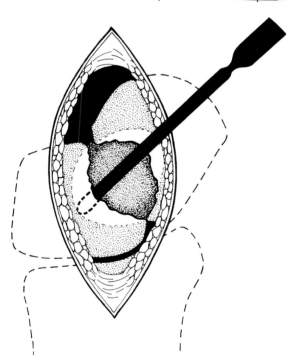

Fig. 48.22. Fractured scaphoid. Impaction of bone graft across un-united fragments.

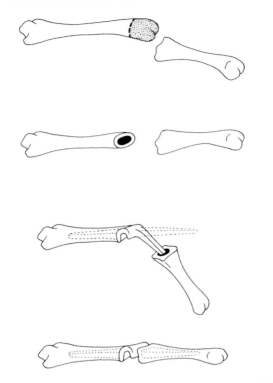

Fig. 48.24. Rheumatoid arthritis. Insertion of Silastic joint implant.

contractures, correction of ulnar drift and excision of the lower end of the ulnar bone.

3. *Late:* where damage is severe. Salvage operations include arthrodesis, e.g. of the wrist, and arthroplasty, especially of the metacarpophalangeal joints.

A combined approach by physician and surgeon is essential. The subject is large and complicated.

Arthroplasty of the Metacarpophalangeal Joints of the Fingers

This is indicated where there is gross destruction of a joint, often with palmar subluxation and ulnar deviation of the proximal phalanx. The joint is approached through a transverse incision, with protection of the dorsal veins, and the eroded metacarpal head exposed and removed. Soft tissue release allows the base of the proximal phalanx to be displaced dorsally and then the appropriate size of Silastic implant (Swanson or Nicolle type) is inserted into the medullary canal of the metacarpal joint and proximal phalanx (*Fig.* 48.24).

A dynamic brace is used postoperatively for 2 weeks to encourage the rapid return of function. Looseness of the 'spacer' prosthesis is inevitable, but the functional result of this operation is usually very good.

FURTHER READING

Beltran J. E., Jimeno-Urban F. and Yunta A. (1976) The open palm and digit technique in the treatment of Dupuytren's contracture. *The Hand* **8**, 73–77.

Bolton H. (1977) Primary tendon repair within the digital theca. In: Pulvertaft R. G. (ed.) *The Hand*; Rob C. and Smith R. (eds) *Operative Surgery*, 3rd ed. London, Butterworths, p. 129.

Bolton H., Fowler P. J. and Jepson R. P. (1949) Natural history and treatment of pulp space infection and osteomyelitis of terminal phalanx. *J. Bone Joint Surg.* **31B**, 499–504.

Boyes J. N. (1970) *Bunnel's Surgery of the Hand*, 5th ed. Philadelphia, Lippincott.

Bruner J. M. (1973) Surgical exposure of flexor tendons in the hand. *Ann. R. Coll. Surg. Engl.* **53**, 88–94.

Carter S. J. and Mersheimer W. L. (1974) The use of catheters in treatment of infections of the hand. In: *Symposium on Reconstructive Hand Surgery, Vol. 9.* St Louis, Mosby.

Ellis J. S. (1974) Peripheral nerve injuries. *The Hand* **6**, 142–147.

Fisher T. R. (1980) Microsurgery in the injured. In: Tubbs N. and London P. S. (eds) *Topical Reviews in Accident Surgery, Vol. 1.* Bristol, John Wright, p.117.

Herbert T. J. and Fisher W. E. (1984) Management of the fractured scaphoid using a new bone screw. *J. Bone Joint Surg.* **66B**, 114–123.

Hueston J. T. (1963) *Dupuytren's Contracture.* Edinburgh, Livingstone.

Hueston J. T. and Tubiana R. (1974) *Dupuytren's Disease.* G.E.M. Monograph. Edinburgh, Churchill Livingstone.

James J. I. P. (1970) The assessment and management of the injured hand. *The Hand* **2**, 97–105.

Kleinert H. L. and Storms A. (1973) Primary repair of flexor tendons. *Orthop. Clin. North Am.* **4**, 865.

Lamb D. W. and Kuczynski K. (1981) *The Practice of Hand Surgery.* Oxford, Blackwell Scientific.

McCash C. R. (1964) The open palm technique in Dupuytren's contracture. *Br. J. Plast. Surg.* **17**, 271–280.

McGregor I. A. (1967) The Z-plasty in hand surgery. *J. Bone Joint Surg.* **49B**, 448–457.

McGregor I. A. (1970) Degloving injuries. *The Hand* **1**, 130–133.

McQuillan W. M. (1970) Nerve repair: the use of nerve isolation. *The Hand* **2**, 19–20.

Michon J. and Moberg E. (1975) *Traumatic Nerve Lesions of the Upper Limb.* G.E.M. Monographs. Edinburgh, Churchill Livingstone.

Millesni H., Meissl G. and Berger A. (1972) The interfascicular nerve grafting of the median and ulnar nerves. *J. Bone Joint Surg.* **54A**, 727–750.

Moberg E. (1972) Differentiation of sensibility as a basis for orthopaedic and hand surgery. Pridie Memorial Lecutre. *J. Bone Joint Surg.* **54B**, 556.

Noble J. and Harrison D. H. (1976) Open palm technique for Dupuytren's contracture. *The Hand* **8**, 272–278.

Pulvertaft R. G. (1956) Tendon grafts for flexor injuries in the fingers and thumb. *J. Bone Joint Surg.* **38B**, 175.

Rank B. U., Wakefield A. R. and Hueston J. T. (1973) *Surgery of Repair as Applied to Hand Injuries*, 4th ed. Edinburgh, Churchill Livingstone, p. 149.

Ratliff A. H. C. (1969) Amputations of the fingers and thumb. *The Hand* **1**, 137–138.

Ratliff A. H. C. (1972) Amputations of the distal part of the thumb. *The Hand* **4**, 190–193.

Richards H. J. (1977) Digital flexor tendon repair and return of function. *Ann. R. Coll. Surg.* **59**, 25–32.

Robins R. H. C. (1952) Infections of the hand: review of 1,000 cases. *J. Bone Joint Surg.* **34B**, 567–580.

Robins R. H. C. (1961) *Injuries and Infections of the Hand*. London, Arnold.

Seddon H. J. (1972) *Surgical Disorders of the Peripheral Nerves*. Edinburgh, Churchill Livingstone.

Sneddon J. (1970) *The Care of Hand Infection*. London, Arnold.

Sneddon J. (1984) Infections. In: Dudley H. and Carter D. (eds) *Operative Surgery: The Hand*, 4th ed. London, Butterworths, p. 108.

Stack H. G. (1977) Amputations. In: Pulvertaft R. G. (ed.) *The Hand*; Rob C. and Smith R. (eds) *Operative Surgery*, 3rd ed. London, Butterworths, p. 352.

Chapter forty-nine

Amputations and Prostheses

K. P. Robinson

An amputation is an operation which results in the severance of part of the body from the patient and is therefore considered to be a mutilating procedure with an inevitable loss of function. However, it is important to accept the philosophy that the production of a satisfactory amputation stump together with a well-designed prosthesis is a method of treatment which may save the patient's life and which may restore or even improve the function of the diseased extremity. Therefore the surgical technique and management of a patient having amputation surgery are of the greatest importance for that patient's future existence. The formation of an amputation stump is an operation to be performed with care, precision and considerable experience if the patient is to have the best result.

INDICATIONS

The indications for amputation may be considered as absolute indications to save life or relative indications to improve function. In trauma, amputation may be life saving if the patient is entrapped by immovable debris when an amputation may be required to release him. This is the only situation in which a guillotine amputation is acceptable. Amputation in trauma may also be required to prevent the crush syndrome and where traumatic gangrene has occurred or is threatened and cannot be averted. In severe burns the limb may be so destroyed that an amputation is required. When gas gangrene occurs amputation may be required despite hyperbaric oxygen and penicillin and may be life saving. Although considerable progress has been made in the treatment of neoplasms by radiotherapy and more recently by chemotherapy, there is still a place for amputation when a sarcoma recurs despite these measures. Marjolin's ulcer and Kaposi's sarcoma may also require amputation if other methods of treatment are not successful.

Acute embolism or intravascular thrombosis may produce peripheral gangrene, although embolectomy should be successful in the majority of patients. Atheroma is principally responsible for chronic occlusion of large vessels to and in the lower limb and the commonest cause of rest pain, ischaemic ulcers and peripheral gangrene which are the indications for amputation if they cannot be relieved by vascular surgery, by sympathectomy or by sympathetic block. Atheroma is encountered prematurely and severely in diabetic patients, but in these patients the additional factors of diabetic neuropathy, diminished resistance to staphylococcal invasion and the diffuse micro-angiopathy must be treated before any decision is taken concerning amputation. In diabetics it is particularly important to control the diabetic state, to counter infection by antibiotics and surgical drainage of deep sepsis. This may involve local resection of osteomyelitis or excision of septic arthroses, usually achieved by ray amputations in the foot; however, without an adequate major arterial blood supply such local procedures are destined to increase the area of local gangrene and precipitate the need for a major amputation. Débridement confined to dead tissue does not involve this rule, but a preliminary local amputation without sutures may be preferred, accepting this as the initial procedure to allow sepsis to resolve before the major amputation is performed.

In the field of vascular surgery established ischaemic gangrene will require amputation and it is not often realized that rest pain is extremely severe and the deterioration which it will produce in an elderly patient will lead to bronchopneumonia and death in a remarkably short space of time if the painful extremity is not removed. In diabetic patients septic gangrene is the precursor of life-threatening septicaemia and amputation cannot be avoided. When combined with ischaemia the level must reach fully vascularized tissue, otherwise a local amputation will be adequate. In Buerger's disease amputation is frequently required, as the scattered nature of the arterial blocks rarely gives the opportunity for vascular surgery.

However, it is where the relative indications are concerned that considerable judgement is required in the decision to make an amputation. The indication is to relieve pain, restore health and restore function. In general it is the informed comparison of the function of the proposed stump and available prosthesis with the existing function that the patient has prior to operation, and it is probably wise for the decision for an elective amputation for relative indications to always be made by more than one surgeon, and where possible with the informed cooperation of the patient who has had the opportunity of meeting other patients in the same situation and can assess their quality of life. Probably in no field is this more difficult than in patients with congenital disorders in whom pressure from parents and the lack of informed decision by the patients, too young to be aware of the full implications of their deformity, put the heaviest responsibility on the medical advisers. In general, an extremely conservative approach using orthoses to a maximum will be the general principle. The indications for amputation where massive trauma to a limb has resulted in infection or gangrene or obvious inability to heal are easy to discern; but there are many limbs damaged by trauma in which non-union or malunion of fractures and joint instability or fixation and extensive soft tissue damage may lead to long-term morbidity and ultimate impairment of function, which at an early stage may be avoided by a well-chosen amputation. Similarly the long-term morbidity of osteomyelitis, fungal infections of the deep tissues of the foot, leprosy and diabetes may all require an amputation procedure at a carefully judged time.

The occasional large benign tumour and the very rare secondary tumour may be an indication for amputation. While arterial ischaemia with rest pain is a clear-cut indication for an amputation, venous ulceration and gangrene due to arteriovenous fistulas may again require considerable judgement, and perhaps in no situation is the decision more difficult than in patients with a neurological deficit after injury or disease to the brachial or sciatic plexus.

SELECTION OF LEVEL FOR AMPUTATION

In congenital disorders the level of amputation can only be determined by a careful study of the individual case. However, in trauma the level of amputation is determined by the most distal level at which sound healing of a well-functioning stump can be obtained. If a guillotine amputation has been required then amputation at a more proximal level will in general be necessary, but where a formal amputation can be performed preservation of all satisfactory tissue should be obtained and no functioning joint should be sacrificed. In neoplastic disease the consideration is the adequate clearance of malignant tissue. Skin tumours should be widely cleared. Soft tissue sarcomas should include the whole of the muscle group in which the tumour is situated and, where neurofibrosarcomas are concerned, frozen sections should be taken of the nerve proximally to ensure adequate clearance. Bone tumours in general require the whole length of the affected bone to be resected as intramedullary spread is not uncommon. In vascular disease there is some controversy in the selection of level; in a non-diabetic patient healing can be assured if the level of amputation is immediately below the most distal palpable arterial pulsation (Taylor, 1967). However, this results in a preponderance of above-knee levels of amputation in elderly patients who may well later become bilateral amputees (Kihn et al., 1972) with a much diminished chance of rehabilitation, although Hall and Shucksmith (1971) report 75 per cent able to walk. Therefore the level of amputation is often

selected at a lower level with an increased risk of delayed wound healing and the need for reamputation.

Many methods of determination of the site of adequate perfusion for healing of the amputation stump have been used; the Doppler ultrasound ankle systolic pressure should exceed 40 mmHg if a below-knee amputation is to succeed and the transcutaneous oxymetry reading in the skin at the amputation site should exceed a partial pressure of oxygen also of 40 mmHg. Isotope clearance studies are of value as are other arterial pressure studies, wave form analysis and dye injection methods but these all have difficulties in routine application.

The author's own preference is for amputation at the below-knee level (Hunter-Craig et al., 1970), provided that there is adequate bleeding from the skin and soft tissue at the time of operation. Others recommend through-knee amputation (Howard et al., 1969; Chilvers et al., 1971; Green et al., 1972; Newcombe and Marcuson, 1972), Gritti–Stokes (Martin et al., 1967) and supracondylar (Weale, 1969) amputations as a compromise giving good wound healing and a longer stump. It is rare for foot and distal amputations to be successful in severe vascular disorders with the exception of patients in whom the blood flow is restored by surgery and in diabetes where the factors of infection, peripheral neuropathy, microangiopathy and bacterial invasion may cause limited wet gangrene regardless of the state of the major arteries. Where amputation has to be performed for clostridial myositis or gangrene due to gas-forming organisms, the level of amputation must be selected above the involved group of muscles.

MANAGEMENT

Once the decision for amputation has been taken with the informed consent of the patient and the knowledge of the patient's doctor, close relatives and sometimes employer, the patient requires a full physical examination taking into account respiratory and cardiac function and the state of the musculoskeletal system. Ideally at this stage the patient should be examined by a limb-fitting surgeon, a physical medicine specialist and, in the elderly, a geriatric specialist. At this stage the social workers and occupational therapist should be informed of the situation. If there is time in the preoperative period a visit to the limb-fitting centre, with a chance to observe other patients in their rehabilitation and to obtain the interest of the prosthetic surgeon, is most helpful. The physiotherapist, who will deal with the patient after operation, should be responsible for the preoperative training. There is much advantage in the admission of the patient to a specialist unit or at least referral to an experienced team in amputation management.

A particular hazard in lower limb amputations is

the development of gas gangrene, usually due to auto-infection from bowel organisms and prophylaxis should begin before operation with culture of a rectal swab. An enema or suppository is given before the operation and thick coverage of the perineum with cottonwool is provided to filter any flatus passed during the operation. In addition systemic penicillin should begin after the operation and continue for 5 days afterwards. The skin of the limb to be amputated should be doubly sterilized with a povidone solution and kept covered with a sterile towel until it is finally exposed in the operating theatre. Where there is an infected extremity enclosing this in an airtight plastic bag before entry to the operating theatre may limit the chances of contamination of the amputation wound.

ANAESTHESIA

Where possible the operation is performed under general anaesthetic as most amputations involve the cutting of bone and despite ear plugs or headphones with music in the conscious patient, the noise can be distressing, but otherwise there is no contra-indication to a regional anaesthetic, and in the lower limb a spinal anaesthetic or epidural anaesthetic provides a highly satisfactory surgical field. In the very frail elderly patient a through-knee amputation is especially suitable for use with a regional anaesthetic as it is silent, speedy and is relatively atraumatic. Where an amputation has to be performed at the site of an accident, a nerve block is most suitable and can be introduced while the patient is inhaling a nitrous oxide–oxygen mixture.

Moderate hypotension with careful blood volume control is advisable for the proximal amputations, and provision of a central venous pressure monitor and of urine output measurement via a catheter is required. Blood should be available for transfusion; 4 units for fore-and hindquarter amputations.

SURGICAL PRINCIPLES INVOLVED IN AMPUTATION

Where an amputation is performed for sepsis, either existing or threatened due to contamination of a traumatized extremity, primary suture should be avoided. A guillotine operation in which all the tissues are incised at the same level will inevitably result in retraction of the skin and muscles and protrusion of the bone end, even if skin traction is applied after the operation, and should be reserved for the release of trapped victims. A modification of this in which the skin is cut distal to the bone as a sleeve is more acceptable but will inevitably lead to a cicatrized terminal scar adherent to the bone with retraction of muscles from the vicinity of the bone end. Both these types of amputation should only be used if the need for a reamputation procedure is accepted. In battle-field amputations the simplest and most distal amputation is accepted but the formation of short equal flaps including muscle closed with delayed primary suture after 5–6 days is very much preferable and on many occasions may avoid the need for a further amputation procedure.

For the elective amputations, whether of the upper or lower limb, it is important that the procedure is conducted as a precision operation with delicate handling of all tissues with adequate assistance to support the limb in the most favourable position. Where ischaemic disease is present a tourniquet is avoided as this may crush a segment of atheroma and precipitate a thrombosis proximal to the stump, but for all other amputations a pneumatic tourniquet should be routinely applied proximal to the amputation site— with safeguards to prevent its inflation to too high a pressure, or for too long a period and with safeguards to avoid it being overlooked at the end of the operation.

The level of amputation should always be carefully measured from the bony landmarks with a rule and the proposed skin incision marked with Bonney's blue dye or other indelible marker and the line of section through the other soft tissues should be repeatedly checked with the rule as the skin will usually retract. The skin flaps are cut and the incision deepened through the fat to the deep fascia. Diathermy is used for haemostasis of the smallest vessels and fine catgut sutures for the remaining vessels. The smallest amount of dead tissue should be retained in the stump and there seems little advantage in using heavy surgical materials. A skin hook should be used to handle the skin rather than dissecting or other forceps. Muscles should be cut cleanly with a scalpel and where a myoplasty is to be performed, that is, the suture of opposing muscles across the bone end to retain their function, then a sufficient length of muscle should be retained from the distal part of the limb to enable this suturing to be effected under natural tension.

An alternative procedure to myoplasty is myodesis—the fixation of muscle to the bone end—and this involves drilling of the bone in order to fix the sutures to the bone end. Where an osteomyoplasty is performed, part of the bone is incorporated in the muscle rearrangement; an example is the fibular bridge which can be employed in the osteomyoplasty of a below-knee amputation. Where muscle is sutured 0 or 1/0 chromic catgut sutures are required. It is important, if muscles are to function within the stump, that their blood supply and innervation are preserved. The presence of active muscles in the stump will ensure that the muscle pump aids venous return, the muscle mass will not waste and the function of the muscle concerned will be preserved. An amputation stump with an adequate myoplasty or myodesis will at rest lie in a natural position as there is no unopposed muscle function to produce a deformity.

The treatment of blood vessels is important. Mass ligature of arteries, veins and nerves should be avoided and the veins should be ligated with fine catgut. If thrombosis is noted within the veins this is an indication to excise more of the muscle mass and to give prophylactic heparin following the operation. Ligature of the veins and arteries together is avoided as arteriovenous fistulas have been described from this technique. The arteries require a fine double catgut ligature and where the arteries are occluded it is sometimes useful to perform a catheter thrombectomy using a Fogarty catheter to increase the blood supply to the stump. The nerves require particular attention and these should be freed from any pressure or ligature and drawn down to be cut transversely with a sharp scalpel so that they will retract 2–3 cm above the scar area; this is important not only for the named major nerve trunks but also for cutaneous nerves and small branches. The formation of neuroma at the amputation site is inevitable, but unless it is in an area of friction or high pressure should not be responsible for symptoms. It is likely that mismanagement of the nerve trunk is responsible for much postoperative and long-term pain in amputation stumps.

The bone requires particular attention. The periosteum should be elevated for the minimum distance and the site of amputation should, if possible, avoid the nutrient vessels to the medullary cavity. The value of leaving a flap of periosteum to cover the open end of the medullary cavity of a bone is of debatable value, but it has been stated that an open medullary cavity prejudices the whole haemodynamic pattern of the shaft of a long bone. A flap of periosteum may be conserved to suture over the open medullary cavity. The bone may be cut with a hand or power saw; the latter allowing for more precise shaping of the bone end. However, the saw cut is always jagged with sharp spicules and careful rounding of all surfaces by a bone rasp and file is required. This process may take 10–15 minutes and is of the greatest importance as the bone end should be able to float atraumatically in the soft tissues within the socket of any prosthesis that is provided.

The general technique should result in a supple stump in which the bone end is covered with an adequate thickness of soft tissue with functioning muscles. The fascia, fat and skin should be mobile over the bone end. The scar should be linear and not attached to the deep tissues. It seems that with modern prosthetic fitting a terminal scar over the bone end is of no disadvantage provided the other criteria are satisfactory. The general shape of the stump should be a cylinder with a hemi-spherical extremity and the diameter of the cylinder should not be wider than the diameter of the contralateral limb. Haematoma, deep infection and muscle necrosis should be carefully avoided by good surgical technique and established infection with a ring sequestrum at the site of bone section should not be encountered. There should be a minimum of foreign material in the stump. The skin and muscles should have a normal vascular supply. Unexplained postoperative pain in the early period is a sign of ischaemic musculature and an unsatisfactory stump.

Following operation the amputation stump is usually covered with a dressing, although in upper limb amputations this is not essential. An absorbent cotton gauze fluffed appears to be the best material and if this is covered with a 10 cm crêpe bandage, applied in a lazy S spiral, it is possible to provide uniform support to the whole stump without producing the proximal constriction which is inevitable in the conventional way of bandaging an amputation stump in which loops of bandage are restrained by a tight proximal turn. However, if the bandage is wider than 10 cm the spiral cannot be made to conform with the stump. There is great controversy about the best way in which an amputation wound should be dressed, with an increasing tendency to avoid anything but the softest net bandage.

There is a natural tendency of a terminal wound to become oedematous and pressure is applied to avoid this, but in many cases a badly applied bandage will itself produce distal oedema due to proximal constriction. A plaster-of-Paris shell applied to the amputation stump will protect it from inadvertent trauma or outside infection and will prevent muscle spasms. This is ideal if it can be rapidly changed should there be any anxiety about the underlying wound, but it may conceal pressure necrosis, ischaemia and infection. A compromise is a wholly split plaster shell retained with bandage.

To avoid these problems intermittent pressure applied in a plastic sleeve with a valvular seal at the top has been used in the technique of the controlled environment chamber, but this apparatus is rather cumbersome and only likely to be available at special centres. A pneumatic sleeve has been applied on the operating table and retained as a dressing with some success. The immediate peroperative fitting of a prosthesis has been successfully used in many centres, a plaster socket being fitted at the completion of the operation to which is applied an upper limb prosthesis or a lower limb foot and extension piece, so that the upper limb patient can use the prosthesis from the moment he or she wakes up and the lower limb patient can make ground contact after 48 hours and partially weight bear at 1 week. It is essential that if a plaster socket is used there are facilities for its immediate removal and replacement if there is any anxiety about the underlying stump, and this is the main limitation to its general usage.

An alternative to plaster is a low-temperature, heat-labile plastic mesh which can be moulded to the stump at operation or shortly after and used as either a rigid dressing or a temporary socket. However, in upper limb amputations immediate prosthetic fitting maintains the cortical representation of the arm which is otherwise very quickly lost, with the result that the patient becomes one-handed and may subsequently reject a prosthesis as cumbersome and of doubtful improvement over a one-handed existence.

In the early postoperative period the nursing care is directed to preventing pressure sores on the sacrum and heels. The lower limb amputee should spend two periods of half an hour in the day lying prone to prevent hip flexion and arm movements should be encouraged in the upper limb amputee from an early stage. As soon as the patient has recovered from the operation, a physiotherapy programme encourages active and passive mobility of the remaining joints and limbs and correction of any postural defect. Lower limb amputees are taught to use a wheelchair from the 2nd postoperative day and should be competent in transfer from bed to chair, chair to toilet by 1 week from the operation. In a limb with normal vascularity soft tissue healing should be complete by 10–14 days, at which time the skin sutures should be removed, but in the lower limb, especially if the amputation has been for ischaemic disease, sutures should be retained for 21 days and for this reason the most satisfactory suture material is either nylon or Prolene, which elicits no inflammatory reaction.

PROSTHETIC MANAGEMENT

Where a plaster socket has been provided on the operating table function can begin within days of the surgical operation, but only partial weight bearing is permitted in a lower limb amputation until the 7th to 10th day and then the degree of weight bearing is progressively increased to full function by 3 weeks. The patient can be taught to grade the pressure using a bathroom scale or pressure-activated biosensor. This represents a great advance over the previous management in which the patient was confined to bed and a wheelchair until his prosthesis was prescribed, sometimes months after the amputation.

The use of an early walking aid pioneered by Devas has considerably reduced this period of delay. The first walking aids were modified pylons, essentially an ischial-bearing device with side-irons, a rocker or foot and a knee hinge with a slide lock. A patient with an amputation at below-knee, through-knee or above-knee level can use one of these from the 10th day after operation and is usually able to walk between parallel bars or with sticks or with a walking frame by the 3rd or 4th postoperative week. Many patients have taken aids of this type home while awaiting their definitive prosthesis.

A considerable advance in early walking aids has come with the pneumatic aid, devised by Little, and modified by Redhead—essentially a pneumatic splint enclosed in a frame with a foot piece. This can be worn from the 7th postoperative day. The patient can wear the appliance for 2 hours at a time, inflated to a pressure of 40 mmHg. It is infinitely adjustable to patients of varying size and can be held in any physiotherapy department in readiness for each new patient. The patient can walk with this aid under supervision until a definitive prosthesis is provided.

In the early weeks after operation the stump is more bulky due to oedema than it will be later on, and the process of shrinkage means that a socket which will fit perfectly on the 14th postoperative day will be much too loose by the 21st, and therefore it is rarely practical to provide a definitive socket until after the 21st postoperative day. The process of shrinkage is much enhanced by the use of a pneumatic prosthesis and slightly delayed by the use of a walking aid in which the stump is not supported. The routine bandaging of an amputation stump is not essential and the traditional method is particularly likely to result in a tourniquet proximal constriction which may cause swelling and breakdown at the suture line. An elastic net sock is much preferred to hold a light fluffed gauze in place. It is unlikely that any amputation stump is fully mature in less than 3 months and it is usual for the first prosthesis to be replaced in this period. Therefore the first definitive prosthesis is usually of a simple type and for manufacturing reasons is often in the nature of a pylon which will allow the patients normal function and the ability to resume their normal environment.

A patient with a lower limb amputation from trauma should be able to return home 4 weeks from the operation and a lower limb amputee for ischaemic disease, even in the geriatric age group, should be able to return home 6–8 weeks after the operation. Upper limb amputees can leave hospital in 10–14 days but will need to attend an arm training school for a much longer period to obtain full rehabilitation.

It is important that before discharge from hospital a home visit has been made to supply special aids, such as hand rails and ramps in the home, to educate the relatives to the needs of the amputee and in the case of employees their employment should be adapted to their ability and this may involve the arrangement of a retraining programme. It is important for the geriatric patient that a geriatrician advises on the best accommodation and the management of the patient after discharge.

Stump Complications

These may be seen in both upper and lower limb amputations and can be considered as follows:

1. Delayed healing may be attributed to local problems particularly ischaemia due to an inadequate arterial supply. In infection, whether auto-infection or cross-infection, what is particularly significant is the lack of cooperation of the patient who may contaminate the wound or traumatize the healing stump or maintain the limb in an unsuitable position applying pressure to the suture line. Delayed healing may also be encountered with intercurrent disease, such

as diabetes in elderly patients, those with uraemia, malnutrition, anaemia and infection at other sites, and these factors should be carefully corrected.

2. An amputation stump may be painful in the early postoperative period and may cause pain throughout the patient's lifetime. In the early postoperative period the most important cause of pain is ischaemia, particularly of the muscles, whether due to pre-existing arterial disease or due to compression of the muscles due to poor operative technique. Deep vein thrombosis may occur in the amputation stump leading to swelling and pain which may not be recognized. Infection is usually apparent by redness, induration and tenderness and osteomyelitis may show by the erosion of the transected bone end. Later pain may be due to incorporation of a nerve trunk in the fibrous scar of the neuroma fortuitously developing in an area exposed to friction or pressure.

If these problems can be excluded it is likely that there is a psychiatric overlay to the problem and depression is frequently encountered. Causalgic pain is sometimes seen in patients who are afraid to use the stump, regarding the phantom sensations, which are an entirely normal phenomenon, as distressing. Psychiatric help may be required in this situation.

3. The scar may be adherent to the bone end and therefore be submitted to tension while the stump is in use, and retrimming is sometimes indicated to free the adherent soft tissue to improve the shape of the bone end.

4. There may be tension of the soft tissues over a prominent bone end. This is a particular problem when an amputation is through a growing bone when the unimpeded epiphyseal lengthening proximal to the amputation causes a conical stump with considerable pain and deformity. The bone end may be prominent due to a poorly judged amputation with tight soft tissues and a badly shaped bone end which may result in osteophyte formation with bony spurs, with sometimes more extensive myositis ossificans. These complications may necessitate a refashioning of the amputation stump.

5. The skin may become thickened and lymphoedematous; sometimes eczema develops due to poor ventilation of the socket and in pressure areas sebaceous cysts may form.

6. Sometimes adventitious bursas are a problem and frequently at the ischium a poorly fitting socket will push a roll of fatty flesh above the socket and cause discomfort. Pressure of the socket in this region may eventually produce arterial and venous thrombosis, although this is often a slow process and usually does not cause any problem in the stump.

7. Otherwise the principal complications of the amputation stump are deformity of the proximal joints progressing to fixation of the proximal joints usually in a flexed position with corresponding loss of function. Flexion deformities may be extremely difficult to treat and prophylaxis is an essential part of the early management of every amputee.

ARM AMPUTATIONS

Forequarter Amputation

Forequarter amputation consists of extirpation of the shoulder girdle including the scapula and most of the clavicle and all the structures of the arm (*Fig.* 49.1). The patient is left with a smooth contour to the rib cage and no projection on which to support a prosthesis. The operation can be performed with the dissection starting either from the front or from behind. In both cases the patient is laid on his or her side with the arm to be amputated upwards and fully towelled. A racquet type of incision is used with the handle of the racquet along the clavicle (*Fig.* 49.1). If the dissection is started from the front the clavicle is divided with a Gigli saw 3 cm from the sternoclavicular joint. The pectoralis major and minor are

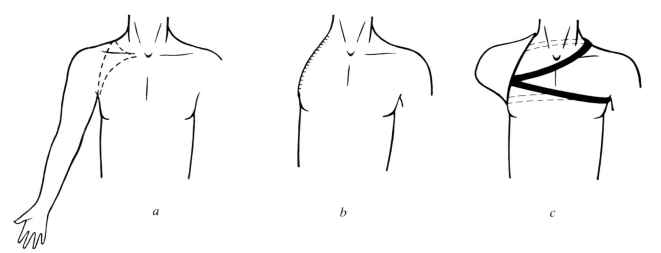

Fig. 49.1. Forequarter amputation. *a*, Skin flaps. *b*, This stump is unsuitable for a prosthesis other than a shoulder pad (*c*).

incised at a distance depending on the pathology and the axillary fascia opened, allowing access to the subclavian vein, the subclavian artery and the trunks of the brachial plexus. These are divided just distal to the tendon of scalenus anterior with double non-absorbable ligatures with special care to avoid retraction before the ligature is secure, and the arm is lifted to bring the muscular attachments of the scapula into view. The levator scapulae, the serratus anterior, the trapezius and rhomboid muscles are divided and finally the latissimus dorsi, resulting in separation of the upper extremity. The serratus anterior and pectoralis major residue can be sutured together to provide additional cover for the exposed rib cage. An alternative approach is to initiate dissection by dividing the trapezius and latissimus dorsi, posteriorly at the start of the dissection, then incising the serratus anterior, lifting the scapula forwards bringing access to the neurovascular bundle from behind. Advantages are claimed for both techniques.

Following operation few patients are able to use a prosthesis and a light shoulder pad is usually all that is used. A prosthetic arm for cosmetic purposes can be supplied but is not found to be satisfactory by the patients.

Shoulder Disarticulation (*Fig.* 49.2)

A racquet or anterior and posterior flap incision is formed at the level of the neck of the humerus and after dissection of the neurovascular bundle the pectoralis major and minor and deltoid are divided close to the humerus. The teres major and minor and the muscles of the rotator cuff are divided, and the anterior capsule with the shoulder joint is incised allowing just the head of the humerus to be dislocated, and incision of the posterior capsule allows the limb to be removed. The pectoralis major, deltoid and rotator cuff muscles are apposed over the glenoid cavity and the skin closed with drainage.

The functional ability of a prosthesis for this amputation is not very satisfactory as despite a large shoulder cap covering the protruding acromion there is some instability and it is difficult to obtain adequate leverage from the opposite shoulder to operate the elbow and the other hand has to be used to lock the prosthesis, either in a flexed or extended position, before shoulder movement can activate a split hook.

Above-elbow Amputation (*Fig.* 49.3)

There is no optimum level for amputation measured from the acromion. The most important factor is that sufficient room must be left below the stump to allow an elbow mechanism in the prosthesis. Therefore a clear 10 cm must be allowed above the elbow joint for this purpose. Otherwise the longest lever that can be retained is best for prosthetic function. In practical terms at least three finger-breadths' (4 cm) length of humerus must project below the axillary fold for a socket to use the humerus as a lever; above this level a prosthesis has all the disadvantages of a shoulder disarticulation although the retention of the head of the humerus and amputation through the surgical neck give a better contour to the shoulder. At whichever level is applicable the skin is incised to make equal anterior and posterior flaps and the muscles are cut transversely inclining inwards and upwards to the line of bone section. The bone is rounded with a bone file and the flexor and extensor muscles are sutured together over the bone end to constitute a myoplasty and the deep fascia closed with fine catgut; the skin is closed with fine sutures, nylon or Prolene, and with Steristrips. This is the ideal amputation for an immediate peroperative fitting of a prosthesis and if the limb has been measured prior to surgery a normal type of prosthesis can be applied on the operating table.

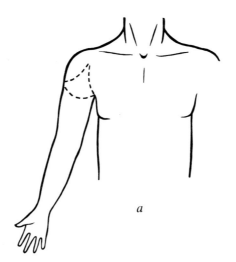
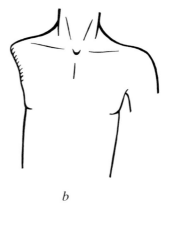

Fig. 49.2. Disarticulation of shoulder. *a*, Skin flaps. *b*, This stump is also unsuitable for a prosthesis.

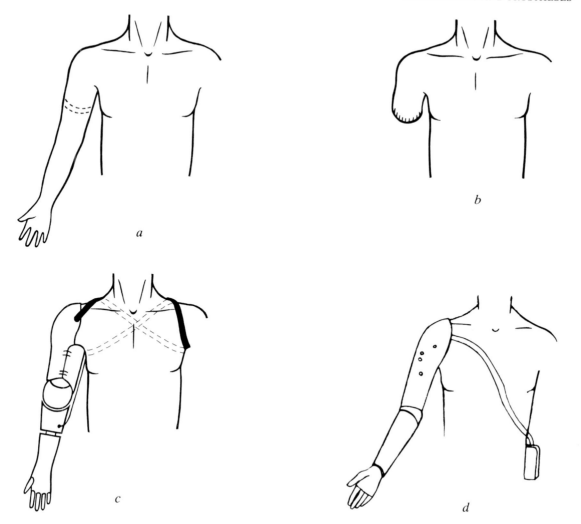

Fig. 49.3. Above-elbow amputation. *a*, Skin flaps. *b*, Stump. *c*, Conventional prosthesis. *d*, Swedish myoelectric arm, with battery pack and triggering detectors on upper arm.

Elbow Disarticulation (*Fig.* 49.4)

If the elbow can be retained disarticulation at the elbow joint is an acceptable procedure. Anterior and posterior flaps are formed based on the medial and lateral epicondyles. Sufficient length of triceps tendon, biceps and brachialis is retained to allow suture over the articular surface of the humerus and the skin is closed with drainage. The prominence of the epicondyles enables the prosthetic forearm to be retained by a leather and lace suspension. The axis of the elbow joint is anterior to the normal elbow but there is no detriment to function.

Elbow flexion can be operated from the opposite shoulder by a cord which on further movement will operate a splint hook; pronation and supination at mid-forearm are effected by the opposite hand.

Below-elbow Amputation (*Fig.* 49.5)

There is no optimal site of amputation below the

elbow but the lever length clear of the biceps tendon should be as long as possible, although sufficient muscle should be available to cover the bone ends to make a myoplastic amputation, and therefore the junction between the lower third and the upper two-thirds of the radius and ulna is ideal. Equal anterior and posterior flaps are formed with suture of the flexor and extensor muscle groups over the transected ulna and radius. At this level an immediate prosthesis can be provided by a plaster socket applied on the operating table carrying a pivot for pronation and supination of either a double hook operated by a cord from the opposite shoulder or a cosmetic hand.

In an attempt to obtain better function at this level Kruckenberg claws have been used, in which the radius and ulna are separated and provided with skin cover, making a lobster claw. This is especially indicated in blind patients and the operation is performed by making an axial incision from four finger-breadths

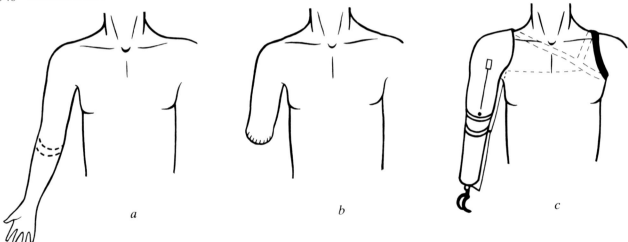

Fig. 49.4. Through-elbow amputation. *a*, Skin flaps. *b*, Stump. *c*, Prosthesis which allows elbow flexion to be operated from the opposite shoulder by a cord. Pronation and supination at mid-forearm are effected by the opposite hand.

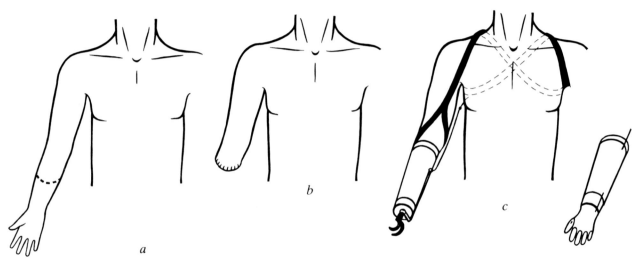

Fig. 49.5. Below-elbow amputation. *a*, Skin flaps. *b*, Stump. *c*, Prosthesis which allows double hook or cosmetic hand operated from the opposite shoulder.

below the elbow joint over the interosseous region on both the anterior and posterior surface of the forearm. The flexor digitorum sublimis is split while the profundus and flexor pollicis longus are removed. The interosseous membrane is divided. The median and ulnar nerves are cut distal to the branches supplying the forearm muscles and the interosseous membrane is divided to within 7 cm of the elbow joint. The lateral part of the flexor digitorum sublimis is attached to the flexor carpi radialis and the medial part is sutured to the flexor carpi ulnaris. The ends of the forearm bones are grooved. The radial extensors and flexors are sutured in the radial groove and the ulnar muscles in the ulnar groove. The skin can be closed around the radius but a graft may be placed to close the inner side of the ulnar jaw. The brachioradialis opens the jaws while pronator teres and the forearm flexors close the jaws.

Wrist Amputations

The wrist can be disarticulated if there is severe and irretrievable hand injury. As much of the carpal structure as is viable should be retained. The operation is essentially performed through anterior/posterior flaps centred on the ulnar and radial styloid processes which, if no carpal bone is retained, may need to be smoothed flush with the articular surface of the radius. The tendons of the flexor and extensor muscles should be left long enough to allow them to be sutured over the bone end and constitute a myoplasty. A plaster shell can be applied at the completion of the operation and a split hook applied to the plaster for immediate function. It is not possible to utilize the patient's own pronation and supination in the prosthesis and this remains a passive function, while activation of a split hook is achieved by a cord from the opposite shoulder.

Amputations in the Hand

This is a particularly difficult problem requiring great experience and should always be managed by a specialist in the field. Part-finger amputations may be unsatisfactory as the release of tendon attachments leads to progressive stiffness and encumbrance due to the rigidity of the remaining portion of the finger. Provided the tendon attachments remain, amputation of the distal phalanx can provide acceptable function, although proximal to this there is a considerable functional deficit, but it is probably always wise to allow the patient to obtain the best use of the remaining digits for a trial period before accepting the need for a more proximal amputation.

Here the problem is whether to leave the patient with an intact metacarpal structure with a wide span across the metacarpophalangeal joints with a strong palm at the expense of a prominent metacarpal head. There is little doubt that heavy manual workers fare best with intact metacarpals, and amputation of a digit should be through the base of the proximal phalanx to preserve the short muscle attachments, but in other patients resection of the metacarpophalangeal joint and part of the metacarpal cut obliquely provides a much more acceptable cosmetic hand. The thumb and index finger are of the greatest practical value and should be preserved if at all possible. The possibility of transference of a digit and its neurovascular connections, as in the procedure of pollicization of an index finger, should be carefully considered before any decision is made to amputate.

A digital amputation can be made either with a racquet incision or by anterior posterior flaps. Considerable care should be taken to avoid ligating the digital nerve. Skin closure with Steristrips and fine 6/0 nylon sutures is recommended.

Where trauma has resulted in extensive digital loss, there should be no attempt to produce any formal amputation, but conservative trimming should aim to produce supple skin cover of smooth bone ends, and provide means of improving function by secondary surgery at a later date.

See also p.726.

Power prostheses for upper limb amputees have made considerable progress in the past decade. There is no limit to the mechanical ingenuity that has been expended on this topic but two problems remain—an acceptable power source and sophisticated control mechanisms. Gas power from cylinders is being superseded by battery-powered electric motors, while actuation of the functions can be triggered by myoelectric potentials, or by pressure detectors over functional muscles. Both require considerable education of, and determination by, the patient in order to achieve acceptable results, but the Swedish arm shows how much can be achieved—finger extension and flexion, wrist rotation and elbow flexion and extension.

AMPUTATION AT VARIOUS LEVELS IN THE LOWER LIMB

Translumbar Amputation (Hemicorporectomy)

Although a dreadful mutilation, amputation at this level has been successfully performed for extensive local tumours in the pelvis and also for extreme trauma to the pelvis and lower limbs (Baker et al., 1970). The amputation is made at the level of the 2nd lumbar vertebra, and the formation of an ileal conduit and the establishment of a left iliac colostomy are necessary. The soft tissues are incised to form two equal anteroposterior flaps, although the best use must be made of the available soft tissue. The aorta and vena cava must be secured at an early stage; while the vena cava may be ligated the aorta is best oversewn with a continuous arterial suture. The spinal theca should also be closed with a continuous catgut suture and some of the muscle of the posterior flap placed over the end of the verebral canal.

The patient is nursed flat in the early days after the operation with active physiotherapy to strengthen the arms and shoulders and to ensure adequate ventilation. Once the soft tissues are healed, the patient can be sat up and a chair-like frame constructed to hold the patient securely by the shoulders while allowing free movement of the abdominal wall and arms. A similar truncal socket can be incorporated in an electric wheelchair with hand controls to provide the patient with mobility.

Hindquarter Amputation

This procedure, which was established by Sir Gordon Gordon Taylor at a time when any major operation carried a considerable hazard, has now developed into a safe elective procedure (Westbury, 1967), which should be carried out with a hypotensive anaesthetic technique and, where possible, with the use of diathermy to cut across the muscle mass and to secure careful haemostasis throughout.

The patient is positioned on the operating table in a half lateral position with the affected leg fully towelled so that its position can be changed. A urethral catheter should be passed. The anterior skin incision runs just distal to the inguinal ligament and the posterior skin flap incorporates most of the skin of the buttock and some of the muscle fibres of gluteus maximus and medius to carry the blood supply. The anterior incision is deepened to the inguinal ligament which is detached from the anterior superior iliac spine and the abdominal wall muscles are erased from the iliac crest back to the ala of the sacrum. In the extraperitoneal plane the peritoneum is separated from the iliac fossa and access can be obtained by retraction to the back of the pubis, which can then be divided with a Gigli saw. This allows the pelvis to open slightly and exposure can be obtained of the common iliac artery and vein. The iliac artery can be ligated without difficulty but the iliac vein must be carefully dissected to safeguard against the small iliolumbar branches emerging from its concealed posterior aspect. By carefully ligating these, the blood loss from the operation is reduced to a minimum and the iliac vein can then be securely ligated and divided.

The dissection is deepened below the pubis to separate the urethral bulb and muscles from the ischium and the levator ani can be detached from the obturator internus fascia. The ischiorectal fat is separated from the pelvic side-wall and the dissection carried into the greater and lesser sciatic notch. Here the superior and inferior gluteal vessels will be secured and the lumbosacral trunk and elements of the sciatic plexus divided, leaving the ala of the sacrum for division with a Gigli saw before the extremity can be detached. Careful haemostasis is obtained and the skin flaps sutured with suction drainage. The patient can be mobilized a few days after the operation and can learn to walk with crutches at the earliest opportunity.

Once the soft tissues are stable and healed, the patient can be measured for a prosthesis which consists of a large socket for the hemipelvis with shoulder straps for stability and a belt embracing the other side of the pelvis. The underside of the socket is flattened and an anterior hinge suspends the leg, which requires a knee joint locking device. The most popular prosthesis is the Canadian pattern tilting table which will allow these patients to walk with an accept-

able gait and to stand and sit with minimal difficulty. Some of these patients are able to walk without the use of any stick or support.

Disarticulation at the Hip Joint (*Fig.* 49.6)

Through an anterior incision, running just below the inguinal ligament, and a posterior flap performed at the lower part of the buttock skin, the femoral triangle is exposed and the femoral artery and vein can be ligated at the level of the inguinal ligament. The posterior skin flap can incorporate a greater or lesser amount of the gluteal muscle mass according to the reason for the amputation. The anterior muscles are erased from the pelvis until the hip joint is exposed; the capsule and iliofemoral ligaments are divided allowing the head to be dislocated and further dissection reaches the sciatic nerve which is divided with a small ligature to secure only the concomitant artery, and the limb can then be detached. Careful haemostasis is secured and the flaps closed with suction drainage.

Early ambulation with crutches can be achieved and the patient can be fitted with a similar prosthesis to the hindquarter amputation, but weight is carried on the ipsilateral ischial tuberosity and the greater stability of the socket on the bony pelvis enables a better gait to be achieved. The patient may walk well with a swing phase control knee joint but usually a knee lock is provided for greater stability.

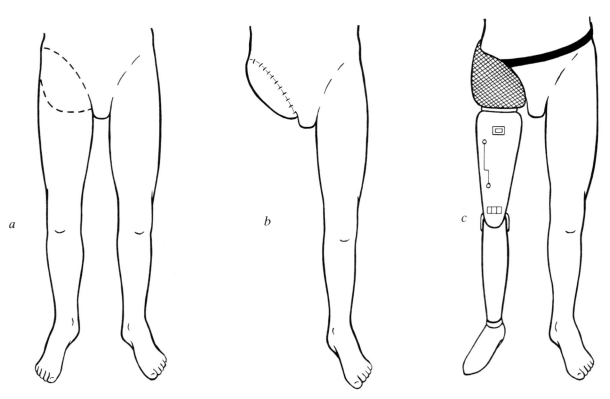

Fig. 49.6. Disarticulation of hip. *a*, Skin flaps. *b*, Stump. *c*, Tilting table prosthesis.

Amputation through the Upper End of the Femur

Through a similar incision to that described for a hip disarticulation, a similar dissection can be performed with the exception that the femur is divided at the junction of the neck and shaft, with the advantage that when the soft tissues cover the bone remnant the stump has a better shape and some weight can be carried by the femoral residue on the ischial tuberosity of the same side. However, with modern cast-resin sockets the prominent femoral remnant may be a disadvantage.

Above-knee Level of Amputation (*Fig.* 49.7)

The exact level of this amputation is not important, but if a sophisticated knee joint mechanism is to be provided then the lower end of the femur must terminate 13 cm above the axis line of the knee joint before operation. At this level the femoral artery and vein are in the lower part of the subsartorial canal. Two equal flaps (*Fig.* 49.7*a*) can be based at this level, 13 cm above the knee joint line, skewed to enable the vertical part of the incision to overly the subsartorial canal to provide early and easy access to the femoral vessels, which are individually ligated as the first stage of the dissection. The incision is deepened through the fascia lata, the lower end of the quadriceps and some of the quadriceps expansion is transected just below the line of bone section, and the hamstring muscles are cut a little longer than the bone end. The iliotibial band is cut 5 cm longer than the line of bone section, as are the adductor, gracilis and sartorius tendons. These transected muscles then constitute four groups. The bone is transected and the edges carefully rounded with a bone rasp and file before the drill holes are made. The adductors can be sutured to the iliotibial band across the end of the femur, but unless the bone end is drilled the attached muscles will slip off and the anchoring effect will be lost. The hamstrings are sutured to the quadriceps mass and again the sutures must be stabilized through drill holes in the bone end.

A full myodesis is then obtained. The fascia lata is carefully repaired and the skin closed with fine nylon sutures, suction drainage being provided as a routine. The above-knee amputation heals readily and is usually stable at 14 days (*Fig.* 49.7*b*). The patient can be supplied with an ischial weight-bearing socket and pylon to facilitate walking training until the stump is sufficiently stable to permit accurate casting for a definitive prosthesis or may use a pneumatic walking aid (*Fig.* 49.7*c–e*). The myoplastic technique described gives a cylindrical stump which is very suitable for the application of a suction socket which can eliminate the need for any straps or buckles and enables the patient with an above-knee amputation to walk with a nearly normal gait (*Fig.* 49.7*f*). The myoplastic amputation requires no special postural treatment as it takes a natural position without hip flexion, although it is advisable for the patient still to lie on his or her face for two periods of half an hour each day to prevent a flexion contracture of the hip developing in the early postoperative period. Physiotherapy is essential to prevent hip flexion, especially prior to the operation.

Supracondylar Amputation (Weale, 1969)

Proposed as an alternative to the Gritti–Stokes amputation, the line of bone section is through the lower end of the femur at the level of the adductor tubercle. Equal skin flaps are formed and the popliteal artery and vein secured posteriorly at an early stage in the dissection. The quadriceps expansion and the hamstring tendons are transected 2·5 cm beyond the bone end so that they can be sutured together and attached over the bone end. The bone end, being square and wide, may not need to be drilled to stabilize the attached tendons. The fascia lata and skin are closed with suction drainage if necessary.

The patients can be allowed to stand with crutches and to walk at an early stage with an ischial weight-bearing pylon and socket. When healed and stable, a prosthesis can be supplied with a simple hinge knee joint and lock which is satisfactory but is inferior to a suction socket and sophisticated knee joint mechanism which can be provided for the slightly higher above-knee amputation.

Gritti–Stokes Amputation (*Fig.* 49.8)

This amputation, popular in some centres, is performed at the same level as the supracondylar amputation. The adductor tendon remains attached to its tubercle. A long anterior skin flap is fashioned, extending to the tubercle of the tibia, so that the patellar tendon is detached from the tibia and the anterior skin flap and the patella and quadriceps expansion are reflected upwards. A short posterior skin flap is deepened to reach the popliteal nerves and the popliteal vessels. The hamstring muscles are divided at the level of bone section. The patella and quadriceps expansion are pulled upwards to obtain access to the supracondylar region of the femur, which is divided transversely and sharp edges rounded with a file. The saw cut should be higher posteriorly so that muscle tension locks the patella in place. The articular surface of the patella is shaved off with a vertical saw cut while the soft tissues are held in a large swab. The patella is then drilled and drill holes are made through the lower end of the femur so that the patella can be attached to the cut surface of the femur by two strong catgut or nylon sutures. The stump of the patellar tendon is secured to the hamstring muscles providing attachment of the flexor and extensor group. The fascia lata and skin are sutured with small stitches. Suction drainage may be required.

This amputation heals readily and provides a

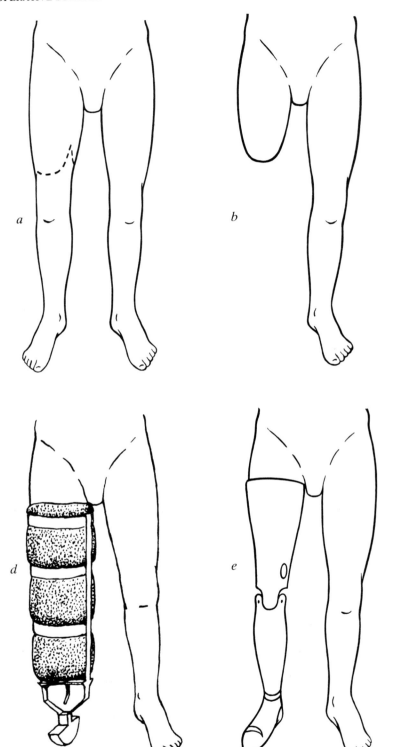

Fig. 49.7. Above-knee amputation.
a, Skin flaps. *b*, Stump.
c, Weight-bearing socket and pylon for
   walking training.
d, PPAM walking aid with inflated air bag
   enclosing stump.
e, Commonly used permanent prosthesis.

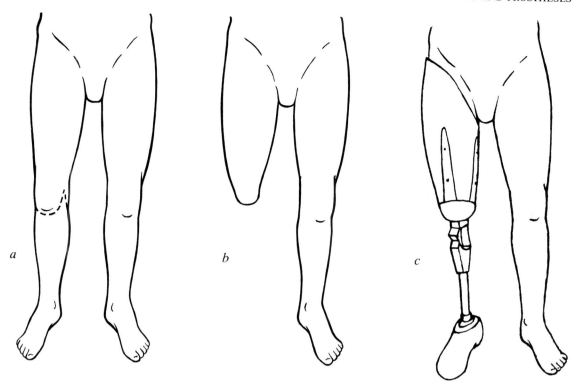

Fig. 49.8. Gritti–Stokes amputation. *a*, Skin flaps. *b*, Stump. *c*, Four-bar modular linkage leg in Gritti–Stokes amputation.

potentially end-bearing stump. Again the patient can have a movable and locking knee joint, but is denied any more sophisticated knee joint mechanism while the tapered stump is not suitable for a suction socket. Nevertheless, the long lever and quick healing characteristics of this amputation make it popular in many quarters. The patient can start walking at an early stage with an ischial-bearing socket and pylon, but many patients continue to use this simple device as detachment and looseness of the patella or avascular necrosis with pain can make end-bearing impossible.

Through-knee Amputation (*Fig.* 49.9)

The wide stump, which is capable of end bearing, that results from this amputation makes it popular with many surgeons. The prosthesis has the disadvantage that the hinged side-irons have to be beside the socket, making it rather wide and cosmetically unacceptable for the younger female patient. However, the stump is durable and painfree and the operation is quick and silent, an advantage in the elderly ischaemic limb, when regional anaesthesia is used. The uncertainties of healing encountered when the conventional anterior flap is used have been avoided by the use of equal lateral skin flaps.

The patient is placed supine on the operating table with the knees hanging over the edge with the end section dropped; some surgeons prefer to lie the patient prone and flex the knee for the anterior dissection. The conventional incision is a long anterior flap extending below the tibial tubercle and a short posterior flap at the level of the knee joint line is made, but the author recommends that equal lateral flaps are formed, from the tibial tubercle descending 4 cm then converging at the joint line posteriorly. Ample skin is needed; the condyles seem very large when the skin is being sutured. With the leg straight the incision is deepened to the tibial periosteum and patellar tendon which is severed from the tibial tubercle and the quadriceps expansion divided so that the knee joint is entered from the front and the patella lifted. With the knee fully flexed the lateral ligaments and the cruciate ligaments may be divided without difficulty. With the leg straight and the foot lifted to flex the hip, the posterior incisions are deepened until the popliteal nerve, the popliteal artery and vein can be individually divided and then the blood vessels ligated. The hamstring tendons are divided 2 cm below the level of the joint line. The patellar tendon is sutured to the cruciate ligaments, which are in turn sutured to the hamstring tendons with heavy chromic catgut. It is important that the patella is not drawn down into the intracondylar notch but is allowed to maintain its natural position on the front of the knee joint, where it prevents rotation of the socket on the stump. The skin is closed with fine sutures and Steri-strips; a crêpe bandage is applied.

Healing is usually rapid and the patient has a firm wide stump capable of end bearing. Until end bearing is possible an ischial-bearing pylon can be worn for the purposes of walking training or a pneumatic walk-

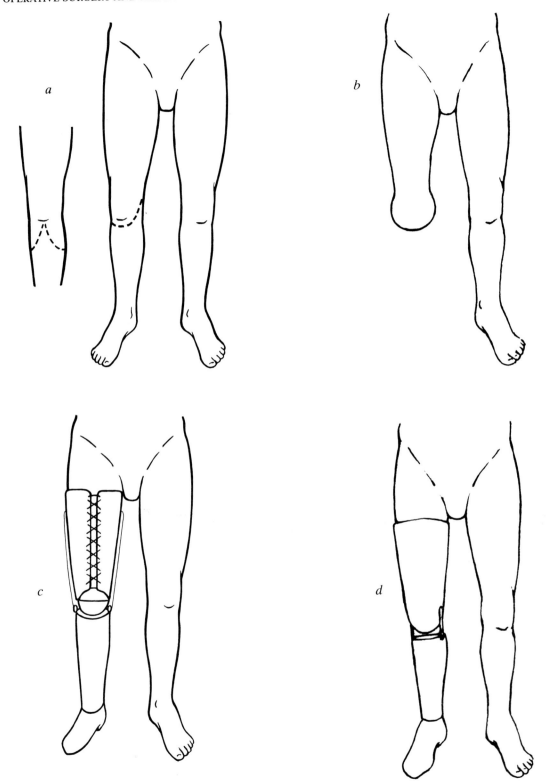

Fig. 49.9. Through-knee amputation. *a*, Anteroposterior or lateral flaps may be used. *b*, Stump. *c*, Close-fitting socket prosthesis with locking knee. *d*, Self-suspending socket using shaped liner.

ing aid, but as soon as the scar is stable a close-fitting socket can be applied. The prosthesis incorporates a simple locking knee joint and the patient is able to walk with an acceptable gait, taking weight on surfaces which normally bear weight.

The through-knee prosthesis has been much improved by the four-bar linkage which puts the joint mechanism below the stump while the axis of movement is in the natural position. The prosthesis is no longer unacceptably wide. An additional development is the use of an inner liner in the through-knee socket which allows the prosthesis to be self-suspending in suitable patients.

Below-knee Amputation

Below-knee amputation is frequently used in ischaemic disease when Doppler ultrasound ankle systolic pressure is 40 mmHg or above. The transcutaneous measurement of oxygen diffusion through the skin 10 cm below the knee is a valuable indication of the ability to heal at this level (Burgess et al., 1982); 40 mmHg oxygen tension is the lowest value compatible with safe healing at below-knee level. Below-knee amputation is contra-indicated in patients who cannot cooperate to extend the knee. Conventionally performed 14 cm below the knee joint line, the anterior skin flap is two-thirds the diameter of the leg and the posterior skin flap is one-third the diameter of the leg. The muscles, nerves and blood vessels are divided at the level of bone section, the fibula being divided 2 cm above the tibia. The bone ends must be carefully rounded, the skin closed with fine sutures and suction drainage.

In patients with vascular disease, it is recommended that the long anterior skin flap is not used as this is frequently ischaemic (Kendrick, 1956), and instead the anterior skin is divided transversely 12 cm below the knee joint line to 2 cm behind the axis of the limb. A posterior skin flap is fashioned from the posterior skin of the limb, extending down to just above the ankle, the excess in order to allow the flap to be secondarily trimmed (*Fig.* 49.10*a*) (Burgess et al., 1969; Hunter-Craig et al., 1970). The anterior tibial muscles are divided and the vessels secured. The fibula is divided 2 cm above the line of bone section, 10 cm from the knee joint line. The tibia is divided transversely with a smooth anterior curve cut with a cantilever blade power saw, then carefully rounded with bone file to leave a smooth contour in all planes.

Once the bones are divided, a plane can be entered between the posterior tibial and the gastrocnemius/soleus mass and these muscles are allowed to remain with the posterior flap, while the posterior tibial itself is divided and the peroneal and posterior tibial muscles and nerves individually divided. The Achilles tendon is cut to free the limb before the long posterior flap is trimmed so that a wedge of muscle extends to its distal end, which can then be folded to meet the anterior tibial periosteum where it is sutured to form a myoplasty of the gastrocnemius/soleus mass.

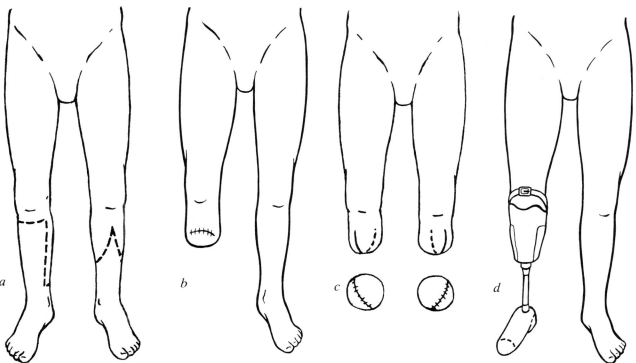

Fig. 49.10. Below-knee amputation. *a*, Long posterior flap on right leg. Skew flap incision on left keg. *b*, Long posterior flap stump. *c*, Skewed sagittal flaps stump. *d*, Californian patellar tendon-bearing socket. Modular (without cover).

Very considerable removal of muscle tissue is needed, especially from the medial and lateral aspects of the flap, if a bulky stump is to be avoided (*Fig.* 49.10*b*). The posterior skin is trimmed to match the anterior incision and sutured with fine nylon or Prolene stitches and Steristrips with suction drainage.

Thermography studies have indicated that skewed sagittal flaps correspond to the distribution of vascular supply better than the long posterior flap, and combined with the gastrocnemius myoplasty produce a stump that requires no secondary shaping and can therefore permit early casting and the supply of prosthesis without any delay (Robinson et al., 1983). The shape which requires no moulding does not require the traditional stump bandage.

This technique often enables healing to occur even when the blood supply is appreciably impaired. The stump is lightly bandaged and the patient may start walking with crutches shortly after the operation and can wear an ischial weight-bearing pylon until the stump is healed and stable or use a pneumatic walking aid (Redhead et al., 1978), until a cast can be taken for a below-knee prosthesis.

A below-knee prosthesis is a nearly total contact socket with a ridge over the patellar tendon, so that the maximum weight bearing occurs at this point, but is also shared by the flare of the tibial condyles. This socket, the California patellar tendon-bearing socket (*Fig.* 49.10*c*), is secured by a single strap above the patella and the lower leg prosthesis carries an ankle joint or a flexible foot and enables a normal gait to be achieved; the young patient is quite able to run. To utilize knee flexion, 4 cm of stump must project beneath the hamstring tendons of the flexed knee. If the stump is unsatisfactory for a patellar tendon-bearing socket, a thigh corset with side-steels and locking knee hinge will allow the stump to be relieved of all stress, in a prosthesis that was the conventional one until 15 years ago.

Syme's Amputation (*Fig.* 49.11)
This has been popular with many surgeons as the patient is able in an emergency to stand and walk without a prosthesis. The original level of amputation was through the ankle joint with the medial and lateral malleolus trimmed. The amputation has been modified to divide the tibia and fibula 1 cm above the joint line and an anterior incision is made over the ankle joint, extending to a point just anterior to the malleoli, when the incision is carried down underneath the heel. The ankle joint is entered from the front and the incision carried to the calcaneum which is carefully enucleated from the posterior tissues, safeguarding the calcaneal vessels which carry the blood supply to the heel skin. When the foot is detached the heel skin can be rotated forwards so that the skin can be sutured across the front of the stump. The stump is bulbous transversely and the skin from the back of the heel forms the lower end of the stump (*Fig.* 49.11*b*).

This heals well, provided the blood supply is not impaired, but it is not recommended where the vascular supply is critical. The bulbous nature of the stump makes it sometimes necessary to fit a 'window' in the socket; alternatively it must be laced throughout its length to enable the stump to be inserted (*Fig.* 49.11*c*). A flexible foot is provided and the patient may walk with a normal gait provided that the heel pad is not displaced.

Wagner has utilized the Syme's amputation in the treatment of septic diabetic gangrene as a two-stage procedure. First, the foot is removed by disarticulation of the talo-tibiofibular joint and suturing the heel flap while providing irrigating suction drainage to the dead space in the heel flap. Six weeks later through vertical, lateral and medial incisions the malleoli are removed with an osteotome and the soft tissues remodelled. The stump is enclosed in plaster, and weight bearing can be achieved in 2 weeks. The viability of the heel skin depends on the integrity of the calcaneal branches of the peroneal and posterior tibial arteries. It is essential that these are not damaged in the surgical procedure.

Other amputations can be performed in the region of the ankle joint, although they are infrequently used in this country at the present time. In the Pirogoff amputation, rather than the calcaneum being enucleated from the heel, the calcaneum is cut across so that its posterior 2 cm remain in the heel flap and this is attached to the lower end of the tibia, making a longer stump than in the Syme's amputation. The difficulties in fixation have led to its infrequent use. The Gunther and Le Fort procedures are similar in principle. If the calcaneum and talus are retained and the amputation performed through the talonavicular joint, the Chopart amputation, the unopposed Achilles tendon and peroneal muscles result in flexion and eversion of the heel, which produce an unstable stump. This can be overcome by arthrodesis of the subtalar joint, as in the Spitzi amputation, or tenodesis to stabilize the peroneal and tibial muscles.

Forefoot Amputation
The Lisfranc amputation is performed with a short distal flap and a long plantar flap of sole skin with bone section along the base of the metatarsals, preserving the navicular and cuboid bones. This makes a stable amputation if the anterior and posterior tibial tendons are preserved and the only prosthesis required is a surgical boot, filling the space for the absent forefoot. The further anteriorly this amputation can be performed the less the disability and a mid-tarsal amputation can be performed in the same way.

Digital Amputation
A single or multiple digital amputation can be performed through a racquet incision or anterior and posterior flaps. Where possible, amputation through

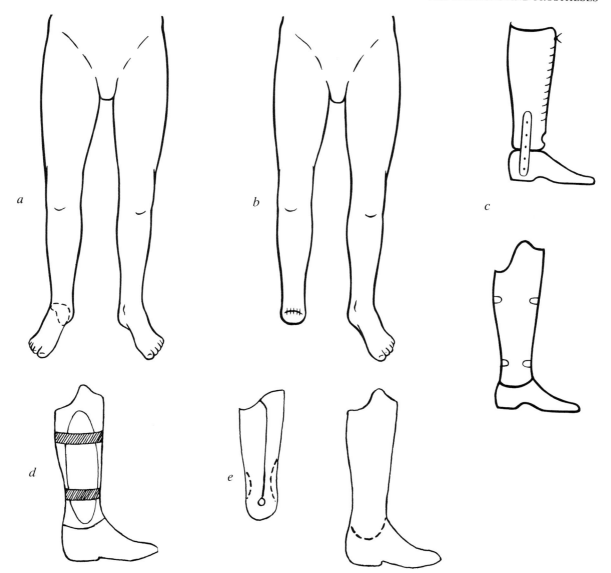

Fig. 49.11. Syme's amputation. *a*, Skin flaps. *b*, Stump. *c*, Lace-up prosthesis with flexible foot. *d*, 'Door' in socket to allow entry of stump. *e*, Split liner to accommodate bulbous end.

the base of the phalanx is preferred to disarticulation at a joint, as the joint capsule can be preserved intact and the tendon attachments can be saved. If there is a septic arthrosis of the metatarsophalangeal joint, as is frequently found in infected diabetic gangrene, it is necessary to resect the greater part of the meta-tarsal, constituting a 'ray' amputation and the skin flaps fall in over the resected bone. Granulation tissue will not cover bare tendon, bone and joint capsules. Therefore enough bone must be resected to give lax skin cover. In the ischaemic foot sutures should be avoided and Steristrips are very satisfactory.

REFERENCES

Baker T. C., Berkowitz T., Lord G. B. et al. (1970) Hemicorporectomy. *Br. J. Surg.* **57**, 471–476.
Burgess E. M., Romano R. L. and Zettl J. H. (1969) *The Management of Lower Extremity Amputations.* 11 TR: 10–6. Prosthetic and Sensory Aids Service, US Veteran Administration.
Burgess E. M., Matsen F., Wyss C. R. et al. (1982) Segmental transcutaneous measurements of PO_2 in patients requiring below the knee amputation for peripheral vascular insufficiency. *J. Bone Joint Surg.* **64A**, 378–382.
Chilvers A. S., Briggs J., Browse N. L. et al. (1971) Below and through-knee amputation for ischaemic disease. *Br. J. Surg.* **58**, 824–826.

Green P. W. B., Hawkins B. S., Irvine W. T. et al. (1972) An assessment of above- and through-knee amputations. *Br. J. Surg.* **59**, 873–875.

Hall R. and Shucksmith H. S. (1971) The above-knee amputation for ischaemia. *Br. J. Surg.* **58**, 656–659.

Howard R. R. S., Chamberlain J. and Macpherson A. I. S. (1969) Through-knee amputation in peripheral vascular disease. *Lancet* **ii**, 240–242.

Hunter-Craig I., Vitali M. and Robinson K. P. (1970) Long posterior flap myoplastic below-knee amputation in vascular disease. *Br. J. Surg.* **57**, 62–65.

Kendrick R. R. (1956) Below-knee amputation in arteriosclerotic gangrene. *Br. J. Surg.* **44**, 13–17.

Kihn R. B., Warren R. and Beebe G. W. (1972) The geriatric amputee. *Ann. Surg.* **176**, 305–314.

Martin P., Renwick S. and Maelor Thomas E. (1967) Gritti–Stokes amputation in arteriosclerosis: a review of 237 cases. *Br. Med. J.* **3**, 837–838.

Newcombe J. F. and Marcuson R. W. (1972) Through-knee amputation. *Br. J. Surg.* **59**, 260–266.

Persson B. M. (1981) Lower leg amputation with sagittal section in vascular diseases—a study of 692 patients. *Beitr. Orthop. Traumatol.* **28** (12), 656–663.

Redhead R. G., Davies B. C., Robinson K. P. et al. (1978) Post-amputation pneumatic walking aid. *Br. J. Surg.* **65**, 611–612.

Robinson K. P., Hoile R. and Coddington T. (1982) Skewflap myoplastic below-knee amputation: a preliminary report. *Br. J. Surg.* **69**, 554–557.

Taylor G. G. W. (1967) Amputation of the lower limb for ischaemic disease. *Proc. R. Soc. Med.* **60**, 69–70.

Weale F. E. (1969) The supra-condylar amputation with patellectomy. *Br. J. Surg.* **56**, 589–593.

Westbury G. (1967) Hindquarter amputation. *Ann. R. Coll. Surg.* **40**, 226–234.

Chapter fifty

Soft Tissue Sarcomas

G. Westbury

Soft tissue sarcomas constitute a relatively rare group of neoplasms which account for less than 0·5 per cent of all cancers registered in England and Wales, though they are proportionately commoner in childhood, ranking third in the Manchester Children's Tumour Registry. They may occur in any anatomical region but are commonest in the lower limb.

PATHOLOGY

The histological classification is somewhat complex and is based on the resemblance of the tumour cells to the various normal components of the soft supporting tissues, e.g. *liposarcoma*, *fibrosarcoma*, *synovial sarcoma* and malignant *fibrous histiocytoma*, the latter being the commonest of all though its identity was recognized only in the 1960s. Malignant tumours of smooth muscle, the *leiomyosarcomas*, arise principally in the gastrointestinal tract and uterus; they are not mentioned further as their management falls within the scope of the general abdominal surgeon and the gynaecologist. Malignant tumours of striated muscle, the *rhabdomyosarcomas*, are extremely rare in the adult. The embryonal rhabdomyosarcomas of infancy and childhood are noteworthy in that they are uniquely responsive to systemic cytotoxic therapy, which plays a major role in their management. For the purposes of tumour staging, prognosis and management the histological *grade* is all important. This depends on an amalgam of factors including histological type, cellularity, mitotic activity and amount of necrosis. The concept of a two- or at the most three-grade classification has the virtues of simplicity and practical clinical value.

The gross appearance of most soft tissue sarcomas is misleading as they often seem to be encapsulated. This is, however, a *pseudocapsule* since it contains tumour cells. Surgical enucleation through this false plane of cleavage will nearly always be followed by local recurrence. Fascial planes, major nerve sheaths and the adventitia of larger arteries are relatively resistant to invasion and sarcomas tend to spread along the lines of least resistance, as is exemplified most clearly within the musculofascial compartments of the limbs. Invasion of major arteries and nerves and of bone occurs relatively late. Lymph node involvement is unusual and is seen mainly in rhabdomyosarcoma and synovial sarcoma. It carries a grave prognosis. Regional node dissection is only rarely indicated.

DIAGNOSIS

Clinical diagnosis of this rare group of tumours depends on a high index of suspicion when a soft tissue mass is encountered in any anatomical site, especially if deep to the deep fascia. Sarcoma must be distinguished from the many benign lesions which can produce similar signs, e.g. lipoma, ganglion, bursa, haematoma, cold abscess.

Plain radiographs of the mass are of limited value but occasionally provide incidental evidence to aid differential diagnosis, e.g. tuberculosis of bone. Computerized axial tomography (CT) usually provides excellent definition of the extent of the lesion and is the most sensitive detector of pulmonary metastases. It is of particular value for tumours of the pelvis and trunk. Arteriography usually (though not always) shows a pathological circulation and demonstrates both the volume of the mass and its relation to the major arteries. Neither CT nor arteriography precludes the need for a tissue diagnosis to exclude other pathology and, if sarcoma is confirmed, to define its histological type and grade of malignancy.

Biopsy

While fine-needle aspiration cytology and large-needle Tru-cut type biopsy yield a high percentage of accurate results for the very experienced interpreter, most pathologists prefer larger tissue samples. Individual soft tissue sarcomas may show wide variation in their histological appearance from one area to another, and needle biopsy can lead to sampling error with regard to type and grade of tumour. Larger tumours usually contain areas of necrosis which may produce false negative findings. Small samples may also lead to false positive reports whereby benign lesions such as the pseudosarcomas (fibromatosis, fasciitis, etc.) or even simple reactive processes can be erroneously labelled as sarcomas.

Excision Biopsy

This is indicated for small, superficially sited lumps. The entire lesion is available for pathological evaluation and should sarcoma be diagnosed this simple surgery will not prejudice subsequent definitive management.

Incision Biopsy

This is the orthodox diagnostic procedure for the larger, deeply placed mass. The incision must always be placed with the possibility of subsequent definitive surgery in mind. It should lie over the midpoint of the mass and run in the direction of the local musculo-fascial planes which in the limbs is *vertical*. Transverse or eccentrically placed incisions, even though sometimes appropriate for access to certain benign conditions, usually prejudice the definitive operation which follows. The tumour surface is exposed with the minimum laying open of tissue planes. Sarcomas are often highly vascular and haemostasis should be meticulous. An adequate sample of solid-looking tumour is taken avoiding the often gelatinous or grossly necrotic areas in the deeper zones as these may be of no diagnostic value. If in doubt frozen section confirmation of a cellular sample is helpful; the delay involved is far preferable to the need for repeat biopsy. The deep fascia is closed. Drainage is avoided where possible but if necessary the drain is placed so as to emerge at one end of the wound; or if of Redivac type the puncture is made close to and in the line of the incision to facilitate subsequent re-excision of all potentially contaminated tissue planes.

Punch Biopsy (Fig. 50.1)

This is the author's usual preference as it is simple, relatively non-traumatic, avoids embarrassing haemorrhage and the opening of tissue planes, and provides adequate material. The apparatus consists of a standard 1·0-cm trocar and cannula together with a pair of Tilley–Heinkel forceps. A stab incision just sufficient to take the cannula is made over the promi-nence of the mass. The trocar and cannula are inserted to the centre of the tumour and the trocar removed; bloody fluid and/or gelatinous material may be released. The forceps are then inserted through the cannula and multiple samples taken from various sites within the tumour. Frozen section control is again helpful in case of doubt. The cannula is removed, gauze pressure applied to the wound for a few moments and the skin closed with one or two sutures. A firm pressure dressing is applied.

GENERAL PRINCIPLES OF MANAGEMENT

The overall management of the soft tissue sarcomas includes the eradication of local disease at the primary site and the control of metastases. The latter aim calls for more effective systemic cytotoxic therapy than is currently available, except in the case of the embryonal rhabdomyosarcomas of infancy and childhood, and is not further discussed except to state that very occasionally selected patients whose primary disease is controlled and who have apparently solitary or few pulmonary metastases may enjoy prolonged disease-free survival following appropriate pulmonary resection. This chapter is concerned principally with the management of the primary disease and to establish a perspective it should be borne in mind that the 5-year survival for the soft tissue sarcomas as a group is approximately 50 per cent, though shorter for larger, fixed tumours of high-grade malignancy than for smaller, low-grade lesions.

Eradication of the primary tumour is therefore of cardinal importance and in the case of the limbs this aim is achieved, wherever possible, without amputation. The available treatment methods of proven value are surgical excision and radiotherapy; these

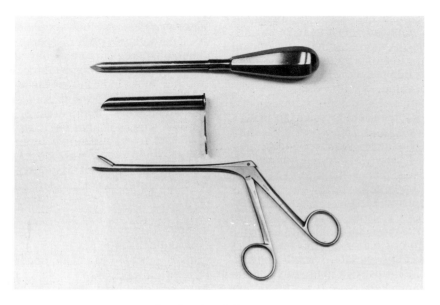

Fig. 50.1. Punch biopsy set.

are often used in combination. Intra-arterial chemotherapy either by isolated, extracorporeal perfusion or by various techniques of intra-arterial infusion produces undoubted anti-tumour effects. Its place in combined management is under study but has yet to be established and is therefore not further considered here.

Surgery

The chances of local cure with surgery alone depend to a major degree on the scale of the operation undertaken. Considerations of pathology (*see* p. 757) indicate that in the case of the soft tissue sarcomas a radical operation is one which encompasses the entire musculofascial compartment in which the tumour is located. This ideal is usually attainable only in the limbs and even then depends on whether the tumour originates within or remains confined to such a compartment. The popliteal fossa and femoral triangle, for example, have very incomplete anatomical boundaries and radical surgery is not possible. The same is true for sarcomas which arise in or involve the skin and subcutaneous tissues. The close confines and anatomical complexity of the head and neck prohibit radical operation for most sarcomas of this area and satisfactory clearance can seldom be achieved in the wide, ill-defined tissue planes of the retroperitoneum. Enneking (1983) has suggested a unified classification of the types of operation for sarcoma which can be applied to any anatomical region. This is shown in modified form in *Fig.* 50.2. Radical excision includes the entire musculofascial compartment. Wide excision implies clearance by several centimetres though less than strictly radical. Marginal excision means enucleation through the pseudocapsule with clear removal of all visible tumour. Intracapsular excision leaves gross residual tumour. Note that even amputation is not a radical cancer procedure if the plane of transection passes through the involved compartment. The validity of these concepts is confirmed by the recorded incidence of local failure following surgery as the sole method of treatment: radical limb-sparing surgery, 30 per cent; wide local excision, 40–60 per cent; marginal excision, 95 per cent.

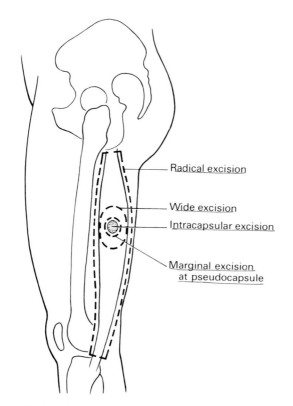

Fig. 50.2. Classification of types of surgery for soft tissue sarcoma (after Enneking).

Radiotherapy

Although it was generally held for many years that the soft tissue sarcomas were radio resistant, they are in fact responsive to a variable degree to irradiation towards the upper end of the therapeutic dose range and a small percentage are totally sterilized. Radiation is therefore useful for palliation of sarcomas which are unresectable by reason of site or fixation. It is also of proved value as an adjuvant to surgery where radical dosage can, for example, reduce the local failure rate following marginal resection from 95 per cent to in the region of 30 per cent or less. It is therefore indicated postoperatively whenever the surgery carried out is for any reason less than radical, and for all high-grade sarcomas. The field of treatment is determined by the same pathological factors as guide the surgeon, i.e. it must cover the compartment at risk and not be restricted to the immediate vicinity of the apparent tumour. Radiotherapy is indicated as a preoperative measure for tumours which are fixed or of dubious mobility; not uncommonly the mass will shrink and become more mobile thus facilitating excision. Such shrinkage may sometimes take several months to become manifest. For this reason the decision to amputate for limb sarcoma should not be taken with undue haste and in any event never without repeat biopsy confirmation of tumour. There is no evidence that such delayed amputation, or amputation following failure of a planned combined surgical/radiation approach, carries a lower chance of survival than does immediate amputation. The prognosis for life is principally determined by the tumour stage at first presentation.

Surgery following radical dose irradiation calls for the usual added caution attached to the tendency to impaired tissue healing. Skin tension and dead space are particularly dangerous, especially in relation to the major arteries.

SURGERY OF SPECIFIC REGIONS

The anatomical ubiquity of the soft tissue sarcomas precludes complete coverage of their operative surgery within a single chapter. Many operations do not conform to classic textbook descriptions because the tumour makes its own rules. The surgeon must always be prepared to extemporize and design each operation to suit the individual sarcoma. Facilities must be available for replacement of involved skin, chest or abdominal wall, major artery or, where necessary, long bone. Skin cover may require Thiersch grafts, pedicled cutaneous, muscle or myocutaneous flaps, or even free flap transfer with microvascular anastomosis. The value of the greater omentum for cover at certain sites should be borne in mind. Sarcomas of the head and neck, which are uncommon, will usually require the services of a specialist surgical team. The embryonal rhabdomyosarcomas of infancy and childhood occur mainly in the head and neck area and in the pelvis; they call not only for specialized surgical skills but should also be managed within the context of a multidisciplinary paediatric oncology unit. Retroperitoneal sarcomas fall within the province of the general surgeon. Their removal, which can seldom be complete, may involve resection of solid and hollow viscera; infiltration of the small bowel mesentery or involvement of the great veins may restrict surgery to a debulking procedure. Sarcomas of the limb girdles may be removable only by forequarter or hindquarter amputation. When, however, the main neurovascular bundle is free, it is possible to perform satisfactory, individually tailored resections of, for example, scapula, the scapula with clavicle and head of humerus (Tikhoff–Linberg operation) or partial resection of the pelvis, with retention of a useful limb.

Two standard operations are illustrated in full which, together with the modifications described, provide a basis in principle for the surgery of most soft tissue sarcomas of the limbs and trunk.

Posterior Thigh Compartmental Resection
(*Figs. 50.3–50.7*)

The skin incision extends in the posterior midline from the gluteal fold to just above the popliteal crease and includes the previous biopsy scar by a 5-cm margin on either side to clear the potentially contaminated subcutaneous fat. The incision will need to be modified if the biopsy has been incorrectly sited (*see* p. 757).

Full-thickness skin flaps are raised widely as far as the mid-adductor plane medially and the corresponding plane laterally. The deep fascia is incised along the length of these two planes. With the ensuing release of tension within the compartment the tumour mass immediately 'loosens' and the extent of the proposed resection becomes more clearly defined.

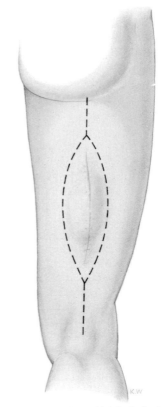

Fig. 50.3. Skin incision which includes biopsy scar.

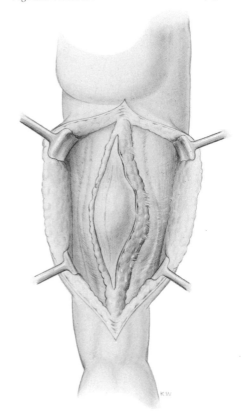

Fig. 50.4. Elevation of skin flaps.

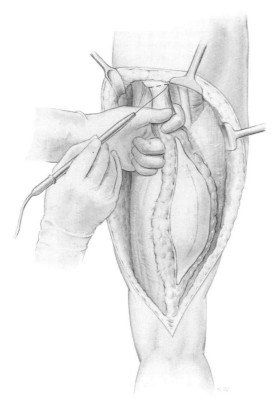

Fig. 50.5. Division of origin of hamstrings.

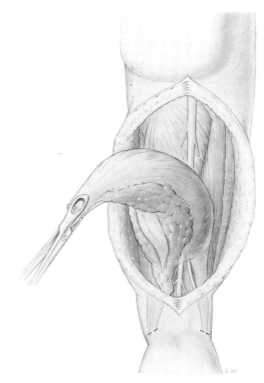

Fig. 50.6. Posterior thigh compartment with contained tumour partially dissected to expose sciatic nerve. Sites for division of hamstring insertions indicated by dotted lines.

The fascia along the lower edge of gluteus maximus is divided and upwards retraction of this muscle exposes the origins of the hamstrings from the ischial tuberosity. The hamstrings are put on the stretch by the encircling index finger and detached flush with the bone; the angled diathermy point is a convenient instrument for this step. For a proximally situated tumour whose upper pole is close to bone more effectively clearance is achieved by dividing the tuberosity horizontally using the osteotome or power saw so that the complete muscle origin, together with its attached plate of bone, is included in the specimen.

The detached muscle origins are grasped with tissue forceps and lifted up so that the relatively avascular medial and lateral planes of separation of the compartment become readily apparent and are cut by running the curved scissors along their length. If the tumour has invaded into the lateral or medial compartments the resection must extend to include appropriate portions of the vastus or adductor muscle groups; in the latter case the superficial femoral artery may be exposed on its posterior aspect.

The proximal end of the sciatic nerve has been uncovered and its relation to the deep aspect of the tumour can now be ascertained. In the case illustrated in *Figs.* 50.3–50.7 the tumour is totally enclosed within a musculofascial envelope and the nerve lies clear. Sometimes the nerve is found closely applied to the tumour pseudocapsule though not grossly

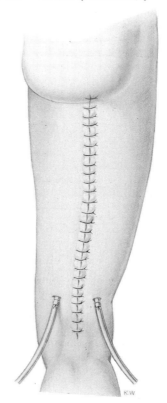

Fig. 50.7. Sutured incision and suction drains.

invaded. It is entirely justified to dissect the nerve off the tumour, if necessary deep to the perineurium, because, provided adjuvant radiotherapy is given, recurrence along the nerve occurs only exceptionally. In the unusual event of frank invasion, or for the rare primary neurogenic sarcoma of the main trunk, the entire sciatic nerve can be sacrificed and, provided there is a good peripheral circulation, the patient retains a useful limb with a foot free from trophic ulceration.

Division of the short head of the biceps close to the linea aspera exposes the perforating branches of the profunda femoris artery and vein, several of which may require division and ligation. The specimen is now attached only by the insertions of the hamstring muscles which are finally divided at the level of the knee joint.

The skin is closed with interrupted sutures placed sufficiently close to secure an airtight wound for effective suction drainage via two large-bore tubes which are laid along the length of the cavity. A firm pressure dressing is applied. Gentle active movements are encouraged from the outset and walking started as soon as the drainage tubes are removed, usually on the 4th or 5th day.

Anterior and Medial Thigh Compartmental Resections

These follow the same lines but the femoral vessels require special consideration. As with the sciatic nerve frank invasion of the wall of the superficial femoral artery is uncommon and it can usually be dissected off the tumour mass in the subadventitial plane (*Fig. 50.8*). A tape is placed under the artery proximal to the tumour and used to apply gentle traction while the vessel is mobilized by serial division of its branches until it lies entirely free along its length. The tumour mass is mainly supplied by the profunda artery and this usually requires division close to its origin from the common femoral artery. Its perforating branches are again encountered close to the linea aspera. The superficial femoral vein can often be dealt with in similar fashion but if this thin-walled structure is adherent to tumour it should be sacrificed and little ultimate disability results. If the femoral artery cannot be readily separated from the tumour the adherent segment is resected *en bloc* and continuity restored, preferably using autogenous long saphenous vein. Residual muscle, if available, is used to cover the exposed femoral artery or graft. If not, and where there is any doubt about the integrity of skin cover, especially after radical radiotherapy, serious consideration must be given to skin or myocutaneous flap replacement for the proximal segment of the limb, or a greater omental flap which will readily reach the knee.

The approach to resections in other limb segments follows the same general guidelines. Loss of the

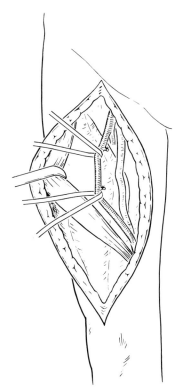

Fig. 50.8. Femoral artery elevated off underlying mass in quadriceps group. Femoral vein still undissected. Sartorius retracted.

gastrocnemius/soleus complex or of the anterior or posterior compartments of the upper limb leaves remarkably little functional disability. The planning of rational surgical excision in the forearm is less straightforward because of the complexity of the muscular anatomy and the proximity of important major nerves. Any resulting disability may be considerably helped by simple splints or by operative measures, e.g. arthrodesis of the wrist or tendon transfers. The surgeon must at all times consider the crucial question: will the residual limb be of greater value to the patient than a prosthesis? The same question applies to the rare soft tissue sarcoma of the hand where, for example, excision of the ulnar three fingers and corresponding palm will leave a more useful functional unit than any artificial limb.

Amputations for Sarcoma

Amputation is indicated when, in the absence of metastases, the tumour is locally irremovable or when its removal would leave a limb of less value to the patient than a prosthesis. Palliative amputation is occasionally required for massive, fungating disease even in the presence of distant metastases.

As mentioned above, amputation must be planned with respect to the potential longitudinal spread of the tumour. This will usually mean section through the site of election proximal to the next joint, e.g. above knee for tumours of the leg. For sarcomas of

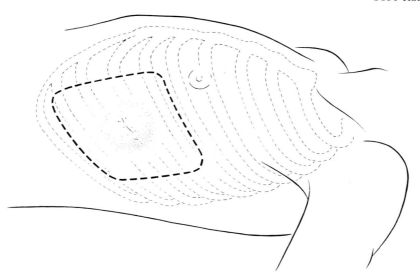

Fig. 50.9. Outline of proposed skin incision.

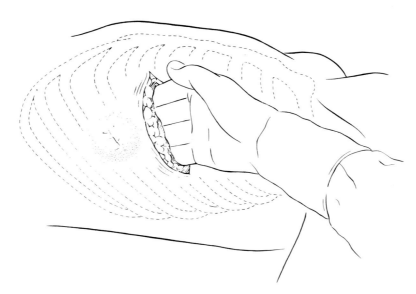

Fig. 50.10. Preliminary thoracotomy to assess deep aspect of lesion.

the proximal arm or thigh forequarter or hindquarter amputation will usually be necessary. Failure to observe these principles carries the risk of stump recurrence.

Full-thickness Resection of Chest Wall (*Figs.* 50.9–50.13)

The case illustrated depicts the operative management of a sarcoma involving the chest wall and overlying skin. The proposed line of incision is outlined with Bonney's blue dye and clears gross tumour by a margin of 5 cm all round. The incision is deepened through the cephalad intercostal space to enter the pleural cavity and allow palpation of the deep aspect of the lesion to confirm operability. The anterior and posterior incisions are then deepened with successive section of the appropriate ribs and the specimen finally freed by division of the muscles and pleura of the caudad intercostal space.

The defect is bridged by a sheet of Marlex (polypropylene) mesh cut to shape and sutured under moderate tension to the surrounding muscles using interrupted, non-absorbable sutures, e.g. monofilament nylon. Added strength is provided by passing a few sutures around the cephalad and caudad ribs, and through drill holes close to the cut rib ends anteriorly and posteriorly. An underwater chest drain is inserted via a separate stab incision prior to the completion of this stage.

Finally, the skin defect is restored by a cutaneous transposition flap and the resulting donor area sur-

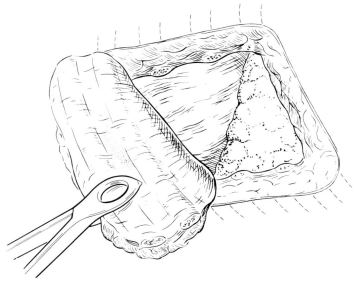

Fig. 50.11. Tumour-bearing segment elevated.

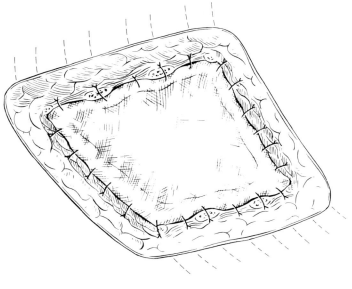

Fig. 50.12. Marlex mesh sutured in place.

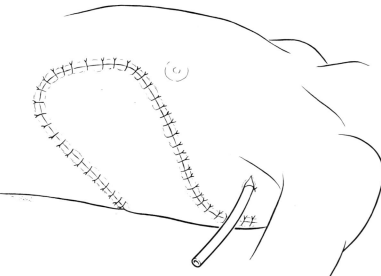

Fig. 50.13. Cover by posteriorly based skin flap.
Underwater chest drain inserted.

faced with split skin which may be applied either at the time or 48 hours later in the ward. It is not necessary to insert drains deep to the flap as this space is drained via the pleural cavity through the interstices of the Marlex. A light dressing is applied which avoids pressure on the skin flap and allows ready inspection of its viability.

Resection of Abdominal Wall

This proceeds as for the chest wall. Peritoneum can be sacrificed with impunity as, like the pleura, it is rapidly reformed on the deep surface of the mesh. The skin may be closed by direct suture provided there is no tension, but in case of doubt an appropriate cutaneous (or myocutaneous) flap should be used. Dead space between the skin and Marlex is obliterated by use of suction drains introduced via separate stab incisions.

FURTHER READING

Das Gupta T. K. (1983) *Tumors of the Soft Tissues*. Norwalk, Conn., Appleton-Century-Crofts.
Enneking W. F. (1983) *Musculoskeletal Tumor Surgery*. New York, Churchill Livingstone.
Enzinger F. and Weiss S. W. (1983) *Soft Tissue Tumors*. St. Louis, C. V. Mosby Co.

Thoracic Surgery

Chapter fifty-one

Tracheostomy

G. Keen

HISTORY

'The evolution of tracheostomy can be divided into five stages. The first and longest period (covering roughly 3000 years from 1500 BC to 1500 AD) begins with references made to incisions into the "windpipe" in the Abers Papyrus and the Rig Veda. However, Alexander the great, Asclepiades, Aretaeus and Galen are all recorded as having used this operation. Between 1546 with the writings of Brassarolo until 1883, the procedure was considered futile and irresponsible and few surgeons had the courage to perform it. The third period starts with Trousseau's report of 200 cases in the therapy of diphtheria in 1833. Tracheostomy became a highly dramatized operation for asphyxia and acute respiratory obstruction. In 1932 Wilson suggested its prophylactic and therapeutic use in poliomyelitis. Tracheostomy was then recommended for a large variety of assorted maladies. This started a tremendous period of enthusiasm' (Frost, 1976) (*Fig.* 51.1).

There are now fewer indications for tracheostomy as the efficient use of endotracheal tubes, which may be left *in situ* for prolonged periods, will usually be adequate to tide most patients over their acute respiratory or airway problem. Nevertheless, should the need for tracheal intubation persist, tracheostomy may become necessary.

Opinions vary concerning the safe maximum period of orotracheal intubation. Certainly in the days of rubber tubes, tracheal damage and stricture formation were frequently recorded. Modern tubes of clear soft plastic seem less traumatic and it is safe to leave such tubes in place for up to 2 weeks before tracheostomy need be considered. In infants and children, however, modern nasotracheal tubes which are made of non-irritant plastic may safely be left in place for periods of 4–6 weeks, frequently avoiding the necessity for tracheostomy. When necessary, tracheostomy should be undertaken optimistically and confidently at a time when benefits are possible and should not be reserved for patients in a terminal state. The more frequent use of tracheostomy and widespread understanding of tracheostomy care has made this operation the safe and useful procedure it now is. Tracheostomy and tracheostomy suction are well tolerated by the patient who needs less sedation than the patient with an orotracheal tube.

INDICATIONS

Tracheostomy is indicated in the following condi-

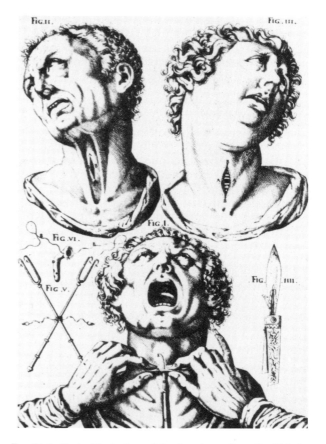

Fig. 51.1. Early illustration of tracheostomy from the Tabulae Anatomicae of Julius Casserius (1627).

tions. It will be resorted to only after an appropriate period of treatment using an endotracheal tube.

1. *In Infants and Children*

When treating severe respiratory or cardiac disease, prolonged ventilation, sometimes for periods of several months, may be necessary and a well-planned tracheostomy using well-designed tubes should be readily tolerated.

2. *Chest Trauma*

The combination of an unstable chest wall and lung damage, perhaps associated with a head injury, frequently requires very long-term airway maintenance with possibly the addition of assisted ventilation. Following a reasonable period of treatment using an orotracheal tube, tracheostomy should be undertaken when it seems clear that long-term treatment is appropriate.

3. *Pulmonary Insufficiency*

In elderly patients with poor pulmonary function complicated by infection, tracheostomy will considerably decrease the anatomical dead space and allow secretions to be removed with less difficulty. This operation should not be undertaken lightly in such patients but from time to time has given some of these a useful and comfortable life when other forms of treatment seem ineffective.

4. *Neurological Problems*

Patients in coma due to head injury or cerebrovascular accidents frequently require long-term maintenance of a good airway and the removal of secretions. In other patients with conditions such as bulbar palsy, poliomyelitis or the Guillain–Barré syndrome, ventilatory support may also be necessary. Tracheostomy is frequently the most comfortable and effective method of dealing with these patients.

5. *Laryngeal and Hypopharygeal Disease*

Permanent end tracheostomy for malignant disease of the larynx and hypopharynx.

THE OPERATION

This should be performed by an experienced surgeon in an operating theatre in good light with adequate surgical assistance and instruments. Although this may be self-evident, one may still encounter the lone doctor attempting tracheostomy in the ward by hand-held lights and with few instruments. That a successful tracheostomy is ever completed under these circumstances is cause for congratulation, but in no way condones such heroic attempts. The availability of adequate endotracheal tubes has almost completely eliminated the need for emergency tracheostomy and the operation should be delayed until good facilities and competent personnel are available. Should the patient be encumbered by splints, intravenous infusions, chest drainage tubes and various electrical leads, it is quite in order to undertake the operation in the bed rather than move the patient on to the operating table, and this is facilitated in those beds from which the head can be removed.

A small sandbag is placed between the shoulders, enabling the neck to be extended. The skin incision is transverse, 2·5 cm above the suprasternal notch and 5 cm in length. The platysma and pretracheal fascia are opened and the strap muscles held aside by the assistant. It may be necessary to retract or divide the thyroid isthmus. The removal of large discs of

trachea or the suturing of tracheal flaps to the skin is unnecessary and furthermore may be followed by stricture formation at the site of this stoma. An adequate opening into the trachea is readily achieved by a simple longitudinal midline incision through the second, third and perhaps fourth tracheal rings, and when this is held apart an appropriate size tracheostomy tube may be readily introduced (*Figs.* 51.2,

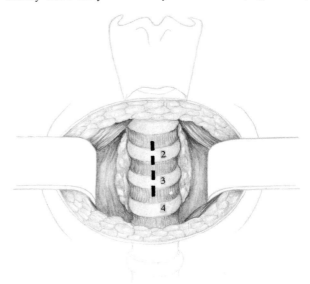

Fig. 51.2. Incision through the second and third rings in tracheostomy.

51.3). One or two skin sutures on either side of the tube are adequate. The tracheostomy tube tapes should be firmly tied by the surgeon using tight knots with instructions that the tapes be left well alone for 48 hours. Tying these tapes with pretty bows invites well-intentioned staff to interfere with these at the earliest opportunity with possible dislodgement of the tube. After 48 hours the tube may safely be changed.

CARE OF TRACHEOSTOMY

Tracheostomy, while of great benefit to the patient, creates its own acute problems:

1. Increased liability to local and pulmonary infection.
2. Decreased ability of patient to clear secretions.
3. Inadequate humidification of inspired air.

All procedures involving handling of the tracheostomy should be undertaken using sterile precautions. The tracheostomy wound should be swabbed with non-irritant antiseptic solutions. Ideally nursing staff should avoid contact with other patients, for cross-infection may become a serious problem in special care units and when, from time to time, several patients become infected with organisms such as *Pseudomonas*, *Escherichia coli* or *Staphylococcus*,

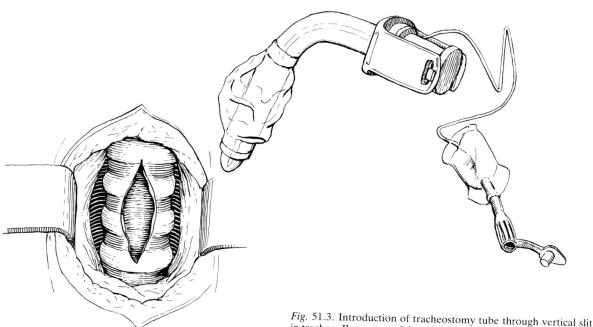

Fig. 51.3. Introduction of tracheostomy tube through vertical slit in trachea. Retractors of the tracheal incision are not shown.

serious generalized infections may threaten the work of the department. Local infections may not only proceed to tracheal stricture formation but in the short term may cause severe and even fatal pulmonary infection. These patients are often debilitated and septicaemia readily occurs.

As with endotracheal tubes, tracheostomy bypasses the vocal cords interfering with the patient's ability to build up that head of pressure within the lungs which is necessary to expel secretions. Weak coughing is possible, which moves peripheral secretions into the central bronchi, but for their further clearance suction is necessary. Furthermore, following the introduction of an endotracheal tube or of a tracheostomy tube it is recognized that within 48 hours the ciliary action of the tracheal mucosa is grossly upset.

Humidification

Humidification is essential, for the nasopharynx which normally provides warming humidification is bypassed. The drying of inspired gases is not only damaging to the tracheal mucosa but encourages thickening of secretions. To ensure adequate humidification it is important that the patient be well hydrated with both oral and intravenous fluids, for general tissue dehydration will eventually affect all mucosal surfaces. It may from time to time be useful to inject small quantities of sterile saline down the tracheostomy tube prior to routine suctioning. This certainly aids both coughing and loosening of secretions. It is important, especially in infants, that this is not overdone or considerable amounts of fluid may be absorbed.

Humidifiers, heated or unheated, saturate the inspired air with water vapour, and recently ultrasonic nebulizers, which add an extremely fine water spray into the inspired gases, have been used with great benefit.

The humidifier and connecting tubes should be frequently sterilized.

Care of the Tracheostomy Cuff

The tracheostomy cuff prevents aspiration of nasopharyngeal secretions and forms an airtight fit, enabling the ventilator to build up an appropriate intrabronchial pressure. A well-designed cuff will position the distal end of the tube centrally within the trachea and it is hoped that the inflated cuff exerts minimal pressure on the tracheal mucosa and the tracheal microcirculation. The most suitable form of cuff seems to combine the characteristics of high compliance, softness and large volume, and although numerous types of cuff are in use it is likely that the large-volume floppy cuff will gain wide acceptance. Cuffs containing plastic foam have been designed and exert low pressure on the tracheal wall. Cuffs may cause complications which include difficulty of insertion of the tube or of occlusion of the end of the tube if badly fitting.

The ideal tracheostomy tube should be smooth and of inert material, polyvinyl chloride tubing being superior to either metal or rubber. The tube should be non-kinking, the internal diameter remaining constant at body temperature. It should have the largest possible diameter together with the smallest wall thickness commensurate with strength, flexibility and non-kinking. Although there is a need for a sensitive indicator of cuff pressures this is by no means readily available. With the cuff just inflated to create an airtight seal very little extra air introduced into the cuff is needed to increase pressure on the tracheal wall to a degree which will cause local necrosis, and perhaps late stricture.

Although it might seem obvious that intermittent deflation of the cuff minimizes the risk of ischaemic damage to the tracheal mucosa, such a programme has its disadvantages. In those patients who require ventilation, deflation of the cuff may deprive the tube of its airtight fit and prevent adequate ventilation, and allow aspiration of nasopharyngeal secretions. On the other hand, an over-inflated cuff will cause ulceration in a very short time, for the tracheal mucosa is soon damaged by pressure necrosis and it is unlikely that any of the currently advised regimens of intermittent inflation and deflation of the cuff will prevent this. It is suggested by some that where possible the cuff should be deflated for 5 minutes in every hour, but it is likely that the adoption of low-pressure floppy cuffs will prove of greater benefit than such arbitrary periods of cuff deflation.

Removal of Tracheostomy Tube

In due course the tracheostomy tube may be dispensed with. As a primary measure the cuffed tube may be exchanged for a smaller-size uncuffed tube, enabling the patient to breathe through the tube and breathe normally. A speaking tube may be used for a time, enabling the patient to cough and speak normally for a trial period, following which the tube may be removed and the wound covered. At this stage it is well worth closing the tracheostomy wound with

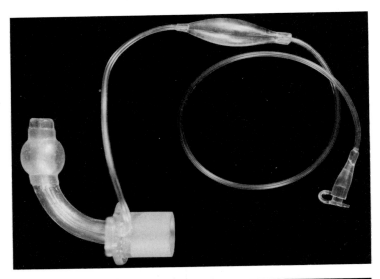

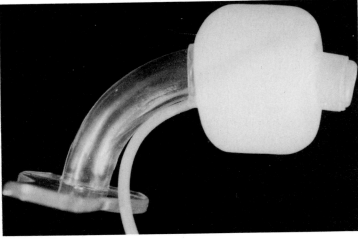

Fig. 51.4. *Top:* Conventional tracheostomy tube with cuff inflated with 3 ml of air. *Bottom:* Tracheostomy tube carrying latex rubber floppy cuff inflated with 8 ml of air. Pressures measured in the cuffs under these conditions indicate that the floppy cuff pressure is about 10 per cent of that within the standard cuff (Grillo et al., 1971).

a few stitches. This will produce a more cosmetic scar.

COMPLICATIONS

These may occur early in the postoperative period; late, following discharge from hospital; or at any other time.

Early Complications

1. *Displacement of Tube*

Displacement of a tube shortly after the operation of tracheostomy is an unforgivable disaster and is related entirely to inadequate fixation of the tracheostomy tube associated with careless nursing of the patient. Should this occur, it is far safer to reintubate the patient using an endotracheal tube passed through the mouth rather than to fumble in the neck of an anoxic, engorged patient. Following the introduction of such a tube, the patient may then be returned to the operating theatre for reintroduction of the tracheostomy tube and its more satisfactory fixation. Some surgeons consider that at the primary operation the tracheal edges should be sutured to the skin wound in order to facilitate reintroduction of a displaced tube, and Björk developed his flap operation to cover this eventuality. The former manoeuvre generally fails in its purpose for the sutures tend to cut out of the tracheal wall which is pulled forward under tension, and the Björk flap is considered unnecessary.

2. *Herniation of Cuff*

In some cases an overinflated cuff may prolapse distally and occlude the end of the tracheostomy tube. This now rarely occurs with the better design of tubes but is diagnosed when attempts at ventilation fail due to an apparent obstruction. The cuff should be deflated which will provide an instant diagnosis, following which the tube should be changed.

3. *Infection*

Infection of the tracheostomy site is a rare occurrence in clean experienced units but it occurs more readily when good surgical and sterile techniques are wanting. The dangers of local necrosis, stricture formation, severe haemorrhage and fistula formation are increased in the presence of infection.

Intermediate Complications

1. *Haemorrhage*

Haemorrhage may occur from the tracheostomy wound shortly following operation, and when control is ineffective by local packing alone it is wise to return the patient to the operating theatre for exploration, when the bleeding point may be ligated or sutured.

A most serious complication is erosion of the trachea and innominate artery, causing tracheoinnominate fistula, usually fatal. Fortunately many of these patients have several small premonitory arterial haemorrhages. These may warn the surgeon of an impending disastrous and terminal event which may, on occasions, be avoided by immediate surgery.

TRACHEO-INNOMINATE ARTERY FISTULA (Grillo, 1981)
Tracheo-innominate artery fistula occurs most commonly from the low placement of a tracheostomy so that the tube lies against the innominate artery at the inferior lateral margin of the stoma and erodes it directly. Less commonly, a high-pressure cuff or the tip of a tracheostomy tube may erode through the anterior wall of the trachea, into the overlying innominate artery. In the latter case the stoma is high and uninvolved in the fistula. The first type of lesion may be controlled acutely by direct pressure at the inferior margin of the stoma against the leaking innominate artery, with concomitant placement of an endotracheal tube through the stoma to seal and maintain the airway. The emergency management of the second type of lesion can only be done by the rapid insertion of an endotracheal tube through the stoma with the inflation of a high-pressure cuff against the leak to tamponade the bleeding. The point of fistulization is not available in this case to a tamponading finger.

Both these lesions must be treated surgically immediately. Anaesthesia is induced through the endotracheal tube which has already been placed. Complete division of the sternum provides maximum access to the artery and arch of the aorta if necessary. A collar incision above provides cervical access. Dissection is done proximally around the origin of the innominate artery, taking care not to injure the artery at this point, and distally beyond the point of leakage, which is just below the bifurcation of the subclavian and common carotid arteries. One may resect the perforated artery, closing both proximal and distal arterial ends with two layers of running arterial sutures.

The stumps of the artery are then carefully buried centrally under thymic tissue and laterally under strap muscles. In the case of a stomal erosion the trachea does not require further treatment except to seal off the tracheostomy from the general incision during the course of the closure. In erosion by a cuff the injured segment of trachea is resected and an end-to-end tracheal anastomosis is performed. Primary arterial grafting is avoided because of the contaminated field.

2. *Tracheo-oesophageal Fistula* (Grillo, 1981

When a tracheo-oesophageal fistula results from the

erosion of an endotracheal tube cuff through the membranous wall, often by compressive action against an inlying nasogastric tube, the problem may be life endangering. Repair of such a fistula is unlikely to succeed if the patient remains on a respirator, since a cuff will be very likely to be adjacent to the suture line. These patients are therefore tided over by placement of a tube with a large-volume, low-pressure cuff seal, the removal of the nasogastric tube, cessation of oral feedings, placement of a gastrostomy tube for gastric drainage to prevent reflux, and jejunostomy tube for long-term feeding. If the patient still suffers excessive contamination of the lungs from salivary excretion, the proximal oesophagus is exteriorized in the neck as an end salivary fistula and the distal end is temporarily closed. This is rarely necessary.

CLOSURE OF TRACHEO-OESOPHAGEAL FISTULA (Grillo, 1981)

The approach to the fistula is very much the same as that of the anterior approach to the trachea for resection. Usually a collar incision alone is sufficient although occasionally an upper sternal vertical incision is also needed. The level of the stoma is usually 1–3 cm above that of the fistula itself since the fistula was due to a cuff. The dissection is carried out as previously described with intubation across the operative field. The diseased segment of trachea is elevated, excising not only it but the fistula in continuity. The oesophagus is closed vertically with two layers of interrupted sutures. A pedicled strap muscle flap is often placed over this because of the contiguity, otherwise, of this suture line with the transverse suture line of the trachea. End-to-end repair of the trachea is next accomplished as described previously.

Late Complications

1. *Stricture Formation*

Most reported series of tracheal strictures indicate that the majority are associated with the use of tracheostomy in the treatment of chest injuries. This may reflect the widespread and perhaps sometimes indiscriminate use of this operation by the less expert in ill-equipped centres, although this complication may follow tracheostomy undertaken with great skill and in a good environment. Apart from clinically manifest tracheal strictures, tracheoscopic and tomographic examination undertaken some months following tracheostomy will in many cases show some degree of tracheal narrowing. Tracheal strictures may complicate tracheostomy or the prolonged use of endotracheal tubes. The stricture may present clinically either shortly after removal of the tracheostomy tube or after a delay of some months. The stricture may be at the site of the inflatable cuff, at the site of the stoma or more distally, when it is due to damage by aspiration catheters. Stomal strictures may be associated with the removal of excessive amounts of tracheal wall at operation or the use of tracheal flaps. The most common aetiological features, however, are pressure necrosis and infection. The adoption of low-pressure cuffs and the insistence on aseptic nursing techniques, together with less destructive surgery, should go some way towards reducing the incidence of this complication.

2. *Failure of Spontaneous Closure of Tracheostomy Stoma*

This complication is considered in Chapter 52.

MINI-TRACHEOSTOMY

Matthews (Matthews and Hopkinson, 1984) has recently introduced an ingenious method of undertaking tracheostomy via the cricothyroid membrane using a fine tube. This apparatus is marketed as a set by Portex Ltd of Hythe, Kent, England and consists of a 4-mm diameter tracheal cannula mounted on an introducer accompanied by a guarded scalpel which can penetrate to a maximum of 0·5 cm (*Fig. 51.5*).

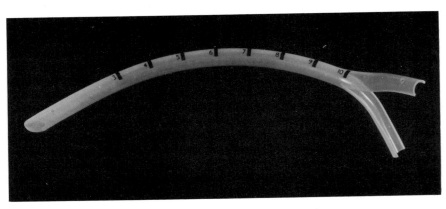

Fig. 51.5. Matthew's mini-tracheostomy tube.

This tracheostomy cannula is readily introduced in the ward in the patient's bed under local anaesthesia and provides a route for adequate suction in those patients who are unable to cough but who nevertheless are able to breath spontaneously. Entry into the trachea is so small that the tight-fitting tube does not allow escape of air around it and consequently the patient is able to cough forcibly and speak normally while this tube is in place (*Fig.* 51.6).

Clearly this tube offers a very successful alternative to the prolonged use of an endotracheal tube or a tracheostomy in patients whose ventilatory ability is adequate but who suffer from the serious effects of sputum retention.

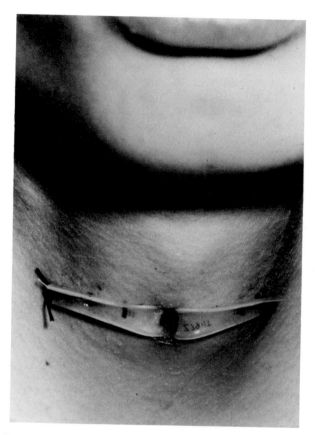

Fig. 51.6. Matthew's mini-tracheostomy tube in place. The tight-fitting tube does not allow escape of air around it.

REFERENCES

Frost E. A. M. (1976) Tracing the tracheostomy. *Ann. Otol.* **85,** 618–624.

Grillo H. C. (1981) *Operative Surgery and Management* (ed. Keen G.), p. 651. Bristol, John Wright.

Matthews H. R. and Hopkinson R. B. (1984) Treatment of sputum retention by mini tracheostomy. *Br. J. Surg.* **71,** 147–150.

Chapter fifty-two

Tracheal Surgery

H. C. Grillo

SURGICAL ANATOMY

The trachea in the average adult measures only 11 cm from the inferior border of the cricoid cartilage to the carinal spur (Grillo, 1972). The carina serves as a definite point of reference although the trachea ends a short distance above this point, and variations in length (approximately 10–13 cm) depend roughly on the individual's height. There are between 18 and 22 cartilaginous rings in the human trachea, approximating two rings in each centimetre. The average internal diameter in the adult is 2·3 cm from side to side and 1·8 cm anteroposteriorly. This results in a roughly elliptical shape. In the infant, however, the anteroposterior diameter is greater. In older patients, with chronic obstructive lung disease, an increase in anteroposterior diameter over the lateral diameter is also seen, particularly in the lower two-thirds ('saber sheath' trachea).

Calcification may occur as the larynx and trachea age and in areas of injury. The limited degree of flexibility present in youth is increasingly lost with age. The trachea may move up and down quite easily in youth, sliding in the connective tissue which surrounds it, and the segmental blood supply also rises and falls with it. The trachea is tethered inferiorly by the arch of the aorta which passes over the left main bronchus. In a thin young person, over 50 per cent of the trachea may rise into the neck with cervical extension, while in an aged, kyphotic, obese person, where the trachea is much more horizontal, the larynx may be fixed in the retrosternal notch.

The blood supply of the trachea comes principally in its upper portion from segmental branches from the inferior thyroid artery and inferiorly from the bronchial arteries (Salassa et al., 1977). Collateral circulation between these nearly end vessels is relatively poor. The vessels enter the trachea laterally, usually after dividing to provide both oesophageal and tracheal branches. Circumferential dissection of any significant length of trachea may easily disrupt this blood supply and lead to necrosis, with either perforation or restenosis of a devascularized trachea.

From a surgical standpoint it must be emphasized that the trachea is short, is an unpaired organ, is relatively non-extensible, is adjacent to the innominate artery and aorta, recurrent laryngeal nerves and oesophagus, and has an essentially segmental blood supply. These facts demand thoughtfulness and caution in surgical approaches.

INDICATIONS FOR OPERATION

1. Benign strictures.
2. Benign and malignant tumours.

Tracheal resection is performed principally for the relief of obstructive lesions with concomitant reconstruction for restoration of an essentially normal airway (Grillo, 1970, 1983b).

1. Benign strictures

The most common indication for such surgery has been for correction of the tracheal stenosis resulting from the cicatricial healing of erosive lesions resulting from intubation for mechanical ventilatory support in respiratory failure (Grillo, 1979b, 1981; Pearson 1974). The most common lesions are circumferential stenoses related to injury by high-pressure sealing cuffs on both endotracheal and tracheostomy tubes or large-volume 'low-pressure' cuffs used within a high enough range of inflation to convert them to high-pressure cuffs. Next most common are stenotic lesions at the site of a tracheal stoma which has been eroded by leverage by equipment attached to the tracheostomy tube. Occasionally both lesions present in the same patient, either separated or confluent.

2. Benign and Malignant Tumours

Primary tumours of the trachea, both benign and malignant, are relatively rare but provide the second most common indication for reconstruction (Eschapasse, 1974; Grillo, 1978; Perelman, 1980; Pearson et al., 1984). The primary tumour that is most often seen is squamous cell carcinoma, the next is adenoid-cystic carcinoma (cylindroma) and after this lesions vary widely with no predominance of a single type. Resection is less often justified for secondary tumours but is indicated for slowly growing papillary and follicular carcinoma of the thyroid gland (Grillo and Zannini, 1986). Less common indications for tracheal reconstruction include: congenital stenosis, post-traumatic stenosis, post-infectious stenosis (tuberculosis, histoplasmosis, diphtheria), idiopathic stenosis, compressive malacia and postoperative stenosis (Grillo, 1983a).

Limitations of Reconstruction

Most patients with benign stenosis of the trachea can

be managed by dilatation of the stenosis and the placement of an appropriate splinting tracheostomy tube or T-tube. Therefore undue risks should not be taken in their surgical resection and reconstruction. The only patients who cannot be maintained in such a fashion are those whose stenosis lies immediately at the carina where airway closure by the stenotic tissue may occur just below the tracheostomy tube. It is rare for inflammatory lesions, however, to be of such length that they cannot be resected and reconstructed at the *initial* operation. This is all the more reason why the initial operation must be well designed, well executed and not done by an occasional operator. If the trachea has been subtotally destroyed by previous surgery and reconstruction is hence not possible, the best available manoeuvre is to place a Montgomery Silastic T-tube (Montgomery, 1964) across the whole length of the damaged trachea internally (*Fig.* 52.1). This will provide a safe, dependable airway which only needs occasional replacement. It does not create the hazards which are attendant on resecting the trachea and attempting to place a prosthesis across the gap so created. The functional effect of a replacement prosthesis is the same as that with a T-tube, but the hazards of erosion of the innominate artery or of granulation tissue obstruction at either end are considerable.

DIAGNOSTIC INVESTIGATIONS

Once a lesion is suspected appropriate roentgenograms of the trachea without contrast medium will suffice to delineate these lesions precisely in their disposition, length and degree of airway compromise (MacMillan et al., 1971; Weber and Grillo, 1978). Equally important are definition of the functional state and involvement of the larynx and the amount of trachea which remains uninvolved by the process. The glottis must be adequate prior to any tracheal reconstruction. CT scanning has proved to be useful only in delineation of the extent of lateral spread of tumours.

Bronchoscopy is frequently reserved for the time of surgical correction, particularly if the degree of obstruction is great. The manipulations performed at bronchoscopy may well precipitate an obstructive episode in such cases. Biopsies of tumours may be done and frozen section diagnosis obtained just prior to resection. Surgery of tracheal tumours requires frozen section control of the margins of resection.

Emergency relief of obstructed airways may be obtained by dilatation of benign stenosis or coring-out of tumours via the rigid bronchoscope under general anaesthesia. Bleeding is usually manageable. Laser treatment offers few advantages.

OPERATIVE TECHNIQUE

Anaesthesia for tracheal resection and reconstruction must be induced with care, preferably with a gentle

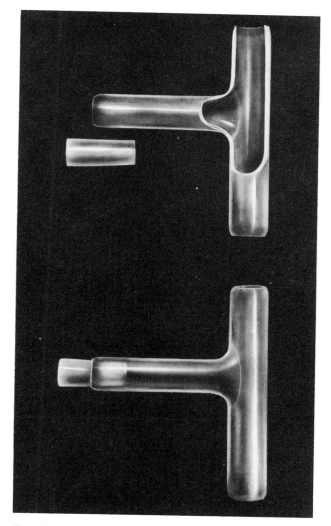

Fig. 52.1. <u>Montgomery tracheal T-tube</u>. This silicone T-tube (E. Benson Hood Laboratories, 575 Washington St., Pembroke, Ma 02359) serves as a <u>tracheal stent and tracheostomy tube</u>. It is available in <u>multiple diameters</u> and <u>lengths</u>, With the <u>side-arm plugged</u> the patient has an <u>inlying tubular stent</u>. (Reproduced with permission from Montgomery W. W. (1973) *Surgery of the Upper Respiratory System*, *Vol. II*. Philadelphia, Lea & Febiger, p. 384.)

inhalation induction to avoid obstruction (Geffin et al., 1969). Bronchoscopy is next performed with a rigid instrument which permits manipulation and adequate biopsy. Endotracheal tubes may usually be passed beside a tumour unless it is a rare circumferential one. Very tight stenoses may be dilated under direct vision using ventilating bronchoscopes serially in size, but with lesser degrees of obstruction an endotracheal tube is positioned above the lesion. The patients breathe spontaneously throughout the operation and ventilation is maintained at all times with judiciously placed endotracheal tubes across the operative field, as indicated later. High-frequency ventilation may be used and is especially applicable in intrathoracic carinal reconstruction. The patient should, in general, be extubated at the conclusion of the procedure and be able to breathe independently. If ventilatory support is needed postoperatively it should be for very brief periods of time only. There is no theoretical need for cardiopulmonary bypass in any but the most complex and unusual cases, and in the most complicated cases, where extensive intrathoracic manipulation is necessary, the anticoagulants required for bypass pose lethal hazards.

Inflammatory stenoses and post-intubation stenoses are operated on through an anterior cervical or cervicomediastinal approach. Upper tracheal tumours are similarly approached. Tumours of the lower trachea or carina are best approached through a transthoracic route. Median sternotomy with exposure between superior vena cava and aorta affords difficult but adequate access for small distal tumours, but is inadvisable for complex problems. Special approaches must be designed for special problems (Grillo, 1970, 1972, 1983a).

Anterior Approach (*Fig.* 52.2)

With the patient supine, the neck is hyperextended with the aid of an inflatable bag placed beneath the shoulders. The field is draped so that the entire neck from the chin down is accessible and also the presternal area. A low collar incision is most frequently employed. After elevation of flaps and retraction of the strap muscles the anterior surface of the trachea is exposed from the level of the cricoid cartilage to the carina (*Fig.* 52.2). The thyroid isthmus is usually divided and reflected laterally. If the lesion is lower in the trachea or if the extent of resection is such that the final suture line will lie quite deeply in the upper mediastinum, it is necessary to obtain wider access to the operative field. The collar incision is extended with a vertical limb over the midline of the sternum. This is carried only 1 or 2 cm below the sternal angle. The sternum is divided to this point and a small spreading retractor is used to separate the sternum. It is not necessary to divide the sternum laterally at the lower end of the sternal incision. The bone always yields at an appropriate point. Complete sternotomy does not aid the exposure and adds nothing but further pain and potential instability. Even partial sternal division is less often needed in young patients since a large portion of the trachea rises into the neck with hyperextension.

Where operation is being performed for a post-intubation stenosis or other inflammatory lesion, dissection is kept very close to the surface of the trachea. Where the resection is being performed for tumour it is preferable to include adjacent overlying tissue with the specimen including a lobe of thyroid gland, if this overlies an area of possibly invasive tumour. If the innominate artery is adherent to an area of inflammatory stenosis the dissection must be kept very much on the tracheal surface, and no effort should be made to isolate the artery itself since this may lead to postoperative haemorrhage from a damaged arterial wall. In inflammatory stenosis the recurrent laryngeal nerves are not dissected, damage to nerves being avoided by keeping the plane of dissection against the trachea. On the other hand, in the case of a tumour, the nerve should be identified and isolated at a distance from the tumour and a decision made on whether or not the nerve should

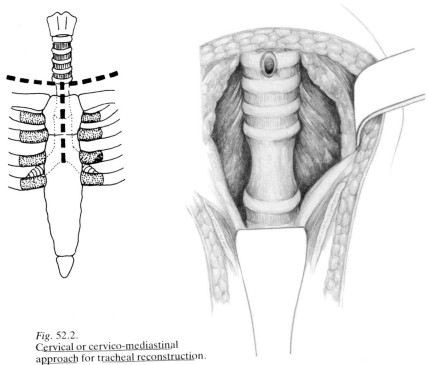

Fig. 52.2.
Cervical or cervico-mediastinal approach for tracheal reconstruction.

be sacrificed because of actual involvement by tumour.

When the level of the lesion is identified the dissection is carried circumferentially around the trachea at a point just below the lesion in most cases. Dissection is not carried circumferentially around the trachea for any distance longitudinally since this will result in destruction of the segmental blood supply which reaches the tracheal wall laterally (Salassa et al., 1977). If the lesion is very low in the trachea, the dissection is sometimes carried around the trachea more simply just above the lesion. With care and patience it is possible then to pass a tape about the trachea without injury either to the membranous posterior wall or to the oesophagus. If the dissection is kept fairly close to the level of the inflammatory lesion, any inadvertent injury to the membranous wall of trachea can be encompassed in the subsequent line of resection. With the approximate line of division now established, lateral traction sutures of heavy material (2/0 Vicryl) are placed in the mid-lateral line on either side, approximately 2 cm distal to the anticipated line of division. These sutures pass through the tracheal wall. An armoured flexible endotracheal tube of appropriate size is arranged in the operative field along with connecting anaesthesia tubing which is passed to the anaesthetist. The trachea is divided below the lesion and the patient is intubated directly across the operative field (*Fig. 52.3*) or a catheter if high-frequency ventilation is elected. Conservatism governs the initial tentative division below or above an inflammatory lesion. Additional rings of trachea may be taken subse-

quently. In the case of a tumour the exploratory opening of the trachea is done on the side opposite the tumour base to avoid crossing tumour tissue. If this exploratory opening of limited extent is not sufficiently distant from the tumour, successive levels may be selected until an appropriate one is obtained.

The lesion is elevated after grasping the ends of the trachea with Allis forceps and the trachea is dissected away from the oesophagus. If there is neoplastic involvement of the oesophageal wall, which usually has been determined preoperatively by oesophagoscopy or barium roentgenogram, a portion of oesophageal wall may also be resected. The specimen is finally removed by transecting the trachea above the level of the lesion or, in the case of low stenotic lesions, completing the division below the lesion. In the latter case the trachea is divided just above the lesion, a tight stenosis is dilated and the endotracheal tube is passed through the lesion. Traction sutures are placed in the mid-lateral position proximal to the upper line of tracheal division. Thus, when resection is completed circumferential dissection of the remaining trachea has extended a distance no greater than 1·5 cm either proximal or distal to the line of division. This prevents devascularization, which could lead to later sloughing of the tracheal cartilages and subsequent stenosis.

If the upper end of the lesion is at the cricoid cartilage the transection must be done at this level. Great care must be taken posteriorly where the recurrent laryngeal nerves are closely applied to the posterolateral angles of the trachea, coursing up behind the cricoid plate just inside the inferior cornua of the thyroid cartilage. In such cases the lateral traction sutures must be passed through the substance of the larynx proximally. Where the lesion is circumferential, the anterior surface of posterior cricoid plate is bared and later covered by advancing a flap of membranous wall of distal trachea.

Ease of approximation is tested after the segment has been resected. The anaesthetist places a hand behind the patient's head and flexes the neck, directing the chin towards the sternum. The surgeon and assistant on each side apply counter-traction between the upper and lower traction sutures drawing the ends of the trachea (or the larynx and the trachea) together. If the ends approximate without significant tension, anastomosis is possible with no other manoeuvre than the already described pretracheal dissection and the addition of cervical flexion. In young adults this may be all that is required even for resection of 50 per cent of the trachea (*Fig. 52.4*). In older patients, however, who are kyphotic, whose trachea is somewhat more horizontal, and in whom the larynx and trachea do not rise on cervical hyperextension, even very limited resection may result in an unacceptable degree of tension. Under these circumstances the next most useful manoeuvre is a suprahyoid laryngeal release (*Fig. 52.5*) (Montgomery, 1974).

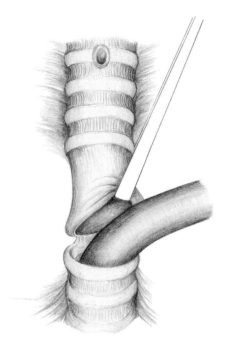

Fig. 52.3. Tracheal stricture. Following division below the stricture the trachea is intubated across the operative field.

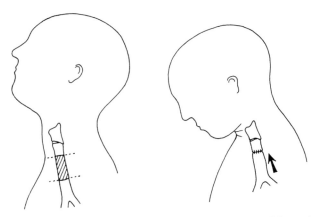

Fig. 52.4. Following tracheal resection extreme flexion of the neck ensures that approximation and suture of the trachea may be done without tension in most cases.

Once it has been demonstrated that approximation may be obtained with safe degrees of tension, the anastomotic sutures are placed. Since the suture line may become relatively inaccessible after major resections, it is best to use strong suture material and to place all of the sutures in serial fashion prior to tying any of them. Although it is attractive conceptually to complete the posterior portion of the suture line and then to place the anterior sutures, it is not really possible to accomplish this satisfactorily after extended resection. Sutures of polyglycolic acid polymer (Vicryl 4/0) are recommended. The use of such absorbable material minimizes the suture line granulomas which occur with non-absorbable material (Grillo, 1979a; Grillo et al., 1985).

The anastomotic sutures are placed so that the knots will lie outside the tracheal lumen. The first suture is placed in the midline of the membranous wall, passing through the wall approximately 3 or 4 mm from the edge, outside to inside and then to the outside again. This suture is grasped with a fine haemostat which in turn is clipped to the drapes of

the field close to the midline superiorly. Additional sutures are placed individually at approximately 4 mm intervals, working out laterally from the initial posterior midline suture. Each suture is grasped and similarly clipped in sequence with fine haemostats. The sutures are placed in series recognizing that they will later be tied starting from the most anterior suture. It is therefore necessary to be certain that each suture will lie anterior to the line of the just previously placed suture. The sutures are placed serially from the posterior midline to a point just anterior to the opposite midline. Two-thirds of the anastomotic sutures have now been placed. The remaining anterior third are placed and then temporarily aligned on the anterior chest wall. It is occasionally necessary to remove the endotracheal tube intermittently from the distal cut trachea while the sutures are placed, although in some patients with an appropriately sized endotracheal tube it is possible to work around the tube (*Fig.* 52.6a). Once all the sutures have been placed the distal trachea is carefully suctioned from across the operative field and the original endotracheal tube, which had been retracted upwards to be out of the way of the operator, is readvanced into the distal trachea (*Fig.* 52.6b). In cases of high lesions it is very helpful to suture a catheter to the tip of the proximal endotracheal tube after tracheal division to guide it back through the glottis at this point.

The patient's neck is sharply flexed and securely supported in this position. The surgeon and assistant draw the lateral traction sutures together, tying them so that the ends of the airway are approximated but not intussuscepted. The anastomotic sutures are thus tied without tension. The anterior sutures are tied first, continuing posteriorly until the midline is reached first from one side and then from the other. The most posterior sutures, particularly if the suture line is near the larynx, cannot be seen at this point even if gentle rotatory force is applied to the lateral traction suture. However, it is possible to feel the

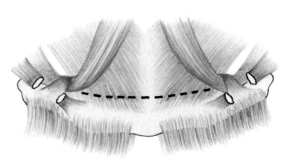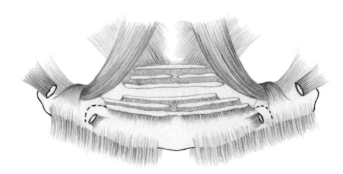

Fig. 52.5. Suprahyoid laryngeal release. The suprahyoid release described by W. W. Montgomery has the advantage of providing 1–3 cm of anterior release without interfering as markedly with the function of the superior laryngeal nerves as does the thyrohyoid release. Exposure is frequently made through a separate horizontal incision. The mylohyoid, geniohyoid and genioglassus muscles are dissected from the superior border of the hyoid bone. The stylohyoid tendons are detached from their points of fixation on the hyoid. The lesser cornua of the hyoid are divided to release the chondroglossus muscles and then the body of the hyoid divided just medial to the sling of the digastric muscles on either side. The pre-epiglottic space is thus opened.

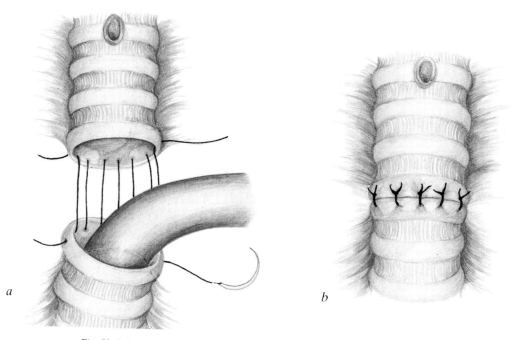

Fig. 52.6. Tracheal stricture. Resuture of trachea following stricture resection.

setting of the knots very accurately. After the anastomosis has been accomplished, the lateral traction sutures are removed, the field is flooded with saline and the anastomosis is tested for airtightness.

Where the entire anterior cricoid cartilage has been removed, the distal trachea is gently bevelled backwards, taking care, however, not to create too small a segment of free cartilaginous ring. An exact fit is not required, and the anastomotic principles otherwise are precisely the same, taking care to correct visually for any discrepancy between larynx and trachea. There is no need to gather the membranous trachea together posteriorly or to create a groove in the cricoid plate, direct suture technique being possible (*Fig.* 52.7). Where the posterior cricoid has been exposed a previously fashioned flap of membranous tracheal wall is advanced to cover it (Grillo, 1980; Pearson et al., 1975).

Closure is made in the usual fashion, wiring the sternum together and approximating the strap muscles in the midline. Suction drains are placed both in the pretracheal and retrosternal spaces. Tracheostomy is hardly ever used following such a reconstruction.

The management of an existing tracheostomy is relatively complicated. Sometimes where it is clearly going to have to be resected it may be included in the line of the original incision. If this forces the incision to be placed in an ungainly spot, the cutaneous stoma may be removed independently leaving a second small incision. Sometimes a tracheostomy may be left in place and allowed to close spontaneously later. If it binds the trachea and prevents its advancement for anastomosis, the skin may require detachment from the trachea and the tracheostomy re-exteriorized through a new opening following the anastomosis, or it may be closed (*Fig.* 52.8). If the tracheostomy ends up in the mediastinum as a result of the advancement, closure is done either by pedicling a strap muscle over it or, if there has been epithelium-to-epithelium healing prior to the reconstruction, the inversion technique may be used (Lawson and Grillo, 1970).

The operation is completed by placing one or two heavy sutures from the horizontal crease just beneath the point of the chin to the skin of the presternal area. This acts as a guardian suture to prevent sudden extensile motions in the 1st postoperative week. It

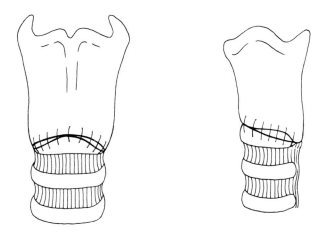

Fig. 52.7. Direct suture of trachea to thyroid cartilage following resection of anterior cricoid. Details of this complex reconstruction are not shown.

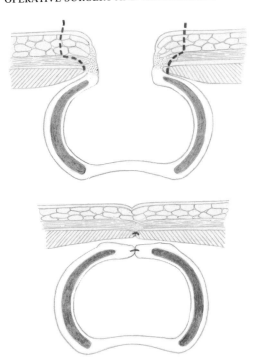

Fig. 52.8. When it is necessary to close a persistent tracheostomy stoma it is essential to separate the trachea from the superficial musculocutaneous layer. If the skin has healed to the tracheal mucosa, the stoma is circumcised and a small margin of skin inverted with a subcuticular suture to provide epithelial closure. This prevents granuloma formation. In other cases, closure with adjacent strap muscle is accepted.

is more effective and much more comfortable than splints or collars.

Transthoracic Approach (*Fig. 52.9*)

Transthoracic Tracheal Reconstruction

The best approach has been through a high right posterolateral thoracotomy, although occasionally sections of the lower trachea and carina are approached through a trapdoor type of incision which consists of a right anterolateral thoracotomy and a median sternotomy up to the neck or, less effectively, through median sternotomy alone. After the trachea and an area of pathology, including carina in some cases, have been mobilized, additional mobilization is performed as is deemed to be necessary. This may consist of division of the inferior pulmonary ligament, dissection of the pulmonary vessels, intrapericardial release of the pulmonary vessels and carinal mobilization. Proximal and distal lateral traction sutures are placed as described earlier. If the point of division below the lesion is just above the carina, intubation is performed into the left main bronchus. The right pulmonary artery is occluded atraumatically only if physiological evidence develops of a shunt into the unventilated lung. Approximation and anastomosis are done as previously described.

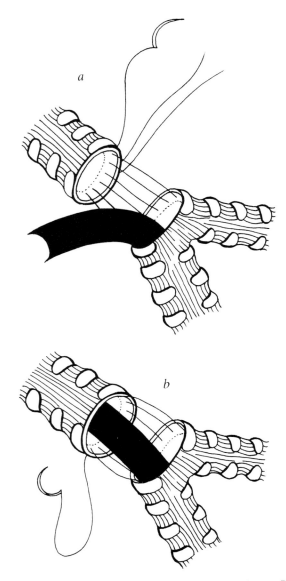

Fig. 52.9. Transthoracic resection of low tracheal stricture. Posterior view (*a*) following resection and while some sutures are placed, the left main bronchus is intubated directly across the operative field (*b*) to be later replaced by an endotracheal tube.

Carinal Reconstructive Methods

When the carina is resected without removal of a large segment of trachea, the reconstruction is performed either by end-to-end anastomosis of trachea to right main bronchus, or to left main bronchus, with then the implantation of either the right or left main bronchus into a lateral opening in the devolved trachea, a short distance above the line of end-to-end anastomosis. Direct reconstruction of the carina itself by approximation of right and left main bronchi presents more difficulties unless the resection has been very limited. This is because the aortic arch anchors and tethers the left main bronchus, and the consequent suturing of right-to-left main bronchus means that the trachea must be devolved even further down for approximation to be accomplished. Carinal reconstruction is complex, difficult and prone to complications even when expertly done (Grillo, 1982; Barclay et al., 1957).

If greater lengths of trachea are resected reconstruction is done by the technique of Barclay et al. (1957), anastomosing the left main bronchus to the side of the right bronchus intermedius, following end-to-end anastomosis of right main bronchus to trachea (Grillo, 1982).

TRACHEAL FISTULAS

1. Tracheo-oesophageal Fistula

When a tracheo-oesophageal fistula results from the erosion of an endotracheal tube cuff through the membranous wall, often by compressive erosion against an inlying nasogastric tube, the problem may be life endangering. Repair of such a fistula is unlikely to succeed if the patient remains on a respirator, since a cuff will very likely be adjacent to the suture line. These patients are therefore tided over by placement of a tube with a large-volume, low-pressure cuff seal, the removal of the nasogastric tube, cessation of oral feedings, placement of a gastrostomy tube for gastric drainage to prevent reflux, and jejunostomy tube for long-term feeding. If the patient still suffers excessive contamination of the lungs from salivary secretion, the proximal oesophagus is exteriorized in the neck as an end salivary fistula and the distal end is temporarily closed. This is rarely necessary and frequently impossible. The oesophago-gastric junction is never ligated.

Once the patient has been weaned a single-stage repair of the tracheo-oesophageal fistula is preferred.

Closure of Tracheo-oesophageal Fistula

The approach to the fistula is very much the same as that of the anterior approach to the trachea for resection. Usually a collar incision alone is sufficient, although occasionally an upper sternal vertical incision is also needed. The level of the stoma is usually 1–3 cm above that of the fistula itself since the fistula was due to a cuff. The dissection is carried out as previously described with intubation across the operative field. The diseased segment of trachea is elevated, excising not only it but the fistula in continuity. The oesophagus is closed vertically with two layers of interrupted sutures. A pedicled strap muscle flap is placed over this because of the contiguity,

otherwise, of this suture line with the transverse suture line of the trachea. End-to-end repair of the trachea is next accomplished as described previously. The interposed muscle flap prevents recurrence of fistula.

2. Tracheo-innominate Artery Fistula

Tracheo-innominate artery fistula occurs most commonly from the low placement of a tracheostomy so that the tube lies against the innominate artery at the inferior lateral margin of the stoma and erodes it directly. Less commonly, a high-pressure cuff or the tip of a tracheostomy tube may erode through the anterior wall of the trachea, into the overlying innominate artery. In the latter case the stoma is high and uninvolved in the fistula. The first type of lesion must be controlled acutely by direct pressure at the inferior margin of the stoma against the leaking innominate artery, with concomitant placement of an endotracheal tube through the stoma to seal and maintain the airway. The emergency management of the second type of lesion can only be made by the rapid insertion of an endotracheal tube through the stoma with the inflation of a high-pressure cuff against the leak to tamponade the bleeding. The point of fistulization is not accessible in this case to a tamponading finger.

Both of these lesions must be treated surgically immediately. Anaesthesia is induced through the endotracheal tube which has already been placed. Complete division of the sternum provides optimal access to the artery and arch of the aorta if necessary. A collar incision above provides cervical access. Dissection is done proximally around the origin of the innominate artery, taking care not to injure the artery at this point, and distally beyond the point of leakage, which is just below the bifurcation of the subclavian and common carotid arteries. The author has resected the perforated artery, closing both proximal and distal arterial ends with two layers of running arterial sutures. The stumps of the artery have been carefully buried centrally under thymic tissue and laterally under strap muscles. In the case of a stomal erosion the trachea does not require further treatment except to seal off the tracheostomy from the general incision during the course of the closure. In erosion by a cuff the injured segment of trachea is resected and an end-to-end tracheal anastomosis is performed. Primary arterial grafting has been avoided because of the contaminated field. Thus far no neurological injuries have been seen, but some hazard exists.

REFERENCES

Barclay R. S., McSwan N. and Welsh T. M. (1957) Tracheal reconstruction without the use of grafts. *Thorax* **12**, 177.

Eschapasse H. (1974) Les tumeurs trachéales primitives. Traitement chirurgicale. *Rev. Fr. Mal. Respr.* **2**, 425.

Geffin B., Bland J. and Grillo H. C. (1969) Anaesthetic management of tracheal resection and reconstruction. *Anaesth. Analg.* **48**, 884.

Grillo H. C. (1970) Surgery of the trachea. In: Ravitch M. M. (ed.) *Current Problems in Surgery*. Chicago, Year Book.

Grillo H. C. (1972) Tracheal anatomy and surgical approaches. In: Shields T. W. (ed.) *Textbook of General Thoracic Surgery*. Philadelphia, Lea & Febiger.

Grillo H. C. (1978) Tracheal tumours—surgical management. *Ann. Thorac. Surg.* **26**, 112.

Grillo H. C. (1979a) Complications of tracheal operations. In: Cordell A. R. and Ellison R. (eds). *Complications in Thoracic Surgery*. Boston, Little, Brown.

Grillo H. C. (1979b) Surgical treatment of postintubation tracheal injuries. *J. Thorac. Cardiovasc. Surg.* **78**, 860.

Grillo H. C. (1980) Primary reconstruction of airway after resection of subglottic laryngeal and upper tracheal stenosis. *Ann. Thorac. Surg.* **33**, 3.

Grillo H. C. (1981) Tracheostomy and its complications. In: Sabiston D. C., Jr. (ed.) *Davis-Christopher Textbook of Surgery*, 12th ed. Philadelphia, Saunders.

Grillo H. C. (1982) Carinal reconstruction. *Ann. Thorac. Surg.* **34**, 356.

Grillo H. C. (1983a) Congenital lesions, neoplasms and injuries of the trachea. In: Sabiston D. C., Jr. *Gibbon's Surgery of the Chest*, 4th ed. Philadelphia, Saunders.

Grillo H. C. (1983b) Tracheal surgery. *Scand. J. Thorac. Cardiovasc. Surg.* **17**, 67.

Grillo H. C., Moncure A. C. and McEnany M. T. (1976) Repair of inflammatory tracheo-oesophageal fistula. *Ann. Thorac. Surg.* **22**, 112.

Grillo H. C. and Zannini P. (1986) Resectional management of airway invasion by thyroid carcinoma. *Ann. Thorac. Surg.* **42**, 287.

Grillo H. C., Zannini P. and Michelassi F. (1985) Complications of tracheal reconstruction: incidence, treatment and prevention. *J. Thorac. Cardiovasc. Surg.* **91**, 322.

Lawson D. W. and Grillo H. C. (1970) Closure of a persistent tracheal stoma. *Surg. Gynecol. Obstet.* **130**, 995.

MacMillan A. S., James A. E., Jr. Stitik F. P. et al. (1971) Radiological evaluation of post tracheostomy lesions. *Thorax* **26**, 696.

Montgomery W. W. (1964) Reconstruction of the cervical trachea. *Ann. Otol.* **73**, 5.

Montgomery W. W. (1974) Suprahyoid release for tracheal anastomosis. *Arch. Otolaryngol.* **99**, 255.

Pearson R. G. (1974) Techniques in the surgery of the trachea. In: Smith R. E. and Williams W. G. (eds.) *Surgery of the Lung*. The Coventry Conference. Norwich, Page Bros.

Pearson F. G., Cooper J. D., Nelems J. M. et al. (1975) Primary tracheal anastomosis after resection of the cricoid cartilage with preservation of recurrent laryngeal nerves. *J. Thorac. Cardiovasc. Surg.* **70**, 806.

Pearson F. G., Todd T. R. J. and Cooper J. D. (1984) Experience with primary neoplasms of the trachea. *J. Thorac. Cardiovasc. Surg.* **88**, 511.

Perelman M. I. and Koroleva N. (1974) Surgery of the trachea. *World J. Surg.* **18**, 16.

Salassa J. R., Pearson B. and Payne W. S. (1977) Gross and microscopic blood supply of the trachea. *Ann. Thorac. Surg.* **23**, 100.

Weber A. L. and Grillo H. C. (1978) Tracheal tumors: radiological, clinical and pathological evaluation. *Adv. Otol. Rhinol. Laryngol.* **24**, 170.

Chapter fifty-three

The Lung, Pleural Cavity and Mediastinum

R. Hurt

PART I

SURGICAL ANATOMY OF THE LUNGS

The two lungs are basically very similar, despite the fact that on the right side there are three lobes and on the left two. The lingular segment of the left upper lobe corresponds to the right middle lobe and is the first branch of the left upper lobe bronchus. Each lobe is divided into segments which function as individual units, each having its own bronchus, artery and vein. The segmental arteries run very close to the bronchi, usually on their superior or lateral aspect, whereas the segmental veins run *between* the segments, from which they receive tributaries. The segments are held together by loose connective tissue and no bronchi or arteries cross the intersegmental plane.

Nomenclature of Bronchopulmonary Segments

The classification adopted by the Thoracic Society of Great Britain (1950) (*see also* Brock, 1950; Boyden, 1955) is as follows:

Right lung

The three lobes have 10 main segments:

RIGHT UPPER LOBE
1. Apical segment.
2. Posterior segment.
3. Anterior segment.

RIGHT MIDDLE LOBE
4. Lateral segment.
5. Medial segment.

RIGHT LOWER LOBE
6. Apical segment.
7. Medial basal (cardiac) segment.
8. Anterior basal segment.
9. Lateral basal segment.
10. Posterior basal segment.

Left lung

The two lobes have nine main segments (segment 7 is omitted in the left lung):

LEFT UPPER LOBE
1. Apical segment.
2. Posterior segment.
3. Anterior segment.
4. Superior division of lingula.
5. Inferior division of lingula.

LEFT LOWER LOBE
6. Apical segment.
8. Anterior basal segment.
9. Lateral basal segment.
10. Posterior basal segment.

Anatomy of the Bronchial Tree

The anatomy of the bronchial tree is illustrated in *Fig.* 53.1. Each lung has an *upper lobe*, which is divided into anterior, apical and posterior segments.

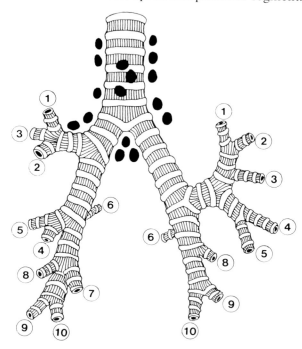

Fig. 53.1. The anatomy of the bronchial tree. The position of the paratracheal, pretracheal, superior and inferior tracheobronchial lymph nodes is shown.

On the right side, these segmental bronchi branch as a trifurcation, but on the left side there is usually an apicoposterior stem bronchus and a separate

785

anterior segmental bronchus. It is important to appreciate that the origin of the right upper lobe bronchus is only just distal to the carina, with the result that the right main bronchus is very short.

The right *middle lobe* lies anteriorly and is a branch of the intermediate bronchus. In the left lung, however, the middle lobe is represented by the lingular segment, the first segmental bronchus of the left upper lobe which passes anteriorly and inferiorly.

The *lower lobe* on each side is composed of three basal segments, together with an apical segment lying posteriorly, which in the right lung arises immediately opposite the middle lobe. In the right lower lobe there is, in addition, a medially placed cardiac segment arising between the apical segmental bronchus and the basal divisions.

Three Surgical Anatomical Points

There are three important surgical points to note:

1. The right main bronchus is situated more vertically than the left; therefore inhaled foreign bodies are more common on the right than on the left.

2. The origin of the right upper lobe is *very* close to the carina. Indeed at bronchoscopy the right upper lobe orifice and the carina appear to be almost the same distance from the upper jaw.

3. The middle lobe and the apical segment of the right lower lobe arise from the intermediate bronchus immediately opposite each other. This is of importance in right lower lobectomy.

Bronchial Vessels

The lung has a systemic as well as a pulmonary blood supply. The bronchial arteries arise from the descending thoracic aorta or upper intercostal arteries and run along the corresponding bronchi. They become very much dilated in chronic infective disease (e.g. bronchiectasis) and also in congenital heart disease when the pulmonary arterial flow is reduced (e.g. tetralogy of Fallot). The bronchial veins drain into the systemic and pulmonary circulation.

Pulmonary Arteries (*Fig.* 53.2)

Each main pulmonary artery gives off lobar and segmental branches corresponding to the lobar and segmental branches of the bronchial tree. Although these usually follow a regular pattern there is no substitute for careful dissection and identification of these arteries, for variations are common.

Pulmonary Veins (*Fig.* 53.3)

The segmental veins run in the planes between the segments, joining to form the lobar veins which drain into the main pulmonary veins. Of particular importance is the middle lobe vein which drains into the right upper pulmonary vein and must be preserved when upper lobectomy is performed.

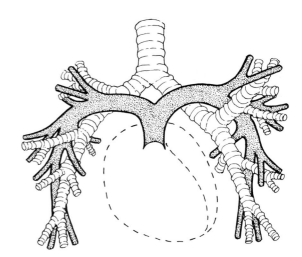

Fig. 53.2. Distribution of the pulmonary arteries. Note that the pulmonary segmental arteries are closely related to the segmental bronchi.

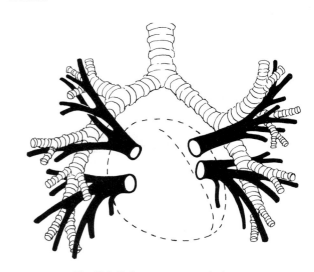

Fig. 53.3. Pulmonary venous drainage.

BRONCHOSCOPY

Therapeutic bronchoscopy may be required to remove secretions from the tracheobronchial tree of severely ill patients suffering from sputum retention (including postoperative sputum retention and lobar collapse) or to remove foreign bodies, which are especially liable to be inhaled by infants and young children. Diagnostic bronchoscopy is one of the most commonly used methods of investigation in the study of chest disease, both to establish the diagnosis and to assess operability and the type of operation to be performed.

Bronchoscopy is preferably done under general anaesthesia. In cases of sputum retention it is important that the patients wake up as rapidly as possible so that they may again be encouraged to cough—it is probably better in these cases to carry out the bronchoscopy under local anaesthesia. The modern

Sanders technique of oxygen jet-injection has made it possible to maintain adequate oxygenation even during a prolonged examination, and this is especially valuable during the removal of foreign bodies in children (Sanders, 1967). No patient is too ill to be bronchoscoped and if necessary the examination may be carried out under local anaesthesia in the patient's bed.

The flexible fibre-optic bronchoscope, more commonly used by physicians, may be passed to view and biopsy upper lobe lesions. It is also of value for forceps biopsy or brush biopsy of peripheral lesions under radiographic control.

Technique (*Fig.* 53.4, 53.5)

The Negus rigid bronchoscope is preferable since its lumen is slightly elliptical and for any given size of

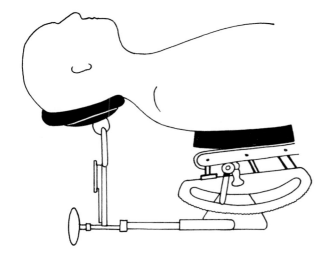

Fig. 53.4. Position for bronchoscopy. Note extension of patient's head.

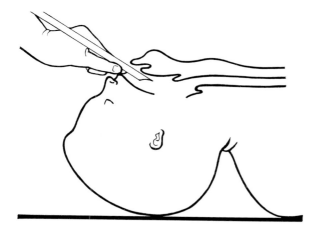

Fig. 53.5. Introduction of bronchoscope. Note the protection of the upper lip, teeth and jaw by the operator's fingers.

instrument there is less pressure on the teeth or gums. The more modern Storz bronchoscope, however, has very much better illumination and a wider range of accessories. Unless the patient is distressed due to sputum retention, superior vena caval obstruction or heart failure, and the examination is therefore being done in the sitting position, the patient lies supine, without pillows and with the head moderately extended.

Complications

1. Haemorrhage

The main complication of bronchoscopy is haemorrhage, which may occur after biopsy of an unusually vascular carcinoma or more commonly a carcinoid tumour (adenoma), for these tumours are often very vascular. It may also occur after a biopsy from the region of the middle lobe or left upper lobe bronchus, to both of which a pulmonary artery branch is closely related. Haemorrhage may be controlled by locally applied swabs soaked in 1 in 1000 adrenaline. This, together with suction, is usually adequate. The bronchoscope should be left in place until the effects of the anaesthetic have worn off and the patient is beginning to cough. The bronchoscope may then be removed and the patient laid on the side from which the haemorrhage is coming, to prevent inhalation of blood into the contralateral lung. Rarely an emergency thoracotomy may be required, in which case a Thompson blocker or Fogarty catheter should be used to occlude the bronchus and prevent inhalation of blood into the remaining lung.

2. Laryngeal Oedema

Laryngeal oedema is not uncommon in infants or children, and is best treated by humidification of the inhaled air or a steam tent, together with systemic steroids. A tracheostomy is only rarely necessary.

MEDIASTINOSCOPY

This investigation, which was first carried out by Carlens in 1959, has proved to be a most valuable procedure for establishing the diagnosis of intrathoracic disease, without embarking on the more major procedure of an exploratory thoracotomy (Pearson et al., 1972; Paulson, 1974; Nohl-Oser, 1976). Positive histology may often be obtained in cases of mediastinal or hilar lymph node enlargement and the diagnosis of bronchial carcinoma, Hodgkin's disease, sarcoidosis, tuberculosis, pneumoconiosis or other disease confirmed. Anterior mediastinal conditions such as thymic tumours cannot be approached by this procedure as they lie in front of the great vessels. In the presence of superior vena caval obstruction there is a special risk of haemorrhage—the operation is best avoided.

Operative Technique

Mediastinoscopy is carried out under general anaesthesia.

The patient lies supine with a sandbag under the shoulders so that the neck is extended and the head turned slightly to the left. The table is tilted slightly foot downwards to reduce venous congestion.

A transverse incision is made through the skin and platysma 5 cm in length just above the suprasternal notch. The pretracheal muscles are separated by blunt dissection in the midline, taking care to avoid the inferior thyroid veins which can usually be retracted laterally but may need to be divided. The pretracheal fascia, which has now been exposed, is incised transversely so that a tunnel may be made by blunt dissection with the index finger down into the mediastinum *behind* the pretracheal fascia immediately in front of the trachea (*Fig.* 53.6). It is absolutely vital for the finger to be in the correct plane,

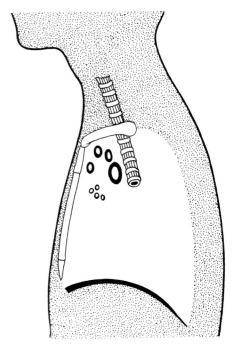

Fig. 53.7. Mediastinoscopy. Major vessels are at risk in the superior mediastinum.

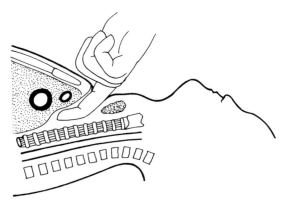

Fig. 53.6. Mediastinoscopy. Creation of plane deep to the pretracheal fascia.

otherwise the great vessels in the mediastium (in particular the left innominate vein) are likely to be damaged (*Fig.* 53.7). If the dissection is in the correct plane immediately in front of the trachea, the area is avascular and, in addition, the pretracheal fascia will protect the great vessels during the subsequent introduction of the mediastinoscope.

The Carlens mediastinoscope has a slit along the whole of the right side and this facilitates the introduction of forceps and suction without obstructing the view of the operator. The surgeon moves to the head of the table and the mediastinoscope is gently introduced into the mediastinal tunnel already made by the index finger (*Fig.* 53.8). The instrument must remain in the midline and the tracheal rings should therefore be visible. At the preliminary digital exploration enlarged glands may have been palpated. These, together with other lymph nodes, are exposed by blunt dissection. It is often difficult to distinguish lymph nodes from veins because of the bluish colour of both structures. Further dissection will often distinguish a node from a vein, but before taking a

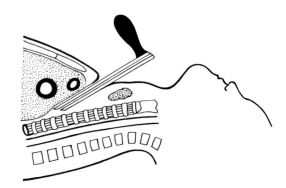

Fig. 53.8. Mediastinoscopy. Introduction of the mediastinoscope anterior to the trachea and posterior to the great vessels.

biopsy it is always wise to carry out a preliminary diagnostic aspiration. A blind biopsy should never the taken.

Complications

The most important complication is haemorrhage. This may well cease on removal of the mediastinoscope, with or without packing the area with gauze. If haemorrhage persists then a posterolateral thoracotomy must be carried out on the side from which the biopsy was taken. It is unwise to use an anterior approach through a midline sternotomy to deal with this problem. Other complications are injury to the recurrent laryngeal nerve and pneumothorax.

ANTERIOR MEDIASTINOTOMY

Diagnostic exploration of the mediastinum may also be carried out by anterior mediastinotomy, the value of which has only recently been appreciated (Evans et al., 1973). Through a short horizontal incision about 10 cm long lateral to either side of the sternum, the 2nd or 3rd costal cartilage is excised and the incision in the rib bed extended laterally along the upper border of the rib (*Fig. 53.9*). The internal mammary

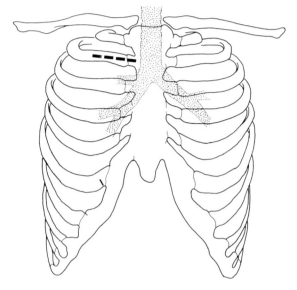

Fig. 53.9. Incision for mediastinotomy.

vessels are ligated and the mediastinum may be explored extrapleurally. Hilar and paratracheal lymph nodes or any anterior mediastinal mass are easily accessible for biopsy. If necessary, the pleura may be opened for inspection and biopsy of the lung or pleural cavity. If the pleura is opened, an underwater drain should be inserted through a separate stab incision. This procedure disturbs the patient very little more than a mediastinoscopy and provides very much more information.

SURGICAL ACCESS IN THORACIC OPERATIONS

Preoperative Assessment

The preoperative assessment of patients undergoing thoracic surgery is most important. There are no definite standards to establish whether a patient is sufficiently fit to tolerate a major lung resection or other intrathoracic procedure. Many factors must be taken into account. An obese, bronchitic, middle-aged patient may not tolerate thoracotomy, whereas a relatively thin man of 75 years may tolerate the procedure very well.

History

A history of recurrent bronchitis or bronchospasm increases the operative risk and the likelihood of the patient becoming a respiratory cripple after operation, especially pneumonectomy.

Clinical Examination

The chest movements and configuration of the chest must be assessed by clinical examination. Patients with a 'barrel-shaped' chest (large anteroposterior diameter) often suffer from chronic bronchitis and emphysema, and this will be confirmed by the radiological signs of lack of lung markings and depressed diaphragms. Excessive obesity increases the operative risk.

Lung Function Studies (Saunders, 1975)

It is customary to undertake extensive lung function studies in patients being considered for lung resection. These tests of respiratory function will provide valuable confirmatory evidence of impaired lung function. They are often very difficult to interpret, however, and do not replace the simple tests of asking the patient how short of breath he is on exercise and of walking with him up two flights of stairs.

Preoperative Treatment

The preoperative preparation of patients for thoracic surgery is most important and 2–3 days' intensive treatment will often shorten the patient's stay in hospital by 2–3 weeks—it may even be life saving.
   Treatment should be directed to:
1. Reduction of bronchial infection by the appropriate antibiotic, together with postural drainage if necessary.
2. Reduction of bronchospasm by antispasmodic drugs such as ephedrine or salbutamol (Ventolin), together with steroids if necessary.
3. Correction of anaemia.
4. Instruction in breathing exercises by the physiotherapist.

Techniques of Thoracotomy

There are five standard approaches for entering the thorax and the anatomical position of the lesion will determine the correct incision. The five approaches are:
1. Posterolateral thoracotomy.
2. Anterolateral thoracotomy.
3. Median sternotomy (*see* Chapter 39).
4. Thoraco-abdominal (*see* Chapter 8).
5. Face-down or Overholt position (obsolete).

1. Posterolateral Thoracotomy

A posterolateral thoracotomy, along the upper border of the 6th rib, is suitable for all lung resections and for many other intrathoracic procedures. Repair of a diaphragmatic hernia is best carried out through the 8th rib bed and operation for coarctation of the aorta or patent ductus arteriosus through the 4th rib bed. The patient lies in the lateral position with a pad under the chest to spread the ribs and with chest and hip supports (*Fig.* 53.10). The knees and hips are flexed. The diathermy pad is under the buttock or strapped to the thigh.

in the neighbourhood of the incision are divided and then a Finochietto type of rib spreader introduced to spread the ribs.

CLOSURE OF CHEST

After almost every thoracotomy an apical (air) or basal (fluid) tube is inserted—very often both. These tubes remain in place for 1–7 days, depending on

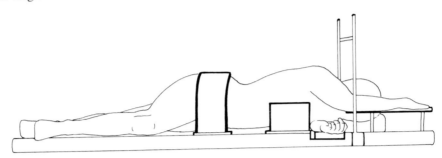

Fig. 53.10. Position on operating table for right thoracotomy. Note position of chest and hip supports. The pad under the chest is hidden by the chest support.

The skin incision (*Fig.* 53.11) begins below the nipple over the 5th or 6th rib, runs backwards 2–3 cm below the angle of the scapula and then turns upwards to a point halfway between the vertebral border of the scapula and the midline. The muscle layers are then divided with the diathermy needle in the line of the incision. The first layer consists of the latissimus dorsi and trapezius, and the second layer, the rhomboids and serratus anterior. It is often possible to retract the serratus anterior and not divide it. The scapula is then elevated using a scapular retractor and the ribs counted from above downwards to select the correct rib. The periosteum is elevated from the upper border of the 6th rib and the pleura entered through the rib bed, taking care not to damage the underlying lung. The costotransverse ligament should be divided with a rougine or grooved chisel. It is not necessary to resect a rib, though in the older patient, whose ribs are more brittle, it is probably wise to divide the back end of the rib. Any adhesions

the amount of drainage (*see* Postoperative Care). The tubes must be of adequate internal diameter—7 mm is recommended—and of adequate rigidity so that they do not kink. They are placed through separate stab incisions below the thoracotomy wound, anteriorly in the axillary line so that the patient will not compress the tubes when sitting up in bed after operation. The tubes are introduced by drawing them through the chest wall from within with a strong clamp (*Fig.* 53.12). The posterior tube is a basal tube

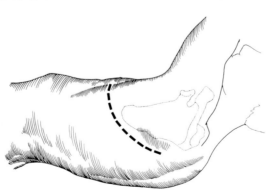

Fig. 53.11. Incision for left posterolateral thoracotomy. The anterior end of the incision should be over the 5th rib.

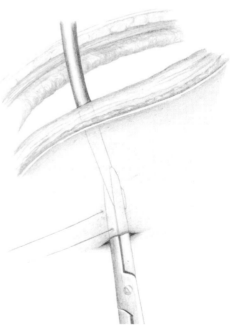

Fig. 53.12. Introduction of pleural drainage tube.

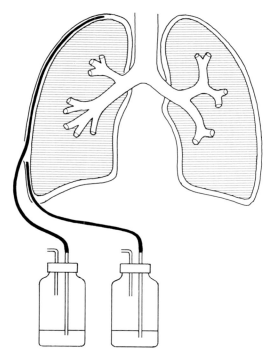

Fig. 53.13. Position of basal and apical tubes following pulmonary resection. The end of the basal tube should be at the level of the dome of the diaphragm.

and its end lies at the level of the dome of the diaphragm. The anterior tube is an apical tube which passes up inside the chest to the apex (*Fig.* 53.13). A stitch should be placed around the tube through the intercostal muscle on the upper border of the thoracotomy incision to prevent it falling away from the apex when the patient sits up. Stitches are placed to fix the tubes to the skin and also to close the stab incision when the tube is removed. Both tubes are connected to underwater seals.

The chest wall is then closed. A rib approximator is useful to bring the ribs together. The rib bed is closed with a continuous non-absorbable suture (using 2/0 nylon), placed through the intercostal muscle parallel to the rib above and below the rib bed incision. It should *not* encircle the rib as this will compress the intercostal nerve and cause persistent postoperative pain. The two muscle layers are then closed separately with continuous Dexon, nylon or catgut. Finally, the skin is closed with a continuous suture.

This standard posterolateral thoracotomy may be enlarged if necessary by extending the incision anteriorly as far as the costal cartilage, and by dividing the back ends of one or more adjacent ribs.

2. Anterolateral Thoracotomy

This incision is used for closed mitral valvotomy and may sometimes be appropriate for anterior mediastinal tumours. It provides poor access to the hilum of the lung. The patient lies on his or her back with a pad under the left shoulder to give a slight tilt to the right. The upper left arm is bent over the head. The incision starts at the 5th left costal cartilage (counting from the first cartilage downwards) and runs along the line of the rib in the submammary groove to end in the mid-axillary line (*Fig.* 53.14).

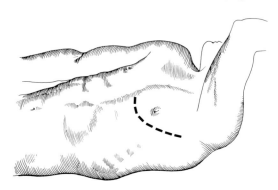

Fig. 53.14. Left anterior thoracotomy.

The pectoralis major is divided over the 5th intercostal space and retracted (with the breast in a female patient) upwards. The dissection is carried well back by splitting the serratus anterior and undercutting the skin incision to expose the ribs as far as the posterior axillary line. The perichondrium and periosteum on the lower border of the 5th rib and cartilage are elevated and the rib bed opened. The internal mammary vessels are divided between ligatures, the 5th costal cartilage divided and a rib spreader and protecting towels introduced. If further exposure is required, the sternum may be transected with a Gigli saw and the incision extended into the right chest, with division of the right internal mammary vessels. Alternatively the 4th left costal cartilage may be divided.

The wound is closed in layers in the same way as a posterolateral thoracotomy, with an underwater-seal drainage tube inserted through a separate stab incision low down in the chest in the line of the axilla. If the sternum has been divided the edges should be brought together with three no. 24 SWG wire sutures inserted with an awl and using a protective spoon.

Postoperative Care

After operation it is important to prevent tracheobronchial infection and its sequelae, and in the case of segmental resection and lobectomy to encourage expansion of the remainder of the lung. Postoperative physiotherapy is vital and may be life saving. The following are most important:

1. Expectoration

This should be encouraged as much as possible, partly

verbally and partly by manual support of the operated side of the chest. This encouragement is extremely effective in helping a patient to maintain a clear airway. If the sputum is thick and tenacious, inhalations are useful.

2. *Analgesics*

These should be given as necessary to relieve the pain of the thoracotomy incision. Sputum retention or lobar collapse may occur as a result of the excessive administration of analgesics, which reduce the cough reflex, but on the other hand the same effect may occur from the *inadequate* relief of postoperative pain.

3. *Postdural Drainage*

Postural drainage ('tipping') should be instituted for 1 hour three times a day, or more often if there is any tendency for sputum retention. If inhalations have been given, then the period of 'tipping' should be immediately afterwards.

4. *Antibiotic Cover*

This should be continued for at least 10 days after operation. It may be necessary to check the bacteriology of the sputum, for sometimes the predominant organism alters after operation, in which case the type of antibiotic may have to be changed. In elderly patients, chloramphenicol is very often life saving.

5. *Ambulation*

The patient should be encouraged to move about in bed as much as possible, and it is a help if there is a cord attached to the foot of the bed for him/her to pull himself or herself up on. Patients should be allowed out of bed as soon as their general condition permits (on the 2nd or 3rd day, if possible), even though a drainage tube is still in position.

6. *Management of Chest Tubes*

The chest tubes drain blood and air from the pleural cavity and are connected to underwater seals to which suction is applied. They are removed after a varying number of days, depending on the amount of drainage of air or fluid, and also on the radiographic appearance.

Complications of Thoracotomy

1. *Sputum Retention*

Collapse-consolidation of a lobe or lung will occur if the patient is unable to expectorate the bronchial secretions adequately, in spite of intensive physiotherapy. Sooner or later respiratory insufficiency will occur, leading to general weakness and still further difficulty in expectoration. The treatment is bronchoscopy or, if this has to be repeated more than once daily, intubation with an endotracheal tube or a mini-tracheostomy (Matthews, 1984).

2. *Atrial Fibrillation*

Most patients undergoing lung resection for a tumour are over the age of 50 years and may develop atrial fibrillation after operation, especially if the pericardium has been opened. This most commonly occurs during the first 10 days, and if the heart rate is fast may produce a shock-like condition. The irregularity should be confirmed by an electrocardiogram and careful digitalization carried out as a matter of urgency.

3. *Bronchospasm*

Bronchospasm may occur, leading to dyspnoea, tachycardia and cyanosis. Ephedrine, salbutamol (Ventolin) or hydrocortisone should be given.

4. *Surgical Emphysema*

Surgical emphysema may occur if the drainage tubes are blocked or, when the tube is functioning, if the air leak from the raw surface of the lung is greater than the suction pump can handle. The treatment is to unblock the drainage tube, introduce a new tube or *remove* the sucker so as to allow the free escape of air.

5. *Haemorrhage*

Excessive haemorrhage will require exploration.

PART II

ACUTE EMPYEMA

The advent of modern chemotherapy has radically altered the natural history of empyema and many cases are now relatively late in their development. The most important factor in the diagnosis of an empyema is an awareness that it may be present. In some cases an empyema may be 'sterile' when first diagnosed, due to use of an antibiotic early in any pulmonary infection, and these patients may be best treated by decortication. In any patient over the age of 40 years, it is important to exclude an underlying carcinoma by examination of the sputum for malignant cells and by bronchoscopy.

The *choice of treatment* depends on the thickness of the pus and the patient's clinical state. Treatment may be by:

1. Aspiration and instillation of an antibiotic.
2. Drainage by rib resection or intercostal tube.
3. Decortication.

1. Aspiration and Instillation of an Antibiotic

Some patients may be treated successfully by this method if the pus is thin *and remains thin*. An arbitrary definition of thin pus is pus that contains less than one-third sediment after 24 hours. Treatment must be carried out under radiological control and aspirations carried out every 2nd or 3rd day until no more fluid is formed. On each occasion as much fluid as possible should be removed. A large dose of the appropriate antibiotic is instilled and in addition the patient must be given systemic chemotherapy, also in high dosage so that the antibiotic reaches the pleural cavity. If this regimen is successful the fluid will become sterile after about 1 week and will become less purulent at each aspiration. The radiograph will show continued expansion of the lung and only minimal residual pleural thickening will remain. Physiotherapy must be given throughout this period to maintain equal movement of both sides of the chest. If pus is still being produced after 10 days, this method of treatment should be abandoned, and tube drainage or rib resection carried out.

It is important to appreciate the limitations of this method of treatment. If the patient remains febrile, if aspirations become increasingly difficult because of frequent needle blockage by fibrin, if the organism is resistant to antibiotics, or if the radiograph shows multiple fluid levels due to loculation, then this regimen must be abandoned and rib resection and drainage instituted. The use of fibrinolytic enzymes such as streptokinase is not recommended. If significant fibrin is present, it is better to proceed to immediate rib resection and drainage in order to prevent the development of a chronic empyema.

Aspiration treatment is especially valuable in children or in the elderly.

2. Drainage

Drainage may be by intercostal tube or rib resection.

Intercostal Tube (*Figs.* 53.15, 53.16)

Intercostal tube drainage may be necessary as an emergency procedure in the patient's bed. It is indicated:

  a. In an acutely ill patient with severe toxaemia.
  b. When an empyema is associated with a bronchopleural fistula and threatens to 'drown' the patient due to inhalation of pus into the contralateral lung.
  c. In a case of delayed diagnosis of a ruptured oesophagus, which is usually associated with severe toxaemia.
  d. In an acute lung abscess associated with an empyema.

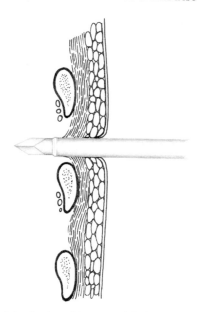

Fig. 53.15. Introduction of intercostal drainage tube. It is important to stay close to the upper surface of the lower rib to avoid damage to the intercostal bundle.

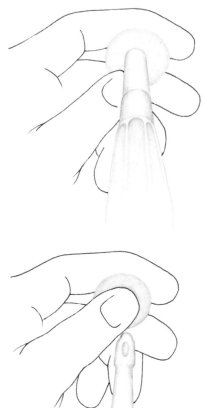

Fig. 53.16. Introduction of intercostal drainage tube.

TECHNIQUE OF INSERTION

If there is a bronchopleural fistula, the patient must be in a sitting position, leaning forwards over a bed-table. The site of drainage is usually the 8th or 9th intercostal space in the posterior axillary line but this must be confirmed by chest radiography, which will include a lateral view.

The site of insertion is infiltrated down to the pleura with 20 ml 0·5 per cent lignocaine with adrenaline. The presence of pus must be confirmed either by aspiration through the needle used for the local anaesthetic or a large-bore needle if the pus is thick. If no pus is obtained another site must be chosen. It is a mistake to aspirate too low. A large-size trocar and cannula should be used, together with the largest Malecot catheter that when stretched will go through the cannula. A small incision is made in the skin and the trocar and cannula introduced into the empyema by a steady, thrusting movement accompanied by rotation. The trocar should be kept as close as possible to the rib below to avoid damage to the intercostal vessels, and the forefinger should be in contact with the patient's chest in order to guard against uncontrolled entry of the trocar. The trocar is withdrawn and the opening in the cannula is immediately closed with the thumb to prevent the entry of air into the chest—this is *most* important (*Fig.* 53.16). The Malecot catheter, held stretched over the introducer, is then introduced simultaneously as the thumb is moved from the opening in the cannula. The cannula is now removed from the chest, *while keeping the catheter stretched on the introducer.* Before finally removing the cannula from the tube, the catheter must be occluded between the index finger and thumb, again to prevent the entry of air into the chest. The catheter, still occluded by finger and thumb, is then connected to an underwater-seal bottle by an assistant. Alternatively, the tube may be clamped first.

The disposable Argyle catheter and introducer may be used instead of the Malecot catheter.

Aftercare: Each day the drainage is measured and a known volume of sterile water replaced. The tube must be clamped while the bottle is being changed. Physiotherapy is most important to encourage both lung expansion and the restoration of chest wall movement.

Rib Resection

Rib resection drainage is indicated if the pus is thick (more than one-third sediment), if aspiration and antibiotic replacement therapy has failed, or as a later procedure following intercostal tube drainage. *It must not be delayed too long*, or the empyema will become chronic. It must also be *adequate and dependent*.

If the empyema is drained at the correct time and proper aftercare is instituted, the lung will soon re-expand and the empyema obliterate. If the drainage has been unduly delayed, it may be preferable to carry out a decortication operation.

TECHNIQUE

Two important facts must be established before the actual rib resection is undertaken.

Is There a Bronchopleural Fistula? A patient who has a bronchopleural fistula *must* be drained in the sitting-up position under local anaesthesia (*Fig.* 53.17). If a rib resection is done under general anaesthesia in the lateral position a 'spill-over' aspiration

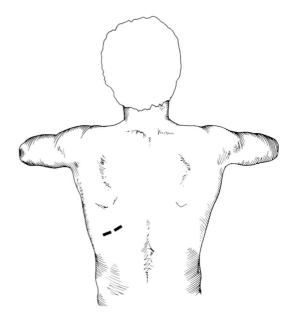

Fig. 53.17. Sitting-up position and incision for rib resection and drainage of empyema.

pneumonia will occur in the contralateral lung, with a probable fatal outcome. A bronchopleural fistula may be excluded by gently turning the patient towards the opposite side—if this causes expectoration a fistula is likely. It may be confirmed by the injection of methylene blue into the empyema. If a fistula is present this will be obvious from the colour of the sputum. A radiological air/fluid level is diagnostic of bronchopleural fistula, unless a previous aspiration has been carried out or gas-forming organisms are present.

Which Rib to Resect? The drainage tube must be placed at the lowest point of the empyema cavity and therefore the rib to be resected must be determined before operation by radiography. Ten millilitres of Lipiodol or Dionosil (propyliodone) are injected into the empyema and posteroanterior and lateral chest radiographs are taken (*with extra penetration*) to show not only the radio-opaque dye at the bottom of the cavity but also the lowermost ribs, and in particular whether or not the 12th rib is short or long (and therefore palpable), for it is from *below upwards* that the ribs are counted at operation (*Fig.* 53.18). The 7th–9th rib in the posterior axillary line

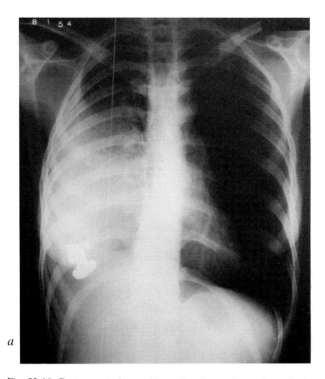
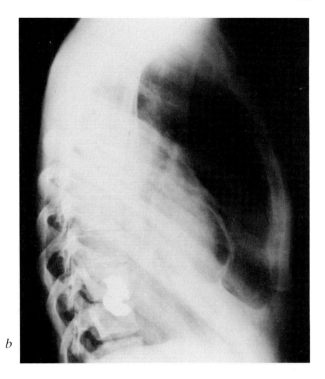

a   *b*

Fig. 53.18. Posteroanterior and lateral radiographs to show the lowermost extent of the empyema cavity which has been demonstrated by injecting Dionosil. It is important that these radiographs are taken with extra penetration.

or the 8th–10th rib in the scapular line is usually the correct site for drainage but each case must be individually assessed by radiographic localization.

Rib Resection: An oblique incision through skin and muscles is made over the appropriate rib, about 5 cm of which should be resected (*Fig.* 53.17). If much fibrin is present a longer segment should be removed to permit adequate inspection and removal of fibrin. A longitudinal incision is made with a diathermy needle in the periosteum, which is then elevated towards the upper and lower borders of the rib (*Fig.* 53.19). The periosteum is cleared from the upper and lower borders of the rib in the direction shown, to avoid damaging the obliquely placed intercostal muscles, and then from the undersurface of the rib, using a Doyen raspatory. The rib is then divided as close as possible to the edge of the elevated periosteum, to avoid leaving any rib denuded of periosteum, which might later develop osteomyelitis. A wide-bore aspirating needle should confirm that the correct rib has been removed. The rib bed is incised keeping towards its upper border to avoid damaging the intercostal vessels. A pleural biopsy should be taken if there is any suspicion of tuberculosis or carcinoma—it is probably wise to take a biopsy in all cases. The empyema cavity is opened the full length of the incision, the fluid sucked out, the cavity inspected with a sterile light, fibrin removed with sponge-holding forceps and a *wide-bore* tube (internal diam-

eter at least 1 cm) inserted well into the cavity. The wound is closed in layers around the tube using catgut for the muscles. The tube should be fixed in place shown in *Fig.* 53.20. Except in a small localized empyema closed drainage to an underwater drainage bottle is preferable since it diminishes the number of dressings and encourages early lung expansion by re-establishing a negative intrapleural pressure (*Fig.* 53.21).

Postoperative Management

The subsequent management is most important—*inadequate postoperative care is the most common cause of a chronic empyema.* Breathing exercises are essential and the patient should get out of bed as soon as possible to walk round the ward. While still on closed drainage the patient should carry the bottle in a special carrier. Closed drainage may be converted to open drainage as soon as the drainage is less than 100 ml daily. Care must be taken that the tube does not become blocked by fibrin, and should this happen the tube will cease to 'swing' with respiration. Serial sinograms should be taken every week and the tube adjusted as necessary. The tube may need to be *lengthened* even though the cavity has become smaller. As soon as the patient is fit enough, he or she may be discharged from hospital and arrangements made for daily dressings as an outpatient and serial radiographs every 2–3 weeks.

Suction is *not* advisable. If suction is applied the

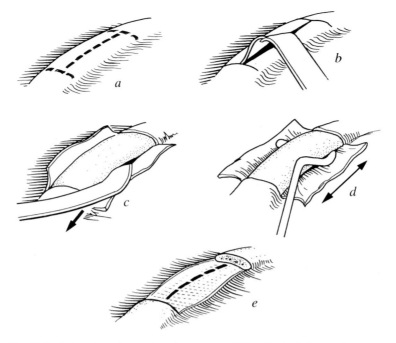

Fig. 53.19. Subperiosteal resection of a segment of rib prior to drainage of empyema.

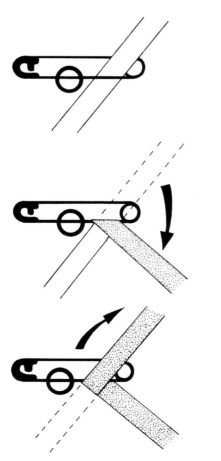

Fig. 53.20. Fixation of drainage tube using adhesive strapping. Note that the adhesive surface faces outwards in the upper diagram.

lower lobe may expand prematurely so that the upper portion of the empyema becomes separated off, requiring a second rib resection higher up.

Irrigations are not necessary for they do nothing to aid recovery.

The drainage tube should *never* be removed from an empyema cavity. While there is still a cavity the tube should remain in place. It should only be removed when the sinogram shows a tube track only. *One of the commonest causes of a chronic empyema is premature removal of the drainage tube.*

3. Decortication

The operation of decortication consists of the complete removal of the fibrous walls of the empyema cavity from both the lung and the chest wall and diaphragm to allow the underlying lung to expand and fill the space previously occupied by the empyema. Originally confined to the treatment of sterile empyema, it is now being increasingly used in the treatment of cases of infected empyema following their near sterilization by intrapleural antibiotics. This is naturally a more extensive operation than a simple rib resection drainage but with the rapid expansion of the lung, the period of convalescence is reduced from many weeks to days.

The operation is a major procedure and should only be undertaken in a previously fit patient whose general condition is still reasonably good. It is not advisable in the elderly.

Operative Technique

Elective hypotension may be provided by the anaes-

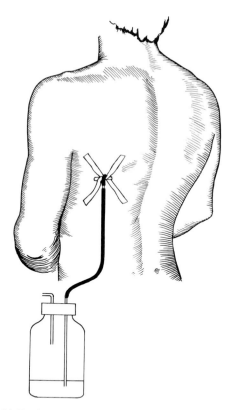

Fig. 53.21. Drainage of empyema cavity into an underwater seal.

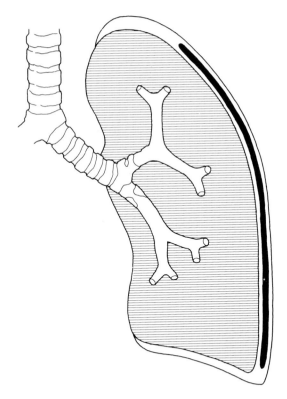

Fig. 53.22. Chronic empyema cavity showing thickened, fibrous layer on its internal and external surfaces.

thetist, as there is always considerable oozing from the lung and chest wall during the removal of the thick layer of fibrin (*Fig.* 53.22).

A posterolateral thoracotomy with resection of the whole of the 5th rib will give good access. The ribs are always very close together and entry into the chest will be very difficult unless a rib is excised. Resection of 2 cm of the posterior ends of the 4th and 6th ribs will provide extra exposure if required. The rib bed is incised and the extrapleural layer entered by blunt dissection with the finger or Roberts forceps. The outer layer of the empyema is stripped off the chest wall by a combination of blunt and sharp dissection (*Fig.* 53.23). Considerable force may be required. The mobilization of the lung is continued over the apex and down the mediastinum to the hilum (*Fig.* 53.24). Great care must be taken not to damage the superior vena cava or azygos vein on the right side or the innominate vein or aorta on the left side, nor the vagus and phrenic nerves, though fortunately the dissection is usually easier in this area. The mobilization should be carried down to and over the diaphragm, though it may prove to be impossible to free the diaphragm completely. The inner wall of the empyema is next peeled off the surface of the lung, starting at a point where there appears to be a good plane of separation.

In practice the empyema cavity itself may be accidentally opened before it has been mobilized from the chest wall and diaphragm or alternatively it may be necessary to open it intentionally if complete parietal mobilization proves to be too difficult. In such a case the empyema cavity should be sucked dry and all fibrin removed. A *long* incision should then be made in the thickened visceral pleura until the normal lung surface can be seen underneath. The thick layer of fibrin can then be 'peeled off' the whole of the lung by a combination of sharp and blunt dis-

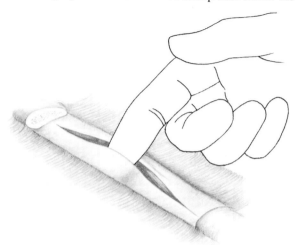

Fig. 53.23. Decortication of empyema. Commencement of extrapleural strip deep to the incised periosteum.

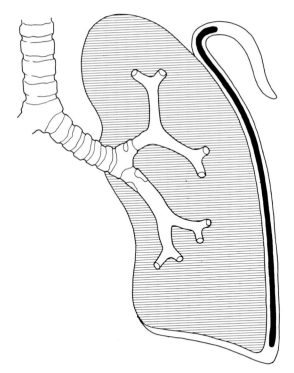

Fig. 53.24. Decortication of empyema. The thick layer of fibrin on the parietal and visceral pleura is excised completely.

section. It is preferable to leave very adherent portions of fibrin on the lung surface rather than produce too many air leaks by their attempted removal.

Finally, and this is important and rewarding, the fissures between the lobes should be opened up. It will be surprising how much invagination of lung has occurred and how much increased expansion of lung will be produced.

After operation there is always considerable drainage and it is therefore wise to insert *three* underwater-seal drainage tubes—one apical, one posterior basal and one anterior basal, all connected to strong suction to encourage rapid lung expansion which reduces bleeding.

Complications of an Undrained Empyema

An undrained persistent empyema may rupture into the lung and result in a bronchopleural fistula or it may rupture onto the skin surface and cause an empyema necessitas.

1. *Bronchopleural Fistula*

This is an acute emergency. The patient will suddenly expectorate large quantities of purulent fluid, which will increase when the patient lies towards the opposite side and will cease almost immediately if laid on the affected side. If untreated the patient will develop an inhalation pneumonia into the contralateral lung or even succumb from 'drowning' if the

empyema is large. It is imperative that the empyema be drained as soon as possible by intercostal tube or rib resection *under local anaesthesia in the sitting position*. Until this is done the patient *must* lie on the affected side, which will immediately prevent further expectoration.

2. *Empyema Necessitas*

An empyema necessitas may not point immediately over the underlying empyema. The pus may track along tissue planes (including the intercostal vessels) and commonly points anteriorly. Radiographical localization must be carried out before rib resection drainage is undertaken.

CHRONIC EMPYEMA

An empyema which persists for more than 2 months may arbitrarily be defined as chronic, and the most common cause of this is imperfect treatment during the acute phase. The drainage may have been too late or inadequate or the drainage tube may be too small or have been removed too early. Another important cause is underlying lung disease—tuberculosis or bronchiectasis in the young or carcinoma in the middle-aged and elderly. It may also be due to a retained drainage tube or swab. A chronic empyema can usually be prevented, though the correct time for surgical drainage in the acute stage requires considerable clinical judgement and experience.

Before embarking on any further surgical treatment, underlying lung disease must be excluded by bronchoscopy, examination of pleural pus for tuberculosis or actinomycosis and histological examination of the pleura or granulation tissue for tuberculosis or carcinoma.

Treatment (if there is no underlying lung disease)

1. *Redrainage*

A chronic empyema will often obliterate if adequate dependent drainage is instituted, together with ardent physiotherapy and activity on the part of the patient.

2. *Decortication*

Redrainage may be somewhat time consuming and because of this a decortication (*see above*) is advisable if the patient is sufficiently fit for this major procedure and the underlying lung is healthy.

3. *Roberts' Flap Operation*

An alternative procedure to decortication is a Roberts' flap operation. It is indicated if it is considered that the lung would not expand sufficiently well after a decortication, perhaps because of old-standing fibrotic changes. In this operation a subperiosteal resection of the ribs overlying the empyema cavity and well beyond the margins of the cavity posteriorly is carried out. This decostalized portion of chest wall (consisting of thickened parietal pleura, periosteum and intercostal muscle) is then made into a U-shaped flap by cutting along its anterior, upper and inferior borders. It is hinged posteriorly to preserve its blood supply (*Figs.* 53.25, 53.26). This flap is then turned

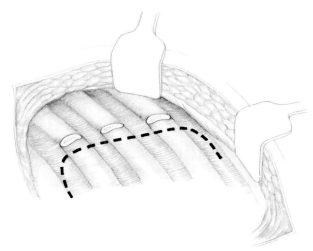

Fig. 53.25. Roberts' flap operation for chronic empyema. Rib resection prior to incision into empyema cavity to produce U-shaped flap, hinged posteriorly.

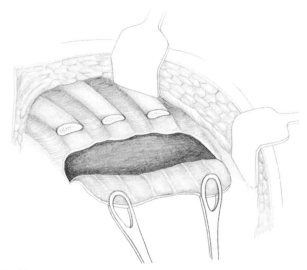

Fig. 53.26. Roberts' flap operation for chronic empyema showing posterior hinged flap.

inwards against the medial wall of the cavity, the whole of which has been freshened by thorough curettage. The two walls of the empyema are maintained in contact by a flavine gauze pack placed outside the

flap. The skin, subcutaneous tissues and chest wall muscle are sutured over the pack and a further pad strapped over the skin surface. Ten days later the pack is removed, a temporary corrugated rubber drain inserted in its place, and the wound resutured. A sinus may persist for a few weeks after this operation but usually it will ultimately heal.

4. *Schede Operation*

A Schede operation is indicated if the empyema cavity is small. The cavity is 'unroofed' by resecting subperiosteally the overlying rib or ribs, excising the thickened parietal pleura over the cavity, and packing the cavity open with dry gauze. The gauze pack is changed regularly until the residual cavity has filled with granulation tissue and is covered by epithelium.

CHRONIC SINUS

A chronic sinus (which implies the discharge of a small amount of pus on the skin surface) must always be examined radiographically following the injection of radio-opaque material. It may be due to an underlying empyema, often surprisingly large. It may also be due to osteomyelitis at the end of the previously resected rib, a retained nylon stitch, infected costal cartilage, a tuberculous gland under a rib, or even a retained drainage tube or swab. These causes will all be apparent on the chest radiograph or at subsequent operation.

Any underlying cause must be treated. An osteomyelitic portion of rib should be excised or infected cartilage removed. If the infected cartilage is part of the 6th–10th cartilage complex, most of the cartilage must be removed and the operation may be much more extensive than had been anticipated. A tuberculous gland should be removed after excision of the overlying rib. If there is no underlying cause and the empyema is small, a Schede type of operation should be carried out. If the underlying empyema is large, an adequate redrainage operation may be sufficient to obtain healing. Alternatively a decortication or a Roberts' flap operation will be required.

RECURRENT AND CHRONIC PNEUMOTHORAX (Smith and Rothwell, 1962; Sengupta, 1963; Killen and Gobbel, 1968)

A chronic pneumothorax implies the persistence of a small bronchopleural fistula which maintains the pneumothorax and causes minimal symptoms. This persisting pneumothorax is usually due to a leaking bleb or bulla, though there may be no apparent cause. It most commonly occurs in the 20–30 year age group due to a congenital bleb, or in the 50–60 year age group due to an emphysematous bulla. In some elderly patients there may also be gross emphysema associated with bronchospasm. At any time, however, the fistula may become valvular, causing an increase in size of the pneumothorax or even a 'tension' pneumothorax.

Although there is wide divergence of views concerning the treatment of recurrent and chronic pneumothorax, ranging from observation alone to bilateral parietal pleurectomy (on the basis that the underlying lung pathology is a bilateral condition), the generally accepted regimen for the treatment of this condition is:

1. Intercostal tube for first and second attack.
2. Parietal pleurectomy for third or subsequent attacks and also for chronic (persisting) pneumothorax, together with ligation of bullae if present.
3. Instillation of a pleural irritant for elderly patients not fit for pleurectomy due to chronic bronchitis and emphysema.

These patients should not be treated conservatively because of the risk of tension pneumothorax or haemothorax.

Differential Diagnosis

It is most important to differentiate a pneumothorax from a large emphysematous bulla—if an intercostal tube is inserted into a bulla, a tension pneumothorax may occur. An unusual but not very rare presentation of a bronchial carcinoma may be by spontaneous pneumothorax—this underlying pathology will usually be apparent on the chest radiograph.

Treatment

1. Intercostal Tube

The tube should be inserted in the 2nd intercostal space in the mid-clavicular line.

2. Parietal Pleurectomy

Parietal pleurectomy should be advised in a patient who has had two or more previous pneumothoraces, who has a persisting pneumothorax, or who has radiological evidence of a bulla, providing the patient is fit for thoracotomy. It is carried out through a small posterolateral or axillary thoracotomy in the 5th space. The plane between the parietal pleura and the endothoracic fascia can easily be developed by blunt dissection and the parietal pleura stripped from the chest wall over the upper half of the thoracic cage above the thoracotomy incision—over the apex and down over the mediastinum to the level of the hilum, anteriorly to the sternum and posteriorly to the paravertebral gutter.

3. Instillation of a Pleural Irritant

This procedure is reserved for patients who are consi-dered unfit for thoracotomy, usually because of age or poor respiratory function. The daily injection through the intercostal tube of 50 ml 50 per cent glucose will almost always seal the air leak. Iodized talc may also be used to produce a chemical pleurisy though the recurrence rate is at least 30 per cent and probably higher. Silver nitrate produces very severe pain and is not now advised, nor is camphor in oil.

CHYLOTHORAX (Gingell, 1965; Roy et al., 1967; Ross, 1978; Milsom et al., 1985)

Anatomy of the Thoracic Duct

The thoracic duct ascends from the abdomen through the aortic opening in the diaphragm to the left of the vena azygos. It passes up the posterior mediastinum, to the right of the midline between the azygos vein and the aorta. At the level of the 7th thoracic vertebra the duct passes obliquely upwards to reach the left side of the mediastinum at the level of the 5th thoracic vertebra. It passes behind the oesophagus at this level and then passes upwards along the left border of the oesophagus to the neck where it enters the junction of the internal jugular and subclavian veins. Occasionally there is an extra terminal branch which enters the veins on the right side of the neck. In about 50 per cent of individuals two or more ducts are present at some stage in its course through the mediastinum. There are, in addition, numerous other connections between the main thoracic duct and the azygos, intercostal and lumbar veins. This collateral circulation is so extensive that the duct may be ligated at any point in its course without any untoward effect.

Aetiology

The cause of the chylothorax must be considered—whether the duct has been damaged during an operation in its vicinity, e.g. Blalock operation, operation for coarctation of the aorta or thoracoplasty (though curiously oesophageal operations are rarely complicated by a leak of chyle), or whether there is any evidence of malignancy or a history of hyperextension injury, which may rupture the duct just above the diaphragm. In many cases no cause can be found. Treatment must be active because 50 per cent of cases are said to die from inanition.

Treatment

The initial treatment is repeated aspiration of the pleural cavity to dryness, in the hope of obtaining full expansion of the lung and cessation of the leak. With this regimen the leak will cease in 50 per cent of cases within 2–3 weeks. The advice regarding diet during this time is conflicting. Some advise a low fat and protein diet in the hope of reducing chyle secretion and therefore aiding closure of the leak. This would seem logical, and it should be combined with supplementary intravenous feeding if necessary. Others advise a high fat and protein diet in order to prevent deterioration of the patient's condition from dietary insufficiency. This will, of course, *increase* chyle production, and tend to keep the leak open.

If chyle production continues unabated, closed intercostal drainage will be necessary to try and obtain complete lung expansion, and if this fails, early thoracotomy is indicated. Cream taken by mouth 4 hours before operation will help to identify the damaged duct. If the cause was a recent operation, then that area should be explored and the injured duct sutured. If no previous operation has been carried out, then a thoracotomy on the side of the effusion should be undertaken. The chyle is aspirated and the pleura will be seen to be covered by a whitish exudate. The mediastinum will look swollen and be exuding chyle. This area should be opened up and an attempt made to identify the duct, which should then be sutured on either side of the tear. If this is not possible the area should be encircled with sutures tied over generous quantities of fibrin foam. If these procedures fail to cure the leak then the duct should be ligated through a low thoracotomy just above the diaphragm. This is much easier through a right thoracotomy, for at this level the duct is to the right of the midline. If a left-sided approach is used, it may be necessary to mobilize the aorta to gain access to the duct. Iodized talc pleurodesis (*see above*) has also been suggested as a treatment for chylothorax.

PART III

TUMOURS OF THE LUNG

The most common tumour of the lung is carcinoma which arises in a main or lobar bronchus, or less often more peripherally. Other tumours, comprising about 4 per cent of cases, may be innocent hamartoma, carcinoid adenoma of low-grade malignancy, or an adenoid cystic carcinoma (cylindroma) of relatively low-grade malignancy.

Resection is the treatment of choice for carcinoma of the lung, by standard pneumonectomy (simple extrapericardial), extended pneumonectomy (radical intrapericardial), lobectomy, or by segmental resection, provided (1) the patient is fit enough to undergo operation, (2) there is no evidence of spread of the growth outside the chest, and (3) there is no clinical or investigatory evidence of inoperability.

Evidence of Spread of Growth Outside the Chest
Metastases may occur in the supraclavicular glands,

liver, lumbar and thoracic vertebras, pelvis, ribs, brain and long bones and these must be excluded as far as possible. Supraclavicular glands may be palpable on the same or contralateral side, and growths in the left lung not uncommonly spread to the right supraclavicular area. Radioactive liver scan may detect secondary deposits but not infrequently the report is equivocal. The place of ultrasound in the diagnosis of liver metastases has not yet been established, but it would appear to be of more value than a radioactive scan. A recent onset of pain in the back must be investigated by appropriate radiographs, including lateral tomography, together with radioactive bone scan. Likewise, a recent onset of headache, muscular weakness in a limb or epileptiform fits must raise the possibility of a cerebral secondary deposit and suggest the need for brain or CT scan.

Clinical or Investigatory Evidence of Inoperability
Superior vena caval obstruction or left recurrent laryngeal paralysis causing a hoarse voice may both be presenting symptoms, usually of upper lobe growths, and both imply inoperability. Bronchoscopic evidence of inoperability includes actual involvement by tumour of the trachea or main bronchus at its origin (not merely distortion by glands or growth *outside* the lumen) or gross widening of the carina or its involvement by growth. The significance of rigidity of a main bronchus is not easy to assess. Phrenic nerve paralysis in the presence of an upper lobe growth implies inoperability, but if the growth is in the middle or lower lobe, resection may still be possible by opening the pericardium, which often seems to act as a barrier to the spread of the growth. Dysphagia must be investigated by a barium swallow—actual involvement of the oesophageal mucosa indicates inoperability. Mere displacement of the oesophagus may only signify para-oesophageal glands which may be removable at operation. The Pancoast syndrome (a small growth in the apex of the lung, which involves the 1st rib, 1st thoracic and 8th cervical nerves and stellate ganglion causing a Horner's syndrome) is usually regarded as inoperable, but Paulson (1974) has treated 26 of these cases by preoperative radiotherapy followed by resection and obtained a 10-year survival in 8. Chest wall involvement is not a contra-indication for it may be possible to resect a large area and replace it with a prosthesis of tantalum gauze or Marlex mesh. A pleural effusion, whether or not bloodstained, is likewise not a contra-indication, for it is not necessarily due to the carcinoma—it may be due to an infarct or infection distal to a carcinoma. Axillary node biopsy, unless the gland is hard and clearly malignant, is generally not rewarding for such nodes are frequently palpable in otherwise normal men.

The value of routine mediastinoscopy in the assessment of patients with bronchial carcinoma is debatable. Some authorities (Nohl-Oser, 1976) are of the opinion that the presence of positive mediastinal lymph nodes contra-indicates thoracotomy but, on the other hand, these nodes are often removable at operation and many such patients are known to have been cured of their growth (Shields et al., 1978). The crux of the matter is 'What is the significance of a positive node obtained at mediastinoscopy?' The answer is not yet known and the problem may well be more complex than it appears. CT scan of the thorax has recently been found to be of considerable value in the assessment of mediastinal gland enlargement, though unfortunately not necessarily of involvement.

Only about one-third of patients with bronchial carcinoma are suitable for thoracotomy, and of these about 10 per cent are found to be unresectable at operation.

Choice of Operation

In patients who so often have some degree of chronic bronchitis, pneumonectomy is often a very disabling procedure, especially in those over the age of 60 years, and many never resume work. Fortunately, lobectomy provides excellent results, both as regards cure rate and the quality of life, and lobectomy for peripheral carcinoma is as effective in curing the patient as is pneumonectomy, and furthermore carries a lower operative mortality (Flavell, 1962; Bates, 1981).

Indications for Lobectomy

1. Patients in whom the growth is relatively peripheral and confined to one lobe (or middle and right lower lobe). In the case of an upper lobe growth, especially on the right, it is possible to obtain almost as good a clearance of lymphatic glands as by pneumonectomy.
2. Patients who are considered unfit for pneumonectomy because of age or impaired lung function.

Indications for Segmental Resection

A localized peripheral tumour in an elderly patient with poor respiratory function.

Operative Technique for Pheumonectomy

This may be 'standard' pneumonectomy with division of the pulmonary vessels outside the pericardium, together with removal of carinal, paratracheal, pretracheal and para-oesophageal lymph nodes if they appear to be involved, or it may be an 'extended' radical operation, with division of the vessels inside the pericardium, and removal of all the involved lymphatic glands described above. This 'extended' operation must of necessity be more limited on the left than the right because of the interposition of the aortic arch.

A posterolateral thoracotomy through the 5th rib bed provides the best exposure and allows the hilum to be approached both from in front and behind. The apex of the lung is mobilized and drawn downwards so that the aortic arch or azygos vein are clearly seen. The rest of the lung is mobilized so that a clear view of the hilum is obtained. If the lung is very adherent to the chest wall, an extrapleural strip should be carried out over the adherent area. Operability is decided by vision and palpation, though a final opinion may not be possible until the pericardium has been opened and a hilar dissection attempted. Mediastinal lymph node involvement must be assessed and a decision made whether to open the pericardium to divide the pulmonary artery and veins. On the right side the liver should be palpated and if necessary the diaphragm opened.

Signs of Inoperability

1. Inability to separate growth from aorta or superior vena cava.
2. Inability to separate tumour from lower end of trachea.
3. Spread of growth along pulmonary veins to involve left atrium to such an extent that the vein cannot be divided, even by 'pinching up' a portion of atrial wall.
4. Spread of growth along pulmonary artery to such an extent that it cannot be divided, even on the left side proximal to the obliterated ductus arteriosus.
5. Inability to separate tumour from vertebral bodies.
6. Involvement of oesophageal mucosa.

In all cases (including lobectomy or segmental resection) it is theoretically advisable first to divide the vein draining the part of the lung containing the carcinoma to prevent tumour embolization during its manipulation. Thereafter it does not matter in which order the hilar structures are divided, though if there is an excessive amount of sputum or haemoptysis it is preferable at least to clamp, if not actually divide, the bronchus first.

The hilar anatomy is shown in *Figs.* 53.27 and 53.28 which demonstrate that on the left side the main bronchus is just below and behind the pulmonary artery, the superior vein is immediately below the pulmonary artery and in front of the bronchus, and below both is the inferior vein. On the right side the pulmonary artery is immediately in front of the bronchus, with the superior vein just below and a little in front, and the inferior vein lower still.

The inferior or superior vein is divided first, according to the position of the tumour.

The *inferior vein* is exposed by retracting the lower lobe upwards and forwards so that the vein is approached from behind (*Fig.* 53.29). The adventitia around the vein is incised, the vein isolated and then

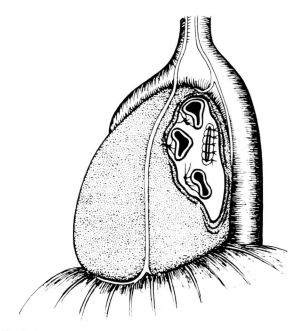

Fig. 53.27. Major mediastinal structures following left pneumonectomy. The pulmonary artery is above and anterior to the left main bronchus. The superior pulmonary vein is immediately anterior to the bronchus and the inferior pulmonary vein lies below.

divided between two strong ligatures proximally and a clamp or another ligature distally, ensuring that an adequate cuff of vein remains. If necessary, the pericardium is opened to obtain greater length, and if still more length is required, an angled Satinsky clamp may be placed on the atrial wall, the vein divided and the atrium closed with a continuous 3/0

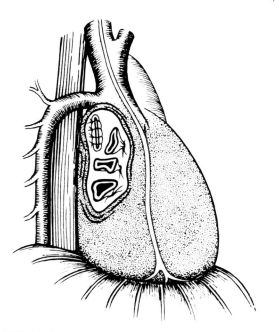

Fig. 53.28. Mediastinal structures following right pneumonectomy. The pulmonary artery is anterior to the right main bronchus and the pulmonary veins lie below the pulmonary artery.

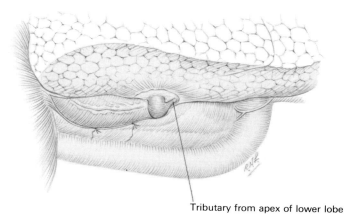

Tributary from apex of lower lobe

Fig. 53.29. Left pneumonectomy. Exposure of inferior pulmonary vein anterior to the oesophagus.

Mersilene stitch. The vein may be approached from in front or behind, or a combination of both. Not infrequently the tributary from the apex of the lower lobe enters the pericardium separately from the main vein to join it inside the pericardium.

The *superior vein* is approached from in front and the lung retracted backwards (*Fig.* 53.30). As with

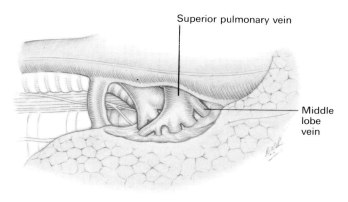

Superior pulmonary vein

Middle lobe vein

Fig. 53.30. Right pneumonectomy. Ligation and division of the right superior vein will expose the right main pulmonary artery and its main branches.

the inferior vein, the pericardium is opened if necessary to obtain greater length on the vein for the ligature or to place a clamp on the atrium itself.

The *pulmonary artery* is next isolated and divided between double proximal ligatures and another ligature or clamp distally. If necessary, the pericardium may be opened and the artery divided and sutured within the pericardium. On the right side, there is a condensation of tissue between the superior vena cava and pulmonary artery which must be deliberately cut with scissors, and when it is divided a considerable extra length of pulmonary artery is obtained. It is then very easy to encircle the artery so that it may be ligated or, better still, sutured.

Finally, the *bronchus* must be defined. The surrounding adventitious tissue containing bronchial arteries and pulmonary branches of the vagus must be divided between clamps. On the left side care must be taken to preserve the recurrent laryngeal nerve as it hooks around the obliterated ductus.

The bronchus must be divided flush with the carina to avoid pooling of pus in a long stump (*Figs.* 53.31, 53.32). If a clamp is used for bronchial closure it

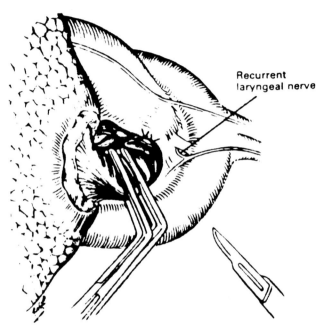

Fig. 53.31. Left pneumonectomy. Following ligation of the left pulmonary artery and left upper lobe vein, the left main bronchus is dissected deep to the arch of the aorta and controlled with bronchial clamps prior to division.

must be of the non-crushing variety. Alternatively, the bronchus may be divided with a knife and interrupted sutures placed in the cut open end as the division proceeds until the bronchus has been completely divided. The author's preferred technique is to use a non-crushing clamp placed on the bronchus with the handles towards the patient's head so that the membranous (posterior) wall of the bronchus is brought against the concavity of the C-shaped cartilage. Care must be taken to avoid placing the clamp too proximal or the opposite main bronchus may be narrowed or the anaesthetist's tube compressed and subsequently caught in the sutures. The bronchus is divided with a long-handled angled knife. The bronchial stump is closed with interrupted figure-of-eight no. 2 SWG stainless steel wire sutures on atraumatic needles, placed so that the proximal loop is inserted under the blades of the clamp (*Fig.* 53.33). It is important to cut the bronchial sutures short to avoid the danger of the ends of the wire suture perforating the

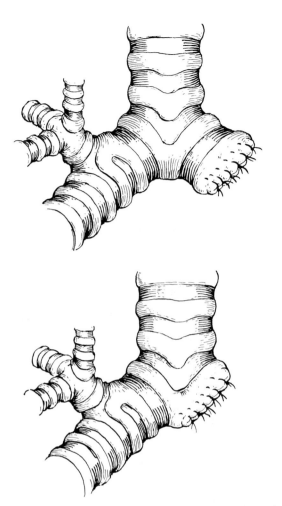

Fig. 53.32. Pneumonectomy. Upper (incorrect) and lower (correct) level of division of the main bronchus.

oesophagus on the right, or the pulmonary artery on the left. Airtight closure may be confirmed by pouring saline onto the stump and requesting the anaesthetist to apply gentle pressure. It is sometimes possible to cover the bronchial stump with adjacent pleura. A pedicled intercostal muscle bundle is recommended by some surgeons.

The bronchus may also be safely closed using the 'Auto Suture' automatic stapler.

Five Points Concerning the Division of the Pulmonary Artery and Veins

1. It is most important to ensure the assistant relaxes on the lung retraction at the moment when the ligatures are being tied.

2. The distal ligatures may be multiple ligatures on the branches or tributaries of the vessel, rather than on the main vessel itself. Alternatively, if there is insufficient length of vessel for a distal ligature, a clamp may be used distally and the vessel divided with a knife flush with the clamp.

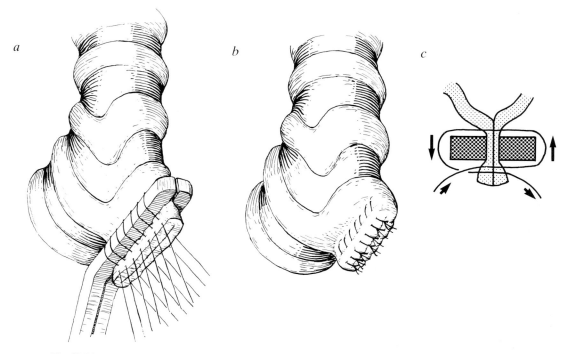

Fig. 53.33. Pneumonectomy. Closure of bronchial stump using figure-of-eight interrupted wire sutures.

3. The ligature material must be reasonably thick—a thin ligature may cut through the vessel.

4. The two proximal ligatures should be tied so that they overlap each other. There should be a cuff at least 1 cm long distal to the two ligatures. If this is not possible then it is wise to apply a Satinsky clamp and after division suture the vessel with a continuous 4/0 Mersilene suture. A transfixion suture may cause problems and is not required if an adequate cuff of vessel is available.

5. The pulmonary artery and veins are all ensheathed in a layer of adventitia. It is most important to pick up this adventitia with forceps and deliberately cut it with scissors, so as to enter the correct layer. It should then be relatively and often surprisingly easy, and certainly much safer, to pass a clamp around the vessel.

Extended (Radical Intrapericardial) Pneumonectomy

If the growth is extensive with considerable mediastinal lymph node involvement, an early decision must be made whether to use the intrapericardial technique. The pericardium is opened around the whole lung root, both anteriorly and posteriorly. If possible, it is preferable to retract the phrenic nerve anteriorly and not divide it. This will avoid the paradoxical movement of the diaphragm which will occur after phrenic division and the consequent difficulty in expectoration during the postoperative period. However, the situation of the growth may make this impossible and the nerve may have to be divided.

On either side the dissection exposes the oesophagus and care must be taken not to damage it on the medial side of the main bronchus or in the region of the inferior pulmonary vein. A small portion of oesophageal muscle may be removed providing the mucosa is preserved. The lung is removed together with the subcarinal lymph nodes. On the right side the azygos vein is divided and the areola tissue containing the paratracheal and pretracheal lymph nodes is removed completely, exposing the side of the trachea, the superior vena cava and ascending aorta. The dissection is carried from the oesophagus behind to the internal mammary vessels in front. On the left side the vagus is divided below the recurrent laryngeal nerve unless there are so many glands in the subaortic fossa that the nerve has to be sacrificed. The lymphatic clearance is of necessity less complete on the left side.

Operative Technique for Lobectomy

The final decision whether to carry out lobectomy or pneumonectomy must remain until the operation because the growth may be more extensive than anticipated. A posterolateral thoracotomy, through the 5th rib bed, is suitable for all lung resections.

In all cases of lobectomy or segmental resection it is wise to request the anaesthetist to inflate the lung after the bronchus has been clamped and *before* it is divided, to ensure that the proposed division is not too proximal—a mistake surprisingly easy to make.

Upper Lobectomy

This is a more difficult operation than lower lobectomy because of the more complex arrangement of the upper lobe arterial branches as they leave the main arterial trunk and the close proximity of the superior pulmonary vein to the main pulmonary artery to the lower lobe. This artery lies immediately posterior to the vein, damage to which will jeopardize the preservation of the lower lobe. The pulmonary vein, which lies in front of the hilum, should be divided first, opening the pericardium if necessary.

RIGHT UPPER LOBECTOMY

The lobe is retracted posteriorly to expose the venous drainage. It is most important to preserve the middle lobe vein, which drains into the superior vein (*Fig. 53.34*). The division of the veins to the upper lobe

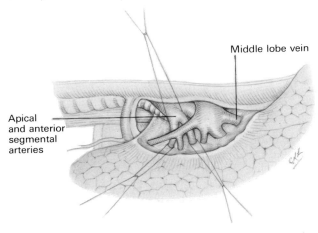

Apical and anterior segmental arteries

Middle lobe vein

Fig. 53.34. Right upper lobectomy. The right upper lobe arteries are mobilized; the right upper lobe veins are ligated and divided. Note carefully that the middle lobe vein, a tributary of the right upper lobe vein, is preserved.

must therefore be distal to the middle lobe vein and this must first be identified. Division of the vein will expose the arterial branches, of which there are two or three. These are divided. The posterior segmental branch arises low down below the upper lobe bronchus and often quite close to the middle lobe artery. It may not easily be visible until the bronchus has been divided. Finally, the lobe is retracted forwards to expose the upper lobe bronchus. The margins are defined, the adventitia containing bronchial arteries divided between clamps and the upper lobe bronchus clamped. The bronchus is divided close to the main bronchus but not so close that the lumen is narrowed. This is most important to prevent postoperative lower lobe collapse. The bronchial stump is closed as described under pneumonectomy, or with simple interrupted 2/0 Ethibond sutures on a 25-mm half-circle eyeless needle. The hilar structures have now all been divided but the lobe may not yet be completely free—it may still be partially attached to the apex of the

lower lobe and there may also be an incomplete fissure or no fissure between the upper and middle lobes. Attachment to the apex of the lower lobe is best managed by division of lung tissue between clamps. The apex of the lower lobe is then closed with a continuous suture over the clamp (*Fig. 53.35*).

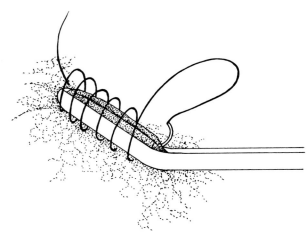

Fig. 53.35. Closure of raw surface of lower lobe using a continuous suture over a clamp.

The lobe is separated from the middle lobe by traction on the divided upper lobe bronchus and gentle blunt dissection with the index finger in the relatively avascular interlobar plane, as in segmental resection, beginning at the hilum and working towards the periphery. Inflation of the lung by the anaesthetist will help in the identification of the correct plane. Small air leaks and bleeding points are controlled by ligation. Finally, the pulmonary ligament should be divided so as to allow the lower lobe to swing upwards to fill the upper part of the chest.

LEFT UPPER LOBECTOMY

After division of the superior pulmonary vein the lobe is retracted anteriorly to expose the arterial branches, of which there are three to five (*Fig. 53.36*). These branches are separately divided. The lingular artery may arise from a basal branch to the lower lobe and not from the main artery itself. The division must therefore not be too proximal. The artery to the lower lobe is retracted posteriorly to expose the upper lobe bronchus. The margins are defined, the adventitia containing bronchial arteries divided between clamps and the upper lobe bronchus clamped with a non-crushing clamp. The bronchus is divided close to the main bronchus but not so close that the lumen is narrowed. This is most important to prevent postoperative lower lobe collapse. The bronchial stump is closed as described under pneumonectomy, or with simple interrupted 2/0 Ethibond sutures on a 25-mm half-circle eyeless needle.

The hilar structures have now all been divided but the lobe may not be completely free—it may still

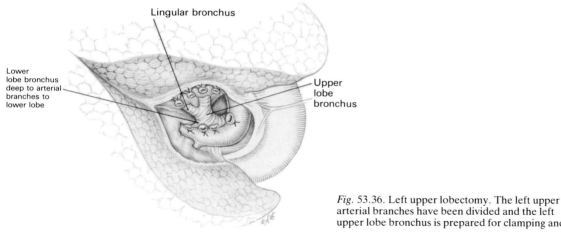

Fig. 53.36. Left upper lobectomy. The left upper arterial branches have been divided and the left upper lobe bronchus is prepared for clamping and division.

be partially attached to the apex of the lower lobe. Attachment to the apex of the lower lobe is best managed by division of lung tissue between clamps. The apex of the lower lobe is then closed with a continuous suture over the clamp. Finally the pulmonary ligament should be divided to allow the lower lobe to swing upwards to fill the upper part of the chest.

Lower Lobectomy

RIGHT LOWER LOBECTOMY

The inferior vein is divided first (*see* Operative Technique for Pneumonectomy). Care must be taken to preserve the right middle lobe artery, which arises opposite the artery to the apex of the lower lobe. The arteries to the apex of the lower lobe and the basal segments must all be divided separately. The bronchus to the middle lobe must also be preserved— it arises opposite the apical lower lobe bronchus. It is necessary in most cases to divide the apical lower segmental bronchus and the lower lobe bronchus separately. If the middle lobe bronchus is more proxi-

mal than usual, this separate division may not be necessary.

If there is an incomplete fissure between the apex of the lower lobe and the upper lobe, the separation is as described under Upper Lobectomy.

LEFT LOWER LOBECTOMY

The inferior vein is divided first (*see* Operative Technique for Pneumonectomy). Care must be taken to preserve the lingular artery, which may arise from a basal branch artery or from the main artery (*Fig.* 53.37). Finally, the bronchus is defined by dividing the peribronchial tissue containing the bronchial arteries. The pulmonary artery is retracted anteriorly so that the upper lobe bronchus is identified. This identification of the upper lobe is important to prevent narrowing of the upper lobe bronchus by too proximal application of the bronchus clamp or even division of the main bronchus itself. The lower lobe bronchus is then clamped and divided close to the upper lobe, taking care not to narrow the origin of the upper lobe bronchus (*Fig.* 53.37). The bronchial

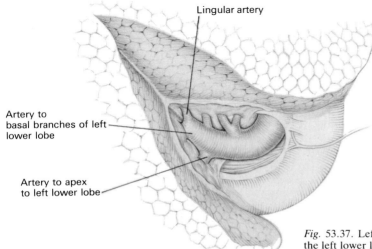

Fig. 53.37. Left lower lobectomy. Note that the apical artery to the left lower lobe lies at a more proximal level than the lingular artery to the left upper lobe, necessitating individual attention to the apical lower artery and the three basal branches.

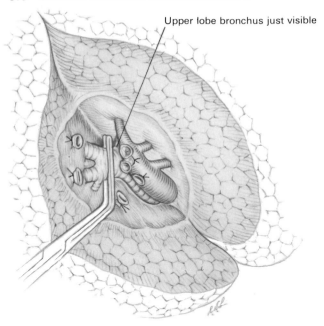

Upper lobe bronchus just visible

Fig. 53.38. Left lower lobectomy. The pulmonary arterial branches to the lower lobe have been secured, preserving the lingular vessels. The left lower lobe bronchus has been clamped prior to division.

stump is closed as in upper lobectomy. A suture line flush with the upper lobe is important—a long stump is the usual cause of a bronchopleural fistula.

If there is an incomplete fissure between the apex of the lower lobe and the upper lobe, the separation is as described under upper lobectomy.

Middle Lobectomy

The middle lobe is retracted posteriorly so as to expose the origin of the middle lobe vein, which is divided between ligatures close to its entry into the superior vein. The lobe is then retracted anteriorly and the oblique fissure between the middle lobe and lower lobe developed so as to expose the arterial branches to the middle and lower lobes. The middle lobe is supplied by one or two arteries which pass anteriorly from the right main pulmonary artery opposite or just proximal to the branch to the apex of the lower lobe. The middle lobe artery is divided between ligatures, and the middle lobe bronchus can then be seen and defined. It is divided and closed as in upper and lower lobectomy. The middle lobe can now be removed by traction on the middle lobe bronchus and gentle dissection with the index finger in the plane between the middle and upper lobes. Inflation of the upper lobe by the anaesthetist will help to define the correct plane. Small air leaks and bleeding points are controlled by ligatures.

Right Middle and Lower Lobectomy

A right middle and lower lobectomy is not infre-

quently required for bronchial carcinoma. The technique for the venous and arterial ligation is as described for middle lobectomy and right lower lobectomy. The bronchial dissection is similar to a left lower lobectomy, i.e. the right upper lobe must be visualized before the bronchus clamp is applied, so as to avoid a long bronchial stump or a narrowed right upper lobe bronchus.

Upper Lobectomy with 'Sleeve' Resection of the Main Bronchus (Johnson and Jones, 1959; Bennett and Smith, 1978)

Upper lobectomy with 'sleeve' resection of the main bronchus is a most valuable procedure in those cases in which the growth involves the actual origin of the upper lobe bronchus at its junction with the main bronchus and where standard upper lobectomy would not provide a complete removal of the growth. In these cases a 'sleeve' of main bronchus is removed with the upper lobe and the two ends of the main bronchus are reanastomosed (Fig. 53.39). This technique may be applied to the left or right upper lobe, though it is technically more difficult to perform on the left side because of the proximity of the aortic arch. The lymphatic drainage area can be removed as completely as by pneumonectomy. In older patients, or in younger patients with diminished respiratory reserve, this technique is most valuable in permitting the tumour to be removed, with preservation of the right lower and middle lobes or left lower lobe. If necessary the resection may be extended to include a 'sleeve' of the main pulmonary artery. The final decision concerning the possibility of 'sleeve' resection must be taken at thoracotomy. The technique is best reserved for squamous carcinoma or innocent tumours.

Anaesthesia into the opposite lung must be by double-lumen tube. If the tumour is localized and it is decided that this technique can be carried out, the venous and arterial dissection is performed as already described. The main bronchus is isolated and up to about 2·5 cm may be resected. The main bronchus is divided proximally and distally. The proximal end of the bronchus may be left open but the distal portion should be temporarily occluded with ribbon gauze to prevent the entry of blood. The upper lobectomy may then be completed as already described. The remaining lobe or lobes must be mobilized by division of the pulmonary ligament. The two ends of the bronchus are anastomosed with interrupted no. 3/0 Ethibond (Ethicon) on an atraumatic needle, with the knots on the outside of the bronchus. The main problem encountered is the discrepancy in size of the two portions of the bronchus. This can generally be overcome by placing the sutures closer together on the distal bronchus. If this does not suffice, the technique illustrated in Fig. 53.40 may be used. Before final closure the lower lobe should be aspirated by a fine catheter. Airtight closure is easily

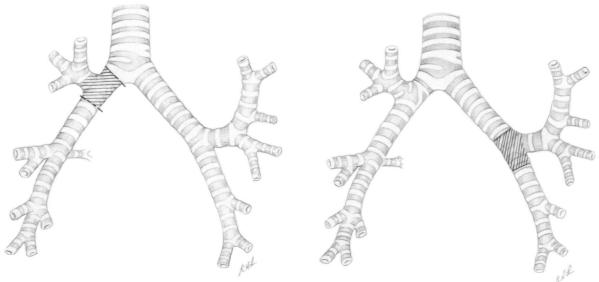

Fig. 53.39. Sleeve resection of right upper lobe and left upper lobe. This is an acceptable method of dealing with malignant tumours situated at the mouth of the upper lobe in those patients with poor lung function who might not tolerate pneumonectomy.

obtained and the lower and middle lobes are readily inflated by the anaesthetist. A flap of pleura should be placed between the bronchus and the pulmonary artery, to prevent the rare but well-recognized late complication of secondary haemorrhage from the pulmonary artery.

Perhaps rather surprisingly there are no special immediate postoperative problems after this operation. The main late complication is a stricture at the site of the anastomosis, but the incidence of this is not high.

Operative Technique for Segmental Resection

Any segment of the lung may be resected, though in the case of carcinoma it is the lingula or apical segment of the lower lobe that is most commonly removed (Le Roux, 1972).

General Principles

Each bronchopulmonary segment has its own individual artery and bronchus. The vein runs *between* the segments in the intersegmental plane, receiving tributaries from both adjacent segments. When a segment is to be resected the appropriate segmental artery and bronchus are divided at the hilum. A clamp is then placed on the distal end of the bronchus. The segment can be separated from the adjacent lung by traction on this bronchus and gentle dissection with the index finger from the hilum outwards in the relatively avascular intersegmental plane. The correct plane is shown by the line of the intersegmental vein which must remain in place undisturbed. Its tributaries from the segment to be removed are divided. Inflation of the remainder of the lung by increased endotracheal pressure by the anaesthetist will assist in defining the correct line of separation.

There is only minimal air leak from the damaged alveoli and these soon seal off with swab pressure. Very little, if any, lung suture is required. The raw

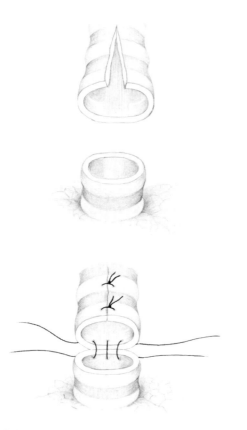

Fig. 53.40. Sleeve resection. Method of tailoring the right main bronchus prior to airtight closure.

surface of the lung should not be oversewn, as any attempt to do this will only increase the air leak. The bronchial stump is closed by an 'open' technique with two or three simple stainless steel or Ethiflex sutures.

Lingulectomy

The lingular vein (situated anteriorly) is first divided. The lingular artery is next divided (for anatomy see Left Lower Lobectomy) and finally the origin of the lingular bronchus is defined prior to its division. It is the first inferior branch of the upper lobe bronchus.

Apical Lower Segmentectomy

The vein is situated posteriorly. It drains into the inferior vein although sometimes it enters the pericardium separately. The artery is approached through the oblique fissue. The artery is divided and immediately underneath the segmental bronchus will be seen and this too is divided.

Other Tumours of the Lung

1. Hamartoma

At operation a hamartoma is freely mobile within the lung substance like a fibro-adenoma of the breast. It can always be removed by grasping the tumour between thumb and forefinger and making a small incision in the overlying lung—the tumour will then 'pop out'. The lung incision is closed by interrupted catgut sutures placed so as to obliterate the cavity. Alternatively a wedge resection can be carried out.

2. Carcinoid (Adenoma)

This is a tumour of very low malignancy (Lawson et al., 1976). It often presents as a well-defined red lobulated mass which protrudes into a bronchus and has a narrow pedicle. It sometimes bleeds profusely on biopsy. Local excision of the tumour by bronchotomy is the procedure of choice, providing the tumour is small and distal bronchiectatic changes have not occurred (see also Hurt and Bates, 1984). Frequently, however, a segmental resection, lobectomy or even pneumonectomy is required.

Complications of Lung Resection

Apart from haemorrhage, bronchospasm, sputum retention, pulmonary collapse and cardiac arrhythmias, the most important complications are persistent air space, empyema and bronchopleural fistula.

1. Persistent Air Space and Empyema Following Lobectomy or Segmental Resection, Uncomplicated by Bronchopleural Fistula

The diagnosis will be suspected by the onset of fever with radiological evidence of increased fluid. There may be discharge of pus at the site of the drainage tube. The diagnosis should be confirmed by diagnostic aspiration and the empyema should be drained. Although an important bronchopleural fistula may not be demonstrated, the majority of these patients do, in fact, have a pinhole leak which is responsible for this complication.

2. Post-pneumonectomy Empyema Without Demonstrable Bronchopleural Fistula

It is sometimes possible to sterilize these empyemas by daily aspiration and the instillation of antibiotics but more frequently rib resection drainage of the empyema will be required. Opening up and marsupialization of the space have been recommended as a method of sterilizing such a cavity but in the presence of persistent infection it is worth while considering a ten-rib thoracoplasty. This major procedure should be reserved only for those patients who appear to be long-term survivors from their carcinoma.

3. Postoperative Bronchopleural Fistula

AFTER LOBECTOMY OR SEGMENTAL RESECTION

This complication is uncommon but must be suspected if the patient expectorates bloodstained sputum and develops an air space with a fluid level. Should this space not obliterate completely with tube drainage and suction, further operation and resuture of the bronchus or leaking lung together with removal of the fibrin peel are advised.

AFTER PNEUMONECTOMY

A bronchopleural fistula following a pneumonectomy is a very major disaster and all too often ultimately leads to the death of the patient or a permanent tube or stoma drainage of the pneumonectomy space. It may be associated from the beginning with infection in the pneumonectomy space, and it almost always occurs on the right side, usually in those cases in which the blood supply to the bronchial stump has been reduced by the removal of enlarged pretracheal or paratracheal lymph nodes. Most cases occur from 4 to 21 days after operation, but a fistula may develop months or even years after operation.

The diagnosis is made by the sudden expectoration of bloodstained sputum, exacerbated by the patient lying towards the contralateral lung and dramatically relieved by lying towards the pneumonectomy side (Fig. 53.41). The development of a fistula is a surgical emergency and the patient must be instructed to lie on the pneumonectomy side (which will immediately abolish the cough and expectoration) until the chest has been emptied of fluid, either by intercostal tube or thoracoscopic suction. If the fistula is small or there is doubt concerning the diagnosis, the instillation of methylene blue dye into the pneumonectomy space

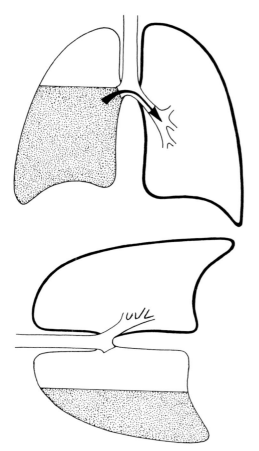

Fig. 53.41. Bronchopleural fistula following pneumonectomy. Lying the patient on the operated side prevents further aspiration of bloodstained fluid.

will confirm the diagnosis. The sputum will immediately change colour.

The elective treatment of the fistula depends on whether or not the pleural fluid is sterile. If the fistula has occurred 3 or more months after the pneumonectomy, bronchoscopy should be performed to determine whether or not there is recurrence of carcinoma.

If the Fluid is Sterile: The bronchial stump should be resutured. The operation should be carried out in the lateral position and it is unwise to rely on a cuffed endobronchial tube to prevent further spillage into the remaining lung, however expert and persuasive is the anaesthetist. The only safe procedure is to aspirate the pneumonectomy space dry through a thoracoscope with the patient in the sitting position immediately prior to induction of anaesthesia. Only by this means is the aspiration of fluid into the contralateral lung and its very serious consequences prevented with certainty.

The chest is opened, the pneumonectomy space evacuated of blood clot and fibrin, and the fistula identified—it is usually obvious. On the right side (which is almost always the side of the fistula—the author has never had a fistula on the left) a longitudinal incision is made behind the bronchial stump in the line of the oesophagus. This plane is then followed around the stump anteriorly until it is completely freed. The azygos vein is divided unless it was previously divided at the time of the pneumonectomy. The superior vena cava and the pulmonary artery stump both lie anteriorly. On the left side the dissection is much more difficult because of the very close proximity of the pulmonary artery and superior pulmonary vein, as they lie anterior to the bronchus which is deep in the mediastinum. It is preferable to open the track of the fistula first and then subsequently to mobilize the bronchial stump.

However tempting it may be, the fistula must not merely be closed by an extra two or three stitches. A recurrence of the fistula will inevitably occur. It is imperative that the whole of the previously sutured stump be re-amputated so as to provide a fresh bronchus for suture. The stump should be covered with a pedicled muscle graft.

If the Fluid is Infected: If the fluid is infected then it is unwise to attempt to resuture the bronchus. Not only will this fail, but it is likely that much of the thoracotomy wound will become infected. It is better to drain the empyema by rib resection and then, about 6 months later when the infection has subsided and the patient's condition has improved, perform a lateral thoracoplasty (with preservation of the first rib) together with a modified Roberts' flap operation in which the decostalized chest wall is sutured onto the open bronchial stump (*see* p. 798). Complete healing will usually occur within a few weeks.

If there is a recurrence of carcinoma at the bronchial stump, then resuture or lateral thoracoplasty are not advisable and the treatment can only be directed to the prevention of aspiration of infected pleural fluid into the contralateral lung. This will usually require rib resection drainage.

PART IV

MEDIASTINAL TUMOURS

Mediastinal tumours occur from infancy to old age in both sexes and are best classified according to their position on the chest radiograph. Neurogenic tumours occur in the posterior mediastinum, foregut duplications and lymphatic tissue tumours in the central mediastinum, while thyroid, thymic and dermoid tumours occur in the anterior mediastinum (Blades, 1941; Morrison, 1958) (*Fig.* 53.42).

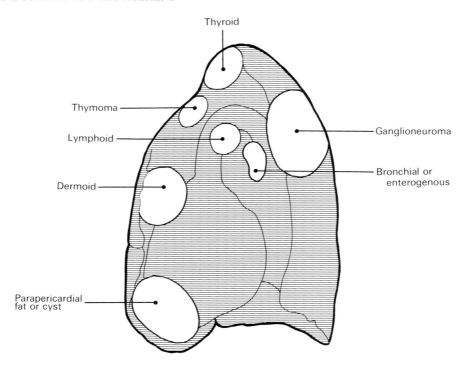

Fig. 53.42. Mediastinal tumours. Those commonly seen are: anteriorly from above down, thyroid, thymus, dermoid, para-pericardial cyst; posteriorly, neurogenic tumours; centrally, bronchial or enterogenous cysts or tumours. A vascular or lymphatic swelling or tumour may occur at any site.

Classification of Mediastinal Tumours

Posterior mediastinum (paravertebral gutter):
　Neurofibroma.
　Ganglioneuroma.
Anterior mediastinum (from above downwards):
　Retrosternal thyroid.
　Thymic tumour.
　Dermoid and teratoma.
　Para-pericardial cyst.
Central mediastinum:
　Foregut duplication cyst (bronchogenic or gastrogenic).
　Lymphatic tissue tumours (including sarcoid).
　Primary tuberculosis.
　Secondary bronchial carcinoma.

Any mediastinal tumour may be an aortic aneurysm or a tumour of lymphatic origin.

Diagnostic aspiration is best avoided and thoracotomy is usually required, both for diagnosis and treatment, for many of these tumours are potentially malignant and may suddenly increase in size if a haemorrhage occurs into them.

A foregut cyst, which is often associated with a vertebral abnormality (hemivertebra), may develop a bronchial communication producing cough and sputum, together with a fluid level on the chest radiograph.

Thymic tumours, unless associated with myasthenia gravis, are usually found on routine radiographic examination, as also are dermoids, neurofibroma and ganglioneuroma, unless they are so large as to cause pressure symptoms.

Posterior Mediastinal Tumours

Surgical Approach

A high posterolateral thoracotomy through the 4th or 5th rib bed, with division of the posterior end of the rib above if necessary, will provide an adequate exposure. If the tumour is large and closely applied to the ribs there may be difficulty in ligating the intercostal vessels. In this event it is best to secure haemostasis after the tumour has been removed. The oesophagus may be displaced by the tumour and must be identified at operation—the passage of a stomach tube may be of great help.

Complications of operation include damage to the sympathetic trunk (causing Horner's syndrome or sympathetic impairment to the upper limb) or thoracic duct (causing a chylothorax).

A neurofibroma may penetrate and enlarge an intervertebral foramen and care must be taken to avoid damage to the spinal cord when ligating the spinal branch of an intercostal artery. There may even be a prolongation into the vertebral canal ('dumbbell' tumour) causing symptoms of cord or root compression. A myelogram is necessary to ascertain the extent of the intraspinal prolongation and laminectomy may be required for its removal.

Anterior Mediastinal Tumours

Surgical Approach

The approach may be by posterolateral thoracotomy on the side to which the tumour mainly projects or by median sternotomy if the tumour is bilateral. An anterolateral thoracotomy does not give an adequate exposure, nor is it so easy to enlarge if this proves necessary. After incision of the mediastinal pleura the tumour may be enucleated from its false sac often without division of a single blood vessel. If there has been malignant change or previous infection, the dissection may be extremely difficult and the great vessels in the mediastinum are at risk.

Central Mediastinal Tumours

Surgical Approach

These tumours should usually be approached through a right posterolateral thoracotomy. Division of the vena azygos will permit a full exploration of the mediastinum, the exposure of which will not be hampered by the aortic arch and its left branches. If the chest radiograph shows that the whole tumour is on the left side, or if the left lung is involved, then clearly a left thoracotomy would be necessary.

A bronchogenic cyst is usually situated high in the mediastinum, has thin walls and is relatively easily excised. A gastrogenic cyst is lined by gastric epithelium, may develop peptic ulceration and become very adherent to adjacent structures, particularly the oesophagus, aorta or bronchus.

Before embarking on a resection of a central mediastinal tumour, it is important to exclude an aneurysm of aorta, generalized disease of the lymphatic system, or secondary carcinoma.

Retrosternal Thyroid

Retrosternal prolongation of a goitre may occur into the chest. It is a potentially dangerous condition because of the possibility of superior vena caval obstruction or stridor from tracheal compression. These symptoms may suddenly increase if a haemorrhage occurs into the retrosternal prolongation. The extension into the chest is usually in the plane immediately behind the sternum and *in front of* the innominate vein, though rarely it may pass behind the vein or even behind the trachea and oesophagus. The blood supply is invariably from the neck.

Operative Approach

Most retrosternal prolongations of the thyroid may be removed through the neck. The thyroid is exposed by a cervical collar incision and the superior, middle and inferior thyroid vessels isolated and divided as described in Chapter 24.

The index finger is then passed down into the mediastinum and gently swept around the gland to free it from adhesions. In almost all cases the gland may be successfully delivered into the neck. It may be helpful to evacuate the contents of some of the cysts. If difficulty is encountered due to abnormal adherence, size or position of the gland, then the manubrium should be split vertically (*see* Chapter 24).

MYASTHENIA GRAVIS

The functions of the thymus are not fully understood and there is considerable controversy concerning its exact relationship to myasthenia gravis. Initiated by Sauerbruch in 1913 and popularized by Blalock et al. in 1939 and Keynes in 1949, thymectomy has nevertheless now become an established procedure in the treatment of myasthenia, though its exact benefit is difficult to define since myasthenia is notorious for its spontaneous remissions. The patients who most benefit from thymectomy are young females with a short history who have a macroscopically normal thymus. The gland, though not enlarged, usually has an excess of germinal follicles.

The diagnosis of myasthenia should be confirmed pharmacologically. The possible presence of a tumour should be ascertained by a lateral chest radiograph and lateral tomography of the mediastinum or, if possible, CT scan. If muscle antibodies are present in the blood it is likely that there is a thymic tumour. The presence of a tumour makes a good operative result much less likely and in these cases the patient should have preliminary radiotherapy.

Thymectomy (Keynes, 1949; Edwards and Wilson, 1972)

The main postoperative complication is respiratory failure from 'cholinergic crisis'. The doses of anticholinergic drugs which will produce the maximum therapeutic response must be determined by trial and error, and care must be taken to avoid overdose.

The operation is carried out through a median sternotomy. The pleura is displaced laterally by blunt dissection to reveal the yellowish-pink H-shaped thymus. The gland is grasped in light artery forceps at its two lower poles and peeled upwards, taking care not to damage either pleural cavity. The gland is gently lifted upwards until the innominate vein is exposed on its deep surface. The thymic veins which drain into the innominate vein are then divided. The upper poles of the thymus are mobilized and it is here that the thymic arteries may be seen, arising from the internal mammary artery. They are divided and the thymus removed. If either pleural cavity is opened it should be drained by an underwater-seal drainage tube inserted through the lateral chest wall.

After operation the patient is best managed in an intensive care unit, for respiratory problems are common. An immediate postoperative chest radiograph is important to exclude pneumothorax or haemothorax. Artificial ventilation through an endotracheal tube for 24 hours is advisable. Thereafter assisted respiration can usually be reduced, provided there is no respiratory infection and the patient's respiratory muscles are strong enough. A nasogastric tube will allow the crushed anticholinesterase drugs to be given into the stomach, which is the most effective route, but they should be withheld until their need is apparent, to prevent the serious complication of a cholinergic crisis. The reader is referred elsewhere for a description of the specific drug and steroid therapy suitable to this condition.

Transcervical Thymectomy (Donnelly et al., 1984)
An alternative approach is the removal of the thymus gland via the collar incision used in thyroid surgery. Several large series of patients have been treated satisfactorily in this way. However, this is a very specialized technique and in the absence of special experience, is likely to result in the thymus being incompletely removed.

CHRONIC SUPERIOR VENA CAVAL OBSTRUCTION

Superior vena caval obstruction is usually due to advanced malignant disease and is best treated by radiotherapy. In a few cases, however, it is due to benign idiopathic mediastinal fibrosis, caseating granuloma or old-standing tuberculous glands and the obstruction may be relieved by the insertion of a conduit between the left innominate vein and the right atrial appendage. Synthetic grafts almost always thrombose due to the thrombogenicity of the graft material and the relatively slow venous flow. An autogenous venous graft is therefore advisable. A preliminary venogram, preferably by CT scan with venous enhancement, is carried out to define the caval obstruction.

A midline sternotomy is performed to confirm feasibility of venous bypass and to biopsy the obstructing lesion. The thymic remnant is excised and the pericardium opened in the midline to expose the right atrial appendage. The innominate vein is ligated as close to its entry into the superior vena cava as possible. A vascular clamp is applied to the jugulo-subclavian junction and the innominate vein divided. The graft is then anastomosed with 5/0 Prolene sutures to the left innominate vein and the right atrial appendage. The graft must not be kinked as this would predispose to later thrombosis. The venous graft may be a composite spiral vein graft fashioned from the long saphenous vein (Doty, 1982) or it may be a segment of common femoral vein. The spiral vein graft is made by opening the segment of saphenous vein longitudinally to form a ribbon which is then wound round a stent as a spiral and made into a tube by suturing its edges together with a continuous 7/0 Prolene suture. Alternatively a segment of common femoral vein is obtained by incising the deep fascia along the posterior border of the sartorius to expose the adductor canal and excising a segment of common femoral vein distal to the profunda femoris vein (the long saphenous vein must be present and normal if this technique is used).

PART V

SURGERY OF PLEURA AND CHEST WALL

Pleural Biopsy

Pleural biopsy may be required for the diagnosis of pleural effusion or diffuse pleural tumours. It may be carried out by a closed 'aspirating' technique or by an open technique.

Closed Technique
The site of the proposed biopsy is anaesthetized with 0.5 per cent Xylocaine (lignocaine) and then a wide-bore needle advanced into the pleural tumour. The needle is gently angulated when the end is judged to be in the tumour so as to cut off a piece of tissue. The needle is withdrawn while suction is continuously applied by means of a 20-ml syringe, and the biopsy is then expelled from the needle into fixative.

A more sophisticated method is to use an Abrams needle which has a side-hole near its end. This hole is wedged against the pleura or tumour and a small piece of tissue cut off by the sliding internal cannula (Abrams, 1958). A Tru-cut needle is also useful.

A high yield is provided by the Steel drill biopsy, in which a rapidly rotating drill 'cores out' a piece of tissue. This was originally designed for lung biopsy but is equally effective for pleural tumours (Steel and Winstanley, 1969).

Open Technique
This is a more certain method of obtaining positive histology. A portion of rib is resected under local or general anaesthetic, the rib bed incised and a wedge biopsy carried out.

Tumours of the Pleura

Primary tumours of the pleura are relatively rare, though secondary invasion from bronchial carcinoma or breast carcinoma is common. The primary tumour may be a fibroma or a mesothelioma.

Fibroma
A fibroma is usually found by chance on a routine chest radiograph, though it may cause a dull chest

pain or hypertrophic pulmonary osteoarthropathy. It is basically an innocent tumour, but should be resected together with a generous portion of adjacent chest wall (rib and intercostal muscle), for it is likely to recur and may behave as a slow-growing, low-grade malignant tumour. If an area of chest wall involving long lengths of several ribs is removed, it will be necessary to close the deficit with Marlex mesh or tantalum gauze in order to prevent respiratory embarrassment after operation. If the deficit is under cover of the scapula, however, a much larger portion of chest wall may be excised without the use of a prosthesis (Thomas and Drew, 1953).

Mesothelioma

A mesothelioma is usually due to exposure to asbestos, often many years previously. It may or may not be associated with a pleural effusion. If no effusion is present it commonly causes multiple pleural opacities. Treatment is unsatisfactory and there is evidence that resection (or even open biopsy) may hasten the growth of the tumour, which is usually much more extensive than appears on the chest radiograph. There is no evidence that radiotherapy, cytotoxic drugs or intrapleural radioactive material influence the prognosis. The duration of life after diagnosis is very variable and may be surprisingly long (Hickman and Jones, 1970; Elmes and Simpson, 1976).

Secondary Carcinoma

If secondary carcinoma from the lung or breast is associated with a recurrent pleural effusion, a pleurectomy will produce adherence of the lung to the chest wall and prevent a recurrence of the effusion and at the same time remove some of the tumour. There is a small risk of implantation of tumour cells into the chest wall. The advice of an oncologist may help the patient.

Chest Wall Tumours

Excision of the chest wall may be required for primary tumours such as chondrosarcoma (the commonest), chondroma (which often becomes malignant) or osteochondroma, or for secondary tumours (e.g. from the breast), provided that the primary growth is adequately controlled. Malignant tumours, especially chondrosarcoma, have a marked tendency to recur and a wide excision must be carried out. The whole length of the ribs involved must be removed together with adjacent intercostal muscle and underlying pleura and part of the diaphragm if necessary. If the lung is involved a lobectomy may be required. It is usually possible to distinguish benign from malignant tumours by a careful study of the radiographs.

The wide excision of chest wall leads to a problem in reconstruction, in which there are two functional considerations:

1. Airtight closure.
2. Restoration of the functional integrity and rigidity of the chest wall.

If the defect is likely to be large it is important to plan the operation in conjunction with a plastic surgeon, who can prepare in advance full-thickness pedicled skin grafts to fill the chest wall deficit.

Lateral Chest Wall Tumours

An elliptical incision is made in the line of the ribs to encircle the tumour. It is deepened to expose the chest wall. If there is doubt concerning the resectability of the tumour, only one half of the elliptical incision should be made. The periosteum of a normal rib above the tumour is incised longitudinally, stripped from its lower border and the pleura opened to ascertain the extent of the tumour and to make sure that scattered nodes are not present throughout the pleural cavity. The presence of multiple nodules would preclude resection, though an intercostal neurectomy should be carried out if the pain is severe. A frozen section is advisable to ascertain the nature of the tumour. If it is malignant the resection will need to be much wider than if innocent, though the tumour may only be malignant in part and this may not be the site of the biopsy. The periosteum is elevated from the involved ribs for a short length anteriorly and posteriorly, so that they can be divided with a costotome. The intercostal muscles and bundle are divided between clamps and longitudinal incisions are made along the adjacent normal ribs above and below so that the tumour and involved chest wall may be removed. If there is involvement of the underlying lung and diaphragm an appropriate resection must be undertaken.

If the chest wall deficit is under cover of the scapula, quite a large opening may be left unclosed. If, however, the deficit is lower down and involves more than two ribs, some type of prosthesis is required to strengthen the chest wall. The most satisfactory materials are Marlex mesh or tantalum gauze. Tantalum gauze should be turned in at its edges to avoid fraying. The edge of the prosthesis should overlap the edge of the defect by 1 cm and be fixed in place outside the chest wall with interrupted wire sutures. If the tumour has involved a wide area of skin and it is difficult to obtain complete skin closure, a pedicled skin graft may be used to cover the defect. The pleural cavity should always be drained by a tube inserted through a separate stab incision posteriorly in the lowest part of the chest.

Sternal Tumours

Tumours of the upper end of the sternum may require the excision of the medial ends of both clavicles. If the tumour is malignant the whole sternum may need to be removed.

The restoration of rigidity of the bony cage

depends on the extent of sternal excision. If a portion of manubrium can be preserved, the rest of the sternum may be excised and the deficit satisfactorily closed by bringing together the attachments of the pectoralis major from each side. If the whole of the sternum has been removed, the ribs must be stabilized by the insertion of a prosthesis of a tantalum plate or acrylic resin.

PART VI

EMPHYSEMATOUS CYSTS

An air-containing cyst in the lung may be a congenital bronchogenic cyst or an acquired emphysematous cyst.

A *bronchogenic cyst*, which is usually diagnosed on a routine chest radiograph, should always be removed as it is prone to become infected.

An *emphysematous cyst* should be excised if:
1. The patient is breathless.
2. There is evidence that the cyst is enlarging.
3. The cyst occupies more than one-third of the lung.
4. The patient is fit for operation—the patient must not be so incapacitated by chronic bronchitis, bronchospasm, the effects of cor pulmonale or ischaemic heart disease that the risk of operation is too high.

Careful selection of patients is most important, for the operative mortality is high in poor-risk patients with bilateral disease. Many patients fall into this group.

Surgical Excision or Obliteration

The method of anaesthesia is most important. The more usual technique of paralysis and manual ventilation is very likely to rupture the cyst and cause a tension pneumothorax before the chest has been opened.

The larger cysts are excised and obliterated while the smaller cysts are simply ligated or oversewn. If the whole lobe is replaced by a cyst, and no functioning lung remains, a lobectomy should be carried out. However, an important aim of the operation is conservation of lung tissue—no functioning lung should be removed. Cysts should be obliterated so that the surrounding compressed lung may expand.

When treating larger cysts the wall is excised, starting at its junction with normal lung and continuing around its base (*Fig.* 53.43). Trabeculae may need to be divided near normal lung. The cyst should then be obliterated by multiple interrupted catgut sutures placed through its wall, including its deepest part (*Fig.* 53.44). Alternatively the cyst is excised and its base closed with the T90 'Auto Suture' stapler applied across normal lung tissue.

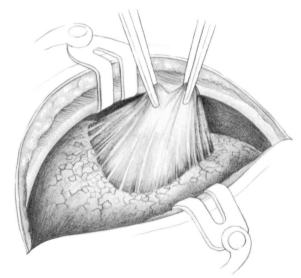

Fig. 53.43. Mobilization of lung cyst prior to excision.

Smaller cysts with a narrrow pedicle are readily treated by ligature and excision.

At the conclusion of operation the anaesthetist should avoid vigorous inflation of the lungs, or new air dissections, or a contralateral spontaneous pneumothorax may be caused.

The chest is closed. Three tubes (apical, basal and anterior) should be inserted, as air leak is always a major problem and it is important to obtain rapid expansion of the lung. Care must be taken that the

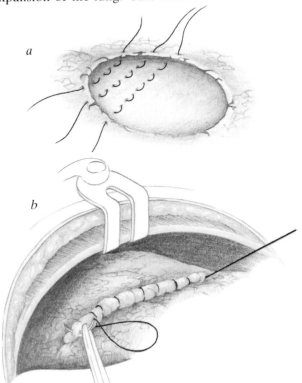

Fig. 53.44. Lung cyst. Suture obliteration of lung cysts. Alternatively the base of the cyst may be stapled

suction is sufficient to deal with the volume of air leak when the patient coughs—otherwise surgical emphysema will occur. Alternatively, one tube should be attached to an underwater seal, without suction, to allow excess air to escape readily.

Postoperatively it is important to make sure that the tubes remain patent, being removed only when all air leak has ceased.

Intracavity Suction (Monaldi Drainage) (Macarthur and Fountain, 1977)

This is a most valuable technique in patients with a large cyst who are severely disabled due to cor pulmonale and very poor lung function and who are unfit for thoracotomy. The cyst may be reduced in size by introducing a Malecot catheter and applying suction. A two-stage operation is required so as to ensure adherence of the two layers of pleura. At the first stage a short length of rib overlying the cavity is resected under local anaesthesia and a gauze pack soaked in 1 per cent iodine placed against the parietal pleura. The wound is closed. Two weeks later the pack may be removed and a tube inserted into the cavity by a trocar and cannula technique. The tube is attached to suction and gradually over a period of 2–3 weeks the cavity will reduce in size. The tube may then be removed and usually the cavity remains small or actually obliterates.

A recent modification enables this operation to be carried out in one stage. A 2·5-cm length of rib overlying the cavity is excised subperiosteally and a purse-string chromic catgut suture is inserted through the parietal pleura into the visceral pleura and underlying cyst wall. The cyst is then opened through the centre of the purse-string and a large self-retaining Foley urethral catheter inserted into the cavity. The balloon is inflated and the purse-string tightened. If a pneumothorax is inadvertently produced a separate underwater-seal drainage is instituted.

Obstructive Emphysema

This term is used to describe two entirely separate conditions.

1. Congenital Obstructive Emphysema

This rare condition occurs in infants and is due to lack of cartilage support in the bronchial wall. A 'ball-valve' mechanism occurs in the affected lobe, usually the upper, which becomes increasingly distended. This causes mediastinal shift to the opposite side and severe respiratory embarrassment. Symptoms occur soon after birth. The treatment is lobectomy.

2. Obstructive Emphysema Due to Bronchial Blockage

The bronchial blockage may not be complete and a 'ball-valve' mechanism may occur due to dilatation and contraction of the bronchus with each respiration, allowing air to enter the lung but to leave less easily. The affected part of the lung gradually becomes distended and is more translucent on the chest radiograph. The cause is an inhaled foreign body or a tumour (usually innocent) blocking the bronchus. This will lead later to complete collapse of the affected lobe or lung and subsequent bronchiectasis. The treatment is that of the causative lesion. If the foreign body has caused bronchiectasis, a lobectomy may be required.

HYDATID CYSTS OF THE LUNG

Hydatid cysts of the lung should always be removed to prevent their subsequent rupture and the consequent spread of the parasite into the pleural cavity or the rest of the lung (Barrett, 1947; Lichter, 1972).

Surgical Technique

This will depend on whether the cyst is still unruptured in the substance of the lung or whether it has developed a bronchial communication and become infected.

1. Unruptured cyst

This is the more common situation. Posterolateral thoracotomy is performed and the lobe containing the cyst packed off from the surrounding lung and pleural cavity by large swabs soaked in 2 per cent formaldehyde solution. Some of the fluid in the cyst is aspirated with a fine needle to make it less tense. Ten millilitres ether or 10 per cent formaldehyde solution may be injected into the cyst to sterilize the contents. Very great care must be taken to avoid any contamination of the pleural cavity. The 'pericyst' (the adventitious layer of fibrous tissue surrounding the cyst itself) is carefully incised and with gentle pressure on the lungs by the anaesthetist, the cyst itself will be extruded intact from the lung substance. The interior of the pericyst is inspected, any bleeding points or bronchial communications are closed, and the lung cavity obliterated by interrupted mattress catgut sutures. If the cyst is less than 3 cm in diameter it is best removed by a wedge resection of the lung containing the cyst.

If the cyst is very large, a lobectomy may be required.

2. Infected cyst

If the cyst has become infected a lung resection must be carried out, either a segmental resection or a lobectomy depending on the size and situation of the cyst.

PART VII

SURGICAL TREATMENT OF PULMONARY TUBERCULOSIS

The management of pulmonary tuberculosis has been revolutionized during the past 30 years by the use of modern chemotherapy. Operation may still be required, however, in patients who have developed drug resistance and are still sputum positive. This is usually due to inadequate initial treatment.

The assessment of these patients for surgery is often very difficult and controversial and note must be taken of the following:

1. The quantity of sputum, the presence of tubercle bacilli and their sensitivity to antituberculous drugs, together with the presence of other organisms and their sensitivity to antibiotics.

2. The extent of lung cavitation and infiltration and its exact location in the upper lobe or apex of the lower lobe, as shown by the posteroanterior and lateral radiographs, including tomograms.

3. Any evidence of tuberculous activity, as shown by weight loss, evening temperature, raised sedimentation rate (ESR) and radiological evidence of recent change. All previous radiographs should be examined if possible for evidence of previous disease.

4. The presence both of bronchitis and bronchospasm.

5. The state of respiratory function, including perhaps differential lung function as shown by bronchospirometry or ventilation/perfusion studies using radio-isotope techniques.

6. The presence of bronchostenosis or endobronchitis, as shown by bronchoscopy.

Surgical Procedures Available

The surgical procedures available for the treatment of tuberculosis comprise resection of a part or the whole of the lung (combined with decortication if an empyema is present), thoracoplasty to obliterate an upper lobe cavity by permanently collapsing the affected lobe, and 'sleeve' resection of a bronchus for a localized bronchostenosis causing distal infection (*Fig.* 53.45). Artificial pneumothorax and phrenic crush combined with pneumoperitoneum are no longer practised.

Indications for Surgery

Tuberculosis which is active must be treated medically by chemotherapy for several months before surgical treatment is considered. By this time the cavity may have closed, the sputum become negative and the disease process arrested. On the other hand the cavity may remain open and the sputum be negative or positive. If the sputum is negative operation is only required if the cavity is large, because in many

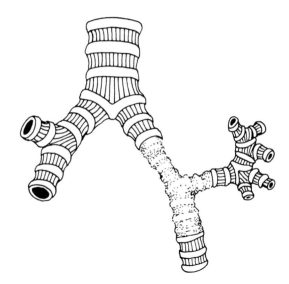

Fig. 53.45. Tuberculous bronchostenosis affecting the region of the left upper lobe orifice. This is an ideal situation for left upper lobectomy with 'sleeve' resection of the main bronchus.

of these cases a fungal infection (Aspergilloma) will develop, leading to repeated haemoptyses, which may threaten life (British Tuberculosis Association, 1970). If the sputum is positive, then surgical treatment is advisable, probably thoracoplasty, for by this time the organisms are almost certainly drug resistant.

Indications for Resection

These are now well established (Crofton and Douglas, 1969).

1. *Persistent positive sputum*, despite adequate chemotherapy.

2. *Persistent cavity* for more than 2 years (so called 'open-negative' case). There is considerable difference of opinion concerning the treatment of this type of patient, and the present tendency is to advise resection if the cavity is thick walled, if there has been only a slow response to treatment, as shown by time taken for sputum conversion, or if the patient undertakes strenuous physical activity, or is likely to be unreliable in follow-up examination (e.g. an alcoholic).

3. *Tuberculoma.* A localized nodule greater than 2 cm in diameter. In older patients, it may not be possible to differentiate this lesion from a carcinoma unless percutaneous needle biopsy under radiological control is available.

4. *Destroyed functionless lung.* If the patient has haemoptyses or considerable sputum a pneumonectomy may be required, provided there is very definite evidence of lack of function (as shown by previous extensive disease), presence of fibrotic changes on tomography, or bronchiectatic changes on bronchography. It must be remembered that such patients

may live without surgical intervention for many years and an estimate must be made of the likely progress of the patient with and without surgery. In these patients a lateral thoracoplasty (ribs 2–7) is often advisable 2 weeks after pneumonectomy, to prevent overdistension of the remaining lung.

5. *Tuberculous empyema.* If there is significant underlying lung disease, lobectomy or pneumonectomy will be required as well as the decortication.

6. *Failed thoracoplasty.* If an adequate thoracoplasty fails to close a cavity and the sputum still remains positive, a resection of the diseased part of the lung should be carried out under the thoracoplasty.

Contra-indications to Resection

The main contra-indications to resection are inadequate cardiac reserve, respiratory insufficiency due to bronchitis and bronchospasm, tuberculous disease in the lung which is too extensive to remove without making the patient a respiratory cripple, and progressive extrapulmonary tuberculosis. In addition, active endobronchitis at the point of the proposed division of the bronchus will almost certainly lead to a bronchopleural fistula and is therefore an absolute contra-indication.

Indications for Thoracoplasty

This operation was devised before the advent of antituberculous chemotherapy and provided a selective permanent collapse of the upper lobe and apex of the lower lobe. The operation causes a greater loss of lung function than does resection and must be carried out as a staged procedure. For these reasons the operation is now rarely performed for tuberculosis, though it may be indicated for a post-pneumonectomy empyema (*see* p. 810). The morbidity and mortality are less than after lung resection and because of this it is still advisable in some poor-risk patients who would not tolerate a resection.

Operative Procedures

1. *Lung Resection*

The operations available are wedge resection, segmental resection, lobectomy or pneumonectomy, together with 'sleeve' resection for a tuberculous stricture of a main bronchus. The segments most commonly excised are the apical and posterior segments of the upper lobe and the apical segment of the lower lobe (often combined with an upper lobectomy). The detailed technique is described in the section on tumours of the lung. Special points to note during resections for tuberculosis are:

a. The avoidance of lung division across tuberculous tissue.

b. Extrapleural separation of the lung where it is adherent to the chest wall.

c. Increased difficulty of hilar dissection because of fibrotic changes around the blood vessels and bronchus.

It is important to obtain complete expansion of the remainder of the lung as soon as possible and in some cases a decortication of the remaining lobe will be necessary. Fortunately the portion of lung to be resected is often atelectatic and the adjacent lung will have already become overdistended. 'Sleeve resection' of the main bronchus, in combination with an upper lobectomy, is indicated if previous tuberculous endobronchitis has caused a stenosis of the main bronchus. In such a case it is necessary to excise the narrowed segment of bronchus in order to prevent the occurrence of non-tuberculous infection and subsequent bronchiectasis in the lower lobe.

2. *Decortication*

This may be required in cases of tuberculous empyema. The initial treatment of such an empyema must always be aspiration and streptomycin injection into the pleural cavity, at first twice weekly and then subsequently once weekly, together with systemic antituberculous chemotherapy. In some cases the empyema will absorb on this regimen, with re-expansion of the lung and obliteration of the pleural cavity.

However, most cases of tuberculous empyema require decortication, the technique of which is described on p. 796. If there is underlying lung disease a lobectomy or pneumonectomy will also be required and the necessity for this must be judged partly on a knowledge of the previous extent of the tuberculosis, as shown by previous radiographs, and partly on the findings at operation. The tuberculous disease is likely to be more extensive at the apex of the lung and the extrapleural strip must proceed with care at this point to avoid damage to the brachial plexus or subclavian artery and vein. On the mediastinal side the dissection is less difficult and the actual hilar dissection may be surprisingly easy.

If a bronchopleural fistula has developed, shown by the expectoration of purulent fluid when the patient lies on the opposite side and confirmed by the injection of methylene blue into the pleural cavity, operation is a matter of extreme urgency in order to prevent tuberculous spread to the contralateral lung. If the patient is sufficiently fit pleuropneumonectomy should be carried out. The empyema must first be aspirated dry through a thoracoscope in the sitting-up position and then thoracotomy performed in the face-down position or in the lateral position with an appropriate blocker or cuffed endobronchial tube to prevent a 'spill-over' into the opposite lung. If the patient is unfit for a resection intercostal tube drainage must be instituted.

3. *Thoracoplasty* (Thomas and Cleland, 1942) (*Fig. 53.46*)

A thoracoplasty, together with an extrafascial apicolysis, mobilizes the chest wall and allows concentric relaxation of the affected lung. This abolishes the bronchial ball-valve mechanism which maintains the distension of the tuberculous cavity, and thus allows healing to take place. The number of ribs resected depends on the extent of the disease and it is usual to carry the resection to one rib below the lowermost area of tuberculosis, as related to the posterior end of the ribs on the posteroanterior chest radiograph. In practice a 5–8-rib thoracoplasty is usually required. A 6-rib thoracoplasty should never be performed, for the inferior angle of the scapula 'rides' on the unresected 7th rib and causes considerable discomfort. The operation must be done in two or three stages or the patient will succumb from the effects of a large mobile portion of chest wall and resultant paradoxical respiration. The transverse processes of

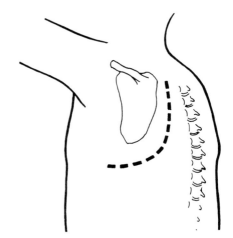

Fig. 53.46. Thoracoplasty showing extended parascapular incision.

the vertebras should not be removed, or a severe scoliosis will develop.

REFERENCES

Abrams L. D. (1958) A pleural biopsy punch. *Lancet* **i**, 30.

Barrett N. R. (1947) The treatment of pulmonary hydatid disease. *Thorax* **2**, 21–57.

Bates M. (1981) Analysis of 2000 resections for bronchial carcinoma. *Ann. R. Coll. Surg.* **63**, 164–167.

Bennett W. F. and Smith R. A. (1978) A twenty-year analysis of the results of sleeve resection for primary bronchogenic carcinoma. *J. Thorac. Cardiovasc. Surg.* **76**, 840–845.

Blades B. (1941) Intrathoracic tumours. *Am. J. Surg.* **54**, 139–148.

Blalock A., Mason M. F., Morgan H. G. et al. (1939) Myasthenia gravis and tumours of the thymic region. *Ann. Surg.* **110**, 544.

Boyden E. A. (1955) *Segmental Anatomy of the Lungs*. New York, McGraw-Hill.

British Tuberculosis Association (1970) Aspergilloma and residual tuberculous cavities. *Tubercle* **51**, 227–245.

Brock R. C. (1950) *The Anatomy of the Bronchial Tree*. London, Oxford University Press.

Carlens E. (1959) Mediastinoscopy: a method for inspection and tissue biopsy in the superior mediastinum. *Dis. Chest* **36**, 343–352.

Crofton J. and Douglas A. (1969) *Respiratory Diseases*. Oxford, Blackwell Scientific Publications, p. 250.

Donnelly R. J., Laquaglia M. P., Fabri B. et al. (1984) Cervical thymectomy in the treatment of myasthenia gravis. *Ann. R. Coll. Surg.* **66**, 305–308.

Doty D. B. (1982) Bypass of superior vena cava. *J. Thorac. Cardiovasc. Surg.* **83**, 326–338.

Edwards F. R. and Wilson A. (1972) Thymectomy for myasthenia gravis. *Thorax* **27**, 513–516.

Elmes P. C. and Simpson M. J. C. (1976) The clinical aspects of mesothelioma. *Q. J. Med.* **45**, 427–449.

Evans D. S., Hall J. H. and Harrison G. K. (1973) Anterior mediastinotomy. *Thorax* **28**, 444–447.

Flavell G. (1962) Conservatism in surgical treatment of bronchial carcinoma—a review of 826 personal operations. *Br. Med. J.* **1**, 284–287.

Gingell J. C. (1965) Treatment of chylothorax by producing pleurodesis using iodised talc. *Thorax* **20**, 261–269.

Hickman J. A. and Jones M. C. (1970) Treatment of neoplastic pleural effusions with local instillation of quinacrine (Mepacrine) hydrochloride. *Thorax* **25**, 226–229.

Hurt R. L. and Bates M. (1984) Carcinoid tumours of the bronchus; a 33 year experience. *Thorax* **39**, 617–623.

Johnson J. B. and Jones P. H. (1959) The treatment of bronchial carcinoma by lobectomy and sleeve resection of the main bronchus. *Thorax* **14**, 48–54.

Keynes G. (1949) Results of thymectomy in myasthenia gravis. *Br. Med. J.* **2**, 611–616.

Killen D. A. and Gobbel W. G. (1968) *Spontaneous Pneumothorax*. Boston, Little, Brown & Co.

Lawson R. M., Ramanathan L., Hurley G. et al. (1976) Bronchial adenoma: review of an 18-year experience at the Brompton Hospital. *Thorax* **31**, 245–253.

Le Roux B. T. (1972) Management of bronchial carcinoma by segmental resection. *Thorax* **27**, 70–74.

Lichter I. (1972) Surgery of pulmonary hydatid diseases. *Thorax* **27**, 529–534.

Macarthur A. M. and Fountain S. W. (1977) Intracavitory suction and drainage in the treatment of emphysematous bullae. *Thorax* **32**, 668–672.

Matthews H. R. and Hopkinson R. B. (1984) Treatment of sputum retention by minitracheostomy. *Br. J. Surg.* **71**, 147–150.

Milsom J. W., Kron I. L., Rheuban K. S. et al. (1985) Chylothorax: an assessment of current surgical management. *J. Thorac. Cardiovasc. Surg.* **89**, 221–227.

Morrison I. M. (1958) Tumours and cysts of the mediastinum. *Thorax* **13**, 294–307.

Nohl-Oser H. C. (1976) Mediastinoscopy. *Br. J. Hosp. Med.* **16**, 33–36.

Paulson D. L. (1974) In: Smith R. E. and Williams W. G. (eds) *Surgery of the Lung*. London, Butterworths.

Pearson F. G., Nelems S. M., Henderson R. F. et al. (1972) The role of mediastinoscopy in the selection of treatment for bronchial carcinoma with involvement of superior mediastinal lymph nodes. *J. Thorac. Cardiovasc. Surg.* **64**, 382–390.

Ross J. K. (1978) In: Rob C. and Smith R. (eds) *Operative Surgery*. London, Butterworths.

Roy P. H., Carr D. T. and Spencer-Payne W. (1967) The problem of chylothorax. *Proc. Mayo Clin.* **42**, 457–459.

Sanders R. D. (1967) A ventilating attachment for bronchoscopy. *Del. Med. J.* **39**, 170.

Sauerbruch F. (1913) *Mitt. Grenzgeb. Med. Chir.* **25**, 746.

Saunders K. B. (1975) The assessment of respiratory function. *Br. J. Hosp. Med.* **15**, 228–238.

Sengupta A. (1963) The treatment of recurrent spontaneous pneumothorax with iodine and talc poudrage. *Br. J. Dis. Chest* **57**, 197–199.

Shields T. W., Humphrey E. W., Higgins G. A. et al. (1978) Long-term survivors of resection of lung carcinoma. *J. Thorac. Cardiovasc. Surg.* **76**, 439–445.

Smith W. G. and Rothwell P. P. G. (1962) Treatment of spontaneous pneumothorax. *Thorax* **17**, 342–349.

Steel S. J. and Winstanley D. P. (1969) Trephine biopsy of the lung and pleura. *Thorax* **24**, 576–584.

Thomas C. Price and Cleland W. P. (1942) Extrafascial apicolysis with thoracoplasty. *Br. J. Tuberculosis* **36**, 109.

Thomas C. Price and Drew C. E. (1953) Fibroma of visceral pleura. *Thorax* **8**, 180–189.

Thoracic Society of Great Britain (1950) The nomenclature of bronchopulmonary anatomy. *Thorax* **5**, 222–228.

The Nervous System

Chapter fifty-four

Intracranial Neurosurgery

H. B. Griffith

GENERAL TECHNIQUE

The consequences of infection or unnecessary tissue damage can be disastrous for the neurosurgical patient. Habits of handling tissue with the fingers, dabbing and wiping subcutaneous bleeding points with hand-held gauzes, and of allowing the fingers to touch the skin of the patient have no place in neurosurgery. Tissues, needles and sutures are handled only with instruments. An intelligently meticulous 'notouch' technique is mandatory. Since the hair follicles of the scalp cannot be sterilized by detergent followed by bactericide, which is the usual skin preparation, exposed skin edges must be covered and separated from the deeper parts of the exposure by on-laid strips of Lintine. Tissue exposed for several hours must be protected from bacterial fallout by tailored guttapercha sheet. Bactericidal powder applied as a light frosting is used in the extradural layers in wound closure. Subcutaneous sutures have their knot-tails cut obsessionally short and buried under the galeal layer. Talking should be kept to a minimum. Hand signals are often more appropriate and more easily understood than a preoccupied mumble. This is an additional reason for keeping the use of instruments to an easily followed sequence.

Investigation

The best way of developing an instinctive knowledge of the internal topography of the brain in relation to the surface of skull and scalp is always to look at radiographs, arteriograms, isotope scans and CT scans in a standard way. For instance, a left-sided arteriogram should invariably be orientated on the screen as if the surgeon were gazing at the left side of the patient's head. Radiographs taken on a standard skull table are usually magnified by a factor of 6:5, whereas linear isotope scans are exactly the same size as the brain. In order to reinforce this three-dimensional idea of the internal architecture of the head on which the surgeon is about to operate, it is important for the surgeon in person to position the patient on the operating table headrest. If possible the surgeon should use transparent plastic drapes so that the major topographical features (nose, ears, external occipital protuberance) are visible during surgery. In this way the surgeon will build up an unconscious awareness of the exact whereabouts of, for instance, the occipital horn, if the time comes during the operation to 'tap the ventricle'. The surgeon who hurries into the operating theatre to

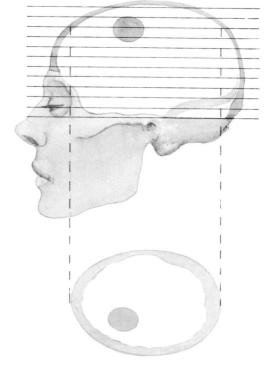

Fig. 54.1. CT scan. Anatomy. To show how, for correct localization, the CT scan must be strictly interpreted according to slice levels.

carry out the allegedly 'important' part of an operation on a patient, whose head has been positioned, prepared and opened by a junior, will fail to acquire this instinctive knowledge of the patient's brain.

Computed tomography (CT) scans occasionally mislead about the position of a mass inside the brain since the plane of cut may be such that a lesion situated almost in the centre of the head may appear to be just beneath the forehead (*Fig.* 54.1).

Anaesthesia

It has been said with only a little exaggeration that neurosurgical anaesthesia consists of 'two aspirins and some oxygen'. A sizeable number of minor operations on the skull are safely performed under local anaesthesia and the history of neurosurgery early in the century is studded with examples of major procedures carried out under local anaesthesia alone. What is usually regarded as premedication for general anaesthesia, namely the injection of an opiate with atropine, is not suitable as a tranquillizing agent for neurosurgical patients. This is because opiates depress respiration leading to the retention of carbon dioxide and the increase of intracranial pressure. The best premedication for a patient about to undergo a procedure under local anaesthesia alone is a clear and confident explanation to a patient who is able to receive the information about what is to occur. The patient should understand that the surgeon will be able to talk to him or her throughout and the patient, if not dysphasic, will be able to talk to the surgeon.

If there are any doubts about the ability of the patient to cooperate, either in understanding or in carrying out instructions, it is better to conduct the procedure under full general anaesthesia with an endotracheal tube. Since intracranial pressure is often high, an increase in cerebral blood flow by unnecessarily prolonged apnoea during induction, venous obstruction due to an awkward position of the head on the shoulders and an increase in cerebral blood flow with a use of vasodilating agents are to be avoided. A reinforced and flexible tube should be used to avoid tube obstruction and in order that the surgeon can reposition the head during operation without provoking a reaction from the patient due to relative movement between the trachea and endotracheal tube.

It is generally preferable to have the patient mechanically ventilated at an adequate gas exchange rather than to rely on the activity of a respiratory centre which may well be compromised by displacement or brain oedema. It is sometimes held that a patient breathing spontaneously will give visible evidence of interference with the respiratory mechanism during surgery in the posterior fossa, but it is far better to be assured of good operating conditions which enable the surgeon to visualize precisely the anatomy involved.

Positioning

For cranial neurosurgery there are three main positions. The *supine* position can be used for all approaches to the anterior three-fifths of the head, neck rotation being minimized by lifting one shoulder with a pad. The *lateral* position can be used for the middle three-fifths of the head, including paramedian incisions for the cerebellopontine angle of the posterior fossa. For the occipital region and the posterior fossa the best position is for the patient's body to lie in a *true lateral* posture with the head turned into the horseshoe rest, a small turn in the neck being permitted. This has the advantage that chest and abdomen are free to move and consequently requires less inflation pressure from the ventilator. A modest head-up tilt deals with the problem of systemic venous pressure without the dangers of the sitting position with respect to air embolism. The prone position is now superseded, since it is inefficient on

three counts: the ventilator has to lift the entire weight of the patient's trunk to ensure an adequate gas exchange, the head tends to be dependent with a tendency to venous bleeding, and access for the surgeon for lesions near the midline can be extremely awkward. The sitting position for the posterior fossa carries with it the dangers of air embolism and of uncontrollable hypotension during brisk blood loss.

Surgery of Access

As the vascular supply and the cranial nerves are concentrated at the base of the brain, together with the pituitary gland, orbit and inner ear, a substantial fraction of the surgery of access to the cranium consists of an approach to the base of the brain. Pathology near the brain convexity, whether above or below the tentorium, is approached through the skull vault. Basal pathology may also be approached via the skull vault with retraction of the inferior surface of the cerebral hemisphere. Alternatively, basal pathology can be approached more directly through the paranasal air sinuses or through the drilled petrous bone. Occasionally, such as for an acoustic neuroma, these approaches may be combined in one operation. Nevertheless, leaving aside this kind of combined approach, the account which follows will be divided into approaches via the skull vault on the one hand and via the skull base on the other.

It is important to have in one's mind a clear idea of the surface markings of the main features of the brain. In addition, the location of the main vault sutures, coronal, sagittal and lambdoid, have relation to the scalp on the one hand and to the brain on the other. The sutures can often be clearly visualized, especially the lambdoid suture, which appears as a visible ridge when the scalp is shaved. This is especially important when operating on infants where the frontal, parietal and occipital bones are still separated.

Skin Incisions

These are basically of two types, namely linear and circumferential. When the approach is a limited one, such as for a burr hole or a trephine, a linear scalp incision will provide an economically large area of exposure of the scalp per unit length of incision. This is because of the shape of the skull and the elasticity of the scalp. When retractors are placed so as to distract and stretch the edges of a linear wound, a diamond-shaped exposure is obtained. When the scalp is very elastic, as in infants, a sizeable osteoplastic craniotomy can be turned via such an exposure. However, when the exposure required is large, a circumferential or scalp flap incision is more efficient. Frequently, as in exploratory head injury surgery, a burr hole to locate a haematoma can be extended into a circumferential incision when it is sited on the circumference of a future flap. Occasion-

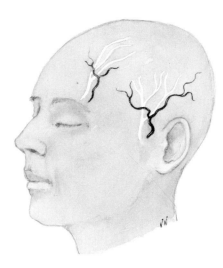

Fig. 54.2. Superficial arteries and veins of the anterior and lateral scalp. Note how the anterior branch of the superficial temporal artery (external carotid circulation) can easily establish an anastomosis with the supraorbital artery (internal carotid circulation).

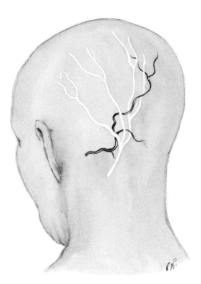

Fig. 54.3. Superficial arteries and nerves of the posterior scalp. Note that the occipital artery (external carotid branch) emerges behind the mastoid process, considerably lateral to the origin of the greater occipital nerve.

ally, as when tapping an otogenic and temporal lobe abscess, the requirement for future surgery may be ignored and the short burr-hole incision will be radial to the circumference of a future osteoplastic flap craniotomy for abscess removal if this subsequently proves to be necessary. Scalp lacerations can usually be extended into an S-shaped incision if a nearby compound depressed fracture needs to be dealt with (*see Fig.* 54.14).

On each side of the head there are three main scalp nerves. These are the supraorbital (V1), auriculotemporal (V3) and greater occipital (C2). Accompanying each of these there are three main arteries

(*Figs.* 54.2, 54.3). The supraorbital artery is a branch of the ophthalmic which, in turn, stems from the internal carotid. The external carotid artery gives rise to the superficial temporal artery which crosses the zygoma to accompany the auriculotemporal nerve. The occipital artery branches posteriorly from the external carotid deep to the mastoid process and runs a little distance from the greater occipital nerve which is more medially situated. Scalp incisions should be placed so as to respect and preserve both innervation and arterial supply, although the latitude given to surgeons by the excellent anastomotic blood supply of the scalp makes almost any incision possible. The shape and size of the flap should respect the general rule of having a sound vascular pedicle and should preferably taper gently from base to apex. Remember that the frontalis and occipitalis muscles and the occasionally well-developed muscles attached to the ear pinna (anterior superior and posterior auriculares) are part of the scalp and are not, as are the temporalis muscles and the suboccipital muscles, attached to the skull.

The major venous sinuses, namely the sagittal sinus, torcula and the transverse (lateral) and sigmoid sinuses, dominate the surgery of the skull. This is because the outer layer of these venous sinuses is composed of flimsy collagen which tears easily. It is possible to lose a large amount of blood in a short time when this occurs. The veins which bridge between the cortex and the superior sagittal venous sinus seriously hamper access to the great longitudinal fissure, and to divide them can lead to damaging venous infarction. Avoid this by utilizing, where possible, the gaps, such as at the occipital pole, which are free of such veins. The supratentorial pineal approach slips through this constant gap. There is another less complete gap in the area between frontal pole and coronal suture.

Surgical Sequences: Basic Steps

Burr Hole

This is the simplest method of gaining access to the brain. The hair is removed by shaving over an area measuring 10 × 12 cm minimum. After preparation and draping, the scalp is infiltrated with local anaesthetic (usually lignocaine 1 per cent with adrenaline 1:200 000 added as a vasoconstrictor) (*Fig.* 54.4). The pointed scalpel incises all layers including pericranium in a single cut of 3 cm length. The pericranium is swept back on either side with a curved Adson's periosteal elevator. A self-retaining retractor is inserted and opened to produce enough tension in the wound edges to stop bleeding (*Fig.* 54.5). A small Hudson's brace with a 15-mm perforator is used. Considerable force is transmitted from the trunk via the left hand of the operating surgeon who stands (as in *Fig.* 54.6) with the legs placed so that the forward foot is safely underneath the head of

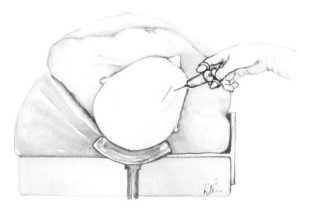

Fig. 54.4. Burr-hole infiltration. A bleb of local anaesthetic raises a substantial wheal in the scalp around the intended burr incision under local anaesthetic.

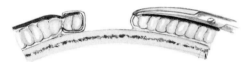

Fig. 54.5. Scalp haemostasis. On the left an encompassing Raney scalp clip; on the right galeal tension by means of curved haemostatic forceps.

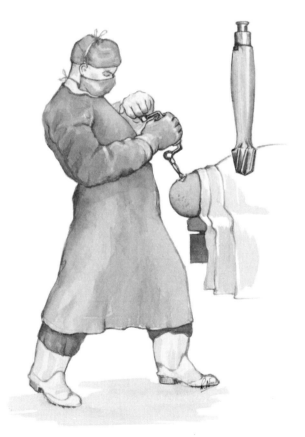

Fig. 54.6. Stance for the Hudson's brace. Note that the left foot, onto which all weight is transferred, provides both a safety factor and for a more sensitive manoeuvre.

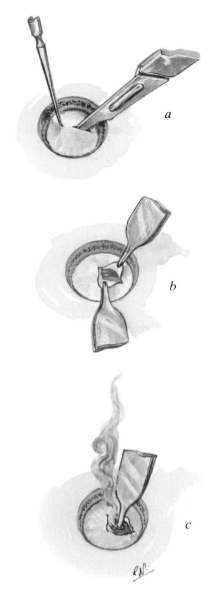

Fig. 54.7. *a*, Dural opening. After burr hole or disc trephine the sharp hook tents up the dura into which a light incision is made. This is then opened by forceps or by scissors (*b*). *c*, A pial spot for ventricular cannulation or an incision is coagulated with the unipolar diathermy.

the patient. The right hand now rotates the brace at speed. It is only necessary for two fingers or the index finger and thumb to grasp the handle of the brace lightly so that the subtle changes of vibration as the perforator shaves through the outer table, diploë and inner table can be detected in sequence by a combination of feel and noise. An assistant drips saline slowly onto the rotating perforator so that it lubricates and cools the sharp cutting edge without irrigating the skin edges. When the inner table is breached over an area 2 mm across, the 16-mm tapered conical burr is used to ream out the hole. Less trunk pressure and more rotary force are used.

is now coagulated lightly with the low setting of the unipolar diathermy connected to a fine non-toothed dissecting forceps held in the right hand (*Fig.* 54.7*c*). A fine sucker held in the left hand keeps the small exposure free of blood and cerebrospinal fluid. As the diathermy sparks coagulate arachnoid, pia and the superficial layers of the cortex, the closed tip of the dissecting forceps is thrust through the coagulated spot to a depth of approximately 3 mm.

If, for example, an abscess is to be aspirated, a glioma biopsied or the ventricle visualized, a slim brain cannula or endoscope is now introduced by thumb and index finger while the heel of the hand rests on the head (*Figs.* 54.8, 54.9). Similarly supported, left-handed fingers grasp the butt of the cannula when the stylet is withdrawn. The syringe is inserted smoothly into the flexible rubber connector, with which all brain cannulas should be fitted. The cannula is held motionless while cerebrospinal fluid (CSF), pus or liquid haematoma or glioma fragments are aspirated. If bleeding is encountered, the cannula is not withdrawn until it stops. When the cannula is withdrawn the dura is not closed but the small dural hole is covered by a stamp of Gelfoam sponge. Scalp closure is accomplished by two interrupted inverted

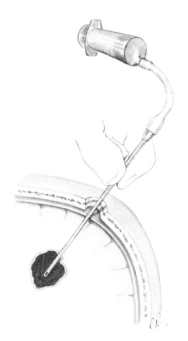

Fig. 54.8. Aspiration of intracerebral abscess. Note the flexible connection to syringe to avoid needle movement.

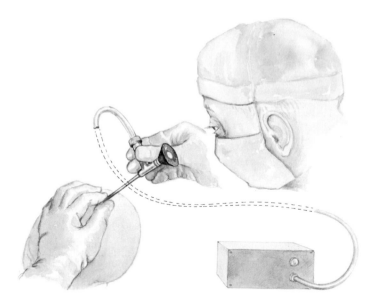

Fig. 54.9. Endoneurosurgery. Note endoscope held with steadying left hand, and manipulating right hand, which should be supported.

The brace becomes difficult to turn as the burr engages in the bone. Bone flakes are now picked off the dura as the surgeon sits down comfortably. Bone dust is irrigated away from the hole. A sharp right-angled fine hook tents up the dura in the centre of the hole (*Fig.* 54.7*a*) and a rounded tenotome (no. 15 blade) incises the dura with one or two deft strokes 5 mm or so in length. This short nick is pulled apart with dissecting forceps into a diamond-shaped exposure (*Fig.* 54.7*b*). A pial spot on the crown of a gyrus

galeal absorbable sutures (3/0) with four through-and-through deeply biting skin sutures (2/0 or 3/0), which under-run the plentiful scalp arteries and accomplish scalp haemostasis without need for diathermization of skin edges (*Fig.* 54.10).

A Trephine Disc (Figs. 54.11, 54.12)
A disc 2·5–5·0 cm in diameter must be removed when the cortical exposure needed is larger than afforded

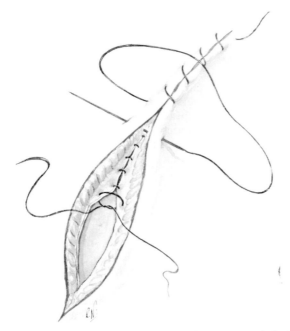

Fig. 54.10. Scalp closure. The deep (galeal) sutures are tied with knots inverted, the superficial scalp being brought together by deep bites of continuous or interrupted sutures round the superficial scalp vessels.

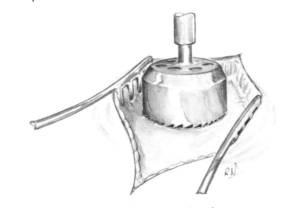

Fig. 54.11. Trephine exploration.

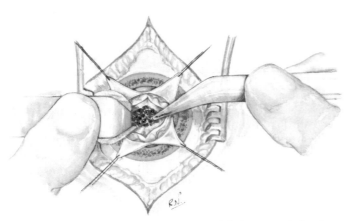

Fig. 54.12. An intracerebral haematoma is being evacuated under direct vision with a retractor working opposite the sucker.

by a burr hole. For example, the aspiration of a solid intracerebral haematoma, the search for a suitable sylvian artery in superficial temporal/middle cerebral microvascular anastomosis, or the taking of a block cortical brain biopsy, usually require at least a 2·5-cm exposure. This can be obtained by the circumferential nibbling enlargement of a burr hole (as in exploration of extradural haematoma—*see Fig.* 54.13 but the resulting skull defect then produces a visibly pulsating indent or bulge which can be upsetting for patients and relatives. A straight all-layer scalp incision about 6 cm in length is distracted by self-retaining retractors (Mollison's are convenient) into a diamond-shaped cranial exposure. In its centre a 2·5-mm twist drill guarded to a 6-mm depth produces a hole which takes the centre pin of the Scoville trephine. Taking care to avoid snagging the trephine cutting teeth on the surrounding pericranium, the trephine begins to cut a disc. An even cut is made to a depth of 3 mm or so. At this stage, the trephine is disengaged from the skull, its centre pin is removed and the trephine cuts again. As the inner table is reached, rotation is more cautious with frequent checks. This will allow the surgeon to cut just through the inner table (without perforating the dura) over approximately half the circumference of the bone disc. Orientation marks to ensure correct reinsertion are now made by a small nibbling bite on inner and outer lips of the cut respectively. Bone elevators prise out the disc, taking care not to allow the disc to jump uncontrollably out of the wound with the final snap.

The dura is usually opened in a cruciate incision with scissors or director with tenotome. When a solid subcortical haematoma is to be removed, the surgeon dons a headlight, sits comfortably and, with sucker in the left hand and dissecting forceps in the right, coagulates the arachnoid and pia over a 2-cm linear incision in the crown of the gyrus. Fine brain scissors are used to divide the cortex and lepto-meninges. The incision is now deepened by strokes of a narrow sucker held in the right hand while the incision is opened by a metal strip brain retractor held in the left. The brain is protected by Lintine strips overlapping the lips of the cortical incision. When the haematoma is encountered, the large sucker is used to evacuate it under direct vision, taking care not to abrade the delicate granulating walls of the cavity. For haemostasis the emptied cavity is lightly packed with cottonwool balls soaked in 10 volume hydrogen peroxide for 4 minutes. During this wait, the surgeon attends to any small cortical bleeding points with the bipolar diathermy.

When haemostasis is complete the four triangular dural flaps are drawn together with a single silk suture through their apices. Gelfoam sponge pledgets are laid over the remaining gaps in the dura. The bone disc is replaced and the pericranium and/or temporalis fascia is closed with interrupted 2/0 silk sutures so as to hold it in position. The scalp is then closed in the usual two layers without suction drainage.

SURGICAL MANAGEMENT OF EXTRADURAL HAEMORRHAGE

Indications for Surgery

The classic picture of a rapidly advancing extradural haemorrhage is well known. A young person, often after a relatively minor head injury, sometimes without loss of consciousness, and after a lucid interval which may vary from minutes to hours, usually first complains of increasing headache, becomes drowsy and then unconscious. Signs of increasing limb paresis may or may not be obvious. With depression of the level of consciousness, which is the most important observation, comes a progressive dilatation of the pupil on the side of the haematoma, slowing of the pulse, and increase in the systolic blood pressure so as to give a bounding pulse and, later, periodic respiration. The pupillary dilatation is due to stretching of a third (oculomotor) nerve by the medial portion of the temporal lobe, which is being squeezed through the tentorial hiatus into the posterior fossa, distorting as it does so the midbrain and producing depression of consciousness by compromise of the ascending reticular activating system. Examination of the head will usually give enough information to enable an alert surgeon to rescue a deteriorating patient. Almost invariably, and particularly in young people, a transverse lateral fracture is present low on the skull, usually in the thin and vulnerable temporal bone. Not only does the fracture lacerate the middle meningeal artery, producing a sizeable lens-shaped haematoma, often several centimetres thick, but the blood under arterial pressure leaks out under the temporalis muscle, producing the characteristic 'boggy swelling'. This feels characteristically different to the exploring finger of a surgeon from the ordinary scalp haematoma which can be indented. Skull radiographs are helpful to delineate the underlying fracture but, particularly in the restless child, indifferent skull radiographs may mislead one into the belief that a fracture is not present.

The immediate treatment is evacuation of the haematoma and hopefully a reversal of the progressive mid-brain and medullary compression, which otherwise will be rapidly fatal. The simplest manoeuvre is to make a burr hole and then enlarge this with nibbling bone forceps so that a sucker can evacuate with the solid haematoma (*Fig.* 54.13). Dealing with the site of haemorrhage itself is not always necessary, since in many cases by the time the surgeon arrives at the haematoma the haemorrhage will have stopped. The main difficulty, however, is to site the exploring burr hole squarely over the haematoma.

The burr hole should be sited: (1) in relation to the boggy swelling; (2) in relation to the skull fracture seen on the radiograph, particularly at the place where the fracture may cross the middle meningeal artery seen on the skull radiographs; (3) in the temporal region if no boggy swelling is present and no fracture can be discerned on the skull radiograph. The side chosen is always the side of the first and larger dilating pupil.

The incision is made 3 cm long at right angles to the skull base and halfway between the bony rim of the orbit and the external auditory meatus, just above the zygoma. The scalpel cut is firmly taken down through the temporalis to the underlying bone, where an unsuspected fracture edge may be felt by the encountering blade. A periosteal elevator scrapes the temporal muscle from its underlying attachment to the bone, and the deep-bladed self-retaining retractor holds the edges of the wound apart. The perforating burr is now used, care being taken when making a burr hole adjacent to a linear fracture (*Fig.* 54.14). Immediately the burr is lifted a tarry haematoma is apparent if the hole has been accurately sited. If dura is encountered, it should be opened if blue, since an acute subdural haematoma can mimic the clinical picture of an extradural haemorrhage. The dura, which will be tightly bulging, should be depressed gently with the periosteal elevator in the direction towards the base of the skull and swept gently round, hard against the inner table of the skull. A spurt of blood will indicate location of the adjacent haematoma and nibbling of the bone in that direction will give access to the edge of the clot. If the dura is slack then cerebral compression is not present and the situation should be reassessed. In this context the presence of fat embolism in the patient with limb fractures should not be overlooked.

When the haematoma is encountered, further bone is nibbled away (*Fig.* 54.13). An extension of the burr-hole incision may be necessary to enable this to be done comfortably. The temporalis muscle is retracted to enable the direction and extent of the haematoma to be seen as it is evacuated with the sucker and periosteal elevator. Usually the clot will track down across the floor of the middle fossa towards the foramen spinosum. If a bleeding extradural artery can be seen it is dealt with by diathermy coagulation. The traditional matchstick plugging of the foramen spinosum is usually unnecessary. There may be multiple oozing points from the dura, and from the bone edge, the latter being dealt with by Horsley's bone wax being squeezed into the narrow diploic spaces. When the haematoma is extensive, the linear burr-hole incision may be extended into a circumferential osteoplastic flap craniotomy incision. Often, however, the application of cottonwool patties or pledgets soaked in peroxide, combined with patience, will allow the extradural space to be closed again by the steadily re-expanding brain. The dura should be inspected for rents which can be closed with interrupted fine black silk sutures.

When the bleeding has been controlled, any patties are removed, and the temporalis fascia is apposed with interrupted black silk sutures. The scalp is then closed with a layer of inverted sutures to the galea.

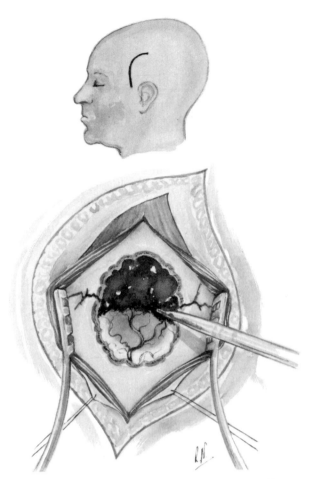

Fig. 54.13. Extradural haemorrhage. Sucker evacuation of haematoma after division of temporalis muscle and enlargement of burr hole.

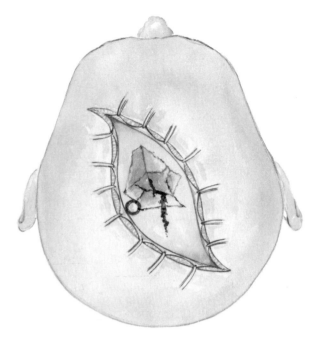

Fig. 54.14. Compound depressed vault fracture. Note extension of laceration into S-shaped exposure. Burr hole placed at margin of fracture, the inner table fracture being larger than the outer table fracture.

aponeurotica, and interrupted black silk or continuous nylon to the skin at 1-cm intervals. Drainage is not usually necessary, but if the ooze is persistent then a suction drainage tube can be introduced gently into the extradural space and let out through a stab wound adjacent to the main incision.

Evacuation of the haematoma is usually followed by a rapid and dramatic reversal of the deteriorating preoperative sequence. If this does not occur, then specialized help should be sought, not forgetting that a CT scan usually discloses rapidly and clearly a fresh intracranial haematoma.

CRANIOTOMY

General Principles

The need for craniotomy is dictated by two considerations. One is the size of the pathology to be dealt with. Clearly, a large tumour will usually require a sizeable exposure, not for the evacuation of the mass intact, but in order to gain access to the planes of cleavage when normal brain must be discretely and carefully separated from tumour boundary such as in the removal of a meningioma. The second reason for craniotomy is to gain access, for instance, at the skull base to an aneurysm which may itself be quite small. Here the base of the cerebral hemispheres must be retracted and although some of the space to be gained can be taken up by the removal of cerebrospinal fluid by lumbar or ventricular puncture, the surgeon needs enough exposure at the surface to enable him or her to deploy instruments and retractors without dangerous overcrowding. Although it is quite possible to carry out basal procedures via a 5 cm trephine, it is on the whole preferable to permit onself the exposure which an adequately sized osteoplastic flap provides.

The siting of the craniotomy naturally will depend on the procedure. Dandy introduced the 'concealed' osteoplastic frontal craniotomy, a scalp flap designed with its incision virtually entirely hidden behind the hairline on one side overlying a modestly sized bone flap sited so as just to avoid the frontal air sinus, yet sufficiently low on the temporal bone to enable the operator to proceed along the sphenoidal ridge in the direction of the brain base. A lateral craniotomy gives access to the temporal lobe and to the tentorial hiatus at the brain base, and an occipital craniotomy, besides being the approach for occipitally placed tumours, may be used with occipital lobe retraction to give access to the pineal region. The main decision to be made when siting a craniotomy is the relation of the flap to the main venous sinuses, mainly the superior sagittal sinus, especially in its posterior portion, and the lateral and sigmoid venous sinuses (*see Fig.* 54.16). The outer wall of the triangular lumen of a large venous sinus may be deficient, especially in the sigmoid region, and a craniotomy whose margin transgresses these structures runs a risk of torrential blood loss during the opening stages. If the medial longitudinal fissure of the brain is to be entered then the craniotomy must go beyond the midline. Special care has then to be taken to preserve and protect the sagittal sinus. Where a bifrontal procedure has to be undertaken, such as for an anterior falx meningioma or bilateral dural repair, then a coronal scalp flap gives an excellent cosmetic result under which either a bifrontal or two separate frontal craniotomies can be turned down. A convexity meningioma may evoke a hyperostosis from the overlying skull at the site of dural attachment and this must be encompassed by the planned flap so that the attachment presents in the middle of the exposure when the skull flap is turned down.

In general it is better to allow a bone flap to remain attached by a thick pedicle of temporalis muscle as this can be conserved without impairing the operator's approach. Occasionally it is difficult to fashion and turn down a flap which does not, by its very presence, somewhat impair the operator's access to the brain base, and in these circumstances there should be no hesitation about stripping the bone from its musculofibrous attachment, to be replaced as a free bone graft at the closure.

A posterior fossa craniotomy is really a craniectomy. The thin bone of the posterior fossa is simply removed piecemeal and not replaced. There are two reasons for this. One is the technical difficulty of fashioning an osteoplastic craniotomy based on the occipital muscles without damaging the underlying cerebellum and venous sinuses, particularly at the torcula. The second is the frequent need for an adequate decompression of the posterior fossa structures after the operative procedure, since room is restricted and any swelling of the cerebellum may lead to medullary compression with dire consequences. The occipital muscle attachment regenerates a thin bony integument of the posterior fossa fairly well over the course of the next 2 or 3 months after the acute period has passed, so that lack of bone over the posterior fossa structures is neither a serious nor a cosmetic defect.

Osteoplastic Craniotomy of the Skull Vault (*Figs.* 54.15, 54.16)

After skin preparation and draping and with the patient under endotracheal general anaesthesia, the incision is made through the outer four layers of the scalp which have been infiltrated with local anaesthetic containing adrenaline. This latter procedure makes it easier to avoid incising the pericranium with the knife. The guide to complete division of the galea

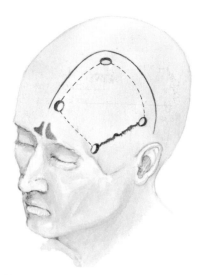

Fig. 54.15. Osteoplastic craniotomy—frontotemporal. Note the scalp incision largely concealed behind the hair line.

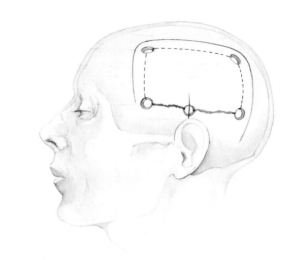

Fig. 54.16. Lateral craniotomy. Note that the two posterior lowermost burr holes are placed above the transverse or lateral venous sinus.

aponeurotica is the parting of the edge of the scalp under the slightly distracting finger pressures of operator and assistant. Scalp bleeding can always be controlled by digital pressure properly applied. Haemostats (curved artery forceps) are applied to the galea or, if preferred, removable haemostatic scalp edge clips of the Raney variety, either metal or plastic, are applied (*see Fig.* 54.5). In infants and in the temporal region the scalp thickness may need to be augmented by folded strips of wet gauze to enable the clip to apply enough pressure to stop edge bleeding. The incision is usually completed in two sweeps of the scalpel. The scalp flap is then picked up with forceps or retractor and the areolar layer of tissue divided by sweeps of the scalpel using the broad edge rather than its point. Any bleeding vessels

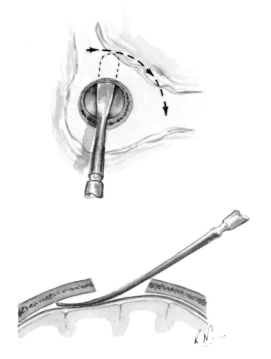

Fig. 54.17. To show method of dural separation from the inner scalp table.

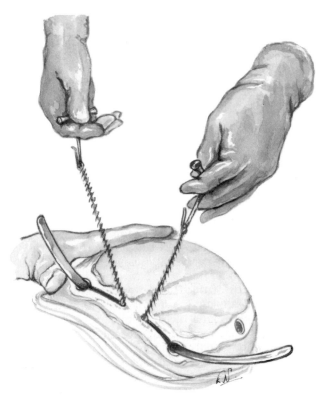

Fig. 54.18. Use of the Gigli saw between burr holes, introduced by means of the De Martel saw guide.

are now picked up with the low coagulating diathermy current directed via fine non-toothed dissecting forceps held in one hand while the sucker is used in the other. This scalp flap is then wrapped in a wet gauze and held back with stay sutures. The pericranium and temporalis, on which the flap is to be based, are now divided by the point of the cutting diathermy. The pericranium is eased back by the flat-ended periosteal rugine lubricated by a thin stream of warm saline. A four-pointed bone flap is usually adequate for most purposes if perforator and burr are to be used. The motor-driven craniotome gives a little more freedom in the shaping and extent of the exposure. Each burr hole is made with perforator, then burr, and a curved Adson's periosteal elevator is used to separate gently the somewhat adherent dura from the inner table of the skull (*Fig. 54.17*). In older patients hyperostosis frontalis interna can promote dural shredding during the lifting of the bone flap due to great adherence of the bone to the outer dural layer.

The Gigli saw guide is now passed between the skull vault and the dura from burr hole to burr hole, except at the base of the flap which is best fractured. The Gigli saw is kept taut while its full length is used, the advancing cut being cooled by a dribble of saline (*Fig. 54.18*). As the base of the flap, usually bridged by temporalis muscle, is thin, a few nibbles across here with a bone rongeur are sufficient to enable the skull flap to be snapped back. Carefully prising the flap will avoid a sharp bone edge penetrating the dura. Often the middle meningeal artery will have been torn as the flap is lifted and the first priority is to stop this bleeding with the bipolar diathermy. The jagged edges of the base of the flap are now trimmed with a bone rongeur and the skull flap held back by a towel clip through enveloping twisted gauze. When the craniotomy nears or encroaches upon the midline, venous bleeding from the superior longitudinal sinus or lacunae laterales is controlled by Gelfoam pledgets under stamps of gutta percha held in place by patties.

The dura is now exposed for the surgeon to make the decision as to how it should be opened (*Fig. 54.19*). If the dura is very tight measures must be taken to slacken it by ventricular tapping, anaesthetic hyperventilation or intravenous mannitol, since cortical herniation through even the smallest incision can produce venous bleeding that is impossible to control. The type of dural opening is dictated by the underlying pathology to be treated. For instance, a vault meningioma will usually have a dural attachment which must be removed with the tumour (*Fig. 54.20*). A cut radial to the circumference of the tumour will bring the surgeon up to its edge. A circumferential cut around the tumour attachment is then made. The hypertrophied dural vessels are controlled with silver or tantalum dural clips. Further radial cuts in the uninvolved dura will enable the boundary of the meningioma and normal brain to

is to be approached, the dura is opened in a curved incision along but 5 mm away from the forward edge of a frontal craniotomy exposure, since there are virtually no bridging veins here. The vulnerable 'corner' of the cerebral hemisphere where convexity becomes base is protected with gutta percha strips overlaid by Lintine. The retractor which now elevates the frontal lobe for access, for example, to a pituitary neoplasm or a basal aneurysm is used to coax the brain away from the base rather than to pull it.

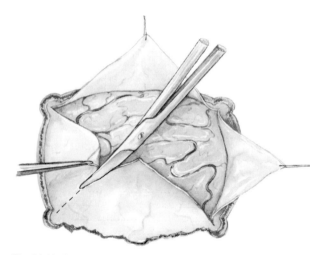

Fig. 54.19. Dural opening for maximum brain exposure.

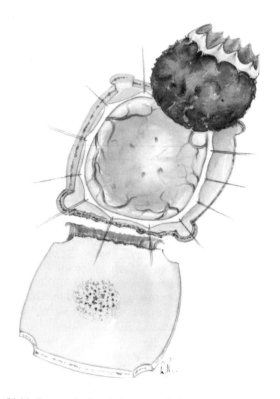

Fig. 54.20. Removal of vault (or convexity) meningioma. Showing hyperostosis on inner table of osteoplastic flap. Method of tumour traction utilizing dural sutures.

be discerned so that the removal can begin. If a glioma is to be approached then there is a choice between turning a dural flap up towards the superior sagittal sinus so as to avoid damaging veins bridging cortex to sinus. Alternatively, the dura can be opened in a cruciate incision, beginning at the site most likely to reveal discernible pathology, so that the dural opening can then be restricted only to what is necessary for the biopsy or removal. When the brain base

Closure

Hitch sutures are often employed to tie dura to pericranium at the edge of the craniotomy exposure in order to discourage the accumulation of extradural blood postoperatively. These should be placed very precisely so that no undue lateral traction on the dura ensues. If there is likely to be an appreciable period of haemostasis, as, for example, in drying up a tumour bed, then placement of these sutures is most profitably left to what would otherwise be a period of waiting. For basal approaches, however, hitch sutures are best put in before the dural opening since haemostasis will have to take place during the time that the brain is still retracted.

When all intradural bleeding points are completely controlled, leaving nothing to chance or probability, the dura is closed. Intermittent 3/0 fine silk sutures spaced at 1-cm intervals are usually sufficient. If brain swelling is thought likely then the dura is left open over the temporal lobe but closed over the convexity and the bone flap is removed. Even without brain swelling, this flap removal is sometimes best in meningiomas which are modest in size but which have provoked a marked oedematous reaction in the surrounding brain. The bone flap is replaced when the intracranial pressure normalizes, usually after 2 or 3 weeks. The flap is stripped carefully from temporalis muscle and periosteum and this layer is then sutured at 2 cm intervals with 2/0 black silk exactly in the position it would have occupied were the bone flap still in place. The elasticity of muscle and periosteum is usually sufficient to accommodate all but the most desperate of swellings.

When the dura is closed, external bleeding points on it are dealt with by very light touches with the bipolar diathermy or, if venous, by pressure on a stamp of gelatin sponge or Surgicel. When haemostasis is complete, the bone flap is fitted in position and, while an instrument wielded by an assistant holds it so, the surgeon places several 2/0 sutures through the pericranium to hold it in place. The closure is then completed with further sutures at 1·5-cm intervals. A powdery mixture of antibiotic and bone dust is compressed into each burr hole so as to prevent an unsightly dent on the forehead. The sutures are placed only in pericranium or temporalis fascia and not through muscle. Unless an air sinus has been opened, a 3-mm polythene catheter for suction drainage is now reverse introduced through the scalp about 2 cm from the craniotomy edge and allowed to lie in the subgaleal space. The scalp is closed with a galeal layer of interrupted absorbable sutures (3/0 in children) inserted so that the knots lie underneath the galea with tails cut no more than 1 mm long. These are put in at intervals of 1–1.5 cm, taking care to approximate galea only and to avoid placing the suture through potentially contaminated deep hair follicles. Alternatively, a continuous absorbable suture can be used to close this layer. The top layer is most speedily closed with a continuous 3/0 nylon suture introduced with a straight needle, but interrupted sutures or a subcuticular Dexon with Steristrip closure may also be used. If continuous sutures are employed it is unnecessary to use diathermy coagulation to control bleeding points in the vessels which lie between galea and skin.

SPECIAL MANOEUVRES

Aneurysm Clipping

Operations to prevent rebleeding from ruptured intracranial basal aneurysms are usually undertaken in the first 3 weeks after bleeding. The common sites for these aneurysms are at the inferior aspect of the internal carotid artery just before it bifurcates into anterior and middle cerebral branches (posterior communicating site), the bi- or trifurcation of the middle cerebral artery and at the anterior communicating artery respectively. The initial approach to all these aneurysms is by retraction of the frontal lobe along the sphenoidal wing (*Fig.* 54.21). A basic tenet of aneurysm surgery is to approach the aneurysm so that control of the vessel feeding it can be speedily undertaken were the aneurysm to rupture during dissection. Consequently, when the middle cerebral aneurysm is to be approached the sylvian fissure is opened just proximal to the aneurysm so that, before the aneurysm base is dissected, the middle cerebral artery can be prepared to take a clip in an emergency rupture. Similarly, the choice of side in the approach to the anterior communicating aneurysm is dictated by the artery which most readily fills it. This will usually give the most advantageous approach since the aneurysm will usually point away from the main feeding artery, thus presenting its neck for clipping advantageously at right angles.

The approach to the aneurysm is a cautious one with adjustments of the retractors and division of arachnoidal bands by sharp-pointed bayonet-shaped micro-scissors. The dissection is directed to the neck of the aneurysm and not to its vulnerable fundus, where the wall is very thin and the leak which produced the intracranial haemorrhage is sealed only by a friable fibrin plug. The expanded base of the aneurysm has to be dissected away from enveloping blood vessels so that the true neck, which may be

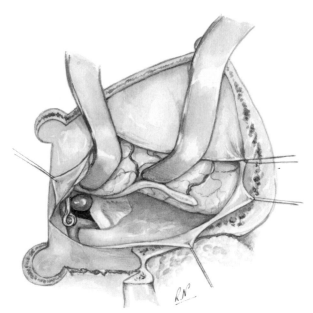

Fig. 54.21. Clipping of basal aneurysm. Note that the olfactory bulb has been avulsed from the cribriform plate (unfortunately). Scoville removable spring clip applied to the neck of the aneurysm.

sizeable, can be discerned. When this has been done, a temporary clipping to lower the pressure in the aneurysm or shrinkage of the neck by brief applications of the bipolar diathermy current sometimes enables an inoperable aneurysm to become operable. Removable spring clips, of which there are many patterns, the Scoville being the most versatile, are used. When an expanded trifurcation and aneurysm of the middle cerebral are dissected, it sometimes is seen that there is no true neck and one has to be 'manufactured' by the act of clipping. When this has been done without compromise of vessels, it may be clear that some of the fundus remains proximal to the clip and further expansion of the aneurysm may yet be possible. In these circumstances the clipped aneurysm and the vessels of origin can with advantage be invested in a quick-setting acrylic resin. This can be introduced around the aneurysm and solidifes in a few minutes. Aneurysms at the posterior communicating site usually point at right angles to the surgeon and the neck is encountered first. Occasionally the arachnoid around the neck has to be divided to allow a clip to slide around it. In turn the clip may impinge on the dura of the cavernous sinus or petroclinoid ligament. Occasionally the posterior communicating artery can be neither easily seen nor dissected and is included in the clip. The anterior communicating artery dissection best takes place through an approach which removes a very small volume of gyrus rectus above the optic chiasm which is bridged by the anterior cerebral artery. Division of the arachnoid 5 mm medial to the olfactory tract, with sucking away of the subjacent brain at the level of the optic nerve, gives access to the anterior communicating region together with the terminal anterior cerebral artery. It is important to see the contralateral anterior cerebral artery and to dissect away the pericallosal arteries from the base of the aneurysm before application of the clip.

Although most aneurysm surgery is straightforward, it occasionally occurs that the clip may compromise the circulation in the distal vessels in a way which cannot be discerned from inspection even under the operating microscope. In these circumstances it has been found advantageous to carry out an operative arteriogram through a flexible catheter introduced retrogradely down the superficial temporal artery as far as the carotid bifurcation. Eight or 10 ml of radiological contrast, together with a single unscreened film under the head, usually give sufficient detail to reassure the surgeon that the clip has not embarrassed the remaining circulation. If the circulation is sparse then the clip will have to be readjusted and a further arteriogram taken. The incision in the superficial temporal artery is closed by a continuous 10/0 nylon microsuture under high magnification.

POSTERIOR FOSSA CRANIOTOMY
(*Fig.* 54.22)

There are three basic surgical approaches to posterior fossa structures. The most commonly practised posterior approach is with a craniectomy via a midline incision. Most intracerebellar tumours and cysts can be dealt with by this approach and it has the added advantage that dangerous posterior fossa herniation through the foramen magnum can be effectively decompressed. In addition, tumours which extend into the spinal canal, such as haemangioblastomas and ependymomas, can be encompassed simply by downward extension of the incision. A second approach used for surgery of tumours of the high cerebellar vermis is an occipital osteoplastic craniotomy with retraction upwards of the occipital lobe after opening the dura above the lateral sinus. The posterior fossa is opened by division of the tentorium. Another more anterior transtentorial access can be gained by a lateral craniotomy so as to lift up the temporal lobe with division of the anterior tentorium along the petrous ridge attachment. This gives good exposure of the upper cranial nerves and to aneurysms of the upper vertebral artery and of the basilar artery. The third route of entry to the posterior fossa is via its anterior wall but as this is formed by the petrous bone, this structure has to be drilled away in the translabyrinthine approach to acoustic neuromas.

Ensuring Good Operating Conditions
Positioning for a posterior fossa craniotomy is very important. The most common position in former times was with a patient lying prone with the head

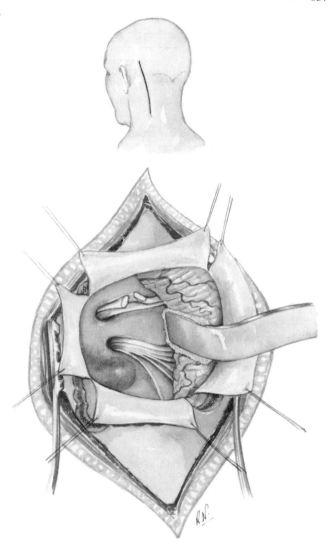

Fig. 54.22. Intracranial (posterior fossa) division of vestibular nerve for Ménière's disease. Note very light retraction of cerebellum and intact jugular group of nerves.

flexed. The position of the operating surgeon was then somewhat awkward and with mechanical ventilation the inflation pressures required from the pump were high since each ventilatory cycle had in effect to lift the weight of the trunk. This makes for somewhat less than ideal operating conditions. The sitting position gives good operating conditions for surgeons as far as pressures are concerned, but there is a small but appreciable mortality in this position from unexpected massive air embolism even though anticipated and guarded against. In addition, hypotension due to substantial blood loss can less easily be countered in this position. The lateral position for approaches to the posterior fossa suffers from none of the disadvantages which have been mentioned. With a slight head-up tilt and the patient lying on the side operating conditions are good, the suregon can sit comfortably in a specially designed chair for microdissection and the anaesthetist has good access to the ventral surface of the patient. The thorax and abdomen are free so that either mechanical or spontaneous ventilation can then be employed.

Many posterior fossa pathologies have secondary effects in precipitating obstructive hydrocephalus. This leads to high intracranial pressure which in turn elevates the intracranial venous pressure. As the intracranial veins are in communication with the diploic veins, the result of breaching the bone, particularly around the torcula, is brisk loss of venous blood at substantial pressure. One way of dealing with this situation is to insert a ventriculo-venous shunt some time before operation, particularly if the patient is in poor nutritional shape and is clearly not fit to face a major posterior fossa operation. However, the benefits of this somewhat complicated manoeuvre can be gained very rapidly by the insertion of a catheter into the lateral ventricle via a frontal burr hole, such as for positive contrast ventriculography. If, as usually occurs nowadays, the diagnosis has been made purely on the CT scan, a parieto-occipital burr hole inserted 3 cm from the midline just above the lamboid suture gives access to the lateral ventricle and intracranial pressure control can be rapidly effected by draining a few millilitres of cerebrospinal fluid.

Approach

The lambdoid suture becomes visible on the shaved and prepared scalp as a slight ridge. This burr hole is marked out just above it. The midline linear incision to the posterior fossa is marked out from some 2 cm above the external occipital protuberance to a similar distance below the palpable spine of the second cervical vertebra (axis). After draping, the cut is made with one sweep of the scalpel and artery forceps are applied to the skin edges to control bleeding. Occasionally in a young person the scalp will be pliable enough for Raney scalp edge clips to be effective. With bleeding controlled, self-retaining retractors of the Mollison type now produce distracting tension to allow the muscles to be split, using the cutting diathermy and keeping strictly to the midline. If this relatively avascular midline plane is not easily apparent it is worth picking it up at the external occipital protuberance first and then following it down into the nuchal musculature. One or two veins are found crossing the midline but these can be dealt with by the coagulating diathermy. The incision is taken onto the truncated spine of the posterior arch of the atlas and below this onto the much stouter midline spine of the axis vertebra. Remember that the posterior arch of the atlas is sometimes deficient in the midline, and because of the circular venous sinus at the foramen magnum it is safer to clear the tissue from the atlanto-occipital membrane with a tenotome than with cutting diathermy.

It is important while elevating the muscles from the posterior fossa bone below the superior nuchal line to use the controlled force of a double-handed grip on the periosteal elevator. With reinsertions of the self-retaining retractor with teeth in the muscle layer together with judicious upward cuts of the diathermy, especially at the superior nuchal line, the muscles can be elevated to display a considerable width of the occipital bone. Clearly if the structure to be approached is to one side of the midline (and this should be the side chosen uppermost when positioning the patient on the operating table) the muscles are cleared more completely on this side. Now, with an extension to the Hudson brace, a burr hole is placed to each side of the midline just below the external occipital protuberance. The Adson periosteal elevator is used to separate the dura from bone and the burr hole is enlarged by nibbling first with narrow and then with broader bone rongeurs until the foramen magnum is reached and opened to the extent of the posterior quarter of its circumference. If the cerebellar tonsils are shown, perhaps in ventriculographic or myelographic studies, to have descended below the foramen magnum, the central 3 cm of the posterior arch of the atlas are removed after elevating the periosteum from this structure. The bony removal superiorly is usually taken upwards to the inferior margin of the transverse venous sinus. This is seen as a blueness of a slightly elevated contour of the dura. The bone, especially near the torcula, is cancellous and may bleed freely from the diploë which is plugged with bone wax.

The dura is now ready for opening but if its tension is excessive, cerebrospinal fluid should be drained via the ventricular catheter. The usual approach to a structure close to the midline is to make a Y-shaped incision in the dura, the junction of the three limbs being approximately 1 cm above the foramen magnum. It is most convenient to make the upper limbs of the incision first, making separate breaches in the dura with hook and tenotome. These are then extended with the long-handled dural scissors. The small cerebellar sinus is found in the midline. The keel of double-folded dura in which it is enclosed extends a variable distance inwards between the cerebellar hemispheres, usually no more than 0·5 cm. To encompass this, a patty is introduced on either side of the structure so as to push away the cerebellum from the advancing dural scissors with which the cut is made. The open upper end of the divided cerebellar sinus is closed either with several haemostatic dural clips of tantalum or silver or by an encircling ligature. Diathermizing it brings about excessive dural shrinkage. The lower limb of the Y is taken through the small venous sinus running circumferentially at the foramen magnum and this bleeding is likewise controlled with dural clips. The dural opening in the midline below the foramen magnum is taken to the lower margin of the cerebellar tonsils but not further unless downward extension of a tumour demands it.

Operative Procedures

The dura is now drawn upwards to expose the cerebellar hemispheres and vermis and is held aside by stay sutures. If the pathology to be encountered is an intrinsic tumour of the cerebellar hemisphere, broadening of the transversely running cerebellar folia is looked for as a sign of an underlying mass. This is sought by exploration with a blunt-ended brain cannula introduced through a coagulated punctum of a pia-arachnoid, so that the increased resistance of a cyst wall or tumour margin can be felt. If an incision into the cerebellum is decided on, this is made in a direction at right angles to the folia, that is to say a cut parallel to the midline. This results in much less bleeding from the pia-arachnoid which is coagulated with successive pincer-like movements of the bipolar diathermy, the more resistant coagulated strands being divided with fine scissors. The incision is opened by either the hand-held or mechanical retractor resting on a protecting patty and deepened by light strokes of a slim metal sucker held in the right hand.

A cyst or tumour is usually encountered as a blue-grey mass looming through the white matter. With a blunt-ended brain cannula the nature of this mass is now explored and, if cystic, the fluid is aspirated. The retractors are now introduced directly into the cyst and, with headlight or operating microscope, the lining and walls are inspected for mural tumour nodules. A haemangioblastoma is usually seen as a reddish-grey nubbin of tissue often on the deep aspect of the cyst wall. There are usually prominent blood vessels running to it and these are taken with the bipolar diathermy and the nubbin removed. Astrocytoma tissue, on the other hand, is greyish-brown, relatively avascular and usually has a clear line of demarcation between it and the surrounding cerebellar white matter. The removal of solid tissue of this kind is accomplished by sweeps of the metal sucker along the line of demarcation between it and white matter with the placement of Lintine and patties so that the tumour is gradually encompassed. Depending on its extent, it can often be completely removed. The most common adult tumour to be encountered in the cerebellum is a metastasis, usually from bronchus, with tissue which is usually friable and vascular and it is removed using a similar technique. The more common childhood tumours not already mentioned are the medulloblastoma which is usually central, softer and more vascular and is best removed with a sucker. The ependymoma usually presents emerging from the foramina of the 4th ventricle and its lobules are removed piecemeal. The tumour grows out of the 4th ventricular floor and when this is the case, having removed the bulk of the tumour, it is unwise to delve too deeply into the medulla and pons, since the opportunity for irremediable damage exists and the tissue plane here is much less clear than elsewhere.

The closure is begun after haemostasis of discernible bleeding vessels with the bipolar diathermy and of an ooze by pledgets of cottonwool soaked in peroxide and introduced into the tumour bed. After 3 or 4 minutes these are removed gently by irrigating a flow of saline between tissue and cottonwool ball as this is then lifted gently out. When haemostasis is complete, the dura is replaced over the cerebellar hemispheres and the upper extremities of the Y are usually then closed by 3/0 black silk sutures. As the dura will usually have shrunk a complete closure would present difficulties even if this were desirable. It is wisest to allow the incision near the midline to remain open in case of cerebellar swelling. To limit the ingress of blood and tissue exudate, strips of gelatin sponge are laid transversely across the dural exposure. Alternatively, a dural graft of artificial dural substitute or gelfilm can be sewn in. However, grafts have the possible disadvantage that they may act as an impermeable film behind which cerebrospinal fluid can leak and become trapped. It then forms a source of compression for the underlying nervous system. The muscles are closed by interrupted sutures of 1/0 silk, taking care to introduce these through the most aponeurotic part of the musculature since this will not only give the most secure closure but will avoid unnecessary muscular necrosis. Antibiotic powder is usually sprayed into the wound at this stage before the muscle closure is quite complete. After the ligamentum nuchae has been reconstituted the superficial tissues are usually drawn together in two layers. The skin is approximated either by a continuous subcuticular Dexon 2/0 suture or by a continuous over-and-over suture introduced by either straight or curved atraumatic needle.

Postoperative Care

The postoperative care of patients after posterior fossa exploration begins in the anaesthetic room. It is desirable for the patient to return to a level of consciousness sufficient to obey commands and to ensure that he or she is capable of speaking, swallowing and of being able to deal with the secretions. If this is not clearly so the patient is retained in the theatre suite recovery bay or room until these functions return. If the patient's ascent to full consciousness is delayed for no good reason connected with anaesthesia, then a postoperative clot is suspected and preparations are made to reopen the wound. The intracranial pressure can be monitored via the ventricular catheter which has been left *in situ*. If the pressure here is found to be raised, preparations are made to redrape and reopen the wound. If progress and recovery are smooth, the main precaution to take is to ensure that when the patient is first offered sips of fluid, swallowing is more likely to function properly if the 'normal' side is disposed downwards when the patient lies in the lateral position. This minimizes the risk of aspiration and pneumonia if the jugular

nerves have been involved in the dissection for, for example, a sizeable acoustic neuroma. The ventricular catheter is usually removed 48 hours after operation.

Cerebello-pontine Angle

For lateral approaches to the posterior fossa, such as into the cerebellopontine angle, a favourite incision is an inverted 'hockey stick' (with the straight limb in the midline) to 1 cm above the superior nuchal line and then sweeping laterally and downwards to the tip of the mastoid process. The muscles are detached from the posterior fossa after dividing the rather tough pericranium just above the superior nuchal line. The whole of the posterior fossa bone on one side is then exposed. The dura is uncovered by enlarging a burr hole so as to remove bone between foramen magnum inferiorly and the transverse and sigmoid sinuses superiorly and laterally. An alternative incision is to make a linear curved cut, convex laterally, which at the midpoint almost reaches the mastoid process. The cutting diathermy is used through muscle to the bone. The edges of this muscle-cutting incision are then distracted with self-retaining retractors. The bony removal is taken laterally to the mastoid air cells which may have to be opened to obtain an adequate exposure. If opened they should be sealed during the closure to prevent Eustachian CSF leakage via the mastoid air cells and middle ear cavity. It is somewhat more difficult to reach the foramen magnum by this method but for operations of short duration and limited exposure, such as division of the glossopharyngeal upper filaments for glossopharyngeal neuralgia, for division of the vestibular division of the 8th nerve for Ménière's disease or of the 5th nerve for trigeminal neuralgia, this incision suffices. The dura is opened in a curved incision 5 mm away from the transverse and sigmoid sinuses so as to uncover the minimum of cerebellum. The cerebellar hemisphere is retracted to one side to expose the inferior cranial nerves and cerebellopontine angle (*Fig.* 54.22).

The removal of an acoustic neuroma by this posterior fossa approach, a procedure which is reserved for the small tumours, is achieved first of all by draining cerebrospinal fluid to allow the cerebellar hemisphere to fall away under gravity rather than be retracted. Gutta percha tissue and Lintine strips are now placed to protect the cerebellum from the mechanical retractor. The skull fixation for this is a 6·5-mm hole drilled into the skull above the lateral sinus, into which is inserted a tapered self-tapping lug from which the retractor takes origin. With the cerebellum held aside the internal auditory meatus is approached and the tumour is seen bulging into the posterior fossa cisterna. The posterior margin of the expanded meatus is now defined and the dura is divided from here backwards parallel with the superior petrosal sinus for a distance of 3 cm. This uncovers the posterior bony lip and wall of the internal auditory meatus which is now drilled away with a high-speed air drill and burrs. By this means the thinned dura lining the meatus (which forms a false capsule for the contained yellow fleshy schwannoma) can be opened with a linear cut. The cuff of dura and arachnoid which expansion of the tumour has formed as a collar at the porus is divided.

Under the operating microscope the lobules of tumour are now tilted gently away from the depths of the meatus, identifying the superior vestibular nerve from which the tumour usually arises. Superiorly and slightly anteriorly the facial nerve is to be found and the tumour is teased gently away from this. When the meatal tumour has been cleared, the arachnoid adhesions at the porus are divided by bipolar diathermy and micro-scissors and the rest of the tumour can now be debulked. It is then again teased away from the facial nerve which runs superiorly and then over the front of the tumour. The nerve here becomes expanded and thinned and greyer than expected, but great pains should be taken to identify it to avoid stretching it. No effort or time should be spared to preserve it intact. When the removal, which is usually piecemeal, is complete, the facial nerve should be traceable intact from the internal meatus to the pons. If the tumour is a large one and the nerve cannot be preserved, it should be reconstituted by laying the divided ends together on a short pledget of gelatin sponge which, with the application of fibrin, soon serves to anchor the oedematous and friable nerve. After small adjustments of the nerve ends are made to maximize close approximation, a second similar pledget of gelatin sponge is used to form a sandwich, nerve ends being the filling. Alternatively, 10/0 microsutures can be used to approximate ends that have been redivided.

The closure, after haemostasis is complete, is usually made with interrupted fine silk to the dura, strips of gelatin sponge over the dural incision to minimize the entry of blood from the muscle layer, which itself is closed with interrupted sutures of waxed 1/0 silk. The galeal and subcutaneous layers are closed with interrupted Dexon and the skin for a linear incision by subcuticular 2/0 Dexon.

TRANSPHENOIDAL PITUITARY SURGERY

The advent of the binocular stereoscopic operating microscope has renewed interest in the transphenoidal approach to the pituitary gland which was employed in the early years of the century by Cushing and others. It was then largely given up by him in favour of the subfrontal approach. Four ways of entering the sphenoidal sinus exist. The original trans-septal approach via sublabial incision was to elevate the mucosa from either side of the nasal septum and then to resect this structure. A bivalved speculum was then opened so as to expose the midline prow of the sphenoid bone which was resected antero-inferiorly to allow entry to the sinus. The transeth-moidal route exploited by Angell James approaches via a curved ethmoidal incision from the medial eyebrow downwards and medially, and then curves a short way onto the cheek. The lacriminal sac and trochlea for the superior oblique muscle are then elevated subperiosteally with the rest of the anterior orbital contents (taking care to avoid breaching the orbital periosteum) to expose the anterior ethmoidal air cells. These are punched away after a specially designed ethmoidal retractor has been introduced to hold aside the anterior orbital contents. The air cells are removed together with the upper posterior square centimetre of nasal septum where this abuts onto the prow of the sphenoid bone. The roof of the ethmoidal cells is seen above and maintained intact, as is the posterior ethmo-orbital wall. As the anterior wall with its ostium of the sphenoidal air sinus is approached, it is opened and punched away from the anterior fossa floor above so as to expose the whole of the anterior sellar wall which may of course be vastly expanded by tumour (*Fig.* 54.23).

The transpalatal and transantral routes to the sphenoidal sinus have not gained the popularity of the two methods described since they do not appear to be as direct and offer no special advantages.

EXTRACRANIAL VASCULAR SURGERY OF THE BRAIN

Eastcott's pioneer operation for reconstitution of the internal carotid artery took place in 1954. In 1969 Yasargil first carried out an operation using a microvascular technique at which the superficial temporal artery was connected end to side with a middle cerebral branch on the cortical surface of the brain. Both

operations have been progressively exploited and now are secure as part of the neurosurgical repertoire.

Carotid Endarterectomy (*Fig.* 54.24)

There is no simple explanation for the siting of atheromatous plaques at the carotid bifurcation although flow eddies may be important. The build-up of atheroma seems to be maximal in the internal carotid at the point approximately 1 cm distal to the carotid bifurcation. Its effect is twofold. Platelet embolization from an ulcerating atheromatous plaque may give rise to stereotyped attacks of ischaemia in the territory of the ophthalmic artery and of the middle cerebral artery. Ophthalmic embolization gives rise to transient blindness sometimes called 'amaurosis fugax'. Middle cerebral embolization produces transient ischaemic attacks (defined as neurological symptoms and signs of less than 24 hours' duration) affecting the face and arm and, on the left side, speech function. Marked involvement of the leg should arouse suspicion that vertebrobasilar ischaemia is present. These transient ischaemic attacks can often be reduced or abolished by formal anticoagulant treatment or by aspirin or Persantin (dipyridamole). If the stenosis is severe then there is the danger of further thrombosis to complete occlusion. This may be silent but is more likely to produce a major infarct in the middle cerebral territory, often with propagating thrombus into the middle cerebral vessels.

Both these consequences of carotid atheroma can be effectively treated by carotid endarterectomy. Although the atheromatous plaque penetrates into the media to a varying degree, atheroma is basically an intimal process. In well-developed plaques a plane between media and plaque can be fairly easily dissected. The principle of the operation consists of

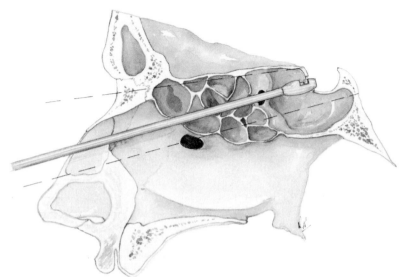

Fig. 54.23. Transethmo-sphenoidal pituitary exposure. The bone punch nibbles out anterior wall of sella turcica.

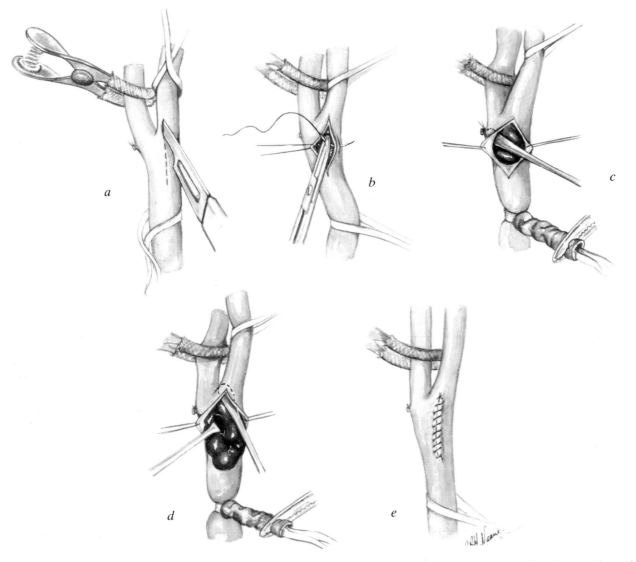

Fig. 54.24. Carotid endarterectomy. This operation is undertaken at normal temperatures, carefully controlling the carotid vessels. (For purpose of clarity the shunt is not shown.)

removing plaque and overlying distorted intima, leaving a fairly smooth bare media with the intimal margins undisturbed in order to promote re-intimalization of the reconstituted channel.

Investigations

These patients frequently have well-developed coronary and other atherosclerosis. Part of the clinical work-up should be specially directed to the clinical assessment of these lesions and in particular to determine whether the cerebral attacks could have a basis in cardiac embolization from mural thrombus consequent on endocardial involvement in myocardial infarction. In addition the femoral arteries should be checked for patency and bruits since much selective cerebral catheterization for arteriography is

nowadays transfemoral. The clinical work-up should include special attention to bruits in the neck and the patency of the superficial temporal arteries.

Selective arteriography is still *sine qua non* for carotid surgery. Pictures of the carotid bifurcation should be obtained in two directions at right angles, including if possible the skull base up to the siphon. Formal cerebral arteriograms in two directions at right angles should be taken since siphon atheroma is common and middle cerebral stenosis, best seen in an anteroposterior view, can produce transient ischaemic attacks. Both right and left bifurcations should be clearly visualized, since the contralateral internal carotid artery will bear the main burden of cerebral blood supply during occlusion of the operated side. If possible the vertebral vessels should be visualized at the same time since these, too, can occlude silently. Pulsed Doppler images of the carotid bifurcation should be obtained and studied in conjunction with the arteriograms. These are especially valuable since they can be useful for follow-up purposes. At present, however, the clarity of the image does not permit sufficient confidence in the investigations to hinge operation on the pulsed Doppler scan alone.

Technique

During operations on the carotid arteries the necessary temporary surgical occlusion of these vessels will reduce the cerebral flow, sometimes appreciably. Nevertheless, the contralateral carotid system and the vertebral arteries are adequate to prevent cerebral ischaemic damage in the majority of patients. Various protective methods have been devised.

1. Hypothermia

Surface cooling to 30 °C using a water bath or ice packs was used for many years and was found to prolong the safe ischaemic time to an acceptable level.

2. Intravascular shunts

The introduction of intravascular shunts, which are manufactured tubes of polyvinyl chloride or Silastic rubber, has superseded hypothermia. The shunts are inserted into the common carotid proximally and internal carotid artery distal to the site of operation at the carotid bifurcation, thus maintaining the cerebral circulation.

During surgery it is necessary to monitor the electro-encephalogram as significant deprivation of cerebral blood supply during carotid clamping is readily detected and will then declare the need for shunting. Measurement of the distal carotid pressure during clamping, so-called 'stump pressure', is also of great use and it is suggested that a distal stump pressure of less than 60 mmHg should be regarded as an indication for temporary shunting.

Although hypothermia was used for many years and intra-arterial shunting is favoured by many, the invariable need for such precautions is questioned and the author has found that provided surgery is undertaken rapidly and that continuity of blood flow is established within 30 minutes the patients come to no harm.

Local anaesthesia is sometimes used for endarterectomy but appears to have no particular merit. General anaesthesia cuts down the oxygen requirement of the brain by its depressing effect on metabolism. The anaesthetist can usually ensure an adequate level of systemic blood pressure for collateral circulation. In addition, inadvertent movement and what must be a somewhat stressful adventure for the patient are avoided.

The position of the patient is supine with the head turned slightly away from the side of the operation with a slight head-up tilt to disengorge the neck veins. The incision is via a collar skin crease taken approximately from the external jugular vein to somewhere near the midline. The incision is deepened through platysma and small bleeding points are picked up precisely with the bipolar diathermy. The dissection is continued towards the carotid bifurcation with the blunt-tipped dissecting scissors, when the carotid sheath can usually be seen shining through the areolar layer of connective tissue. Bifurcating veins running from the thyroid gland are ligated flush with the jugular vein and a length of 1 or 2 cm of vein is taken in case a repairing patch is needed after the endarterectomy. The carotid bifurcation is now exposed and the hypoglossal nerve and digastric posterior belly are reflected upwards. The adventitia is stripped from the lateral aspect of the bifurcation and internal carotid, the extent of the stripping being guided by palpation of the hard atheromatous plaques through the wall of the artery. This clearance is taken at least 2 cm below the carotid bifurcation. Encircling tape ligatures are now passed around the common carotid as low as possible, usually 3 cm below the bifurcation and around the main trunk of the external carotid, just above the superior thyroid artery take-off. The superior thyroid is occluded by a small bulldog clip. The internal carotid is encircled but a small curved vascular clamp is used here for occlusion.

The anaesthetist is now told that all is ready for the incision and the tapes on the common carotid and external carotid are tightened to occlusion. The clamp on the internal carotid is closed and a count started by the anaesthetist, this being for record purposes. The times are not called out as the surgeon will clearly work as rapidly as is possible with safety. An incision is made with a tenotome and no. 15 blade smoothly on the surface of the internal carotid and taken down a smooth line well into the common carotid. (*Fig. 54.24a*). Usually this will penetrate the lumen and the atheromatous plaque can be visualized. The sucker is used to empty the vessel and the plane between plaque and media is now picked up carefully and the dissection proceeds upwards and downwards to the full extent of plaque. Care is taken with the dissection to maintain the cleavage plane and, where this deepens into the media to avoid perforation, especially of the medial wall. As the dissection proceeds anteriorly it will usually be seen that a sleeve of atheroma can be disengaged from the mouth of the external carotid artery. With fine sharp-pointed scissors this sleeve is cut off flush with the intima, taking care to leave no tags or intimal fringe which could lift and form an occluding dissection between media and intima. The same principle holds for the dissection down into the common carotid but here, due to the direction of blood flow, the risk of postoperative flap occlusion is less. As the sleeve of atheroma is gently disengaged from the internal carotid, it is vitally important here to guard against later intimal lifting. Special care is necessary here. As the dissection is completed the entire atheromatous cast is lifted intact from the artery. The bed can now be inspected for tags of intima or ulcers. These are dealt with. The margin of intimal dissection in the upper internal carotid is now inspected again and any intimal lifting is dealt with by either retrimming or a through-and-through loop tacking suture inserted from without inwards and in the reverse direction again (*Fig.* 54.24*b–d*).

The closure is made with a 5/0 Prolene single-ended arterial needle beginning at the upper end of the arteriotomy. The sutures are placed continuously without locking approximately at 1·5–2-mm intervals. It is important to have equal bites of media on either side of the incision. The assistant maintains steady tension on the suture line, taking care to hold the suture either between finger and thumb or with a forceps protected so as to avoid damage to the suture. This closure is best done under magnification, by either loupes or operating microscope. The last three passages of the needle are not drawn tight, although the assistant maintains tension on the rest of the suture line (*Fig.* 54.24*e*). The internal carotid clamp is now released and a backflow of arterial blood obtained. This briefly washes out the arteriotomy, then the arterial clamp is closed again. The remaining loops of suture are now drawn tight and the suture is securely knotted. The internal carotid clamp is now released followed by the external carotid and common carotid snares in that order. This attempts to ensure no residual fibrin or clot is delivered into the internal carotid circulation. As the clamps are removed the suture line usually leaks. This is dealt with by laying a gutta percha strip over the suture line and packing wet saline swabs over this. Firm pressure is maintained with the fingers for 10 minutes by the clock, after which the leaks will usually have ceased. The gutta percha tissue is removed and antibiotic powder is lightly sprinkled into the wound. The neck closure is by buried 2/0 interrupted sutures to the platysma at 1·5-cm intervals with a continuous 3/0 Dexon subcuticular suture to the skin. If wound drainage is needed a short length of corrugated drain emerges through the centre of the incision and clips are used for skin closure.

As anaesthesia is terminated and dressing is applied, the patient should be awake for neurological testing before return to the recovery bay or ward. Observations about manual strength and, in the case of left-sided operations, the ability to speak clearly should be continued at hourly intervals for the first 48 hours after operation. Blood pressure is charted so as to guard against hypotension. Unexplained events, even those which do not at first seem to have a direct neurological cause, such as sudden severe breathlessness, should arouse suspicion of a postoperative occlusion of the artery at the arteriotomy site. Naturally hemiplegia or hemiparesis occurring

under these circumstances on the appropriate side merits immediate reexploration of the wound. Digital palpation of the internal carotid reveals thrombotic occlusion. In these circumstances the arteriotomy should be reopened and resutured again after clot removal. Secondary haemorrhage is uncommon but can occur at the period of maximum fibrinolysis at the end of the 1st week. In these circumstances the neck must be re-explored to remove the haematoma and the suture line inspected for its origin. For this reason patients must be kept under observation in hospital for over 1 week after operation. A check arteriogram is carried out to ensure patency and an adequate operation. It should not be assumed that in the absence of any neurological signs, the reconstituted artery is necessarily patent. Silent occlusion can and does occur. If, as occasionally happens, occlusion is detected only at late arteriography a decision has then to be made as to whether a superficial temporal-to-middle cerebral bypass should be performed.

EXTERNAL CAROTID/INTERNAL CAROTID ANASTOMOTIC SURGERY (*Fig.* 54.25)

The most common form of bypass surgery for complete occlusion of the internal carotid or vertebral vessels is end-to-side anatomosis of the posterior branch of the superficial temporal artery to one of the larger middle cerebral branches emerging from the sylvian fissure. The indications for this operation are still not entirely clear. Complete occlusion of the internal carotid followed by transient ischaemic attacks which persist despite anticoagulants, severe stenosis of the internal carotid artery between its origin at the common carotid bifurcation in the neck and the intracranial branching into the anterior and middle cerebral arteries or severe middle cerebral stenosis with persistent symptoms are indications for this procedure. It has also been invoked in established stroke either in the acute phase of the 1st week or in the recovery phase if this seems not to be proceeding rapidly. In addition, a prophylactic bypass may be constructed prior to aneurysm surgery (for instance, at the intracranial internal carotid bifurcation) in cases where occlusion of major branches is to be feared. The main contra-indication to the operation is swelling of the underlying cerebral hemisphere as revealed by a CT scan. Lucency of cerebral tissue, often regarded as cerebral oedema in the scan, is not necessarily a contra-indication. The presence of haemorrhage in the hemisphere in stroke is, however, a direct contra-indication.

Arteriography preoperatively should reveal precisely the state of the neck and intracranial vessels on both sides. Four-vessel arteriography is a desideratum. Late films will often reveal a substantial intracranial anastomotic circulation via the anterior branch of the superficial temporal artery which connects with the ophthalmic artery via the supraorbital

ficial temporal vessel is dissected under the low magnification of the operating microscope from its origin to the major branches near the vertex, This usually displays approximately 8 cm of artery, not all of which need be used. The minor side-branches of the first 5 cm of this vessel are coagulated by the bipolar diathermy and divided close to the parent vessel. A sleeve of adventitia is left on the artery.

When a sufficient length of artery has been mobilized but not yet divided distally, the incision is deepened through temporalis and this muscle is retracted so as to expose the temporal bone lying above the sylvian fissure. A 4·5-cm trephine disc is now drilled and removed, taking great care not to breach the dura. The dura is now opened with a cruciate incision and a search is made for a suitably sized middle cerebral branch emerging from the sylvian fissure. Further extension of the bony removal may need to be taken if a large enough vessel does not immediately present itself. The vessels emerging over the upper lip are used for preference. With the high magnification of the microscope the arachnoid over the selected vessel is now cleared for approximately 1 cm and the very fine-tipped bipolar diathermy is used to coagulate perforating vessels which run down into the subjacent cortex directly from the selected vessel, After division of these coagulated vessels, a strip of gutta percha tissue is inserted so as to lie under the selected arterial segment, Specially weakened arterial spring clips are readied for occlusion. Patties and Lintine are placed so as to limit the brain exposure to the small segment of interest. Any bleeding is dealt with at this stage.

The superficial temporal artery is now divided with sufficient length to bring the end without tension to the site for anastomosis. This is usually just over 5 cm. The vascular clip is reapplied more proximally over a part of the vessel covered by adventitia. The extreme distal end of the artery is grasped firmly and the adventitia is pulled proximally for about 0·5 cm. This cuff of excess adventitia is then trimmed away. The arterial termination is then retrimmed with an oblique cut at approximately 45° to the long axis of the vessel so as to present an undamaged and unhandled media and intima for suturing.

The magnification of the operating microscope is now increased. The 1-cm segment of recipient middle cerebral branch is now isolated by application of the vascular clips at either end. A longitudinal incision in this vessel approximately 3 mm long (to correspond with the length of the obliquely cut end of the superficial temporal artery) is now made with a diamond knife or sharp scalpel. It is important to ensure that media and intima are cut together and it is often best to do this with sharp micro-scissors and with one definitive cut. Taking more than one cut usually results in fraying and disparity between media and intima. With no. 3 watchmaker's forceps in the left hand and a slightly curved micro-needle holder in the right, a 10/0 monofilament microsuture is trimmed to

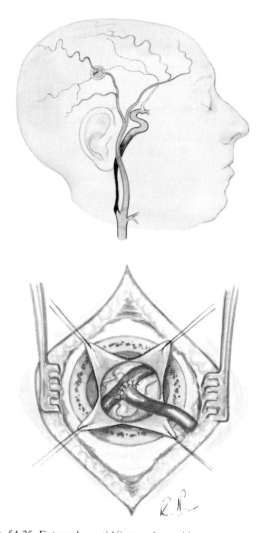

Fig. 54.25. External carotid/internal carotid anastomotic surgery. The posterior branch of the superficial temporal artery is anastomosed to the middle cerebral artery or one of its branches.

vessels. This should not be disturbed. Even in the absence of this angiographic demonstration effective collateral circulation can be demonstrated by Doppler change of phase of flow on compression of the superficial temporal artery over the zygomatic arch. For these reasons the posterior branch of the artery is used.

The operation can be caried out under local anaesthesia but general anaesthesia is preferable if there is any doubt about the patient's cooperation. The scalp is shaved over the side of the head and the continuous wave Doppler probe is employed to map out the course of the superficial temporal artery and branches in the scalp. The point of maximum echo should be marked by Bonney's blue pricked into the skin through a sharp needle so that, after the scalp is prepared and draped, the course of the vessels can be clearly seen, The incision, after scalp infiltration with 1 per cent lignocaine without adrenaline, is made over the posterior branch of the artery. The super-

approximately 8 cm in length. The anastomosis begins by passing this needle from without in at one end of the arteriotomy cut, taking care to include both media and intima. The suture is now passed in the reverse direction through the much thicker-walled superficial temporal artery, selecting either the shorter or longer end of the obliquely cut vessel as appropriate. This suture is now tied with the microvascular technique, having deposited the needle on a nearby patty. A convenient method is to zoom the microscope to a smaller magnification and increased field for tying the suture. This suture is then cut and a corresponding suture at the other extremity of the anastomosis is again placed in a similar way, after zoom up to a higher magnification.

An important point of technique is that the edges of the vessels to be sewn are not grasped by the watchmaker's forceps as this would damage seriously the delicate endothelium. The function of the forceps is to pick up the needle and to support with counterpressure the tissue through which the needle is being introduced. When the end sutures are tied the two sides of the anastomosis are constructed with interrupted sutures, an average number being 10 or 12 in a vascular reconstruction of this size. An alternative technique is to insert and tie two separate microsutures at each end of the anastomosis. The suturing is then completed with a continuous suture, each tied to the tail of the other. Care is taken during the reconstruction to avoid fibrin accumulating inside or near the cerebral vessel. A micro-sucker is used to ensure this.

The anastomosis is now wrapped in gutta percha tissue and mild pressure by saline-soaked patties is applied. The vascular clips are now removed, first from the middle cerebral branch, then from the superficial temporal artery. Unless there is uncontrollable bleeding the anastomosis is not disturbed for 10 minutes. When the patties are removed and the gutta percha peeled back, the suture line is usually secure and arterial pulsation can be discerned in all three segments of vessels. Unlike an end-to-end anastomosis, the test for patency is difficult without a radiographic or fluorescein angiogram which may be carried out by an injection into a specially prepared and cannulated small side-branch of the superficial temporal vessel.

The bone disc is now trimmed so as to allow appropriate access for the entering superficial temporal vessel. The dura is closed and Gelfoam pledgets placed on any gaps. The bone disc is replaced. It is held in place by sutures of 2/0 silk through the temporalis fascia, again allowing an appropriate gap for the entry of the superficial temporal artery. The scalp is closed with interrupted sutures at 1-cm intervals to the galea, with a continuous suture to the skin, taking care at the lower end of the incision to avoid traumatizing the superficial temporal vessel. Patency of the anastomosis is tested in the early days by Doppler, the vascular ultrasonic signal being fairly readily followed into the small craniectomy, where a change in the character of the signal is usually detectable. Arteriography for patency should usually be delayed since a patent anastomosis will occasionally not fill immediately.

Chapter fifty-five

Neurological Disorders of the Spine

B. H. Cummins

The operative management of neurological disorders of the spine and peripheral nerves demands much common sense, some expert knowledge and limited investigation. Careful history taking and meticulous examination will suggest the diagnosis and the choice of treatment in the majority of cases.

SURGICAL ANATOMY OF THE REGION

The *spinal cord* is an extension of the brain anatomically and functionally, dependent on a very adequate blood supply. Rich anastomoses within the cord protect it from ischaemia. The main arterial inflow arrives at C7 and D9 and occlusion of the latter frequently precipitates paraplegia (*Fig.* 55.1).

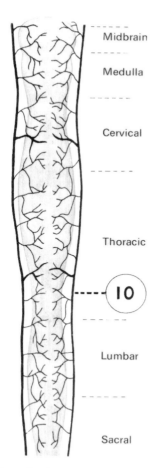

Fig. 55.1. Arterial supply of spinal cord. The critical level (D10) is indicated. At this level interference with the blood supply readily produces paraplegia.

Midbrain

Medulla

Cervical

Thoracic

10

Lumbar

Sacral

The cord is moored throughout its length along either side of the equator by the denticulate ligaments, which appear flimsy but are strong enough to hold a stitch for gentle rotation of the cord. They separate the dorsal sensory from the ventral motor roots, and are an important landmark when cordotomy is undertaken.

The cord is naturally expanded in the cervical and dorsolumbar regions, where much of the integration of limb control occurs. In adults, the conus of the cord ends at the top of the 1st lumbar vertebra, rising to that position from infancy when it is close to L5. Thus the lumbar sac of cerebrospinal fluid is much smaller in children, which should be borne in mind when performing lumbar puncture or myelography. The conus is held longitudinally at its tip by a string-like filum terminale to the dura of the sacrum. In adults it may develop a tumour, in children be thick and short, tethering the conus unduly low, with consequent gait and micturition disorders.

The spinal cord is bathed in *cerebrospinal fluid* (CSF) in direct communication with that of the cranium, unless there is pathological obstruction. The arterial pulsation of the brain is transmitted through the spinal CSF, causing the intact dural tube to pulsate in time. This is a valuable guide to the presence of obstruction at operation and the adequacy of surgical decompression. The pressure of the spinal CSF reflects the intracranial pressure plus the hydrostatic pressure of difference in height. It fluctuates normally with changes in venous pressure (the Queckenstedt test) and rhythmically with ventilation. Normally CSF is clear and colourless with a low protein (less than 50 mg per cent), less than 3 white cells/mm^3 and no red cells. In subarachnoid haemorrhage it is obviously bloodstained with a xanthochromic supernatant. Below an obstruction it is at low pressure and yellow, with a high protein.

The CSF is contained by the arachnoid and dura in a tube which ends in a rounded funnel in the sacrum. The arachnoid mater is filmy but surprisingly tough so that with care the dura mater can be opened widely without perforating it, allowing atraumatic surgical inspection of the cord.

The *dura mater* is a fibrous tube enveloping the arachnoid and extruding out to sheath each collection of nerve roots which form spinal nerves. These sheaths are well demonstrated in water-soluble contrast radiographic studies (radiculography) which is particularly important in the diagnosis of extruded lateral invertebral discs. The dura mater is firmly attached only to the circular rim of the foramen magnum; elsewhere it is loosely moored by the sheaths along the peripheral nerves, and encased in epidural fat and veins, so that considerable mobility is possible longitudinally within the flexible spinal canal. Rapid variations in calibre occur with changes of venous or CSF pressure.

The fibres are predominantly longitudinal, so that the dura can be torn gently lengthways with two pairs of forceps, while requiring to be cut transversely. It is an effective barrier to tumour and infection; the common extradural secondary carcinoma rarely spreads through the dura.

The *epidural fat* allows easy slippage of the dural sheaths through the intervertebral foramina—it is lost where there is constriction or postoperative scarring, leaving the sensitive dura anchored to the adjacent fibrous tissue or bone. A well-preserved epidural layer allows the skilled anaesthetist to perform reginal anaesthesia or inject steroids to alleviate back pain; after laminectomy, however, this plane is lost.

The *epidural venous plexus* is not valved and transmits secondary carcinoma readily to the epidural space from bronchus, prostate and breast, and infection from the pelvis and abdomen. Useful to compensate for volume changes within the spinal canal, these thin-walled veins can be a considerable nuisance if severed at laminectomy.

The lower down the spinal column, the more massive must be the *vertebra* to support the accumulated weight of the body. The uneasy compromise between stability and mobility takes its toll late in life when osteophytes encroach on the spinal canal, usually where a more mobile part of the spine joins a stable one, as in the lower cervical and lumbar regions. Hard manual labour builds heavy bone, the penalty for which is often stenosis of the spinal canal. The canal is usually capacious in the cervical region: in the adult the lumbar region contains only the roots of the cauda equina, but in the thoracic spine the canal is snugly close to the cord; laminectomy here demands great care.

SURGICAL DISORDERS OF THE CERVICAL SPINE AND CORD

These may be classified as follows:
1. Traumatic—acute.
2. Degenerative—cervical spondylosis.
3. Neoplastic:
    a. Extrinsic to the spinal cord:
        i. Extradural, usually metastatic.
        ii. Intradural, usually neurofibroma or meningioma.
    b. Intrinsic to the spinal cord—astrocytoma or ependymoma.
4. Congenital anomalies:
    a. Spina bifida.
    b. Chiari malformation with syringomyelia.
5. Vascular—angioma of the spinal cord.

Trauma

A broken neck may declare itself immediately with tetraplegia or more insidiously by the slow development of 'electric shocks' in the limbs, continued pain in the neck and spastic weakness of the legs. Acute hyperextension of the neck in the middle aged with osteophytic encroachment onto the spinal cord produces a contusion of the spinal cord typically at C5–C6 and C6–C7. This may happen to patients intubated for anaesthesia, to occupants of cars run into from behind and to those who are thrown out of public houses.

The management of trauma to the cervical region centres around the preservation of spinal cord function, and the provision of the right environment for the recovery of the damaged cord. In general, traction and skilled conservative handling win in the end; the contused cervical cord does not take kindly to enthusiastic reduction under anaesthesia or open operation. There are, however, occasional instances where operation is indicated.

Conservative Management

This demands skilled and patient care from the time the diagnosis is made; it is not a recipe for idleness.

At the site of the accident, if the patient has severe pain in the neck or weakness of the limbs, he or she should be treated as if the neck was broken, being lifted en bloc with the head held neutral in position, and supported thus in transit. Similar vigilance must be exercised in the accident and particularly in the X-ray departments.

IN THE ACCIDENT DEPARTMENT
1. Record a careful neurological examination.
2. Diagnose and treat other injuries causing severe blood loss:
    a. Haemothorax, with or without pneumothorax.
    b. Fractured limbs.
    c. Fractured pelvis.
    d. Ruptured spleen or other viscus.
3. Take radiographs of:
    a. Cervical spine, including odontoid views.
    b. Chest.
    c. Other parts as indicated.
4. If the fracture is stable and there is no neurological deficiency, put to bed in a collar. Mobilize early but record progress.
5. If the fracture is unstable, or there is severe crushing or slipping of the vertebras, insert skull callipers.

Insertion of skull callipers:
1. Place on operating table with care.
2. Shave areas of scalp about halfway between the ear and the vertex on each side.
3. Clean skin and instil local anaesthetic where the

callipers will fit, having held them open, close to the cleaned skin.

4. Nick the skin with a scalpel.

5. Drill through the outer table of the skull only. Deeper drilling invites extradural abscesses.

6. Insert callipers and screw up tightly. Tighten the screw each day for the 1st week.

7. Transfer to a prepared motorized Stoke Mandeville bed or Stryker frame. Use 2·7–3·6 kg (6–8 lb) traction.

IN THE WARD:

1. Turn every 2 hours to protect skin.

2. Catheterize if incontinent or paraplegic.

3. Watch for the first signs of pneumonia. In the completely paralysed elderly it is kinder not to treat this, except with euphoriants.

4. Monitor temperature and blood pressure. Both are labile in high spinal cord lesions.

5. Preserve joint function with physiotherapy.

6. Encourage occupational therapy and visitors.

7. Excise bed sores, if they occur, and treat anaemia.

Indications for Operation

1. UNSTABLE 'HANGMAN'S FRACTURE' OF C1 WITH INADEQUATE REDUCTION BY TRACTION (*Fig*. 55.2)

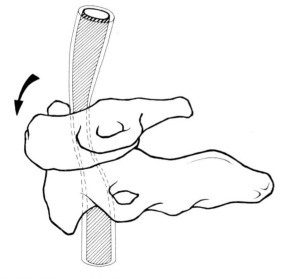

Fig. 55.2. Atlanto-axial subluxation. The spinal cord is compressed between the odontoid process and the arch of the unstable atlas.

McGraw's method is very useful for this fracture and for rheumatoid arthritic atlanto-axial dislocation.

Operation:

a. Induce anaesthesia very carefully with endotracheal intubation.

b. Lay patient prone, prepare the back of neck and one posterior iliac crest. Check reduction

of the fracture with image intensifier or lateral radiograph.

c. Incise from the occipital protuberance to the spinous process of C7, and, keeping in the avascular midline, using the cutting diathermy like a pencil, expose the occipital bone and the spinous processes of C2–C5.

d. Keeping close to the bone of the spinous processes, lay bare the laminas of these vertebras and the posterior arch of the atlas. Remove part of the large spinous process of C2, and gently remove some of the cortical bone of C1 and C2.

e. Very gently, using two hands, separate the extradural tissue from the undersurface of C1 and C2.

f. Prepare a 2·5-cm square graft of bone from the posterior iliac crest. Cut notches in each side.

g. Place a single loop of 18 SWG wire beneath the laminas and secure the graft (*Fig*. 55.3).

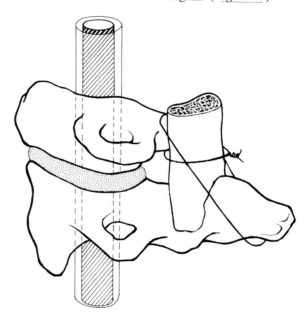

Fig. 55.3. Fixation of atlanto-axial subluxation using bone graft and wire.

h. Close with continuous sutures, preferably absorbable.

i. Mobilize within a few days.

2. LATE DEVELOPING PROGRESSIVE WEAKNESS

Unrecognized unstable spine: This may be due to relatively mild trauma, such as forced flexion or extension while surfing, when the patient complains only of electric shocks while moving the head some time later.

Physical signs may be few at rest, although the plantar responses are usually extensor.

Lateral radiographs of the cervical spine in flexion

and extension confirm the diagnosis, with widening of the angle between the spinous processes of the affected vertebras in flexion, with often a little slip forwards of the body of the upper vertebra.

Operation:
  a. A simple midline incision, as above, baring the spinous processes.
  b. Establish the exact level by counting (C1 has no spinous process) or by lateral radiograph.
  c. Wire the spinous processes together in a simple figure-of-eight using malleable steel wire (18 SWG).
  d. Close with continuous suture.
  e. Mobilize immediately.

3. EXTRUDED DISC FROM HYPEREXTENDED SPONDYLOTIC SPINE

There is usually a clear history of trauma, although the circumstances may be lost in the post-traumatic amnesia of the associated head injury. A frontal scalp laceration or contusion is excellent evidence of the injury sustained, commonly from contact with the windscreen frame of a crashing car. There is usually evidence of at least mild cord contusion, increased leg reflexes and extensor plantar responses which may progress to weakness of the hands, spasticity of gait and incontinence of urine, accompanied by nerve root pain down the arms from the neck.

Straight radiographs may show only cervical spondylosis with osteophytes intruding into the spinal canal, usually at C5–C6. Myelography is essential. If present at the screening, the operator will appraise the situation better than by examining selected films alone.

Operation: Anterior fusion with removal of disc (*see below*). Substantial extradural and subdural collections of blood occur rarely after trauma of the spine. Haematomyelia rarely repays operation.

Cervical Spondylosis

Over the age of 50, 50 per cent of the population suffer with cervical spondylosis, with degenerative discs and osteophytic encroachment into the spinal canal. The spondylosis is usually symptomless or produces only occasional neck pain, relieved by rest, a soft collar and heat.

A minority will develop radiculopathy or myelopathy resistant to all forms of treatment except operation.

Brachial neuralgia is caused by the compression of the nerve roots by lateral extrusion of the intervertebral foramen (*Fig. 55.4*). The pain is often dull and ill defined, from the neck to the arm and hand, but paraesthetic tingling localizes the lesion well. Tingling in the thumb and forefinger is usually from

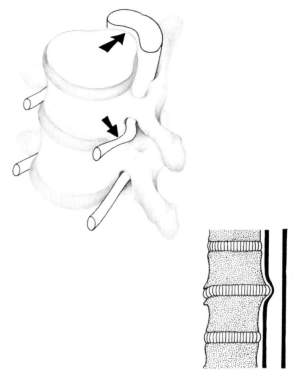

Fig. 55.4. Cervical spondylosis. Central protrusions of the disc will induce myelopathy while lateral protrusions cause brachial neuralgia.

a C5–C6 disc prolapse, while tingling in the other fingers presages a C6–C7 lesion.

The pain may be abrupt in onset and be related to mild trauma, when an acute soft disc prolapse is common, with relatively normal plain radiograph findings, except loss of lordosis and narrowed disc space. More commonly, the pain comes gradually associated with obvious spondylitic radiographic changes.

Physical signs may be few, although weakness, diminished reflexes and dermatome sensory loss characterize the severe cases.

Myelography shows a laterally placed indentation at the disc space with truncation of the nerve root.

Occasionally, in a case with well-established clinical signs myelography is normal. *Discography* can then be performed. Although often disappointing, as a last resort, it may show a disc disorder, particularly if followed by computerized axial tomographic (*CT*) scanning.

CT scanning is useful in the neck particularly for bony disorder of the canal or foramina.

In brachalgia, good plain X-ray oblique views of the foramina may hint at the best surgical approach— a very constricted foramen in unilateral brachalgia may favour posterior foraminotomy. There is frequently more than one level involved and often both sides.

In the management of brachial neuralgia operation should be recommended only after conservative measures have failed or when there is rapidly progressive weakness of the arm or legs.

Conservative Treatment

1. Rest, a firm plastic collar and mild analgesics tide most patients through an attack which may last for a few weeks only.

2. Halter traction in bed with 2·7–3·6 kg (6–8 lb) may abort a severe episode.

3. A lightweight Minerva collar (a plaster-of-Paris cast encasing the thorax, back of the neck and the forehead in one piece) is successful in long-term relief of pain in 50 per cent of intractable cases if worn for 3 months. Most patients find this to be very cumbersome, and unpleasant in hot weather.

Operative Management

On the whole, anterior fusion is more effective than cervical laminectomy, provided the cause of the pain, whether soft disc or bony osteophyte, is removed. Cloward's operation provides good access for this to be done (see below). Lateral foraminotomy, a limited posterior approach through facet joint, is useful particularly for lateral osteophytic compression of the root in brachial neuralgia.

Myelopathy due to Spondylosis

Long-standing compression of the spinal cord from spondylosis is common in the elderly. Whereas spondylitic brachial neuralgia usually affects a single level, myelopathy is commonly the result of severe constriction of the spinal canal at centrally multiple levels (Fig. 55.4).

The average true anteroposterior diameter of the narrowest part of the cervical spinal canal is 13 mm. This is reduced to 11·3 mm in brachial neuralgia and to 10 mm in myelopathy. Measurements from lateral cervical spinal radiographs should be multiplied by 5/6 to compensate for magnification.

Progressive spastic weakness of the legs, with preserved joint sensation, clonus of the ankles and extensor plantar responses, usually suggests a spondylitic myelopathy. Sensory loss to pain may be slight, or confined to one side, as in the Brown–Séquard syndrome. Continence is usually preserved.

Motor neurone disease and disseminated sclerosis may present a similar picture and may indeed coexist with spondylitic myelopathy.

Plain radiographs of the cervical spine show narrowing of the canal at one or more levels. Myelography shows central barring of the contrast column, most commonly at C3–C4, then C4–C5, C5–C6, C6–C7 in descending frequency. The contrast tends to run to either side of the central protrusion, so that the lateral views may mask a marked protrusion unless the classic double shadow (X-ray) is observed. Posterior indentations from the ligamentum flavum are often seen, and may contribute to the compression of the cord.

Management

Conservative management rarely produces reversal of spasticity. A Minerva collar improves only 30 per cent.

If the patient is to improve, operation is indicated before irreversible changes occur in the spinal cord. The patients are often frail and elderly, with bronchitic chests and prostatic hyperplasia. Nevertheless, with good anaesthesia, competent surgery and attentive postoperative care, recovery of function is surprisingly rapid, even in octogenarians.

Cervical laminectomy has its adherents, particularly if there is widespread stenosis of the spinal canal, as shown on CT scanning, but frequent success is achieved by the anterior approach with removal of the osteophytes and fusion of the appropriate levels, when 65–70 per cent will show a marked improvement in walking.

Operation: Anterior Fusion of Cervical Spine (Cloward's Operation)

Blood is rarely required. A microscope aids training in the operation, but the majority of surgeons prefer a headlight. The relevant myelogram should be available.

1. Induce anaesthesia with great care to avoid hyperextension of the neck.

2. Place patient face up on the table with a halter attached to the head and good support to the back of the neck. Slightly raise the right hip on a sandbag (Fig. 55.5).

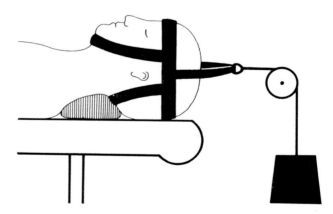

Fig. 55.5. Halter traction for Cloward's operation of cervical fusion. Adequate neck support is essential.

3. Prepare the neck and the right iliac crest.

4. Plan a collar incision from the external jugular vein to the midline, at the upper edge of the thyroid cartilage for C3–C4 and at the cricoid cartilage for C6–C7. Incise platysma.

5. Using scissors, cut the fascia along the anterior border of sternomastoid muscle and enter medially to the carotid sheath, using blunt dissection to open the avascular planes. the omohyoid muscle, the larynx and the oesophagus are retracted, exposing the anterior longitudinal ligament and the medial borders of both longus colli muscles to establish the disc spaces and the midline. Insert a lumbar puncture needle into the most likely disc space. Occasionally a breaking anterior osteophyte identifies the space by palpation, and may occlude the space itself. This should be removed with bone forceps.

6. Establish the exact level with a lateral radiograph, taking care to include C1 and C2 on the film.

7. While the radiograph is developing, expose the right iliac crest and remove as many bone dowels as are necessary from the crest.

8. Excise a narrow rectangle of anterior disc capsule at the appropriate level, and exenterate such disc material as is easily available with rongeurs.

9. Measure the body of the appropriate cervical vertebra on the lateral radiograph, correct for magnification ×5/6, and measure the amount of protrusion of the drill from the drill guide.

10. Set the drill guide with its equator on the disc space and hammer it home. Drill a core of bone to either side of the disc space. Insert the self-retaining retractor (*Fig.* 55.6)

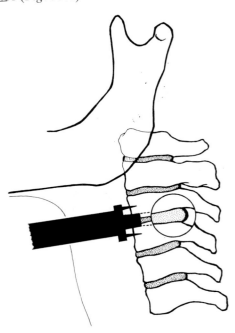

Fig. 55.6. Cloward's anterior cervical fusion showing insertion of drill guide and bit.

11. Place 10·8–12·7 kg (24–28 lb) weight on the head halter traction.

12. With the high-speed air drill, under good illumination, remove the posterior osteophytes from the cervical bodies.

13. Carefully removed extruded fragments of disc with hook, curette, punch and rongeurs, and control oozing from epidural veins.

14. Place shaped bone dowel in the hole; tap in until just under flush.

15. Suture platysma and skin.

Postoperative Care

1. Give physiotherapy to chest on night after operation.

2. Mobilize after 2 days after check radiograph of cervical spine.

3. Remove neck stitches in 5 days, iliac in 7 days.

Before discharge, gentle rotatory exercises of the neck should be taught, to combat the frequent tense ache in the back of the neck.

In younger patients, allow clerical work in 1 month, light manual work in 6 weeks and heavy manual labour in 3 months.

Rheumatoid Arthritis

The appearance of cervical spine radiographs is often more alarming than the clinical signs in this deforming disease, and over-adventurous surgery should be avoided, if only because the poor quality of the tissues makes grafting and wiring uncertain and the instability of the joints precludes laminectomy. Also the cardiovascular prognosis of disabled patients in the active phase of their disease is poor. Pain in the neck and occiput is best treated with a collar or very gentle traction.

Two conditions reward careful surgery to the cervical spine in this disease:

1. Atlanto-axial Dislocation

This may induce unconsciousness from vertebral artery occlusion on head flexion or profound tetraparesis. Lateral radiographs of the flexed neck show more (sometimes much more) than 4-mm separation between the back of the anterior arch of the atlas and the front of the odontoid process. Recently, magnetic resonance imaging (MRI) has revealed the considerable intrusion made by the soft tissue behind the odontoid, deforming the uppermost part of the spinal cord.

Operation

Posterior fusion is effective if the posterior arch of the atlas is not too attenuated; otherwise the occiput should be included in the fusion. Where MRI has shown major distortion of the anterior cord and brainstem, transoral removal of the odontoid process of C2 may be required after posterior stabilization.

2. Spontaneous Dislocation of the Mid-cervical Vertebras

Usually C3 slides forwards on C4, sharply narrowing the spinal canal. One or more other levels may be involved.

Operation should be reserved for definite weakness of the limbs, although this is frequently difficult to assess in deformed limbs, and reflex activity is often impossible to elicit.

When the signs do not fit in with the plain radiograph findings, a myelogram may be justified, since large soft extrusions can occur in this disorder from the more normal-looking spaces.

Operation

1. *Wiring of the spinous process* (q.v.) has the benefit of simplicity, where forward slip of the upper vertebra is the main feature. The wire may cut through the bone within a few weeks.

2. *Anterior fusion* is useful when a large protrusion compresses the spinal cord. Since the vertebral bodies are often small and disordered, a large keystone graft spanning three or more vertebras placed in a midline channel is more effective.

Neoplasms Affecting the Cervical Spine

Extradural Tumours

These are almost entirely metastatic lesions, predominantly from bronchus, breast and prostate. They are the most common tumours of this region of the spine, although the thoracic region is a more frequent site.

Occasionally, myeloma presents as an extradural lesion spreading from the body of a cervical vertebra, and this should be considered even in the absence of the characteristic plasma protein changes when no primary source can be discovered.

Root pain precedes paralysis, often by months. Paraplegia may occur after trivial trauma, and is probably the consequence of the collapse and extrusion backwards of the diseased body of the vertebra, with ischaemia and compression of the cord.

If complete paralysis of the limbs and bladder has been present for several hours, little is to be gained from decompressive laminectomy. The outlook for secondary carcinoma of the bronchus is particularly forlorn, and these patients should be spared unnecessary operations.

Where movement remains and the patient's general condition is good, decompressive laminectomy should be performed as an emergency. The diagnosis is clear if there is a known primary cancer, less so if this is occult.

Careful examination will establish the level of the lesion both by weakness and sensory loss extending to the dermatomes of the upper limbs.

Plain radiographs usually establish the diagnosis with loss of the crisp view, and wedging collapse of the body of the vertebra on the lateral. Myelography is not often required, but a chest radiograph is essential. CT scanning will reveal the extent of the tumour, not only within the spine but into the surrounding soft tissues.

Operation: Cervical or Dorsal Laminectomy (Figs. 55.7–55.9)

1. Extradural spinal tumours may bleed severely.

2. Use controlled ventilation anaesthesia and intubate carefully on account of the unstable neck.

3. Gently place the patient in the prone position with the face in a horseshoe rest, the neck slightly flexed and the chest support at the clavicular level and the iliac crests on blocks so that the abdomen hangs slack to allow easy ventilation with reduced venous pressure. Tilt the table slightly head-up, again to reduce venous pressure. The sitting position is sometimes used, but bears a high risk of air embolism. Ensure an adequate intravenous line.

4. Make a midline incision centred over the lesion, erring on the generous side. Using the cutting diathermy like a pencil, keeping close to bone, expose the spinous processes and the laminas, holding the muscles away with Mollison's self-retaining retractors. The muscle may be involved with tumour and may bleed (*Fig.* 55.7).

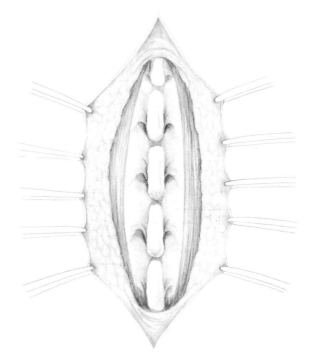

Fig. 55.7. Standard laminectomy. (The principles of this operation are similar at all levels.) The muscles have been separated from the spinous processes and laminas.

5. With the laminas bared, inspect for overt tumour; if none is apparent, gently rock the spinous

processes; where the pedicles have been invaded these are excessively mobile.

6. The laminas of the spinal canal are like slates on a roof; it is easier to remove them safely from below. Remove the spinous processes with Horsley's broad bone forceps, which have a slight curve to their long axis with a thinner underlip. Gently nibble away the lower margin of the chosen lamina across its whole width, biting the lamina away in small morsels, holding the bone forceps almost vertically in two hands (*Fig.* 55.8).

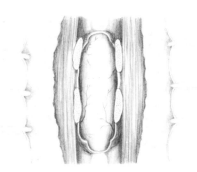

Fig. 55.8. Standard laminectomy. Removal of laminas exposes the dural tube.

7. In the ideal situation, deep to the lamina will be epidural fat and a slack, non-pulsatile dural tube. Often the extradural tumour extends below the collapsed vertebra and a solid cuff of firm tumour will be immediately encountered. Proceed upwards, removing the laminas until the upper limit of the cuff of tumour is passed; where are again seen epidural fat and a pulsating dura, Hijak punches may be used to extend laterally. Blood loss may be heavy from the disordered bone; adequate suction is essential, and a headlight often helpful. Bone wax or hydrogen peroxide packs control most of the bleeding. Unipolar diathermy near the cord should be avoided, and bipolar diathermy, which must be exact, is ineffective since there is rarely a well-defined vessel bleeding.

8. With the wound dry, the superficial portion of the firm cuff of tumour can be gently removed from the dura, which it rarely penetrates. Only limited success is possible, for the bulk of the tumour is in front of the cord in the body of vertebra, which may be apparent as a sharp hump under the dura. Remove only that which is easily accessible, without disturbing the dura.

9. Occasionally no tumour will be found on removing the first two laminas, although this is rare when a myelogram has been performed and the radiologist confirms the level of the block. When too high the dura pulsates freely and is full; when too low it is slack and pulseless. Confirmation of the site of block can be made by making a small nick in the dura, and passing a soft rubber catheter in the subdural space in the expected direction.

10. Ensure haemostasis and close the wound with a few stitches to hold the muscles together and close the space, and a firm continuous stitch to the tough fascia investing the muscles. A drain is rarely needed. Subcutaneous and skin stitches are also continuous.

Postoperative Management

1. These operations are acutely *painful*. Adequate potent analgesia is essential.
2. *Urinary retention* is common, requiring catheter drainage.
3. *Paralytic ileus* is common and distressing. Intravenous fluids will be necessary until absorption is re-established. Gastric dilatation may require a nasogastric tube.
4. *Pressure areas* must be protected if the patient is both weak and in pain on movement. A ripple bed is valuable but no substitute for 2-hourly turning.
5. *Returning limb function* should be encouraged by physiotherapy, and mobilization achieved as soon as possible.
6. *Anaemia* is common. Routine postoperative blood count is essential.
7. *Radiotherapy* is indicated for myeloma, lymphoma and solitary metastases.
8. *Hypophysectomy* often produces dramatic relief of pain and slows progression of tumour in metastases from the breast and prostate.

Intradural Tumours

These are usually benign; those extrinsic to the spinal cord usually removable by surgery, those within the cord rarely so.

Extrinsic Tumours

Neurofibromas and meningiomas predominate in the cervical and dorsal spine; neurofibromas, lipomas and dermoid cysts in the lumbar.

The history of cervical and dorsal tumours is usually of slowly progressive spastic weakness of the limbs for many months with little sensory loss and preserved bladder function. When the lesion is in the lumbar region, there is back pain which is worse at night; frequency and uncertainty of micturition are commonly associated with reduced lower limb power with diminished reflexes.

NEUROFIBROMAS

Neurofibromas may be obvious in von Recklinghausen's disease; more commonly they are solitary, or hinted at by a few inconspicuous subcutaneous lumps and *café-au-lait* patches. *Oblique* views of the appropriate spinal level often show an enlarged intervertebral foramen.

MENINGIOMAS

Meningiomas occur in the elderly.

OPERATION: CERVICAL OR DORSAL LAMINECTOMY FOR INTRADURAL TUMOUR

1. Proceed as described in steps 2–6 (p.853).

2. Incise the epidural fat in the midline, coagulating the cut epidural veins with *bipolar* diathermy; peel back the fat to expose the dural tube. The tumour may be apparent:

   a. As a deficiency (from pressure) in the fat.

   b. By a bulge, particularly laterally in neurofibromas.

   c. By a little patch of congested vessels in a meningioma.

   d. By a failure of dural pulsation.

   e. To very gentle palpation by the moistened finger.

3. A careful study of the myelogram will determine the site of opening of the dura, midline for laterally placed neurofibromas and eccentric to avoid the base of the vascular meningioma.

4. Using a sharp hook in the left hand (if right-handed), lift the dura by its outer layer. Nick the two layers of the dura with a tenotome until the clear arachnoid bulges through. Take two pairs of fine-toothed forceps and split the dura longitudinally by pulling it apart, preserving the arachnoid, and thus the spinal cord. Inspect for the tumour. Cut lateral incisions to make a flap to display the tumour and hold it back with stay sutures on forceps (*Fig.* 55.9).

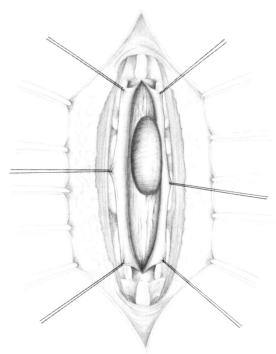

Fig. 55.9. Standard laminectomy. The dural tube is opened to reveal intradural pathology.

5. The position of the spinal cord is now crucial, since it must be preserved at all costs. If the tumour is superficial to the cord then it is readily removed with gentle dissection and bipolar diathermy.

Neurofibromas push the cord sideways, and extrude out through the intervertebral foramen as a dumbbell. It is often wise then to incise into the tumour and eviscerate it, allowing the periphery of the tumour to fall in, and enabling safe dissection from the spinal cord. Only the affected nerve root of the tumour must be sectioned.

Meningiomas may be lateral or in front of the cord. The cord can be very gently rotated by the insertion of a 3/0 atraumatic stitch into the denticulate ligament above and below the tumour, then cutting the ligament at its dural attachment. It is safer to leave some tumour than to damage the cord.

6. After removal of the tumour, suture the dura with a 3/0 atraumatic continuous stitch. A small Silastic patch, glued on with cyanomethyl acrylate, may be necessary to close a deficiency caused by meningioma attachment.

7. Close the wound.

POSTOPERATIVE MANAGEMENT

This should be uncomplicated. Mobilization should occur after the 2nd day, with the physiotherapist urging active exercise. Full recovery of cord function may take 6 months.

Intrinsic Tumours

These tumours are uncommon and are, in general, gliomas and ependymomas of low-grade malignancy. They are frequently cystic and produce slowly progressive weakness of the limbs. Myelography shows a fusiform swelling of the cord rather than a discrete block.

Operation usually confines itself to laminectomy, biopsy and aspiration of a cyst and dural decompression with a Silastic gusset sewn in. Radiotherapy is valuable in ependymomas. Rarely these can be excised from the centre of the cord, using the operating microscope and bipolar diathermy. A CO_2 laser may vaporize an intrinsic tumour without disturbing the thin shell of viable spinal cord surrounding it. An ultrasonic aspirator can perform much the same feat.

EXTRADURAL ABSCESS OF THE SPINE

Acute pyogenic infection of the spine is fortunately uncommon, but constitues a surgical emergency when it occurs. There is usually a history of infection, which may be simply a furuncle on the back, usually staphylococcal.

Severe pain in the back is almost universal, and the toxic symptoms of systemic infection are common. Weakness of the limbs is followed within hours by paraplegia, which may be irreversible. Lumbar myelography may be impossible, and cisternal myelography necessary unless the clinical diagnosis is clear, in which case laminectomy should be undertaken forthwith.

Operation

1. Proceed as for standard laminectomy. A generous incision should be made.
2. After the removal of one lamina, a gush of pus is usual, and this should be sent immediately for Gram stain and culture. Rarely the pus is subdural, when this layer should be incised.
3. Adequate decompression of the cord may require four or five laminas to be removed.
4. Soft rubber catheters are placed into the extradural space and the area irrigated with 1 mega unit (1M) of penicillin in 10 ml of saline. Appropriate antibiotics are started after the bacteriology report.
5. The wound is closed with the catheters *in situ* extending through the skin.

Postoperative Management

1. Treat with the appropriate bacteriocidal antibiotic, both intravenously and into the catheters.
2. Keep in bed until the infection is settled. Retention, ileus and paralysis may need the care outlined above.
3. Deal with the primary focus of infection.

VASCULAR LESIONS OF THE SPINAL CORD

Ischaemic strokes of the cord are common in the elderly. Surgically remediable vascular lesions are rare.

Spontaneous Extradural Haematoma

This uncommon cause for rapid paraplegia is a surgical emergency. It occurs in middle-aged hypertensives and the young with small angiomas. There is an abrupt onset of severe spinal pain followed by weakness developing usually within a few hours. Urgent myelography and laminectomy will restore function in the majority. An angioma can be excised and is often only apparent as a small collection of bleeding vessels.

Spinal Cord Angioma

This may present as a subarachnoid haemorrhage, with sudden severe pain, or as a progressive loss of cord function, with step-like deterioration. Occasionally a stroke-like episode occurs, with a stable plateau thereafter. The arteriovenous malformation invests the cord, fed from one or more main arterial sources, which must be identified by painstaking selective spinal angiography, if operation is to be usefully performed. It is a matter of judgement whether this is indicated.

Operation

This consists of laminectomy and identification of the feeding vessels, ligation of those arteries and removal of the redundant vessels.

DISORDERS OF THE THORACIC SPINAL REGION

Tumours

Both extradural and intradural tumours are more common in this area than in the cervical. Their treatment is identical.

Thoracic Disc Protrusion

The thoracic spinal canal is narrow, the spinal cord tight within it and thoracic discs calcified. This dangerous combination renders simple laminectomy unsafe. The most common levels are D9–D10, D10–D11, where the main arterial supply to the lower cord enters.

Diagnosis is by plain radiograph, which shows degeneration and calcification, tomography (plain and CT) and myelography.

Operation

This is usually achieved through the thorax, taking care to identify the exact level by on table radiography. The calcified disc is allowed to fall back into a cavity made in the adjacent vertebral body by a high speed drill.

Kyphoscoliosis with Cord Compression

The management of this condition is primarily orthopaedic. Rarely an uncorrectable kyphosis will require a long laminectomy and longitudinal incision of the dural tube which has bow-stringed across the curve compressing the cord. A generous Silastic gusset is used to enlarge the dural tube capacity.

SURGERY OF THE LUMBAR SPINE

Spina Bifida

Few surgical manoeuvres have been more prey to enthusiasm and fashion as the correction of spina bifida aperta. The closure of the sac is relatively simple, but the selection of the patient is difficult. Well-defined criteria for operation have been worked out, and their application will allow surgery in only about 10 per cent of cases. The majority of the remainder should be allowed to die of meningitis within a few weeks.

Criteria for Operation

The infant should have:

1. Either a meningocele without a mural plaque (*Fig.* 55.10).

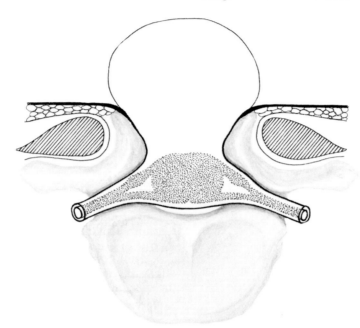

Fig. 55.10. Meningocele.

2. Or a meningomyelocele (*Fig.* 55.11).
   i. Reasonable movement in the lower limbs.
   ii. No gross skeletal deformity.
   iii. No severe hydrocephalus (2 cm beyond the 90th percentile).
   iv. No other severe congenital disorder.
   v. No infection.

The closure of the defect in these babies is the first operation of many in the overall management, which frequently requires correction of supervening hydrocephalus, joint deformity and ureteric reflux. Multidisciplinary spina bifida units are now common.

Sites

The most common is lumbosacral, followed by thoracolumbar and finally cervical.

Type

MENINGOCELE

The laminas are splayed apart, and the dural tube opens out into a wide sac, tenuously covered with arachnoid mater. The neural elements remain unharmed deep within the sac.

MENINGOMYELOCELE

This, unfortunately the most common congenital deformity in Western countries (up to 4 per 1000 live births), consists of the opening out of the spinal cord like a filleted kipper, so that the nerve roots dangle from the undersurface of the neural plaque, which may be slight or voluminous. The size of the defect in the skin may be very large.

Surgical Tactics

Where operation is indicated, it should proceed within the first 36 hours of life, or infection may supervene. Neurological disorder will not be improved by operation. The object is to fashion a dural tube around the defect and to cover it with viable skin, even at the expense of skin cover elsewhere. Commitment to close the defect logically imposes surgical treatment of other disorders and the parents must understand and agree to this before the first operation is embarked on.

Operation

1. PREPARATION

a. The infant should be kept in an incubator until placed on a heated blanked in the operating theatre, and wrapped in tinfoil. Maternal blood may be grouped for cross-matching, but blood loss should be minimal.

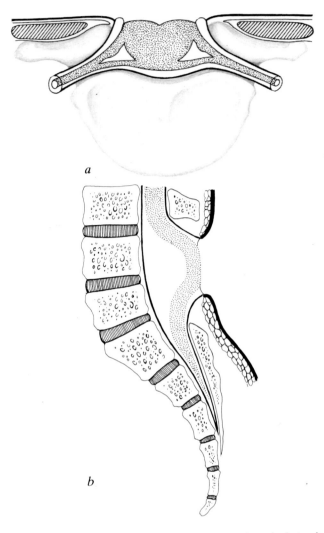

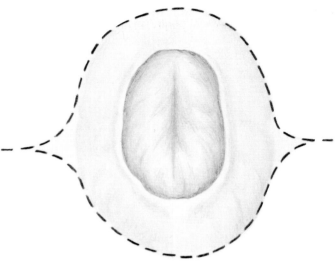

Fig. 55.12. Incision for raising skin flaps which will close meningomyelocele.

Fig. 55.11. Meningomyelocele. *a*, Transverse view. *b*, Lateral view.

b. In experienced hands, general anaesthesia is possible; the operation can proceed easily under local anaesthesia using 5 ml of 0·5 per cent Xylocaine (lignocaine) subcutaneously where the incision is made. Local anaesthetic into the sac can cause a considerable drop in blood pressure. A teat filled with dilute sweetened brandy keeps the baby well sedated.

c. Place the baby face down with small pads under the iliac crest to allow easy breathing. Plan the incision carefully to minimize skin loss and allow for one or more relieving incisions if necessary. Clean the back carefully, preserving the exposed neural element, if present. Drape with enough skin exposed to allow for a relieving incision.

2. EXCISION (*Fig.* 55.12)

a. Incise normal skin and close to the neck of the sac, to produce ultimately a linear closure under no tension. Coagulate bleeding points with bipolar diathermy or low-power unipolar diathermy.

b. Define the neck of the sac with its opened-out dural tube, exposing the lumbar fascia, heaped over the splayed-out cartilaginous ends of the laminas.

With a *meningocele*, incise the sac leaving an ample collar to fashion a dural tube, encasing the intact neural elements, by a continuous vertical atraumatic 4/0 or 5/0 silk suture. Reinforce the dural tube with a waistcoat of lumbar fascia flapped across from either side, if necessary.

With a *meningomyelocele*, skirt around the perimeter of the neural plaque, allowing it to drop with its roots into the dural groove. If possible, fashion a dural tube from a layer superficial to the lumbar fascia, continuous with the dura. Reinforce the tube with a fascial waistcoat, if necessary, excising extruding cartilaginous spears.

3. SKIN CLOSURE

Undermine the skin widely along the lumbar fascia and over the gluteal muscles, leaving the thick fat adherent to the skin. If the wound will close without tension, suture the skin with a subcuticular absorbable material (e.g. Dexon) and adhesive strips to the skin. If there is, as is usual with a big defect, too much tension (shown by blanching of the skin), fashion one or more relieving incisions parallel to the proposed line of skin suture, and far enough away not to expose the dural tube or endanger the viability of the skin bridge. Undermine the skin bridge completely. Then close the defect as indicated. Leave the relieving incision open, and dress with water-soluble gauze.

Postoperative Care

1. Replace the baby immediately into a warm incubator.
2. Watch for development of hydrocephalus and urine retention.

THE LUMBAR DISC

Lumbar Disc Prolapse

Prolapse is common. Although many lay people, and some doctors, vaguely refer to back pain as 'slipped disc', the clinical syndrome of an acute lumbar disc prolapse is usually crisp and recognizable. The majority of lumbar disc prolapses occurs at the two lower spaces, namely L4–L5 and L5–S1, and usually only one disc is involved as a cause of the present symptoms. However, a prolapse at the adjacent space, often many years previously, may lead to loss of disc height, loss of mobility and joint sclerosis at that space, throwing extra strain on the adjacent space. This extra range of movement, coupled with a localized annular weakness which is a necessary precondition for disc prolapse, is more likely to lead to prolapse than if the adjacent space had been able to carry out its full movement range.

Diagnosis

The diagnosis depends on the complaint of sciatica, which is a pain down the back of the leg, in buttock, thigh, and outer calf to heel. The pain itself rarely goes into the foot. In disc prolapse back pain is usually outweighed by the pain in the leg. If the pain in the back is worse than the pain in the leg, the diagnosis is unlikely to be one of disc prolapse. The pain is usually severe, made worse by coughing, sneezing, straining at stool, lying on the side of the sciatica and by travelling in motor cars or sitting on low chairs. It is usually improved by bedrest, lying on the side opposite to the pain, lying on the floor or an extremely hard bed perhaps with underlying boards, and sometimes by walking about, often at night. The patient may say that flexing the straight leg on the side opposite to that with the pain produces contralateral pain.

This picture is sufficient to make the diagnosis of a prolapsed disc very likely. However, the surgeon needs to know which nerve root is involved, namely the L5 nerve root at the L4–L5 interspace or the S1 nerve root at the L5–S1 interspace. This information is often provided by careful enquiry about numbness or tingling, usually in the foot. The L5 territory usually involves the big toe, or at least the medial

side of the foot and toes. The S1 territory comprises the lateral sole on the little toe side. Similarly, on the motor side eversion and dorsiflexion of the foot and toes are an L5 function, whereas plantarflexion is an S1 function. The best test for these motor functions consists in making the patient walk on tiptoe and on the heel when minor degrees of weakness, sometimes missed on bed testing, will emerge. Beware, however, of interpreting movement limitation due to pain as that due to weakness. Reflex change is not often found with a L5 nerve root lesion but absence of the ankle jerk (S1) or depression compared with contralateral fellow. Do not forget to inspect the perineum, for involvement of perineal nerves is an absolute indication for speedy (within hours) intervention as the function in the cauda equina compressed acutely by a central disc prolapse recovers poorly with desperate long-term consequences in sphincter and sexual function.

The diagnosis of disc prolapse is confirmed by lumbar CT scanning. The prolapse can often be seen when cuts sufficiently thick to give good radiological contrast on low noise (4 or 5 mm) are used. Plain radiographs are carried out just as much to exclude unexpected alternative disease of the lumbar spine as to indicate the involved space since disc narrowing is not a reliable guide to the presence of the prolapse. If there is still doubt about the diagnosis after CT scanning, then myelography (radiculography), nowadays using water-soluble contrast (Niopam, Omnypaque, Amipaque), will sometimes reveal a disc which is not apparent on CT scan. However, the reverse is often true, namely that a CT scan will reveal a disc which is not visible even on careful and expert myelography. This is especially true of the lateral prolapse which may take place into the intervertebral foramen, and which causes root compression at one segmental level higher than expected.

Conservative Treatment

The treatment is determined by the clinical course. It is conventional to prescribe bed rest with analgesics for a short time. If the patient improves conservatism should be persisted with, except in one circumstance. This is where the severe sciatica is suddenly succeeded by loss of pain and the onset of severe foot drop or paralysis of plantarflexion. The interpretation here is that the prolapse has moved out further and has abolished nerve function in the stretched nerve root, overwhelming the pain mechanisms. The indication here is for immediate operation to preserve nerve root function. Patients who are disabled by pain, and who are worsening or not improving, deserve surgical treatment (microdiscectomy). Traction is usually ineffective, epidural anaesthesia is capricious and irrelevant, and manipulation is absolutely contra-indicated.

On *examination* the signs are on the one hand of movement limitation, and on the other of impairment of nerve root function (neurological signs). Movement limitation is usually immediately obvious when the patient enters the consulting room. He or she will wish to sit on a high rather than a low chair, will have a stiff lumbar spine on forward bending often with a scoliosis, straight-leg raising will be impaired to less than 40°, sometimes with exacerbation of sciatica on raising the contralateral straight leg. The patient will be unable to sit on the couch to a right angle and the ability to turn over, except by holding himself or herself extremely stiffly, is visibly absent. The neurological signs are as already described.

Operative Treatment: Microdiscectomy

The operation of choice for neurosurgeons for lumbar disc prolapse is a microdiscectomy which supersedes the hemilaminectomy which has been the standard procedure since the description of disc prolapse in the early 1930s. This is as applicable to the emergency of acute central disc prolapse as to the less urgent lateral prolapse.

The operation of microdiscectomy is usually carried out under general anaesthesia and in the prone position. Local anaesthesia is surprisingly efficacious until one comes to manipulate the stretched nerve root. Even by injecting local anaesthesia into it, it is extremely difficult to produce analgesia, so that the exposure of the offending disc may be compromised by the patient's discomfort. The lateral position (offending side uppermost) is favoured by some. When prone, the patient is raised on blocks to elevate thorax and anterior superior iliac spines above the level of the operating table to avoid compression of the abdominal contents and great veins, which produces a high venous pressure inside the spinal canal. The level of the superior margin of the iliac crests laterally is marked, the interval between the spines of L4 and L5 being approximately 1 cm below this. A midline incision approximately 4 cm long is drawn on the skin after preparation and towelling, and a thick lumbar puncture needle is introduced just to one side of the midline to act as a radiological marker in a lateral horizontal beam radiograph taken to make quite certain of the level of the incision. After local anaesthetic infiltration a skin incision is made to the level of the lumbar fascia and retractors are inserted. The lumbar fascia is divided approximately 1 cm lateral to the midline, and the small flap of lumbar fascia held back over the contralateral side with stay sutures. This incision runs from the junction of the upper third and lower two-thirds of the spine above, to a similar situation on the vertebra below. The muscle is then detached from the midline by blunt dissection either with the finger or a slim osteotome, dividing the muscular insertions with scissors. The osteotome then scrapes muscle and fascia from the lower margin of the vertebral lamina above, from the ligamentum flavum between the two neural arches, and from the upper margin of the vertebra lamina below. A special self-retaining retractor is now inserted into the interspace and opened. The remainder of the operation is carried out using the operating microscope.

The bone is removed with an angled punch. Approximately 0·5 cm of the lateral inferior hemilaminar fringe is removed, stopping just short of the upper margin of the ligamentum flavum. With a sharp tenotome and hook this ligament is divided until the appearance of greyish-yellow extradural fat, being the signal that the spinal canal has been opened. With the sharp hook now putting the ligament on the stretch, the ligamentum flavum is divided as laterally as possible, laterally and inferiorly to the upper border of the lamina below, and is turned posteromedially as a flap and preserved. The nerve root is now explored with a slim metal sucker/retractor in the left hand and a dissector in the right. The nerve root is usually stretched tightly over the subjacent prolapse which, if it has penetrated the posterior longitudinal ligament, is referred to as a 'sequestrum' or 'free' prolapse. More frequently, however, the stretched and thinned posterior longitudinal ligament has confined the disc prolapse which has emerged through the hole in the annulus fibrosus, which is an invariable condition of the prolapse. This hole is usually penetrable by the dissector thrust without undue force through the thinnest portion of the posterior longitudinal ligament. By drawing the nerve root medially with the retractor/sucker the breach in the posterior longitudinal ligament which the dissector has made is enlarged, and out through it bulges the fibrocartilaginous degenerate nuclear disc fragments which form the prolapse. These are evacuated by hooks and curettes. When the superficial disc fragments have been removed it is usually possible to see into the disc space through the annular rent. Curettes and disc rongeurs are now used to exentrate the disc, stopping short of disturbing the cartilaginous end plates. The aim is to make certain that there are no further loose disc fragments to emerge through the same annular hole to compress the suprajacent nerve root. Great care is taken to seek any remaining disc fragments elsewhere in the canal or under the posterior longitudinal ligament. The nerve root should now be quite slack and the wound is closed.

The ligamentum flavum is allowed to fall back into place, the retractors are withdrawn, the lumbar fascia is closed with heavy interrupted silk sutures, and the superficial fatty layers are apposed with interrupted polyglycolate sutures. The skin is closed with subcuticular polyglycolate which does not need a removal.

POSTOPERATIVE CARE

Postoperative discomfort with a small incision and by this technique using the operating microscope is usually slight. This is not always the case, however, but the majority of patients will wish to be up and about by the 3rd postoperative day, and will not be averse to returning home on the 4th or 5th day after operation. The operation has been carried out on day cases with satisfactory results.

COMPLICATIONS

These are few. The first is re-prolapse. This can be early or late. Early prolapse (in the first year after surgery) is almost certainly due to more disc material emerging through the same annular hole at the same disc interspace. If the latter, especially after several years, it is worth while making certain that the symptoms are identical. Even if they are there is no guarantee that prolapse at the same space is responsible for these and it would be wise to reinvestigate thoroughly. Infection is rare. A more common source of postoperative discomfort is what is known as a 'closed disc syndrome'. This is a well-defined clinical picture, coming on at any time in the first 4 postoperative weeks and characterized by a movement-related transverse backache of agonizing spasms often radiating into the groins. Sciatica is not a feature. ESR, blood viscosity measurements and full blood count are performed to make sure than an infection is not present. The treatment is bedrest, sometimes for several weeks. These patients eventually make an excellent recovery.

Clinical Course

The sciatica is usually relieved at once by operation. Rehabilitation usually needs no special physiotherapy beyond instructions in how to excercise weak back muscles. However, as wound strength reaches maximum only after 6 weeks, it is prudent to advise against severe muscular activity before this time. Violent or contact sports are discouraged for at least 3 months after surgery.

The major problem in surgery for prolapsed lumbar disc is in patient selection, together with a recognition that some patients may be made worse by disc surgery. These are patients who have an interesting and largely unstudied condition called 'non-disc sciatica', which is sometimes impossible clinically to differentiate from true disc prolapse. Happily, these patients do very well with exploration so long as the essentially normal disc is not interfered with in any way. Equally, a disc bulge is not a prolapse. A prolapse is a condition where degenerate nuclear disc fragments prolapse through an annular hole. It is extremely doubtful whether nerve root compression is ever produced by a bulging disc, since the disc bulges are mostly over the central portion of the annulus, and nerve root symptoms arise from compression of the nerve roots laterally. Certainly, a bulging disc should never be incised. It is not a pathological condition, and sciatica in these cases is due to 'non-disc sciatica'. Sometimes patients with this condition are explored since the clinical picture, CT scan and myelogram all misleadingly indicate a disc which is not, in fact, prolapsed. It is the duty of the surgeon to recognize when this is the case, and to refrain from incising a perfectly normal disc, having first made certain that he or she is, in fact, exploring the correct interspace.

Lumbar Stenosis

In any population there is a wide spectrum of the internal diameters of the spinal canal. In later life osteophytic overgrowth, due to osteoarthropathy particularly at the posterolateral synovial articulations and also at the disc margins, may produce a narrowing of the spinal canal generally, and also in the lateral angles in particular. This degenerative process usually produces a trefoil-like spinal canal in which there is insufficient room for the cauda equina to flourish. The symptoms produced are those of leg pain, sometimes like a classic sciatica. The syndrome of 'intermittent claudication of the cauda equina' is one such clinical group. Others are the patients who develop leg pain on walking, but who can cycle in the flexed position for many miles. Walking with a forward stoop sometimes helps the pain. In others there is movement limitation of marked degree. The clinical picture is quite unlike disc prolapse in this respect, the patients with narrow canals usually have objective weakness and wasting with sensory loss and reflex change, and very little movement limitation to the tests of forward bending of the spine and straight-leg raising. The picture is often asymmetrical. The disease is not due to disc prolapse. Lumbar stenosis is a mid-lumbar disease, the L4–L5 level common to both prolapse and stenosis.

Treatment

Treatment is by a laminectomy, the bony removal being taken out laterally in order to open up the lateral canals formed by encroachment on nerve roots by osteophytes from behind. The anterior osteophytes are not interfered with. To do so would hazard the wellbeing of the immediately adjacent nerve roots. The laminas and posterior osteophytes are removed with laminectomy rongeurs, but for the lateral canals containing the nerve root, judicious shaving with a sharp osteotome and a cautiously wielded hammer is the best and safest method. Guided by the myelogram or CT scan it is usually unnecessary to do a full laminectomy of the whole of the lumbar spine, but best simply to select the levels at which compression is taking place and deal with these.

Postoperative Care

Postoperative care of these patients is straightforward. If there has been little structural interference with the stability of the spine, mobilization can be governed entirely by the postoperative discomfort in the wound. For instance, in elderly males and females there may be postoperative difficulty in emptying the bladder voluntarily. If unable to void in bed, with analgesics and good nursing, they can be helped to a bedside commode which often obviates the need for a catheter. Further mobilization proceeds in the same way. Despite their age these patients are often ready to leave hospital after 1 week, but some need a rather longer period. They are not encouraged to bend the back, or carry out extension exercises but simply to readopt ordinary life gradually over the next 3–6 weeks. Walking range dramatically increases, and power and sensation in the legs improve, although more slowly over the months.

The results of this kind of surgery are normally extremely gratifying and long-lasting. However, it is necessary to be precise about the site of compression and the bone removal needed to relieve it. If a patient with intermittent claudication is not relieved after surgery, it is wise to check the levels operated on and check the diagnosis. One group of patients particularly is difficult to treat, namely those with achondroplasia in whom the spinal canal from top to bottom is of very constricted diameter and in whom degenerative cord and cauda equina compression can arise in early middle rather than in later life.

Trauma to the Lumbar Spine

This most frequently takes the form of crushing of the vertebral bodies in falls landing on the feet, or of rupture of the transverse processes. Operation is rarely required.

Occasionally, an unstable fracture dislocation of the thoracolumbar junction requires stabilization, with plates across the spinous processes, but the majority of these lesions can be managed conservatively.

Tumours of the Lumbar Spine

Extradural Tumours

The most frequent tumours are metastases from carcinoma of the bronchus, breast and prostate. Root pain often precedes neurological disorder by several weeks and may be intractable, since the tumour arises in the body and spreads in a cuff around the dural tube and roots, being largely irremovable.

The signs are those of conus medullaris of cauda equina compression, with flaccid weakness and sensory loss of the lower limbs and overflow incontinence of urine and faeces.

If these signs have persisted for more than a day, decompressive surgery is of little avail.

Straight radiographs (including chest) usually make the diagnosis; myelography may be unnecessary or impossible because of the tumour.

Decompressive laminectomy (as for stenosis) should be performed if there is residual movement and if the patient is not moribund.

Radiotherapy is indicated in myeloma and may relieve pain in metastatic cancer.

Hypophysectomy may induce dramatic and prolonged pain relief, as may stilboestrol in prostatic carcinoma.

Intradural Tumours

These are, in general, benign and, depending on their nature and position, may or may not be removable.

1. *Tumours Associated with Congenital Anomalies*

DERMOID CYSTS

Mild back pain associated with slowly progressive weakness of the legs and urinary incontinence in predominantly young patients characterizes this lesion. A midline sinus which may cause infection and even meningitis is common.

The straight radiographs show enlargement of the spinal canal with thinned pedicles. Myelography may be hazardous.

Surgical Management:
   a. Treat the infection if present with specific antibiotics.
   b. Excise the lesion, if possible, by judicious laminectomy, expose enough dura to remove the cyst from the roots of the cauda equina. Close the dura, using a graft if necessary.

2. *Lipomas*

These may be heralded by a subcutaneous lipoma in the midline over the lumbar region, and they may have a dumbbell shape, with an isthmus at the laminas and an intradural extension. From time to time, the lipoma involves the conus medullaris so intimately that no place of cleavage can be made.

OPERATION

Excise the lipoma, following it down through the laminas. After opening the dural tube, great care is advised to identify and save the conus of the spinal cord and the roots of the cauda equina. Close the dural tube.

3. *Extrinsic Intradural Tumours*

A. EPENDYMOMAS

These glial tumours arise typically in the filum terminale, and present with dull back pain, often while lying in bed at night, and progressive incontinence, with mild limb weakness. The pain may exist for years before physical signs unequivocally demonstrate that this is not yet another patient with nondescript backache. Often in retrospect, the canal is seen to be a little wide and the pedicles narrow on a straight radiograph. Occasionally these tumours erode bone, producing enormous cavities in the bodies of the vertebras or the sacrum, reminiscent of a haematogenous bone cyst.

Operative Management: Laminectomy with total excision should be the aim, but if the tumour has widely eroded into bone, or if it extends upwards to involve the conus, total excision is impossible. Radiotherapy is then beneficial.

i. Prepare and carry out laminectomy as for stenosis, sparing all but the laminas overlying the tumour.

ii. Open the dura with a tenotome and then, by pulling the sides apart, achieve a vertical slit. Place hitch stitches in the dura. Identify the elliptical tumour, tethered in the midline by the filum terminale, which should be cut below the tumour. Lift the lower pole out by the filum and gently free it from its bed. Carefully delineate the upper pole, and if separate from the conus of the cord, excise the whole tumour. If there is no plane between cord and tumour, excise what is safe, leaving the rest for radiotherapy.

iii. Close the dura and the wound.

B. NEUROFIBROMAS (SCHWANNOMAS)

These present in a similar fashion to ependymomas, although they do not grow so large, may be associated with multiple neurofibromatosis, or at least with *café-au-lait* patches, and cause discrete areas of anaesthesia or weakness from the affected roots.

Operative Management: This is the same as for ependymoma except that excision is usually total, sacrificing the nerve root involved. Radiotherapy is not required.

POSTOPERATIVE MANAGEMENT

For all major lumbar laminectomies, there should be gradually increasing mobility over the course of 10 days. Postoperative retention of urine is the most frequent complication, which usually clears after 3–4 days' catheterization, unless delayed by infection.

SURGICAL TREATMENT OF PAIN

Surgery for pain can be readily divided into that which seeks to remove the cause of the pain and that which deals with the pain alone. The former is more frequently successful. Assaults on the nervous system to provide pain relief are characterized by high failure rate and short-lived effectiveness. Analgesics are improving continually.

Three pain-relieving procedures have stood the test of time and warrant description in a general text:

1. Treatment of trigeminal nerve lesion.
2. Percutaneous cordotomy.
3. Open cordotomy.

Trigeminal Neuralgia

Tic douloureux is a lancinating pain arising from a discrete area of the face, often by the angle of the mouth, of excruciating severity sufficient to drive sufferers to the brink of suicide or starvation, since the act of talking or chewing will precipitate an attack. On examination there is no objective neurological impairment.

In recent years carbamazepine (Tegretol) has controlled the majority of episodes, although some patients develop a troublesome ataxia, which prevents them taking the drug. There are remissions, often of long periods.

In intractable cases, selective destruction of the appropriate part of the trigeminal nerve is useful, in general beginning peripherally and working centrally if no gain is made. The corneal reflex should be preserved if possible. Denervation can be unpleasant, and the wooden feeling of numbness (anaesthesia dolorosa) is, at times, bitterly resented and has little hope of cure. This should be discussed with the patient before an apparently minor procedure is undertaken.

Local injection

a. A remission may be precipitated by the simple injection of local anaesthetic into the appropriate foramen (supraorbital, infraorbital, mental, inferior dental and ovale).

b. Longer-lasting relief may ensue from the injection of a small quantity of absolute alcohol (0·2–0·5 ml).

Local Avulsion

The supraorbital and infraorbital nerves may be avulsed by exposing them (through the upper gingival sulcus in the case of the infraorbital), grasping them with artery forceps and winching them out like rolling up a sardine can lid. This produces profound analgesia of long standing, but protects the cornea.

A transitory complication is the development of herepes simplex in the denervated area lasting a few days.

Trigeminal Ganglion and Mandibular Division Lesion

Chemical ablation with absolute alcohol or phenol (0·1 ml of 3 per cent phenol in glycerin) has long been practised but is relatively non-discriminatory. A modern refinement of this needle technique is the radio-frequency lesion.

TECHNIQUE

a. Premedicate the patient with an analgesic.

b. Provide intravenous anaesthesia sufficient to induce sleep with rapid reversal.

c. Insert 18 G needle, insulated except for 3-mm tip, along the plane of the illustration until the foramen ovale is penetrated through the base of the skull (*Fig.* 55.13).

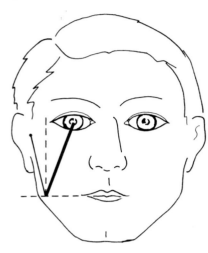

Fig. 55.13. Surface markings and direction of needle for injection of trigeminal ganglion via the foramen ovale.

d. Check position of needle with base and lateral skull radiograph. The tip of the needle should be at the back of the clivus.

e. Wake up the patient. Stimulate with 50 Hz seeking to get an exact reference to the trigger area at 0·1–0·2 V.

f. After adjustment of the needle tip, make a 60-sec lesion, with a temperature probe inserted, seeking 65 °C.

This technique frequently produces long-lasting pain relief with no loss of sensation.

Intracranial Operations

Intracranial operations are rarely needed.

Spinal Cord Lesions

In general, cordotomy can be relied on to give pain relief for a maximum of 2 years, and frequently provides less. Consequently, it is of maximum benefit in the intractable unilateral pain of cancer, when it may be exceptionally effective, allowing freedom of movement and abandonment of opiates.

Recent work has shown the astonishing heterogenicity of cord anatomy, so that it is not surprising that cordotomy, open or closed, has only a 70 per cent success rate. The spinothalamic tract crosses

early to the opposite anterolateral column of the cord, in most cases. Open cordotomy tends to last longer, but is a more major procedure and cannot easily be repeated.

Percutaneous Cordotomy Technique

1. Lay the patient face up on a radio-translucent headrest. Provide intravenous anaesthesia for rapid reversal.

2. With image intensification, insert an 18 G needle laterally between the laminas of C1 and C2 to enter the CSF just above the midline, on the opposite side of the neck to the pain.

3. Instil a few drops of emulsified Myodil to identify the ligamentum denticulatum at the equator of the spinal cord. Establish the tip of the guide needle on anteroposterior viewing at the lateral border of the odontoid.

4. With the 18 G needle in position, insert a fine electrode with a 3-mm bare tip into the spinal cord.

5. Check the impedance (if 600–900 ohm, there is no CSF leak).

6. Stimulate at 50 Hz, seeking a tingling feeling in the painful area at 0·2–0·4 V. Adjust position as necessary.

7. When a satisfactory position has been achieved, test and make a radio-frequency lesion at 70 °C for 60 sec. This achieves an elliptical necrotic area of about 4 mm wide and 5 mm long. Test sensation again.

Postoperative Care

The patient is often weak for a day or so, with headache from CSF loss, relieved by lying flat. Mild weakness of the ipsilateral limbs occurs in 30 per cent of cases lasting for some days. Sensory loss may be slight.

The major danger is depression of ventilation, and patients with carcinoma of the lung may die in their sleep from failing respiration. If all is well, the patient is home in 3 days.

Open Cervicothoracic Cordotomy

This operation achieves the same results as percutaneous cordotomy. It cannot control as high a level of pain, since it is effective a few segments below the cord incision. The recovery period is longer than percutaneous cordotomy.

Technique

1. Prepare as for laminectomy. Check with cervicothoracic radiographs that there is no obvious spinal metastasis. Blood is rarely needed.

2. Remove the laminas of T2–C7.

3. Open the dura. Identify the denticulate ligament of the side opposite to the pain, and hitch with

a 4/0 atraumatic silk stitch. Cut the ligament off the inner surface of the dura and gently rotate the cord.

4. Incise with a cordotomy knife or tenotomy 4 mm in and destroy the appropriate anterolateral column of the spinal cord.

5. Close the dura and the wound.

Postoperative Care

The care is as for standard laminectomy, and the patient should be home in 10 days. Sensory loss is more marked than with percutaneous cordotomy and patients should be warned that they may not feel hot water with the foot.

Other forms of surgical pain relief such as subdural and extradural stimulation, midline section of the spinal cord and intracerebral implanted electrodes have not given long-standing benefit in sufficient cases to warrant their general use.

The account of Lumbar Disc Prolapse and of Lumbar Stenosis in this chapter was contributed by H. M. Griffith.

Chapter fifty-six

The Autonomic Nervous System

R. C. N. Williamson

The autonomic nervous system supplies the viscera, glands and non-skeletal muscles of the body. The system comprises independent sympathetic and parasympathetic moieties, whose functions are generally antagonistic. The operative procedures described in this chapter involve ablation of various efferent sympathetic pathways (sympathectomy), usually to reduce vasoconstrictor tone or sweating in the extremities.

Upper thoracic and lumbar sympathetic ganglionectomy denervates the upper and lower limbs respectively. Division of the superior hypogastric plexus (presacral neurectomy) may control pain arising from diseased pelvic viscera. Although obsolete, extended upper thoracic sympathectomy has been performed for angina pectoris, and thoracolumbar sympathectomy (plus splanchnicectomy) has been performed for essential hypertension or the relief of

pain from chronic pancreatitis. Vagotomy, however, which produces parasympathetic denervation of most of the abdominal viscera, is traditionally a part of surgical gastroenterology and is described in Chapters 12 and 13.

ANATOMY OF THE SYMPATHETIC NERVOUS SYSTEM

The Thoracolumbar Outflow (Fig. 56.1)

Efferent sympathetic (visceral) pathways, unlike those of the somatic nervous system, are interrupted by a peripheral synapse; two neurones are thus interposed between the central nervous system and the effector organ. Cell bodies of the primary (connector) neurones are located in the lateral grey column of

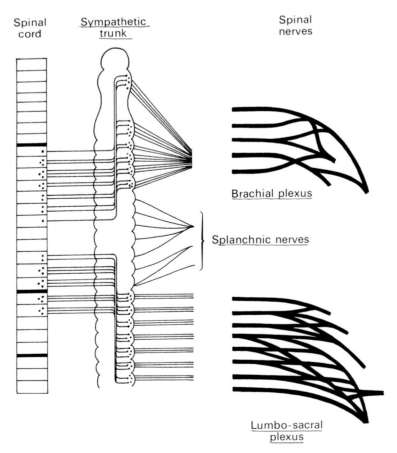

Fig. 56.1. Efferent sympathetic pathways to the upper and low limb. The splanchnic nerves are also shown.

the spinal cord from the 1st thoracic to the 2nd lumbar segments. Myelinated preganglionic axons pass by the anterior spinal nerve roots and their white rami communicantes to relay with secondary (excitor) neurones in ganglia, lying either at different levels of the sympathetic trunk or in one of the major visceral plexuses.

Non-myelinated postganglionic fibres either return by grey rami communicantes, to be distributed with the spinal nerves, or pass directly to the effector organs by visceral and vascular branches. As several postganglionic fibres synapse with a single connector fibre, the sympathetic output is diffused.

The Sympathetic Trunks

These ganglionated nerve chains extend on either side of the vertebral column from the base of the skull to the front of the coccyx, where they join to form the terminal ganglion impar. Within the chest each trunk lies anterior to the heads of the ribs, and within the abdomen it lies anterolateral to the vertebral bodies. Though variable in number, there are usually 3 cervical, 11 thoracic, 4 lumbar and 4 sacral ganglia. The inferior cervical and the 1st thoracic ganglia are normally fused to form the cervicothoracic (stellate) ganglion which lies in front of the neck of the 1st rib on either side, and through which passes the entire sympathetic supply to the head and neck.

Innervation of the Limbs

Preganglionic fibres supplying the upper limb arise from the upper six thoracic segments of the spinal cord and ascend the sympathetic trunk to synapse in the cervicothoracic and middle cervical ganglia. Incomplete sympathetic denervation of the arm follows stellate ganglionectomy alone, however, because of additional postganglionic fibres that pass to the nerves of the brachial plexus from the 2nd and 3rd thoracic ganglia. Complete denervation is achieved by removal of the lower portion of the stellate ganglion and the sympathetic chain down to and including the 3rd thoracic ganglion. Additional excision of the 4th ganglion denervates the breast and axillary region, and of the 5th ganglion, the heart. Preservation of the inferior cervical ganglion and the white ramus arising from T1 prevents the development of Horner's syndrome.

Preganglionic fibres supplying the lower limb arise from the 10th thoracic to the 2nd lumbar segments of the spinal cord and relay segmentally in the lumbar (and sacral) ganglia of the trunk. Thereafter, postganglionic fibres are distributed by the spinal nerves as in the upper limb. Removal of the upper three lumbar ganglia will denervate the lower limb, but bilateral damage to the 1st lumbar ganglion often interferes with ejaculation.

The sympathetic nerve supply to the arm and leg comprises vasoconstrictor fibres to blood vessels in the skin and skeletal muscles, vasodilator fibres to blood vessels in muscle only, secretomotor fibres to the eccrine sweat glands and motor fibres to the arrector pili muscles. Neurotransmission is adrenergic at vasoconstrictor and pilomotor nerve endings, but cholinergic for vasodilator, sudomotor and all preganglionic fibres.

PHYSIOLOGICAL EFFECTS OF SYMPATHECTOMY

In cases of peripheral vascular insufficiency sympathectomy is undertaken to release the physiological component of the peripheral resistance. By abolishing vasoconstrictor tone in cutaneous resistance vessels (arterioles), sympathetic denervation produces a rapid and substantial increase in blood flow to the skin, provided that the distal vascular tree is capable of undergoing dilatation. Skin temperature is also increased, but augmented flow more than compensates for the associated increase in metabolic activity. If sympathectomy is complete, the affected limb is warm, red and dry, irrespective of the ambient temperature, and gooseflesh cannot be provoked by local cooling.

After hyperaemia lasting 2–3 days, there is usually a transient rebound phase of decreased blood flow followed by a return to initial flow levels and then a gradual decrease over the next few weeks. Digital skin temperature generally remains elevated for several months, especially in the lower limb, and sweating is permanently abolished. Possible reasons for the transience of the vasomotor response include incomplete denervation, recovery of intrinsic vascular tone, increased alpha-receptor sensitivity to circulating catecholamines and progression of occlusive disease. Certainly initial postoperative hyperaemia is reduced in proportion to the fixed resistance of the proximal vascular tree. Sympathectomy does not affect arteriolar spasm, which is a local vasoconstrictive response arising independently of autonomic tone.

In contrast to the skin, blood flow to the skeletal musculature either at rest or during exercise is virtually unaffected by sympathetic denervation. Vasodilatation of muscle vessels probably depends more on local metabolic factors than on sympathetic innervation which, in any case, includes both constrictor and dilator fibres. In the presence of vascular occlusion, sympathectomy might actually divert some of the remaining blood from muscle to skin. The effect of sympathetic ablation on blood flow in collateral vessels is uncertain.

INDICATIONS FOR SYMPATHECTOMY

Atherosclerosis

Sympathectomy alone is of limited value because

vasoconstrictor tone normally makes an insignificant contribution to the fixed resistance offered by narrowed atheromatous vessels. By itself the operation has no place in the management of acute or chronic arterial insufficiency resulting from a major proximal occlusion, nor can it save a severely ischaemic limb; but in milder cases sympathectomy may provide relief from rest pain or assist healing after digital amputation for gangrene, especially where disease predominantly affects the distal arterial tree.

Sympathectomy may be indicated if the patient is too frail for arterial reconstruction or if arteriography shows that reconstruction is not practicable. It is also a useful adjunct to arterial reconstruction, since it enhances distal blood flow following removal of the fixed proximal resistance. In such cases postoperative hyperaemia, though transient, may help to ensure healing of ischaemic ulcers or areas of distal gangrene.

Sympathectomy alone is of no value in intermittent claudication. This failure might be predicted from its lack of effect on muscle blood flow.

Careful assessment of patients with frank or threatened gangrene of the lower limb is essential and should start with a full history and clinical examination to detect anaemia, heart disease, diabetes and other medical conditions common in this elderly population. Palpation of peripheral pulses and auscultation for bruits may be supplemented by the use of a Doppler ultrasound probe or a pulse-volume recorder. If arterial reconstruction is contemplated, arteriography is necessary for accurate delineation of occlusive lesions (*see* Chapter 37).

Thrombo-angiitis Obliterans (Buerger's disease)

This condition classically arises in 30–50-year-old men who are heavy cigarette smokers and is characterized by patchy gangrene of the toes resulting from distal arterial thrombosis. The arterial disease may have a vasospastic component and is often associated with migratory superficial thrombophlebitis. Marked improvement is obtained following lumbar sympathectomy, but progressive bilateral ischaemia of the extremities is the rule unless the patient stops smoking.

Raynaud's Syndrome

Raynaud's *disease* is a primary vasospastic disorder, generally affecting the hands of young women and resulting from an abnormal sensitivity of arterial smooth muscle to cold. It is a benign condition, rarely causing trophic changes. Symptoms can usually be controlled by sensible precautions to avoid cooling of the fingers, but sympathectomy may be required in severe cases to increase digital temperature and prevent triggering by cold. Long-term improvement can be anticipated after operation in no more than 50 per cent of cases.

Raynaud's *phenomenon* of episodic digital ischaemia may result from structural arterial disease (atherosclerosis, embolism, trauma, arteritis) or from haematological disorders affecting blood viscosity (polycythaemia, leukaemia, cold agglutination syndrome, cryoglobulinaemia, sickle cell disease, use of the contraceptive pill). Serious trophic changes in the fingers, often due to systemic sclerosis, may necessitate upper thoracic sympathectomy, but long-term results are disappointing owing to the extent and progression of the disease. Intra-arterial injections of reserpine offer an alternative means of therapy.

Hyperhidrosis

Local excision of skin and subcutaneous tissues often controls excessive sweating in the axilla, and topical antiperspirants and anticholinergic drugs may alleviate symptoms here or in the extremities, but sympathectomy is warranted for disabling hyperhidrosis, especially of the hands or feet.

Cold Injury

Severe cooling of the extremities can produce actual tissue freezing and local circulatory arrest; during the recovery phase inflammation and haemoconcentration may provoke secondary arterial thrombosis. Dry cold at high altitude (frostbite) particularly affects the fingers, whereas prolonged cooling at ground level typically affects the feet ('trench foot'). Besides their occasional application during the acute recovery phase, sympathetic block or surgical sympathectomy may be used to treat later sequelae of pain, hyperhidrosis or Raynaud's phenomenon.

Causalgia

First described in Union casualties of the American Civil War, causalgia is a burning pain in the extremity associated with marked hyperaesthesia, and sometimes with vasomotor and trophic changes. Artificial synapses at the site of incomplete nerve section may allow inappropriate mingling of autonomic and somatic impulses. Sympathectomy can produce dramatic relief.

Post-traumatic Dystrophy (Sudeck's atrophy)

This disabling condition occasionally complicates distal limb fractures or even minor trauma and resembles causalgia in causing pain, sympathetic dysfunction and trophic changes in the extremity. Sympathectomy may again be curative.

Other

Sympathectomy may be used to treat circulatory depression accompanying prolonged disuse of a limb, for example in spastic paralysis or old poliomyelitis.

Other occasional indications include primary acro-cyanosis, erythromelalgia, traumatic neuroma, phantom limb pain and non-union of fractures.

SYMPATHETIC BLOCK

Paravertebral ganglion blockade using local anaesthetic helps to predict the likely result of surgical sympathectomy, if the indications for operation are in doubt. Permanent sympathetic block using 6 per cent aqueous phenol or 50 per cent alcohol (*chemical sympathectomy*) is a valuable alternative to surgery in poor-risk cases, particularly in the management of lower limb ischaemia. However, these powerful neurolytic agents can produce devastating side-effects if injected without care, and chemical sympathectomy should not be undertaken casually by those inexperienced in the technique.

Sympathetic blockade of the upper limb is achieved by injection of 5 ml 0·5 per cent lignocaine into each of the four upper thoracic ganglia, these structures lying close to the side of the vertebral body and about 3 cm deep to the transverse process. Before injection at each site the needle should be aspirated to exlude the presence of air, blood or cerebrospinal fluid, and accurate placing of the needle is particularly important before injection of phenol or alcohol.

Lumbar sympathetic block (*Fig.* 56.2) is obtained

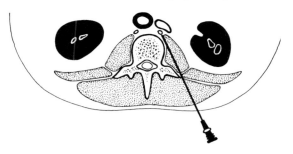

Fig. 56.2. Transverse section of the trunk at the level of the 2nd lumbar vertebra, showing the technique of lumbar sympathetic block.

by insertion of the needle at two points 10–12 cm from the midline at the level of the 2nd and 3rd lumbar spines. The needle is advanced just lateral to the transverse process and through the psoas fascia to abut against the side of the vertebral body. Injection of 15 ml local anaesthetic or 4 ml phenol produces either temporary or permanent blockade at this level.

Complications of sympathetic block include haemorrhage, somatic neuritis, spinal anaesthesia or paraplegia following accidental intrathecal injection, and pneumothorax, which is usually self-limiting.

UPPER THORACIC SYMPATHECTOMY

Choice of Route

Although several different approaches have been described, the upper thoracic sympathetic trunk can best be explored by either the cervical (supraclavicular) or the transaxillary route. The cervical approach causes less disturbance to the patient but may present technical difficulties; the patient should be warned of the possible risk of Horner's syndrome. The axillary transpleural approach permits a lower dissection of the sympathetic chain, but should be avoided in patients likely to have apical pleural adhesions (e.g. those with old pulmonary tuberculosis).

Cervical Route

The patient is placed supine with the head raised slightly and rotated to the opposite side. A transverse incision is made 8 cm long and 1 cm above and parallel to the medial half of the clavicle. The incision is deepened through platysma, and the external jugular vein, clavicular head of sternomastoid and posterior belly of omohyoid are divided. Dissection of the subjacent prescalene fat pad will now expose scalenus anterior, crossed obliquely by the phrenic nerve, with the internal jugular vein lying at its medial border (*Fig.* 56.3).

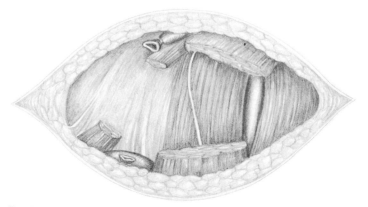

Fig. 56.3. Upper thoracic sympathectomy (cervical approach): division of the clavicular head of sternocleidomastoid reveals the phrenic nerve crossing scalenus anterior.

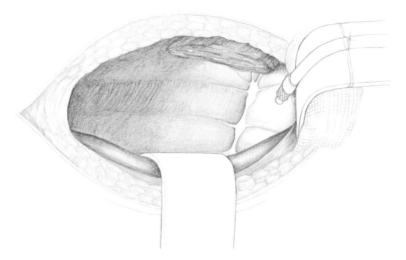

Fig. 56.4. Upper thoracic sympathectomy (cervical approach): retraction of the apex of the lung and the subclavian artery to display the cervicothoracic (stellate) ganglion and sympathetic trunk on the right-hand side.

After medial retraction of the nerve and vein, the scalenus muscle is clearly defined and is divided carefully a few fibres at a time to expose the suprapleural membrane (Sibson's fascia), traversed by the brachial plexus above and the subclavian artery below. The artery, now freed by division of scalenus anterior, is gently retracted either upwards or downwards, with ligation of the small branches that pass across the suprapleural membrane.

The extrapleural space is opened and the apical pleura is stripped gently away from the side of the vertebral column and costovertebral joints by digital dissection. A lighted retractor is inserted into the extrapleural space to help identify the ganglionated sympathetic trunk as it crosses the necks of the ribs (*Fig.* 56.4).

The cervicothoracic (stellate) ganglion is divided below the entry of the highest white ramus communicans (arising from the first thoracic nerve); the 2nd and 3rd thoracic ganglia are gently mobilized and the sympathetic chain is divided caudally at the appropriate point (i.e. below the 3rd or 4th ganglion), care being taken to avoid damaging adjacent veins. Any haemorrhage should be controlled initially by firm pressure and thereafter as necessary, either by diathermy or by application of a Cushing's clip to the bleeding point.

The lung is re-expanded and maintained fully inflated during closure of the wound; a small breach of the pleura can safely be managed in this way, without the need for underwater seal drainage. Sternomastoid, platysma and skin are resutured in layers.

Axillary Route

The patient is placed in the lateral position with the arm abducted to a right angle and supported in a sling. An oblique incision (*Fig.* 56.5) is made across the medial wall of the axilla in the line of the 3rd rib, extending forwards for about 15 cm from the posterior border of the axilla to terminate just behind the anterior axillary fold. After deepening of the incision through the fibro-fatty tissue of the axilla, retraction of the adjacent muscles and long thoracic nerve will expose the periosteum, which is incised throughout the length of the wound and is elevated from the underlying bone. Subsequent exposure is facilitated by removing a short length of the rib (*Fig.* 56.6).

Following incision of the pleura, the chest is opened using a rib-spreading retractor. The lung is displaced downwards to expose the mediastinal pleura, beneath which the sympathetic chain is easily seen and palpated. The pleura is incised vertically along the chain and dissected back for a short distance on either side by gauze pledgets (*Fig.* 56.7).

The sympathectomy is carried out as in the cervical operation, except that the first thoracic ganglion is

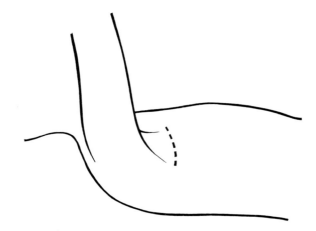

Fig. 56.5. Upper thoracic sympathectomy: incision for transaxillary approach.

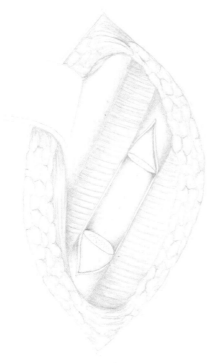

Fig. 56.6. Upper thoracic sympathectomy (axillary approach): resection of the right 3rd rib. The dotted line marks the line of incision of the subjacent periosteum and pleura.

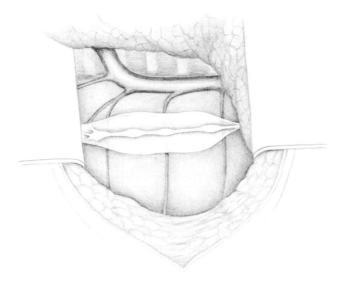

Fig. 56.7. Upper thoracic sympathectomy (axillary approach): incision of the mediastinal pleura to reveal the ganglionated (right) sympathetic trunk, running lateral to the azygos vein.

much less easily accessible, whereas the 4th (and 5th) ganglion can readily be excised. Haemostasis is secured as above. An intercostal drain is then inserted, the lung is reinflated and the ribs are approximated. The periosteum and intercostal muscle layer is sutured with continuous nylon before

closure of the subcutaneous tissues and skin. The intercostal drain is removed after 24 hours.

Complications

Surgical emphysema or a small pneumothorax may occur whenever the pleura is opened, but usually the air is rapidly absorbed. If in doubt, a chest radiograph should be obtained while the patient is in the recovery room, and this is a wise precaution in any event. A larger pneumothorax, from failure to keep the lung inflated during wound closure, or a haemothorax, owing to inadequate haemostasis, requires the insertion of an intercostal drain. Bilateral sympathectomy should not ordinarily be attempted at the same operation if the axillary route is chosen, or if the pleura is accidentally opened during the cervical approach.

Temporary or permanent Horner's syndrome results from damage to the cervicothoracic ganglion. Traction injuries to the brachial plexus and phrenic nerve or (on the left side) injury to the thoracic duct are other rare complications of the cervical operation.

LUMBAR SYMPATHECTOMY

Choice of Route

Removal of the 2nd and 3rd lumbar sympathetic ganglia, generally performed for lower limb ischaemia, is carried out through an anterior extraperitoneal approach. Ganglionectomy performed as an adjunct to aorto-iliac surgery is readily accomplished by a transperitoneal approach through the laparotomy incision. Complete sympathetic denervation of the lower limb and buttock, though rarely indicated, requires the additional removal of the 11th and 12th thoracic and 1st lumbar ganglia via a posterolateral approach through the bed of the 12th rib.

Anterior Route

A transverse incision is made at the level of the umbilicus, just crossing the linea semilunaris and extending laterally towards the tip of the 11th rib. External oblique is divided in the line of the wound and the muscular incision is continued medially for a short distance into the anterior rectus sheath. Internal oblique and transverse abdominis are divided, care being taken to avoid entering the peritoneum at the lateral edge of the rectus muscle.

The peritoneum is stripped off the parietes by progressive dissection with gauze and fingers, starting in the lateral part of the wound and extending downwards and then in front of the psoas muscle to reach the vertebral column. The ureter will be lifted up with the peritoneum during the dissection. If the peritoneum is opened, the defect should be closed immediately before proceeding.

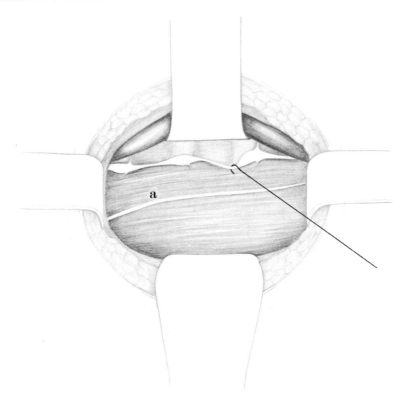

Fig. 56.8. Left lumbar sympathectomy: medial retraction of the aorta to display the sympathetic trunk. The genitofemoral nerve (*a*) runs more laterally on the surface of the psoas.

Deep retractors are now inserted. On the right side the sympathetic trunk is covered by the inferior vena cava; on the left side it lies in loose areolar tissue alongside the aorta. The trunk can be palpated as a tight cord against the sides of the vertebral bodies and its ganglionated appearance distinguishes it from the genitofemoral nerve which runs further laterally on the surface of the psoas muscle.

The trunk is lifted forwards using a nerve hook (*Fig.* 56.8), and the 2nd and 3rd lumbar ganglia are identified and excised together with the intervening sympathetic trunk. The dissection usually extends from the tendinous crus of the diaphragm to the sacral promontory, where the trunk may divide into several smaller strands. Care must be taken to avoid injury to the lumbar veins close by. Previous chemical sympathectomy makes dissection of the sympathetic trunk more difficult because of fibrosis.

The wound is closed by accurate apposition of the three muscle layers and the skin. The sympathetic trunk may be sent for histological confirmation.

Complications

There are few postoperative problems with this extra-peritoneal approach, although transient ileus may be anticipated. Prolonged ileus may accompany retro-peritoneal haematoma. Bilateral removal of the 1st lumbar ganglion frequently interferes with the mechanism of ejaculation, causing dry orgasm. Worsening of chronic ischaemia (paradoxical gangrene) is occasionally seen after lumbar sympathectomy. It is probably caused either by extension of the original disease process, or by atheromatous emboli dislodged by retraction of the aorta or the haemodynamic disturbance of operation.

PRESACRAL NEURECTOMY

This operation has been performed for spastic dysmenorrhoea or an irritable unstable bladder. The pelvis is approached through a transverse or midline lower abdominal incision. The peritoneum lying between the common iliac arteries is incised and a block of tissue is excised down to the bodies of the 5th lumbar and 1st sacral vertebras.

SPLANCHNICECTOMY

Removal of the three splanchnic nerves together with the lower thoracolumbar sympathetic chain is rarely undertaken to relieve the pain of chronic pancreatitis.

Previous splanchnic block will indicate the likely response. The use of this operation (on both sides) for uncontrolled hypertension is virtually obsolete.

The sympathetic trunk is approached transpleurally through the bed of the 9th rib, with diaphragmatic splitting to provide access to the upper lumbar ganglia. Postoperatively, wound pain and postural hypotension may be particularly troublesome.

FURTHER READING

Atkins H. J. B. (1954) Sympathectomy by the axillary approach. *Lancet* **i**, 538–539.

Baddeley R. M. (1965) The place of upper dorsal sympathectomy in the treatment of primary Raynaud's disease. *Br. J. Surg.* **52**, 426–430.

Barcroft H. (1952) Problems of sympathetic innervation and denervation. *Br. Med. Bull.* **8**, 363–370.

Birnstingl M. A. (1967) Results of sympathectomy in digital artery disease. *Br. Med. J.* **2**, 601–605.

Birnstingl M. A. (1973) *Peripheral Vascular Surgery*. Philadelphia, Lippincott, pp. 350–383.

Callow A. D. and Simeone F. A. (1978) The Grimonster Symposium on the occasion of the 50th anniversary of the first lumbar sympathectomy. *Arch. Surg.* **113**, 295–296.

Challenger J. H. (1974) Sympathetic nervous system blocking in pain relief. In: Swerdlow M. (ed.) *Relief of Intractable Pain*. Amsterdam, Excerpta Medica, pp. 176–194.

Eastcott H. H. G. (1973) *Arterial Surgery*, 2nd ed. Philadelphia, Lippincott, pp. 192–200.

Ellis H. (1972) Hyperhidrosis. *Br. J. Hosp. Med.* **7**, 641–644.

Gillespie J. A. (1960) Late effects of lumbar sympathectomy on blood-flow in the foot in obliterative vascular disease. *Lancet* **i**, 891–894.

Greenhalgh R. M., Rosengarten D. S. and Martin P. (1971) Role of sympathectomy for hyperhidrosis. *Br. Med. J.* **i**, 332–334.

Patman R. D. (1977) Post-traumatic pain syndromes: recognition and management. In: Rutherford R. B. (ed.) *Vascular Surgery*. Philadelphia, Saunders, pp. 477–483.

Peacock J. H. (1960) The effect of changes in the local temperature on the blood flows of the normal hand, primary Raynaud's disease and primary acrocyanosis. *Clin. Sci.* **19**, 505–512.

Reid W., Watt J. K. and Gray T. G. (1970) Phenol injection of the sympathetic chain. *Br. J. Surg.* **57**, 45–50.

Rob C. (1968) Sympathetic nervous system. In: Rob C. and Smith R. (eds) *Operative Surgery*. London, Butterworths, pp. 212–241.

Rutherford R. B. (1977) *Vascular Surgery*. Philadelphia, Saunders, pp. 477–483.

Strand L. (1969) Lumbar sympathectomy in the treatment of peripheral obliterative arterial disease: an analysis of 167 patients. *Acta Chir. Scand.* **135**, 597–600.

Taylor G. W. (1973) Chronic arterial occlusion. In: Birnstingl M. A. (ed.) *Peripheral Vascular Surgery*. Philadelphia, Lippincott, pp. 211–234.

Terry H. J., Allan J. S. and Taylor G. W. (1970) The effect of adding lumbar sympathectomy to reconstructive arterial surgery in the lower limb. *Br. J. Surg.* **57**, 51–55.

Warwick R. and Williams P. L. (ed.) (1973) *Gray's Anatomy*, 35th ed. Edinburgh, Longman, pp. 1068–1083.

Gynaecology and Neonatal Surgery

Chapter fifty-seven

Gynaecology and the General Surgeon

D. McCoy

This chapter has been written for the general surgeon. No attempt has been made to describe specialized gynaecological techniques, but the routine operations that the general surgeon may need to undertake have been illustrated and detailed. Emphasis has been placed on the indications, complications and diagnostic difficulties that may be encountered. Details of material pre- and postoperative management have been given only if differing from accepted surgical techniques.

MINOR GYNAECOLOGICAL OPERATIONS

Dilatation of the Cervix and Curettage of the Uterus

1. *Dilatation of the Cervix*

It is not usually necessary or desirable to dilate the cervix to more than 8 Hegar. A sound should always be passed prior to passing the cervical dilators in order to ensure that the dilators themselves are passed in the curvature of the cervical canal.

INDICATIONS

  a. Prior to curettage.
  b. Prior to insertion of radium.
  c. In cases of cervical stenosis.
  d. Occasionally to treat dysmenorrhoea—excess dilatation should be avoided for fear of causing cervical incompetence in the nulliparous patient.

2. *Curettage*

INDICATIONS

  a. Dysfunctional uterine haemorrhage—this occasionally helps the symptoms but is more useful in checking the pathology of the uterine curettings.
  b. Bleeding occurring 1 year or more after the cessation of regular menstruation at the menopause.
  c. To exclude intrauterine pathology at any age.

It is not necessary to illustrate the operation but the surgeon should be careful to:
  i. Complete a proper bimanual examination and assess the size and position of the uterus accurately before passing any instruments.
  ii. Sound the uterus and confirm the size of the cavity and its direction.
  iii. Having dilated the cervix, to introduce small intrauterine polyp forceps before doing the curettage.
  iv. Send any material obtained for pathological studies.

Evacuation of the Uterus

Indications

  1. Incomplete abortion.
  2. Missed abortion.
  3. Hydatidiform mole.
  4. Secondary postpartum haemorrhage.

Once again there should be a careful bimanual assessment of the size and position of the uterus. If the uterus is over 12 weeks in size evacuation should be digital in the case of retained products, or carried out by other means in the case of hydatidiform mole or missed abortion. Three points may be noted:

  a. Ergometrine 0·5 mg intravenously can be given before the onset of cervical dilatation as this in no way impedes dilatation of the uterine cervix but helps to make the uterus contract, thus decreasing the chances of perforation.
  b. The uterus is first evacuated either digitally, with sponge-holding forceps or suction curette.
  c. Evacuation is then completed with a sharp curette. It is not necessary to use only blunt curettage as there is no greater risk of perforation with a sharp curette used intelligently.

Cautery of the Cervix

Indications

  1. Cervical erosion causing symptoms, e.g. recurrent or excessive vaginal discharge.
  2. Large cervical erosions.
  3. Chronic cervicitis.

The cervix is cauterized either with a heated ball or loop under general anaesthesia. Alternative methods are to use a triangular 'cheese-cutting' wire to perform a diathermy conization. Smaller erosions can be treated by cryosurgery, as an outpatient procedure.

When using cautery care should be taken to avoid any preparation containing surgical spirit during the preoperative toilet of the vagina. This avoids the risk of severe burning should the spirit become ignited by the cauterization.

Shirodkar-type Suture

Cervical incompetence may occur following forceful dilatation of the cervix during a previous operation. Many cases would now seem to follow previous vaginal termination of pregnancy.

The typical history of cervical incompetence is of either mid-trimester abortion or premature labour, and in both cases the labour starts with spontaneous rupture of the membranes in the absence of either bleeding or uterine contractions. Cervical suture will not cure premature labour, or recurrent miscarriages for other reasons, and selection of cases is therefore of the greatest importance.

The operation is best performed at about 14–16 weeks' gestation when the pregnancy is relatively stable, and after the 'at risk' period for spontaneous abortion.

Technique

This should be as simple and atraumatic as possible. A braided nylon tape is inserted with quadrantic bites at 12, 3, 6, 9 and 12 o'clock by means of a trocar pointed needle with a large eye, at the level of the internal cervical os. The tape is tied tightly with the knot anteriorly and both ends of the tape are left long. There would seem to be no need to reflect the bladder or incise the vaginal epithelium as such. The patient remains in bed for 48 hours postoperatively under sedation. She is then allowed home. The suture is removed at 38 weeks.

Conization of the Uterine Cervix

In this operation the squamocolumnar junction of the cervix is removed in a cone of cervical tissue.

Indications

1. As a diagnostic procedure in the presence of a positive smear to confirm or exclude carcinoma *in situ*.
2. Used by some surgeons as a definitive treatment of carcinoma *in situ*.

It must be stressed that conization of the cervix is not without its risks, mainly from haemorrhage at the time of the operation or secondary haemorrhage about the 10th day. Postoperatively further permanent damage may result with cervical stenosis leading to difficulties in subsequent labour. It is for this reason that the practice of colposcopy and limited punch biopsy of the cervix has grown in popularity.

Cone biopsy is not necessary or desirable in frank carcinoma of the cervix when a wedge biopsy is adequate.

Procedure

1. Dilatation of the cervix should not be performed prior to cone biopsy as this may remove the endocervical epithelium and destroy the evidence of carcinoma *in situ*.
2. The cervix is marked with a suture to help in orientation of the specimen.
3. Using a sharp scalpel (no. 11 blade), a cone of cervix is removed to include the squamocolumnar junction and the lower third of the endocervical canal.
4. A dilatation and curettage is performed after this procedure.
5. Haemostasis may be obtained either with quadrantic catgut sutures or by diathermy.

Marsupialization of Bartholin's Cyst or Abscess

Either a cyst or abscess of Bartholin's gland may be treated by this method. Marsupialization has the advantage of being a relatively minor operation, and avoids the risk of haemorrhage or scarring with subsequent dyspareunia which may attend excision of a Bartholin's gland. Furthermore, as the cyst or abscess is usually in the duct of the gland, after marsupialization the gland can continue its normal secretory function.

The Operation

The swelling is opened by a cruciate incision placed so that resulting stoma will open on the inner aspect of the labium and at the posterior aspect of the introitus. The flaps between the limbs of the incision are removed leaving an opening into the cyst, preferably big enough to take the tip of a finger. The walls of the cyst are identified and sutured to the skin edges of the incision with a few fine 3/0 catgut sutures. The roof of the swelling has therefore been removed like the top of an egg, but the floor of the swelling remains. A ribbon gauze pad soaked in proflavine emulsion is inserted into the cavity and removed the next day.

OPERATIONS ON THE TUBES, OVARIES AND ROUND LIGAMENTS

The Fallopian Tubes

The general surgeon is often confronted with a diagnosis between a general surgical emergency or a gynaecological emergency. The commonest problem is probably to differentiate between acute salpingitis, ruptured ovarian cyst, appendicitis or ectopic pregnancy. Many of these difficulties can be aided by the use of laparoscopy when the pelvic viscera can be inspected directly, and the general surgeon should be encouraged to use this relatively simple technique.

On clinical grounds it is worth remembering that:

1. Salpingitis is usually bilateral and accompanied by a higher temperature and tachycardia than appendicitis. There may be a history of sexual contact, vaginal discharge or surgical interference.

2. In appendicitis the pain is usually localized to one side, there is a history of gastrointestinal disturbance, the temperature is usually not grossly elevated and the patient has a fetor.

3. There is no sign that is diagnostic of ectopic pregnancy. The pregnancy test is unreliable, as is aspiration of the pouch of Douglas. There may be a history of having missed one or even two periods, but usually the symptoms develop fairly soon after missing a period and may be confusing. The signs are of blood loss, i.e. tachycardia and low blood pressure, with severe peritoneal irritation and occasionally shoulder-tip pain. Blocking the foot of the bed may elicit this sign.

If any doubt as to the diagnosis exists, a laparotomy should be performed.

Ectopic Pregnancy

While resuscitation by blood transfusion is vital, the surgeon should not delay laparotomy. Once the bleeding points have been clamped the patient's general condition will often improve rapidly.

Examination under anaesthetic is not reliable. An ectopic pregnancy may not only be missed but ruptured during the course of the examination, with disastrous results in the patient who is lying unconscious in the recovery room.

Once the peritoneal cavity has been opened, the uterus and both tubes should be visualized. The affected tube is mobilized, and provided that the other Fallopian tube is present the tube is removed in its entirety by clamping its mesosalpinx and its medial end flush with the uterus. The vessels are tied, those at the uterine end being transfixed and doubly tied. The ovary of the affected side is normally preserved if possible. Occasionally if the Fallopian tube of the opposite side is missing, or if the ectopic is sitting in the fimbriated end of the tube, the ectopic can be milked out and the tube preserved. It should be remembered that ectopic pregnancies tend to occur in diseased tubes and the value of such tubes is debatable unless the circumstances are exceptional.

Should the ectopic pregnancy involve both the tube and ovary, difficulty may be experienced with haemostasis. In such cases a salpingo-oophorectomy should be performed, provided that the presence of an ovary on the opposite side has been confirmed. The peritoneal cavity should be cleared of excess blood clot but not drained.

Bilateral Salpingectomy

This may be done for:

1. Chronic salpingitis causing severe symptoms in patients who have failed to respond to repeated courses of antibiotics and in whom the tubes are clearly grossly diseased.

2. Rare conditions, e.g. torsion of the tube.

3. A method of sterilization.

The Ovaries

Oophorectomy

REMOVAL OF THE OVARY

1. The indications to remove one ovary may be multiple providing the other ovary is healthy, for example a large benign ovarian cyst in which the cyst has completely destroyed all normal ovarian tissue. If a significant part of healthy ovarian tissue remains, the cyst alone may be dissected from the remaining tissue—ovarian cystectomy.

2. As part of another operation, for example hysterectomy, when better haemostasis may be assured.

Bilateral oophorectomy, while technically simple, is a much more serious operation and the indications may be:

3. Routinely with hysterectomy on all postmenopausal women, or women over the age of 50 to exclude the small risk of a carcinoma developing in a remaining ovary.

4. As an adjunct to treatment for advanced malignant disease, e.g. carcinoma of the breast.

5. For ovarian carcinoma—any tumour showing obvious signs of malignancy. Clinically this may be suggested by:

   a. Large bilateral tumours.

   b. Where the capsule is perforated by tumour.

   c. Any tumour associated with ascites or obvious deposits in the pouch of Douglas.

   d. Grossly irregular multilocular tumours with large dilated vessels.

Such cases are best treated by hysterectomy and bilateral salpingo-oophorectomy. Difficulties may arise in a younger woman of reproductive age, and sadly it is not unknown for both ovaries to be removed for completely benign ovarian cysts. In doubtful cases, if facilities are not available for frozen section, the surgeon is best advised to remove the offending ovary and then be prepared to operate at a later date after paraffin sections have been taken which confirm the diagnosis, and after having had a chance to explain the situation to both the patient and her relatives.

Wedge Resection of the Ovary

In this operation wedges of ovarian tissue are removed from the antimesenteric border in order to reduce the ovarian mass by about one-third. After haemostasis has been secured the ovary is reconstructed with a continuous catgut suture on a trocar pointed needle. The operation is used in cases of Stein–Leventhal syndrome, which is usually found in patients complaining of infertility. The mechanism by which the operation is effective seems uncertain but with the greater use of drugs to stimulate ovulation its use may become less frequent.

The Round Ligaments

Ventrosuspension of the Uterus

Retroversion of the uterus is not uncommon, but is often blamed for many symptoms from backache to infertility. It may be:

1. Secondary to some other condition—the treatment is then of that condition.
2. Primary—the uterus is otherwise healthy and mobile.

Surgical correction should only rarely be undertaken as a primary operation for deep dyspareunia and very occasionally for low backache. Before subjecting the patient to surgery it is wise to antevert the uterus with a Hodge pessary, as a temporary measure, to show that once the retroversion is corrected the symptom disappears.

Plication of the round ligaments by means of an over-and-over stitch of silk or some other unabsorbable suture is effective. When the ends of the stitch are tied the uterus is anteverted by the concertina-like effect of the round ligament.

Sterilization

Interruption of the patency of the Fallopian tubes is becoming an increasingly popular operation as a form of contraception. It is important that:

1. The patient realizes that the operation is, from a practical point of view, always irreversible.
2. The patient and her husband consent.
3. Any material removed is sent for histology.

The operation may be performed either through a laparoscope, vaginally or abdominally.

Through a Laparoscope

This is an increasingly popular method in that there is minimal scarring of the abdomen and the patient's stay in hospital is usually no more than 48 hours. Readers are referred to standard textbooks for operative details. With the aid of the laparoscope, the Fallopian tubes are identified and then either diathermied or diathermied and cut. They may also be occluded with small plastic clips. The disadvantages of the technique are: that damage to other viscera may occur from the trocar or diathermy point, failure of the operation due to poor visualization of the Fallopian tubes and cardiac arrhythmia due to the pneumoperitoneum induced with carbon dioxide.

Vaginal Sterilization

This is done through the posterior vaginal fornix with the patient in the lithotomy position. The pouch of Douglas is opened, the tubes divided and tied. The advantage is that abdominal scarring is avoided; the disadvantage would seem to be the difficulty of access, operating through a potentially infected passage. The patient cannot have sexual intercourse for some 6 weeks until the vaginal scar has successfully healed.

The Abdominal Approach

There are numerous ways of sterilizing the patient through the open abdomen which is the method of choice in the puerperal patient.

All would seem to have a failure rate of 0·5–1 per cent and there would be seem to be no better results from complicated techniques, such as burying the tubes. The most simple and popular is the Pomeroy method in which the tubes are picked up and a segment is isolated between clamps. The segment is removed and the ends tied and left as widely separated as possible. The tubes are then returned to the peritoneal cavity.

Tubal Reconstruction

As the demand for sterilization grows, so does the demand for tubal reconstruction. Techniques employed are very refined and do not fall within the scope of this book.

ABDOMINAL HYSTERECTOMY AND ITS MODIFICATIONS

It is intended to describe total hysterectomy in detail and to explain the differences between the various operations, illustrating the main operational points.

Total Abdominal Hysterectomy

This involves removal of the body and cervix of the uterus.

Indications

Indications are: symptomatic benign uterine disease, preferably after child-bearing has been completed, e.g. uterine myomas, dysfunctional uterine bleeding, chronic pelvic sepsis, endometriosis, carcinoma *in situ*, and increasingly when sterilization has been requested in the presence of menorrhagia.

Operative Details

A Pfannenstiel incision is usually used but if difficulties are expected owing to the size of the uterus, previous adhesions or obesity, a paramedian incision may be wiser.

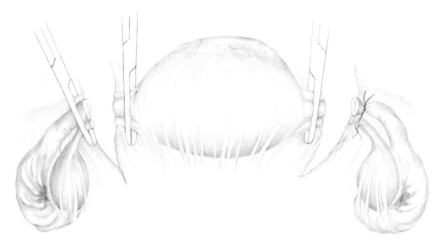

Fig. 57.1. Abdominal hysterectomy. Division of broad ligaments.

1. DIVISION OF BROAD LIGAMENTS (*Fig.* 57.1)

Parallel haemostatic clamps are applied across the broad ligaments to include the round and ovarian ligaments with the Fallopian tubes. The tissues are divided and the lateral pedicle transfixed and doubly ligated.

2. MOBILIZATION OF THE BLADDER

The peritoneum is picked up at its reflection from the bladder to the uterus and divided transversely with scissors enabling the bladder to be pushed down from the anterior wall of the uterus and cervix, taking the ureters with it. The bladder and ureters are mobilized until the longitudinal fibres of the anterior vaginal wall are clearly identified, and the bladder and ureters are free of them.

3. DIVISION AND LIGATION OF THE UTERINE ARTERIES

The uterine vessels now exposed are secured by either straight or curved hysterectomy clamps. The tip of the clamp should reach some halfway down the cervix and be applied as closely to the cervix as possible. The tissue medial to the clamp is divided and the pedicle ligated and doubly tied.

4. SECURING OF THE VAGINAL ANGLE AND UTEROSACRAL LIGAMENTS (*Fig.* 57.2)

Angled Kocher's forceps are now applied to include the vaginal angle and uterosacral ligaments in their grasp. The tip of the instrument should reach just below the cervix. The tissues medial to the clamp are divided and the pedicle tied. The ligature is left long and used as a second tie around the uterine pedicle, thus doubly securing this vessel and preventing any bleeding from the vessels between the vaginal angle and the uterine artery.

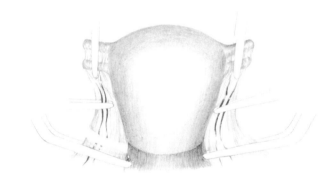

Fig. 57.2. Abdominal hysterectomy. Clamping of uterine arteries and uterosacral ligaments prior to division.

5. OPENING THE VAGINA

The vagina will have been entered with the last incision. The incision is continued transversely across the anterior vaginal wall to expose the cervix which is grasped with volsellum forceps, the posterior vaginal wall is divided transversely and the uterus removed.

6. CLOSURE OF THE VAGINAL VAULT

The vaginal valult is now closed either by a continuous suture uniting anterior and posterior walls or by interrupted mattress sutures.

7. CLOSURE OF PERITONEUM (*Fig.* 57.3)

Starting at either side, the anterior peritoneum is picked up, then the round ligament, ovarian ligament and posterior peritoneum. This suture is tied to invert the ovarian pedicle within the peritoneum leaving the ovary free within the abdominal cavity. The long end of the suture is used as a continuous stitch to

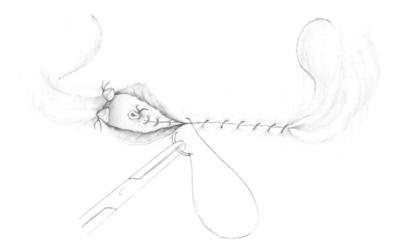

Fig. 57.3. Abdominal hysterectomy. The peritoneum is reconstituted over the previously sutured and closed vaginal vault.

close the peritoneum until the pedicle on the opposite side is dealt with in the same way.

Subtotal Hysterectomy

The body of the uterus is removed leaving the cervix intact.

Indications

The principal indication is benign uterine disease where removal of the cervix may be technically too difficult or lead to damage of the bladder or ureters.

Operative Details

The operation is similar to total hysterectomy until division of the uterine arteries. The incision is continued between the two uterine clamps to transect the cervix. The cervical remnant is then sutured with a trocar pointed needle and interrupted figure-of-eight sutures to secure haemostasis.

Total Hysterectomy and Bilateral Salpingo-oophorectomy

Indications

The operation is indicated where the ovaries themselves are the site of malignancy which is operable, in cases of endometrial carcinoma, and in menopausal patients in whom any doubt of ovarian abnormality exists. Every attempt should be made to conserve ovaries in young women.

Operative Details

DIVISION OF THE BROAD LIGAMENT

The round ligament and the infundibulo-pelvic ligament are clamped and divided lateral to the fim-briated outer end of the Fallopian tube and ovary. Care is taken not to damage the ureter on the side-wall of the pelvis.

Extended and Wertheim's Hysterectomy

Total hysterectomy with the removal of a vaginal cuff is usually reserved for cases of malignancy where the vaginal vault is a common site of recurrence. In order to remove a reasonable vaginal cuff the bladder and ureters must be further mobilized to prevent their damage. This requires the division of the uterine artery lateral to the ureters so this may be best achieved—an extended hysterectomy. Should this procedure be combined with dissection of the lymphatic nodes from the obturator fossa, around the iliac and presacral vessels and all lymphatic tissue as far as the pelvic brim, the operation is termed a 'Wertheim's hysterectomy'.

Indications

Wertheim's hysterectomy is indicated for carcinoma of the cervix either as a sole treatment or in conjunction with pre- or postoperative radiotherapy. Its use is now usually confined to stage I or early stage II carcinoma of the cervix.

PELVIC FLOOR REPAIR OPERATIONS

Fothergill Operation (Manchester Repair)

In this operation the uterine cervix is amputated in order to expose the cardinal ligaments so that they may be used to support the vaginal vault. The uterus is left *in situ*. The bladder (cystocele) and rectum (rectocele) are also supported. Any enterocele is sought for and repaired. The perineal body is also refashioned (perineorrhaphy). A posterior repair is usually required as this helps to support the anterior wall, unless the patient is very young or there is a risk of excessive narrowing of the vagina.

Indications

Forthergill repair has to some degree been replaced by vaginal hysterectomy and repair. Its place would seem to be:

1. Where the uterus is enlarged, is held in the abdomen by adhesions, or is itself asymptomatic.
2. Where the uterus does not descend sufficiently for vaginal hysterectomy to be a safe operation.
3. In a young woman with a prolapse who wishes to retain the ability to have children.

Operative Details

1. THE INCISION

The site of incision is infiltrated with 1 : 400 000 adrenaline solution. A dilatation and curettage should be done to exclude any uterine disease. The urethra is marked with tissue forceps and the cervix grasped with downward traction by volsellum forceps. The incision may be either a vertical midline incision from the volsellum to the tissue forceps, or a diamond incision using the urethra as its apex to a point laterally either side of the cervix, and joined by a transverse incision across the posterior aspect of the cervix at the level of the internal os.

Starting at the apex of the incision the skin is removed to expose the bladder, either aided by blunt gauze dissection or a few deft strokes of a scalpel. The bladder is then pushed up to expose the anterior aspect of the cervix and the lower extremity of the cardinal and uterosacral ligaments (*Fig.* 57.4).

2. DIVISION OF COMBINED CARDINAL AND UTEROSACRAL LIGAMENTS (*Fig.* 57.5)

The ligaments are then clamped, divided and transfixed, the ends of the suture being left long.

3. SEARCH FOR ENTEROCELE

Opportunity is taken at this stage to open the pouch of Douglas and to search for any hernial sac which should be excised, the defect being corrected by uniting the uterosacral ligaments.

4. AMPUTATION AND THE CERVIX (*Fig.* 57.6)

The cervix is now amputated at the level of the division of the cardinal ligaments.

5. RE-EPITHELIALIZATION OF THE CERVICAL STUMP

The cervical stump is covered with vaginal skin.
a. Posteriorly—by the Sturmdorf suture. The

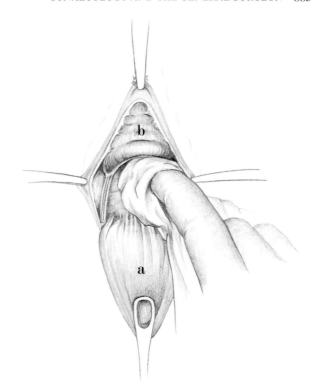

Fig. 57.4. Manchester repair. The skin flap (a) is pulled posteriorly and the bladder (b) brushed forwards anteriorly away from the cervix which is beneath the swab.

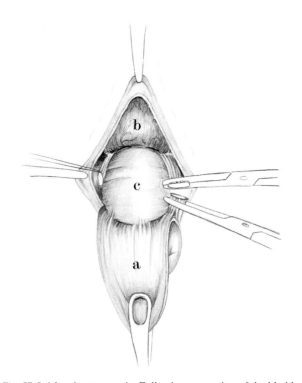

Fig. 57.5. Manchester repair. Following separation of the bladder (b) from the vagina and cervix (c) the combined cardinal and uterosacral ligaments are clamped, divided and transfixed.

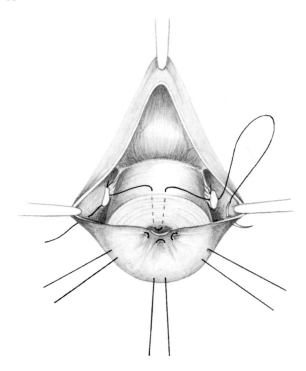

Fig. 57.6. Manchester repair. The cervix is amputated and its stump is covered with vaginal skin.

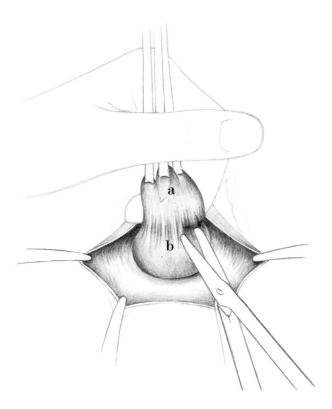

Fig. 57.7. Manchester repair. The vaginal skin (a) is separated from the anterior aspect of the rectum (b) and the redundant vaginal skin of each flap is excised.

centre of the posterior skin incision is transfixed and the suture tied at its midpoint. Both ends are introduced on a trocar pointed needle consecutively down the cervical canal and out through the posterior aspect of the cervix and the skin flap, each slightly on opposing sides of the midline. The posterior skin flap is pulled into the canal covering the posterior aspect of the amputated cervix with skin. The stitch is tied.

b. Anteriorly—the Fothergill stich picks up the vaginal edge, cardinal ligament, enters and exits the canal to pick up the identical structures on the other side. Tying the suture apposes the cardinal ligaments and covers the anterior aspect of the cervix with skin.

6. ANTERIOR COLPORRHAPHY

Following excision of redundant vaginal skin the incision anterior to the cervix is now closed either by continuous or interrupted sutures, care being taken to pick up both skin and pubovesical fascia.

7. POSTERIOR COLPOPERINEORRHAPHY

A triangular area is marked out in the vaginal skin over the rectum, the apex being as near the cervix as possible and the base marked by two tissue clamps applied to the lower extremities of the labia minora at the vaginal introitus.

8. REMOVAL OF THE TRIANGLE (*Fig.* 57.7)

A transverse incision is made at the base of the triangle and the vaginal skin is dissected from the rectum, using both blunt and sharp dissection to the apex of the triangle. The redundant vaginal skin of each flap is excised, care being taken not to remove too much skin and overtighten the vagina.

9. REPAIR OF THE VAGINAL EPITHELIUM (*Fig.* 57.8)

The trimmed edges are approximated with a continuous suture working from the apex downwards.

10. INSERTION OF THE LEVATOR ANI SUTURES

Before completing the posterior vaginal epithelial repair sutures are placed to approximate the medial edges of the levator ani muscles. Two or three interrupted sutures usually suffice.

11. REPAIR OF PERINEAL BODY

Once the vaginal skin has been repaired, the resulting defect in the perineal body is closed with two or three deep sutures and similarly two or three sutures close the skin.

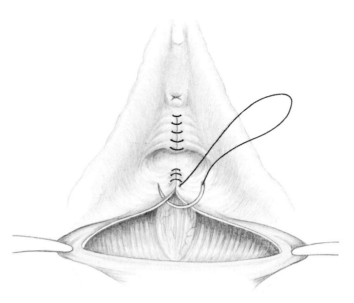

Fig. 57.8. Manchester repair. The vaginal epithelium is repaired. Before completing the posterior vaginal epithelial repair, sutures are placed to approximate at the medial edges of the levator ani muscles.

12. POSTOPERATIVELY

A vaginal pack is inserted and removed after 24 hours. The bladder may be drained, either by urethral or suprapubic catheters, from between 2 and 5 days until the urethral oedema has settled.

Vaginal Hysterectomy

This entails removal of the uterus per vaginam.

Indications

1. Vaginal vault prolapse with or without a malfunctioning uterus.
2. Surgical preference rather than a Manchester repair.

This operation is usually combined with the repair of a vaginal prolapse. For the sake of brevity the details of the repair will be omitted and reference should be made to the section on Fothergill repair. Contra-indications for vaginal hysterectomy are dealt with in that section.

Operative Details

The operation is similar to the Manchester repair until subsection 2. At this stage the pouch of Douglas should be opened.

1. A finger is now passed up behind the uterus and introduced over the fundus to help demonstrate the uterovesical pouch of the peritoneum which is opened transversely, care having been taken to ensure that the bladder has been pushed upwards, well clear both in the midline and laterally.

2. DIVISION OF THE UTERINE VESSELS (*Fig.* 57.9, 57.10)

Once the combined uterosacral and cardinal ligaments have been divided, a finger is passed up behind the broad ligament and the uterine vessels identified.

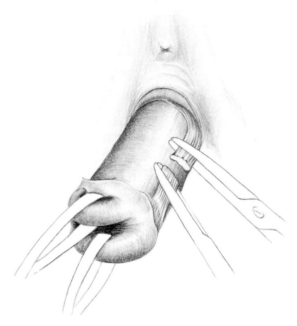

Fig. 57.9. Vaginal hysterectomy. After opening the pouch of Douglas, the cervix is drawn down with volsellum forceps, exposing the cardinal ligaments which may then be clamped, divided and ligated.

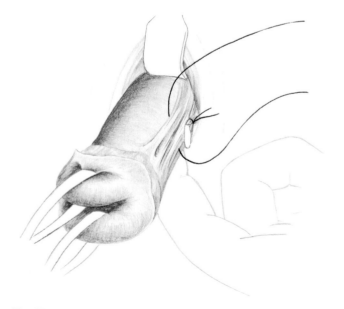

Fig. 57.10. Vaginal hysterectomy. After division of the cardinal ligaments, the uterine vessels may be mobilized, ligated and divided.

These are either transfixed or clamped and the pedicle divided medial to the clamp. The pedicle is then transfixed and doubly tied, the ligature being cut.

3. DIVISION OF THE FALLOPIAN TUBES, ROUND LIGAMENTS AND OVARIAN LIGAMENTS (*Fig.* 57.11)

If there is gross descent, traction on the uterus will now demonstrate these structures and they can readily be secured by a strong clamp. Should there be difficulty, a finger should be introduced behind the uterus before applying the clamp to ensure that no other viscus is included in the clamp. The pedicle is divided, transfixed and doubly tied, both ends of the ligature being left long and clamped to the drapes. Following this procedure on the opposite side, the uterus is removed and haemostasis carefully checked.

4. CLOSURE OF THE PERITONEUM (*Fig.* 57.12)

Starting on one side the three pedicles are demonstrated and the peritoneum closed and tied to exteriorize these pedicles. The suture continues transversely across the vault and ends by a similar closure on the other side.

5. APPROXIMATION OF PEDICLES AND THE UTEROSACRAL LIGAMENTS

The two lowest pedicles (cardinal) are tied together in the midline and one suture on either side left long. The upper pedicles are also tied together and both ends of the suture left long. Any potential gap between the uterosacral ligaments which may allow enterocele formation is now obliterated with interrupted sutures.

6. FIXATION OF THE VAGINAL VAULT

The sutures used to tie the uterosacral ligaments are now used to transfix the middle of the skin flap made when the skin was divided on the posterior aspect of the cervix. When tied, these obliterate the dead space and help support the new vaginal vault. Similarly, both ends of the suture used to tie the combined tubo-ovarian pedicles are used to transfix the vaginal skin edge of the same side at the point marking the base of the original diamond incision. This obliterates dead space but also helps to support and widen the new vaginal vault. The repair of the bladder and rectum now continues as described under Manchester Repair.

OPERATIONS FOR INCONTINENCE OF URINE

It is important before attempting any surgical correction or urinary symptoms to obtain an accurate his-

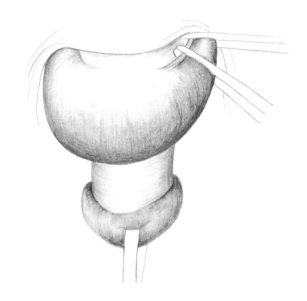

Fig. 57.11. Vaginal hysterectomy. With further traction on the cervix, the Fallopian tubes, round ligaments and ovarian ligaments will be brought into view, when they may be clamped, divided and ligated.

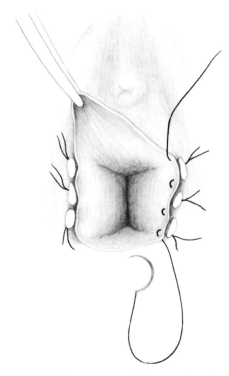

Fig. 57.12. Vaginal hysterectomy. After removing the uterus, the peritoneum is carefully closed, following which the pedicles of the cardinal ligaments and the uterosacral ligaments are brought together in the midline and sutured.

tory. Stress incontinence can be cured by operations which are designed to:

1. Elongate the urethra, and restore it to its place behind the pubic symphysis.
2. Restore the posterior vesical urethral angle.
3. Support the bladder and urethra with the anterior vaginal walls and associated fascial tissues.

Many patients may complain of symptoms of urge incontinence or of urinary infection. These are not cured by surgery and may even be made worse.

Urge incontinence is relatively common compared to stress incontinence and must account for many of the so-called failures of surgical repair for stress incontinence. It is wise, therefore, before contemplating any repair to ensure that the symptoms are amenable to surgery by bladder pressure studies and to make sure the urine itself is sterile.

There are many operations for stress incontinence but two types are commonly performed—the vaginal repair and the abdominal repair.

The Vaginal Repair (Kelly Type) (*Fig.* 57.13)

1. The incision is as for an anterior colporrhaphy.
2. The bladder and urethra are carefully identified and mobilized from any adhesions. Attention is paid to freeing the bladder neck.
3. The tissues on either side of the bladder and the urethra are approximated below the urethra and

bladder neck by interrupted sutures placed about 1 cm apart from below upwards.

The nature of the tissues used by this method varies according to how far laterally they are sought. Usually the pubovesical fascia is used as a buttress, but if a very wide dissection is performed laterally the anterior border of the levator ani may be drawn across.

Any redundant vaginal skin is trimmed away and the vaginal wall closed with interrupted sutures. A pack is inserted for 48 hours and the bladder drained either with a urethral catheter for 5 days or a small suprapubic catheter which allows the patients to void urine spontaneously when they are able.

The Abdominal Repair
(Marshall–Marchetti–Krantz) (*Fig.* 57.14)

The patient is placed supine with the legs slightly apart and the head tipped downwards. A 30-ml Foley catheter is placed in the bladder and the balloon distended. A tape is tied over the end of the side-tube and runs down between the patient's legs to hang over the end of the table. When pulled on, this helps to identify the vesico-urethral junction by the site of the balloon in the bladder.

1. The abdomen is opened through a transverse incision.
2. The peritoneum is not opened but the retropubic space is opened by blunt dissection with either a swab on a holder or the surgeon's fingers. The bladder neck and the urethra are identified. Any large veins that might bleed are diathermized.
3. Nonabsorbable black silk sutures are placed on either side of the vesico-urethral junction and urethra on a no. 4 J-shaped needle carrying 2/0 silk. The sutures are placed as low as possible and run from the paraurethral and paravesical tissues through the periosteum on the back of the pubic symphysis. The sutures are left long until they have all been inserted and then tied starting with the lowest on each side and working upwards. If much bleeding is evident, the retropubic space should be drained. The wound is closed. The catheter is left in for 5 days, the patient being placed on a suitable antibiotic while the catheter is *in situ.*

VULVECTOMY

Simple vulvectomy is removal of the vulva itself. Radical vulvectomy includes removal of the vulva with its lymphatic drainage, i.e. the superficial and deep inguinal and femoral lymph nodes.

Simple Vulvectomy

Indications

1. Non-malignant lesions of the vulva causing severe symptoms, usually itching, when conservative treatment has failed, i.e. leucoplakia, lichen sclerosis.

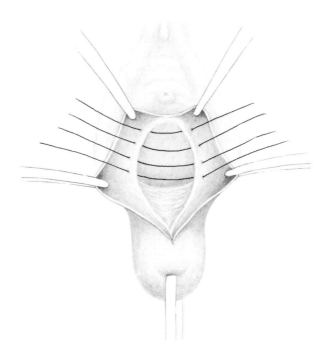

Fig. 57.13. Stress incontinence. Vaginal repair (Kelly operation). Following removal of vaginal skin, the deep fascia is secured with interrupted catgut sutures which, when tied, raise and thrust forwards the bladder neck.

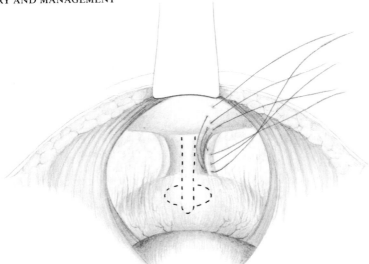

Fig. 57.14. Stress incontinence. Abdominal approach (Marshall–Marchetti–Krantz). Retropubic space is dissected via a transverse incision. Non-absorbable silk sutures are placed on either side of the vesico-urethral junction and the urethra. The sutures are placed as low as possible and run from the paraurethral and paravesical tissues through the periosteum on the back of the pubic symphysis. When these sutures are tied the bladder neck is drawn upwards and forwards.

2. Preinvasive changes in the above lesion, i.e. excision biopsy.
3. Carcinoma of the vulva when the patient is too unfit to stand more radical surgery. This may be combined with radiotherapy to regional lymph nodes or excision of lymph nodes at a later date when the patient has recovered from the vulvectomy.

Operative Details
The patient is placed in lithotomy and catheterized. Either a diathermy cutting needle or a scalpel may be used to incise the skin.

1. VAGINAL INCISION
The incision runs anterior to the urethra around the introitus on both sides to the posterior fourchette.

2. VULVAL INCISION
The incision runs on both sides from the pubic symphysis downwards along the line of the junction between the thigh and the vulva. The incisions meet on the perineum just anterior to the anus. The primary incision is deepened to demonstrate the deep fascia.

3. REMOVAL OF THE VULVA
The vulva is now removed by a diathermy cutting needle, care being taken to keep in the plane of the deep fascia. It is wise to identify the crura of the clitoris and electively clamp this with transfixation

of the pedicle to secure haemostasis. The whole area is very vascular and careful haemostasis with fine catgut sutures and diathermy coagulation is of prime importance. Constant care must be taken not to damage the urethra anteriorly.

4. CLOSURE OF THE INCISION
Primary closure should usually be possible with fine 0/0 catgut on a cutting needle to the vaginal/skin edge. Black silk sutures should be used to close the skin edges anterior to the urethra.

5. POSTOPERATIVELY
It is advisable to leave a self-retaining Foley catheter *in situ* with continuous drainage of 48 hours until acute discomfort has passed. A sterile gauze dressing should be applied to the area and held in place with a T-bandage.

Radical Vulvectomy

Indications
1. Carcinoma of the vulva.
2. Other malignant conditions of the vulva, e.g. melanoma.
3. Adenocarcinoma of Bartholin's gland.

The Operation
Dissection of the lymphatic glands is carried out with the patient in the dorsal position and the legs slightly separated. Preferably two surgical teams work syn-

chronously, one on either side for the lymphatic dissection, and once the groin incisions have been closed, as far as is practical, the area is covered with sterile towels and the patient placed in the modified lithotomy position while vulvectomy is performed as previously described.

1. MARKING OUT THE SKIN FLAPS

Postoperative morbidity is a greater risk to the patient than the operation. It is important that primary skin closure is achieved without tension on the suture line if at all possible, so that early mobilization of the patient may be achieved. Bearing this in mind, it is wise to plan the skin incision very carefully before starting the operation, and it is sometimes helpful to draw these on the skin of the anaesthetized patient with methylene blue on a cottonwool bud.

2. THE INCISION (*Fig.* 57.15)

A curved incision runs from one anterior superior iliac spine to the opposite side, reaching the upper

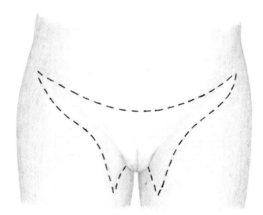

Fig. 57.15. Incision for radical vulvectomy.

border of the pubic symphysis in the midline. A second incision on either side runs from the anterior superior iliac spine along the lower border of the inguinal ligament with a triangular extension over the femoral triangle running medially to join the proposed vulval incision.

3. DISSECTION OF THE INGUINAL AND FEMORAL LYMPH NODES (*Figs.* 57.16–57.18)

Starting laterally, the incision is deepened to show the aponeurosis of the external oblique and the inguinal ligament. The skin, fat and lymph nodes are now reflected medially to uncover these structures. Over the femoral triangle the borders of the triangle are defined, i.e. the sartorius laterally and the pectineus medially. The long saphenous vein is isolated at the apex of the triangle, clamped and tied. The vein is

now followed until it turns down to join the femoral vein. It is carefully isolated, clamped and divided at this junction. The vein is doubly tied, care being taken not to stenose the femoral vein.

Further venous tributaries, i.e. the superficial external pudendal and the superficial circumflex iliac

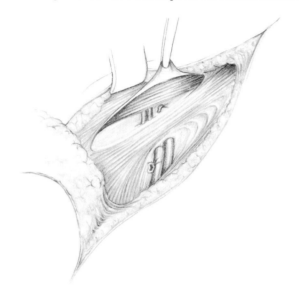

Fig. 57.16. Radical vulvectomy. Block dissection of inguinal nodes.

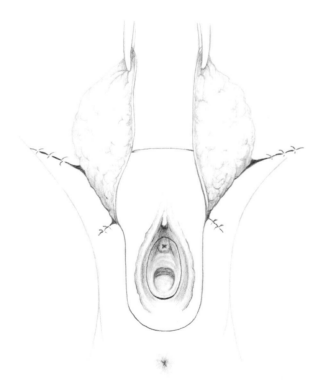

Fig. 57.17. Radical vulvectomy. Following clearing of nodes in both inguinal and femoral regions, the mons pubis is cleared and the whole block of tissue turned forwards. The inguinal and femoral skin incisions are closed at this stage.

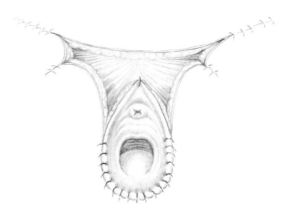

Fig. 57.18. Radical vulvectomy. The skin of the perineum is now sutured directly into the vagina.

veins, are demonstrated, clamped and tied at the extremities of the incision.

The whole block of glands, fat and vessels is now removed from the femoral triangle, clearing the femoral vessels up to the inguinal ring. The gland of Cloquet is removed from the femoral canal medial to the femoral vein.

If there is clinical or pathological (frozen section) evidence to believe that these glands are involved in neoplastic disease, the surgeon may choose to remove the external iliac lymph nodes by opening the inguinal canal from external to internal ring, dividing the internal oblique and transversus abdominis muscles in the line of the incision, and by peritoneal retraction exposing the lymph nodes around the external iliac vessels. These nodes and those in the canal can now be removed, the defect being closed by interrupted sutures.

Once the nodes have been cleared in the inguinal and femoral region of both sides, the mons pubis is cleared and the whole block of tissue turned downwards. The inguinal skin incisions are now closed along with their femoral extensions by black silk sutures. It will not be possible to close the medial part of the incision until the vulvectomy has been performed.

Great attention is paid to haemostasis but it is useful to insert suction drainage tubes under the skin of the groin incisions, the area then being covered with sterile towels and the patient placed in lithotomy for completion of the vulvectomy.

Postoperative Care

The area is dressed with tulle gras and cottonwool. The groin incisions can be dressed separately from the vulval incision. The drains are left until all drainage has ceased. Great attention is paid to mobilization of the patient. The silk sutures are removed on the 10th day. The bladder is drained for 5 days with an indwelling catheter.

CAESAREAN SECTION

There are two methods of performing Caesarean section:
1. Incising the lower segment of the uterus.
2. Incising the upper segment of the uterus.

Lower segment Caesarean section is the most commonly performed.

Lower Segment Caesarean Section

Indications (*Fig.* 57.19)

These are many and varied. Caesarean section should be considered for good clinical reasons only as it car-

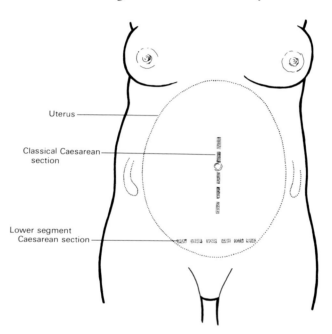

Uterus

Classical Caesarean section

Lower segment Caesarean section

Fig. 57.19. Incisions for classic and for lower segment Caesarean section.

ries an increased risk to the mother, not only at the time but in future pregnancies. Greater awareness of fetal wellbeing has, however, increased recourse to Caesarean section in place of either difficult labour or difficult instrumental delivery.

1. Placenta praevia—in all but the most minor forms of placenta praevia.
2. Cephalopelvic disproportion—either in absolute disproportion on erect lateral pelvimetry, or after a failed trial of labour.
3. Failure to progress in labour judged by:
    a. Descent of fetal head in relationship to maternal pelvic spines.
    b. Failure of the cervix to dilate.
    c. Excessive caput and moulding of the fetal skull.
4. Fetal distress diagnosed by:
    a. Clinical grounds.
    b. Changes in the fetal heart trace.

c. Changes in the pH of a sample of fetal scalp blood.

A combination of fetal blood sampling combined with use of the fetal heart trace can do much to lower an increasingly high Caesarean section rate for apparent fetal distress.

5. Malpresentation—brow or shoulder presentation. Caesarean section is used increasingly in the delivery of breech presentations.

6. Prolapse of umbilical cord.

Other indications finding increasing favour are severe pre-eclampsia and eclampsia.

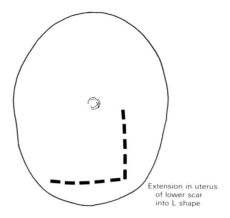

Extension in uterus of lower scar into L shape

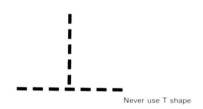

Never use T shape

Fig. 57.20. Lower segment Caesarean section. If found to be too small or inappropriate, the transverse incision should be extended into an 'L' shape, and not a 'T' shape.

The Operation

This may be undertaken under general anaesthesia or epidural anaesthesia. The advantages of epidural anaesthesia as regards more rapid maternal recovery and the experience of instant bonding are self-evident.

1. The patient is placed as for any abdominal operation with a diathermy pad *in situ* and the bladder draining freely from an indwelling catheter.

2. The abdominal incision may be transverse (Pfannensteil) or vertical (midline or paramedian) depending on the speed of the operation or surgeon's performance.

3. The rectus muscles are separated and the peritoneum opened longitudinally. The paracolic gutter may be packed to absorb spilled liquor or blood. The uterus is corrected for rotation and deviation to the right.

4. The reflection of peritoneum from the bladder to the uterus is identified and the peritoneum divided transversely just above it.

5. The lower flap of peritoneum is pushed downwards with a gauze swab exposing the lower uterine segment. A Doyen retractor is used to keep the bladder clear of the operating site.

6. The lower segment is incised transversely and the incision extended either with the fingers or by surgical incision to make an opening big enough to deliver the baby—care must be taken not to extend the incision too far, or tearing may occur into the uterine vessels.

7. The baby's head is delivered either with a hand inside the uterus or with Wrigley's forceps. Fundal pressure by the assistant will help to deliver the body of the baby.

8. Once the baby is delivered the cord is clamped, the baby handed to an assistant and the placenta and membranes delivered through the incision by cord traction. Digital exploration is used to confirm that the uterine cavity is empty.

Note: Should the transverse incision be found to be too small or inappropriate, the incision should be extended from one extremity converting it into an 'L' not a ' ⌐L' incision (*Fig.* 57.20).

9. Following delivery of the placenta and membranes the lower segment is repaired with two layers of continuous catgut (no. 1). The first layer is haemostatic and the second varying the first layer and restoring the constitution of the myometrium. Great attention must be paid to this as the safety of future pregnancies depends on this reconstruction of the uterine wall.

10. The peritoneum is closed on the uterine incision, the packs removed, the paracolic gutters cleaned and the abdomen closed in the usual way.

11. The vagina should also be swabbed out to ensure that there is no excessive vaginal bleeding.

Classic Caesarean Section

This operation is seldom done as the risk of the scar rupturing in subsequent pregnancies is 10 times greater than that of lower segment Caesarean section. It is a much easier operation, however. The incision is vertical on the anterior wall of the uterus and the bladder is undisturbed.

The indications would seem to be:

1. The completely inexperienced surgeon performing a Caesarean section for the first time with little skill in delivery of the baby in order

to avoid the hazards of the lower segment Caesarean section operation.

2. Where the lower segment is inaccessible due to large pelvic veins, fibroids or previous bladder surgery.

3. When the baby could not be delivered through a lower segment, e.g. transverse lie with prolapsed arm.

4. In extreme haste, e.g. postmortem Caesarean section.

Chapter fifty-eight

Surgery of the Newborn

J. D. Atwell

INTRODUCTION AND GENERAL PRINCIPLES

The scope of paediatric surgery is wide and the needs vary depending on the age of the neonate, infant or child. In the neonatal period the successful outcome of surgery depends on many factors such as surgical techniques, expert paediatric anaesthesia, nursing skills and staffing on intensive care units, the availability of micro-methods for haematological and biochemical investigations, full paediatric radiological services and specialized equipment.

It has been shown that one of the most important results of the concentration of such cases in neonatal units is a fall in the operative mortality from 72 to 24 per cent (Rickham, 1952; Forshall and Rickham, 1960). In recent years, with the improvements in neonatal resuscitation and the use of expensive monitoring equipment, together with advances in surgical technique and parenteral nutrition, the average mortality has decreased to about 10 per cent. Therefore only if these services are available can neonatal surgery be safely undertaken and achieve results that are acceptable.

The nature of neonatal surgery has changed over the past 15 years. Factors such as the policy of treating neonates with spina bifida and hydrocephalus, intensive care of the premature infant and antenatal diagnosis by cytology, biochemical estimations and ultrasonography have brought about these changes. The decrease in the number of admissions with spina bifida is partly due to the estimation of alpha-fetoprotein in maternal serum and amniotic fluid and to a decrease in its true incidence. These improvements in antenatal care allow the recommendation of a therapeutic abortion. Antenatal diagnosis can now identify conditions such as oesophageal atresia, Down's syndrome with duodenal atresia, diaphragmatic hernia, exomphalus and gastroschisis. Anomalies of the urinary tract, in particular the obstructive uropathies, are commonly seen on ultrasonography and allow early postnatal treatment. The role of intra-uterine interference in obstructive uropathy has been proposed but is *not* recommended in the majority of patients as adequate early post-natal surgery is successful. A comparison of the admission to the author's unit of 1970/1971 and 1983/1984 reflects these changes (*Table* 58.1).

1. Anaesthesia

The advances in neonatal anaesthesia have largely been responsible for the progress of neonatal surgery.

Table 58.1. Neonatal surgical admissions 1970/71 and 1983/84

Diagnosis	1970	1971	1983	1984
Spina bifida	51	44	12	8
Oesophageal atresia	6	13	6	5
Diaphragmatic hernia	4	6	5	8
Necrotizing enterocolitis	—	—	8	14
G.U. system	6	7	13	13

First, in the neonate the surface area available for gaseous exchange is reduced in relation to body weight compared to the adult. Therefore any loss of functioning pulmonary tissue, e.g. diaphragmatic hernia or increased oxygen requirement due to cooling, will produce a pulmonary deficiency in an infant with minimal pulmonary reserves. Second, the small calibre of the airway passages means that the airway resistance will become critical with the accumulation of any secretions, especially as in the neonate the cough reflex is depressed. These factors may cause hypoventilation and the risks of aspiration pneumonia are increased. The newborn is also prone to other pulmonary disorders often related to prematurity and the need to establish a separate existence following birth. The respiratory distress syndrome, apnoeic attacks, aspiration of meconium and pulmonary and ventricular haemorrhage are such examples which may complicate the pre- and postoperative course of the surgical neonate.

Principles of Management

Analgesics are avoided pre- and postoperatively. Atropine is the only premedication used and is given intramuscularly at a dosage of 0·2 mg. Postoperatively the humidity in the incubator is kept at maximal levels and may be increased by the use of an ultrasonic nebulizer. All the nurses are instructed in routine chest physiotherapy. Aspirations may be reduced by nursing babies in the prone position, aspirating the pharynx at regular intervals and keeping the stomach empty by nasogastric aspiration until evidence that peristalsis and adequate gastric emptying are occurring (absence of bile in the aspirates). Death resulting from aspiration of a vomit or from secretions should be considered as an avoidable cause of death. The nursery should be fully equipped for resuscitation. Following the repair of a diaphragmatic hernia or exomphalos it may be necessary to maintain the newborn on positive-pressure ventilation.

2. Nursing Care

The successful outcome of neonatal surgery is dependent on constant nursing supervision by nurses skilled and experienced in neonatal care throughout the 24 hours of each day. Failure of this provision will result in unnecessary deaths. Unfortunately due to the shortage of nurses such ideals are not always fulfilled. Expensive monitoring equipment may assist in recording the vital parameters of the sick neonate, but these should be considered as an aid to nursing rather than a replacement of nursing skills.

Principles of Management

As stated above, the nursing care is the most vital aspect in the management of the surgical neonate. The observations made on such an infant are many (Appendix I) but probably the most important are the care of the airway and prevention of the aspiration of vomit. Nasogastric aspiration is used routinely following surgical procedures on the gastrointestinal tract. It is essential to use an adequate sized tube (no. 10 Fr. gauge) with 1- or $\frac{1}{2}$-hourly aspirations with free drainage into a receptacle between aspirations. Oral feeding is not started until the aspirates are clear, i.e. non-bile stained. Oral feeding is always introduced gradually, and in the full-term infant with 5 per cent dextrose at 5·0 ml/hr and then with increasing volumes and a change to half and finally full strength feeds. This transitional period may take several days or even weeks in infants with prolonged gastrointestinal problems, e.g. after the repair of a gastroschisis, or surgery for necrotizing enterocolitis.

3. Temperature Control and Regulation

The surface area of the infant per total body mass is greater than that of an adult, therefore the infant is more prone to heat loss than the adult. In the premature infant the heat losses are correspondingly greater due to the lack of subcutaneous tissue. Exposure to cold results in heat production and an increased oxygen consumption which may be harmful to the infant if it is already under stress. Sclerema neonatorum is a condition seen in neonates and premature infants where the subcutaneous tissue and skin undergo a change resulting in a very characteristic 'hardened' feel to the tissues, especially in the extremities. It is related to cooling and infection and is commoner in the premature infant. The incidence may be reduced by careful measures to prevent heat loss during transport, investigations, operation and postoperative care of the infant.

Principles of Management

PREVENTION OF HEAT LOSS

The infant requiring surgery is transported in a suitable portable incubator. In patients with a condition such as gastroschisis, when the heat loss may be severe, it can be reduced by wrapping the infant in aluminium foil. On arrival in the neonatal surgical unit the infant is nursed in an incubator preheated to the correct temperature. Exposure of the infant for radiological investigation, collection of blood and intravenous infusion is kept to a minimum and any exposed areas should be wrapped in warm padded gauze. Heat loss at the time of induction of general anaesthesia may be rapid and can be reduced by the use of water blankets and additional overhead heating. Similarly during the operation the temperature in the theatre is kept higher than in the normal operating theatre. The neonate's temperature is monitored throughout these procedures with an electrical thermometer with either a skin electrode or with oesophageal or rectal probes. Every attempt is made to maintain the body temperature between 36 and 37 °C as oxygen consumption is minimal at this level.

4. Homeostasis

a. Fluid and Electrolytes

BASIC DATA

The total body water of the neonate is higher than that of the adult (80:60 per cent); the distribution between the intracellular and extracellular spaces is 35 and 45 per cent respectively in the infant and 40 and 20 per cent in the adult. Changes of fluid balance with increased losses or decreased intake therefore have a greater effect in the neonate compared to the adult (*Fig.* 58.1). A comparison of the daily gastrointestinal fluid turnover in a 70-kg adult and a 3·5-kg neonate is seen in *Fig.* 58.2.

PRINCIPLES OF MANAGEMENT

Maintenance Fluid: A neonate requires 150 ml/kg/day if being fed orally. In the premature infant this is increased to 200 ml/kg/day. Following intestinal surgery when fluid is given intravenously and the bowel is aspirated regularly the transfers shown in *Fig.* 58.2 are reduced; therefore the maintenance intravenous fluid requirements are less. In such circumstances the infant needs 70 ml/kg/day unless there is jaundice or urinary complications such as obstruction. The newborn infant in the 1st week of life requires even less fluid and this can be administered on a regimen of 10 ml/kg/day in the 1st day of life, increasing to the full 70 ml/kg/day by the 7th and subsequent days. The maintenance fluid should be isotonic and N/5 saline in 4·3 per cent dextrose is suitable.

Replacement of Fluid Losses: Initial assessment of fluid losses in an infant is difficult but depends on the degree of dehydration as assessed by the loss of

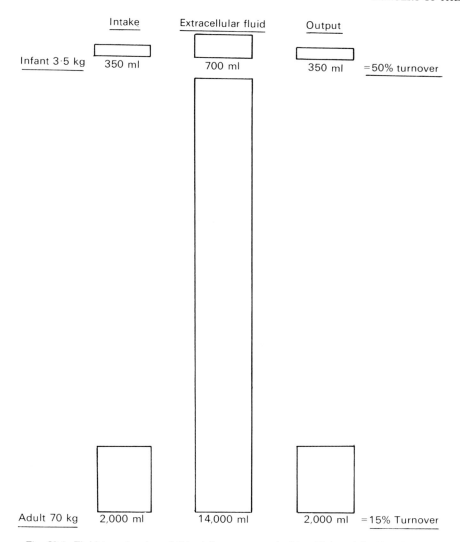

Intake   Extracellular fluid   Output

Infant 3·5 kg   350 ml   700 ml   350 ml   =50% turnover

Adult 70 kg   2,000 ml   14,000 ml   2,000 ml   =15% Turnover

Fig. 58.1. Fluid transfers in a 3·5-kg infant compared with a 70-kg adult. Note how increased losses or decreased intake have a more marked effect on the homeostasis of the infant.

weight (difference between birth weight and weight on admission), loss of skin elasticity, depression of the anterior fontanelle, pulse rate and results of biochemical estimations. Later losses following surgical procedures are usually easier to estimate as they are recorded accurately on an hourly basis, e.g. nasogastric aspiration. The composition of intestinal aspirates in the newborn averages 100–120 mmol/L of sodium, 5–15 mmol/L of potassium and 100–120 mmol/L of chloride (Young, 1966, 1968). Therefore, the ideal solution for replacement purposes is N saline given on a volume-for-volume basis.

Correction of Acid Base Balance:
i. *Acidosis:* A metabolic acidosis is the commonest acid base disturbance found either due to disturbance of gastrointestinal or renal physiology or due to cardiorespiratory arrest. In the first instance it may be

corrected by the intravenous administration of 1/6th molar lactate solution; correction is slow due to the need to metabolize the lactate in the liver, which may take up to 2 hours (3·0 ml/kg 1/6 M lactate raise the HCO_3 1 mmol). Immediate correction of acidosis can be achieved with intravenous 8·4 per cent sodium bicarbonate (1·0 ml/kg $NaHCO_3$ raises the HCO_3 1 mmol).

ii. *Alkalosis:* This occurs when the obstruction is proximal to the opening of the bile ducts such as in duodenal atresia and congenital hypertrophic pyloric stenosis. The alkalosis can be corrected by the intravenous administration of N saline (3·0 ml/kg N saline will lower the HCO_3 1 mmol). Only in exceptional circumstances is the use of ammonium chloride needed.

iii. *Potassium:* Intravenous replacement of potassium losses is restricted for the first 24 hours following

DAILY GASTRO-INTESTINAL TURNOVER

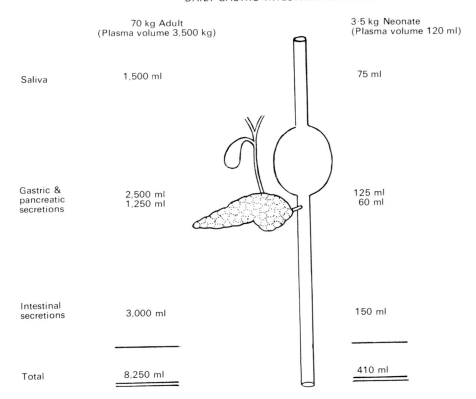

	70 kg Adult (Plasma volume 3,500 kg)	3·5 kg Neonate (Plasma volume 120 ml)
Saliva	1,500 ml	75 ml
Gastric & pancreatic secretions	2,500 ml 1,250 ml	125 ml 60 ml
Intestinal secretions	3,000 ml	150 ml
Total	8,250 ml	410 ml

Fig. 58.2. Daily gastrointestinal fluid turnover of a 3·5-kg infant compared with a 70-kg adult.

the birth of the infant or surgery. The neonate requires 3–5 mmol potassium per day. The easiest way to administer this is to add 1 g potassium chloride (13·4 mmol) to the maintenance and replacement fluids, i.e. the potassium is diluted in 500-ml units; the patient then receives the appropriate aliquot of potassium.

b. Blood Transfusion

BASIC DATA

The normal haemoglobin of a neonate is 19 g/100 ml and falls to a level of 11 g/100 ml at 3 months of age. This fall is due to the fetal haemoglobin being replaced by adult haemoglobin.

The normal white blood cell count in a neonate is 12 000 with a predominance of lymphocytes (70 per cent). These values fall to normal adult levels by 1 year of age.

PRINCIPLES OF MANAGEMENT

A sample of the infant's and mother's blood is required for grouping and cross-matching. In assessing the need for a blood transfusion it must be realized that the blood volume for a neonate varies between 70 ml/kg (full-term infant) and 85 ml/kg

(premature infant). For example, an 8·5-ml blood loss in 1-kg premature infant represents a 10 per cent loss and requires a replacement transfusion; similarly a blood loss of 28 ml in a 4-kg infant represents a 10 per cent loss and requires replacement.

In view of the significance of small losses of blood in neonatal surgery careful measurements of these losses is essential; this is achieved by accurate weighing of the swabs in the operating theatre.

c. Total Parenteral Nutrition

BASIC DATA

The full-term infant requires 100 cal/kg/day rising to 150 cal/kg/day in the premature infant. Intravenous feeding may be given by either a peripheral or a central vein.

PRINCIPLES OF MANAGEMENT

i. *Peripheral Intravenous Feeding:* A suitable regimen includes the consecutive administration of three solutions changing at hourly intervals, i.e. Vamin, Intralipid and 10 per cent dextrose. These may be administered at the rate of 6·0 ml/hour for a 1-kg infant, 12 ml/hour for a 2-kg infant and 18 ml/hour for a 3-kg infant (Puri et al., 1975).

ii. *Central Intravenous Feeding:* This requires a central line with the tip of the catheter in the right atrium. The internal jugular vein is usually used and the catheter is led subcutaneously to a distal site either on the anterior chest wall or above and behind the ear; the former is the preferred site. As hypertonic parenteral solutions can cause tissue damage unless given directly into large veins with a high flow it is important to check the position of the catheters by radiological methods before treatment starts. The solution should be made up daily in the pharmacy under strict aseptic conditions. The composition of a suitable solution is calculated from the electrolyte and calorie requirements of the infant.

iii. *Monitoring of Parenteral Nutrition:* Regular estimations are needed for haemoglobin, plasma proteins, urea and electrolytes, calcium, magnesium and phosphate and screening of the plasma to check that the intralipid has been cleared. The infants are weighed daily.

d. Specific Metabolic Problems

I. JAUNDICE

All newborn babies have a rising level of bilirubin in the serum for the first 3 days of life. Jaundice which persists and becomes more severe requires full investigation and treatment in order to prevent brain damage due to kernicterus. Premature and infected infants are more susceptible to jaundice. Haemolytic disease of the newborn is suspected if the mother is rhesus negative with detectable rhesus antibodies. Careful monitoring of the level of bilirubin in the serum is therefore required to prevent brain damage and rising levels will require treatment with either phototherapy or an exchange transfusion.

II. HAEMORRHAGIC DISEASE OF THE NEWBORN

The liver in the newborn is immature and may be inefficient at synthesizing blood clotting factors. In order to prevent bleeding all infants are given an intramuscular injection of vitamin K_1 prior to operation. In the majority of paediatric medical and obstetric units this drug will have been given routinely in order to prevent this complication.

III. HYPOCALCAEMIA

The level of calcium may fall after birth and is related to immaturity of the parathyroid glands. It is particularly prone to occur in premature infants, the infants of diabetic mothers and infants fed on cows' milk with the increased phosphate content which interferes with absorption of calcium. Operations in the neonatal period and infection increase the risk of this condition. Treatment is by the intravenous administration of 5–10 ml calcium gluconate. This may be

given orally diluted in 100 ml per day to prevent further signs of hypocalcaemia.

IV. HYPOMAGNESAEMIA

This diagnosis should be confirmed when fits occur in the absence of hypoglycaemia and hypocalcaemia (Atwell, 1966). Treatment consists of magnesium acetate 2·5 mmol intravenously to be followed by a daily oral intake of 5·0 mmol of magnesium chloride.

V. HYPOGLYCAEMIA

Hypoglycaemia is often found in the neonatal period. At risk are premature and dysmature infants, infants of diabetic and prediabetic mothers, twins and infants of mothers with toxaemia of pregnancy. Other factors which increase the risks are infection, anoxia, birth and surgical trauma. The level considered important is 1·6 mmol/L in the neonate. Levels below this require treatment although symptoms are usually delayed until the level falls below 1·0 mmol/L. Hypoglycaemia may be prevented by early oral feeding but this is often impossible in infants following an operation in the neonatal period. The incidence of hypoglycaemia is reduced by using N/5 saline in 4·3 per cent dextrose as the standard maintenance intravenous fluid and monitoring of blood levels with the Dextrostix (Ames) at 4-hourly intervals. Hypoglycaemia can be treated by the intravenous administration of 5·0 ml/kg of 20 per cent dextrose or 10–20 ml 10 per cent dextrose.

e. Zinc and Copper Deficiencies

In infants on parenteral nutrition the plasma level of zinc begins to fall within 2 weeks and increases with time. Supplements of 40 µg/kg/day prevent this fall in full-term infants but high levels are required in premature and infants with increased losses with an enterostomy. In these patients the requirement is increased up to 300 µg/kg/day. Copper losses through faecal fistulas occur after 4 weeks of parenteral nutrition. Careful monitoring of zinc and copper levels in infants on parenteral nutrition and with enterostomies is required with adequate replacement in order to prevent deficiencies occurring (Suita et al., 1984).

5. Infection

After and during delivery the newborn is exposed to the risks of infection. The immune response of the newborn infant is low and is further reduced if breast feeding is not established. This is due to the failure to transfer maternal antibodies which are present in high concentrations in the colostrum and breast milk. The incidence of infection has an adverse effect on surgical results and increases neonatal morbidity and mortality.

Principles of Management

Prevention of infection and cross-infection is the key-note of success and depends on strict nursing techniques. Neonatal units should have a controlled environment for temperature and humidity and ideally a positive-pressure system as recommended for operating theatre suites. The infant is nursed in an incubator with its own positive pressure system and barrier nursing techniques are used. The routine care of the umbilicus with spirit swabbing and powdering is essential. Bacteriological screening of infants in the unit is done on admission and at regular intervals with umbilical, nose, throat, skin, stool and rectal swabs. Blood culture, urine culture and lumbar puncture are carried out if infection is suspected. Administration of antibodies is usually required in neonates undergoing surgical corrective procedures because of the possible complications related to the primary condition, e.g. aspiration pneumonia with oesophageal atresia, septicaemia with necrotizing enterocolitis.

6. Equipment

The management of a newborn infant following major surgery requires the use of specialized equipment, e.g. incubators, apnoea alarm blankets, oxygen monitors, temperature, pulse and respiratory rate monitors, etc. Essential items which are required for equipping a neonatal surgical unit are listed in Appendix II.

7. Results

In any infant with a severe congenital anomaly there is an increased incidence of other congenital defects. There is the well-known example of the association of rectal atresia with oesophageal atresia and duodenal obstruction with Down's syndrome. Renal and vertebral anomalies may coexist. These associated defects will have an adverse effect on the management of any congenital anomaly requiring surgery, thus increasing the operative mortality. Similarly the mortality of any operative procedure in the neonatal period is dependent on the maturity of the neonate, the full-term infant withstanding surgery better than the premature infant.

These factors are important when assessing the results of surgical treatment and have been incorporated into a classification used routinely by most neonatal surgical centres. Grade A infants have a birth weight above 2·5 kg and there are no associated congenital defects. In Grade B infants the birth weight may range between 1·8 and 2·5 kg or higher and there is a second moderately severe associated congenital defect. In Grade C infants the birth weight is less than 1·8 kg or higher and there is a second severe associated congenital defect, e.g. oesophageal atresia and congenital heart disease such as the tetralogy of Fallot.

CONGENITAL DEFECTS OF THE ANTERIOR ABDOMINAL WALL

Surgical Embryology

Closure of the omphalocele in the fetus with the return of the midgut contents to the true abdominal cavity (*Fig.* 58.3) will allow the normal development

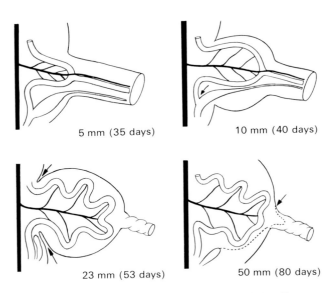

5 mm (35 days)　　10 mm (40 days)

23 mm (53 days)　　50 mm (80 days)

Fig. 58.3. Embryology of the anterior abdominal wall.

of the anterior abdominal wall. Initially the membrane of the omphalocele is thin and transparent but at a later stage it becomes invaded by the ventro-lateral portion of the myotomes and dermatomes. These structures differentiate to form the abdominal musculature. A strip of muscle is found in the free ventral edge which will become the rectus abdominis (*Fig.* 58.4). Fusion of these free edges in the midline closes the abdominal cavity. Fusion first occurs in the upper abdomen, then in the suprapubic region and finally in the umbilical region (Duhamel, 1963). Development of the anterior abdominal wall is complete by the 80th day of intrauterine life (50-mm embryo). Failure of the closure of the abdominal folds will result in a series of different congenital defects. If the proximal fold is deficient a syndrome of ectopia cordis, diaphragmatic hernia and exomphalos results (Cantrell et al., 1958). Failure of the mid-lateral folds results in a defect at the umbilicus, i.e. an exomphalos. Failure of fusion of the distal folds will result in the formation of either an exomphalos or ectopia vesicae and more rarely, when associated with absence of the hindgut, a vesico-intestinal fissure (Rickham, 1960). Failure of the ribbon of muscle in the free edge of the lateral folds on one side will allow a normal insertion of the umbilical vessels but with a defect adjacent to the umbilical ring. This, together with loss of the covering membrane, will result in a gastroschisis (Bernstein, 1940).

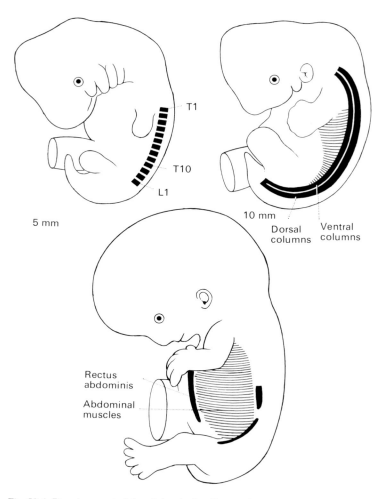

Fig. 58.4. Development of the abdominal wall musculature from the myotomes.

Surgical Anatomy and Pathology

There are differing classifications in use for the description of abdominal wall defects; these depend on the size and position of the defect at the umbilicus and the presence or absence of the covering membrane (*Fig.* 58.5).

If the defect is less than 2·5 cm in diameter at the umbilicus it can be called either a 'hernia into the cord' (*Fig.* 58.5) or a 'type I non-syndrome omphalocele'. If the defect is between 2·5 and 5·0 cm it is called an 'exomphalos minor' or a 'type II non-syndrome omphalocele'. These defects are often grouped together as exomphalos minor as the surgical treatment of such defects is very similar. If the defect at the umbilicus is larger than 5·0 cm it is called 'exomphalos major' (*Fig.* 58.5) or 'type III non-syndrome omphalocele' (Shuster, 1967).

The high incidence of associated anomalies with exomphalos allows certain ones to be classified as 'syndrome omphaloceles': namely the 'upper midline syndrome' with sternal, diaphragmatic pericardial and cardiac defects; the 'lower midline syndrome'

with bladder exstrophy and vesico-intestinal fissure and the 'Beckwith–Wiedemann syndrome' with macroglossia and gigantism.

In 'gastroschisis' (*Fig.* 58.5) the defect is usually small, i.e. less than 2·5 cm, and is to the right of the normal insertion of the umbilical vessels. The sac is absent and the abdominal viscera have protruded through the defect to lie on the anterior abdominal wall. They are usually swollen and oedematous having been bathed in the amniotic fluid prior to delivery. This swelling may be extreme to produce apparent shortening of intestinal length. Occasionally larger defects are found in association with gastroschisis (2·5–5·0 cm and greater than 5·0 cm), but these are extremely rare.

The incidence of associated anomalies with gastroschisis is low and is usually confined to anomalies of the gastrointestinal tract, such as an intestinal atresia.

A universal mesentery and anomalies of intestinal rotation are common to both gastroschisis and exomphalos. Prematurity is not often found in infants with

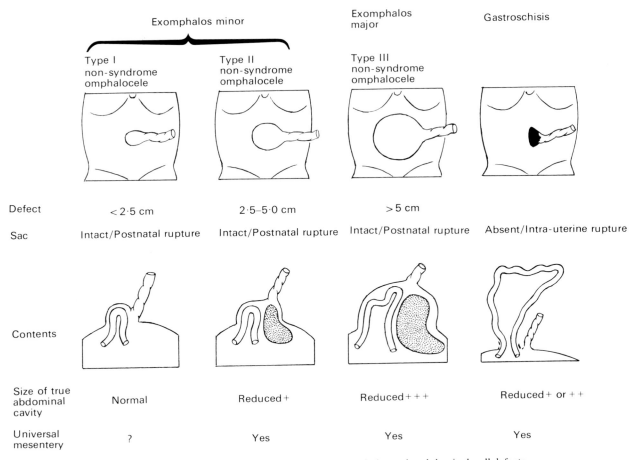

Fig. 58.5. Classification of the common types of congenital anterior abdominal wall defects.

exomphalos but there is a statistically significant difference in the birth weights of infants with exomphalos and gastroschisis, the latter usually being less than 2·25 kg compared to birth weights of over 3·0 kg (Moore, 1977).

The size of the defect and rupture or absence of the sac will determine the timing and type of any surgical repair. In large defects the true abdominal cavity is small (*Fig.* 58.6) and immediate closure with its resultant increase in intra-abdominal pressure results in interference with venous return to the heart and limits respiratory movements. This combination of complications in the past has often resulted in a cardiorespiratory death.

Surgical Management

Clinical Features

Diagnosis is immediate and visual and treatment is determined by the size of the defect or whether the sac is intact or has ruptured.

Preoperative Care

The immediate management is to cover the defect

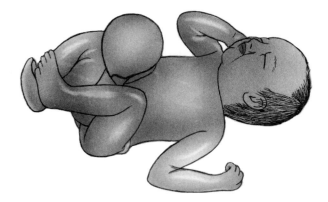

Fig. 58.6. Exomphalos major. Note the umbilical cord insertion to the left and inferiorly. The contents of the sac will include the liver and the small bowel on a universal mesentery.

with a sterile warm and moist dressing to prevent drying of the sac. Loss of body temperature in infants with a ruptured sac or gastroschisis can be minimized by wrapping the infant in aluminium foil and transferring in a portable incubator to a neonatal surgical unit.

Radiographs of the chest and abdomen are taken

to exclude any associated cardiac and diaphragmatic defects and atresia of the intestine. Maternal and infant blood is sent for grouping and cross-matching. A nasogastric tube is passed and aspirated at 1-hourly intervals and left on free drainage. If primary closure is considered impossible without a dangerous rise of intra-abdominal pressure a catheter should be passed into the inferior vena cava to monitor the pressure during the operation.

Operative Repair of Exomphalos

1. PRIMARY CLOSURE

This is only suitable for small defects, i.e. less than 5·0 cm diameter. The incision is made at the junction of the skin with the amniotic membrane and continued circumferentially around the defect. Entering the correct plane may be easier with an incision at right angles to the skin margin which will allow curved dissecting scissors to be passed under the skin edges (*Fig. 58.7*).

The peritoneum is then opened and incised around the neck of the sac. The umbilical vein is ligated and divided. Similarly the umbilical arteries and the urachus are divided between ligatures.

In small defects a formal laparotomy is not undertaken, but in larger defects an associated malrotation may require treatment. A Meckel's diverticulum with or without a band passing to the umbilicus should always be looked for and removed if present. In the larger defects the liver may be adherent to the wall of the sac. The contents of the sac are then returned to the abdominal cavity.

The repair of the defect is then completed with interrupted non-absorbable sutures to approximate the free edges; the skin is closed with interrupted sutures (*Fig. 58.7*).

2. STAGED REPAIR OF EXOMPHALOS MAJOR

a. The 'Gross' Operation (Gross, 1948): The aim of this operation is to convert the intact exomphalos sac into a skin-covered ventral hernia which can be repaired at a second-stage operation when the infant is older.

At operation the umbilical vessels are ligated and divided as close to the wall of the sac as possible. The skin is mobilized in a similar manner as described for primary closure. The incision is in the midline at the upper margin of the defect and at right angles to the junction of skin and the coverings of the sac. The skin is then undermined and mobilized except at or above the costal margin, thus preventing later herniation and moulding of the liver within the sac. The skin is then closed with interrupted sutures over the convexity of the exomphalos. Lateral relieving incisions may be required to allow sufficient freeing of the skin to cover the defect (*Fig. 58.8*). The repair of the ventral hernia thus formed is delayed until the abdominal cavity can safely accommodate the visceral contents of the sac.

b. Silastic 'Bag' or 'Silo' (Shuster, 1967): This opera-

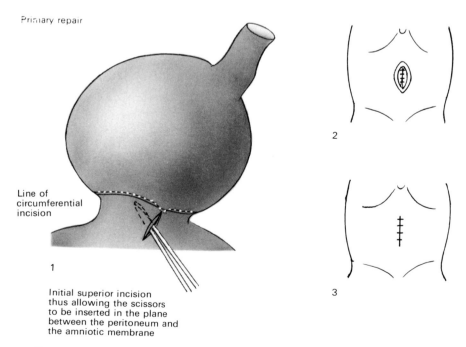

Primary repair

Line of circumferential incision

Initial superior incision thus allowing the scissors to be inserted in the plane between the peritoneum and the amniotic membrane

1

2

3

Fig. 58.7. Primary repair of exomphalos minor. The contents are easily reduced in such patients as the true abdominal cavity contains the liver and is relatively normal in size. Vitello-intestinal remnants should be checked for carefully at operation.

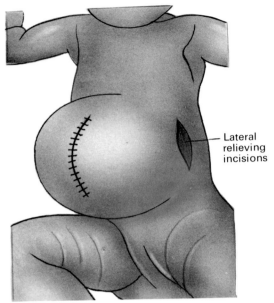

Fig. 58.8. Repair of exomphalos major by the Gross technique. Note the lateral relieving incisions to allow the skin to cover the defect and to be sutured in the midline.

tion is suitable for exomphalos major and gastroschisis if primary skin closure is impossible. It has resulted in an improvement in the operative mortality as it allows a staged reduction of the contents of the sac over a period of 2–3 weeks and removes the need for a second-stage repair of the ventral hernia which follows other forms of operative treatment.

The principles of the operative technique are similar whether used for repair of a gastroschisis or exomphalos major. A Silastic pouch is fashioned and sutured to the free edges of the defect with a continuous 2/0 silk suture (*Fig.* 58.9). The two halves are then sutured in the midline superiorly and inferiorly to form a bag which contains the contents of the sac. Finally, the bag is closed by a continuous suture.

In patients with a gastroschisis no attempt is made to cleanse the surface of the oedematous bowel as this may well prolong any recovery period and lead to a localized perforation and peritonitis. It is important to exclude an intestinal atresia in neonates with gastroschisis and to correct any malrotation and atresia in neonates with an exomphalos. Care must be taken when freeing the liver from the sac as the bare area is adherent to it. Elongation of the inferior vena cava to the level of the wound margin is also found and it may kink on returning the liver to the abdomen, thus interfering with venous return. Over succeeding days, usually at 48–72-hourly intervals, it is possible to reduce the size of the Silastic pouch. This should be done under a general anaesthetic. This procedure is repeated until final closure can be achieved. Closure within 2 weeks is the aim as infection and separation of the Silastic at the margins of the defect may become troublesome.

c. The 'Grob' Technique (Grob, 1963): In exomphalos major skin is often seen growing onto the surface of the sac; the extent is variable. If the surface of the sac can be kept clean the skin will grow over

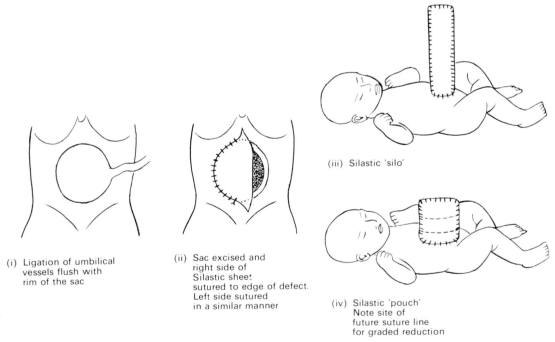

(i) Ligation of umbilical vessels flush with rim of the sac

(ii) Sac excised and right side of Silastic sheet sutured to edge of defect. Left side sutured in a similar manner

(iii) Silastic 'silo'

(iv) Silastic 'pouch' Note site of future suture line for graded reduction

Fig. 58.9. Staged repair of exomphalos major and for gastroschisis using a Silastic sheet to fashion either a 'silo' or a 'pouch'. Reduction in the seize of these is then performed every 48–72 hours, thus allowing skin closure by the 10th–14th postoperative day.

the sac by secondary intention, converting it into a skin-covered ventral hernia. This healing can be assisted by the use of 2 per cent mercurochrome or antibiotic sprays to reduce the incidence of infection. Unfortunately this method of treatment is lengthy and a large defect may take 3–4 months for epithelialization. Mercury poisoning has been described as a complication of this treatment and therefore its use has been discontinued and has largely been replaced by the use of a Silastic prosthesis for staged repair of this defect.

Operative Repair of Gastroschisis

1. PRIMARY CLOSURE

'One-stage' repair operations are not often possible in this condition as it is feared that the subsequent rise in intra-abdominal pressure will lead to cardio-respiratory embarrassment.

2. TWO-STAGE REPAIR

At operation the bowel is inspected carefully to exclude an associated intestinal atresia. The defect is then extended in the midline to the xiphisternum (*Fig.* 58.10). The abdominal wall is then stretched by inserting fingers under the free edge of the defect in order to increase the capacity of the abdomen. Skin closure over the abdominal contents is all that is required. This leaves a small ventral defect which may require repair at a second-stage operation (Thomas and Atwell, 1976).

3. SILASTIC SAC

This operation, described under the repair of exomphalos major, is only rarely required in gastroschisis. Its use should be limited to those patients in whom skin closure would result in a need for mechanical ventilation. A pouch or silo may be fashioned (*see* Fig. 58.9). In deciding on management an order of priorities is useful: namely, skin is better than Silastic, Silastic is better than mechanical ventilation.

Operative Repair of the Secondary Ventral Hernia

This may be necessary after the operative repair of either exomphalos major or gastroschisis. The operation of choice is the extraperitoneal 'keel' operation of Maingot (Maingot, 1961).

The margins of the defect are incised to leave an ellipse of skin (*Fig.* 58.11). The skin is then dissected free from the underlying fibroperitoneal layer which is left intact. This extraperitoneal approach avoids the complication of an ileus leading to a rise in the intra-abdominal pressure which interferes with wound healing. The edges of the sheath covering the rectus abdominis muscle are seen and closed with a continuous monofilament nylon suture. This is repeated until closure of the defect is obtained by the formation of a midline keel. The skin is closed with interrupted non-absorbable sutures, leaving a suction drain subcutaneously (Redivac).

Postoperative Care

The standard nursing care has been described in the section on general principles. The main aims of treatment are to prevent respiratory failure, to feed the infant and to prevent infection. Thus the success of postoperative care depends on the efficient management of assisted ventilation, if required, parenteral nutrition, which may be prolonged for a number of weeks in patients with gastroschisis, and the use of antibiotics.

Complications

EARLY

Associated Anomalies: These have already been described, but malrotation, intestinal atresia, diaphragmatic hernia and cardiac defects may cause problems in the postoperative period.

Prematurity: Low birth weight is well recognized in association with gastroschisis but is less common in exomphalos unless associated with chromosomal defects. Whether the low birth weight is due to pre-

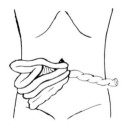

a. Umbilical vessels ligated.
  Enlargement of the defect superiorly in the midline up to the xiphisternum

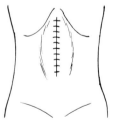

b. Abdominal cavity closure
  after stretching:
  skin closure only

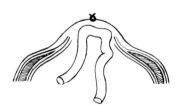

c. Coronal section to show separation
  of divided linea alba and skin—
  covered ventral hernia

Fig. 58.10. Repair of gastroschisis. Defect enlarged by dividing skin and linea alba in the midline superiorly to the xiphisternum. Abdominal cavity enlarged by inserting the fingers under the margins of the defect and stretching the abdominal muscles. Skin closure only with interrupted sutures. Resultant residual ventral hernia is repaired at a later date.

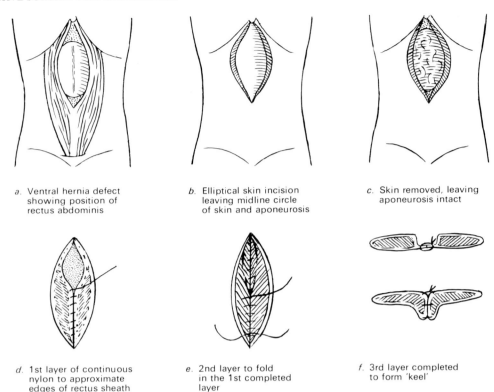

a. Ventral hernia defect showing position of rectus abdominis

b. Elliptical skin incision leaving midline circle of skin and aponeurosis

c. Skin removed, leaving aponeurosis intact

d. 1st layer of continuous nylon to approximate edges of rectus sheath

e. 2nd layer to fold in the 1st completed layer

f. 3rd layer completed to form 'keel'

Note extraperitoneal principle of the operation, thus reducing incidence of postoperative distension

Fig. 58.11. Maingot 'keel' operation for the secondary repair of the ventral hernia following successful repair of a gastroschisis.

mature delivery, intra-uterine growth retardation or a combination of such defects is uncertain. Pre-term infants tolerate surgery poorly and develop complications due to their respiratory immaturity or relative immunological enzymatic and haematological insufficiency. Mature but 'small for dates' babies are particularly prone to hypoglycaemia.

Respiratory Failure: Increase in intra-abdominal pressure following operative repair interferes with respiratory exchange and assisted ventilation may be required for a period postoperatively. Superadded complications may be the respiratory distress syndrome in a premature infant and congenital heart disease.

Infection: Prophylactic broad-spectrum antibiotic cover is an essential adjunct to surgery in these infants as septicaemia is now the second most common cause of death.

Prolonged Ileus: The duration of the postoperative ileus in infants with gastroschisis is related to the rate of resolution of the pre-existing inflammatory changes. The reduction in length of the bowel is secondary to inflammatory thickening and is not a primary anomaly. Subsequent operations and radiological studies (Touloukian and Spackman, 1971) have shown a normal length and mucosal pattern of the bowel thus confirming that the changes seen in the bowel at birth are reversible.

LATE

Growth and Development: The growth and development in infants with exomphalos and gastroschisis have been normal in the majority of patients (Thomas and Atwell, 1976).

Ventral Hernia: A ventral hernia following repair of exomphalos or gastroschisis may be planned or unplanned. The repair of such defects has been described; the extraperitoneal 'keel' operation (Maingot, 1961) is the operation of choice.

Inguinal Hernia: Subsequent development of inguinal hernias is not uncommon and is probably related to a pre-existing peritoneal sac and the raised intra-abdominal pressure following repair of the umbilical defect.

CONGENITAL DIAPHRAGMATIC HERNIA

Surgical Embryology

The development of the diaphragm is completed by the 10th week of intra-uterine life, thus dividing the coelomic cavity into its abdominal and thoracic compartments. The diaphragm is formed by a fusion of mesoderm from different origins (*Fig.* 58.12). The in the development of the diaphragm may be contributory factors in the aetiology of diaphragmatic hernia. This is reflected in the very high incidence of a universal mesentery and malrotation of the intestine in these patients.

Associated malformations of the lungs are a common finding in diaphragmatic hernia and include extralobar sequestration (Berman, 1958), aplasia and

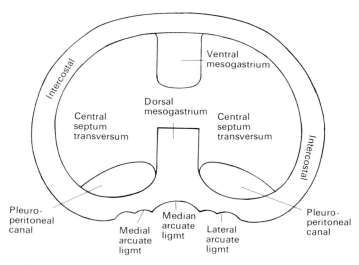

Fig. 58.12. Embryological development and origins of the diaphragm.

peripheral part develops from the intercostal muscle and the central part from the septum transversum and the dorsal and ventral mesogastrium. The posterolateral spaces are then closed by the pleuroperitoneal folds. This latter component is initially membranous but later muscle fibres grow between these layers to complete the formation of the diaphragm.

The development of the right side of the diaphragm is completed before the left which may account for the high incidence of left-sided defects. The pleuroperitoneal folds in the posterolateral position (foramen of Bochdalek) are the last to form which may account for the high incidence of defects at this site. Failure of fusion of the central and lateral portions of the diaphragm may result in a defect in the anterolateral portion of the diaphragm (foramen of Morgagni). Central defects are extremely rare and may be associated with other serious congenital malformation such as congenital aplasia of the spleen and congenital heart disease. Aplasia of the diaphragm may be found in association with any of the defects, resulting in the partial or complete absence of the hemidiaphragm.

The midgut is developing at the same time as the diaphragm with an increase in length followed by the closure of the omphalocele with return of its contents to the abdominal cavity. The intestine then undergoes rotation and fixation to take up its adult anatomical position. Early return of the midgut or a delay

hypoplasia of the lungs (Sabga et al., 1961). The causation of these associated malformations is obscure, but if the intestine entered the pleural cavity between the 75th and 90th days of intra-uterine life causing compression of the lung it would coincide with the stage of development of the airways within the lung (Kitagawa et al., 1971). A reduction in the airway number and alveolar counts has been reported in pathological studies on one infant dying with a diaphragmatic hernia. The alveolar numbers were almost normal when related to the number of terminal bronchioli in the lung.

After operative correction of a diaphragmatic hernia many lungs which appear small and hypoplastic will expand and fill the pleural cavity. The method of postnatal growth of a hypoplastic lung is debatable; it is unlikely that any new airways or new arterial branches would develop in this region (Kitagawa et al., 1971). Alveolar multiplication together with intra-acinar multiplication would be expected but whether this would proceed until the normal total alveolar number is reached is unlikely. The most likely result would be multiplication to give the normal alveolar number supplied by each terminal bronchiolus. As the lung expands to fill the pleural cavity there will be compensatory emphysema.

The association of congenital heart disease with diaphragmatic hernia is common and the main contributory cause of death. In our series of 44 patients 18 died and 11 of these were found to have congenital heart disease. The most common finding was a widely patent ductus arteriosus (10), coarctation of the aorta (2), hypoplastic left heart and aorta (1), ventricular septal defect (1), right-sided aortic arch (1) and a single ventricle (1). The high incidence of a widely patent and high flow ductus may be related to the severe hypoxia and raised pulmonary vascular resistance leading to persistence of the fetal type of circulation (Collins et al., 1977). The mesonephros also contributes to the closure of the diaphragm and renal ectopia has been recorded with diaphragmatic hernia (Bulgrin and Holmes, 1955). Other congenital defects found in association with diaphragmatic hernia include congenital absence of the spleen, pericardial defects, ectopia cordis, exomphalos, undescended testes, de Lange syndrome, vertebral and musculoskeletal anomalies, spina bifida cystica and inguinal hernias.

Surgical Anatomy

1. *Types of defect*

A. POSTEROLATERAL DEFECT (FORAMEN OF BOCHDALEK)
This is the commonest defect found in the neonatal period (over 75 per cent). The defects can be subdivided into two subgroups (Harrington, 1948), those with the defect confined to the pleuroperitoneal canal and those with an additional aplasia of part of the adjacent diaphragm (*Fig.* 58.13). The aplasia of the diaphragm may involve one-half of the whole diaphragm or more commonly is partial to produce a hemi-absence of one side of the diaphragm.

B. ANTEROLATERAL DEFECT (FORAMEN OF MORGAGNI)
This is a rarer defect in the newborn but in a similar manner to posterolateral defects aplasia of the diaphragm may be found in association with it to produce a larger defect (*Fig.* 58.13).

C. OTHER DEFECTS
These are rare and often found in association with multiple congenital defects (*Fig.* 58.13). Two such patients have been seen in our series of 44 and in both it was impossible to reduce the contents and repair the defect; both patients died. In one of our two patients the defect was bilateral and associated with the syndrome of congenital absence of the spleen, multiple congenital heart defects, a midline liver with anomalous portal venous return and a midline stomach. The second patient was associated with a thoracic meningocele. Occasionally a true anterior or retrosternal costochondral defect is found.

2. *Side of Defect*
Left-sided defects (60 per cent) are more common than right-sided defects. Whether this is related to the later closure of the left side of the diaphragm or to the liver protecting the right side remains unanswered. Central defects are very rare and in our experience are impossible to repair. Bilateral diaphragmatic hernias are extremely rare and in 1965 a search of the surgical literature yielded only nine such patients (Fitchett and Tavarez, 1965).

3. *Hernial Sac*
In the majority of defects the hernial sac is absent (65 per cent). Diaphragmatic hernia with a hernial sac must be differentiated from eventration of the diaphragm. In the former there is no muscle tissue between the folds of the pleura and peritoneum whereas in eventration muscle and fibrous tissue are found between the layers.

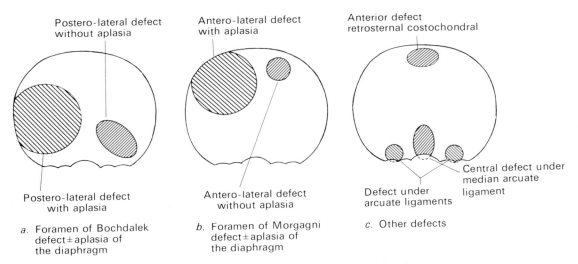

Fig. 58.13. Types of congenital diaphragmatic hernia.

Surgical Management

Clinical Features

The diagnosis of a congenital diaphragmatic hernia must be suspected in any newborn with respiratory difficulties, an apparent dextrocardia due to a shift of the mediastinum and a scaphoid abdomen.

Preoperative Care

The diagnosis is confirmed by a single radiograph of the chest and abdomen. This shows displacement of the mediastinum by gas-filled loops of intestine in the chest. It is important to include the abdomen on the film as confirmatory evidence of the diagnosis will be provided by an abnormal gas pattern below the diaphragm. Occasionally the hernial sac, if present, can be seen on the radiograph.

In the differential diagnosis multiple staphylococcal lung cysts, congenital cystic adenomatoid malformation of the lung and haemorrhagic disease of the newborn have caused mistakes and in some patients unnecessary operations. In these conditions the gas pattern below the diaphragm is normal, thus providing the most helpful diagnostic sign. There is *no* need for the use of contrast studies which may be harmful.

Administration of oxygen by a face mask is *harmful* as this will merely increase the gaseous content of the bowel in the chest, leading to a further shift of the mediastinum and compression of the contralateral lung. The oxygen content of the incubator may be increased, but if there is no improvement an endotracheal tube is passed and positive-pressure respiration established. Arrangements are made for an anaesthetist or doctor experienced in endotracheal intubation of a neonate to accompany the infant on transfer to a neonatal surgical unit.

A nasogastric tube (no. 10 Fr. gauge) is passed into the stomach and aspirated. The tube is left open on free drainage into a gallipot and is aspirated at half-hourly intervals.

The infant is nursed in an incubator, lying on the side of the defect and with the head slightly elevated. These measures may improve the expansion of the lung on the contralateral side.

Samples of the mother's and infant's blood are sent for grouping and cross-matching and an intravenous drip is established. Levels of electrolytes in the serum and blood gases are determined.

The successful management of a congenital diaphragmatic hernia depends on early diagnosis, resuscitation, correction of acid base disturbances and rapid effective surgical treatment. In some centres operation is delayed to allow resuscitation; in others the surgery is rapid and combined with resuscitation. The results of this change in policy have not yet been fully evaluated but the mortality remains high in patients with symptoms and signs developing in the first 6 hours following delivery (Bloss et al., 1980; Bohn et al., 1983; Vancanti et al., 1984).

In the preoperative period a tension pneumothorax may require urgent treatment. Insertion of a needle through an intercostal space allows the air to escape; the needle is then connected to an underwater-seal drainage bottle.

Operation

An abdominal approach is preferred as it is easier to reduce the contents and treat the associated universal mesentery and malrotation. The infant is placed flat on its back and a curved subcostal incision is made 2·0 cm below the costal margin (*Fig.* 58.14).

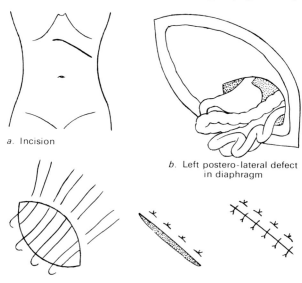

a. Incision

b. Left postero-lateral defect in diaphragm

c. Repair with interrupted linen sutures

Fig. 58.14. Operative repair of a posterolateral diaphragmatic hernia.

The abdomen is opened and the defect is inspected. The stomach and loops of small and large bowel are seen entering the pleural cavity (*Fig.* 58.14). The spleen, lobes of the liver and kidney may also be contents of the hernial sac.

The contents are gently reduced into the abdominal cavity. Close inspection is necessary to find if a hernial sac is present. This can easily be missed as it is thin walled and subject to the negative intrathoracic pressure and covers the chest wall and the unexpanded lung. If a sac is present it is excised from the free margin of the defect in the diaphragm, taking extreme care about haemostasis. This manoeuvre is made easier if the sac is opened at one point to reduce the negative intrathoracic pressure. The sac is then easily pulled into the abdominal cavity.

The lung is inspected. It is often small and hypoplastic. The anaesthetist should be dissuaded from attempting to inflate it. An underwater pleural drain is then inserted through a lower intercostal space in the posterior axillary line.

The defect in the diaphragm is then repaired (*Fig.*

58.14). In small hernias the edges are approximated with a layer of 2/0 or 3/0 non-absorbable interrupted mattress sutures. These are tied and the free edge is then sutured with a row of interrupted 2/0 or 3/0 sutures. In larger defects, especially if the posterior rim of diaphragmatic muscle is absent, the repair is more difficult. Under these circumstances the anterior free edge of the diaphragm may be sutured to the intercostal muscles or to the periosteum of the ribs or even to the posterior layer of perirenal fascia. In extreme cases either a Silastic prosthesis is tailored and sutured into the defect or a reverse latissimus dorsi flap is used (Bianchi et al., 1983).

Attention is then turned to the abdomen and any associated malrotation is corrected by dividing Ladd's band and mobilizing the bowel to leave the small intestine on the right, and the large bowel on the left side of the abdomen (Ladd's operation).

The closure of the abdomen is often the most difficult part of the operation due to the small size of the true abdominal cavity. The range of alternative procedures used to ease this stage of the operation is as follows:

1. Normal closure in layers.
2. Stretching of the abdominal wall with the fingers inserted under the free edge of the wound.
3. Skin closure only leaving a planned ventral hernia which will require a secondary repair at a later date.
4. Insertion of a Silastic patch into the wound with or without skin cover. This is then repaired within the first 2 postoperative weeks (cf. repair of exomphalos, p. 901).
5. The use of a respirator in the postoperative period to maintain a satisfactory respiratory exchange until the abdominal cavity enlarges sufficiently so that normal respiration may be established.

In patients who have presented within the first 24 hours of life it is advisable to insert an underwater drain to the contralateral pleural cavity. This will prevent any mortality due to the contralateral lung developing a tension pneumothorax in the immediate postoperative period (Young, 1968). Hypoplasia of the lung and assisted ventilation may be predisposing factors for the development of this complication.

Postoperative Care

NURSING CARE

This is intensive and the infant is 'specialed'. Observations of pulse and respiratory rate are constantly monitored or measured at regular intervals. Temperature is monitored or measured at 1-hourly intervals. Peripheral circulation is checked by pressure on the finger pulp space and the time taken for the return of the colour is measured and recorded. The head is kept slightly elevated within the incubator. Hypoglycaemia is checked for by Dextrostix tests at 4-hourly intervals, or more frequently if the infant is premature. Care of the mouth and frequent aspiration of any secretions are essential.

The pleural drains are watched carefully and clamped at any time before moving the infant. Physiotherapy and suction are performed hourly.

The nasogastric tube is aspirated at half-hourly intervals for 12 hours and then at hourly intervals, and in between aspirations is left on free drainage. Abdominal girth measurements are recorded 4-hourly. Oral feeds are not introduced until the aspirates are minimal and non-bile stained, meconium has been passed and the abdomen is soft.

Routine nursing care is given to the wound and to the care of the umbilicus. Intake and output charts are accurately kept and intravenous drips are maintained on a standard regimen.

Many of these infants will be maintained on a ventilator postoperatively for a variable time and require the intensive management that such a regimen needs.

Antibiotic cover is given as a routine because of the risks of infection and because of the poor immunological response of the newborn.

Complications

EARLY

Tension Pneumothorax: This complication should be prevented by the routine insertion of bilateral underwater chest drains.

Pulmonary Hypoplasia: In some infants it is impossible to achieve a satisfactory pulmonary exchange. The hypoxia may be the cause of the persistence of the fetal circulation with widely patent high-flow ductus arteriosus which is so often found at a postmortem examination.

Infection: This should be minimized by strict barrier nursing, intensive physiotherapy and antibiotic care.

Associated Malformations: Congenital heart disease and other malformations are often found in infants with a diaphragmatic hernia and increase the mortality.

Gestational Age: Prematurity and 'small for dates infants' have specific complications such as hypoglycaemia, hypocalcaemia and hypomagnesaemia which require careful monitoring and treatment.

LATE

Recurrence: Whether this is due to the difficulties in achieving a satisfactory repair, or the poor expansion of the lung on the affected side, or to raised intra-abdominal pressure due to difficulties in closing the abdomen, is open to conjecture.

Ventral Hernia/Inguinal Hernia: The factors listed above predispose to the development of these complications.

Undescended Testis: This associated defect is probably related to the primary defect and will require surgical treatment at a later date.

EVENTRATION OF THE DIAPHRAGM

Only rarely does this condition present in the neonatal period. Whether it is due to a failure of migration of muscle fibres into the developing diaphragm, atrophy or hypoplasia of part of the diaphragm is uncertain. The presenting features are similar to those of a diaphragmatic hernia, but in the older infant or child there is often a history of recurrent chest infections. Treatment is surgical with plication of the diaphragm.

OESOPHAGEAL ATRESIA AND TRACHEO-OESOPHAGEAL FISTULA

Surgical Embryology

The oesophagus and trachea develop from the primitive foregut and their differentiation is completed between the 3rd and 5th weeks of intra-uterine life. The ingrowth of the ventral ridges of the foregut (laryngotracheal sulcus) starts at 21–23 days and has finished by 27–32 days of intra-uterine life (3–8 mm-embryo). This process starts caudally and eventually with fusion of the lateral ridges the oesophagus becomes separated from the developing tracheo-oesophageal tree (*Fig. 58.15*). Failure of fusion of the tracheo-oesophageal septum at some point will lead to the formation of a tracheo-oesophageal fistula.

The causation of oesophageal atresia is more obscure and remains unknown. Many theories have been suggested such as inflammation and ulceration, deficiency of material where the lung primordium uses up the common material available, relative pressure changes either from an enlarged cardiac primordium or from external pressure, malposition of the large vessels, vascular insufficiency or compression of the oesophagus due to external pressure of the developing pneumo-enteric processes (Rickham and Johnston, 1969). The development of oesophageal atresia could be due to other factors related to segmentation of the embryo. The segmentation of para-axial mesoderm on each side of the notochord and the formation of the sclerotomes and myotomes and formation of the membranous vertebras on an inter-segmental plane occurs at a similar time. As the upper oesophagus contains striated muscle the foregut may be susceptible to vascular changes caused by segmentation, and this may be important in the causation

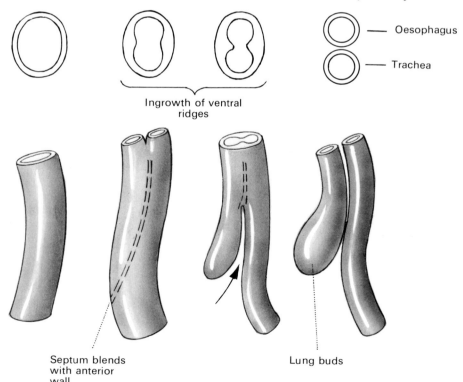

Ingrowth of ventral ridges

Oesophagus

Trachea

Septum blends with anterior wall

Lung buds

Fig. 58.15. Development of the trachea and bronchial tree from the foregut.

of oesophageal atresia (Bond-Taylor et al., 1973). The high incidence of vertebral and other associated anomalies with oesophageal atresia lends support to this hypothesis. Similarities occur in anorectal malformations where there is a high incidence of vertebral and associated anomalies; striated muscle is present and the vertebral column is in close approximation to the developing bowel.

Surgical Pathology and Anatomy

Oesophageal atresia occurs in a variety of differing forms but can be conveniently subdivided into three basic types, namely oesophageal atresia with and without a tracheo-oesophageal fistula and tracheo-oesophageal fistula without an oesophageal atresia (*Fig.* 58.16). These basic types account for 95 per cent of the patients. The other 5 per cent of patients with congenital anomalies of the oesophagus have additional fistula and other defects superimposed on this basic pattern.

The blood supply of the oseophagus is poor when related to other parts of the alimentary tract. The upper oesophagus receives its supply from the inferior thyroid arteries, the middle third of the oesophagus from the intercostal and bronchial arteries and by branches from the aorta and the lower third from the left gastric and phrenic arteries. The

middle third of the oesophagus therefore has the poorest blood supply and this may have been one of the causes of anastomotic leaks and operative failure in the past.

In oesophageal atresia there is usually a wide disparity in size between the upper hypertrophied pouch and the lower distal oesophageal segment which is thin walled and has a narrow lumen. The blood supply to the lower oesophageal segment is poor when compared to the rich blood supply of the hypertrophied upper oesophageal segment. Variations occur in the degree of separation of the blind upper pouch of the oesophagus and the distal lower segment whether associated or unassociated with a tracheo-oesophageal fistula. In the latter group of patients there is usually wide separation which makes any primary repair using the oesophagus impracticable. In patients with a tracheo-oesophageal fistula the segments may overlap or be separated by up to 4 cm. Prematurity is a complicating factor in oesophageal atresia, particularly in the patients without a tracheo-oesophageal fistula.

Associated anomalies are found in 50 per cent of infants with oesophageal atresia and tracheo-oesophageal fistula. These range from vertebral and musculoskeletal (40 per cent), genito-urinary (30 per cent), gastrointestinal (25 per cent), cardiovascular (20 per cent) and other miscellaneous defects (5 per

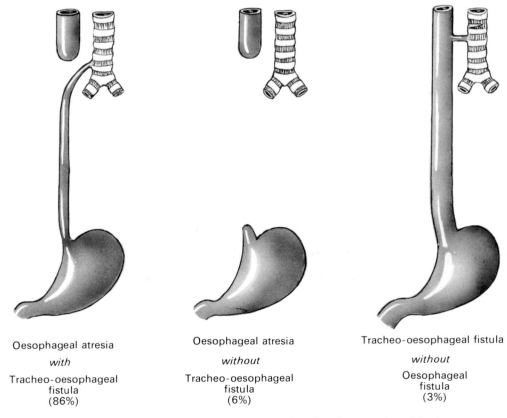

Oesophageal atresia

with

Tracheo-oesophageal
fistula
(86%)

Oesophageal atresia

without

Tracheo-oesophageal
fistula
(6%)

Tracheo-oesophageal fistula

without

Oesophageal
fistula
(3%)

Fig. 58.16. Types of congenital oesophageal atresia and tracheo-oesophageal fistula.

cent). The associated anomalies are often life threatening and may modify surgical treatment in addition to altering the morbidity and mortality of the primary condition.

Surgical Management

Clinical Features

A history of hydramnios should alert the clinician to the possible diagnosis of oesophageal atresia as it is found in half of the cases. The inability to swallow saliva results in aspiration into the tracheobronchial tree and may interfere with respiration and lead to pneumonia. Early diagnosis at this stage will reduce the risks of these complications. Reflux of acid juices from the stomach through a tracheo-oesophageal fistula causes a serious and often fatal pneumonitis.

The diagnosis of oesophageal atresia is confirmed by passing a radio-opaque no. 10 catheter which is held up 10 cm from the lip margins. Lateral and posteroanterior radiographs of the chest and abdomen are taken; the presence or absence of gas below the diaphragm thus differentiates the patients into those with or without a tracheo-oesophageal fistula.

The diagnosis of a tracheo-oesophageal fistula without an oesophageal atresia should be suspected in any infant who has difficulties in feeding—in particular, cyanotic attacks with the feed or recurrent chest infections affecting the right upper lobe. In some infants air passes from the tracheobronchial tract into the gastrointestinal tract to cause abdominal distension similar to that found in Hirschsprung's disease. The diagnosis is confirmed by demonstrating the fistula with contrast material on ciné radiology. In some cases the fistula may be seen and cannulated with a ureteric catheter during oesophagoscopy or bronchoscopy. If the infant is oesophagoscoped and intubated, anaesthetic gases can be detected passing through the fistula and into the eye of the examiner!

Preoperative Care

The infants are nursed level in an incubator. Additional oxygen and humidity are often required. Periodic aspiration of the upper oesophageal pouch at half-hourly intervals will reduce the incidence of an aspiration pneumonia. Antibiotics are given and blood is sent to the laboratory for estimations of haemoglobin and urea and electrolytes in the serum and grouping and cross-matching.

Choice of Operation

1. OESOPHAGEAL ATRESIA AND
TRACHEO-OESOPHAGEAL FISTULA

a. Fit Full-term Infant: Primary anastomosis is the operation of choice, with either a gastrostomy or transanastomotic tube for feeding in the postoperative phase. A gastrostomy is safer.

b. Premature Infant: Staging of the procedures may improve the operative results. Various operations and sequences of operation are possible:
   i. Gastrostomy and suction of the upper pouch with a Replogle tube, followed at a later date by primary anastomosis. An alternative to gastrostomy is parenteral nutrition.
   ii. Ligation and division of fistula and gastrostomy followed by primary anastomosis at a later date.

c. Widely Separated Upper and Lower Oesophageal Segments: Either (i) ligation of tracheo-oesophageal fistula, gastrostomy and cervical oesophagostomy, or (ii) ligation of tracheo-oesophageal fistula, gastrostomy and continuous suction of the upper oesophageal pouch. This second procedure, if successful, may avoid the need for oesophageal reconstruction as a delayed primary anastomosis may be possible.

d. Infant with Severe Pulmonary Complications: In these infants treatment should be delayed or staged until the chest condition improves.

e. Infant with Multiple Congenital Anomalies: Careful staging of the various operations is vital for a successful outcome.

2. OESOPHAGEAL ATRESIA WITHOUT
TRACHEO-OESOPHAGEAL FISTULA

a. Fit Full-term Infant: Either (i) gastrostomy and cervical oesophagostomy and later oesophageal reconstruction, or (ii) a primary oesophageogastrostomy (Ivor Lewis operation) (Atwell and Harrison, 1980) or colonic replacement of the oesophagus (Sherman and Waterston, 1957). (*See* Chapter 9.)

b. Premature Infant: Either suction of the upper segment or a cervical oesophagostomy. This can be combined with either a gastrostomy or total parenteral nutrition until the infant reaches a weight suitable for either staged operations and early or late oesophageal reconstruction.

3. TRACHEO-OESOPHAGEAL FISTULA WITHOUT
OESOPHAGEAL ATRESIA

Ligation of the tracheo-oesophageal fistula is performed through a left cervical approach, cf. cervical oesophagostomy. Preoperative oesophagoscopy and cannulation of the fistula with a ureteric catheter will make the identification of the fistula much easier at the operation.

Gastrostomy (*Fig.* 58.17)

A transverse left upper abdominal muscle-cutting incision is made. The body of the stomach is delivered into the wound by placing Babcock tissue forceps

Gastrostomy   (Stamm.)

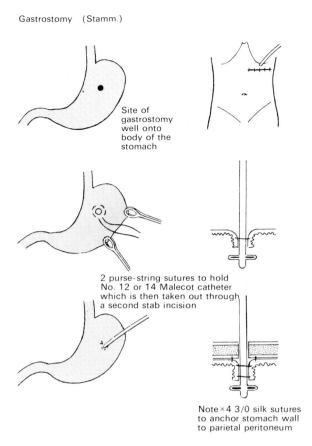

Site of
gastrostomy
well onto
body of the
stomach

2 purse-string sutures to hold
No. 12 or 14 Malecot catheter
which is then taken out through
a second stab incision

Note × 4 3/0 silk sutures
to anchor stomach wall
to parietal peritoneum

Fig. 58.17. Operative technique for fashioning a Stamm gastrostomy in the newborn.

REPAIR of oesophageal atresia: primary anastomosis

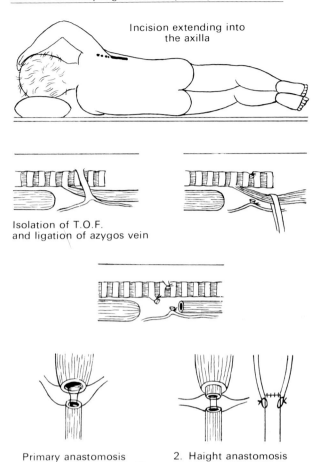

Incision extending into
the axilla

Isolation of T.O.F.
and ligation of azygos vein

Primary anastomosis
with single layer 4/0 silk

2. Haight anastomosis

Fig. 58.18. Transpleural method of primary anastomosis of oesophageal atresia after ligation of tracheo-oesophageal fistula.

onto the greater curvature, taking care to avoid any injury to the gastro-epiploic vessels.

A seromuscular purse-string suture is then inserted at the site of the proposed gastrostomy which is well up into the body of the stomach. The stomach is opened with the cutting diathermy and a no. 12 latex Malecot catheter is introduced and the purse-string suture of 3/0 chromic catgut is tied. A second purse-string is then inserted and tied. The catheter end is then passed out through a second stab incision 1 cm above the wound. Four non-absorbable silk sutures (3/0 silk) are then placed in position in the N.S.E. and W. positions. These seromuscular and peritoneal sutures, when tied, hold the anterior wall of the stomach firmly against the abdominal wall, thus reducing the risk of leakage. The wound is then closed in layers.

Ligation of Tracheo-oesophageal Fistula and Primary Anastomosis *(Fig. 58.18)*

1. TRANSPLEURAL ROUTE

The patient is positioned on the table as shown. The vertical incision is anterior to the midaxillary line and extends from the axilla to the 8th rib. The serratus anterior is incised down to the rib cage and the shoulder girdle is displaced posteriorly. Care is taken to preserve the nerve supply of the serratus anterior. Anteriorly the pectoral muscles are freed from the rib cage with the cutting diathermy to the line of the nipple. Superiorly care must be taken as the incision extends to the floor of the axilla. The chest is then opened through the 4th intercostal space using cutting diathermy to divide the muscles down to the pleura. As the lung collapses the incision is extended anteriorly to the nipple line and posteriorly to the angle of the rib. Straight and curved mastoid retractors are suitable in the newborn period to keep the chest open. The edges of the curved retractor are placed under the rib margins and then a straight retractor is used to separate the skin margins.

The lung is then retracted inferiorly and anteriorly to expose the mediastinal surface of the right pleural cavity. The azygos vein is identified and divided between ligatures. The vagus and phrenic nerves are identified. The tracheo-oesophageal fistula is seen passing upwards and merging with the posterior wall of the trachea and is closely related to the vagus nerve. The fistula is isolated with a sling, taking care to preserve the small blood vessels supplying the lower segment of the oesophagus. The fistula is then transfixed and ligated with 3/0 silk as close to the tracheal wall as possible. If a gastrostomy is not established it is important to pass a fine tube into the stomach to deflate it. This reduces the risks of forceful regurgitation of gastric contents in the early postoperative period, leading to possible breakdown of the anastomosis.

The upper pouch is identified. It may be seen in relationship to the posterior wall of the trachea and may overlap the site of the previously ligated tracheo-oesophageal fistula. Often the upper pouch is widely separated and identification is difficult. This is simplified by asking the anaesthetist to pass a no. 10 catheter into the pouch. A no. 2 polyvinyl tube has previously been passed into the no. 10 catheter. Once identified the upper pouch is mobilized, held with a stay suture and its fundus is opened.

Interrupted silk sutures (4/0) are used for the anastomosis. On completion of the posterior layer of the anastomosis the catheter in the upper pouch is gently advanced into view; the end of this tube is then cut off and the inner polyvinyl tube is pulled into the chest and the anaesthetist withdraws the outer catheter. The polyvinyl tube is passed into the lower oesophageal segment and on into the stomach. The anterior portion of the anastomosis is then completed over the tube. If a gastrostomy has been performed the polyvinyl tube is passed into the lower segment, to facilitate the completion of the anastomosis, but it is then withdrawn.

An underwater pleural drain is inserted (no. 12 latex Malecot catheter with the limbs cut off). The open end of the cathether is left as near as possible to the anastomosis.

The chest is closed in layers. Three chromic catgut (3/0) rib sutures are inserted and used to approximate the ribs. The intercostal muscles are closed with continuous 3/0 absorbable sutures. The serratus anterior is closed with interrupted 2/0 or 3/0 chromic catgut. The skin is closed with a 3/0 cubcuticular nylon suture and held with beads and aluminium stops at each end.

Specific Problems:

a. Disparity in Size: The disparity in size of the upper and lower oesophageal segments may make the anastomosis difficult.

b. Avascularity of Lower Segment: This should be avoidable by taking extreme care in handling the tissues and keeping mobilization of the lower segment to a minimum.

c. Aberrant Right Subclavian Artery: This anomaly is often found in association with oesophageal atresia and may increase the technical difficulty of the anastomosis.

d. Tension on the Anastomosis: If the ends of the

upper and lower oesophageal segments are widely separated primary anastomosis may be impossible. In some patients the anastomosis is completed under increased tension with a much higher risk of breakdown and an increased mortality. Careful judgement is required in making the decision of whether to complete the anastomosis or to ligate the fistula and leave the upper pouch for either repeated aspiration and stretching or performing a cervical oesophagostomy.

Two other procedures are useful in overcoming the technical problem of widely separated oesophageal segments (*Fig.* 58.19):

    i. Circular Myotomy (Livaditis operation): Circular myotomy of the upper pouch down to the submucosal layer may increase length and allow completion of the anastomosis.

    ii. Anterior Flap (Gough operation): An anterior flap may be fashioned from the wide upper oesophageal segment and folded down, thus providing additional length. The anastomosis is completed without tension.

Oesophageal atresia: Modifications of primary anastomosis

a. Circular myotomy (Livaditis opn)

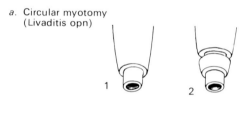

b. Anterior flap (Gough opn)

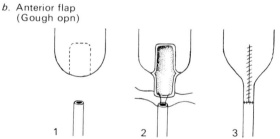

Fig. 58.19. Operative procedures to assist in achieving a primary anastomosis with widely separated upper and lower oesophageal segments.

2. EXTRAPLEURAL ROUTE (Holder, 1964)

Stages in this operation are similar to the primary repair and ligation of the tracheo-oesophageal fistula. Technically it is more difficult and time consuming and the pleural cavity is often opened inadvertently. The advantage of the extrapleural route is that if an anastomotic leak occurs it can be treated successfully by conservative measures.

Cervical Oesophagostomy

This operation allows saliva to escape onto the surface of the neck and thus reduce the incidence of pneumonia. It can be used as a preliminary procedure or following complications of a primary repair. The incision is made in a skin crease along the left clavicle extending from the sternal head of the sternomastoid to the midpoint of the clavicle. The clavicular head of sternomastoid is divided with cutting diathermy. The sternal head is left attached but may be divided at its periosteal attachment and reflected upwards. The omohyoid muscle is divided and the great vessels in the neck are retracted laterally. The lateral wall of the oesophagus and trachea are seen. The lateral lobes of the thyroid are retracted anteriorly. The oesophagus is then identified and mobilized, care being taken to avoid damaging the left recurrent laryngeal nerve. The fundus of the oesophagus is then opened and sutured to the skin with interrupted silk sutures. If the sternal head of sternomastoid was divided it is then sutured to its periosteal attachment.

Ligation of Isolated Tracheo-oesophageal Fistula

The incision is above the left clavicle extending from the midline of the neck to the mid-clavicular line. The clavicular head of sternomastoid is then identified and divided with cutting diathermy. The sternal head can be divided at its periosteal attachment and reflected upwards to expose the omohyoid and the great vessels in the carotid sheath. The belly of omohyoid is divided.

The oesophagus can be approached from either behind or in front of the great vessels, the latter being the method of choice. The oesophagus and trachea are identified together with the left recurrent laryngeal nerve. The fistula is identified. Slings placed around the oesophagus above and below the fistula often make its identification easier. The fistula is transfixed on the tracheal side with a 3/0 silk suture and divided. The oesophageal side of the fistula is repaired with 3/0 non-absorbable sutures. The wound is closed in layers with an infant Redivac drain down to the site of the fistula.

Postoperative Care

NURSING

Observations for the routine postoperative care of the newborn are as previously described. The infant is nursed level.

UNDERWATER PLEURAL DRAIN

This is left *in situ* for 10 days, i.e. until the infant has been fed orally for the first time.

GASTROSTOMY

The gastrostomy is left on free drainage into a gallipot at the level of the infant. This reduces intragastric pressure and decreases the possibility of gastro-oesophageal reflux which can cause disruption of the anastomosis.

The gastrostomy tube is aspirated at 1-hourly intervals. Dextrose followed by milk feeds can be introduced any time after 4–5 days until the critical initial healing phase is over.

If the gastrostomy tube becomes dislodged in the first 10 days postoperatively the infant must be taken to the operating theatre for reintroduction of the tube. This may be done without an anaesthetic, but during this early phase it is possible to push the stomach off the anterior abdominal wall on reintroducing the catheter resulting in peritonitis. After the first 10 days it is usually safe to replace the gastrostomy tube on the ward; delay is to be avoided as the opening can close very quickly. When the infant is on full oral feeds the gastrostomy tube is removed.

PREVENTION OF INFECTION

Chest physiotherapy and antibiotics are used to reduce pulmonary complications.

PARENTERAL FLUID AND CALORIES

Intravenous fluid is administered to maintain the internal homeostasis of the infant. Parenteral nutrition is not used initially but reserved for use in the complicated patient.

Complications

EARLY

Anastomotic Leak: This is the most dangerous complication especially when it occurs between the 3rd and 5th day. It is heralded by the appearance of saliva or bile-stained fluid in the tubing of the underwater pleural drain. If disruption occurs early the chest is reopened and either a second repair is attempted or the lower segment is transfixed and ligated and a cervical oesophagostomy is established. A gastrostomy is required for feeding if not already established at the primary operation.

Anastomotic leaks which occur later than 7 days can usually be treated conservatively with antibiotics and suction. Oral feeding is delayed until healing is complete. Any leak from the anastomosis predisposes to stricture formation and the development of a recurrent tracheo-oesophageal fistula.

Pneumonia: This complication affects the mortality of the primary treatment. It is not possible to differentiate whether this is a postoperative complication or a continuation of preoperative aspiration problems but is largely preventable by early diagnosis. Physiotherapy, antibiotics and aspiration of secretions are all that is usually required. Other patients will need assisted ventilation and possibly a tracheostomy.

Prematurity: The association of oesophageal atresia

with prematurity is accompanied by an increased mortality and in such patients staging of operations is necessary to ensure a successful outcome (Koop and Hamilton, 1965).

Associated Anomalies: The high incidence of associated malformations may complicate the management of oesophageal atresia. Often congenital heart disease may become apparent in the postoperative period and be a cause of late death. An intravenous pyelogram is performed before discharge in all patients to exclude associated renal anomalies (Atwell and Beard, 1974).

Tracheomalacia: This complication, although rare, can cause severe respiratory problems and a tracheostomy may be required. It should be differentiated from subglottic stenosis which may be an associated congenital defect.

LATE

The late complications are stricture, recurrent fistula, hiatus hernia and dysmotility of the oesophagus. All of these complications may present in a similar manner with respiratory and feeding difficulties.

A barium swallow will exclude stricture and hiatus hernia with reflux. Recurrent fistula and dysmotility of the oesophagus are difficult to demonstrate without ciné radiology.

CONGENITAL HYPERTROPHIC PYLORIC STENOSIS

Surgical Pathology and Anatomy

Congenital pyloric stenosis is a relatively common condition of early infancy; males are more often affected than females (sex ratio 5:1). The aetiology remains unknown but genetic factors are important as the incidence is increased in siblings of affected persons ($\times 15$) and in the offspring of affected persons (affected father: risk 1 in 10; affected mother: risk 1 in 4). Thus it appears that a mother may transmit the condition more strongly to the next generation although the condition is commoner in the male.

Although called 'congenital' this is not strictly true as it has never been reported in a stillborn infant. Similarly the stomach has been noted to be normal at a laparotomy performed for vomiting; in such an infant at a later laparotomy for persistence of symptoms a classic pyloric tumour has been found and treated by pyloromyotomy. Recent investigations have suggested that the gastrointestinal hormones such as gastrin (Janik et al., 1978) and secretin are involved but whether this is cause or effect remains uncertain. It seems likely that the cause of congenital

hypertrophic pyloric stenosis is multifactorial (Carter, 1961). One possible explanation is that hypertrophy of the pylorus occurs in everyone after birth but only in a few are the changes severe enough to cause symptoms.

There is hypertrophy of all of the muscle layers which is maximal in the region of the pylorus; this hypertrophy may be severe enough to produce a duodenal fornix. The obstruction is also aggravated by the pyloric mucosa and submucosa which become oedematous and appear as an obstructive element proximal to the sphincter (*Fig.* 58.20).

Surgical Management

Clinical Features

The onset of symptoms is usually gradual in an infant who has given no previous cause for concern. The majority of patients present at 3–5 weeks of age, although this can range between 1 week and 5 months. Vomiting of feeds occurs, initially small amounts but later the vomit becomes forceful and projectile; the vomit is never bile stained. The infant fails to gain weight. As the vomiting increases in amount the baby becomes dehydrated and alkalotic. The diagnosis is confirmed by palpating the pyloric tumour during a test feed and by noting visible peristalsis from left to right across the upper abdomen. Constipation and rarely jaundice may be additional signs. Radiological confirmation of the diagnosis demonstrates separation of contrast in the duodenal cap from that in the stomach—the 'gap' or 'rat tail' sign (*Fig.* 58.20).

Preoperative Care

The degree of dehydration and metabolic alkalosis is assessed and corrected by an intravenous infusion of normal saline with added potassium. A urinary infection as the cause of symptoms should be excluded by routine bacteriological examination of a clean-catch specimen of the urine. One or two gastric washouts with normal saline are used to remove retained curds from the stomach and for treatment of the associated gastritis. Time spent in adequate preparation of the infant prior to surgery reduces the morbidity and mortality. Congenital hypertrophic pyloric stenosis is no longer an emergency needing immediate surgery.

Operation: Rammstedt's pyloromyotomy (*Fig.* 58.20)

General anaesthesia is usually used although if expert anaesthesia is not available local anaesthesia is satisfactory. A transverse incision is made in a skin crease midway between the umbilicus and costal margin and

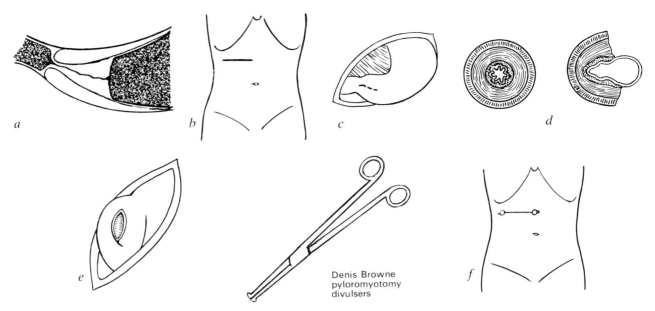

Fig. 58.20. Congenital hypertrophic pyloric stenosis. *a*, The shaded area shows the 'rat tail' sign of congenital pyloric stenosis. In later stages the 'tail' disappears leaving a gap consisting of hypertrophied muscle and redundant mucosa and submucosa. *b*, Skin crease transverse incision and rectus split. *c*, Incision through the pylorus down to the submucosa which bulges out. *d*, Release of mucosa and submucosa shown schematically following division of the pyloric sphincter thus increasing the size of the lumen. *e*, The incision in the pylorus changes direction at a right angle as the duodenal fornix is approached. When this change of direction is seen the distal incision is adequate. *f*, Skin closure with a continuous subcuticular nylon with beads and stops.

overlies the full width of the right rectus abdominis muscle. The skin edges are undermined to expose the anterior rectus sheath which is then incised vertically to expose the muscle fibres of the rectus abdominis; these are then split to expose the peritoneum. The peritoneum is then opened and four artery forceps are left on the lateral, upper and lower margins of the peritoneum. The liver is usually seen first and is displaced upwards with a finger and then the tumour is palpated. A moist gauze swab opened out into a single layer is helpful in holding the body of the stomach and makes the delivery of the pyloric tumour easier. The gastroduodenal junction is identified and the line of the proposed incision into the pylorus is planned. The tumour is then incised through the longitudinal and circular muscle fibres down to the submucosa taking care not to open this layer. Denis Browne pyloromyotomy divulsers are used to push through the last innermost layer of circular muscle, then rotated through 90° and opened. The muscle separates proximally onto the antrum and distally towards the pylorus. Sufficient separation is achieved when it is noted that the line of splitting begins to change direction at a right angle to the incision at the gastroduodenal junction. Care must be taken to ensure that the mucosa has not been opened inadvertently at the duodenal fornix; if opened it must be closed with a horizontal mattress suture of 3/0 chromic catgut. The pylorus is returned to the abdomen and the wound closed in layers using continuous 3/0 chromic catgut for the peritoneum and interrupted for the anterior rectus sheath. The skin is closed with a subcuticular nylon suture with beads and aluminium stops.

Postoperative Care

Initially the infant is given one or two small dextrose feeds but feeding is then regraded rapidly over 24–48 hours, especially if breast fed. The infant is discharged home on the 3rd or 4th postoperative day. If vomiting persists postoperatively the regrading of feeds may have to be slower and further gastric washouts may be required. The postoperative vomiting may be due to an oesophagitis secondary to the gastric outlet obstruction.

Complications

EARLY

Peritonitis due to failure to recognize that the mucosa was opened at the time of pyloromyotomy. Wound infection and wound dehiscence occasionally occur. Persistent vomiting due to an inadequate pyloromyotomy, gastritis or oesophagitis may require treatment. Rarely a second operation is required.

LATE

Intestinal obstruction due to adhesions may be a late complication, especially if peritonitis was a complication of the initial operation.

NEONATAL INTESTINAL OBSTRUCTION

Surgical Embryology

The development of the intestine and its fixation in the peritoneal cavity is completed by the 10th week of intra-uterine life. Initially, the vitello-intestinal duct is the main part of the midgut. Up to the 5th week of intra-uterine life the primitive intestine consists of a hollow tube. This is followed by an active phase of proliferation of the intestinal mucosa which fills the lumen of the developing intestine. The midgut then increases in length and vacuolization of the epithelium is said to occur thus restoring the lumen of the bowel. It has been suggested that failure of the vacuolization (Tandler, 1902) would cause an intestinal atresia (Tandler theory). Other workers have shown by serial sectioning of the fetal intestine that a lumen always persists. This phase of development occurs before the closure of the omphalocele and obliteration of the vitello-intestinal duct.

The development of the duodenum, pancreas, fixation of the intestine and the development of the midgut occur at about the same time.

Duodenum and Pancreas

The liver and pancreas develop as two large extramural glands from the duodenum. The combined hepatopancreatic bud grows ventrally and the pancreatic bud dorsally into the mesoduodenum (*Fig. 58.21*). The dorsal outgrowth is proximal to the ventral outgrowth and forms the body and tail of the pancreas with its own duct (Santorini). The ventral outgrowth subdivides into an hepatic component and a pancreatic component which forms the head of the pancreas with its own duct (Wirsung). The duodenum then rotates on its long axis so that the ventral outgrowth lies in the region of the dorsal mesoduodenum. The mechanism causing this rotation remains obscure. As both components continue to grow they fuse to form the adult type of pancreas. A communicating duct joins the two outgrowths, although separate openings of both outgrowths may persist (*Fig. 58.21*).

Fixation of Intestine

Closure of the omphalocele with disappearance of the vitello-intestinal duct is complete by the 80th day of intra-uterine life. Before this the true abdominal cavity enlarges to accommodate the returning midgut. Rotation of this gut occurs so that the intestine comes to lie in the adult position. This U-shaped limb of the midgut does not return as an upper and lower limb but as a left (distal) and right (proximal) limb (*Fig. 58.22a*). This may be due to the rapid develop-

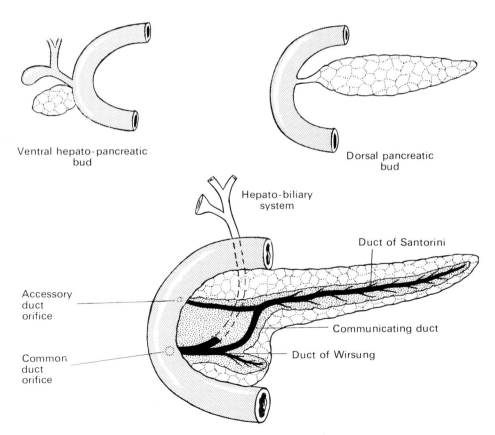

Fig. 58.21. Development of the pancreas from dorsal and ventral outgrowths from the duodenum.

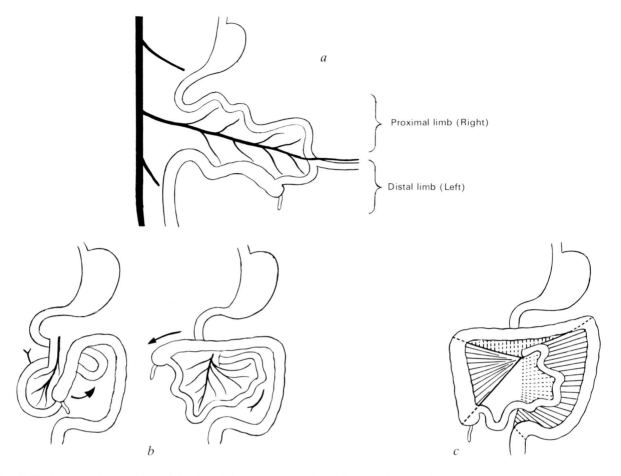

Fig. 58.22. Stages in the rotation and fixation of the intestine. *a*, The midgut lengthens on the axis of the superior mesenteric artery into a proximal and distal limb. *b*, Anticlockwise rotation and descent of the caecum. *c*, Fixation of the ascending and descending colon to the posterior abdominal wall by zygosis of adjacent layers of peritoneum.

ment of the liver which forces the duodenum inferiorly. The return of the intestine occurs in an orderly manner and rotation of the gut occurs in an anticlockwise direction. This is associated with descent of the caecum (*Fig.* 58.22*b*,*c*) and the zygosis of the visceral and parietal peritoneum of the ascending and descending colon; the colon then becomes fixed to the posterior abdominal wall by zygosis of adjacent layers of peritoneum.

Rectum and Anal Canal

The hindgut comes down to join the proctodeum. The allantoic diverticulum joins the hindgut to form a common cloaca at the junction of the endoderm and ectoderm (*Fig.* 58.23). The cloaca consists of a narrow strip of cells in the anteroposterior plane (*Fig.* 58.23). The separation of the anterior urogenital structures from the posterior hindgut proceeds by the downgrowth of the mesodermal urogenital septum (*Fig.* 58.23). This downgrowth divides the cloacal membrane into two parts, anteriorly the urogenital

orifice and posteriorly the anus. Failure of this downgrowth results in a congenital fistula between the anterior and posterior components, i.e. either a recto-urethral fistula, as in the male, or a high recto-vaginal fistula in the female.

Classification

The various forms of neonatal intestinal obstruction are suitably subdivided on a positional basis (*Table* 58.2). Other rare causes of intestinal obstruction in the neonatal period such as Meckel's diverticulum, intussusception and congenital bands are excluded in this account, also the more common inguinal hernia which may cause neonatal obstruction in the neonatal period, especially in the premature infant.

General Principles of Surgical Management

Clinical Features

The classic signs and symptoms of intestinal obstruc-

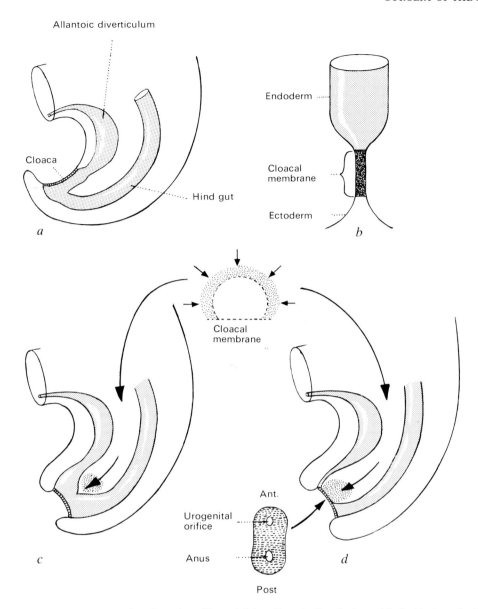

Fig. 58.23. Development of the rectum and anal canal. *a*, Cloaca joining allantoic diverticulum with the hind gut. *b*, Cloacal membrane in the anteroposterior plane joining ectoderm and endoderm. *c*, and *d*, Urogenital septum separating the cloacal membrane into anterior and posterior portions (urogenital and anal orifices).

tion are either primary, such as abdominal pain, vomiting and absolute constipation, or secondary (*Fig.* 58.24). Variations in the pattern of presentation occur depending on whether the obstruction is either complete or incomplete and the level of obstruction within the alimentary tract (Atwell, 1971).

GROUP I

In duodenal atresia the obstruction may be either proximal or distal to the opening of the bile ducts and in some patients bile may enter above and below by the persistence of an accessory duct. The absence of bile in the vomit in duodenal atresia proximal to

the bile ducts may cause delay in diagnosis (Young, 1966) but vomiting is usually within the first 48 hours. In high intestinal obstruction a history of hydramnios is often obtained and some of the patients are jaundiced. Abdominal distension and visible peristalsis are confined to the upper abdomen and diagnosis is confirmed by a straight radiograph demonstrating a double bubble. Associated anomalies such as congenital heart disease, Down's syndrome and other defects are often found in this group of patients. In patients with partial duodenal obstruction, such as an annular pancreas, malrotation or volvulus, the clinical presentation is different. The vomiting in these patients may be intermittent and bile or non-

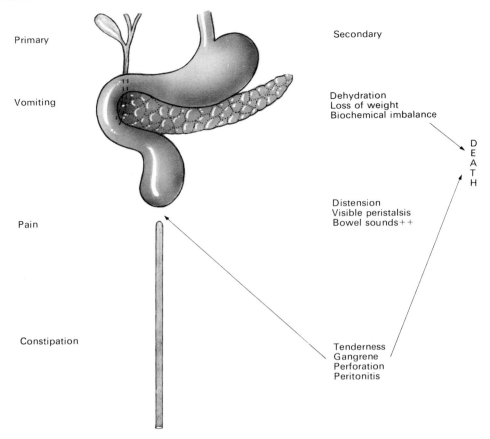

Primary

Vomiting

Pain

Constipation

Secondary

Dehydration
Loss of weight
Biochemical imbalance

Distension
Visible peristalsis
Bowel sounds++

Tenderness
Gangrene
Perforation
Peritonitis

DEATH

Fig. 58.24. Signs and symptoms of intestinal obstruction.

Table 58.2. Causes of intestinal obstruction in the newborn

I. *Duodenal*

    Atresia: stenosis
    Annular pancreas
    Malrotation ± volvulus

II. *Jejuno-ileal*
    Inguinal hernia
    Meckel's   Atresia: stenosis
      diverticulum Meconium ileus
    Congenital bands Volvulus neonatorum

III. *Colo-rectal*

    Hirschsprung's disease
    Atresia: stenosis
    Anorectal anomalies

IV. *Idiopathic Intestinal Obstruction*
    Meconium plug
    Milk plug
    Faecal plug
    CNS
    Hypothyroidism
    Necrotizing enterocolitis
    Exchange transfusion
    Infection
    Pseudo-Hirschsprung's
    Hypoganglionosis
    Hypoplastic left colon
    Drugs
    Cooling

bile stained. Distension of the abdomen with volvulus of the small bowel is extremely rare. Blood in the stool is an important sign of impending gangrene of the intestine. The intermittent nature of these signs and symptoms causes difficulty in diagnosis and if associated with volvulus there is an increase in the morbidity and mortality. Straight radiographs of the abdomen show either malposition of loops of intestine, a double bubble with some air in the bowel distally or a homogeneous area in the centre of the film which represents the base of the volvulus.

GROUP II

There is seldom any delay in the diagnosis of jejuno-ileal atresia or meconium ileus. In jejuno-ileal atresia bile-stained vomiting, abdominal distension and fluid levels on a straight radiograph confirm the diagnosis. In incomplete obstruction, such as a jejuno-ileal stenosis, such signs are often masked with minimal vomiting and distension. This is particularly so in ileal stenosis where alterations in the bacterial flora and transport of water and electrolytes may cause the neonate to present with gastroenteritis. Fortunately an isolated stenosis at this level of the intestine is a rare finding.

In patients with meconium ileus and with meconium peritonitis delay in the diagnosis is extremely rare. Abdominal distension is a striking finding and occurs early and may even cause obstructed labour. The vomiting is often minimal in meconium ileus which contrasts markedly with the degree of distension. Volvulus of the bowel may occur pre- or post-natally in approximately 60 per cent of patients and evidence for this may be found in repeated radiographs. On rectal examination the rectum is empty and tight (cf. Hirschsprung's disease). In some infants there is a family history of fibrocystic disease. Confirmation of the clinical diagnosis is made by finding an elevated level of sodium in the sweat obtained by iontophoresis.

GROUP III

In this group the diagnosis is either simple or extremely difficult. In the newborn with an anorectal malformation the diagnosis is confirmed by inspection and a rectal examination, thus there is no excuse for delay in diagnosis. There are difficulties, however, in differentiating the different types of anorectal malformation which may be found. In infants with Hirschsprung's disease subacute intestinal obstruction is the commonest method of presentation and vomiting occurs within 48 hours of delivery in 75 per cent of patients. Abdominal distension, delay in the passage of meconium, a tight and empty rectum on rectal examination and explosive decompression of the bowel on removal of the finger occurs in over 50 per cent of patients. Diagnosis is difficult in some patients due to the intermittent nature of the symptoms, which may be related to difficulty in evacuating meconium or to changes in the consistency of the stool, i.e. because of being breast fed or bottle fed. The subacute obstruction of Hirschsprung's disease may cause diarrhoea especially after the age of 7 days. Perforation of the caecum causing a pneumoperitoneum and faecal peritonitis is a rare presentation but is accompanied by a high mortality and usually occurs in the first 2 days of life. Diagnosis and management are more difficult in this group.

GROUP IV

Diagnosis and management are more difficult in this group due to the multiplicity of causes, the high incidence of prematurity and the dangers and complications of perforation of the intestine with a resultant pneumoperitoneum and faecal peritonitis. There is often a sequence of events which may assist in diagnosis. Prenatal factors such as a complicated pregnancy and delivery, e.g. multiple births, prematurity, early rupture of the membranes and difficulties with resuscitation are common. Perinatal factors are also important, e.g. exchange transfusion (Corkery et al., 1968), cooling, infection and composition of the feeds. These factors all interact to produce an infant with signs of subacute intestinal obstruction with vomiting, abdominal distension, visible peristalsis, tenderness, loose stools often containing blood or constipation. Later perforation may lead to gross abdominal distension with a pneumoperitoneum. Radiographs show distended loops of bowel with fluid levels, and either evidence of a gradient from the level of the obstruction or the presence of intramural air, a diagnostic feature of necrotizing enterocolitis. Serial radiographs at 6- or 12-hourly or daily intervals are invaluable in assessing the progress of the condition and increasing dilatation of isolated loops of bowel (toxic dilatation) is a sign of impending gangrene and perforation.

Preoperative Care: General

The principles of preoperative management are the same irrespective of the cause or level of the obstruction. The prevention of the aspiration of vomit is of paramount importance. A No. 10 Fr. gauge nasogastric tube is passed into the stomach and then aspirated at $\frac{1}{2}$–1-hourly intervals. It is left on free open drainage in between aspirations. The degree of dehydration is assessed and intravenous replacement of fluid and electrolytes is started with careful monitoring of the biochemical state of the infant. Samples of the infant's and of the maternal blood are sent for grouping and cross-matching. Radiological examination with straight radiographs of the abdomen in the erect supine and erect lateral position are taken. On rare occasions contrast studies are required such as a barium meal to demonstrate duodenal obstruction of an incomplete type or a barium enema to demonstrate the transitional area in Hirschsprung's disease or malposition of the caecum in malrotation.

Duodenal Atresia: Stenosis: Annular Pancreas

Surgical Pathology

Atresia, stenosis and annular pancreas may cause an intrinsic obstruction of the duodenum either proximal (25 per cent) or distal to the opening of the bile ducts (75 per cent). Extrinsic factors are significant in some patients with evidence of intra-uterine volvulus or extrinsic bands. The high incidence of associated anomalies (*Table* 58.3) in this group suggests that in the majority of patients the obstruction occurred in early intra-uterine life.

The level of obstruction is usually found in the second part of the duodenum in close relation to the ampulla of Vater. The bowel above and below the obstruction is often in continuity especially in patients with a duodenal diaphragm producing a windsock type of deformity. In annular pancreas a constricting ring of pancreatic tissue is found surrounding the duodenum to produce a stenosis or complete obstruction (*Fig.* 58.25).

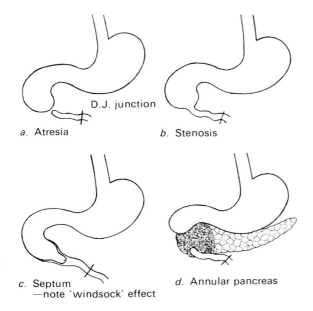

Fig. 58.25. Types of duodenal atresia, stenosis and annular pancreas.

Table 58.3. Associated anomalies in 40 patients with duodenal atresia and stenosis

I. Trisomy 21		14
II. Gastrointestinal tract		17
Malrotation	6	
Oesophageal atresia and tracheo-oesophageal fistula	3	
Anorectal atresia	1	
Jejuno-ileal atresia	2	
Meckel's diverticulum	2	
Meconium peritonitis	1	
Ectopic pancreas	1	
Congenital bands	1	
III. Congenital vascular disease		3
IV. Vertebral anomalies		6

Surgical Management

The Operation

The operation of choice is a duodeno-duodenostomy, thus restoring continuity. A gastrostomy and transanastomotic feeding tube are useful additions and aid the postoperative care. In some patients a duodenojejunostomy (retrocolic), gastrostomy and transanastomotic feeding tube are easier but less satisfactory. Gastroenterostomy should be avoided.

The abdomen is opened through a transverse supraumbilical muscle-cutting incision (*Fig.* 58.26). The hepatic flexure is mobilized to expose the duodenum and the site of the intrinsic obstruction is inspected. The bowel proximal and distal to the obstruction is approximated with several seromuscu-

lar sutures which are then tied (*Fig.* 58.26). The bowel is opened with cutting diathermy on the hypertrophied proximal bowel and with iridectomy scissors on the collapsed distal bowel. The posterior part of the anastomosis is completed using interrupted mattress sutures of 4/0 silk and each corner is turned in using a Connell suture (*Fig.* 58.26).

The anastomosis is then left at this stage and a gastrostomy is established (cf. oesophageal atresia). In this operation it is essential to pass the transanastomotic feeding tube (no. 2 polyvinyl tubing or a no. 3·5 Fr. gauge umbilical vein catheter) through the gastrostomy opening before inserting the Malecot catheter and tying the purse-string suture. The feeding tube is then pulled through the pylorus and into the wound at the site of the partially completed duodeno-duodenostomy. Then 15 cm of this feeding tube are passed into the upper jejunum. This is difficult and while doing this it is essential to keep the position of the tube constant at the anastomosis. The anterior part of the anastomosis is completed with interrupted Connell sutures of 4/0 silk. On completion of the anastomosis the colon is replaced into the normal anatomical position and the wound is closed in layers.

If a duodenojejunostomy is preferred, a window is made in the transverse mesocolon between the right and middle colic arteries and the dilated duodenum is pulled into view. The anastomosis, gastrostomy and transanastomotic feeding tube are completed in an exactly similar way. The proximal duodenum is sutured to the mesocolon to prevent invagination of the jejunum at this point (*Fig.* 58.26). In patients with a duodenal diaphragm the duodenum is exposed and opened longitudinally.

The diaphragm with its central aperture is often found prolapsed distally. The diaphragm is then excised, either by using cutting diathermy or by overrunning the cut edges with a continuous 4/0 catgut suture. The duodenum is closed transversely with interrupted silk sutures.

Postoperative Care

The gastrostomy is left on free drainage and aspirated at 1-hourly intervals. The volume of aspirate is usually 100–150 ml per day, and gradually decreases as the anastomosis opens up. Initially these aspirates are replaced by an equal volume of normal saline intravenously. After 24–28 hours, however, the aspirates may be injected slowly down the transanastomotic feeding tube at a maximum rate of 1 ml/min. Similarly milk feeds can be started down the feeding tube and are increased until the infant is on full oral requirements. After a time the quantity of gastric aspirate decreases and the catheter may then be spigotted. If this is successful the transanastomotic feed can be reduced in 5·0-ml stages, and instead is given orally. Then, when the infant can manage full oral feeds without vomiting, the gastrostomy and

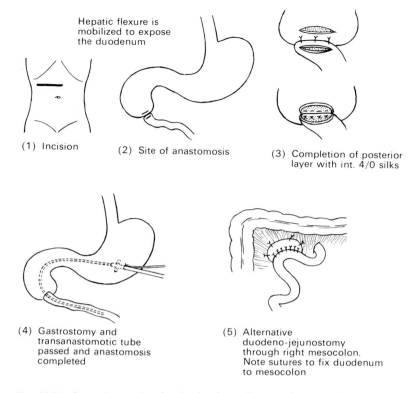

Hepatic flexure is mobilized to expose the duodenum

(1) Incision

(2) Site of anastomosis

(3) Completion of posterior layer with int. 4/0 silks

(4) Gastrostomy and transanastomotic tube passed and anastomosis completed

(5) Alternative duodeno-jejunostomy through right mesocolon. Note sutures to fix duodenum to mesocolon

Fig. 58.26. Operative repair of a duodenal atresia, stenosis or annular pancreas by duodeno-duodenostomy, gastrostomy and transanastomotic feeding tube. Alternative duodeno-jejunostomy.

transanastomotic tubes are removed. The transition from tube to full oral feeds may take several days.

Complications

EARLY

An anastomotic breakdown is unusual but may result in a localized or subphrenic abscess. Duodenal ileus may occur due to the gross dilatation and hypertrophy proximal to the atresia. This delay at the anastomosis may persist for a long time postoperatively. Adhesions can form and cause subacute obstruction with vomiting or, combined with duodenal ileus, cause diarrhoea and secondary disaccharide intolerance. The complications of the gastrostomy are listed (*see* p. 914) under 'Oesophageal Atresia'. The management of the transanastomotic feeding tube is difficult. The tube may become displaced back into the stomach and if this occurs intravenous fluids or parenteral nutrition are required until full oral feeds can be tolerated. Perforation of the intestine may occur if the tubing is not polyvinyl, or if the feeds are given too rapidly, i.e. maximum rate 1 ml/min.

LATE

Blind Loop Syndrome: Chronic obstruction at the anastomosis may lead to progressive dilatation and the development of a blind loop syndrome. In these infants there is an iron deficiency anaemia, failure of normal growth and complete loss of appetite. Contrast studies are used for diagnosis and a further laparotomy and either refashioning or excision of the anastomosis is required.

Associated Anomalies: Congenital heart disease, Down's syndrome and other gastrointestinal malformations may complicate the initial and late management of duodenal obstruction. Radiological investigations are undertaken to exclude associated renal and vertebral anomalies, e.g. radiograph of the spine and an intravenous pyelogram.

Malrotation: Volvulus Neonatorum

Surgical Pathology

'Malrotation' is the term used to cover a variety of conditions in which there is a failure of the normal rotation of the midgut on returning from the omphalocele to the true abdominal cavity. In many cases there is an associated volvulus. If the caecum lies high and to the left a condensation of parietal peritoneum (Ladd's band) may cross the duodenum and cause obstruction (*Fig.* 58.27). In our experience this component of the obstruction is relatively rare; a much more common finding is volvulus due to the

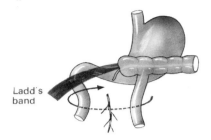

Fig. 58.27. Note the narrow base for the attachment of the mesentery of the small bowel thus predisposing to a volvulus. Ladd's band crossing the duodenum may be a cause of obstruction.

narrow pedicle formed by the attachment of the mesentery. Such a volvulus may endanger the blood supply of the small bowel. In some patients the duodenum and colon may be normal in position but the whole of the small intestine has undergone a volvulus (volvulus neonatorum).

Other predisposing factors to abnormalities of intestinal rotation are exomphalos, gastroschisis, intrinsic duodenal obstruction, congenital diaphragmatic hernia, duplications of the intestine and abdominal masses such as pelvi-ureteric hydronephrosis or renal tumour (*Fig.* 58.28).

Surgical Management

Operation

The abdomen is opened through a supraumbilical transverse muscle-cutting incision. The intestines are delivered into the wound and inspected carefully. The intestine must be delivered completely into the wound otherwise it will be impossible to recognize the variety of the malrotation that is present. The volvulus, if present (usually clockwise), is untwisted, which will immediately improve the blood supply to the intestine if it had been threatened. Ladd's band is divided and the duodenum mobilized with the proximal small intestine being left to the right. The adhesions to the caecum are divided to widen the base of the pedicle; the caecum is placed to the left with the large bowel; thus the bowel is left in the primitive non-rotated position. No attempt is made to fix the intestine. In patients with a normally fixed intestine and volvulus neonatorum simple untwisting of the volvulus is insufficient. The duodenum and caecum must be mobilized to produce the non-rotation situation in order to prevent a recurrent volvulus.

Appendicectomy should not be performed but the parents must be told of the abnormal position of the appendix in order to prevent confusion if an acute abdomen develops at a later date.

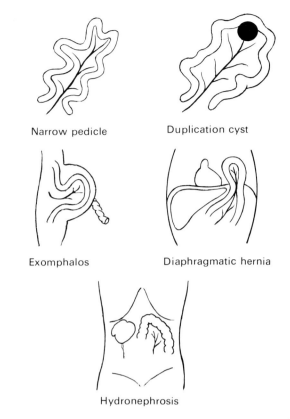

Fig. 58.28. Congenital defects which affect the normal rotation and fixation of the intestines during intra-uterine life.

In some patients the intestine is gangrenous and a resection and end-to-end anastomosis are performed. Rarely the whole of the midgut is considered non-viable and intestinal resection in such cases is associated with a high mortality and morbidity. In such patients a second look 48 hours after a Ladd's operation may allow a more limited resection.

Postoperative Care

Duodenal ileus may require nasogastric aspiration and intravenous fluid and calorie replacement until full oral feeds can be tolerated.

Complications

Recurrent volvulus rarely occurs unless one has inadequately treated a volvulus neonatorum. Adhesions causing an intestinal obstruction at a subsequent date may occur in up to 10 per cent of cases and are associated with a mortality. Malabsorption and failure to thrive often follow a massive intestinal resection. This 'short gut' syndrome will need careful monitoring of the biochemical state and replacement of fluid, electrolytes and calories. An anastomotic leak may occur if a resection has been necessary, especially if large lengths of bowel are ischaemic and there has been an attempt to preserve intestinal length.

Jenuno-ileal Atresia: Stenosis

Surgical Pathology

There are two main theories for the pathogenesis of intestinal atresia. In the first (Tandler, 1902) there is a failure of recanalization of the bowel following the proliferation of the intestinal epithelium which occurs in the 6–7-mm embryo. This theory does not explain the findings in patients with absence of part of the bowel and in some of these lanugo, epithelial squames and bile may be detected in the meconium distal to a complete atresia. These findings led to the 'vascular accident theory' for the causation of intestinal atresias.

In this second theory it is suggested that intestinal ischaemia during intra-uterine life will lead to resorption of the affected intestine (*Fig.* 58.29) if it is empty,

born 12–14 days after an intra-uterine operation lesions were found similar to those found in the human. Thus for jejuno-ileal atresias the vascular accident theory has more support than the failure of vacuolization proposed by Tandler in 1902. Further evidence in support of this conclusion is the low incidence of other congenital malformations in infants with jejuno-ileal atresia.

Surgical Management

Operation

1. RESECTION: END-TO-BACK ANASTOMOSIS (Nixon)
The abdomen is opened through a transverse supraumbilical muscle-cutting incision. The site of the atresia, which may be single or multiple, is identified and any predisposing factor such as volvulus or bands is corrected. The grossly dilated and hypertrophied bowel proximal to the atresia is resected and an end-to-back anastomosis using interrupted 4/0 silk sutures is used to restore continuity (*Fig.*

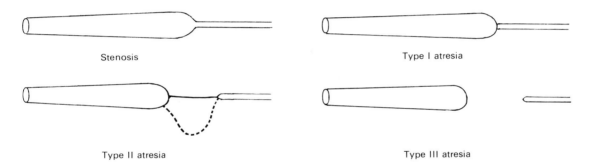

Stenosis

Type I atresia

Type II atresia

Type III atresia

Multiple/Single

Fig. 58.29. Types of jejuno-ileal stenosis and atresia.

to produce either a septum (type I), fibrous cord (type II) or a complete gap (type III). If the bowel lumen was full of meconium at the site of an intra-uterine perforation it will cause a chemical peritonitis resulting in a meconium peritonitis. Calcification seen on preoperative plain radiographs allows early diagnosis of this complication. In patients with intestinal atresias the pathologist can often establish evidence of meconium peritonitis on microscopical examination of the resected specimen.

The vascular accident theory has been subjected to experimental proof in studies with pregnant bitches (Louw and Barnard, 1955; Louw, 1959). Between the 45th and the 55th day of their pregnancy the uterus was opened and the fetal abdomen of the puppy explored. The blood supply to a segment of intestine was interrupted and the bowel replaced in the abdomen. Finally the maternal uterus was closed and the bitch allowed to go to term. A normal delivery was obtained in 38 animals and in those puppies

58.30). Prior to the anastomosis the patency of the collapsed distal bowel is confirmed by injecting normal saline into the bowel lumen and watching the fluid content pass down to the ileocaecal valve. Colonic atresias are so rare that it is not necessary to check for the patency of the colon in these patients.

2. LIMITED RESECTION: GASTROSTOMY: TRANSANASTOMOTIC FEEDING TUBE
In some patients with a high jejunal atresia it is impossible to resect the grossly dilated bowel proximal to the atresia. It is therefore safer to restore continuity and to establish a gastrostomy and transanastomotic feeding tube (cf. duodenal atresia).

3. REFASHIONING OF JEJUNUM (JEJUNAL TAPERING)
An alternative operation in high jejunal atresia is to reduce the calibre of the jejunum proximal to the

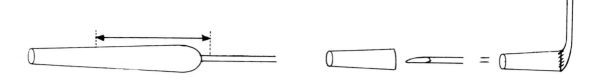

Nixon end-to-back anastomosis

Fig. 58.30. End-to-end anastomosis (Nixon) for restoring continuity in jejuno-ileal atresia. Single-layer anastomosis with 4/0 silk sutures.

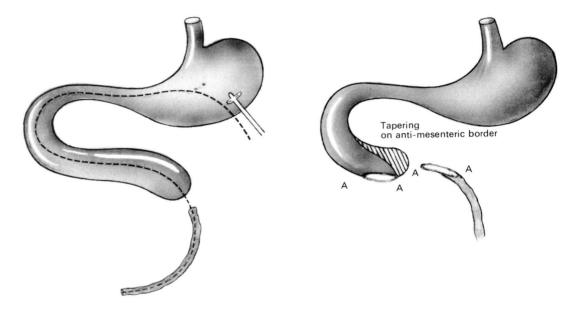

Tapering
on anti-mesenteric border

Fig. 58.31. Tapering jejunoplasty used for restoring continuity in high jejunal atresia when resection of the proximally dilated bowel is impracticable.

atresia by refashioning (*Fig.* 58.31) and then to restore continuity by end-to-end anastomosis.

Postoperative Care

Prolonged nasogastric aspiration, replacement of fluid and electrolytes and parenteral nutrition are required until full oral feeding can be tolerated.

Complications

EARLY

Aspiration pneumonia should be avoidable by efficient nasogastric aspiration and nursing care. An anastomotic breakdown may be due to the disparity in size between the proximal and distal bowel which increases the technical difficulty of the anastomosis. At re-exploration the anastomosis can be either refashioned or oversewn. Metabolic complications are common and are related to the initial dehydration and prolonged therapy in the postoperative period. Hypokalaemia, hypocalcaemia and hypomagnesaemia may require urgent treatment.

LATE

Malabsorption may be due either to loss of intestinal length or to the development of a secondary disaccharide intolerance. Adhesions can cause an acute intestinal obstruction or be a contributory factor in the causation of malabsorption. Failure to thrive may cause delayed growth and development in these patients. Growth often returns to normal by 1–2 years of age as compensation for loss of intestinal length occurs.

Meconium Ileus

Surgical Pathology

Fibrocystic disease of the pancreas is genetically determined by an autosomal recessive gene with a recurrence risk in future pregnancies of 1 in 4. In 10–15 per cent of such patients the abnormal viscid meconium and deficient pancreatic secretions cause a bolus type of intestinal obstruction in the neonatal period. The level of the obstruction is usually in the distal ileum but may occur at jejunal and colonic levels. Proximally the bowel is distended and hypertrophied. Distally the bowel is small and collapsed to produce a 'microcolon' effect. Volvulus and perforation of the distended loop of intestine may occur prenatally or postnatally, leading to either meconium peritonitis, intestinal atresia or bacterial peritonitis (*Fig.* 58.32).

Koop, 1957) (*Fig.* 58.33). The bowel is inspected and any volvulus is untwisted. The grossly distended bowel is resected proximal to the apex of the obstruction caused by the rabbit-type pellets of abnormal meconium. The distal end of the bowel is brought out as an ileostomy in the right iliac fossa after anastomosing the end of the proximal bowel to the side

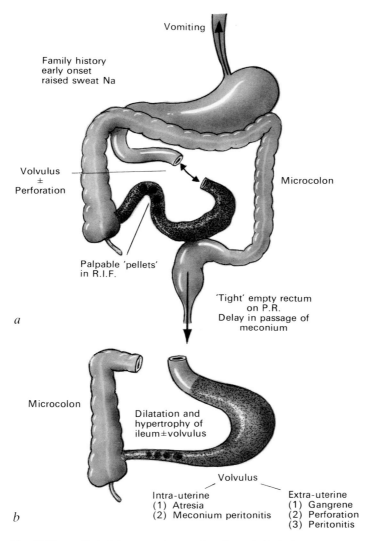

Fig. 58.32. *a*, Clinical features of meconium ileus. *b*, Pathological findings in meconium ileus.

Surgical Management

Operation

The abdomen is opened through a transverse supraumbilical muscle-cutting incision. The findings are as described above and only rarely is there any difficulty in diagnosing the condition. The operation of choice is the Bishop–Koop ileostomy (Bishop and

of the distal ileum. No attempt is made to clear the intestinal content from the bowel lumen except immediately adjacent to the line of the resection.

Conservative treatment is possible in some patients as the obstruction can be relieved by the hygroscopic effect of a Gastrografin enema. It is not suitable in patients with a volvulus and it is unfortunate that this complication is so common (60 per cent).

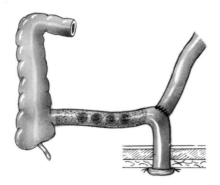

Fig. 58.33. Bishop–Koop ileostomy.

Postoperative Care

Postoperatively the infant is on intermittent naso-gastric aspiration and replacement and maintenance intravenous fluids. Oral Pancrex (pancreatin) (125 mg in 5 ml N saline) is given 4-hourly after aspirating the stomach. Similarly, Pancrex is instilled into the ileostomy stoma using a syringe and a short soft catheter. Initially this is started 24 hours after the operation and given at 2-hourly intervals. Within 48–72 hours the meconium distal to the stoma liquefies and is passed per rectum. Oral feeding is then started using 5 per cent dextrose and followed by half- and full-strength milk feeds. Specially prepared predigested feeds are well tolerated in such infants (Pregestimil). By the 7th–10th postoperative day the stools should be normal and the fluid losses from the ileostomy will decrease: this now acts as a mucous fistula.

Intraperitoneal closure of the ileostomy is under-taken at a second-stage operation prior to discharge home or is deferred to a later date. Final confirmation of the diagnosis is made either by measuring the tryptic activity of duodenal juice or by measuring the sodium content of a sample of sweat obtained by iontophoresis.

Complications

EARLY

Anastomotic leak may occur as the blood supply to the bowel is reduced in some patients and exploration with further intestinal resection may be required. Failure to thrive is due to multiple factors related to the primary pathology, operation and infective complications.

LATE

Pulmonary complications eventually result in the majority of these patients becoming respiratory cripples. The patients often die in childhood or early adult life from the sequelae of their fibrocystic disease, including complications such as intestinal malabsorption, portal hypertension and liver failure.

Hirschsprung's Disease

Surgical Pathology

Hirschsprung's disease is due to the congenital absence of ganglion cells (*Fig.* 58.34) from the myen-

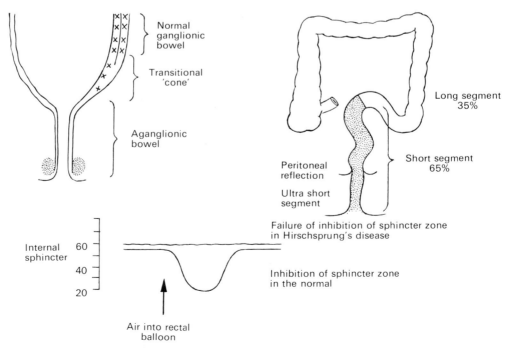

Fig. 58.34. Surgical pathology of Hirschsprung's disease.

teric (Auerbach's) and submucosal (Meissner's) plexus of the bowel wall. The aganglionosis is always distal, involving the sphincter zone, and extends proximally: the length of this proximal extension varies from patient to patient. If the disease is confined to the bowel distal to the apex of the sigmoid loop it is known as 'short-segment' disease (65 per cent of patients). Extension of the disease proximal to this point is called 'long-segment' disease (35 per cent of patients). Occasionally the disease extends upwards to involve the small bowel and in rare cases up as high as the stomach. 'Ultra-short segment' disease is used as a subdivision of short-segment disease, the segment between the normal and aganglionic bowel (transitional zone) lying below the reflection of the pelvic peritoneum. Skip lesions have been reported but must be extremely rare and should not be considered in the day-to-day management of an infant with Hirschsprung's disease. The innervation of the bowel is from neuroblasts which migrate down the vagal trunk; this embryological feature may therefore account for the rarity of skip lesions.

In the affected intestine the characteristic histological and histochemical findings are absent ganglion cells, an increase in the number of abnormal medullated nerve fibres and an excess of cholinesterase. Inflating a balloon in the rectum of a normal subject causes relaxation of the anal sphincter. In the patient with Hirschsprung's disease the response is different as there is no recordable inhibition or relaxation of the sphincter. It has been possible to use these differences of anorectal physiological response for the clinical diagnosis of Hirschsprung's disease (*Fig. 58.34*).

Surgical Management

Clinical Features

The incidence of Hirschsprung's disease varies between 1 in 2000 to 1 in 5000 live births. It is more common in boys (M:F, 5:1) but in long-segment disease the sex ratio is equal. Genetic factors are important in the aetiology of the disease as a family history may be elucidated in up to 20 per cent of patients. There is a higher incidence of Down's syndrome and urinary tract disorders in patients with Hirschsprung's disease.

It is essential to here an early diagnosis if the lethal complications of the disease are to be avoided. The commonest method of presentation is with subacute intestinal obstruction in the neonatal period (75 per cent); there is vomiting, abdominal distension and rectal signs such as delay in the passage of meconium and a tight and empty rectum on digital examination and explosive decompression of the bowel on removal of the finger. Diarrhoea commonly occurs after the 1st week of life (25 per cent) and may become severe with its own associated mortality. Distension, leading to perforation of the caecum, is an unusual presentation and is probably associated with competence of the ileocaecal valve. The classic presentation described of the infant with severe constipation and a megarectum is unusual in modern paediatric practice with the emphasis on early diagnosis. Only in this way can the mortality be reduced.

Operations

POLICY

Intestinal decompression with a colostomy or enterostomy is the treatment of choice and if performed in the 1st week of life reduces the incidence of enterocolitis. Histological confirmation of the diagnosis can be obtained by combining this operation with intestinal biopsy above and below the cone or transitional zone. Definitive surgery should never be undertaken until histological confirmation of the diagnosis has been obtained, either by rectal or intestinal biopsy.

Radiological examination with straight films and contrast studies may assist in establishing a diagnosis. Care must be taken in interpreting the results of barium enema examinations to demonstrate the transitional zone (cone), as false positives and false negatives may be obtained. Measurement of the alterations in anorectal physiology with pressure transducers and recorders can assist in diagnosis.

In some patients it is possible to perform the definitive operation as a primary procedure, after suitable preparation with rectal washouts and correction of dehydration and infection. More commonly, and often safer, is careful staging of the surgical operations, i.e. preliminary colostomy or enterostomy. The definitive operation is then delayed until the infant weighs at least 5 kg. In some patients the colostomy closure is performed at this time, but in others it is closed as a third stage. There are three standard definitive operations for the surgical treatment of Hirschsprung's disease, an abdomino-perineal pull-through (Swenson), a double barrelled pull-through using the enterotome (Duhamel) and the mucosal stripping operation, leaving a muscular tunnel through which normal bowel is pulled and anastomosed (Soave) (*Fig. 58.35*).

1. TRANSVERSE COLOSTOMY: ENTEROSTOMY (*Fig. 58.36*)

It is vital to choose the correct site for the colostomy or enterostomy. First it must be in normal ganglionic bowel. Second, the positioning of the colostomy depends on the length of aganglionic intestine, e.g. in short-segment disease a right transverse colostomy will allow resection of the aganglionic segment without disturbing the colostomy, i.e. it protects the distal anastomosis following the definitive corrective surgery. In long-segment disease the colostomy should always be positioned in normal bowel immediately adjacent to the cone, thus preserving intestinal length for use at the definitive operation.

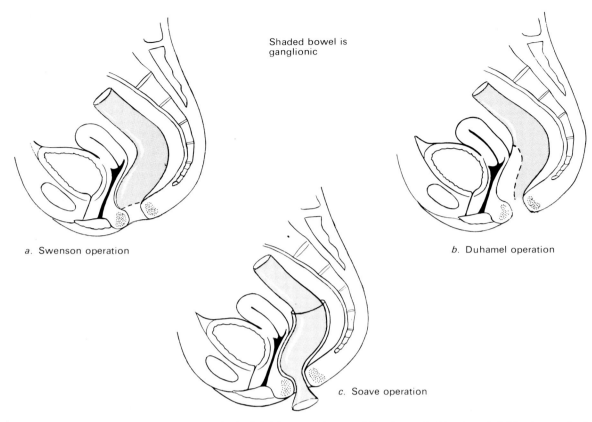

Shaded bowel is
ganglionic

a. Swenson operation

b. Duhamel operation

c. Soave operation

Fig. 58.35. Schematic representation of the three basic definitive operations used for the surgical treatment of Hirschsprung's disease. (Shaded bowel is ganglionic.)

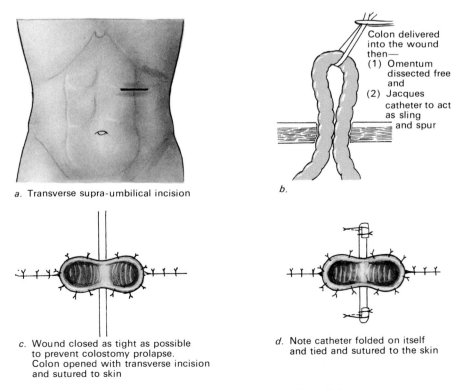

a. Transverse supra-umbilical incision

b.

Colon delivered
into the wound
then—
(1) Omentum
    dissected free
    and
(2) Jacques
    catheter to act
    as sling
    and spur

c. Wound closed as tight as possible
to prevent colostomy prolapse.
Colon opened with transverse incision
and sutured to skin

d. Note catheter folded on itself
and tied and sutured to the skin

Fig. 58.36. Transverse colostomy: operative technique.

A transverse supraumbilical incision either to the left or right of the midline is used. Inspection of the bowel reveals dilatation and hypertrophy proximal to the transitional zone, the bowel distal being collapsed and of normal calibre. The intestine is then biopsied above and below the cone and the site for the colostomy is selected.

The colostomy is usually sited to the right of the middle colic artery, as the bowel will depend on this blood vessel after excision of the aganglionic intestine. The flimsy greater omentum is dissected free from its attachment to the area chosen for the colostomy. A catheter sling is then passed through the mesocolon and the wound is closed around the loop of transverse colon.

Six non-absorbable sutures are used to anchor the colostomy, being seromuscular on the bowel wall and peritoneal on the abdominal wall side. This is important in order to prevent prolapse of the colostomy, which is one of the commoner complications. The incidence of this complication can be reduced by making the colostomy extremely 'tight' at the time it is established.

The colostomy is opened with cutting diathermy and sutured to the skin with interrupted mucocutaneous non-absorbable sutures. The ends of the rubber catheter acting as the spur are then folded on themselves and tied. This prevents the spur slipping out, but these ends should be sutured to the skin to prevent rotation of the spur, which is likely to occur in an active infant. A full-thickness piece of colon from the colostomy is sent for histology to confirm the presence of ganglion cells.

2. CLOSURE OF THE COLOSTOMY

A full intraperitoneal closure is required. The skin is incised circumferentially around the stoma and extended along the line of the previous incision. The muscle of the abdominal wall is then separated from the bowel wall and mesocolon by careful dissection and with upward traction the afferent and efferent limbs of the colostomy are delivered into the wound. In the infant it is then necessary to excise the stoma and restore continuity with end-to-end anastomosis using a single layer of interrupted silk sutures. The wound is then closed in layers leaving a fine sliver of a corrugated drain down to the site of the anastomosis.

3. BIOPSY OF THE INTESTINE AND RECTUM (*Fig.* 58.37)

This may be done as an elective operation, e.g. rectal biopsy, or as part of a laparotomy to relieve intestinal obstruction from Hirschsprung's disease, i.e. intestinal biopsy.

Intestinal Biopsy: The site for the biopsy is selected and is linear along the taenia coli. The bowel is held between the finger and thumb to compress the linea leaving the taenia uppermost. Then using iridectomy scissors the seromuscular layer is excised in a strip. With care and practice the mucosa and submucosa are left intact. The edges of the seromuscular wound are then closed with interrupted silk sutures. It is usually necessary to biopsy the bowel above and below the cone, thus confirming the diagnosis and delineating the extent of the disease.

Rectal Biopsy: The methods are available using either a suction biopsy technique or a linear strip of mucosa and submucosa from the posterior wall of the rectum. The former of these methods is better as it avoids tearing of the mucosa, which may occur at the time of the definitive procedure. Both methods require careful histological examination by a pathologist experienced in this type of work; serial sections and specific histochemical techniques are helpful in most patients in confirming the diagnosis.

4. SWENSON'S OPERATION (*see also* Chapter 19 and *Fig.* 58.35*a*)

The infant is positioned in the extended Trendelenburg lithotomy position using a special table (Stephens') which is strapped in position on the normal adult operating table (*Fig.* 58.38). The abdomen is opened through a long left paramedian incision from the costal margin to the pubic symphysis. Any adhesions are divided and the small intestine is packed away into the right upper abdomen. The colon is inspected and the 'cone' identified by the marker sutures at the site of the previous intestinal biopsies. The splenic flexure, descending colon and sigmoid colon are mobilized onto their own mesentery by dividing their peritoneal attachments.

The rectum and sigmoid are pulled upwards and initially to the right, in order to incise the peritoneum just medial to the left ureter; this incision is carried forwards in a curve anteriorly to the posterior wall of the bladder. It is important to display the whole course of the left ureter. Similarly with the rectum and sigmoid pulled upwards and to the left, the peritoneum is incised medial to the right ureter and extended anteriorly to meet the opposite incision on the surface of the bladder. The incision in the right mesocolon is extended upwards towards the third part of the duodenum exposing the inferior mesenteric artery and vein which are ligated and divided. This leaves the left side of the colon dependent on the blood supply through the marginal artery from the middle colic artery.

The posterior pelvic dissection is started by identifying the presacral nerve and freeing the superior pedicle from the lower aorta and down to the sacral promontory. The presacral space is entered with the finger in the midline and the rectum is separated from the sacrum down to the level of the coccyx.

Anteriorly the posterior surface of the bladder is identified together with the vasa and seminal vesicles,

Intestinal Biopsy

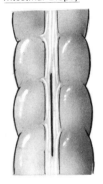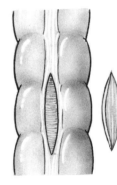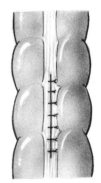

Longitudinal incision
down to submucosa

Linear strip of
circular and longitudinal
muscle removed

Closure with
int. silk sutures

Rectal Biopsy

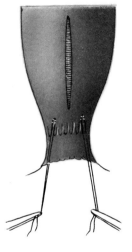

Mucosa and submucosal
biopsy through anus in the
midline posteriorly.
Note stay sutures and
retractors will aid exposure.
Linear incision closed
with continuous 3/0 chromic

Fig. 58.37. Diagnosis of Hirschsprung's disease by intestinal and rectal biopsy.

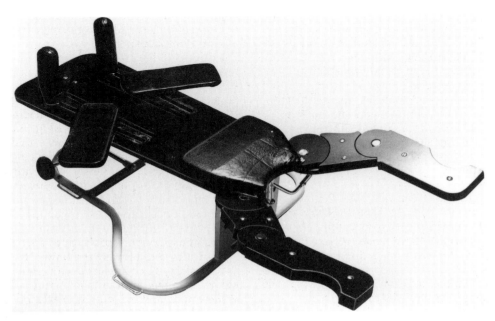

Fig. 58.38. Stephens' table for operation on infants in the Trendelenburg–lithotomy position.

which are held anteriorly with a malleable copper blade retractor of the appropriate size. Gentle dissection with pledgets on straight forceps is used to separate the anterior structures from the rectum. It is important at this stage to stay as close to the rectal wall as possible.

In the female the anterior dissection can be made easier by suturing the uterus to the wound edges with stay sutures. The plane between the rectum and posterior vaginal wall is incised with scissors and opened by blunt dissection with a pledget on straight forceps; this plane between the rectum and the posterior wall of the vagina is opened down to the floor of the pelvis.

Finally the lateral ligaments on each side are identified and as these contain the middle haemorrhoidal artery it may either be divided between ligatures or diathermized, keeping close to the rectal wall. The ligaments can be made taut on the rectum upwards and towards the opposite side of the pelvis.

It is extremely important to ensure that the dissection down to the pelvic floor is complete circumferentially around the rectum before proceeding to the final stage of the operation which requires transection of the bowel and everting it through the anus.

The bowel is divided at the level previously determined and a straight vascular clamp is applied proximally. Distally the bowel is invaginated and is closed with interrupted silk sutures. Care at this stage must be taken to ensure that the blood supply to the normal ganglionic bowel, which will be brought down for the anastomosis, is adequate, and that there is sufficient length so that the anastomosis will not be under tension. The operator goes to the lower end of the table with a separate scrub nurse and assistant, the first assistant being left to complete the abdominal part of the operation. At the lower end the buttocks are separated to expose the anus (Joll's thyroid self-retaining retractor is useful for this purpose). Sponge-holding forceps are inserted into the anus and passed upwards into the rectum, being guided by the abdominal operator. The forceps are opened and closed in order to grasp the invaginated end of bowel just below the level of the transection. The distal rectum and anal canal can be evaginated by gentle traction and left hanging freely. Inspection of the everted bowel mucosa should reveal the anal valves in the anterior, lateral and posterior position, thus confirming that the pelvic dissection was adequate.

The everted bowel is divided longitudinally in the anterior position to expose and open the rectal wall; this is extended to 1 cm from the anal valves. Curved ductus arteriosus forceps are passed through this opened bowel to grasp the prepared ganglionic bowel. It is important to ensure that the vascular pedicle is lying posteriorly and that the bowel is not twisted. This proximal bowel is pulled and guided from above so that it appears below through the incised everted rectum and anal canal.

The anastomosis is now completed. Initially the bowel is sutured with a single non-absorbable suture in the anterior position, which is used as a stay suture. The everted rectum is pulled laterally and is divided with cutting diathermy to just beyond the left lateral position and a further stay suture is inserted. The procedure is then repeated for insertion of the right lateral stay suture. The everted rectum is now left attached posteriorly and the bowel anastomosis is held by the anterior and lateral sutures. The final part of the bowel is then divided and the proximal and distal bowel are held by inserting a posterior stay suture. The anastomosis is now completed by placing interrupted sutures between adjacent stay sutures. When the anastomosis is complete the stay sutures are divided but left long; the anastomosis is pushed gently through the anus with a finger to take up its normal position.

The abdominal part of the operation is completed with closure of the peritoneum of the pelvic floor. A small infant suction drain (Redivac) is left in the presacral space and taken out lateral to the wound by an extraperitoneal route. The pelvic floor is then closed with a continuous 3/0 chromic suture. The intestines are then replaced into their normal position and the wound is closed.

Specific Pre- and Postoperative Care

PRELIMINARY ENTEROSTOMY: COLOSTOMY
The specific feature after this procedure is that nasogastric aspiration and intravenous fluids may be required for several days as the stoma is made tight in order to prevent subsequent prolapse.

CLOSURE OF COLOSTOMY
Blood is always required for the closure of a loop colostomy in the neonate and in infancy. Preoperative bowel preparation with neomycin or cephradine and metronidazole is advisable.

RECTAL BIOPSY
Careful observation must be made postoperatively for evidence of continuing hidden haemorrhage. This can usually be prevented by closing a posterior linear biopsy with a continuous chromic catgut suture. This complication is less likely to occur if a suction biopsy technique is used. Similarly the incidence of pelvic cellulitis and peritonitis is reduced by this technique.

SWENSON'S OPERATION
Preliminary washouts of the bowel distal to the colostomy are used to prepare the bowel. In long-segment disease the gut flora is sterilized with neomycin given orally over the preceding 48 hours. The bladder is catheterized and emptied immediately prior to surgery. This catheter is not required postoperatively as micturition in the infant is reflex and retention

of urine is not seen as a complication. A presacral suction drain (Redivac: infant) is left *in situ* and removed after 48 hours. Broad-spectrum antibiotics are given for 7 days.

Complications

PRELIMINARY ENTEROSTOMY: COLOSTOMY

The persistence of the pre-existing enterocolitis may be life threatening. Prolapse of the colostomy is not uncommon and occasionally a cutaneous fistula is seen at the site of one of the seromuscular and peritoneal sutures. Wound infection is common.

CLOSURE OF COLOSTOMY

Nasogastric aspiration and intravenous fluids are required until the anastomosis opens up. An anastomotic leak is rare. Wound infection is common.

RECTAL: INTESTINAL BIOPSY

Haemorrhage which may be hidden. A localized intraperitoneal abscess or peritonitis may complicate an intestinal biopsy, especially if the mucosa and submucosa were opened. In some patients this complication may follow a local perforation from enterocolitis.

SWENSON'S OPERATION

An anastomotic leak is the most serious complication and needs a defunctioning colostomy or enterostomy to control the pelvic cellulitis: stricture as a sequelae is often seen. Haemorrhage into the presacral space also acts as a focus for infection. Wound infection and postoperative ileus are not uncommon. Errors in assessing the length of aganglionic intestine should not occur if adequate intestinal biopsies have been obtained and carefully examined. Damage to the autonomic nerves during the pelvic dissection may cause urinary incontinence and impotence as a late sequelae. These complications are largely avoidable by meticulous surgical technique.

Anorectal Malformations

Surgical Pathology

Congenital anorectal anomalies are subdivided into two main groups (Santulli et al., 1970). In high anomalies the rectum ends above the level of the pelvic floor and usually has a fistulous communication with the viscus lying anteriorly, i.e. the posterior urethra in the male and the vagina in the female. In low anomalies the rectum has passed through the pelvic floor and opens onto the surface in an abnormal position which is usually anterior to the normal anus, e.g. vestibular ectopic anus in the female, 'covered' anus

in the male (*Fig.* 58.39). A very rare intermediate type of anomaly is caused by a membranous obstruction at the junction of the developing proctodeum and hindgut. In classifying anorectal malformations a plea is made for the use of descriptive terminology rather than the use of numerical classifications, also to avoid the term 'imperforate anus' unless used to describe the rare intermediate type.

Congenital anomalies are often found in association with anorectal malformations such as vertebral anomalies, urinary tract malformations, gastrointestinal and cardiovascular defects. These associated defects are often serious and adversely alter the prognosis for the infant (Stephens, 1963).

Surgical Management

Clinical Features

The diagnosis of a congenital anorectal malformation is easy; it is all too apparent, provided the anus has been inspected and examined as an essential part of the routine examination of the newborn. There can be no excuse for delay in diagnosis.

Differentiation between the different types of anorectal malformation is more difficult and is dependent on experience and further investigation. It is vitally important to determine whether the lesion is a high or low one as the surgical treatment and results, particularly concerning continence, are largely dependent on this fact.

The standard method used to establish the diagnosis is to take a straight lateral radiograph of the infant upside down centred on the greater trochanter (Wangensteen method) and with a radio-opaque marker on the anus. A line is then drawn between the symphysis pubis and the tip of the sacrum (Stephens' pubococcygeal line). If a shadow of gas in the rectum is seen above the pubococcygeal line the anomaly is a low one, if below the anomaly is a high one (*Fig.* 58.40). False positives and false negatives may occur with this simple investigation; variations may occur due to the age of the patient (unreliable under 24 hours of age), sacral anomalies and the viscosity of the meconium. Despite these reservations the technique is easy and reliable for diagnosis in the majority of patients.

Another method used to differentiate the type of anomaly requires the use of contrast material. The perineum is explored with a needle and syringe; if air or meconium is obtained some radio-opaque contrast is injected into the space (20 per cent Hypaque) and lateral views taken to determine the relationship of the viscus to the pelvic floor.

Air in the bladder or meconium on the tip of the penis are indicative of high defects with a rectourethral fistula. Similarly in the covered anus in the male white or green meconium may be seen anterior to the anus which is covered with an inverted V fold of skin which merges with the median raphe on the scrotum. In the female a careful search must be made

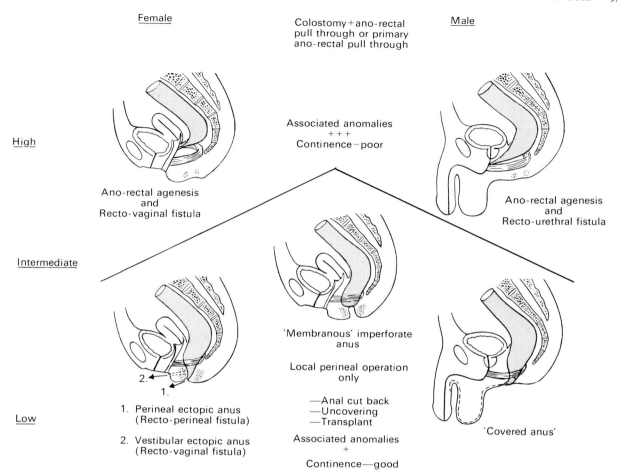

Female

Colostomy + ano-rectal
pull through or primary
ano-rectal pull through

Male

High

Associated anomalies
+ + +
Continence – poor

Ano-rectal agenesis
and
Recto-vaginal fistula

Ano-rectal agenesis
and
Recto-urethral fistula

Intermediate

'Membranous' imperforate
anus

Local perineal operation
only

—Anal cut back
—Uncovering
—Transplant

Associated anomalies
+
Continence—good

Low

1. Perineal ectopic anus
   (Recto-perineal fistula)

2. Vestibular ectopic anus
   (Recto-vaginal fistula)

'Covered anus'

Fig. 58.39. Schematic representation of the different types of congenital anorectal malformations. The classification depends on the relationship of the anomaly to the level of the pelvic floor (levator ani).

for any ectopic opening in the vulvar, vestibular or perineal regions.

Operations

POLICY

The correct surgical treatment requires accurate diagnosis. High anomalies are treated with a temporary colostomy, followed by a definitive operation which includes either an abdomino-anorectal pull-through or a posterior sagittal anoplasty. The colostomy is closed as a third-stage procedure. Argument exists about the optimum time and type of operation for the definitive operation but early operation in the first few months of life is recommended. In selected patients a primary single-stage abdomino-anorectal pull-through operation is satisfactory. In patients

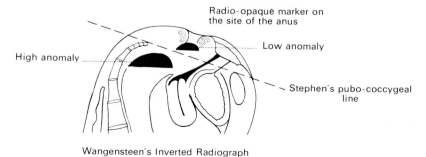

Radio-opaque marker on
the site of the anus

High anomaly

Low anomaly

Stephen's pubo-coccygeal
line

Wangensteen's Inverted Radiograph

Fig. 58.40. Diagnosis of high and low anorectal anomalies by observing the position of gas in the distal bowel when the infant is radiographed in the inverted position. A lateral radiograph is taken centred on the greater trochanter.

with low anomalies a colostomy is not required as surgical treatment with a local perineal operation gives excellent results in the majority of patients.

TRANSVERSE COLOSTOMY

With high anorectal anomalies a left transverse colostomy is the standard treatment. Operative details have already been described (*see* p. 929).

ABDOMINO-PERINEAL ANORECTAL PULL-THROUGH

This operation is either performed in the neonatal period as a primary procedure or is deferred until the infant is 1 year of age if a preliminary colostomy has been used. The principle of the operation is to ligate the fistula and to pull the bowel through the pelvic floor into the perineum to form a new anus. The success of the operation depends on the bowel being pulled through anterior to the puborectalis sling which is closely wrapped around the posterior urethra at the site of the fistula. Failure to achieve this will impair results as continence in the high anomalies is largely dependent on an efficient anorectal angle due to the sling effect of the puborectalis muscle.

The infant is placed in position in the Trendelenburg–lithotomy position using a special table designed for the purpose (*Fig.* 58.38). The bladder is catheterized and an efficient scalp vein infusion is established. The incision is a left long paramedian. The bladder is mobilized by dividing the urachus and applying traction. In the female the uterus may be pulled forwards by stay sutures between the skin edge and around the Fallopian tube. These manoeuvres will allow adequate visualization of the pelvis and in the male will help to lift up the prostatic urethra.

The abdominal phase starts with an incision in the peritoneum medial to the course of the right and left ureters. These incisions meet anteriorly on the posterior part of the bladder. The presacral space is entered by blunt dissection taking care to leave the pelvic autonomics either in the mesentery of the rectum or laterally, so that the bladder innervation is not jeopardized.

The fistula to the posterior urethra or vagina is identified and ligated after transfixation. It is important to ligate the fistula as close to the urethra as possible without damaging or narrowing the urethra. This is facilitated by passing a metal bougie into the bladder before transfixing the fistula.

The rectum is mobilized so that there is sufficient length to bring the bowel down to the perineum without any tension.

The perineal dissection starts with the excision of an ellipse of skin (or a cruciate incision) over the site of the anus. The external sphincter is identified in the subcutaneous tissues and is split in the midline. A metal bougie is passed into the urethra which acts as a guide in making the tract from the anus upwards to the site of the ligated fistula. Curved artery forceps or divulsors are passed along this tract which can then be gently stretched with graduated Hegar's dilators. The bowel can then be grasped and pulled through this tract and down to the perineum. The rectum is sutured to the pelvic floor with chromic catgut sutures in the midline and laterally. The rectal mucosa is sutured to the skin edges using interrupted silk sutures.

The abdominal wound is closed leaving an infant suction drain into the presacral space (Redivac).

POSTERIOR SAGITTAL ANORECTOPLASTY

A preliminary colostomy is established. A course of preoperative irrigations distal to the colostomy are given. The bladder is catheterized with a No. 8 Fr. gauge Foley and the site of the anus identified using an electrostimulator. The infant is operated on in the frog position.

The midline skin incision extends from the mid-sacrum through the site of the anus to the perineum. The sphincteric muscle is identified and the coccyx is split in the sagittal plane. The levator ani is split in the midline and dissected from the smooth longitudinal muscle coat of the rectum. The bowel is then mobilized by sharp and blunt dissection.

The bowel is opened in the midline to identify the associated fistula to the bladder, prostate or bulbar urethra. The submucosal plane is used to identify the fistula which is then transected and closed. The bowel is mobilized to obtain sufficient length to suture it to the site of the anus. The sphincters are repaired and the wound is closed. Occasionally tapering of the distal bowel is required (de Vries and Pena, 1982; Pena and de Vries, 1982).

ANAL CUTBACK

This operation is suitable for low anomalies in the female, e.g. ectopic anus, rectovestibular fistula or rectoperineal fistula.

The newborn is held in the lithotomy position and a sound is passed into the ectopic opening to ascertain its direction and size. The blade of straight scissors is then inserted and a cut is made in the midline posteriorly to enlarge the opening. The mucosa and skin margins of the enlarged opening are sutured with interrupted silk sutures.

'LAYING OPEN' A COVERED ANUS

This operation is a minor modification of the anal cutback procedure. The fistulous tract on the scrotum is identified and a probe passed backwards along the tract to pass through the anus and into the rectum. The ridge of skin with the apex lying anteriorly covers the normal site of the anus. This is excised using straight scissors in the horizontal plane, thus exposing the normal anus with its identifiable anal columns and valves. The anus is dilated up to a No. 12 or 14 Hegar and mucocutaneous silk sutures are inserted.

Postoperative Care

TRANSVERSE COLOSTOMY

See under Hirschsprung's disease.

ABDOMINO-ANORECTAL PULL-THROUGH

Blood transfusion may have been required at the time of operation, further loss should be watched for by regular inspection of the infant Redivac drainage bottle. Nasogastric aspiration and intravenous replacement are continued until the aspirates are non-bile stained, abdominal distension is absent and bowel sounds have returned. Oral feeding can start after the first colostomy action or bowel action. Antibiotics are used for the first 7 postoperative days.

Dilatation of the new anus and rectum are started after the 10th postoperative day and continued daily or at regular intervals until the healing is complete and the anus is supple; this may take several months.

ANAL CUTBACK

Apart from the anal dilatations no specific treatment is required.

'LAYING OPEN' A COVERED ANUS

Regular dilatations are required after the 7th postoperative day. Following this and after discharge home these are continued by the mother who has received careful instruction in performing this procedure.

Complications

In all anorectal malformations close supervision is required for some years because some children will develop a secondary megarectum as a late complication. This complication is preventable if adequate long-term follow-up care and assessment are undertaken.

TRANSVERSE COLOSTOMY

See under Hirschsprung's disease.

ABDOMINO-ANORECTAL PULL-THROUGH

Early: Retraction of the bowel may be due to inadequate mobilization of the bowel and is therefore preventable. Peritonitis due to contamination can cause postoperative ileus, localized abscess formation and adhesions. Stricture may be ischaemic in origin or due to inadequate preparation of the pathway for the bowel through the pelvic floor.

Late: Stenosis occurs at the mucocutaneous junction and may require dilatations or operative correction by an anoplasty. Mucosal prolapse and bleeding require similar treatment. Incontinence is the main problem as the results of this operation are disappointing in at least 50 per cent of the patients. The degree of continence is dependent on accurate technique, which results in the bowel being pulled through anterior to the puborectalis sling. If the puborectalis sling is palpated anterior to the pulled-through rectum some improvement may be obtained by a secondary pull-through operation. In some patients the best results are obtained with a terminal left iliac colostomy. Calculi can form in a small pocket at the site of the recto-urethral fistula. Rarely an abscess forms at this site and may rupture intraperitoneally.

ANAL CUTBACK

Either stricture or stenosis may occur if the cutback has been inadequate. Occasionally the levator ani may be damaged if the cutback has been too radical. Secondary megarectum due to inefficient defaecation can be prevented in most patients by careful supervision, regular rectal examinations and with the help of a sensible and cooperative mother. Aesthetic complications occur in adolescence due to the appearance of the perineum. The 'shotgun' perineum described by Sir Denis Browne is aesthetically displeasing but functionally adequate. Further surgery in such patients should be resisted as bowel control may suffer.

'LAYING OPEN' A COVERED ANUS

Either stenosis of secondary megarectum may occur. Both are preventable and bowel control in these patients is normal.

'Idiopathic' Neonatal Intestinal Obstruction

Surgical Pathology

A newborn infant presenting with subacute intestinal obstruction may mark the onset of further complications such as gangrene and perforation of the bowel secondary to ischaemia or inflammation. Advances and changes in obstetric and paediatric care and resuscitation of premature infants may account for the increased incidence of such cases in recent years.

The pathological findings in these infants (*Fig. 58.41*) depend on many factors including the timing of exploratory laparotomy. Simple necrosis leading to perforation with little inflammatory response is seen in some patients; in others the necrosis is associated with inflammation in the bowel wall immediately adjacent to the site of the perforation. Necrosis, inflammation and widespread haemorrhagic exudate maximal in the submucosa and mucosa may be seen

a. Simple necrosis – Perforation   *b.* Simple necrosis + Inflammation – Perforation

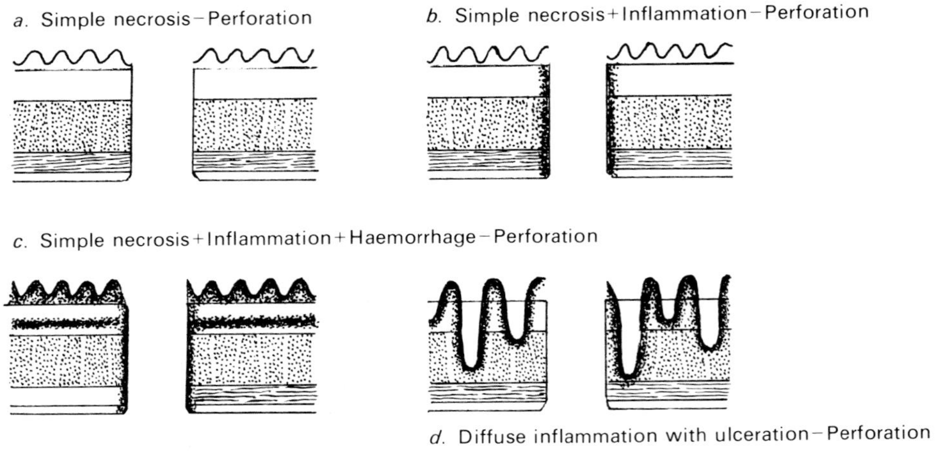

c. Simple necrosis + Inflammation + Haemorrhage – Perforation

d. Diffuse inflammation with ulceration – Perforation

Fig. 58.41. Surgical pathology of necrotizing enterocolitis.

in others with more widespread changes (disseminated intravascular coagulation). In the final subgroup similar findings are associated with diffuse acute inflammatory changes and pneumatosis of the bowel wall (necrotizing enterocolitis).

These pathological changes may result in gangrene and perforation of the bowel, localized abscesses or generalized peritonitis. Septicaemia is common and accounts for the high mortality. Active medical and surgical treatment can result in full recovery but in others the recovery is complicated by subacute or acute intestinal obstruction secondary to adhesions and stricture formation. The operative findings resemble the different types of intestinal atresia found in the newborn (*see Fig.* 58.29), thus suggesting that ischaemia is a significant factor in their causation. At operation the bowel is found to be gangrenous with patent pulsatile vessels up to the margin of the intestine. Thus it appears that the changes seen are secondary to alteration in blood flow through the intrinsic intramural vessels lying in the submucosa

of the bowel. Severe anoxia and other stressful factors may cause intense vasoconstriction of these intramural vessels ('diving reflex'). Many factors may initiate this physiological response in the newborn which leads to mucosal damage, stasis, infection and their sequelae (*Fig.* 58.42). Breast feeding has been shown to provide a protective effect in the experimental animal but necrotizing enterocolitis is sometimes found in the breast-fed infant.

Surgical Management

Clinical Features

Different antenatal and perinatal factors are important in these infants, e.g. prematurity, anoxia, multiple births, cold injury, exchange transfusion, alteration in feeding regimens (milk plug syndrome: Cook and Rickhan, 1969; faecal plug syndrome: Zachary, 1957), stercoral ulceration, infection, particularly with *Clostridium difficile*, drugs, hypothy-

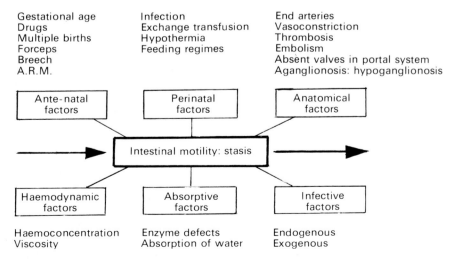

Gestational age   Infection   End arteries
Drugs   Exchange transfusion   Vasoconstriction
Multiple births   Hypothermia   Thrombosis
Forceps   Feeding regimes   Embolism
Breech   Absent valves in portal system
A.R.M.   Aganglionosis: hypoganglionosis

| Ante-natal factors | Perinatal factors | Anatomical factors |

Intestinal motility: stasis

| Haemodynamic factors | Absorptive factors | Infective factors |

Haemoconcentration   Enzyme defects   Endogenous
Viscosity   Absorption of water   Exogenous

Fig. 58.42. Factors of aetiological significance in necrotizing enterocolitis.

roidism, hypoplastic left colon syndrome, abnormal meconium (meconium plug syndrome), the use of intra-arterial cannulas and leaching of polymers from such catheters. Similarly it can be seen as a complication secondary to stasis, cf. Hirschsprung's disease and congenital anal stenosis. Stasis or hypomotility of the bowel is therefore an important common denominator and the infection found in some of these patients is endogenous rather than exogenous in origin (*Fig.* 58.42).

There is often a prodromal phase: the onset of such changes may be marked by jaundice, apnoea and cyanotic attacks in premature infants during the first 2 days of life. Then signs of subacute intestinal obstruction develop with abdominal distension and vomiting of bile. The signs at this stage will be intermittent and resemble those seen in patients with Hirschsprung's disease. It is very rare to find a premature infant with Hirschsprung's disease. Later, as signs advance, the obstruction becomes more obvious as the distension increases. The umbilicus may become everted and inflamed with a red flare radiating from it. Tenderness on palpation and abdominal masses may develop. Diarrhoea and blood in the stool become apparent and are serious signs. Perforation of the bowel with a dramatic increase in the size of the abdomen due to a pneumoperitoneum is not uncommon; finally, faecal peritonitis and abscess formation occur.

Treatment

POLICY

The clinical problem in the management of these patients is to decide whether they need an operation or whether they can be safely treated by conservative measures. It is better to resect gangrenous bowel before perforation occurs rather than to find faecal peritonitis on exploratory laparotomy. Faecal peritonitis in the premature infant is associated with complications which may adversely affect the morbidity of the condition and severely limit the choice of operative procedures.

CONSERVATIVE TREATMENT

The principles of management are to rest the bowel, treat the infection, maintain the internal environment, feed the infant and monitor carefully the changes which herald perforation of the intestine.

All oral feeding is stopped and a nasogastric tube is passed (No. 8 Fr. or No. 10 Fr. gauge), aspirated at regular intervals and left on free drainage. The aspirates are replaced intravenously with an equal volume of normal saline.

Antibiotics are given intravenously; either cephalosporins or gentamicin and Pyopen (carbenicillin). Gentamicin is also given orally to reduce the bacterial flora in the lumen of the bowel.

Replacement infusions of fresh blood and plasma are required in severe cases. Low molecular weight Rheomacrodex (dextran) can be used to improve the blood flow in the small vessels in the wall of the intestine (10–20 per cent of the blood volume may be administered over 2 hours).

Observations of temperature, pulse and respiratory rate are monitored and also regular measurements of the abdominal girth are recorded (*see* Appendix I).

Serial straight radiographs of the abdomen are taken and repeated at 12 hours, 24 hours or longer intervals depending on the clinical response of the patient. Careful note is taken of distended loops, fluid levels, faecal content and intramural gas and any alterations seen on repeated radiographs. Progressive dilatation of the same loop of intestine suggests toxic dilatation and impending gangrene and perforation. Pneumoperitoneum with gross abdominal distension producing respiratory embarrassment is an absolute indication for surgery. Localized perforations may become walled off by adjacent loops of bowel and are not absolute indications for surgery, but at a later date adhesions, strictures and abscesses may require surgical treatment.

Conservative measures can be performed for long periods with the aid of parenteral nutrition, thus allowing reparative healing to occur. In some patients oral feeding can be re-established, in others subacute obstruction persists and is associated with failure to thrive which is a further indication for surgery.

OPERATIONS

Operation is reserved for patients in whom conservative treatment has failed or when complications develop.

Laparotomy: The abdomen is opened through a transverse supraumbilical muscle-cutting incision. It is important to examine carefully the length of the gastrointestinal tract, looking for areas of gangrene, focal areas of necrosis, haemorrhages and perforation. The bowel wall is like wet tissue paper and great care in handling is necessary.

Intestinal Resection and Primary Anastomosis: Nonviable bowel is resected and continuity restored by primary anastomosis. Resections may be single or multiple and involve jejunum, ileum and colon.

Intestinal Resection and Exteriorization: Resection and primary anastomosis are not always possible due to the extent of the disease, the degree of peritoneal soiling and doubts about the viability of the bowel. In such patients a proximal stoma is established (ileostomy, colostomy), the bowel is resected and the distal bowel is brought out as a mucous fistula through a separate stab incision. At a second-stage operation continuity can often be restored.

Colostomy: Ileostomy: In some patients the bowel is considered to be viable but doubts may exist about the precise diagnosis, e.g. Hirschsprung's disease. It is then necessary to biopsy the wall of the intestine and rectum and defunction the bowel by a proximal stoma. After recovery and if the biopsy is normal the stoma is closed at a second-stage operation when the infant is thriving and weighing about 5 kg.

Drainage of Intraperitoneal Abscess: Occasionally localized abscesses in the right iliac fossa or subphrenic space may require treatment and drainage.

'Second-look' Operations: In some patients the length of bowel involvement is so extensive that surgical resection is incompatible with survival. Under such circumstances the abdomen is closed and intensive conservative measures are indicated. After an interval of 2–4 days the abdomen can be explored and a more limited resection may be possible in some patients. The average length of the intestine for the duodeno-jejunal junction to ileocaecal valve in the neonate is 200 cm. Loss of intestinal length of up to two-thirds of this can still result in survival and reasonable growth and development.

Postoperative Care
The principles of postoperative care are the same as for the preoperative conservative management of such patients and have been outlined in this section and in the introduction.

Complications

EARLY
Septicaemia and overwhelming infection may cause death of the patient early in the course of the disease. Clostridial infections are found in this group of patients and gas in the biliary tree on the straight radiograph is a serious prognostic sign but is not invariably fatal as was originally thought. Peritonitis and abscess formation occur. Wound infection and dehiscence and faecal fistula secondary to a breakdown of an intestinal anastomosis or a further perforation are not unusual.

LATE
Adhesions and strictures producing subacute obstruction, failure to thrive and secondary disaccharide intolerances are seen. Later acute intestinal obstruction from bands is seen. Loss of intestinal length (short gut syndrome) may interfere with growth and development.

APPENDIX I
Routine nursing observations of the surgical newborn
Either: (1) Nurse in a warm room temperature (27 °C)
Or: (2) Nurse in an incubator, temperature 30–33 °C or overhead heated cot.

Temperature recorded at 1-hourly intervals.
Pulse rate observation at ½–1-hourly intervals by listening to apex beat.
Respiratory rate at ½–1-hourly intervals.

Inspection of i.v. site at 1-hourly intervals.
Measurement of abdominal girth at 2–4-hourly intervals.
Nasogastric aspiration at ½–1-hourly intervals and to be left on free drainage in between. Check position of end of catheter at 2-hourly intervals.

Change position of newborn at 2-hourly intervals.
Care of the mouth 2–4 hourly.
Care of eyes 2–4 hourly.
Restraining mittens to be checked every 4 hours to prevent a cotton thread causing a ring constriction gangrene.
Care of the wounds and dressings.
Observations of urine stream, volume and frequency.
Meconium passed is saved for inspection and recorded.
Daily weighing.
Measurements of skull circumference (occipito-frontal) at weekly intervals.
Testing for phenylketonuria with the Guthrie test before discharge home.
The neonate should have been on normal feeds for 8 days before testing.

Regular cleansing with cottonwool when in incubator and daily bath when in cot.

Chest physiotherapy 1-hourly. Careful suction of mouth and nasopharynx.

Care of chest drains, gastrostomy tubes and transanastomotic feeding tubes.

Nursing care of a neonate on a ventilator
1. Infant is specialed throughout the 24 hours.
2. Nurse flat with head extended.
3. Careful fixation of ventilator tubes.
4. Prevention of blockage of endotracheal tube by:
   a. Instil 0·5 ml normal saline ½-hourly and immediately after endotracheal aspiration. The nurse wears sterile gloves for the procedure. Disposable catheter used once only.
   b. Any rise in ventilator pressure is indicative of blocking or kinking.
   c. Emergency trolley for reintubation should be immediately available.
5. Care to eyes and mouth.
6. Use special care chart to record:
   a. Infant's TPR on a graph.
   b. Incubator temperature.
   c. Room temperature.
   d. Oxygen concentration.
   e. Peripheral circulation.
   f. Position of infant.

7. Observations of the ventilator:
   a. Rate.
   b. Inspiratory pressure.
   c. Expiratory pressure.
   d. Blow-off valve.
   e. Oxygen concentration.
   f. Oxygen and air (litres per minute).

APPENDIX II
Essential equipment for a neonatal surgical unit
Respirators (Vickers Neovent).
Apnoea alarms (Vickers Mk III).
Oxygen monitor (Hudson).
Roberts' pumps.
Paediatric (90 ml) underwater pleural drainage sets.
Cardiorators (Hewlett Packard).
Incubators: overhead heaters (Ohio): Bassinets.

Intravenous infusion pumps (Ivac Corporation).
Chest vibrator (Pifco).
Electric thermometers.
Oxygen and CO_2 cutaneous monitor (Radiometer).
Oxygen cutaneous monitor (Kontron).
Phototherapy unit (Vickers).
Handley constant infusion pumps.
Doppler blood pressure equipment (Sonicaid).
Electric heating blankets.
Infant inflating bags (Penlon Cardiff).
Electronic nebulizers (Mistogen Equipment).
Portable oxygen cylinders for incubators (BOC).
Anaesthetic resuscitation equipment.
Blood gas analyser.
Bilirubinometer.
Osmometer.
Blood glucose analyser (Ames).

References

Atwell J. D. (1966) Magnesium deficiency following neonatal surgical procedures. *J. Pediatr. Surg.* **1**, 427–440.
Atwell J. D. (1968) The early diagnosis and surgical treatment of Hirschsprung's disease in infancy. *Proc. R. Soc. Med.* **61**, 339–340.
Atwell J. D. (1971) Pitfalls in the diagnosis of intestinal obstruction in the newborn. *Proc. R. Soc. Med.* **64**, 374–377.
Atwell J. D. and Beard R. C. (1974) Congenital anomalies of the upper urinary tract associated with oesophageal atresia and tracheo-oesophageal fistula. *J. Pediatr. Surg.* **9**, 825–831.
Atwell J. D. and Harrison G. S. M. (1980) Observations on the role of oesophagogastrostomy in infancy and childhood with particular reference to the long-term results and operative mortality. *J. Pediatr. Surg.* **15**, 303–309.
Berman E. J. (1958) Extralobar (diaphragmatic) sequestration of the lung. *Arch. Surg.* **76**, 724–731.
Bernstein P. (1940) Gastroschisis, a rare teratological condition in the newborn. *Arch. Pediatr.* **57**, 503–505.
Bianchi A., Doig C. M. and Cohen S. J. (1983) The reverse latissimus dorsi flap for congenital diaphragmatic hernia repair. *J. Pediatr. Surg.* **18**, 560–563.
Bishop H. C. and Koop C. E. (1957) Management of meconium ileus: resection, Roux-en-Y anastomosis and ileostomy irrigation with pancreatic enzymes. *Ann. Surg.* **145**, 410–414.
Bloss R. S., Turmen T. and Beardmore H. E. (1980) Tolazoline therapy for persistent pulmonary hypertension after diaphragmatic repair. *J. Pediatr.* **97**, 984–988.
Bohn D. J., Filler J. R. M., Ein S. H. et al. (1983) The relationship between $Paco_2$ and ventilation parameters in predicting survival in congenital diaphragmatic hernia. *J. Pediatr. Surg.* **18**, 666–671.
Bond-Taylor W., Starer F. and Atwell J. D. (1973) Vertebral anomalies associated with oesophageal atresia and tracheo-oesophageal fistula with particular reference to the initial operative mortality. *J. Pediatr. Surg.* **8**, 9–13.
Bulgrin J. G. and Holmes F. H. (1955) Eventration of diaphragm with high renal ectopia; case report. *Radiology* **64**, 249–251.
Cantrell J. R., Haller J. A. and Ravitch M. M. (1958) A syndrome of congenital defects involving the abdominal wall, sternum, diaphragm, pericardium and heart. *Surg. Gynecol. Obstet.* **107**, 602.
Carter C. O. (1961) Genetic factors in pyloric stenosis. *Proc. R. Soc. Med.* **54**, 453–454.
Collins D. L., Pomerance J. J., Travis K. W. et al. (1977) A new approach to congenital postero-lateral diaphragmatic hernia. *J. Pediatr. Surg.* **12**, 149–155.
Cook R. C. M. and Rickham P. P. (1969) Neonatal intestinal obstruction due to milk curds. *J. Pediatr. Surg.* **4**, 599–605.
Corkery J. J., Dubowitz V., Lister J. et al. (1968) Colonic perforation after exchange transfusion. *Br. Med. J.* **4**, 345–349.
de Vries P. and Pena A. (1982) Posterior sagittal anorectoplasty. *J. Pediatr. Surg.* **17**, 638–643.
Duhamel B. (1963) Embryology of exomphalos and allied malformations. *Arch. Dis. Child.* **38**, 142–147.
Fitchett C. W. and Tavarez V. (1965) Bilateral congenital diaphragmatic herniation: case report. *Surgery* **57**, 305–308.
Forshall I. and Rickham P. P. (1960) Experience of a neonatal surgical unit. *Lancet* **ii**, 751–754.
Freeman N. V. (1974) Hirschsprung's disease. *Update* 177–190.
Grob M. (1963) Conservative treatment of exomphalos. *Arch. Dis. Child.* **38**, 148–150.
Gross R. E. (1948) New method for surgical treatment of large omphaloceles. *Surgery* **24**, 277–292.
Harrington S. W. (1948) Various types of diaphragmatic hernia treated surgically; report of 430 cases. *Surg. Gynecol. Obstet.* **86**, 735–755.
Holder T. M. (1964) Transpleural versus retropleural approach for repair of tracheo-oesophageal fistula. *Surg. Clin. North Am.* **44**, 1433–1439.
Janik J. S., Akbar A. M., Burrington J. D. et al. (1978) The role of gastrin in congenital hypertrophic pyloric stenosis. *J. Pediatr. Surg.* **13**, 151–154.
Kitagawa M., Hislop A., Boyden E. A. et al. (1971) Lung hypoplasia in congenital diaphragmatic hernia. *Br. J. Surg.* **58**, 342–346.

Koop C. E. and Hamilton J. P. (1965) Atresia of the oesophagus. Increased survival with staged procedures in the poor-risk infant. *Ann. Surg.* **162**, 389–401.

Louw J. H. (1959) Congenital intestinal atresia and stenosis in the newborn. Observations on its pathogenesis and treatment. *Ann. R. Coll. Surg. Engl.* **25**, 209–234.

Louw J. H. and Barnard C. N. (1955) Congenital intestinal atresia: observations on its origin. *Lancet* **ii**, 1065–1067.

Maingot R. (1961) Operations for sliding herniae and for large incisional herniae. *Br. J. Clin. Pract.* **15**, 993–996.

Moore T. C. (1977) Gastroschisis and omphalocele: clinical differences. *Surgery* **82**, 561–568.

Pena A. and de Vries P. (1982) Posterior sagittal anorectoplasty: important technical considerations and new applications. *J. Pediatr. Surg.* **17**, 796–811.

Puri P., Guiney E. J. and O'Donnell B. (1975) Total parenteral feeding in infants using peripheral veins. *Arch. Dis. Child.* **50**, 133–136.

Replogle R. L. (1963) Esophageal atresia: plastic sump catheter for drainage of the proximal pouch. *Surgery* **54**, 296–297.

Rickham P. P. (1952) Neonatal surgery: early treatment of congenital malformations. *Lancet* **i**, 332–339.

Rickham P. P. (1960) Vesico-intestinal fistula. *Arch. Dis. Child.* **35**, 97–102.

Rickham P. P. and Johnston J. H. (1969) *Neonatal Surgery.* London, Butterworths, p. 201.

Sabga G. A., Neville W. E. and Del Guercio L. R. M. (1961) Anomalies of the lung associated with congenital diaphragmatic hernia. *Surgery* **50**, 547–554.

Santulli T. V., Kiesewetter W. B. and Bill A. H., Jr (1970) Ano-rectal anomalies: a suggested international classification. *J. Pediatr. Surg.* **5**, 281–287.

Sherman C. D. and Waterston D. (1957) Oesophageal reconstruction in children using intrathoracic colon. *Arch. Dis. Child.* **32**, 11–16.

Shuster S. R. (1967) A new method for the staged repair of large omphaloceles. *Surg. Gynecol. Obstet.* **125**, 837–850.

Soave F. (1977) Megacolon: long-term results of surgical treatment. In: Rickham P. P., Hecker W. Ch. and Prévot J. (eds) *Progress in Pediatric Surgery*, Vol. 10. Munich, Urban & Schwarzenberg, pp. 141–149.

Stephens F. Douglas (ed.) (1963) *Congenital Malformations of the Rectum, Anus and Genito-urinary Tracts.* Edinburgh, Livingstone.

Suita S., Ikeda K., Hayashida Y. et al. (1984) Zinc and copper requirements during parenteral nutrition in the newborn. *J. Pediatr. Surg.* **19**, 126–130.

Tandler J. (1902) Zur Entwicklung des menschlichen Duodenums im fruehen Embryonalstadium. *Morphol. Jahrb.* **29**, 187–216.

Thomas D. F. M. and Atwell J. D. (1976) The embryology and the surgical management of gastroschisis. *Br. J. Surg.* **63**, 893–897.

Touloukian R. J. and Spackman T. J. (1971) Gastrointestinal function and radiographic appearance following gastroschisis repair. *J. Pediatr. Surg.* **6**, 427–433.

Vacanti J. P., Crone R. K., Murphy J. D. et al. (1984) The pulmonary hemodynamic response to perioperative anaesthesia in the treatment of high risk infants with congenital diaphragmatic hernia. *J. Pediatr. Surg.* **19**, 672–679.

Venugopal S., Zachary R. B. and Spitz L. (1976) Exomphalos and gastroschisis: a 10 year review. *Br. J. Surg.* **63**, 523–525.

Young D. G. (1966) Neonatal acid–base disturbances. *Arch. Dis. Child.* **41**, 201–203.

Young D. G. (1968) Contralateral pneumothorax with congenital diaphragmatic hernia. *Br. Med. J.* **4**, 433–434.

Young W. F. (1964) Practical management of the newborn in regard to their water and electrolyte needs. *Maandschr. Kindergeneesk.* **32**, 316–334.

Zachary R. B. (1957) Meconium and faecal plugs in the newborn. *Arch Dis. Child.* **32**, 22.

Transplantation Surgery

Chapter fifty-nine

Renal Transplantation

H. J. O. White

Renal transplantation is a well-established therapy for patients with irreversible renal failure and offers many of them an alternative to life supported by maintenance dialysis. Dialysis and transplant units work closely together, as is shown in *Fig.* 59.1. A patient rejecting a graft may return to dialysis to later receive a second or even third transplant, the outcome of which may be more successful than the first.

Certain patients on maintenance haemodialysis are unsuitable for transplantation but represent the minority. In this group are those with primary malignant disease of the renal tract, renal tuberculosis, chronic renal tract infection that persists despite bilateral host nephrectomy, active chronic glomerulonephritis, established renal osteodystrophy, and those with uncorrected bladder neck obstruction.

Patients selected for renal transplantation will usually be established on a dialysis programme, but occasionally diabetic patients have been transplanted without prior haemodialysis. Bilateral host nephrectomy will be required in those patients whose hypertension cannot be adequately controlled by dialysis and hypotensive drugs, for those with persistent renal tract infection, and lastly for those with large polycystic kidneys. Anaemia is a constant feature in patients on maintenance dialysis and a haemoglobin of approximately 7 g per cent is common. Blood transfusion will only temporarily correct such anaemia and is rarely practised for this reason. There is, however, evidence now that pretransplant blood transfusion may benefit the potential transplant recipient, rejection in these patients being less frequent.

All patients will have been blood grouped, tissue typed and shown to be Australia antigen negative. Their names, with personal details and availability, will be kept on some form of register, possibly a computer, so that when a cadaver donor kidney becomes available, it can be offered to the most suitable recipient. Many such national organ-sharing programmes exist to achieve this aim.

OPERATIVE DETAILS

1. Bilateral Host Nephrectomy

Although bilateral loin or lumbotomy incisions have been used to remove small kidneys, a generous transverse upper abdominal transperitoneal approach is preferred (*Fig.* 59.2). Very large polycystic kidneys can be removed by this technique. The left kidney is approached having incised the phrenico-colic ligament and the splenic flexure mobilized medially. The individual renal vessels are then doubly ligated before removing the kidney and the ureter is divided as low as possible, at or below the level of the pelvic brim. On the right a similar procedure is carried out incising the peritoneum over the right kidney, lateral to the second part of the duodenum. The wound is closed in layers without drainage and the next dialysis delayed for 2 or more days, if this be practicable.

2. Live Donor

If a close blood relative offers to donate a kidney, it is essential that his or her ABO blood group is

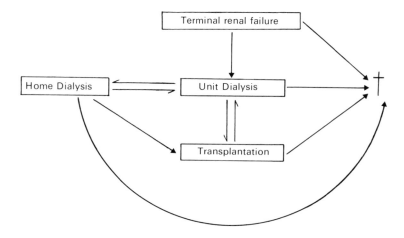

Fig. 59.1. Progress chart of patient with renal failure.

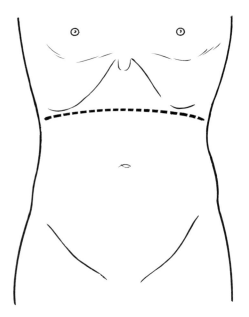

Fig. 59.2. Incision for bilateral host nephrectomy.

compatible with the recipient's. Second, the donor's HL-A tissue typing must show a close match, indicating a good chance for a successful outcome, and, third, a mixed lymphocyte culture of recipient and donor cells should show a low level of stimulation as further evidence of compatibility. The potential donor must be in good health and certain investigations are carried out, including haemoglobin, blood urea, creatinine clearance and intravenous pyelography. Following this initial assessment, it is wise to hand over the further management of the potential donor to a surgeon independent of the transplant team, so that there may be no conflict between the needs of the recipient and of the donor. The ultimate preoperative investigation must include an aortogram to outline the renal arteries, as it is only practical to transplant a live donor kidney with a single artery.

The donor operation is a planned procedure, carried out in an adjacent theatre to synchronize with the recipient's operation and take approximately $1\frac{1}{2}$ hours until the time when the donor kidney is ready for removal. The standard loin exposure for nephrectomy is made. It differs from nephrectomy for a diseased organ in that the renal vessels are dissected out with considerably more care, dissection in the hilum being avoided and concentrated where the renal artery arises from the aorta and the renal vein from the vena cava. On the left, it is necessary to ligate and divide the left adrenal and left gonadal veins. The ureter together with the peri-ureteric vessels is dissected out and divided at the level of the brim of the bony pelvis. Heparin, 10 000 units, together with a systemic diuretic, either mannitol or frusemide, are then given. A few minutes are then allowed to elapse so that these drugs may become

effective and the donor kidney is then removed after cross-clamping and individually ligating the renal artery and renal vein. It is perfused in the same manner as for a cadaver kidney and is then immediately taken to the adjacent recipient theatre, usually in a bowl of ice-cold saline.

3. Cadaver Donor

A good supply of cadaver kidneys involves much hard work, canvassing and liaison on behalf of the transplant team, and requires them to be available to travel to other hospitals within their region to remove these. Donor cadaver kidneys are now virtually only removed from suitable donors maintained on a ventilator with an established diagnosis of brain death. Their removal is frequently part of a multiple organ donation and may be carried out by the heart or liver donor team. Permission for their removal must be obtained as appropriate and is required by law. Certain investigations should be carried out in advance to establish the suitability of the donor. Blood tests should be taken for haemoglobin, blood urea, serum creatinine, Australia antigen testing, as well as ABO grouping and tissue typing, and urine should be sent for culture. The patient's urine volume and blood pressure should be monitored frequently. Potential donors should be free of transplantable carcinoma, tuberculosis and other transmissible infectious diseases. The majority of potential donors will be dying of brain trauma, cerebral vascular accident or a primary brain tumour. Pretreatment with a systemic antibiotic is desirable, particularly in those with an indwelling urethral catheter and/or those who have been maintained on a ventilator for more than a few hours. A systemic steroid will often have been given

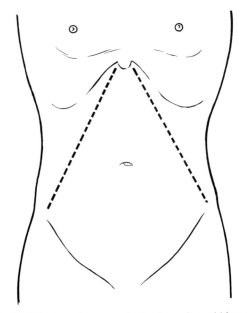

Fig. 59.3. Incision for removal of cadaver donor kidneys.

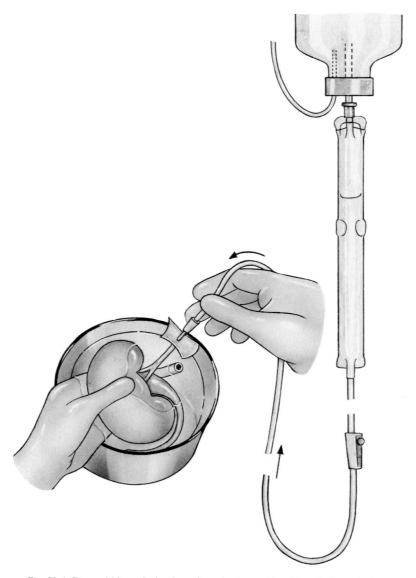

Fig. 59.4. Donor kidney. Irrigation of renal artery with cold perfusion solution.

already for the treatment of cerebral oedema, but should be requested if this has not already been given. If premortem hypotension becomes a problem, a dopamine drip may be necessary to correct this. Once the diagnosis of brain death has been established, certain additional drugs are given, usually in the operating theatre. These include intravenous heparin and certain membrane-stabilizing drugs including phenoxybenzamine, Largactil (chlorpromazine) and curare.

The abdominal skin is cleaned with iodine solution and draped to allow a generous exposure from nipple to groin. Although there are several techniques for removing cadaver donor kidneys, the method described below (Bewick) is that practised by the author. It has the advantage of a monoblock excision of the two kidneys, together with the abdominal aorta

and inferior vena cava, and is therefore less likely to damage any unsuspected multiple or aberrant renal vessels than removal of either kidney individually. An extensive inverted V incision (*Fig.* 59.3) of the abdominal wall is made, with the apex of the V held down by tissue forceps over the symphysis pubis. The peritoneum along the right paracolic gutter is incised and the caecum and right colon mobilized to the left. This exposes the front of the inferior vena cava, right kidney and right renal vein, together with the right ureter, which is dissected down to the pelvic brim but not too cleanly, leaving the periureteric vessels adherent to the ureter. Similarly, on the left, the left colon is mobilized to expose the left ureter to the pelvic brim.

The free edge of the lesser omentum is now clamped between a pair of Kocher's forceps and

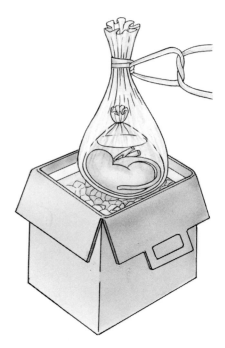

Fig. 59.5. Donor kidney. Enclosure in two sterile plastic bags and preservation in unsterile ice.

divided to expose the superior mesenteric vessels and the coeliac axis which lie immediately above the left renal vein. A finger is passed in front of the left renal vein to isolate the superior mesenteric and coeliac vessels above, which are also cross-clamped between stout Kocher's forceps and divided to expose the front of the abdominal aorta up to the level of the diaphragm. Both kidneys can now be mobilized with all four fingers of each hand meeting behind the vena cava and the abdominal aorta. The abdominal aorta and inferior vena cava can now be clamped opposite the 4th lumbar vertebra and then the aorta above just within the chest at the level of the aortic opening of the diaphragm. Clamping lower than this level may damage one or other renal artery. The inferior vena cava is also clamped above as it enters the undersurface of the liver. Both ureters are now divided at the pelvic brim and the two kidneys, together with the abdominal aorta and vena cava, can be removed monoblock and placed in a bowl of ice-cold saline.

The aorta is then incised vertically along its posterior wall and each renal artery can now be cannulated with the tip of a sterile-giving set (*Fig.* 59.4) and flushed with a suitable ice-cold perfusion solution, i.e. hyerosmolar citrate (Marshall's) or Euro-Collins being in common usage. If there is more than one renal artery on either side, then a smaller cannula can be attached to the end of the giving set and inserted into each arterial orifice. After cooling each kidney with a perfusion of approximately 200 ml of fluid until the venous effluent is clear of blood, further dissection takes place to divide the aorta vertically along its anterior wall and then the inferior vena cava

along its anterior and posterior walls so that the two kidneys are now separated. Each kidney is now placed in an individual sterile plastic bag and then that bag within another (*Fig.* 59.5) and transferred into a polystyrene box containing unsterile ice.

Static cold preservation is satisfactory up to 24 hours, particularly if the kidneys have been removed without premortem hypotension and before cardiac arrest has occurred. Cadaver donor kidneys can be transported to recipient centres at a considerable distance and transplanted within this period of time. Alternatively there are machines, e.g. Gambro, Belzer, which provide hypothermic continuous perfusion and permit longer preservation periods in excess of 48 hours.

Donor lymph nodes and spleen are also removed and sent together with the kidneys, so that further tissue typing can be carried out on these tissues, as well as on peripheral blood. An appropriate form should accompany the donor organ giving full details of the donor kidney, its preservation and any anatomical abnormality found at the time of donor nephrectomy.

4. Recipient Operation

Most potential recipients will be well maintained on dialysis and immediately fit for operation. Occasionally a further short dialysis following admission may be required to correct a dangerously elevated blood urea, serum creatinine or serum potassium or fluid overload. A Resonium A enema to counteract post-transplant hyperkalaemia is given in every case.

The anaesthetist will need to carefully monitor the patient with a central venous pressure line and an ECG. To reduce the risk of thrombosis of an arteriovenous fistula, an axillary or brachial plexus block is requested in the relevant arm.

The recipient is placed supine on the operating table, a Foley catheter inserted into the bladder and the abdomen prepared with a suitable antiseptic. A long curved supra-inguinal incision is made on the relevant side. It is usual practice to transplant a kidney with the renal artery end to end to the internal iliac artery on its contralateral side, and end to side to the external iliac artery on its ipsilateral side (*Figs.* 59.6, 59.7). The end-to-end anastomosis has the advantage that should the kidney subsequently require removal, then ligation of the internal iliac artery can be carried out with total removal of all donor arterial tissue and avoid the danger otherwise of secondary haemorrhage from the suture line. It has the disadvantage that further dissection is required of the internal iliac artery in preparation for this anastomosis, and it is unsuitable where there are two or more donor arteries on a Carrell patch of donor aorta which must then be anastomosed end to side to the external iliac artery. The incision is deepened by muscle cutting through all layers but remaining extraperitoneal to expose the iliac vessels,

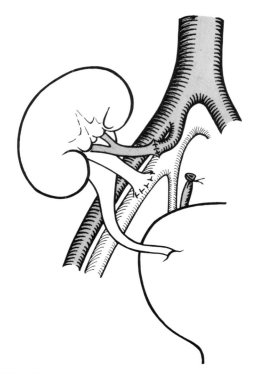

Fig. 59.6. Recipient operation. The renal artery may be united end to end with the internal iliac artery.

which are now dissected out to expose and free the full length of the external iliac artery, the distal inch of the common iliac and the internal iliac artery to its trifurcation, if it is to be used. The external iliac vein is freed from the inguinal ligament below to its junction with the internal iliac vein above. A suitable venotomy is now made vertically in the external iliac vein, between clamps.

The kidney having been removed from its sterile plastic bag, the renal vein is anastomosed end to side to the external iliac vein (*Fig.* 59.6) using stay sutures at both ends and a third stay suture at the midpoint on the medial side, while the lateral border is first sutured with running 5/0 Prolene. The medial side is then sutured to complete the anastomosis. A bulldog clamp can then be applied across the renal vein and so venous blood from the recipient is prevented from refluxing into the donor kidney following removal of the clamps from the external iliac vein. The arterial anastomosis is then carried out either by an end-to-side anastomosis in a similar manner to the venous above (*Fig.* 59.7), using a Carrell patch of donor aorta, or by an end-to-end anastomosis to the divided proximal inch of the internal iliac artery. Running 5/0 Prolene sutures are used, but should the vessels for the end-to-end anastomosis be narrow then a number of interrupted equally placed sutures are preferred to avoid stenosis. The arterial anastomosis being complete, the vascular clamps are removed and the anaesthetist then gives intravenous azathioprine, 5 mg per kg body weight, 200 ml of 20

per cent mannitol and a second 100 mg of hydrocortisone, a similar dose of this drug having been given at the start of the operation. Additional vascular sutures may be required, but once satisfactory haemostasis has been achieved then attention is turned to the uretero-neocystostomy.

The indwelling catheter placed in the bladder at the start of the operation can now be used to inflate and distend the bladder with a sterile solution. This allows the bladder to be easily identified and the donor ureter to be anastomosed to the mucosa of the bladder from without (*Fig.* 59.7). The technique described (Vernon Marshall) is used by the author. An incision is made in the upper outer quadrant of the anterior wall of the bladder on the same side as the transplant to expose the bladder mucosa, which then bulges outwards. A tunnel is made using a pair of suitable curved artery forceps, pushing them upwards and laterally in the submucosal plane for approximately 2 cm, and the ureter is then led in along this tunnel. A small fishmouth incision is made in the lower end of the ureter, which may require shortening. Interrupted 3/0 catgut sutures are used to anastomose the full thickness of the ureter to the mucosa of the bladder, and this is splinted with a Tizard catheter led in through the anterior abdominal and bladder walls and out again through the ureteroneocystostomy. The bladder muscle is then closed over this anastomosis. A renal biopsy is now taken

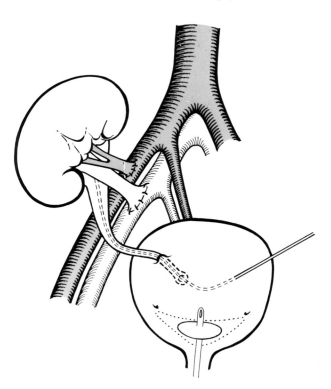

Fig. 59.7. Recipient operation. End-to-side anastomosis of renal artery and renal vein to external iliac artery and external iliac vein with anastomosis of donor ureter to the mucosa of the bladder from without.

and the wound closed in layers with at least two extra-peritoneal suction drains.

Blood transfusion may be required during the operation, but overtransfusion, with the danger of congestive heart failure in the oliguric patient, should be avoided and the need for transfusion judged on blood loss and central venous pressure. The patient then returns to a specialist transplant area or unit where the vital signs, fluid balance and biochemistry are carefully monitored. In the majority the renal transplant will function at once, with a good urine output, and fluid balance is maintained by replacing all fluid losses, volume for volume, together with an allowance for insensible loss. Additional fluid may be required to maintain a positive central venous pressure. In the minority the urine output will be minimal and a condition of acute tubular necrosis be presumed in the graft. Such a patient's fluid requirement will be kept only to that necessary to maintain a positive central venous pressure and replace the patient's insensible and other losses. In these circumstances postoperative dialysis will be required every 2 or 3 days until the function of the graft recovers sufficiently to avoid this.

Immunosuppresive therapy involves the use of either azathioprine and steroids, or cyclosporin A. Some centres use cyclosporin A routinely, while others reserve this more expensive and potentially nephrotoxic drug for highly sensitized patients, recipients of second transplants, and diabetics.

Should there be any anxiety arising over possible leakage of urine from the uretero-neocystostomy, then an injection of radio-opaque dye into the Tizard catheter can be undertaken to check this. The ureteric catheter is usually removed on the 4th or 5th post-transplant day and the urethral catheter 1 day later.

The more immediate postoperative complications include the possibility of threatened rejection, which is usually treated by additional steroids, having excluded the possibility of ureteric obstruction. Its detailed management is really beyond the scope of this chapter. However, certain postoperative complications may require surgical intervention. These include reactionary or secondary haemorrhage and urinary fistulas. Transplant nephrectomy for the irreversibly rejected kidney is best preceded by adequate dialysis, and cross-matched blood should be available for transfusion during this operation.

Chapter sixty

Transplantation of the Liver and Pancreas

Sir Roy Calne

LIVER TRANSPLANTATION

Liver transplantation was first performed in the human by Starzl et al. (1963). The operation has been slow to develop due to the formidable assault that the patient has to suffer. There is nothing comparable in terminal liver disease to dialysis for patients with kidney disease, which is the safety factor that has made kidney grafting a routine procedure. When patients in severe liver failure are referred for consideration of a liver transplant, the odds are stacked against a successful outcome. For a reasonable chance of a safe operation the patient must be referred before the liver failure is advanced. One important advantage that the liver has is a lower incidence of uncontrollable rejection than any other organ or tissue that has been grafted, apart from the cornea. The incidence of fatal liver disease is much less than that of kidney disease, therefore the numbers of centres practising liver grafting is likely to remain small.

The procedure fits most easily into an active renal transplantation programme where organ removal and preservation are routinely practised. The surgery and patient care require a large team of strongly motivated doctors, nurses and technicians and the active participation of hepatologists, on whom lies the chief burden of responsibility in assessing the prognosis and therefore the timing of the liver transplant operation. Continuing laboratory experience of successful orthotopic liver grafting in experimental animals is an essential technical background to performing the operation in man.

Recipient Selection

Patients with primary cancer of the liver and non-malignant parenchymatous liver disease may be considered for transplantation. In Denver the best results have been in children suffering from biliary atresia. We had been reluctant to transplant children because of the stunting and deforming effects of steroids. With, however, the advent of cyclosporin A (CyA) as an immunosuppressant and favourable media publicity for organ donation it has been possible in the United Kingdom to develop liver transplantation in children in the past 18 months with encouraging early results. Metastatic cancer is not an indication for liver transplantation. Patients who have been transplanted for secondary growth in the liver have all rapidly developed further metastases. Acute liver failure has

an uncertain prognosis and there is a significant proportion of patients who will recover completely with modern intensive care. Liver transplantation is not suitable for such patients, who are, moreover, desperately ill and unlikely to survive the operation, but the young patient in subacute liver failure temporarily stabilized can do well following liver grafting.

Of the primary liver tumours, liver cell cancer has been the best indication for grafting, although even in this condition 70 per cent of cases have developed recurrent tumour. Biopsy is essential to determine that the lesion is malignant. Fifty per cent of our cases have had raised alpha-fetoprotein levels. One of our patients with a hepatoma lived for more than 5 years after grafting without evidence of recurrent growth at postmortem examination. Our longest current survivor, who had a hepatoma, has lived more than 11 years after operation.

For parenchymatous liver disease, the timing of the operation is critical. Suitable cases are patients with hepatic encephalopathy and variceal bleeding, where there is insufficient residual liver function for a portacaval shunt. Patients who have developed encephalopathy after portacaval shunting may also be suitable. Patients with terminal liver disease frequently have pulmonary arteriovenous shunts and toxic myocarditis and they may also suffer from renal failure. If the patient's systolic blood pressure is below 100 mmHg then it is unlikely that he or she will survive a liver transplant operation.

Alcoholic cirrhotics often have unstable personalities and will be unsuitable for grafting due to the fact that they are poor attenders for follow-up and may not take their immunosuppressive drugs. Australia antigenaemia is a hazard to hospital staff and other patients. We consider e antigen-positive patients to be unsuitable for grafting due to the danger of the disease occurring in the new liver, but patients with only the surface antigen marker are accepted. Great care is taken in operating on such cases and we give large doses of hyperimmune gamma globulin during the anhepatic and postoperative phase. One of our patients is still free from Australia antigen more than 9 years after grafting.

Chronic sepsis, even confined to the liver, is a relative contra-indication to operation since following immunosuppressive therapy septicaemia is likely to develop.

Preoperative assessment includes full liver function tests, but especially evidence of synthetic function. The serum albumin and prothrombin levels after injection of vitamin K are helpful. Recurrent en-cephalopathy and variceal bleeding indicate a poor prognosis, as do jaundice and ascites in the presence of cirrhosis. Splenoportography and the venous phase of mesenteric angiography may be important to determine that the portal vein is patent. In malig-nant cases CT scanning of the lungs, intravenous uro-graphy, barium meal, enema, sigmoidoscopy, bone scanning, angiography of the hepatic and superior mesenteric arteries and inferior vena cava are per-formed. A liver tumour confined to one lobe is treated by hepatic lobectomy unless there is coinci-dent cirrhosis, in which case transplantation may be considered. A limited laparotomy is part of the assessment to exclude small peritoneal deposits and nodal metastases.

The Donor

The criteria of the liver donor are the same as those required for suitable kidney transplantation, namely the patient with complete and irreversible death of the brain, whose circulation is maintained artifically by means of a ventilator.

Systemic malignancy or infection are contra-indications. The liver must not be too large in relation to the recipient, but small livers can be transplanted into larger recipients.

Immunological selection is seldom possible beyond avoiding incompatibility of red blood cell groups. We do not pay attention to HL-A tissue typing. This is performed for retrospective analysis. Cytotoxic cross-matching of recipient sera against donor lym-phocytes is performed, but the liver seems to be able to withstand the immunological disadvantage of being transplanted when there is cytotoxic killing of even 100 per cent of donor lymphocytes. It is impor-tant to ensure that the donor is not an alcoholic. If there is any doubt of the appearance of the liver a frozen section needle biopsy is performed before starting the operation on the recipient.

The Donor Operation and Liver Preservation

An incision is made across the abdomen below the costal margins with a vertical extension up to the xiphoid, while mechanical ventilation is continued and the circulation is intact (*Fig.* 60.1). The liver and both kidneys are skeletonized. The common bile duct is ligated and divided near the duodenum and both ureters are divided at the pelvic brim. If the heart is to be removed the vertical component of the inci-sion is extended to the manubrium and the sternum is split.

Dissection continues until all three organs are con-nected only by their blood vessels. The hepatic arter-ial dissection can be tedious due to the dense sheath of nerves of the coeliac plexus and anomalous vessels

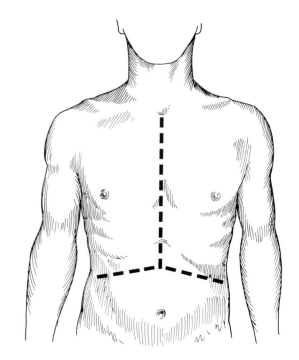

Fig. 60.1. Diagram of standard incision for donor and recipient operations. An extensive subcostal incision with extension up to the xiphoid is continued up to the manubrium if the heart is to be removed.

which are common. Seventeen per cent of cases have a main right hepatic artery arising from the superior mesenteric and 23 per cent a main left hepatic artery arising from the left gastric (*Fig.* 60.2). All branches of the hepatic artery are carefully preserved and if there is a branch arising from the superior mesenteric this is dissected from behind the portal vein as far as the parent vessel, which is removed in continuity with this branch and is later anastomosed to the ori-fice of the splenic artery of the donor specimen. A left hepatic artery is kept in continuity with the left gastric which is preserved at its origin from the coeliac artery. The aorta above and below the coeliac artery is controlled with slings. In children the thoracic aorta is removed with the coeliac axis so that it can be used for anastomosis to the recipient right common iliac artery (*Fig.* 60.3).

Ten thousand units of heparin are given systemi-cally and cannulas are inserted into the aorta and vena cava via the right common iliac vessels. A third cannula is passed into the portal vein via the superior mesenteric vein. The aortic and caval cannulas are declamped and perfusion of the portal vein begun with 1 litre of Hartmann's solution at 4 °C from a drip stand 1 metre above the patient (*Fig.* 60.4). While this perfusion is in progress both kidneys are removed with their vessels intact and Carrel patches of aorta, including any accessory renal arteries. The kidneys are perfused in a standard way. When the Hartmann's solution perfusion has finished the portal perfusion is continued with plasma protein fraction

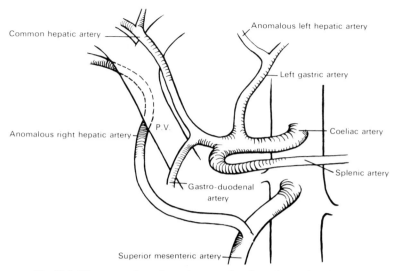

Fig. 60.2. Diagram to show the main anomalous hepatic arteries, the right hepatic artery coming from the superior mesenteric and passing posterior to the portal vein (17 per cent) and the left hepatic artery coming from the left gastric (23 per cent). (By courtesy of Pitman Medical from *Oncological Operations* (Eds. R. Raven and I. Burn), *Operations on the liver,* R. Y. Calne, in press.)

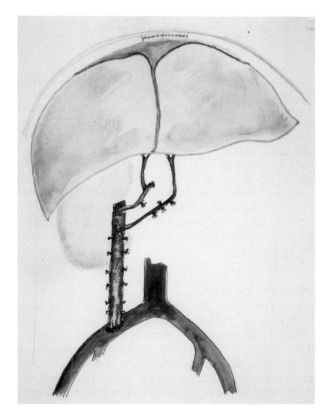

Fig. 60.3. Diagram showing use of the donor thoracic aorta. The proximal end is closed beyond the orifice of the coeliac or the superior mesenteric if there is an anomalous right hepatic artery. The proximal aorta, passed under the posterior parietal peritoneum, in anastomosed to the side of the right common iliac artery. (*Figure* 176 from *A Colour Atlas of Liver Transplantation. Single Surgical Procedures*—27, R. Y. Calne, 1985. Wolfe Medical Publications Ltd.)

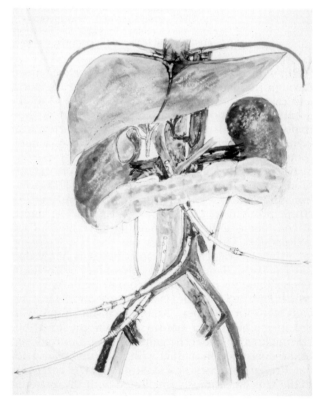

Fig. 60.4. Diagram of the dissection of the liver and two kidneys so that the three organs are attached by their blood vessels only. The ureters and common bile duct have been divided. Cannulas have been inserted into the inferior vena cava and aorta through the right common iliac vessels and into the portal vein via the superior mesenteric for cooling of the liver. (*Figure* 23 from *A Colour Atlas of Liver Transplantation. Single Surgical Procedures*—27. R. Y. Calne, 1985. Wolfe Medical Publications Ltd.)

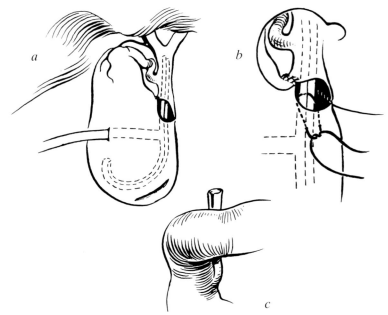

Fig. 60.5. Diagram of biliary drainage most often used in the author's series. The 'bench' technique: after the liver has been cooled the gallbladder is mobilized leaving its blood supply intact. Hartmann's pouch is anastomosed to the common duct (*a,b*). The fundus of the gallbladder will be anastomosed to the recipient common duct after the liver has been transplanted (*c*). (By permission of J. B. Lippincott Co. from Calne R. Y. (1976). A new technique for biliary drainage in orthotopic liver transplantation utilizing the gall bladder as a pedicle graft conduit between the donor and recipient common bile ducts. *Ann. Surg.* **184**, 605.

(PPF) with additives* until 400 ml of this have passed through the liver. If the heart is removed the aorta and cava are not cannulated. Instead, after the abdominal dissection is completed the heart is then removed and perfusion of the liver through the portal vein begins immediately after the aorta has been clamped in the chest.

The organ is then removed and inserted into a bowl of ice-cold saline. One hundred ml of the PPF solution is now infused into the hepatic artery and another 50 ml through the gallbladder and main bile ducts, after an incision has been made in the fundus of the gallbladder. This is to wash out the bile from the main biliary collecting system, since it is likely that bile can cause damage to the cold biliary epithelium. The gallbladder is mobilized from its bed taking care not to interfere with the cystic artery and its accompanying vein, and then, as a 'bench' technique with the liver cold either before or after preservation, Hartmann's pouch of the gallbladder is anastomosed to the donor common duct with interrupted adventitial Prolene stitches and continuous 4/0 catgut or PDS. This anastomosis is splinted with the guttered horizontal limb of the T-tube, the long limb being taken out through the body of the gallbladder and

* To each litre of plasma protein fraction (PPF) is added: 2000 i.u. of heparin, 250 mg of hydrocortisone, 500 mg of ampicillin, 6 ml of 0·1 N HCl, 5 ml of 10 per cent magnesium sulphate, 250 mg dextrose, 15 mmol of potassium phosphate.

the other horizontal limb through the fundus to splint the anastomosis to the recipient common bile duct (*Fig.* 60.5). The liver is then placed in another bowl of ice-cold saline and this is inserted into a sterile plastic bag which is surrounded by a similar plastic bag. The outside bag is surrounded by ice in an insulated polystyrene box. Livers can be transported by car or by air, and periods of preservations have extended to $10\frac{1}{2}$ hours with successful immediate post-transplant function, but it is preferable to limit the time to a minimum and we aim to revascularize the liver within 6 hours after the cessation of circulation in the donor.

Recipient Operation

This is based on that of Starzl et al. (1963). Since the operation imposes rapid and severe interference with the cardiovascular system, it is essential that care of the patient is in the hands of an experienced anaesthetist with sufficient technical help in monitoring and blood transfusion. Light general anaesthetic is used. The timing of the operation is extremely important; special care is taken not to have the patient operated on before the liver is available to be used. Large intravenous lines are inserted into the territory of the superior vena cava. Arterial and central venous pressures, ECG and pulse rate are recorded continuously. Serum levels of potassium, calcium, blood gases and pH are determined frequently.

The incision is the same as that in the donor (*see*

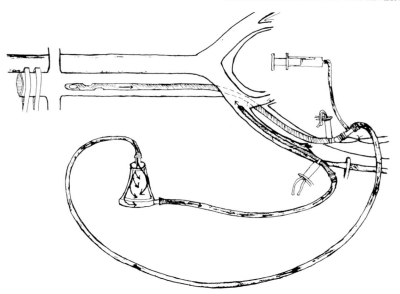

Fig. 60.6. Diagram of the veno-arterial bypass circuit. Blood from the vena cava is removed via the long saphenous vein and pumped into the right common iliac artery. Prostacyclin is infused through the side-arm on the venous limb. (By courtesy of The Editor, *The Lancet.* Calne R. Y. et al. (1985) Use of veno-arterial bypass in orthotopic liver grafting. *Lancet* **i**, 1269.)

Fig. 60.1). The operation is done entirely through the abdomen. Dissection may be very difficult and tedious due to portal hypertension and coagulopathy. Meticulous suture ligation of all tissue to be cut is the only satisfactory method of managing the bleeding tendency, especially from high-pressure venules. The structures in the free edge of the lesser omentum are separated from each other and controlled. Dissection behind the liver is the last part of this phase of the operation, since bleeding in this area cannot be controlled until the liver is removed.

In very sick patients, especially cirrhotics with renal impairment, vena caval clamping may not be tolerated. In such cases and also in patients with severe portal hypertension with coagulation defects, we assist the circulation. Of several techniques used we now favour simple veno-arterial bypass without systemic heparin, oxygenation or a heat exchanger. We use the Biomedicus centrifugal action pump and heparin bonded tubing. Low-dose prostacyclin can be infused in the venous limb of the circuit (*Fig.* 60.6).

The vena cava is temporarily clamped below the liver. If this severely impairs cardiac function the clamp is removed. More blood is transfused and when the heart is capable of withstanding clamping of the vena cava, removal of the liver is proceeded with as quickly as possible. The hepatic artery is ligated and divided, the portal vein clamped and divided and the vena cava similarly dealt with above and below the liver. It is very important that the interval during which the liver is devascularized should be as short as possible, while the organ is still connected to the systemic venous system via the hepatic veins. Manipulation of the liver in this state can lead to massive flooding of the circulation with potassium ions, leading to cardiac arrest. Very rapid transfusion of stored blood should be avoided if possible because this can impair cardiac activity by causing an increase in the serum potassium level and cooling of the heart. The central venous pressure is kept positive to avoid air embolus. A special clamp is applied to the vena cava above the liver. This takes a small cuff of diaphragm and has a screw clip on it to prevent slipping (*Fig.* 60.7). Following removal of the diseased liver the hepatic fossa is inspected for bleeding and any haemorrhagic points are suture ligated.

The donor liver is then removed from its ice-cold environment and the upper inferior vena caval anastomosis is performed with a 2/0 Mersilene stitch, the posterior wall being sutured from within. The bulk of the donor liver may obscure vision and this anastomosis can be difficult. Retraction of the right costal margin is thought to be the cause of a high incidence of temporary right pleural effusion postoperatively. The portal venous anastomosis is then constructed with a 5/0 Prolene stitch. A catheter is inserted into the portal vein through the anterior wall before this layer is finished. Four hundred ml of PPF at room temperature are perfused through the portal vein, to wash out potassium ions present in the original cooling fluid and accumulating from anoxia. The effluent runs out of the inferior vena cava below the liver. The portal venous anastomosis is then completed and the cava below the liver is clamped. The suprahepatic IVC clamps are removed. This is a critical movement since, despite administration of bicarbonate and calcium intravenously, potassium from the mesenteric circulation and liver may lead to cardiac irregularities, hypotension and even asystole.

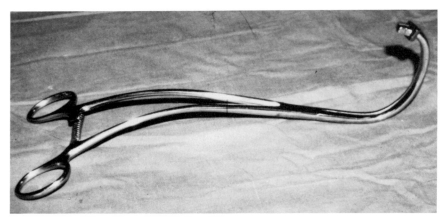

Fig. 60.7. The special clamp used for the suprahepatic inferior vena cava. This takes a bite of the diaphragm and its blades are secured by a little clip that slides over their ends to prevent the vena cava slipping out. (*Figure* 77 from *A Colour Atlas of Liver Transplantation. Single Surgical Procedures*—27. R. Y. Calne, 1985. Wolfe Medical Publications Ltd.)

Once the heart is functioning satisfactorily, the operation continues with a running 4/0 Prolene stitch to anastomose the donor and recipient venae cavae below the liver. The main hepatic and gastroduodenal arteries of the recipient are clamped. An oblique incision is made to include the orifice of the gastroduodenal artery. The Carrel patch of donor aorta containing the coeliac artery is trimmed so as to fit this orifice. The anastomosis is constructed with a running 6/0 Prolene stitch. On release of the arterial clamp there is usually evidence of a good blood supply to the mobilized gallbladder. Bleeding points are diathermied. The fundus of the gallbladder is anastomosed to the recipient common duct using interrupted adventitial 5/0 Prolene and continuous 4/0 PDS stitches through all coats (*Fig.* 60.8). The long arm emerges through the body of the gallbladder. A Tru-cut needle biopsy is taken from the liver. The falciform ligaments of donor and recipient are sutured together. Drains are brought out from the subdiaphragmatic and subhepatic spaces on both sides via the extremities of the main wound. The long arm of the T-tube is brought out through a separate stab incision. If the donor liver has no gallbladder or the gallbladder is unsatisfactory for anastomosis, then a duct-to-duct anastomosis is constructed and the T-tube brought out through the recipient common bile duct (*Fig.* 60.9). If the recipient common bile duct cannot be used, then the gallbladder fundus is anastomosed to a Roux loop (*Fig.* 60.10).

The monitoring used during the operation is continued postoperatively. Urine output and body temperature are recorded. The patient usually requires warming as the blood transfusions and a long operation reduce the body temperature. If the patient has good lung function usually after 24 hours, extubation is done as soon as possible. With severe cirrhotics who often have arteriovenous pulmonary shunts, at least 48 hours of ventilation are undertaken before the endotracheal tube is removed.

Drain removal begins on the 2nd day, one drain each day. The patient is given preoperative antibiotics prophylactically. If, however, there is evidence of organisms resistant to gentamicin appropriate antibiotics are given. The antibiotics are continued for

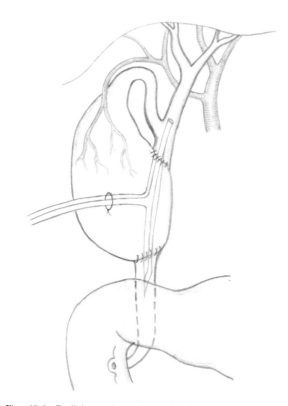

Fig. 60.8. Pedicle graft conduit with donor gallbladder. Hartmann's pouch is anastomosed to donor common ducts and fundus anastomosed to recipient common duct. Irrigating T-tube is inserted with irrigating arm through upper anastomosis. Blood supply to gallbladder is carefully preserved. (By courtesy of Roger Williams and The Editor, *British Medical Journal*, from R. Y. Calne and R. Williams (1977), **1**, 471–476.)

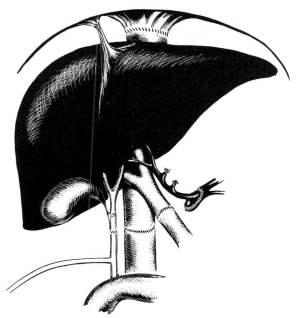

Fig. 60.9. Diagram of orthotopic liver transplantation, with drainage of bile via a choledochodochostomy over a T-tube. (From R. Y. Calne *British Journal of Surgery* (1969), **56**, 729.)

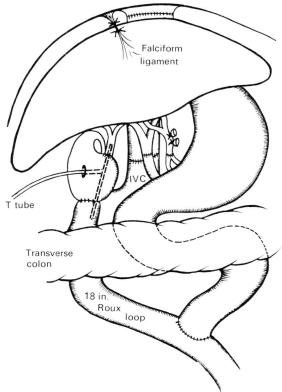

Fig. 60.10. Diagram of the use of the vascularized gallbladder as a conduit between the donor common duct and a long Roux loop of jejunum in patients whose own common ducts cannot be used, for example children with biliary atresia and cases of sclerosing cholangitis. Hartmann's pouch is anastomosed to the common bile duct of the donor and the fundus of the gallbladder to the Roux loop. (By courtesy of the *World Journal of Surgery*, from R. Y. Calne (1977), **1**, 172.)

48 hours. Cultures are taken from the blood, wound, T-tube, mouth and perineum daily.

If cholangiography shows satisfactory biliary drainage at 2 weeks, the T-tube is spigotted but left in place for 3 months. If cholangiography is still satisfactory the T-tube is removed at this time.

Immunosuppression

Immunosuppressive agents will predispose the already weak patient after a major procedure of liver transplantation to infection. We try to avoid large doses of steroids in the 1st week after operation and our current policy is to start immunosuppression with azathioprine and prednisolone 1·5 mg/kg and 1 mg/kg respectively daily, and then start CyA on the 2nd or 3rd day when renal function has been shown to be adequate at a dose of 2 mg/kg/day intravenously, rising to 4 mg/kg/day intravenously if the blood levels are low. It is important that the CyA is not given through a central line as this may lead to alveolar membrane damage and adult respiratory distress syndrome (Powell-Jackson et al., 1984). When the T-tube is clamped at about 15 days, CyA is given orally and it can now be absorbed since there will be bile salts in the intestine; 10 mg/kg/day are given. The azathioprine and steroid doses are both tailed down with careful monitoring of the patient's blood levels of CyA and liver function. Deterioration in liver function which is common between the 7th and 10th day may be due to acute rejection in which case three daily doses of 1 g of Solu-medrone (methylprednisolone) are given intravenously. The diagnosis of rejection can be difficult. Biliary obstruction is excluded by cholangiography. Hepatotoxic drugs and infection may also cause impaired liver function. We try to do an early biopsy before clotting is deranged by the liver damage. If we cannot definitely prove rejection, we assume that this is the cause of the liver impairment and give a trial of Solu-medrone.

Results

In the early days of liver transplanation there were a few long-term survivors and many early deaths, particularly in the perioperative period. Of the complete series of 305 liver allografts in 288 patients, between May, 1968, and October, 1986, 100 patients are alive up to 10·5 years, 78 lived more than 1 year and rehabilitation has been excellent in most. Many of the patients returned to full-time work and it has been particularly gratifying for women to return to run a household and look after their families, having been reduced to an invalid state before operation. Fifty-five of the 78 1-year survivors are still alive, 11 are more than 5 years after grafting and results are improving (*Table* 60.1). The late deaths have not been due to recurrence of the original disease. One patient died from a myocardial infarct, another of colonic carcinoma and a third from cirrhosis follow-

Table 60.1. Survival of patients with liver allografts: May 1968–September 1986

	Up to 1yr	1yr+	2yr+	3yr+	4yr+	5yr+	6yr+	8yr+	9yr+	10yr+
First Grafts										
Alive	44	22	8	4	5	4	2	1	3	1
Dead	157	9	3	1	4	3				
Re-transplants										
1st graft	14	2		1						
2nd graft										
Dead	11									
Alive	1	3	2							

ing acquired non-A non-B hepatitis virus infection. Our longest survivor is nearly 11 years after grafting. His original disease was hepatocellular carcinoma with familial hepatitis B viral infection, his brother having died from a hepatoma and his mother also being HbsAg positive. During the anhepatic phase of his operation and postoperatively he was given high-titre anti-Hbs immunoglobulin and remains well at work as a mechanic (Johnson et al., 1978).

In Starzl's experience the best results have been obtained in children (Iwatsuki et al., 1985). Following the NIH consensus meeting in Washington on liver transplantation there has been a surge of interest in this procedure in the United States and to a lesser extent in Europe. It is important that centres embarking on this form of treatment should benefit by the errors made by those with longer experience, especially in the logistics of organ donation, patient assessment, the actual operation and postoperative care.

Some patients have had excellent therapy and continue to do well years after transplantation. Starzl's longest patient is surviving 16 years after grafting, and has been through school and college. In the history of surgery once an operation can be shown to produce excellent results, for reasons that are difficult to analyse, the procedure usually becomes progressively safer. A good example in recent years has been the extraordinary improvements in open heart surgery, although the techniques currently used were developed at a time when the operative and postoperative mortality was high.

Further improvements in immunosuppression can be expected in the future, which should make the management of patients with liver transplants easier. Liver transplantation after many troubles and disappointments has come of age.

PANCREATIC TRANSPLANTATION

The most serious complication of diabetes in young patients is renal failure and blindness due to microangiopathy. Uraemic diabetics do badly on dialysis; retinopathy progresses and shunt sites are liable to infection. Kidney transplantation for these patients is also disappointing, mainly due to steroids which aggravate the diabetes and make control more difficult. For these reasons much experimental work has been devoted to transplantation of insulin-secreting tissue in the hope that this might prevent progress of the microangiopathy. Separated islets have been injected into the bloodstream or spleen but have tended to be aggressively rejected. Of more than 130 attempts there is only one report of a temporarily successful take in a human (Largiader et al., 1980).

Therefore, for the present, attention will be directed to transplanting the vascularized pancreas where there have been some good results. The 1-year functional survival of vascularized pancreas grafts is just under 30 per cent, whereas in good units the 1-year survival of cadaveric kidney grafts is about 80 per cent. Since the vascularized pancreas appears to be less susceptible to rejection than the kidney, the difference between the results of transplanting the two organs depends mainly on technical factors. A number of different surgical techniques for transplanting the pancreas have been described. We have used the segment of the body and tail of the pancreas vascularized on the splenic vessels, rather than the whole organ, which requires a complicated dissection in the donor to preserve the dual blood supply and drainage without damage. It appears that the body and tail of the pancreas can provide sufficient endocrine function to maintain the patient in good health. One difficulty concerns the management of exocrine secretion, since leakage of digestive enzymes may cause breakdown of anastomoses and sepsis.

We have transplanted 31 segmental pancreatic grafts in 29 patients. In 11 cases the duct was occluded according to the technique of Dubernard et al. (1978), which is a safe way of managing the exocrine secretion but which results in intense fibrosis of the gland, and we suspect in some cases this can compromise endocrine secretion. Only 1 of these 11 grafts is functioning and the patient is off insulin more than 6 years after transplantation, although the kidney from the same cadaver donor has been rejected and the patient is back on dialysis.

We then changed our technique to drainage of the pancreatic exocrine secretion into a Roux loop of small bowel according to the method of Gliedman et al. (1970) and Groth et al. (1982). Of seven transplantations, two are functioning well and one has diminished function. One of the disadvantages of this technique is that, in addition to the patient's own pelvic organs, the pelvis has to accommodate an extra kidney, pancreatic segment and loop of bowel which is draining against gravity. One of the theoretical disadvantages of most techniques described is that the venous drainage of the pancreatic graft is into the systemic circulation instead of the portal system, which is the normal physiological arrangement. In order to try to improve the technical results we have, for the past 18 months, been using a new technique in which the pancreatic segment is transplanted between the spleen and the stomach with the splenic vessels of the graft being anastomosed end to side of the splenic vessels of the recipient between the tail of the recipient pancreas and the hilum of the spleen. The graft therefore lies close to the normal position of the pancreas and has therefore been called the 'paratopic' technique.

One of the main causes of failure of vascularized pancreatic allografts has been early thrombosis of the major vessels. This may be partially due to the relatively sluggish flow in the large splenic vessels when there is no splenic circulation. In order to speed the flow through these vessels, we perform a small side-to-side arteriovenous fistula between the distal end of the graft splenic artery and vein, and since such a high flow into the vein might cause portal venous hypertension, a small casein ameroid ring is placed around the splenic artery just proximal to the fistula. This ring takes up water and should close the fistula after 1 or 2 months.

The Paratopic Technique

The Donor Operation

Most cases which are suitable for kidney donation are also satisfactory for donation of pancreas. The donor will have died from a head injury or a cerebro-vascular catastrophe with irreversible death of the brainstem, demonstrated according to accepted guidelines. Of course, diabetes must be excluded in the donor. This is an important consideration since patients who are diabetic may have head injuries during hypoglycaemic attacks. The pancreatic segment can be removed without interfering with the blood supply of any other organ and it can be done first through a bilateral subcostal incision with a vertical extension to the xiphoid, as is used for liver removal. The structures in the free edge of the lesser omentum are dissected from each other and the common hepatic artery is followed to the trifurcation of the coeliac and a sling is passed around the splenic artery at its origin from the coeliac artery. The splenic vein is approached by following the portal vein in the caudal direction. The short gastric vessels are then ligated and divided so that the spleen can be removed from its bed and an assistant holds the spleen like a handle, as described by Gliedman et al. (1970), which lifts

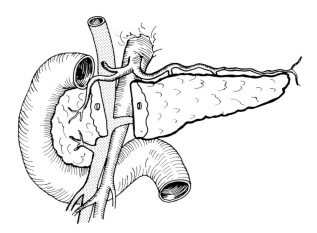

Fig. 60.11. Diagram showing plane of dissection between the superior mesenteric and the portal vein. (By courtesy of *Transplantation Proceedings*.)

up the tail of the pancreas so that connective tissue passing between the body and tail of the pancreas and surrounding structures can be divided. A plane is followed between the pancreas and the posterior parietal peritoneum to demonstrate the superior mesenteric vein in a similar approach as is followed during standard Whipple's operation for a pancreatico-duodenectomy (*Fig.* 60.11). A tape is passed around the pancreas at this level and then it is possible to see the whole specimen of tail and body of pancreas attached to the spleen and splenic vessels. A Crafoord clamp is placed across the pancreas in the line of the superior mesenteric vein and the organ is divided transversely just to the left side of the clamp. A paediatric vascular clamp is placed on the splenic artery close to the coeliac and the vessel is divided adjacent to the clamp. The splenic vein is similarly clamped close to the superior mesenteric vein.

The specimen of pancreas with the splenic vessels and spleen is now inserted into a bowl of ice-cold saline. The preservation technique is similar to that of the kidney. A short plastic cannula is introduced into the splenic artery and hypertonic citrate solution at 4° from a drip stand 1 m above the patient is infused until the effluent from the splenic vein is no longer bloodstained. Then using a bench technique with the cooled organ and loupe magnification a side-to-side arteriovenous fistula is constructed between the splenic artery and the vein using a 7/0 Prolene to produce an orifice approximately 3×1 mm. An ameroid casein ring of appropriate diameter is then placed over the splenic artery just adjacent to the arterio-venous fistula and a nylon ligature is tied around it so that it will not slip off. The splenic vessels are ligated distal to the shunt and the spleen excised. A no. 5 gauge Silastic feeding tube of 1 mm diameter is inserted into the pancreatic duct after cutting the end off obliquely and smoothing it in a flame. It is sutured with 6/0 Vicryl suture passed through the

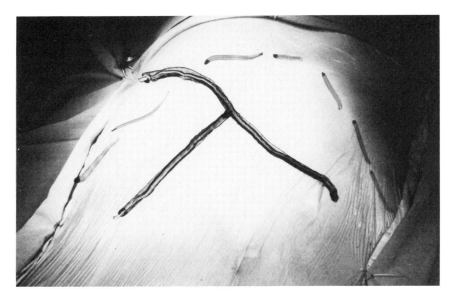

Fig. 60.12. Extension of the incision across the costal margin so that the apearance is of a T. The dashes indicate the costal margin. (*Figure* 45 from *A Colour Atlas of Liver Transplantation. Single Surgical Procedures*—27. R. Y. Calne, 1985. Wolfe Medical Publications Ltd.)

pancreatic duct wall and the tube. The pancreatic segment to be grafted is now wrapped in two sterile bags with cold saline and packed outside with ice.

The limit of preservation has not been defined for the human pancreas but from animal experiments and empirical information in humans it would appear that the pancreas is similar in its tolerance to ischaemia to the liver and one should not exceed 10 hours if possible, and preferably transplant the organ within 6 hours, so that auto-digestion from liberation of exocrine enzymes does not occur.

Recipient Operation (*Fig.* 60.12, 60.13)

The pancreas and usually kidney transplants from the same donor are performed at the same operating session. The incision for the pancreas is left subcostal which can be extended with a right-angled component to the incision across the costal margin and even, if necessary, into the chest to provide adequate exposure (*Fig.* 60.12). The short gastric vessels are ligated and divided and the spleen gently lifted forwards. If the spleen is extremely adherent, splenectomy is performed at this time. The splenic artery will be palpated between the tip of the tail of the pancreas and the hilum of the spleen. Dissection at this point permits separation of the splenic artery and vein from surrounding structures for approximately 2·5 cm leaving room for clamping and anastomosis. The patient is systemically heparinized and fine vascular clamps are used, first on the artery, in which a longitudinal incision is made which is appropriate for anastomosis to the donor splenic artery. The donor graft is now placed so that the artery and vein lie close to the point of anastomosis. An end-to-side anastomosis of the donor splenic artery to that of the recipient is performed with 6/0 Prolene. The splenic venous anastomosis is similarly constructed. When the clamps are removed there should be rapid change of colour of the pancreas with free bleeding from the cut surface. Bleeding points are suture ligated.

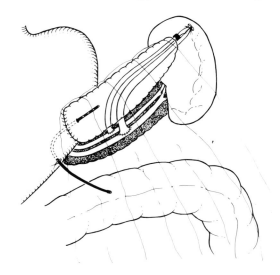

Fig. 60.13. Diagram of paratopic pancreas allograft. The splenic vessels of the donor are anastomosed end to side to those of the recipient between the stomach and the spleen. The pancreatic duct is drained into the anterior wall of the stomach and this anastomosis is protected with a stent brought out through the lumen of the stomach and then out through the skin. The cut surface of the pancreas is sutured to the stomach, the omentum is wrapped around the pancreas, an arteriovenous fistula has been constructed between the distal splenic artery and vein of the allograft, and an ameroid ring, just proximal to the fistula, is placed so that it will swell and close the fistula after between 1 and 2 months.

Table 60.2. Graft survival: paratopic segmental pancreas with simultaneous kidney grafting, January 1984–July 1985

| Patient no. | Allograft Survival (months) | | | Outcome |
| | Kidney | Pancreas | | |
		Full function	Reduced function	
1	>19	>19		
2	>19	8	>11	Reduced exogenous insulin
3	>17	>17		
4	>17	16	> 1	Reduced exogenous insulin
5	>14	>14		
6	>14	>14		
7	5	Removed at 10 days		Thrombosis, died from aspergillosis 5 months later with functioning kidney
8	>12	Removed at 14 days		Thrombosis
9	> 9	> 9		
10	> 9	Removed at 14 days		Thrombosis
11	+	+		Died from leakage of pancreatic fluid with functioning allografts
12	> 5	> 5		
13	> 1	> 1		
14	> 1	> 1		

A stitch is placed in the seromuscular layer of the anterior wall of the stomach adjacent to the cut surface of the pancreatic graft and an incision made around the stitch to allow for a submucous plane to be developed so that a pouch of mucosa can be drawn up like a small tent of approximately 2 cm from base to apex. The apex is now amputated and haemostatic forceps are passed through the stomach lumen and pressed against the anterior gastric wall, distal to the first incision using a scalpel blade to cut onto the tip of the forceps. A further set of forceps is railroaded along the track of the first forceps and the feeding tube that drains the pancreatic duct is pulled through the apex of the mucosal tent into the lumen of the stomach and out through the anterior wall of the stomach. A 4/0 Prolene running stitch is now inserted between the posterior cut edge of the pancreas and adjacent stomach wall. The stitch is left loose so that 4/0 Prolene stitches can be inserted between the pancreatic duct and the orifice of the mucosal pouch. These are tied and then the 4/0 Prolene stitch is pulled tightly posteriorly and continued along the front of the cut edge of the pancreas, sealing the cut edge from the rest of the peritoneal cavity and approximating it to the wall of the stomach (*Fig.* 60.13). A catgut stitch is inserted as a purse-string around the emerging feeding tube from the distal incision in the stomach. The greater omentum is wrapped around the pancreatic segment and the anterior wall of the stomach is sutured to the anterior parietal peritoneum so as to form a tunnel at the lowermost point. An incision is made through the abdominal wall and the feeding tube is brought out to the exterior at this point. It is most important that the pancreatic segment lies satisfactorily and there is no twisting or kinking of the anastomoses, especially the venous anastomosis. A drain is brought out through the lateral extremity of the wound which is closed in the usual way with continuous nylon, interrupted catgut, the subcutaneous tissue is sprinkled with ampicillin powder, and interrupted nylon is used for the skin closure.

The duct can be demonstrated radiographically by injection of contrast through the feeding tube which otherwise is left on continuous free drainage onto a sterile bag. Pancreatic juice can be collected and inspected microscopically for cells. The tube is removed after 21 days.

Immunosuppression has been with cyclosporin A intravenously 4 mg/kg/day for 2–4 days and then, when the patient's bowel sounds return, 17 mg/kg orally reducing slowly over the next 3 months to a maintenance dose of 6–8 mg/kg.

The patients have also been treated with a monoclonal antibody called Campath 1, 25 mg b.d., starting on the day of transplantation. The results are shown in *Table* 60.2. Thrombosis has been the main complication causing failure of the graft, although one patient developed leakage of pancreatic juice and died as a result of peritonitis. Otherwise the results of both the renal and pancreatic allografts have been encouraging and although the follow-up is short the quality of life of the patients with functioning grafts has been transformed by this procedure.

REFERENCES

Calne R. Y. and Williams R. (1977) Orthotopic liver transplantation: the first 60 patients. *Br. Med. J.* **i,** 471–476.

Calne R. Y. and Williams R. (1979) Liver transplantation. *Curr. Probl. Surg.* **16**, 3–44.

Dubernard J. M., Traeger J., Neyra P. et al. (1978) A new method of preparation of segmental pancreatic grafts for transplantation: trials in dogs and in man. *Surgery* **84**, 633–639.

Gliedman M. L., Gold M., Whittaker J. et al. (1970) Clinical segmental pancreatic transplantation with ureter-pancreatic duct anastomosis for exocrine drainage. *Surgery* **74**, 171–180.

Groth C.-G., Collate H., Lundgren C. et al. (1982) Successful outcome of segmental human pancreatic transplantation with enteric exocrine diversion after modifications in technique. *Lancet* **ii**, 522–524.

Iwatsuki S., Shaw B. W., Jr and Starzl T. E. (1985) Five-year survival after liver transplantation. *Transplant Proc.* **XVII**, 259–263.

Johnson P. J., Wansborough Jones M., Portmann B. et al. (1978) Recurrence of primary biliary cirrhosis after liver grafting. *N. Engl. J. Med.* **i**, 216–219.

Largiader F., Kolb Edith and Binswanger U. (1980) A long-term functioning human pancreatic islet allotransplant. *Transplantation* **29**, 76–77.

Powell-Jackson P. R., Carmichael F. J. L., Calne R. Y. et al. (1984) Adult respiratory distress syndrome and convulsions associated with administration of Cyclosporine in liver transplant recipients. *Transplantation* **38**, 341–343.

Starzl T. E. (1986) Personal communication.

Starzl T. E., Marchioro T. L., von Kaulla K. N. et al. (1963) Homotransplantation of the liver in humans. *Surg. Gynecol. Obstet.* **117**, 659–676.

Chapter sixty-one

Cardiac Transplantation

J. C. Baldwin, N. E. Shumway, E. B. Stinson and W. A. Baumgartner

The first human cardiac transplant operation was performed more than 20 years ago, when Hardy and his associates transplanted a chimpanzee heart into a patient dying of left ventricular failure (Hardy et al., 1964). However, poor clinical results in the early worldwide experience after 1967 relegated the technique to an investigational status for many years. Through continued investigation and improvement in surgical technique, postoperative care and pharmacological immunosuppression, cardiac transplantation has emerged during the past few years as a standard mode of clinical therapy for patients with end-stage congestive heart failure.

Alexis Carrel's report in 1905 of a successful canine cervical heterotopic procedure was the first published report of cardiac transplantation (Carrel and Guthrie, 1905). There was gradual refinement in surgical technique, as evidenced in the work of Mann and Priestly in the 1930s (Mann et al., 1933). The advent of safe cardiopulmonary bypass through the work of Gibbon and others transformed the possibilities for cardiac transplantation, as it did those for cardiovascular surgery in general (Gibbon, 1954). Drawing on the accumulating body of knowledge in cardiovascular surgical technique and transplantation technique in particular, safe cardiopulmonary bypass and hypothermic myocardial preservation, Lower and Shumway reported the first successful series of orthotopic cardiac transplantation procedures in dogs in 1960. Subsequent work in graft preservation, electrocardiographic diagnosis of rejection, and prevention and treatment of rejection, using agents borrowed from cytotoxic chemotherapy and renal transplantation, provided the foundation for subsequent efforts in clinical cardiac transplantation.

The first human orthotopic cardiac allograft transplantation was performed in South Africa in 1967 (Barnard, 1967). This operation generated widespread interest and enthusiasm for clinical application, and more than 100 cardiac transplant operations were performed during the following year. However, dismal clinical results brought about a precipitous decline in interest world wide. The clinical programme at the Stanford University Medical Center, begun in January 1968, has continued without interruption, and more than 450 cardiac transplant operations have now been performed.

from the group of patients with end-stage congestive heart failure, with New York Heart Association Class IV symptoms. These are patients for whom life expectancy is judged to be measured in weeks or months, and for whom conventional modes of therapy have been exhausted. An upper age limit of 60 years is currently applied. No lower age limit exists, and potential applications of this technique in selected congenital abnormalities, such as the hypoplastic left heart, are currently being investigated.

Recipients for cardiac transplantation should have no other life-threatening systemic illness, such as malignancy or collagen vascular disease; there should be no active infection present; and recent pulmonary infarcts contra-indicate transplantation, because of difficulties with heparinization and potential for infection in the infarcted pulmonary tissue. Insulin-requiring diabetes mellitus is usually a contra-indication because of the likelihood of exacerbation of the condition with postoperative steroid therapy.

Elevated pulmonary vascular resistance complicates cardiac transplantation, and we currently observe an upper limit of approximately 8 Wood units. The inability of the normal donor right ventricle to sustain circulation with fixed pulmonary hypertension is well established, and the difficulties in treating entities associated with this degree of pulmonary vascular disease prompt consideration of combined heart and lung transplantation. It is important to evaluate preoperatively the degree of reversibility of elevated pulmonary vascular resistance, using sodium nitroprusside and other vasodilator agents. In cases of moderate or reversible elevation of pulmonary vascular resistance, it may be possible to increase the chances of success with use of an on-site donor with short graft ischaemic time and a donor with larger body mass than the recipient's. In addition, there may be a role for temporary right ventricular afterload reduction using pharmacological as well as mechanical manoeuvres.

Currently, most recipients accepted for cardiac transplantation fall into the two broad categories of cardiomyopathy and coronary artery disease. These indications, as well as other more unusual indications for cardiac transplantation, are indicated in *Table 61.1*.

RECIPIENT SELECTION

Recipients for cardiac transplantation are selected

DONOR SELECTION

The factor which limits the number of cardiac trans-

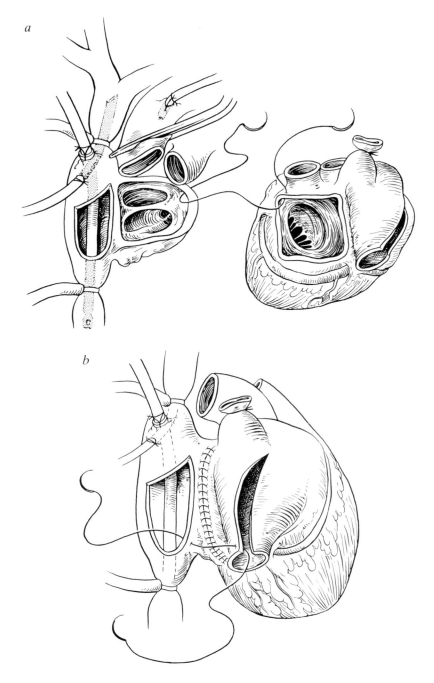

Fig. 61.1. Operative technique for human cardiac transplantation.

  a. Cannulation technique is similar to routine cardiac procedures utilizing central cannulation. Tapes have been placed around the superior and inferior venae cavae and the aorta has been cross-clamped to exclude the heart from the circulation. The recipient heart has been excised at the atrioventricular groove. The superior vena cava of the donor heart has been ligated. The left atrial anastomosis has been started.

  b. The left atrial anastomosis has been completed. The incision in the donor right atrium is curved away from the superior vena cava and the adjacent sinoatrial node. The right anastomosis is begun at the inferior border of the atrial septum.

  c. The right atrial anastomosis is completed. A perfusion catheter has been inserted into the left atrium through which cold (4 °C) normal saline is infused to further cool the left ventricular cavity as well as to displace air. The aortic anastomosis is being completed.

  d. The aortic cross-clamp has been released following completion of the aortic anastomosis. The perfusion catheter has been removed from the left atrium and the pulmonary anastomosis is completed with the heart fibrillating.

  e. The bypass cannulas have been removed. Pacing wires have been inserted on the donor right atrium.

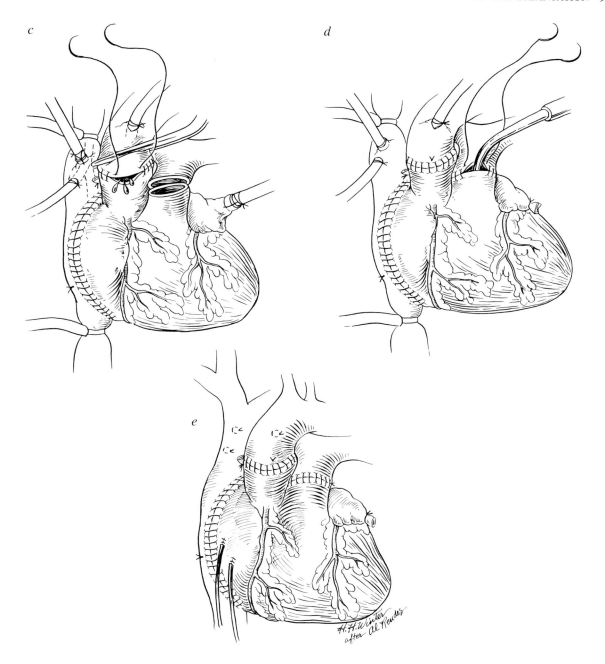

	No. of patients
Coronary artery disease	114
Cardiomyopathy	155
Valvular disease	19
Congenital heart disease	5
Coronary artery emboli	2
Cardiac tumour	1
Post-traumatic aneurysm	1
Myocarditis	1
	325

plantation operations which can be performed at present is donor availability. Cardiac allograft donors are selected from among brain-dead patients who are less than 35 years of age. Prospective cardiac donors should have no prior history of cardiac disease and should be haemodynamically stable on little or no vasopressor support. The achievement of this status frequently requires aggressive fluid replacement and treatment of diabetes insipidus with intramuscular vasopressin. There should be no evidence of external chest trauma likely to have resulted in significant cardiac contusion, and when this consideration arises, measurement of serial cardiac isoenzymes and electrocardiograms may be of value. There should be no active infection present. Aetiologies of brain death resulting in successful organ procurement for cardiac transplantation are listed in *Table* 61.2.

Table 61.2. Aetiology of brain death among cardiac donors, January 1968–May 1985

	No. of cases
Cranial trauma	288
Cerebrovascular accident	60
Anoxia leading to brain death	13
Other	5
	—
	366

Since 1977, the majority of cardiac transplant operations performed in our institution have been accomplished using distant organ procurement and graft preservation techniques. Distant procurement of the cardiac graft has provided several advantages. Most important, this technique facilitates the personal needs of donors' families and physicians, who may prefer that the body not be moved from the institution where the patient died. In addition, the overall donor pool has been increased, and the ability to cooperate with other organ procurement teams has been enhanced.

OPERATIVE TECHNIQUE

The technique used for orthotopic cardiac transplantation varies little from the paradigm established in the report by Lower and Shumway in 1960 (*Fig.* 61.1). Meticulous attention to detail in both the donor and recipient operations is essential to the successful outcome of any transplant effort.

The donor operation is carried out without cardiopulmonary bypass. Standard median sternotomy incision is employed, and the heart and great vessels are carefully inspected. This represents the last opportunity for haemodynamic evaluation and anatomical inspection of the graft. The heart and great vessels are dissected out in the usual fashion, and the donor is fully heparinized. Inflow occlusion is achieved through ligation of the superior and inferior venae cavae, and the aortic cross-clamp is applied near the take-off of the innominate artery. Cold (4°C) potassium crystalloid cardioplegic solution is administered via the aortic root, and the superior vena cava and right superior pulmonary vein are immediately incised, to eliminate the possibility of distension of either the right or left side of the heart. Topical saline (4°C) is applied concurrently with instillation of cardioplegia, and the graft is transported in normal saline at 4°C.

Graft dysfunction related to procurement is most often explained by the occurrence of distension or inadequate cooling. Although laboratory experience indicates the possibility of much longer ischaemic times, we believe that graft dysfunction is related to length of ischaemic time, with associated intramyocardial oedema and depletion of high-emergy phosphate stores. In the clinical programme, we currently limit ischaemic times to approximately 4 hours.

The recipient operation is carried out via median sternotomy, using cardiopulmonary bypass. Cannulation of the aorta is accomplished near the take-off of the innominate artery. Cannulation of the venae cavae is performed selectively, using a lateral approach on the atrium, to maximize the amount of residual right atrial cuff. Snares are placed around the venae cavae to exclude air. After institution of cardiopulmonary bypass and systemic cooling to 28°C, the aorta is immediately cross-clamped, to reduce the possibility of thrombo-embolic phenomena. The heart is excised beginning in the right atrium, just lateral to the right atrial appendage. The incision is carried out inferiorly along the atrioventricular groove through the coronary sinus and across the atrial septum into the left atrium, to empty the left side of the heart of blood. The aorta and pulmonary artery are then transected at the immediate supravalvular level, and the excision is completed, via incision of the left atrium, just posterior to the left atrial appendage.

The donor heart is then brought into the field and prepared for implantation. The left atrial anastomosis is performed first, beginning in the area of the recipient left superior left pulmonary vein and the donor left atrial appendage. The left atrial anastomosis is carried out using a running 3/0 Prolene technique. Topical saline (4°C) is used for graft preservation throughout the ischaemic portion of the transplant, and after completion of the left atrial anastomosis, a second tubing, for infusion of cold saline, is placed into the tip of the left atrial appendage. This technique accomplishes enhanced endomyocardial cooling, as well as exclusion of air from the left side of the graft during the remainder of the transplant operation. The right atrial anastomosis is begun in the area of the mid-septum and carried out using a continuous Prolene technique.

The aortic anastomosis is performed next, using end to end Prolene technique. At the time of institution of the aortic anastomosis, systemic warming is begun. After completion of the aortic anastomosis, the aortic cross-clamp is removed, and spontaneous defibrillation usually occurs. It is quite possible to perform the pulmonary arterial anastomosis with the aortic cross-clamp removed and the heart beating. This manoeuvre allows for reduction of the graft ischaemic time and may be particularly helpful in instances of distant organ procurement.

After discontinuation of cardiopulmonary bypass, patients are ordinarily left on inotropic support for 4–5 days, based on clinical observations of significant graft dysfunction when pressor support is weaned earlier. Isoproterenol is used to maintain heart rates in the range of 110–120 beats per minute. Early extubation and ambulation are emphasized.

Heterotopic transplantation has received considerable attention in some centres, and several advantages have been cited. The native heart remains in place and continues to function, should there be graft dysfunction. Furthermore, in unusual cases where native heart function might return (e.g. myocarditides), this technique would provide for interval removal of the transplanted heart. Most notable and compelling has been the application of the heterotopic technique in cases of end-stage heart failure with elevated pulmonary vascular resistance.

The disadvantages of the heterotopic technique include persistent risk of thrombo-embolic complications from the dilated ventricle of the native heart and frequent requirement for long-term anticoagulation, persistent angina pectoris in cases of coronary artery disease, technical difficulties with venous inflow anastomoses and occasional requirement for synthetic graft material in the pulmonary arterial anastomosis, and dual electrocardiograms.

IMMUNOSUPPRESSION AND DIAGNOSIS OF REJECTION

The current immunosuppression regimen is built around the fungal metabolite cyclosporin A, which has been associated with considerable improvement in survival after cardiac transplantation.

Preoperatively, patients are given a loading dose of cyclosporin (18 mg/kg orally). Immediately after discontinuation of cardiopulmonary bypass, methylprednisolone (500 mg intravenously) is administered. Methylprednisolone is continued for 24 hours postoperatively (125 mg every 8 hours, for three doses). Recent findings regarding adverse side-effects of cyclosporin, particularly renal toxicity, have prompted introduction of a low-dose cyclosporin protocol. Use of lower doses of cyclosporin has prompted adjunctive therapy with azathioprine (2 mg/kg/day, according to WBC count) and equine anti-thymocyte globulin (10 mg/kg/day for 7 days, depending on rosette T-lymphocyte counts). As indicated in *Table* 61.3, our current protocol involves two arms, one including maintenance oral prednisone, and the other not employing steroid maintenance therapy.

The diagnosis of rejection is based on the endomyocardial biopsy. Percutaneous introduction of the endomyocardial bioptome using the Seldinger technique under local anaesthesia is well established, and the first endomyocardial biopsy is ordinarily obtained on the 7th postoperative day. Endomyocardial biopsy is repeated on a weekly basis during the initial postoperative hospitalization, unless rejection intervenes. When rejection does occur, endomyocardial biopsy is repeated 4 days after administration of anti-rejection therapy, based on the observation that

Table 61.3. Immunosuppression protocols with reduced cyclosporin dosage

Protocol #1
  Cyclosporin: 18 mg/kg p.o. preoperatively, 9 mg/kg/day p.o. postoperatively, with target levels of 200–300 mg/ml for first 6 weeks.
  Azathioprine: 2 mg/kg/day, according to WBC count.
  Equine anti-thymocyte globulin: 10 mg/kg/day (dose adjusted by rosette counts) for first 7 days postoperatively.
  Steroids: methylprednisolone 500 mg i.v. at discontinuation of CPB, and 125 mg i.v. q 8-hourly for three doses. Maintenance prednisone 0·2 mg/kg/day p.o.
Protocol #2
  Same as Protocol #1, without maintenance prednisone.

histological resolution usually occurs within this time. Heterogeneity of involvement of the endomyocardium with rejection histology in the cyclosporin-treated patient requires sampling from several areas of the interventricular septum, using fluoroscopic guidance.

When rejection with myocyte necrosis occurs, treatment consists of pulse steroid therapy with intravenous methylprednisolone (1000 mg intravenously per day for 3 days). If rejection persists on a second biopsy, the 3-day pulse of intravenous methylprednisolone is repeated. Should rejection persist on a third biopsy or should rejection be particularly severe and clinically significant, intravenous methylprednisolone therapy is combined with intramuscular rabbit antithymocyte globulin therapy. The latter agent is ordinarily administered over a 3-day period concurrently with methylprednisolone, and serial T-cell rosette determinations are obtained.

In rare instances when rejection is particularly severe or persistent, consideration for retransplantation must be made. Six repeat cardiac transplant operations have been carried out for acute rejection in our programme.

COMPLICATIONS

As indicated in *Table* 61.4, the principal causes of mortality after cardiac transplantation are rejection

Table 61.4. Causes of death after cardiac transplantation among cyclosporin-treated patients, December 1980 to May 1985

	No. of patients
Infection	4
Rejection	6
Malignancy	3
Coronary artery disease	4
Acute graft failure	3
Pulmonary hypertension	1
Stroke	1
Cerebral oedema	1
Liver failure	1
	33

and infection. Rejection occurs in half the patients treated with cyclosporin by the 4th week after transplantation, and the incidence of rejection is not significantly lower among cyclosporin-treated patients than among those who are treated with conventional immunosuppression. However, it has been appreciated that the clinical severity of rejection episodes tends to be less among patients treated with cyclosporin and that their response to treatment is generally more salutary.

Cyclosporin itself has been associated with an array of adverse side-effects, including renal failure with acute tubular injury and chronic development of interstitial fibrosis, hepatotoxicity, hypertension, hirsutism and malignancy. The latter complication has been principally manifested by the occurrence of large-cell immunoblastic lymphomas with apparently short induction periods and predisposition for central nervous system involvement. A recent retrospective analysis of the quantitative degree of immunosuppression among cardiac transplant recipients with lymphomas suggested that this complication was related to overall degree of immunosuppression. During our initial experience with cyclosporin, 6 of 41 patients developed lymphoma. The overall immunosuppressive regimen was then modified, with elimination of prophylactic rabbit antithymocyte globulin and adjustment of cyclosporin dosage according to serum levels. In the last 100 patients in our series, there has been no incidence of lymphoma.

Infection in the cardiac transplant patient is protean in its aetiology and manifestations, as suggested by the organisms involved and sites of infection, shown in *Table* 61.5. As in the case of rejection, cyclosporin-based immunosuppression has not significantly reduced the incidence of infection, but it has altered the clinical characteristics, in that the severity of illness associated with a given infection is less, and response to appropriate antimicrobial therapy is more efficacious than was seen with conventional immunosuppression.

A disturbing complication which persists in clinical cardiac transplantation is that of graft atherosclerosis. More than one-third of patients will have angiographically demonstrable lesions 3 years after transplantation, and the likelihood of this complication appears to be as high among patients undergoing transplantation for cardiomyopathy as among those transplanted for coronary artery disease. In view of the denervated state of the heart, this problem is usually occult, presenting with insidious onset of congestive heart failure or sudden death. The disease is usually diffuse, with involvement of distal vessels, precluding consideration of coronary artery bypass grafting. When the process is severe, retransplantation must be contemplated, and we have performed 18 repeat transplantations for coronary artery disease.

RESULTS

As of this writing, more than 450 cardiac transplant operations have been performed in more than 400 patients in our programme. There has been steady improvement in survival, from 22 per cent 1-year survival in the 1st year of our programme to more than 80 per cent 1-year survival at present.

Actuarial survival is shown in *Fig.* 61.2. The curve designated as #1 indicates survival among patients

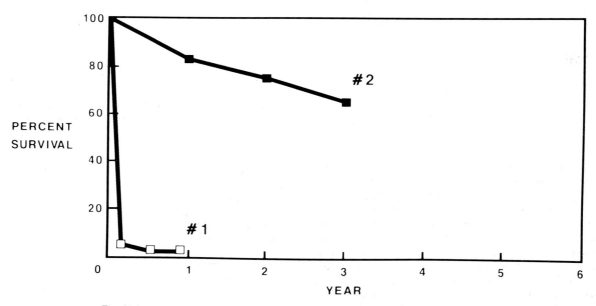

Fig. 61.2. Actuarial survival following cardiac transplantation. (Stanford University.)

Table 61.5. Infections after cardiac transplantation among cyclosporin-treated patients, December 1980 to December 1984

Organisms	No. of patients	Sites of infection	No. of patients
Bacterial	74	Pulmonary	40
Viral	77	Septicaemia	18
Fungal	20	Urinary	23
Protozoan	3	Mediastinum	8
Nocardi	3	Retinitis	2
		Empyema	1
		CNS	1

for whom no donor is found, and curve #2 indicates survival among cyclosporin-treated patients, since December 1980. The dramatic improvement in survival offered by this form of therapy is evident. It is also encouraging to note that among 1-year survivors, rehabilitation, as defined by ability to return to school or work, currently exceeds 80 per cent. This factor reflects the great improvements that have been achieved in this form of therapy, as well as the fact that these patients are relatively young people, with illnesses confined to the cardiac axis and its direct ramifications.

REFERENCES

Barnard C. N. (1967) The operation. *S. Afr. Med. J.* **41,** 1271.

Baumbaugh J. et al. (1985) Quantitative analysis of immonsuppression in cyclosporin-treated cardiac transplant patients with lymphoma. *Heart Transplant.* **4,** (3), 307–311.

Carrel A. and Guthrie C. C. (1905) The transplantation of veins and organs. *Am. J. Med.* **10,** 1101.

Gibbon J. H., Jr. (1954) Application of a mechanical heart and lung apparatus to cardiac surgery. *Minn. Med.* **37,** 171.

Hardy J. D., Chavez C. M., Kurrus F. D. et al. (1964) Heart transplantation in man: developmental studies and report of a case. *JAMA* **188,** 1132.

Lower R. R. and Shumway N. E. (1960) Studies on orthotopic transplantation of the canine heart. *Surg. Forum* **11,** 18.

Mann F. C., Priestly J. T., Markowitz J. et al. (1933) Transplantation of the intact mammalian heart. *Arch. Surg.* **26,** 219.

Index